MEDICAL ASPECTS OF HARSH ENVIRONMENTS
Volume 2

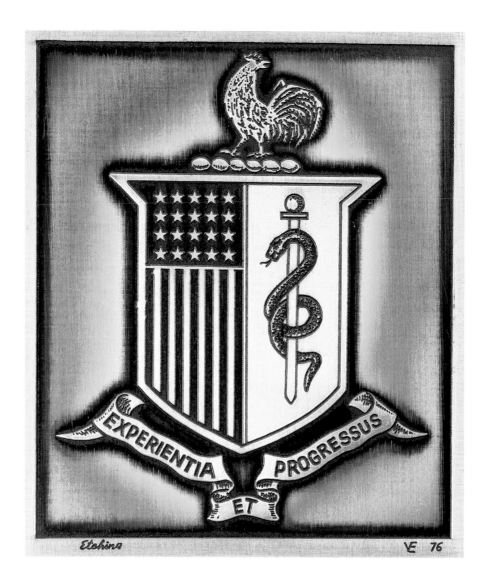

The Coat of Arms
1818
Medical Department of the Army

A 1976 etching by Vassil Ekimov of an
original color print that appeared in
The Military Surgeon, Vol XLI, No 2, 1917

For sale by the Superintendent of Documents, U.S. Government Printing Office
Internet: bookstore.gpo.gov Phone: toll free (866) 512-1800; DC area (202) 512-1800
Fax: (202) 512-2250 Mail: Stop SSOP, Washington, DC 20402-0001

ISBN 0-16-051184-4

The first line of medical defense in wartime is the combat medic. Although in ancient times medics carried the caduceus into battle to signify the neutral, humanitarian nature of their tasks, they have never been immune to the perils of war. They have made the highest sacrifices to save the lives of others, and their dedication to the wounded soldier is the foundation of military medical care.

Textbooks of Military Medicine

Published by the

Office of The Surgeon General
Department of the Army, United States of America

Editor in Chief and Director
Dave E. Lounsbury, MD, FACP
Colonel, MC, U.S. Army
Borden Institute
Assistant Professor of Medicine
F. Edward Hébert School of Medicine
Uniformed Services University of the Health Sciences

Military Medical Editor
Ronald F. Bellamy, MD
Colonel, U.S. Army Retired
Borden Institute
Associate Professor of Military Medicine
Associate Professor of Surgery
F. Edward Hébert School of Medicine
Uniformed Services University of the Health Sciences

Editor in Chief Emeritus
Russ Zajtchuk, MD
Brigadier General, U.S. Army Retired
Former Commanding General
U.S. Army Medical Research and Materiel Command
Professor of Surgery
F. Edward Hébert School of Medicine
Uniformed Services University of the Health Sciences
Bethesda, Maryland

The TMM Series

Published Textbooks

> Medical Consequences of Nuclear Warfare (1989)
>
> Conventional Warfare: Ballistic, Blast, and Burn Injuries (1991)
>
> Occupational Health: The Soldier and the Industrial Base (1993)
>
> Military Dermatology (1994)
>
> Military Psychiatry: Preparing in Peace for War (1994)
>
> Anesthesia and Perioperative Care of the Combat Casualty (1995)
>
> War Psychiatry (1995)
>
> Medical Aspects of Chemical and Biological Warfare (1997)
>
> Rehabilitation of the Injured Soldier, Volume 1 (1998)
>
> Rehabilitation of the Injured Soldier, Volume 2 (1999)
>
> Medical Aspects of Harsh Environments, Volume 1 (2002)
>
> Medical Aspects of Harsh Environments, Volume 2 (2002)

Upcoming Textbooks

> Medical Aspects of Harsh Environments, Volume 3 (2003)
>
> Military Preventive Medicine: Mobilization and Deployment, Volume 1 (2002)
>
> Military Preventive Medicine: Mobilization and Deployment, Volume 2 (2002)
>
> Military Medical Ethics, Volume 1 (2002)
>
> Military Medical Ethics, Volume 2 (2002)
>
> Ophthalmic Care of the Combat Casualty (2002)
>
> Combat Injuries to the Head
>
> Combat Injuries to the Extremities
>
> Surgery of Victims of Combat
>
> Military Medicine in Peace and War

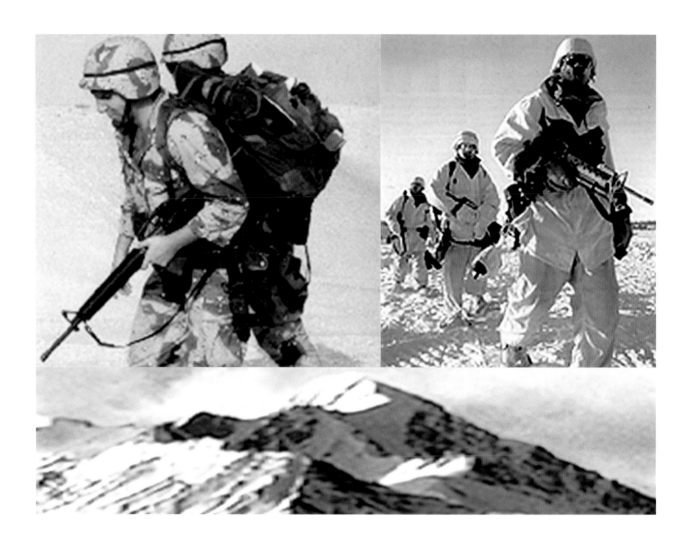

The environments that face combatants on modern battlefields.

Art: Courtesy of US Army Research Institute of Environmental Medicine, Natick, Massachusetts

MEDICAL ASPECTS OF HARSH ENVIRONMENTS VOLUME 2

Specialty Editors

KENT B. PANDOLF, PhD
Senior Research Scientist
US Army Research Institute of Environmental Medicine

ROBERT E. BURR, MD
Formerly, Medical Advisor
US Army Research Institute of Environmental Medicine

Office of The Surgeon General
United States Army
Falls Church, Virginia

Borden Institute
Walter Reed Army Medical Center
Washington, D.C.

United States Army Medical Department Center and School
Fort Sam Houston, Texas

Uniformed Services University of the Health Sciences
Bethesda, Maryland

2002

Editorial Staff: Lorraine B. Davis
Senior Production Manager

Colleen Mathews Quick
Developmental Editor

Douglas Wise
Senior Page Layout Editor

Bruce Maston
Desktop Publishing Editor

Andy C. Szul
Desktop Publishing Editor

This volume was prepared for military medical educational use. The focus of the information is to foster discussion that may form the basis of doctrine and policy. The volume does not constitute official policy of the United States Department of Defense.

Dosage Selection:

The authors and publisher have made every effort to ensure the accuracy of dosages cited herein. However, it is the responsibility of every practitioner to consult appropriate information sources to ascertain correct dosages for each clinical situation, especially for new or unfamiliar drugs and procedures. The authors, editors, publisher, and the Department of Defense cannot be held responsible for any errors found in this book.

Use of Trade or Brand Names:

Use of trade or brand names in this publication is for illustrative purposes only and does not imply endorsement by the Department of Defense.

Neutral Language:

Unless this publication states otherwise, masculine nouns and pronouns do not refer exclusively to men.

Published by the Office of The Surgeon General at TMM Publications
Borden Institute
Walter Reed Army Medical Center
Washington, DC 20307-5001

Library of Congress Cataloging-in-Publication Data
Medical aspects of harsh environments / specialty editors, Kent B. Pandolf, Robert E. Burr.
    p. ; cm. -- (Textbooks of military medicine)
  Includes bibliographical references and index.
    1. Medicine, Military. 2. Extreme environments--Health aspects. I. Pandolf, Kent B., 1945- II. Burr, R. E. III. United States. Dept. of the Army. Office of the Surgeon General. IV. Series.
  [DNLM: 1. Environmental Medicine. 2. Military Medicine. 3. Altitude Sickness. 4. Environmental Exposure--prevention & control. WA 30.5 M489 2002]
RC971 .M43 2002
616.9'8023--dc21

                                             2002024814

PRINTED IN THE UNITED STATES OF AMERICA

09, 08, 07, 06, 05, 04, 03, 02   5 4 3 2 1

Contents

Foreword

Earth's environments have always influenced the planning and conduct of military operations. Past campaigns have been impacted by heat, cold, and altitude, as well as the changes in barometric pressure that divers face in special operations. During the 20th century alone, US armed forces have been involved in terrestrial military operations in hot climates in the North African campaign and Pacific theater operations during World War II, the Vietnam and Persian Gulf wars, and military and humanitarian operations in Panama, Haiti, Grenada, Rwanda, and Somalia. Our major military operations involving cold climates during the past century include World War I and World War II, the Korean War, and most recently in Bosnia and Kosovo. *Medical Aspects of Harsh Environments, Volume 1,* treats the major problems caused by fighting in heat and cold.

The topics of *Medical Aspects of Harsh Environments, Volume 2,* are the effects of altitude, especially as experienced in mountain terrain and by aviators, and the complex interactions between humans and the special environments created by the machines used in warfare. Our warfighters were exposed to mountain terrain during World War II, the Korean War, in military and humanitarian efforts in South America, and most recently in the Balkans. Military action has also occurred in some of the environments considered "special" (eg, on and below the water's surface) in every war that this country has fought, whereas other special environments (eg, air—flights not only within Earth's atmosphere but also beyond it, in space) have become settings for the havoc of war only as a result of 20th-century technology. The second volume also contains a discussion of the personal environment within the protective uniforms worn by service members against the fearsome hazards of chemical and biological warfare. This microenvironment—created by the very encapsulation that protects the wearer—is in some ways different from but in others similar to all closely confined, manmade environments (eg, the stresses that divers face in coping with the changes in barometric pressure). Whatever the environment, this point needs to be kept in mind: indifference to environmental conditions can contribute as much to defeat as the tactics of the enemy.

Medical Aspects of Harsh Environments, Volume 3, emphasizes the need for a preventive approach to decrease attrition due to harsh environments, such as predicting the likelihood of its occurrence and stimulating awareness of how specific factors (eg, gender, nutritional status) are sometimes important determinants of outcome. The third volume concludes with reproductions of two of the classics of environmental medicine: the lectures given by the late Colonel Tom Whayne on heat and cold injury, respectively, at the Army Medical School in 1951; for decades these have been unavailable except as mimeographed handouts to students attending specialized courses.

Military and civilian experts from the United States and other countries have participated as authors of chapters in this three-volume textbook, *Medical Aspects of Harsh Environments.* The textbook provides historical information, proper prevention and clinical treatment of the various environmental illnesses and injuries, and the performance consequences our warfighters face when exposed to environmental extremes of heat, cold, altitude, pressure, and acceleration. The contents are unique in that they present information on the physiology, physical derangements, psychology, and the consequent effects on military operations together in all these harsh environments. This information should be a valuable reference not only for the physicians and other healthcare providers who prepare our warfighters to fight in these environments but also for those who care for the casualties. Military medical personnel must never forget that harsh environments are great, silent, debilitating agents for military operations.

Lieutenant General James B. Peake
The Surgeon General
U.S. Army

Washington, DC
December 2001

Preface

Over the centuries, battles have often been won by innovation: cavalry prevailed over infantry, elephants frightened horses, and mechanized vehicles dispersed chariots. Today, aircraft and rockets seem to make victory possible from a safer distance, but we are learning that even overwhelming airpower is not enough. Sooner or later, a war must be fought on the ground. Ground forces often face harsh environmental conditions—hot or cold, wet or dry—and often the terrain is rugged. The high mountain environment is cold and the air deficient in oxygen. Space travel and underwater operations also pose new and difficult problems.

Alexander the Great lost hundreds of men to mountain hazards. Napoleon's attack on Moscow was broken by winter. Mountain combat during both World War I and World War II caused many avoidable casualties from cold and altitude. In the 1962 Sino–Indian conflict, these mountain conditions cost the unacclimatized Indian troops more loss than fighting did. And the winter retreat of the US forces during the Korean War was nearly identical—except for altitude—to that which the British Army had experienced in Afghanistan a century earlier.

As this second of three volumes devoted to *Medical Aspects of Harsh Environments* goes to press, US and Allied forces are preparing to mark the first anniversary of their deployment to the windswept terrain of the Afghan plateau. The reality of American troop operations at 5,000 to 10,000 feet above sea level brings an unexpected timeliness to this volume. For the first time in history, the US military has had to wage sustained combat at high altitude. Troops have had to confront, and overcome, the hobbling effects of altitude sickness while encumbered with 80 lb of gear and negotiating their way across steep snow-covered slopes. One firefight in March 2002 between US Army Rangers and Afghan Taliban took place at 10,200 ft.

In conjunction with *Medical Aspects of Harsh Environments, Volume 1* (comprising Sections I and II, Hot and Cold Environments), this second volume provides a compendium of human biomedicine in the austere, and often overlapping, environments of heat, cold, and high altitude. In the first half of this textbook (Section III, Mountain Environments, Paul B. Rock, DO, PhD, Colonel, Medical Corps, US Army [Ret], section editor), the US Army Research Institute of Environmental Medicine (USARIEM) presents a comprehensive review of the history, physiology, pathophysiology, and management of altitude illness. The latter half of this volume (Section IV, Special Environments, Sarah A. Nunneley, MD, section editor) examines biomedical aspects of four special environments: aboard ship, the hyperbaric world of diving, supersonic aviation and spaceflight, and unique considerations of 21st century land warfare as it relates to Special Operations and protection from chemical and biological warfare.

USARIEM—particularly Kent B. Pandolf, PhD, and Robert E. Burr, MD, the specialty editors of the three volumes that compose *Medical Aspects of Harsh Environments*—is to be congratulated on the depth and thoroughness of their examination of nearly every aspect of deployed medicine. These volumes are a welcome and overdue contribution to the Textbooks of Military Medicine series.

Charles S. Houston, MD
77 Ledge Road
Burlington, Vermont

Dave Ed. Lounsbury, MD
Colonel, Medical Corps, US Army
Director, Borden Institute, and
Editor in Chief, Textbooks of Military Medicine
Washington, DC

October 2002

The current medical system to support the U.S. Army at war is a continuum from the forward line of troops through the continental United States; it serves as a primary source of trained replacements during the early stages of a major conflict. The system is designed to optimize the return to duty of the maximum number of trained combat soldiers at the lowest possible level. Far-forward stabilization helps to maintain the physiology of injured soldiers who are unlikely to return to duty and allows for their rapid evacuation from the battlefield without needless sacrifice of life or function.

MEDICAL ASPECTS OF HARSH ENVIRONMENTS
VOLUME 2
SECTION III: MOUNTAIN ENVIRONMENTS

Section Editor:

PAUL B. ROCK, DO, PHD
Colonel, Medical Corps, US Army (Ret)
Associate Professor of Medicine, and Acting Director, Center for Aerospace and Hyperbaric Medicine
Oklahoma State University Center for the Health Sciences
Tulsa, Oklahoma

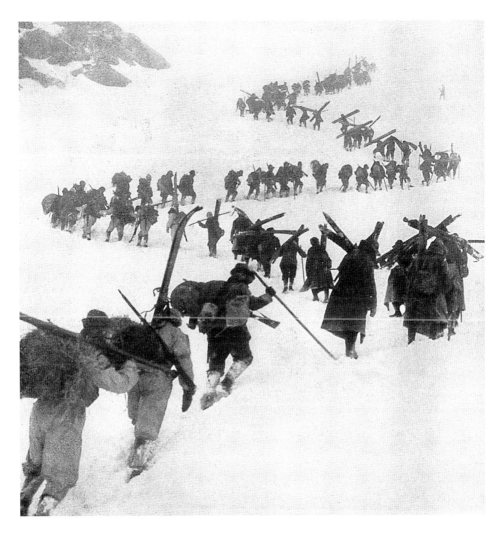

Italian soldiers carrying their skis marching up snow-covered mountain trails. Some of the most ferocious mountain warfare to date occurred during World War I between Italian and Austrian armies, far outstripping mountain battles in other wars. This photograph was taken in April, when the snow had been softened by the warmer rays of the sun and the path made almost impassable by the slush. The difficulty of the march is seen in the step of the men in the rear. Photograph: Comando Supremo, Italian Army (World War I). Reproduced from Bagg EM. Letters from the Italian front. *National Geographic*. 1917;32(1):50.

Chapter 19

MOUNTAINS AND MILITARY MEDICINE: AN OVERVIEW

PAUL B. ROCK, DO, PhD[*]

[*]Colonel, Medical Corps, US Army (Ret); Associate Professor of Medicine, Director, Center for Aerospace and Hyperbaric Medicine, Oklahoma State University Center for Health Sciences, Tulsa, Oklahoma 74132; formerly, US Army Research Institute of Environmental Medicine, Natick, Massachusetts 01760

INTRODUCTION

The Mountain Environments section of this textbook discusses medical concerns associated with military operations in the high mountains (Figure 20-1). Although the focus of the section is limited to military operations, the range of issues addressed is wide, reflecting the broad extent of potential consequences generated by the interaction of activities that military units engage in and the relative complexity of mountain environments. The goal of the section is to provide a comprehensive picture of this interaction that will help military medical personnel prepare to accomplish their mission to conserve the fighting force. This introductory chapter briefly describes the essential aspects of mountains and military operations, and the problems of both that shape their interaction.

Inherent in the concept that medical consequences can result from military activity in mountain terrain are the premises that

1. military operations do take place in mountain terrain, and
2. the interaction between military activity and the environment is of sufficient magnitude as to have discernible consequences.

Houston's excellent review of the history of military campaigns in mountains from ancient times to the present (Chapter 20, Selected Military Operations in Mountain Environments: Some Medical Aspects) illustrates the reality of mountain environments as a legitimate arena for military activity. As Houston points out, this arena has often bestowed considerable success on commanders who had the insight and daring to use the terrain to their tactical advantage. He also notes the large toll that was often extracted from the units involved in those campaigns by the mountain environment itself.

The lengthy border dispute between India and Pakistan at altitudes over 20,000 ft in the Karakorum region of the Himalayan range (still ongoing at the time of this writing [2002]), and the illicit-drug interdiction activities of various military forces in mountain regions of South America suggest that the mixture of soldiers and mountains is not a historical aberration. The United Nations, in designating 2002 as the "International Year of the Mountains," noted that 23 of the 27 armed conflicts ongoing in the world at the beginning of 2002 were being fought in mountain areas.[1] It is likely that as long as war remains a means of settling disputes, tacti-

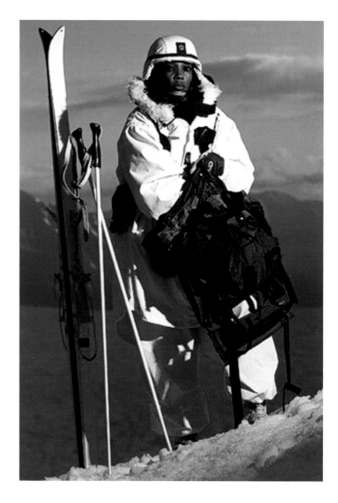

Fig. 19-1. Those involved in providing medical support for military operations in high terrestrial environments are subjected to the same physical and emotional demands that combatants face. The physical rigors of traveling (often on foot) through mountain terrain, combined with the physiological challenges of hypoxia, are exacerbated and made even more dangerous by the emotional decrements (eg, on cognizance and mood state) that are part of life at high altitudes. Although problems such as acute mountain sickness can be resolved by descending to lower altitude and waiting there to acclimatize, this option is not usually available during combat. Military medical officers deployed to high terrestrial environments must therefore insist that the troops receive proper high-altitude training and be aware of the prophylactic pharmacological measures available.

Major Janet Lawrence, Medical Corps, US Army Reserve, seen here in mountain gear during a reserve hospital training exercise in Alaska, typifies the well-equipped Army arctic-mountain soldier. Having served in the Persian Gulf War (1990/91), Dr Lawrence has also experienced the environmental hazards of deserts. Photograph: Courtesy of Rhonda Richards, US Army Reserve Recruiting Command, Fort Knox, Ky.

cal considerations, whether perceived or real, will occasionally thrust military activity into the mountains. Even in the modern era of remote sensing, which lessens the possibility that large forces will use mountain terrain to gain the element of surprise, mountains remain an excellent refuge and a good

---

EXHIBIT 19-1

CATEGORIES OF MOUNTAIN VISITORS APPLICABLE TO HIGH-ALTITUDE MILITARY MEDICINE

Sojourners are persons living at low altitude who travel to altitude and return to low altitude. The meaning is that of a temporary resident, in this case, a temporary resident at high terrestrial altitude. For instance, Nepalese porters *from low altitude* who travel to high altitude to work as porters for a tourist trek (there is a group of low-altitude, native-born Nepalese people who do this), then return to their low-altitude homes, are altitude sojourners—as are the tourists for whom these porters carry supplies. Interestingly, these porters from low altitude are as likely as other unacclimatized individuals are to get altitude maladies.

Trekkers, in the context of mountain medicine, are persons who undertake a prolonged (ie, more than 1 day) journey in the mountains *on foot*. In general, they have a specific geographical goal to visit and then return from (ie, Mount Everest base camp), although both circuit and one-way treks are also popular. Trekkers are sojourners, but sojourners *on foot* as opposed to traveling by vehicle. (NOTE: they can use a vehicle to arrive at the start point of their trek but become "trekkers" when they dismount and walk a significant distance.) They may or may not carry their equipment with them; therefore, they may or may not also be considered "backpackers." When they do not carry their own equipment, they could be considered "hikers," except that trekkers hike for a more prolonged period (days) than do hikers (see below).

Trekkers today tend to be wealthy individuals who can afford to pay large sums of money to be guided through regions of the Himalaya Mountains on foot by commercial concerns that specialize in organizing treks. It was not always so. The word "trek" comes from the Afrikaner language in South Africa and originally referred to the migration of Dutch settlers from the coast into the interior highlands by ox cart. The "on foot" context comes from the fact that the Afrikaners walked beside the oxen to drive them. Oxen pulled the household goods and tools but not the people. In contemporary trekking, human porters carry most of the equipment and the people still walk; the trip is arduous in terms of both physical effort and the complexity of organization that it requires.

Both of these identifying characteristics are probably involved in modern commercial trekking, but the characteristic of interest to military mountain medicine is the traveling through the mountains on foot. Because military units may be required to move through mountain terrain on foot, the data collected on civilian trekkers may be used to approximate disease and nonbattle injury estimates for those military personnel.

Backpackers travel in the mountains on foot for more than 1 day but carry their equipment with them in backpacks. Hikers may or may not also carry equipment but they carry less than backpackers do. The energy requirements of backpackers may be similar to those of military personnel, given that both categories carry their own equipment, although military personnel may carry more weight per person, owing to carrying their own weapons and ammunition.

Hikers also travel on foot but for less than 1 day.

Climbers use their arms and legs to ascend a geological structure (usually a mountain but also cliffs, ice walls, pinnacles, spires, and, recently, indoor climbing walls). They must hang on to the structure to keep from falling. "Technical climbers" employ climbing equipment to keep from falling; "free climbers" do not. For purposes of mountain medicine, the constellation of diseases and injuries differs between these categories of climbers.

Depending on their mission, military personnel who deploy to mountain environments can experience activities equivalent to each of the categories described above. Consequently, military medical officers and other healthcare providers must familiarize themselves with all of them.

arena for small-unit tactical maneuvers. If the history recounted by Houston in Chapter 20 is any guide, it is probable that the mountain environment itself will remain a threat to military units operating there—one capable of causing a significant reduction in force through altitude illness, injury, and hypoxia-induced performance decrements.

Most human activity in mountain regions is not for military purposes. In addition to large indigenous populations in the mountain regions of South America and Central Asia, millions of lowlanders travel into high mountains every year for recreational or economic pursuits (Exhibit 19-1 and Figure 19-2). These civilians are subject to environmentally related medical problems, of course, but the constellation of medical problems arising out of military operations in mountain terrain differs to some extent from those related to civilian activities. The difference is due to the way in which certain inherent aspects of military activity alter the "human-to-mountain" interaction. To appreciate and, more importantly, anticipate the pattern of potential problems, we must be cognizant of the particular characteristics of mountains and military operations that can interact.

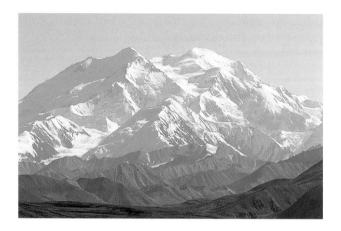

Fig. 19-2. Each year from April to July, many civilians fall victim to altitude illness, hypothermia, and freezing cold injury and are rescued from Mount McKinley, Alaska. Even experienced climbers fail to appreciate how dangerous Mount McKinley is, with its severe cold, raging storms, and avalanches. Military and civilian medical research camps at 7,300 and 14,000 ft make the mountain one of the great physiological and clinical outdoor laboratories. Photograph: Courtesy of William J. Mills, Jr, MD, Anchorage, Alaska.

CHARACTERISTICS OF MOUNTAIN ENVIRONMENTS

Mountain environments are not simple. Although the general geomorphological form known as a "mountain" is universally recognized, it encompasses a variety of actualities. To a small child, especially one with imagination, the dirt pile excavated from a small construction site is as valid a "mountain" as 8,530-m (29,028-ft) Mount Everest (called in Tibet *Chomolungma*, which means "the goddess mother of the Earth"). To someone familiar with only the East Coast of North America, "mountains" range between 150 and 1,525 m (500–5,000 ft) in height, while to someone from the central Rocky Mountains of North America, anything under 5,000 ft is a hill and not a proper mountain at all. The two more-or-less flat regions of Earth that occupy huge chunks of what should be sky from a sea-level perspective (ie, the Andean altiplano and the Tibetan plateau) bear remarkable superficial resemblance to deserts or plains, yet many of the medical problems seen in those regions are the same as those found in the surrounding snow-covered peaks. Such medical problems are not seen in the child's dirt pile or, to any great extent, in the low mountains of the North American eastern seaboard. What then is the difference? The difference is hypobaric hypoxia.

Hypobaric hypoxia (ie, the decrease in oxygen available for metabolic processes due to the progressive decrease in ambient barometric pressure that occurs with increasing elevation) is the most defining characteristic of mountain environments, because it is both unique to and ubiquitous within mountain environments. It causes a host of medical problems, which are usually classified under the general rubric of "altitude illness." It also interacts synergistically with other environmental factors to exaggerate the problems that those factors cause. Young and Reeves present an extensive discussion of hypobaric hypoxia and its physiological effects in Chapter 21, Human Adaptation to High Terrestrial Altitude. Understanding the human body's normal adaptive response to chronic hypobaric hypoxia, a process termed "altitude acclimatization," provides a framework for understanding altitude illness. In one sense, altitude illness results from either failure to acclimatize (inadequate adaptation) or from overcompensation of the acclimatization response (maladaptation).

Although hypobaric hypoxia is the most defining feature of mountain environments in terms of medical significance, it is not the only factor that can affect military personnel operating there. Mountain regions are complex in both space and time. Rugged terrain features that contain a significant and often dangerous vertical component are a nearly constant feature of mountains, one that can present significant obstacles to military operations, including medical evacuation of wounded. Mountains can also make their own weather, in the form of ferocious storms. Although mountains are often thought of as being cold and snowy, they can also be very dry and hot. Ultraviolet (UV) light is filtered less well by the thinner atmosphere in high mountains, creating the possibility for significant UV radiation exposure.

Each of the many terrain and climatic factors that mountains have in common with other environments can constitute a threat to the health and well-being of military personnel, and the medical consequences of many of these conditions are the subjects of the first four sections of *Medical Aspects of Harsh Environments* (eg, Section I, Hot Environments, and Section II, Cold Environments, and their injuries are contained in *Volume 1*).[2] Mountain environments are unique in that hypobaric hypoxia is ubiquitous there, and other potentially harmful conditions interact with it. Depending on the degree of hypoxia, the interaction may significantly alter the effect of the other environmental factor. The alteration is virtually never in a direction that would seem favorable for the soldier deployed there. Rock and Mader discuss the problem of synergy between environmental factors in mountain environments in Chapter 26, Additional Medical Problems in Mountain Environments.

CHARACTERISTICS OF MILITARY OPERATIONS

Two characteristics of military operations are particularly important in shaping the interaction with mountain environments:

1. the wide range of activities associated with military operations, and
2. the frequent lack of choice as to when and where to participate in those activities.

Both are a consequence of the fact that the purpose of military operations is to engage in successful combat when necessary. Both of these aspects function to increase the potential for adverse consequences in the exposed personnel.

The spectrum of activities encompassed by military operations is very broad. It ranges from operation of weapons to operation of computers, from first-aid to lifesaving surgery, from preparation of field rations by individual soldiers to preparation of hot meals for hundreds of soldiers. Further, the contingencies of combat may force an individual soldier to perform multiple different tasks within a relatively short time. Each of those tasks changes the way in which the soldier interacts with the environment: sometimes subtly, often dramatically. In combat, the proficiency with which a task is per-

formed may affect mission accomplishment and have life-and-death consequences, not only for the individual soldier but also for the rest of the unit.

The other characteristic of military operations that shapes the soldier–environment interaction is that the time and place of exposure are often dictated by tactical considerations rather than the presence of favorable or even benign environmental conditions. For soldiers in the forward echelons, virtually everything they do is associated with exposure to environmental hazards on the most basic level. When deployed in the field, they eat, sleep, train, and fight in an immediate and intimate relationship with physical and biological terrain features, hazards, and weather. Unlike the recreational climber or skier, who can choose to wait for better weather or travel a different route, a soldier may not have the option to wait. Unlike a miner who works in a high-altitude mine or an astronomer using a telescope on a high mountain peak, the soldier may not have the choice of staying home from work if the weather is bad or the route only marginally passable. The potential result of these two characteristics of military operations is an increase in the soldier's environmental exposure in the mountains.

MILITARY MEDICINE IN MOUNTAIN TERRAIN

Because mountains are complex environments, they pose a broad spectrum of potential threats to health and well-being. Add to that the potential for military operations to increase the environmental exposure, and a wide array of potential problems can be anticipated. From a military standpoint, those problems are most usefully classified in terms of their impact on unit function (ie, mission accomplishment), and it is this classification that serves to organize the material presented in the chapters in the Mountain Environment section. For a military unit operating in the mountains, environmental problems cause either a decrement in unit force or a decrement in soldier performance. Both can jeopardize the unit's mission.

Altitude illness and other medical conditions related to the mountain environment are best viewed as causing decrement in unit force. Based on their etiology, they can be classified into three groups: (1) hypoxia-related conditions, (2) conditions that are not directly related to hypoxia, and (3) conditions that result from the interaction of hypoxia with other environmental factors.

Hypoxia-Related Conditions

The hypoxia-related conditions are unique to high-mountain environments, and they receive the most attention in this section. These conditions can be further classified into (*a*) hypoxia-induced edemas and (*b*) nonedematous conditions.

Hypoxia-Induced Edemas

Altitude edemas run the gamut from acute mountain sickness (AMS), a common and usually self-limited condition that can cause incapacitating symptoms, to high-altitude pulmonary edema (HAPE) and high-altitude cerebral edema (HACE), usually relatively rare conditions that can rapidly be fatal. AMS can cause a large, temporary decrement in fighting force because it affects large numbers of personnel. Both HAPE and HACE cause permanent decrements by their high mortality. Although HAPE and HACE are considered relatively rare in the civilian recreational setting, the limited data from military conflicts suggests that these deadly conditions may be a much bigger problem in the setting of ongoing hostilities, due either to increased incidence from the specific circumstances of exposure generated by deployment or to battle-related impediments to adequate care and evacuation. It is important to note that all hypoxia-related conditions will resolve if the casualty can be evacuated to a lower altitude in a timely fashion. AMS and HACE are discussed by Roach, Hackett, and Stepanek in Chapter 24; HAPE by Roach and Schoene in Chapter 25; and altitude-related peripheral edema by Rock and Mader in Chapter 26.

Nonedematous Conditions

While the edemas of high altitude are probably considered the quintessential altitude syndromes, other hypoxia-related but nonedematous conditions can cause significant morbidity and, thereby, impact on military operations. These include physical and cognitive performance decrements and

changes in mood states, high-altitude retinal hemorrhages, sleep disturbances, and progressive physical deterioration and weight loss (known as climbers' cachexia). Hypoxia-induced physical performance decrements in mountain terrain can be profound and severely affect overall unit performance. To the affected soldier or commander, hypoxia-related decrements in cognitive function and mood state are often less apparent than physical effects, such decrements also have the potential to compromise unit function. Because hypoxia is ubiquitous, medical officers must remember that command personnel are just as susceptible as other unit personnel. Both physical and cognitive performance decrements must be anticipated so that measures can be taken to lessen their impact. Physical performance decrements are discussed by Fulco and Cymerman in Chapter 22, Physical Performance at Varying Terrestrial Altitudes, and psychological performance is discussed by Banderet and Shukitt-Hale in Chapter 23, Cognitive Performance, Mood, and Other Psychological Effects at High Altitude.

Additionally, the chronic hypoxia of high-mountain environments can also interact with preexisting medical conditions to cause significant morbidity. While this might not be thought of as a major problem for military units, which are traditionally composed of young, relatively healthy individuals without significant pathological conditions, the upper echelons of command generally comprise older individuals who may have conditions of "normal" aging (eg, coronary artery disease, emphysema) that cause them to be at increased risk from hypoxia. Additionally, conditions such as sickle cell trait, which are often unrecognized in young military personnel, can result in life-threatening pathology at high altitude. Nonedematous conditions caused by hypoxia and the interaction of hypoxia with preexisting medical conditions are discussed by Rock and Mader in Chapter 26, Additional Medical Problems in Mountain Environments.

Conditions Not Directly Related to Hypoxia

Illness or injury caused by factors other than hypoxia are not unique to mountain environments, but they can be a significant component of the constellation of medical problems seen during military operations there. Cold injury is the most obvious of these, but dehydration, malnutrition, and even heat injury are also important at high altitude. Although most of these conditions are discussed in detail in *Medical Aspects of Harsh Environments, Volume 1*,[2] they are also listed in Chapter 26, Additional

Medical Problems in Mountain Environments, along with other nonhypoxic conditions such as lightning strikes and constipation, to provide an accurate picture of the medical problems associated with deployment to high mountains. Appreciation of the complete spectrum of possible medical problems is necessary for planning adequate medical support to deploying units.

Interaction of Hypoxia and Environmental Factors

The solutions to the hypoxia-related medical problems and performance decrements experienced during military operations in the mountains fall into two broad categories: Mother Nature's and military or man-made. Nature's solution is "altitude acclimatization," a process of hypoxia-induced changes in physiological processes that regulate homeostasis around a lowered set point of blood oxygen content. Although there are limits to the altitude to which people can successfully acclimatize (eg, < 18,000 ft), the beneficial effects of acclimatization are so well recognized that the absence of altitude illness and improvement in submaximal physical performance are generally accepted to be evidence of the acclimatized state. In many ways, the acclimatization of personnel would be the ideal solution to the medical threats posed by altitude exposure for the military, but some potential problems lurk:

- The biggest problem is that time and exposure to high altitude are needed to achieve and maintain the acclimatized state. This need potentially limits the flexibility for rapid maneuver, which can offer tactical advantages.
- Reliance on acclimatization would necessitate stationing troops more or less permanently at high altitude to maintain the acclimatized state, an option that is not always available or practical. (As previously noted, the physiology of acclimatization is discussed in Chapter 21, Human Adaptation to High Terrestrial Altitude.)

If altitude acclimatization is not possible, then other (man-made) solutions to prevent altitude illness and increase military performance in the mountains must be considered. If military operations in mountain environments could be avoided, these particular problems would cease to exist. Such is not the case, however, so the military must rely on solutions that are more practical, including training and pharmacological prophylaxis against altitude illness. Various options for preventing illness and increasing performance are described in Chapters 22 through 26. Their specific applications to the military situation, and the role of the unit medical officer in implementing medical support for mountain operations is addressed in by Rock and Iwancyk in Chapter 27, Military Medical Operations in Mountain Environments.

SUMMARY

Military operations in mountain terrain can be associated with environmentally related medical problems and performance decrements that can have significant impact on mission attainment. Military personnel may be more at risk for problems than civilians, because military operations can increase exposure to harsh conditions. Hypobaric hypoxia is unique to high-mountain environments and is responsible for altitude illness and physical and cognitive performance decrements. Because hypoxia is ubiquitous, all unit personnel, including command and medical support, are equally susceptible to its effects. Altitude acclimatization can prevent altitude illness and improve performance, but the time and circumstances to achieve acclimatization may not always be available to units in a rapidly changing tactical situation.

REFERENCES

1. Associated Press. Mountains in danger, UN says. *Tulsa World.* 2002;97(134):28 Jan 2002.

2. Pandolf K, Burr RE, Wenger CB, Pozos RS, eds. *Medical Aspects of Harsh Environments, Volume 1.* In: Zajtchuk R, Bellamy RF, eds. *Textbook of Military Medicine.* Washington, DC: Department of the Army, Office of The Surgeon General, and Borden Institute; 2001. Also available at www.armymedicine.army.mil/history/borden/default.htm.

Chapter 20

SELECTED MILITARY OPERATIONS IN MOUNTAIN ENVIRONMENTS: SOME MEDICAL ASPECTS

CHARLES S. HOUSTON, MD[*]

[*]77 Ledge Road, Burlington, Vermont 05401; formerly, Professor of Medicine, and Chairman, Department of Environmental Health, University of Vermont, College of Medicine, Burlington, Vermont 05401

INTRODUCTION

In war, victory often depends on skillful use of the high ground, so hills and mountains have been central to warfare for thousands of years. Gentle hills, like those at Marathon and Gettysburg, give tactical advantage with few obstacles from environment or geography. On higher mountains like the Alps or the Caucasus, the greater is the tactical advantage for offense or defense, but the problems are also greater. The mountain environment poses dangerous medical problems including frostbite, hypothermia, hypoxia, hypoglycemia, and dehydration. Of these, cold injuries (eg, frostbite and hypothermia) have been the most frequent and serious, but altitude illnesses and malnutrition have also caused many casualties (Exhibit 20-1).

Because of the obstacles to men and equipment, few military operations have taken place above 2,400 m (8,000 ft), where the environmental, geographical, and medical obstacles are more significant and often dramatic. On most mountainous terrain below 1,000 m, environment does not cause problems not encountered anywhere else, but armies that have campaigned at elevations higher than 2,500 m have sometimes suffered more casualties from the mountain environment than from enemy action. Military medicine has an obvious need to study basic altitude physiology. In 1946 the US Navy did a pioneer study of human physiological adaptations to extreme altitude, and in 1985 the US Army expanded that study: these are called Operation Everest and Operation Everest II (Exhibit 20-2).

History offers many lessons that, when heeded, can minimize military losses in mountain environments; selected examples are the theme of this chapter.

EXHIBIT 20-1

COLD-, ALTITUDE-, AND NUTRITION-RELATED CONDITIONS EXPERIENCED IN MOUNTAIN ENVIRONMENTS

Frostbite	Air temperature falls one degree Centigrade with every 100 m of altitude, and the dangers of freezing cold injury (frostbite) and hypothermia are compounded by hypoxia, hypoglycemia, and dehydration. Cold also causes problems for animals and equipment.
Hypothermia	Whenever heat is lost faster than the body can generate it, core temperature falls proportionally to the temperature difference and rate of loss, causing weakness, confusion, hallucinations, coma, and death.
Hypoxia	The available oxygen in air decreases in parallel to the decrease in barometric pressure with increasing altitude, resulting in subnormal levels of oxygen in arterial blood or tissue (short of anoxia). Hypoxia impairs judgment, slows reflexes, causes a spectrum of illnesses, and decreases work capacity and will.
Hypoglycemia	Both physical and mental exertion require fuel. Carbohydrate is the most readily available; protein and fat are used later. Owing to difficulties with transport, soldiers often do not have enough food, which may cause a debilitating decrease in blood sugar with symptoms similar to those caused by hypoxia and hypothermia. Hungry troops lose strength and weight, and are slow to respond.
Dehydration	In cold areas, water is usually scarce because it must come from melting ice, and fuel for melting is scanty. Mountain air is dry, and excessive water is lost by the increased ventilation due to work and to hypoxia. Although sweating is insensible, water is lost during strenuous work at altitude.
Injury	Higher mountains are generally more rugged, steeper, and more fraught with danger from rockfalls and avalanches, which are common causes of injuries or death. Transport for the injured or wounded is difficult, and triage is complicated by cold and altitude.
Illness	Sanitary measures are limited, and infectious diseases and malnutrition are problems.

EXHIBIT 20-2

OPERATION EVEREST AND OPERATION EVEREST II

Control of the heights has long been important in war. Two centuries ago the Montgolfier hot air balloon took this to a new dimension—high in the air. When Benjamin Franklin saw one of the first flights, he envisioned an armada of thousands of balloons carrying airborne troops to battle. France formed the first air force—the "Compagnie d'Aerostiers"—and on 2 June 1794 two French soldiers were taken high above gunshot to observe and report the disposition of the Austrian army ranged against them. For many decades such balloons did not ascend more than a few thousand feet. However, in 1875, a huge balloon carried three men to over 25,000 ft; two were dead from hypoxia when they landed. The danger of great altitude was thus dramatically proven: if men were to fight in the air, the hazards of high altitude must be overcome.

By 1920, powered aircraft could reach altitudes that incapacitated pilots if they did not breathe extra oxygen. Twenty-five years later, aircraft could go even higher, beyond the level where pure oxygen, delivered under ambient pressure, sufficed. Pressurized cabins were thought impracticable for battle; other approaches were sought.

By then it was clear that exposure to gradually increasing altitude enabled men to survive, whereas the unacclimatized soon lost consciousness. Some air forces kept pilots for weeks at moderate elevations in the mountains to enable them to fly higher than their adversaries. This was somewhat effective but impractical, and it suggested that aircrews might become acclimatized by repeated exposure to simulated altitude in decompression chambers.

Operation Everest

To examine this concept, in 1946 the US Navy authorized a study of acclimatization called Operation Everest, which was conducted at the Naval Air Station, Pensacola, Florida. Four men were taken to a simulated altitude of 8,800 m (29,000 ft) during 35 days of slow ascent. Samples of arterial and venous blood, expired air, and urine, taken at rest and after exercise, were analyzed, and subjects were examined repeatedly during the ascent. Electrocardiograms and occasional chest roentgenograms monitored cardiac function.

Finally two of the four reached a simulated altitude of 8,800 m, where they were able to do light work for 20 minutes. Next day, breathing 100% oxygen, they were taken slowly from 8,800 to 15,200 m (50,500 ft), where they were able to exercise, although only lightly. This portion of the study showed that when breathing pure oxygen, these partially acclimatized men could go much higher than could the unacclimatized; at the time, this proved that acclimatization could give a small edge to the fighting pilot at extreme altitude. Soon, however, the use of pressurized cabins made moot the issue of acclimatization. Today, for military purposes, the altitude ceiling of the aircraft, rather than the pilot's tolerance, is the limiting factor.

Of more general medical interest were the clinical and laboratory data obtained throughout Operation Everest. Pulmonary ventilation increased the most in the men least affected as the altitude was increased, suggesting the benefits of a strong hypoxic ventilatory drive. The alveolar–arterial oxygen pressure gradient decreased with increasing altitude but increased with exercise. The pH of arterial blood increased in parallel with increasing ventilation but leveled off and slowly fell toward normal as acclimatization matured. The increased alkalinity of blood altered the shape of the oxyhemoglobin dissociation curve, enhancing delivery of oxygen to the tissues. Although blood oxygen saturation fell, oxygen content of arterial blood did not because of the increased hemoglobin. The heart showed no sign of strain. Operation Everest confirmed earlier impressions that acclimatization was accomplished by many integrated changes that tended to restore cellular oxygen toward normal.

The data from Operation Everest also had more general clinical interest by outlining how acclimatization to hypoxia helps persons with chronic heart, lung, or blood disorders. Many such patients may live for months or years with arterial blood oxygen content almost as low as that experienced by a healthy mountaineer as high as some of the Rocky Mountains.

Operation Everest II

Troops often need to campaign in mountainous environments. The experience of armies fighting in the Himalayan Mountains has shown that unacclimatized troops taken too rapidly to altitude will suffer attrition from mountain sickness. To further study acclimatization, Operation Everest II was carried out in 1985 by the US

*(**Exhibit 20-2** continues)*

Exhibit 20-2 *continued*

Army at the US Army Research Institute of Environmental Medicine (USARIEM), Natick, Massachusetts. Like Operation Everest in 1946, this was to be a study of "pure hypoxia" absent the confounding stresses of cold, dehydration, and heavy work encountered on high mountains.

Eight healthy and athletic young men lived in a large decompression chamber for 40 days while atmospheric pressure in the chamber was slowly decreased to that found at 8,800 m. Cardiac catheterizations were done at three altitudes (sea level, 20,000 ft, and 25,000–29,000 ft) to assess heart function at rest and during and after exercise. Using special gas mixtures, pulmonary function and diffusing capacity were also measured at increasing altitude. Muscle biopsies were studied for structure, intracellular adaptations, and biochemical changes. A variety of hormone and electrolyte studies were done. Daily physical examinations, alveolar air sampling, and measurement of caloric intake and output, as well as occasional psychometric tests, were also done.

A slightly slower rate of ascent than in the first study was used, hoping that more complete acclimatization could be achieved. New technology enabled collection of far more data than had been possible 40 years earlier. During ascent, pulmonary ventilation increased, cardiac output decreased, and pulmonary artery pressure increased, but the heart functioned well. Although the alveolar–arterial oxygen gradient decreased, mixed-gas analyses of pulmonary function showed evidence of significant interstitial pulmonary edema, increasing with altitude in all subjects. This suggested that the lung, rather than the heart, may be the factor limiting tolerance for extreme altitude. Alveolar, arterial, and mixed venous blood analyses added to projections made by others. Muscle chemistry and structural analyses cast more light on cellular metabolism. Despite free choice of nutritious and appetizing food, caloric intake fell as the subjects lost appetite, and their weight decreased. Maximal work capacity decreased with altitude and did not approach that found at sea level over the period at altitude.

The findings enlarged the data obtained from the 1946 US Navy study, but suggested that the rate of ascent had been too fast to enable full acclimatization. The 1985 US Army study had special relevance to military forces that must travel, fight, and live at moderate elevations. By demonstrating the decrease in work capacity at high altitude but showing the benefits of slow ascent acclimatization, soldiers and civilians alike have benefited from this ambitious study.

RECOMMENDED READING

Jackson DD. *The Aeronuts: The Epic of Flight.* Alexandria, Va: Time Life Books; 1980.

Houston CS, Cymerman A, Sutton JR. *Operation Everest II 1985.* Natick, Mass: US Army Research Institute of Environmental Medicine; 1991.

ASIA

The vast continent of Asia, including the Middle East, contains the highest and most complicated mountains, the largest and most hostile deserts and plains, and the most difficult terrain for warfare. Yet these areas have has been arenas for battles for many thousands of years.

Ancient Greece: Xenophon

Exiled from Athens for his opposition to democracy in 397 BC, Xenophon[1] joined the army as a foot soldier. His troops elected Xenophon leader of the disorganized Greek army, later known as the Ten Thousand, when it was hard-pressed in central Armenia during the campaign against the Persians. Xenophon's detailed day-by-day account describes the hardships and dangers of warfare in the mountains and deserts of Kurdistan and Armenia and gives an intimate picture of the life of an ordinary foot soldier. In contrast to the well-balanced force that Alexander would lead in the same region many decades later, Xenophon had 10,000 foot soldiers but only 50 cavalry. This limited his mobility and his timely appraisal of the enemy and slowed the advance of his army, exposing the troops to prolonged cold, hunger, and altitude.

In a chapter of his *Anabasis,* or *Persian Expedition,* entitled "Marching Through the Snow," Xenophon describes the hardships that his soldiers encountered while crossing a high plateau in the Taurus mountains, which range from 1,800 to 4,000 m (6,000–13,000 ft) in height:

Next came a three days' march of 45 miles over level ground and through deep snow. The third day's march was a hard one, with a north wind blowing into their faces, cutting through absolutely everything like a knife and freezing people stiff. One of the soothsayers then proposed making a sacrifice to the wind and his suggestion was carried out. It was agreed by all that there was a distinct falling off of the violence of the wind. The snow was six feet deep and many of the animals and slaves perished in it, as did about thirty of the soldiers.

. . . .

The whole of the next day's march from here was through the snow and a number of the soldiers suffered from bulimia. Xenophon who, as he commanded the rearguard, came upon men who had collapsed, did not know what the disease was.[1(pp196–197)]

The elevation of this plateau and the passes that Xenophon crossed are not clear from his account nor are they easily ascertainable from the maps showing his route, but the depth of snow and the cold suggest that much of the route was higher than 2,400 m (8,000 ft). Food, fuel, and water were limited in this harsh, frozen terrain. Some soldiers fell senseless to the ground from what Xenophon calls "bulimia," which was probably a combination of hunger, cold, and exhaustion. Xenophon was told that bulimia should be treated with food, so he personally went among the troops collecting and distributing food to the victims. Xenophon wrote of his troops:

> As soon as they had something to eat, they stood up and went on marching.[1(p197)]

During the day the troops suffered greatly from snow blindness, but some prevented this by holding something black before their eyes. Their feet often froze to the soles of their makeshift sandals of undressed oxen skins.

In the next chapter, entitled "They Capture a Pass by a Manoeuvre," Xenophon describes how, after traversing this difficult terrain, the troops finally reached a pass that led down to the fertile plains where the Ohasis River ran. The pass was held by a strong enemy force, and the generals disagreed how best to proceed. After a powerful address by Xenophon, the Ten Thousand surprised the enemy outposts; after several sharply fought engagements, they attacked the enemy's rear. Then, after securing the pass,

> they offered sacrifices and ... descended into the plain and came among villages full of plenty of good food,[1(p206)]

where his soldiers regained their strength.

This extraordinary military campaign shows how a brilliant and determined commander can successfully lead an army through unknown territory and across mountains and deserts, facing severe weather and all the problems of a mountain environment. Xenophon's leadership places this campaign among the great military operations in history.

Ancient Greece: Alexander the Great

Sixty years after Xenophon's march through this area, Alexander of Macedon followed part of Xenophon's route during his campaign against the Persians and his subsequent invasion of India (Figure 20-1). Accounts of this long and arduous campaign (although often conflicting) describe the hardships encountered in mountainous country.[2–4]

Xenophon had shown restraint as he moved through the western part of this wild and little-known region, but Alexander, when his passage was opposed, ruthlessly destroyed cities, slaughtered inhabitants, and burned crops. Alexander felt compelled to leave only scorched earth behind him because he had insufficient troops for garrisons to protect his long and tenuous supply line. As a result, obtaining water and food was one of his worst problems.

For more than 10,000 miles from Macedonia, through Greece, Egypt, and Asia Minor, it was not unusual for Alexander's troops to march 100 or 150 miles in 4 days over ordinary terrain. Their progress was much slower in the mountains, however, which were often higher than 1,800 m (6,000 ft).[3]

In November 331 BC, driving northward from Kandahar, Alexander crossed the highlands of central Afghanistan, where his army suffered severely from altitude, cold, and snow blindness. Many soldiers died before he descended to the more hospitable environment of Kabul, at 1,800 m (6,000 ft) above sea level. Before him were the imposing Hindu Kush mountains (known in that time as the Caucasus Indicus), north of which his enemy Bessus waited, arrogant and confident that his army could whip Alexander should he attempt to cross these fearsome mountains.

Anticipating that Bessus would expect him by the lowest and easiest of the seven passes, Alexander chose the most easterly Khawak Pass (4,500 m, or 15,000 ft high), the steepest, highest, and most treacherous because of snow and avalanches. He set out from Kabul in 329 BC, too early in the spring to cross such a high pass because, although the snow was beginning to melt in Kabul, winter still raged

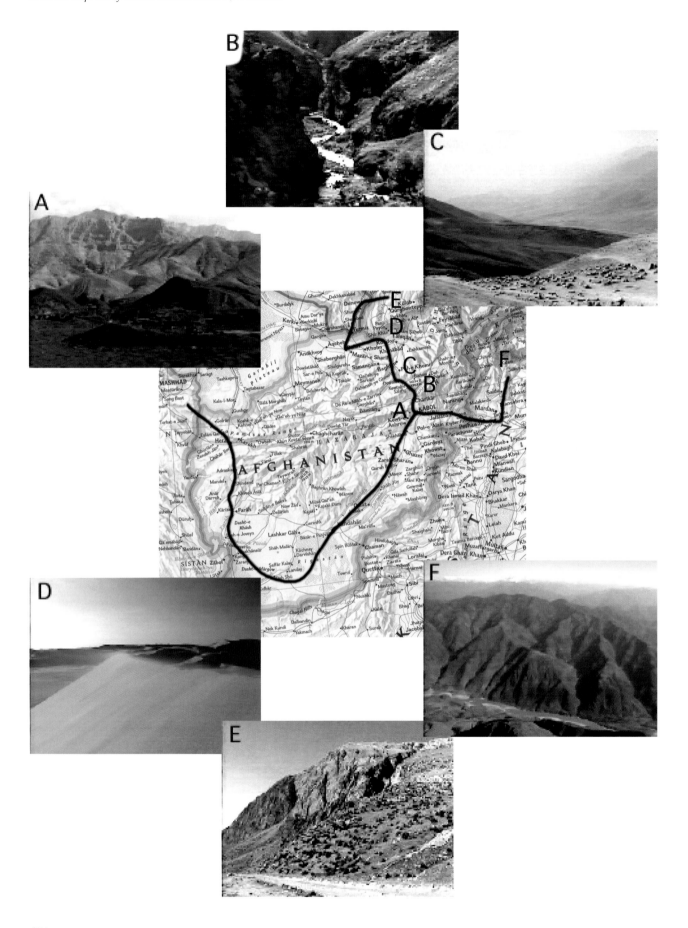

Fig. 20-1. When Alexander's route through central Asia is superimposed on a map of modern Afghanistan, his army is seen to have marched through many populated locations that have recently assumed great importance: Herat, Kandahar, Kabul, and Mazar-e Sharif, to mention a few. The geographical sites that Alexander is renown for traversing are equally impressive. (**a**) A view of the Hindu Kush Mountains from north of Kabul; this range had to be crossed if Alexander were to reach central Asia. (**b**) The Panjshir Valley is seen at a point before the entrance to the Khawak Pass is reached. (**c**) The view looking north from the summit of Khawak Pass (11,000 ft); Alexander's army of approximately 50,000 crossed here in the spring, before the snows had melted. (**d**) The desert that Alexander had to cross before reaching the Oxus River (now, the Amu Darya) and present-day Tajikistan. (**e**) The likely Sogdian Rock in Tajikistan; Alexander's mountain troops are believed to have scaled the rock face to the left. (**f**) The probable site of the last of Alexander's great mountain warfare campaigns, the Aornos Rock in modern northwestern Pakistan. Alexander's mountain troops scaled the deep couloir on the extreme left and traversed the ridge line to his enemy's base camp on the extreme right. Map: Adapted from National Geographic Society, Washington, DC. Video frames: Reproduced with permission from Dobbs R, producer. *In the Footsteps of Alexander the Great.* Maya Vision International, London, England.

in the mountains.

The snow line began 20 miles before the actual pass, and the snow drifts became deeper the higher his army climbed. The weather was severe. (There are several different versions of the story, but they all describe extreme difficulty.) Hundreds of men froze to death, others became snow-blind and wandered away. Altitude illnesses had not been recognized in that era, but it is probable that Alexander's losses were a classic example of the synergism of hypoxia, cold, hunger, and dehydration. After reaching the summit of the pass, the long baggage train, including Alexander's full court, and the surviving thousands of camp followers labored another 40 miles down the northern side to below the snow line. The army was starving and exhausted as it reached a desolated land: Bessus had destroyed everything.

That 60 miles took 15 days and cost Alexander an unknown number of lives, unknown because only battle deaths were recorded.[2] Some reports say that half of Alexander's fighting men died from the altitude and cold, the effects of which were increased by inadequate food and water. This famous campaign is one of the most costly and difficult in the history of mountain warfare.

Many historians describe Alexander's assault on a famous mountain citadel, the Sogdian (or Ariamazes) Rock. (Quintus Curtius Rufus's version is slightly different from that of other historians. He writes that the soldiers drove their wedges into cracks between the rocks, as modern climbers do, and states that the rock was 30 furlongs [2,000 m] high.[5]) Although altitude was not a factor, the rock was said to be at least 1,000 m (3,300 ft) high and precipitously steep on all sides. Its exact location is hard to trace but it is probably in modern Tajikistan, near the Oxus River (now called Amu Darya). It is said to have had persistent snow on the flat summit, which gave the 35,000 inhabitants ample water. Confident of their impregnable position, the Sogdians scoffed at Alexander's demand for their surrender. "To reach us your men will have to fly like birds," they replied. According to Arrian, Alexander was furious and determined to capture and sack the castle. So at night, in midwinter, he asked for volunteers:

> There were some 300 men who in previous sieges had had experience in rock-climbing. These now assembled. They had provided themselves with small iron tent-pegs, which they proposed to drive into the snow, where it was frozen hard, or into any bit of bare earth they might come across, and they attached to the pegs strong flaxen lines ...; then, driving their pegs either into bare ground or into such patches of snow as seemed most likely to hold under the strain, they hauled themselves up, wherever each could find a way. About thirty lost their lives during the ascent—falling in various places into the snow, their bodies were never recovered ... —but the rest reached the top just as dawn was breaking.[2(pp233–234)]

The awestruck defenders, seeing this small band on the high cliffs across from but overlooking their town, believed that Alexander's men had indeed "flown like birds" and immediately surrendered. This must be among the first records of such direct aid climbing in warfare; much later it would become part of the training for troops intended for fighting in the mountains. Alexander killed most of the people; spared their king, Oxyartes; and married the king's beautiful daughter, Roxana.[4]

As was the case with his predecessor, Xenophon, strong leadership inspired Alexander's army to fight its way through uncharted hostile lands despite inadequate supplies, and across high mountains despite extreme cold and altitude. Much later, when Alexander's leadership faltered, the campaign fell apart; after his death, disaster followed.

EUROPE: THE ALPS AND THE CAUCASUS

During the centuries of the Roman Empire, hundreds of roads were built across several dozen passes over 2,000 m (6,500 ft) high through the Alps north of Italy. Some roads were paved and their traces remain today. Some were trade routes, but most were originally military roads over which the Roman armies marched to conquer northern tribes and to police their vast empire. The passes were easily defended, and the Alps provided a strong barrier to invading barbarians from the north. Gibbon, the comprehensive historian, does not describe the environmental problems that Roman soldiers

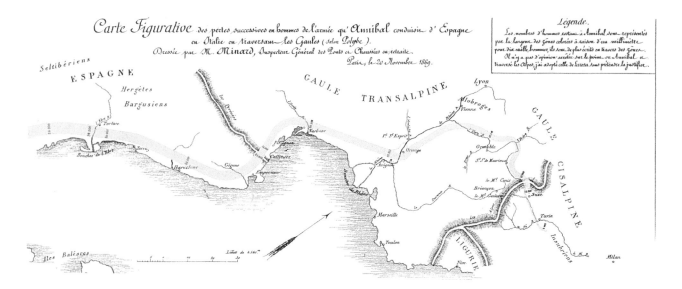

Fig. 20-2. This classic 1869 map drawn by Charles Joseph Minard, Inspector General of Bridges and Roads, depicts the successive losses of men from Hannibal's army as he crossed from Spain to Italy, through Gaul (according to Polybe). Translated, the legend reads, in part:

> The number of men accompanying Hannibal is represented by the thickness of the colored line (1 mm = 10,000 men [at the start, Hannibal's army numbered about 50,000 men]). Geographical landmarks are also shown on or near the colored line. Because it is uncertain where Hannibal crossed the Alps, I have adopted the opinion of Larosa without attempting to defend it.[1]

Confusion still reigns over the exact route that Hannibal took, but it is known that his men and animals suffered greatly from hunger and the cold, wintry conditions. For example, according to the Greek statesman and historian Polybius (ca 200–118 BC),

> [the] conditions were so unusual as to be almost freakish. The new snow lying on top of the old, which had remained there from the previous winter, gave way easily, both because it was soft, having only just fallen, and because it was not yet deep. But when men and beasts had trodden through it and penetrated to the frozen snow underneath, they no longer sank into it, but found both their feet slipping from under them, as happens when people walk on ground which is covered with a coating of mud. What followed made the situation even more desperate. In the case of the men, when they found they could not get a foothold on the lower layer of snow they fell, and then, as they struggled to rise by using their hands and knees, slid downwards even faster on these, no matter what they clutched on the way, since the angle of the slope was so deep.
> As for the animals, when they fell and struggled to rise they broke through the lower layer of snow, and there they stayed with their loads, as though frozen to the earth, because of their weight and the congealed state of the old snow.[2(pp227–228)]

1. Lounsbury D, trans. Colonel, Medical Corps, US Army; Director, Borden Institute, Office of The Surgeon General, Walter Reed Army Medical Center, Washington, DC; March 2002.
2. Polybius; Scott-Kilvert I, trans. *The Rise of the Roman Empire.* New York, NY: Penguin Books; 1979: Book III: The Second Punic War.
Map: Reproduced from Minard CJ. *Tableaux Graphiques et Cartes Figuratives de M. Minard, 1845–1869.* Held at Bibliothèque de l'École Nationale des Ponts et Chaussées, Paris, France.

faced while crossing these mountains.

The Caucasus ranges were quite different from the Alps: scarcely settled, larger in scale, and with only primitive tracks or trails. Until recently, few armies had attempted to cross or to fight on them.

Second Punic War: Hannibal

Among the many battles for these passes, Hannibal's crossing of the Alps is the best known (Figure 20-2). There are many different versions of this feat and the details differ. What is clear is that Hannibal was an imaginative and charismatic leader who had many tricks up his sleeve. Although much of the story may be myth, it is clear that the critical part of the invasion took less than 3 weeks and included all the elements that make fighting in the mountains so perilous.[6] Few Roman mountain campaigns are so well described.

At the age of 28, in 221 BC, Hannibal was elected by the army to head the forces of Carthage. Within 3 years he had consolidated an amphibious attack from Carthage on the Gulf of Tunis in North Africa across the Straits of Gibraltar into Spain. During the summer of 218 BC, Hannibal marched his army of about 50,000 men across Spain, along the Mediterranean coast and over the foothills of the Pyrenees, and on to the Alps of southern France, fighting most of the way. Next, he led the army over small hills and across a plain, from which they would have to find a pass over which they could climb before descending into Italy.

There is little agreement over which pass Hannibal crossed. This, and what hazards he encountered, have been debated for centuries. The most reliable information is from Polybius, who wrote 60 years after the fact, but the contemporary place names have been lost in myth. Recently De Beer[6] examined all the available evidence and concluded that the most likely crossing place is the Col de la Traversette, which is over 3,000 m (10,000 ft) high. Its northern approach is through a narrow gorge, very steep and difficult. Hannibal's army spent 15 days fighting its way up through this gorge, hemmed in by almost vertical cliffs, along narrow trails, and over large boulders. The elephants found the boulders insurmountable. Legend has it that Hannibal built huge bonfires around these boulders, and when they were red hot, poured red wine on the boulders to split them into fragments. Improbable though this may seem, it had already been described by Pliny and Vitruvius. Much later, in the early 19th century, this practice (but using water) was carried out on rocky New England farms. Today's armies would use explosives.

The army was constantly attacked by hostile tribes, who rolled great rocks down the cliffs to block the way. But the tribes attacked only by daylight and returned to their homes at night so that Hannibal was then able to restore the passage. The men suffered terribly from the cold, but the effect of altitude hypoxia probably was slight because the men had gained altitude gradually. The elephants and horses had a dreadful time on the steep, broken tracks, which were often ice-covered. Above the tree line they came onto fresh snow lying treacherously over deep slush near the top of the pass, and this gave them great trouble. From the pass Hannibal showed his men the plains of Italy, although they would still confront problems while making the steep descent.[6]

Hannibal's army crossed the Alps in October or November 218 BC, and descended on Italy with 20,000 infantry and 6,000 cavalry (of his original army of 50,000). Although many elephants may have survived the passage, historians believe they did not tolerate the lower Apennine hills, and most died. Although Hannibal's daring passage through the mountains caught the Romans by surprise, they rallied and—with their much larger armies—forced Hannibal to maneuver around Turin for many months. During this period, Hannibal twice scored significant victories over the much stronger Roman army, crushing it in 216 BC at the decisive Battle of Cannae.

Despite Hannibal's bold and brilliant crossing into Italy, the privations of the mountain environment left him barely enough power to win at Cannae. Thereafter, in a strange and hostile land he faced attrition from the continuously reinforced Roman armies. He had no secure supply line through the Alps or from the sea. Nor could he adequately replenish his supplies from the countryside, which was protected by the Romans. After the Battle of Cannae, Hannibal's leadership weakened. He left Italy several times only to return for years of skirmishing against stronger Roman armies, which slowly exhausted the Carthaginians. Hannibal took poison and died in 183 BC.

Here again, strong and daring leadership enabled a small army to prevail against the difficult barriers of high mountains and, initially, to defeat a much larger force. Owing to increasing problems with supplies and reinforcements during many years of fighting, Hannibal's leadership failed and the decades of war ended in defeat for Carthage.

Two thousand years later, when the French were challenging all of Europe, in May 1800 Napoleon led some 40,000 troops across the Great Saint Bernard Pass (2,500 m, or 8,200 ft, in the Alps between Switzerland and Italy), along an ancient Roman road that Napoleon rebuilt—and which is the major highway in use today. Few altitude-related problems have been recorded. The monks and their huge rescue dogs in the 800-year-old monastery on the summit of the pass received him with impartial hospitality, and in return, Napoleon promised the monks perpetual custody of monasteries there and on the neighboring Simplon Pass.

World War I

Although the years of slaughter and stalemate on the western front are the best-known part of World War I, some of the most desperate battles were fought elsewhere, in mountain environments.

In December 1914, Enver Pasha led a strong Turkish army against a smaller Russian army in the high Caucasus Mountains. His first attack surprised and overwhelmed the Russians but the following counterattack defeated the Turks, who lost 78,000 of Enver's original 90,000 men. Bitter winter cold and altitude contributed heavily to this month-long debacle. Troops on both sides came close to starvation, and scurvy disabled many.[7]

Between 1915 and 1917, many major battles were fought in the Alps between the Italians, who sided with the Allies, and the Austrians, who sided with the Germans. Much of the fighting took place on the frontier mountains at 2,000 m (6,500 ft), and many troops lived for weeks and months at much higher altitudes.[8] More than half a million men were engaged along a 600-mile front but concentrated within 20 miles along the crests or slopes of the steep Italian Alps and the Dolomites (a subsidiary Alpine range in northern Italy), in terrain consisting of steep mountains, ravines, waterfalls, and turbulent streams (Figure 20-3). Ten thousand soldiers fell at the Col di Lano, the most fought-over pass in the Dolomites. Troops fought at an altitude of 3,000 m (10,000 ft), and some 600 injured soldiers arrived daily in Milan, most suffering from frozen feet and hands.[9]

This was terribly difficult terrain, even for the experienced mountaineers who had been professional guides in civilian life and needed only a little military training. Food, ammunition, arms, and supplies of all kinds had to be carried from the roadhead in the foothills to the front line, often on men's backs. Only occasionally could mountain

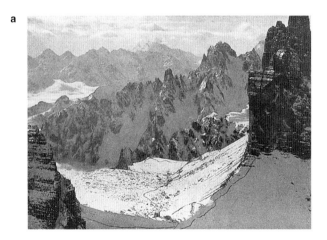

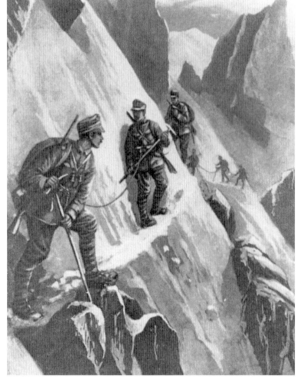

Fig. 20-3. These illustrations give some idea of the arduous terrain in which fighting between the Italians and the Austrians took place during World War I in the Dolomites. (**a**) The first line of Italian trenches in the Cadore district. The dark line across the snow is not the trench itself but the barbed wire entanglements stretched in front. In summer, the wire, which is fastened to posts cemented into the rock, serves its purpose; but in winter, when the deep snow covers it, the enemy could readily advance over the top. To prevent this, little wooden sawhorses are constructed in the trenches, the wire attached, and the portable entanglements pushed out on the hard snow surface. (**b**) An Austro-Hungarian night patrol makes its way cautiously along a ledge in the Dolomite Alps. Photographs and legends: (a) Reproduced from Bagg EM. Letters from the Italian front. *National Geographic.* 1917;32(1):47. (b) Reproduced from Gregory B. *Mountain and Arctic Warfare.* Wellingborough, Northamptonshire, England: Patrick Stephens Ltd. Thorsons Pub Group; 1989: 18.

mules be used. In places, long ropeways were constructed up which loads were hauled.

Most of the engagements were fought between specially trained mountain troops—the brigades or divisions of the Austrian Bersaglieri and the Italian Alpini. Both sides were equipped with white camouflage clothing, skis, and machine guns mounted on skis. The Alpini on Monte Ciove were under continuous attack for 3 weeks, losing 4,000 of their 6,000 men. Frequently the fighting was hand to hand, with bayonets. These elite mountain troops used advanced rock techniques to scale steep cliffs, establish ropeways, and fortify almost impregnable summits. The strong points were vulnerable to long-range artillery so the soldiers lived in snow caves and tunnels, inadequately protected and provisioned.[9,10]

This was the first time that two great armies had faced each other on extended mountainous terrain. Artillery barrages, machine gun attacks, and hand-to-hand bayonet battles caused less damage to both sides than did injuries from rockfalls, avalanches, and cold. The mountains were rugged and access very difficult; blizzards often dumped many feet

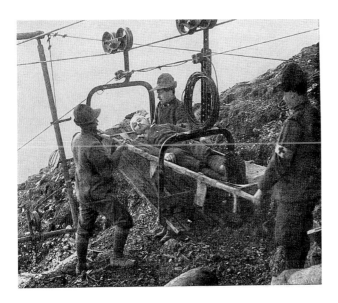

Fig. 20-4. Transporting Italian casualties in the Alps. The teliferica car provided the most comfortable vehicle for the men wounded at the front, and this stage was said to be the easiest of their long journey back to the base hospitals. The teliferica car was also used to carry bodies of Italy's Alpine soldiers to their snowy graves. If time and opportunity permitted, the dead were sent back whence they came, but more often they were buried with full military honors in the ice and snow of the glaciers. Photograph: Reproduced from Bagg EM. Letters from the Italian front. *National Geographic.* 1917;32(1):55.

of snow on slopes too steep to hold it, and avalanches buried many men. At night the great cold froze rocks in place, but as the sun melted the ice, there were dangerous rockfalls. The climbing was difficult, and falls by men and equipment caused many casualties. Some of the fiercest battles took place on skis, often hand to hand.

Food was poor and scanty, and malnutrition and abominable sanitary conditions weakened the soldiers. The effects of altitude hypoxia are not recorded but were probably minimal owing to the acclimatization the men developed. Although casualties could usually be evacuated to a hospital, many were lost (Figure 20-4). Between the mountaineers on both sides a certain chivalry prevailed (what climbers call "the fellowship of the rope"), unlike on any other front. But disputes among the leaders decreased morale, and the years of fighting ended in stalemate when the two huge armies disengaged—except for small battles fought from summit to summit in the Dolomites.

Such campaigns in World War I convinced many countries that special training was important for troops who would fight in the mountains (Figure 20-5). Not so much altitude sickness but steep, broken, and dangerous terrain, and storms, snow, ice, and cold posed then and will always pose major problems for fighting in the mountains, despite advances in supplies and equipment of modern times. Strong, united leadership would be particularly important in such harsh environments; however, not all countries acted on these lessons.

World War II

In 1938 the German mountain troops, or *Gebirgsjäger*, were reconstituted into three divisions, but except for their battles in Italy and the Caucasus, most of the fighting was not in mountains, although their mountain training was invaluable in winter conditions.

The Gebirgsjäger fought in Norway for 8 weeks in 1940, facing bitter cold, deep snow, and long darkness with little food and shelter. Finally they prevailed and drove the British from Narvik. Other Gebirgsjäger fought in the Balkans and Macedonia and captured Athens.[10,11]

After the terrible winter of 1941/42 outside of Moscow, the German Army was slow to recover but in August 1942 began a drive into the Caucasus ranges, the first chance the Gebirgsjäger had to fight in terrain for which they had been specially trained. The southern prong of the 1942 German offensive would cut southward across the Caucasus to the Black Sea to seize the seaport city of Batum, near the Turkish border, and the oil-rich south. (The

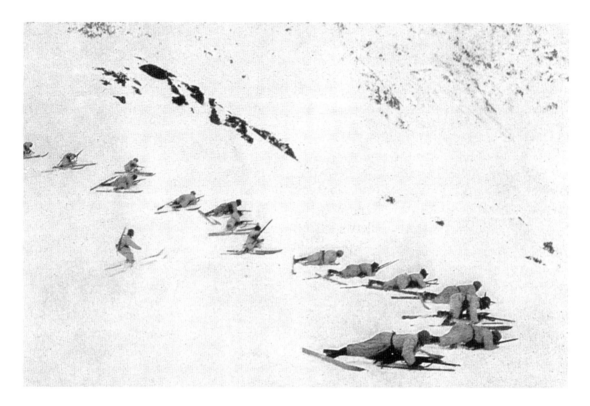

Fig. 20-5. The skirmish line of Italian skimen advancing in attack. These troops, mounted on skis, can descend on an enemy position like a flock of great white birds, bringing a message of disaster to their foe. In this photograph, they are creeping forward in skirmish formation, firing as they go. Photograph and figure legend: Reproduced from Bagg EM. Letters from the Italian front. *National Geographic.* 1917;32(1):61.

northern prong was directed toward Stalingrad.) They fought their way over many passes 2,000 to 3,200 m (6,500–10,500 ft) high, in bitter summer blizzards and cold, and on into the fall and winter.[7]

Throughout the Caucasus campaign the Gebirgsjäger were extremely short of food and adequate winter clothing. They were harassed by thousands of native men and women, who had improvised fortifications in the mountains. German casualties were heavy, but the natives were inured to the mountain environment and suffered less. Here once again, more casualties were due to cold, hunger, and privation than to enemy action. Although trained for mountain warfare, the German Army was inadequately equipped; they had little knowledge of the geography or climate in the Caucasus and were forced to gather information hastily, from 15-year-old sources in Moscow, just as the campaign started.

In both world wars, which were largely European and Middle Eastern wars, too little forethought was given to the problems that troops would face in the mountain environment: extreme cold, lack of oxygen, insufficient food, and the difficulties of providing timely medical care. Some of these lessons

of the past were not entirely ignored in the United States as the storm clouds gathered over Europe in the 1930s. In 1939 several groups of American mountaineers and skiers pressed for the formation of a special Mountain Division. After months of planning, the 10th Mountain Division was commissioned in 1942 and composed of volunteer mountain climbers and skiers. Training began in early 1943 at Camp Hale, Colorado, at 2,700 m (9,000 ft) and included rock and ice climbing, survival in cold weather, ski combat, avoidance of rockfalls and avalanches, and travel in dangerous terrain. The division was originally intended to attack the Germans, who had survived difficult winter months in Denmark and controlled the country. But it was soon apparent that their effort would be too late and inadequate against the large, entrenched German armies.

After 8 months of training at Camp Hale, detachments moved to Camp Swift, Texas, or to the Aleutian Islands, southwest of mainland Alaska, awaiting the invasion of Italy, where they were expected to be most valuable. They arrived in Italy in early 1945, 18 months after the invasion had started, fought notably at Riva Ridge, and moved northward until the war ended.

The main Allied forces had already landed and were fighting north toward Rome. In January 1944 these forces confronted a formidable barrier, Monte Cassino, the center of the Gustav line, which the Germans held across Italy.[12,13] The monastery of Monte Cassino had been built in AD 524 by Saint Benedict, on a high, steep mountain chosen to be impregnable against assault from any side. Although destroyed several times over the centuries, the monastery was always rebuilt more strongly; in 1944 Monte Cassino, rising 500 m (1,600 ft) from the plains, dominated the road to Rome. Although the elite German *Jaegergebirge*, the specially trained and highly experienced mountain troops, had stockpiled armaments and other supplies to repel repeated attacks or a long siege, Monte Cassino was defended by paratroopers of the German 1st Parachute Division. Trained mountain troops from France, Morocco, Turkey, and India, along with regular infantry from England and the United States, attacked again and again, forcing routes up the steep cliffs almost to the summit before falling back with heavy losses from firepower above them. Winter conditions prevailed: mud, slush, snow, and sleet caused casualties comparable to some of the terrible injuries received by troops in the trenches of France in World War I.

The US Quartermaster Corps had been developing a special boot for cold weather warfare, and a few hundred were field-tested in Italy in the closing months of that campaign. The troops who did not have this special boot suffered a special type of cold injury—immersion foot—that caused thousands of casualties and necessitated many amputations. This boot would be nicknamed the Korean boot (or, affectionately, the Mickey Mouse boot) af-

ter it was used in the Korean War 5 years later, although it arrived too late to prevent many amputations for frostbite.

The Italian campaign was bitter. Some German troops said that the winter of 1944 on Monte Cassino was as bad as anything on the Russian front. Allied troops fought four major battles in the next 5 months before the Germans retreated from the monastery, which was by then almost totally destroyed.[12,14]

Monte Cassino fell in May 1944 and Rome was taken 10 days later. In 1945, the 10th Mountain Division had its baptism of fire in an assault on a series of strong points on Riva Ridge and surrounding peaks. The trained mountain division forced routes up steep cliffs, fixing ropes much as Curtius[5] says that Alexander's men had done in Sogdiana. Casualties were heavy, but the mountain training paid off and the German line was broken. The 10th Mountain Division moved northward.

Many of the lessons from World War I had been ignored or forgotten in the following decades and mistakes were repeated in the Italian campaign of 1944–1945. Some top leaders disliked each other and failed to cooperate at important times. They disagreed over tactics at critical times. They led troops who came from many countries and therefore had language problems as well as different cultures and military traditions. The US Army 10th Mountain Division trained for 2 years to fight in the mountains but did not arrive until the bitterest fighting (at Monte Cassino) was over. The military leadership and the US mountain troops, too, had not expected a long winter campaign, and their clothing, footwear, shelter, and even food were inadequate. New commanders for all troops repeated the mistakes of those they replaced. In many respects it was déjà vu all over again, at least in Italy and in the Caucasus.

TRAVELERS' TALES

Most military operations in Europe and the Middle East were conducted below 3,000 m (10,000 ft), where altitude hypoxia is seldom a problem because most troops acclimatize rapidly to these elevations. However, Asian mountain ranges (including the Hindu Kush, Caucasus, Karakoram, and Himalaya) and the South American Andes are high enough to cause serious altitude problems for troops, especially since supply problems limit the time that can be spent on acclimatization. The first reports of altitude or mountain sickness came from travelers in Asia and the Andes, and at least a few military campaigns in Asia have also experienced these problems.

Asia

Some of the earliest accounts of the dangers of high mountains come from the mountains of Asia. For example, in 156 BC, General Du Qin advised Chinese Emperor Wudi not to send envoys to Kashmir because the mountains along the way were too perilous. The general described the dangers of the journey in terms suggesting altitude illness (he and others also mentioned the risks from dragons among the mountains):

> [T]ravellers have to climb over Mount Greater Headache, Mount Lesser Headache, and the Fever Hills. … [T]hey must support each other by ropes.[15(p10)]

An early example of a serious altitude problem was described in the 5th century AD. After crossing the Safed Koh, a subsidiary range of the Hindu Kush, on the way to the higher Kohat Pass near Peshawar, in modern Pakistan,

> Fa Hsien and the two others proceeding southwards, crossed the Little Snowy Mountains. On them the snow lies accumulated both winter and summer. On the north side of the mountains, in the shade they suddenly encountered a cold wind which made them shiver and unable to speak. Hwuy Kung could not go any farther. A white froth came from his mouth and he said to Fa Hsien, "I cannot live any longer. Do you immediately go away, that we do not all die here"; and with these words he died.[16(p10)]

Like Alexander's men, the 5th-century party also experienced snow blindness, and they noted another unusual mountaineering peril, as well:

> The snow reflects a white light so strong that the traveller has to shut his eyes and cannot see anything. Only after he has made sacrifices to the King of the Dragons will his eyesight be restored.[16(p10)]

South America

Soon other travelers noted problems due to altitude. In 1590, Father Jose de Acosta astutely blamed "thinne aire" for the acute sickness he experienced while crossing the high Pariacaca Pass in the Andes Mountains.[17(p10)] His contemporary, Father Alonzo de Ovalle, agreed:

> When we come to ascend the highest point of the mountain, we feel an aire so piercing and subtile that it is with much difficulty we can breathe, which obliges us to fetch our breath quick and strong and to open our mouths wider than ordinary, applying to them likewise our handkerchiefs to protect our mouth and break the extreme coldness of the air and to make it more proportionable to the temperature which the heart requires, not to be suffocated; this I have experienced every time I have passed this mighty mountain.[18(pp46–47)]

A century later, Gruber repeated Acosta's "subtile aire" theory, but added:

> In summer certain poisonous weeds grow there which exude such a bad smell and dangerous odor that one cannot stay up there without losing one's life.[19]

Not until the end of the 19th century would the true cause of altitude illnesses be proven to be due to decreased barometric pressure and the resulting lack of oxygen. The various forms of mountain sickness would be experienced by armies that campaigned above 2,500 m (8,000 ft).

MILITARY CAMPAIGNS

Asia: The Mongols

From 1200 to 1400 AD the tribal peoples from a remote corner of central Asia—the Mongols—dominated the political and military life of the known world except for western Europe.[20] Genghis Khan (also known as Temujin), perhaps the greatest military genius of all time, initiated these conquests; his forces and those of his successors were known as the Golden Hordes. For 200 years the Hordes roamed and conquered much of China, all of central Asia, and Europe to the Adriatic and the Black seas, in bitter winter cold and debilitating desert heat. Although little information describing their health has survived, their standard diet of grains and curd gave them adequate nutrition, and their woolen dress minimized cold injuries.

Their military success as well as their resistance to hostile environments was because of their mobility. Genghis Khan learned very early in his career that speed meant victory. His only fighters were mounted cavalry, each man with a string of relief horses. Men and horses alike were incredibly tough and fast. Living on the grasslands of the Asian steppes, advancing on a very broad front but able to concentrate forces rapidly when faced with battle, the Hordes were brilliantly trained, disciplined, and led. After some years they spread out to form other Hordes, whose cavalry also terrified their opponents by ruthless slaughter and plunder, massacring all the people in the cities they conquered and then razing them to the ground.[21] It was a scorched earth policy in the extreme, like Alexander's.

One Mongol chieftain, Mirza Muhammad Haider, filled a book with detailed descriptions of the campaigns in which he participated. This account, written in 1544 near the end of his long life, is a record of incessant fighting between infidels and Moslems, between members of a family, and between rival clans.[22] Much of the action took place around Samarkand, Tashkent, Yarkand, Khotan, and Kashgar, now largely arid desert. Considerably more rain fell during those years, so that parts of the now-almost-barren high desert were fertile enough to provide fodder for the horses and grain for the people, ensuring the Hordes' mobility. Nevertheless, campaigning was incredibly difficult for these armies (large and small), and their total dependence on horses adds special relevance to the following selection from Haider:

> It is clear that Tibet is a very high-lying country, since its rivers run in all directions. Anyone wishing to enter Tibet must first ascend lofty passes, which do not slope downward on the other side for on the top the land is flat. ... On account of the height, Tibet is excessively cold. ... Having reached this point in my narrative it is necessary for me to give some account of the land of Tibet, for this country is so situated that very few travellers have been able to visit it. On account of the difficulties of the route, which from every point of view is most dangerous whether by reason of its hills and passes, or the coldness of the air or the scarcity of water and fuel, or the shameless and lawless highwaymen, who know every inch of the way and allow no travellers to pass—no one has ever brought back any information concerning this country.

> Another peculiarity of Tibet is the *damgiri* [literally, breathtaking], which the Moghuls call Yas and which is common to the whole country, though less prevalent in the region of forts and villages. The symptoms are a feeling of severe sickness (*nakhushi*). And in every case one's breath so seizes him that he becomes exhausted, just as if he had run up a steep hill with a heavy burden on his back. On account of the oppression it causes it is difficult to sleep. Should, however, sleep overtake one, the eyes are hardly closed before one is awake with a start caused by the oppression of the lungs and chest.

> . . . .

> When overcome by this malady the patient becomes senseless, begins to talk nonsense, and sometimes the power of speech is lost, while the palms of the hands and the soles of the feet become swollen. Often, when this last symptom occurs, the patient dies between dawn and breakfast time; at other times he lingers on for several days.

> . . . .

> This malady only attacks strangers; the people of Tibet know nothing of it, nor do their doctors know why it attacks strangers. Nobody has ever been able to cure it. The colder the air, the more severe is the form of the malady.

> . . . .

> It is not peculiar to men but attacks every animal that breathes, such as the horse, as will be presently instanced. One day, owing to the necessity of a foray, we had ridden faster than usual. On waking next morning I saw that there were very few horses in our camp and on inquiring, ascertained that more than 2,000 had died during the night. Of my own stable there were twenty-four special riding horses, all of which were missing. Twenty-one of them had died during the night. Horses are very subject to *damgiri*. I have never heard of this disease outside of Tibet. No remedy is known for it.[22(pp412–413)]

This account is important because it is an early and very detailed description of the problem of altitude sickness, and of acclimatization, which affected a powerful and resourceful leader campaigning in a high and hostile environment.

The Mongol Hordes were among the most efficient, ruthless, and powerful fighting machines the world has ever experienced. They were an early model for modern mobile forces, living on the land, traveling light and fast, with minimal supplies but able to fuel their transport (horses) as they went. By contrast, tank offensives in World War II were often halted because fuel could not be obtained. The Mongols crossed high mountain passes, fought through severe sand and snow storms, in drought and famine-stricken areas, always moving. During the first decades the strong and brilliant leadership of Genghis Khan brought seemingly impossible successes. Later, as the original Horde split into several smaller ones, most of the leaders were still able and strong. But unbelievable success and booty led to corruption and internal quarrels between leaders. After 2 centuries, all of the territories they had conquered were lost.

Asia: The Great Game

For thousands of years military campaigns have been fought in Asia among the harshest mountains on Earth between bitter enemies. Since the 18th century, these have attracted attention to what Rudyard Kipling called "the Great Game." Sometimes only a few men were involved, but small armies were engaged at others.[23]

Several great and discrete mountain ranges run for 2,000 miles from northwest to southeast across Asia, forming a nearly impassable barrier between the Russian confederation, Mongolia, and China to the north and Iran, Afghanistan, Pakistan, and India to the south. For most of their length the summits are from 6,000 to 8,000 m (20,000–26,000 ft) high. This formidable barrier is breached in many places, but few of the passes are lower than 5,000 m (16,400 ft) and all are covered by perpetual snow and ice. Yet for many centuries, invaders have crossed these passes from the inhospitable north to the warmer, richer, and softer south.[23,24]

Ever since the British Empire gained control of India 300 years ago, the English have been major players in the Great Game against the Russians. Both played for high stakes: the British to retain the riches of India, and the Russians to claim them. Both sought passes by which an army from the north might invade India, and where such an invasion could be halted, even though few places on Earth are less suited to war because of the terrain, extreme cold, great altitude, and lack of food and often of water. The area was unexplored and almost unknown until both sides sent intrepid soldiers, usually disguised as Muslim traders or priests, to penetrate this wild country, map the great rivers, and locate villages and oases. The Oxus and Indus rivers were thought to offer possible routes for an army, ones where bitter cold and altitude would not be problems, but even to reach the rivers involved crossing high mountains.

Not only were these early travelers seeking routes for armies and for traders, they were also trying to win the support of the rulers of the many petty, often warring states. Many of the covert agents took 6 months even to reach their destinations—often being executed if one ruler or another was offended or suspicious. They crossed high mountain passes and endured severe privation on snow and in barren deserts. Their instructions were dictated from India or Britain, took many months to arrive, and were often unclear or contradictory. It is not surprising that, given greatly delayed and wavering leadership from London or Delhi, the hardships they experienced are not as frequently mentioned in their reports as are the political and personal confrontations and frustrations. Although these intrepid agents were few in number, the maps and information they brought from central Asia should have improved strategy and tactics for generations—but unfortunately did not—both because of the long delays in communication and because of vacillating policies and incompetent generals.

In Afghanistan, a climax came in 1843 when Shah Shuja, the Afghan premier, was forced by a revolutionary group to expel the British mission that had installed him as Prime Minister and was negotiating a peace between the two parties.[25] Although promised safe conduct during their retreat from Kabul, the British were treacherously attacked by Shah Shuja's Afghan soldiers and suffered horrible losses. British troops returned a year later and took savage revenge. The Great Game played on for another hundred years, but prior to 1970, the incessant intrigues and struggles for power did not attract much international attention.

Then in 1978, for complicated reasons still being debated, Russia, by then loosely consolidated as the dominant member of the USSR, decided to intervene in the chronic political struggles between Afghan rebels and their government. Without warning, Russian troops invaded Afghanistan through a tunnel that Russia had built beneath Pamirs (the high-altitude region of central Asia, which contains numerous mountain peaks higher than 6,100 m [20,000 ft]) to encourage, as they claimed, free trade.[26] This invasion was what the British had feared and had tried to prevent for a century, but when it happened they were able to do little about it. Using the tunnel enabled Russian troops to avoid many of the problems due to cold and altitude encountered on the peaks and passes that hampered the Afghans, even inured as they were to these hazards. The Russians also used air support, but this was effective only at first.

In Afghanistan the land is high, wild, and barren—frozen or scorched—and dry, with scattered oases along rivers that flow from high and impregnable, snow-clad mountains to disappear in sandy wastes. Ragged, tortured, rocky ridges provided sanctuary for ground forces and gave some shelter from air attack. Russian ground transport was hampered by heat or cold, endless rocky spurs and outcrops, and sand or snow. Supplies had to come by air. The Russians were trying to restore a disheveled government, torn by deceit and murder, as well as many independent guerilla factions, often operating independently and at odds with one another. Despite superior equipment and unopposed air assaults, the Russian armies did not tolerate the mountain hardships, and finally the Afghan rebels, poorly disciplined and led though they were, used the mountainous wasteland better than the Russian troops, and forbade them ground control. After 10 years the Russians could not prevail and, after an ignominious stalemate, withdrew.

The struggles in Afghanistan demonstrate the obstacles that make mountain warfare so difficult and costly. Most of the land is parched and water is available only from the few large rivers, making agriculture possible only in irrigated areas; food is always scarce. The mountains are from 2,500 to 6,000 m (8,200–19,700 ft) high and are always covered with ice and snow. The temperature varies from above 40°C to –30°C (> 104°F to –22°F). Sandstorms, rockfalls, and avalanches are frequent. Cold injury and altitude sickness are major hazards in the high mountains. Belatedly, the Russians recognized that their troops had not been adequately prepared for the terrain and the extreme climate encountered in Afghanistan, and they established a mountain warfare training center in Russia.

Tibet: Geopolitical Machinations

The Great Game was played in another region at the start of the 20th century as Russia increased its efforts to acquire Tibet, at that time still an aloof and little-known country. The British, determined that no other power should control this high, wild land, matched Russia's diplomatic overtures until, in 1904, the delicate negotiations collapsed, and the British monarch sent a small army to escort a diplomatic mission to Lhasa, the principal city in Tibet.[27,28]

Colonel Francis Younghusband was chief of mission, with General Macdonald and 2,000 troops in support. Their orders were ambiguous and fluctuating in an effort to persuade rather than to force the lamaistic theocracy to accept relations with Britain and to lock the door against Russia. When the last polite exchanges failed, Younghusband's party marched from the lowlands of India up into the Himalayas in February 1904 in battle array, dragging artillery along rough and stony tracks and over passes higher than, and almost as difficult as, those that Hannibal's elephants had crossed. After a few minor skirmishes, they faced a Tibetan force of several hundred men armed with ancient firearms and large knives, sheltering behind a formidable stone wall at an altitude of 5,500 m (18,000 ft). One of the party described the difficulties:

> Climbing over boulder strewn surfaces would be bad at sea level; here where the air is so thin it soon becomes a burden. ... The lungs seem foolishly inadequate to the task imposed on them ... the heart goes on beating with increasing strokes until it shakes the walls of the body ... speech comes with difficulty. ... The brain seems cleft in two and a wedge, all blunt and splintery, is hammered into it by mallet strokes with every pulsation of the heart. ... Here too the wind exacts its toll and drives a cold aching shaft into your liver.[27(pp52–53)]

The first battle was joined at the strongly defended wall, which ran across a barren plain between hills that were prelude to immense snow peaks. A strong force of Tibetans was routed and several hundred were killed. Six weeks later, in a narrower valley at 5,600 m (18,500 ft), the Tibetan

forces were larger, and after the battle, the Tibetan dead were estimated at 2,000. The terrain was extremely difficult. A dozen men under a native officer were sent up the almost-vertical face of the 460-m (1,500-ft) southern scarp to outflank the enemy at 18,500 ft—incredibly difficult work even for experienced mountaineers.

Apparently, altitude hypoxia—so vividly described by Landon,[27] who was there—did not halt or greatly impede the comparatively unacclimatized British forces. The Tibetans had lived at altitude all their lives and were fully adapted, an important factor favoring indigenous people meeting freshly arrived invaders anywhere in the mountains. The benefits of acclimatization were very clear when the Chinese invaded Tibet 50 years later, and were even more dramatically illustrated when they were ignored by the Indian armies when they faced the Chinese in 1962.

Younghusband's British party eventually forced its way through to Lhasa at 4,000 m (13,000 ft) and concluded a treaty with the Tibetans. The British force, although smaller than the Tibetan, was better trained, disciplined, and led; they had superior equipment that enabled them to prevail despite the great difficulties of altitude, cold, terrain, supply, and transport. Their advance was slow enough to enable the troops to acclimatize partially to the high altitude. This small military campaign should serve as a model for other larger operations in the mountain environment.[27]

China: The Long March

Perhaps the longest and most grueling campaign fought partly in the mountains was the Long March of the Chinese Communist party. In 1934, about 100,000 Chinese Communist troops and camp followers (85,000 soldiers, 15,000 administrators, and 15 women) were greatly outnumbered and encircled by the Chinese Nationalist armies. The Communists managed to break through the besieging armies and began their journey in October 1934. For the next 18 months the ragged, underfed, underequipped soldiers fought their way across western and northern China over rugged, almost-unknown country.[29,30]

Soldiers and civilians alike suffered their greatest hardships from cold and altitude while crossing the Snowy Mountains, possibly the same range on which Fa Hsien[16] had first recorded a case of high-altitude pulmonary edema many centuries before. Because the Chinese Communists were constantly harassed from the air, they often traveled at night despite the intense cold. Their clothing was inadequate for the glaciers and snow they had to cross. They had little food. Despite acclimatization, their malnourished and weakened conditions increased the adverse effects of altitude, which, together with the cold, killed many thousands. After this high-mountain travel they had to cross a few hundred miles of swampland at 2,000 m (6,500 ft) elevation. They had few medical supplies, and disease and trauma took a heavy toll. They crossed 18 mountain ranges and 24 rivers in 1934 and 1935. Of the 100,000 who had begun the Long March, only 8,000 survived.[30]

Korea: The Retreat From the Chosin Reservoir

Another brutal campaign was fought in Korea in very harsh mountain terrain, although altitude was not a factor. During an intense period beginning 1 November 1950, US Army and Marine troops, recovering lost ground, were attacked by Chinese forces north of the Yalu River near the Chinese border. For 3 weeks the Americans retreated from the Chosin Reservoir along mountain roads, through narrow passes, in heavy snow and blizzard conditions. Although the campaign was described as a "strategic retreat," morale and military discipline deteriorated and there were heavy casualties. The terrain forced the battered troops into narrow defiles, where they were attacked on both sides from steep mountain ridges, reminiscent of the attacks suffered by Hannibal in similar terrain.

The roads were in such bad condition that wheeled transport was almost impossible, and even tracked vehicles had great difficulties. The resulting traffic jams compounded the problem. The wintry cold was extreme and clothing and footwear were inadequate, causing hundreds of cases of hypothermia, frostbite, and ensuing amputations. The greatly hampered transport made food and water scarce, so the troops became weak from hunger and dehydration in the dry cold air, perhaps suffering what Xenophon had called "bulimia." Throngs of civilian refugees clogged the roads and hindered retreat and rearguard action. In this campaign it was the *mountain environment*, although not including altitude, that caused the many casualties.[31] (For more about the Chosin Reservoir retreat, interested readers should also see Chapter 10, Cold, Casualties, and Conquests: The Effects of Cold on Warfare; and Chapter 14, Clinical Aspects of Freezing Cold Injuries, particularly Exhibits 14-7 and 14-8; in Section IV, Cold Environments, in *Medical Aspects of Harsh Environments, Volume 1*.[32])

This tragic operation is almost a replica of the British Army's retreat from Kabul a hundred years before. Then, in January 1842, British forces, expelled from Kabul with a safe conduct, were betrayed by Shah Shuja and attacked from all sides by Afghans. The British fought their way through 50 miles of the narrow Kabul River gorge in bitter cold and heavy snow. Most of the horses were killed, making wheeled transport impossible. Clothing was completely inadequate for the weather, although it had been suitable for garrison duty in Kabul. The 4,500 British soldiers were handicapped by the presence of some 15,000 wives, children, servants, and camp followers. Little or no medical care was possible. The horse-drawn artillery was abandoned when the Afghans shot the horses and blocked the road through the Khyber Pass. One man survived to gallop, badly wounded, into the fort at Jallalabad bringing word of the disaster to the horrified and beleaguered British garrison. Some weeks later, 65 more officers and men, most of whom had been held hostage in Kabul at the start of the journey, found their way around the Afghans to Jallalabad. Only that handful survived the cold and the fighting.[15] The Americans retreating from the Chosin Reservoir a century later, although badly hurt, fared much better.

These two 19th- and 20th-century "campaigns" were disasters in which the forces suffered all the handicaps imposed on military operations in the mountains except for altitude: bitter cold; heavy snow; long winter darkness; and limited food, water, and other supplies. Difficult and constricted terrain for maneuver, vulnerability to ambush and attack from high ground, fearful roads for vehicles, and the heavy handicaps of accompanying refugees or noncombatants made the retreat from the Chosin Reservoir a terrible ordeal for US troops. One of the worst medical problems for the US troops was injury from cold. Most of the survivors had frostbite injuries often requiring amputation. These could have been avoided if the suitable footwear, already field-tested in the Italian campaign 5 years before, had been provided in time. Inappropriate leadership before the Chinese attack laid the base for the Allied retreat, but leadership during the retreat was brilliant and undoubtedly prevented more casualties from enemy action.

South America: Liberation and Continuing Conflict

The valleys and high plateau (altiplano) of the Andes mountains that rim the Pacific coast of South America are relatively hospitable to human habitation. The Amerindian cultures who settled these mountains developed an effective agriculture and high-nutrition crops (eg, high-protein grains, potatoes, fruits) that allowed the altiplano to support very large populations before Europeans arrived in the 16th century. The mineral wealth of the Andes attracted the conquistadors, and Spain colonized the area and subjugated the indigenous populations. Throughout history, the presence of large numbers of people with often-conflicting economic and political interests has provided tinder for armed conflict, and intermittent warfare has occurred in the Andes Mountains from the beginning of human settlement there and continues to this day.

The history of Amerindian societies in the Andes was one of frequent warfare between various tribes until the Quechua-speaking Incas conquered most other tribes and consolidated a sophisticated, mountainous empire during the last half of the 13th century; it stretched from northern Ecuador to the middle of Chile. Owing to the lack of a written language, historical account of the battles was by spoken word; much of that history was lost when the Spanish conquest destroyed the Inca culture. The high altitude of the Andean region probably had little effect on Amerindian warfare because the combatants, who resided there permanently, were acclimatized to the altitude. The rugged topography probably did *shape* the warfare, however. Because there were no ballistic weapons, combat was mostly hand to hand and had to take place in the relatively flat areas where combatants could face each other. Further, the battles were somewhat formalized, with the location and timing chosen to avoid the geographical and climatic impediments of hand-to-hand combat. Some of the battles were immense, with thousands of combatants. The Spaniards were able to conquer and subjugate the Inca in 2 years (1531–1533) with a very small number of soldiers, owing to the following factors[33]:

- the devastating effects of European diseases, which rapidly decimated the Amerindian populations in both North and South America,
- their use of guns and horses, which were advanced technology at that time and intimidated the Inca, and
- the effective exploitation of political unrest in the Inca empire and use of blatant treachery by Spanish conquistador Francísco Pizzaro.

Spanish rule of South America ended with the Wars of Liberation, a series of revolutionary movements and military campaigns that began in 1808 and continued until 1824. Two men are credited with liberating the continent: José de San Martín and Simón Bolívar. To achieve the element of surprise in their campaigns, they used mountain cross-ings by their armies (similar to Hannibal and Alexander before them), but they also fought many battles in the mountains.

Wars of Liberation

José de San Martín, called the Liberator of the South, was born in Argentina but grew up in Spain, where he trained as a military officer; he fought in North Africa and on the Spanish peninsula before the Napoleonic Wars. When the independence movements began in South America, he returned to Argentina and fought for its independence. He became convinced that the stability of the liberation from Spain depended on removing the Spaniards from their main stronghold in South America, which was centered in Lima, Peru. To invade Peru from Argentina, an army would have to cross part of the Amazon basin and then a wide stretch of the Andes Mountains. To circumvent those formidable geographical barriers, San Martín conceived a different plan: to cross the Andes from Argentina into Chile, liberate that region, and then move up the Pacific coast to Peru. To accomplish his plan, he moved to the Cuyo province of Argentina on the east side of the Andes, where he raised and trained an army near Mendoza; from there, San Martín and his Army of the Andes set out to cross the mountains into Chile in 1817. He provisioned his troops with large amounts of garlic and onions to combat mountain sickness and dismantled his artillery pieces to be packed by mules over the rough mountain passages.

To confuse the Spanish and colonial Royalist forces in Chile, San Martín divided his army into three columns, each of which crossed the Andes Mountains by a different route. He led the largest force over the 4,575-m (15,000-ft) Uspellata Pass near Cerro Acongagua (6,960 m; 22,836 ft), the highest mountain in South America. The crossing took 3 weeks and, as had happened with previous armies crossing mountain ranges, the mountain environment and terrain extracted a heavy toll of men and equipment. San Martín lost about one third of his troops to cold, altitude illness, and injury; more than half of his horses and mules; and most of his artillery and ammunition. Despite his losses, however, the element of surprise worked in his favor: the Spanish and Royalist army was divided because its leaders were unsure where San Martín planned to cross. He defeated the Spanish and Royalist forces at Chacabuco, a battle in which San Martín's use of features of the terrain (he had surveyed potential battle sites in Chile before crossing the Andes with his army) and the inspired leadership of his Chilean subordinate, commander Bernardo O'Higgins, carried the day.

San Martín and O'Higgins later defeated the remaining Royalists in the Maipú Valley near Santiago, Chile. San Martín then raised another army, which, with the help of British Admiral Lord Cochrane, he transported by sea to Peru in 1820. There he blockaded Lima, forcing the Spanish military to retreat into the Andes east of Lima. San Martín then attempted to set up a stable independent government and did not immediately pursue the Spanish and Royalist troops, which were between his own force and those of Simón Bolívar fighting in Colombia and Ecuador to the north. San Martín and Bolívar met privately in Ecuador in 1821 to discuss the final campaign to eliminate Spanish rule. What was said during the meeting is unknown, but afterwards San Martín resigned as head of the Peruvian government and returned to Argentina, leaving Bolívar to drive the last of the Spaniards from the Peruvian highlands and, thus, from South America.[34,35]

Simón Bolívar, known as the Liberator of the North, also used mountain warfare to his advantage during his campaigns to free northern South America from the Spaniards. In his early struggles to free Venezuela, he fought in the lowlands but had only intermittent and transient success. Several times his armies were defeated, forcing him to flee to Caribbean islands to find funds for munitions and supplies and to recruit new soldiers. In 1819, after forcing the Spanish and Royalist sympathizers out of many areas in Venezuela, he was joined by a large group of soldiers from Europe who were looking for employment after the Napoleonic wars had ended. These expatriate soldiers constituted about a third of Bolívar's troops and stayed with him throughout the remaining wars, although their numbers were considerably reduced by combat casualties. With his reinforced army, Bolívar set out from Angostura, Venezuela, on the Orinoco River in the interior of the country to help liberate Colombia. He marched his troops through the lowland jungles and pampas of Colombia to the base of the Andes Mountains and then across a 4,880-m (16,000-ft) pass to surprise and defeat the Spanish and Royalist forces at the Battle of Boyacá. The army crossed the Andes as a single unit over a pass that was 1,000 feet higher than the passes that had been used 1 year earlier by San Martín's army in Chile. As with San Martín's crossing, Bolívar's army suffered tremendous losses of men and equipment to the high-mountain environment, especially to the cold, for which his soldiers were poorly provisioned. Bolívar

marched at the head of his troops during this crossing; his strong leadership held the army together and inspired it during a series of battles over the subsequent weeks, culminating in the Battle of Boyacá, which allowed him to claim the city of Bogatá.[36]

Following Boyacá, Bolívar's subordinate general, Antonio José de Sucre, fought a series of battles in the mountains of Colombia and Ecuador that resulted in the final liberation of that region. The last battle there was fought on the slopes of the Pichincha Volcano, near Quito, Ecuador, in 1822. The battlefield was so steep that neither side could deploy its cavalry, and the battle was fought entirely by infantrymen, who struggled up and down the difficult terrain.

That same year, Bolívar turned his attention south to Peru, where the last Spanish and Royalist troops in South America were caught in the mountains between Bolívar's army to the north and San Martín's army in Lima on the Pacific coast. When San Martín left Peru after their meeting in Equador, Bolívar moved his own army nearly 1,000 miles through the Andes Mountains into the Peruvian altiplano. Like his previous crossing of the Andes into Colombia, the long march through the mountains was difficult, and hundreds of troops were injured, died, or deserted the army. The first battle took place in 1823 on the high (4,270 m; 14,000 ft) altiplano in the Junín region of Peru (near the present-day city of Huancayo). There, units of Bolívar's army, led by General Sucre, routed the Spaniards in a short, intense cavalry battle fought entirely with lances and sabers. The Spanish forces fled southward into the mountains, pursued by Bolívar's forces commanded by General Sucre.

The last battle of the Wars of Liberation was fought between these forces in 1824 in the mountains near the present-day city of Ayacucho, Peru. The rugged mountain topography hindered effective lines of artillery and rifle fire, and much of that battle was fought with bayonet and saber. Sucre's use of the rugged topography and the inspired fighting by legendary units of Bolívar's army carried the day and ended Spanish dominion in South America.[36,37]

Continuing Conflict

Following the Wars of Liberation, South America has been (and is still) the site of frequent revolts, violent changes of government, and border conflicts within and between the newly independent countries. Of particular significance in terms of mountain warfare were the Wars of the Pacific (1879–1883) fought between Bolivia and Peru on one side and Chile on the other. The conflict started in a dispute between Bolivia and Chile over nitrate-rich guano deposits in the Atacama Desert on the Pacific coast. Peru was drawn into the conflict through an alliance with Bolivia. Early on, however, Bolivia withdrew from the conflict and subsequently lost its only access to the ocean. Peru and Chile continued to fight. After the Peruvians lost fierce battles on their southern border, the Chileans invaded Peru from the sea, and in more fierce fighting, defeated Peruvian defenses and occupied the Peruvian capital, Lima. Like the Spanish forces before them, the surviving Peruvian forces retreated into the mountains and high altiplano in the interior of the country to regain strength and carry on the resistance. There, under the leadership of Colonel Andrés Cáceres, the Peruvian forces fought a series of engagements known as the Breña Campaign (1881–1882) against the Chilean forces that had been sent to destroy them.

The fighting was part guerrilla and part conventional warfare, and the mountain environment adversely affected both sides at different times. For example, after a victory at Pucara, Peru, Colonel Cáceres marched his forces toward Ayacucho, intending to finally drive the Chilean forces out of the Peruvian mountains. However, he and his troops were caught by a storm in a high Andean pass between Acobamba and Julcamarca, where he lost approximately half his men and all his horses and mules and was unable continue to Ayacucho to capitalize on the momentum from his previous victory. Despite many small victories, the Peruvians were never strong enough to make a serious attempt to take back their capital, Lima.[38]

The war was eventually settled through diplomatic negotiations led by outside countries, but the determined resistance of Colonel Cáceres was a notable demonstration of the concept of the use of mountains for refuge by forces who know how to survive and fight there. This principle was again demonstrated in the same region during the last half of the 20th century, when the Sendaro Luminoso guerillas fought the Peruvian government there for more than 2 decades.

Modern Border Wars

China and Tibet

Since long before the Great Game began, China has claimed sovereignty over Tibet, and exact borders have long been disputed. In 1950, Chinese armies invaded Tibet and soon controlled the entire country. Although much of the action occurred on the high, inhospitable plateau, the Tibetans' acclimatization advantaged them only for the first few months: soon the lowland Chinese adjusted to the altitude and acclimatized fully during the following years.

However, among the occupying Chinese a previously unreported medical syndrome called subacute mountain sickness, appeared in Han (Chinese) infants who were either born at altitude or taken there when very young. This cardiac problem is a form of right ventricular enlargement and failure due to the pulmonary hypertension caused by hypoxia.[39] This is truly an environmental illness and is apparently an infantile form of a syndrome later described among Indian troops fighting at even higher elevations in the Karakoram mountains. Both the adult and the infantile forms are reversed after a few months by descent to lower altitude, but they are often fatal if descent is delayed.

China and India

In 1962 Chinese armies suddenly attacked India, crossing the Himalayan mountain ranges in half a dozen places from the southeastern end (Assam) to the northwestern section (Ladakh). Much of the fighting was between small patrols and pickets, but these engagements were no less bitter because relatively few men were involved in any one place. For the Indian forces, it was not military might but environmental forces that ultimately brought stalemate.[40] Because the Chinese troops had occupied the Tibetan highlands at 4,000 m (13,000 ft) for over a decade, they were well acclimatized to altitude. By contrast, most of the Indian troops were taken up hastily from the low, hot, plains only a few hundred feet above sea level. They were not clothed for the cold mountain environment and were unaware of, and unprepared for, the hazards of altitude hypoxia.[41]

In Ladakh, at the northern end of the Himalayan ranges, many men were taken up by truck and even more were flown up, to defend difficult positions at 5,000 to 5,500 m (16,000–18,000 ft) above the low plains of India. The Indian troops promptly suffered severely from the altitude and cold, whereas the Chinese, well acclimatized and also cold adapted, were unaffected.[42,43]

In Assam at the southeastern end of the Himalayan ranges, cold was somewhat less a problem than altitude, which incapacitated men at crucial periods. Indian regiments moved into the mountains rapidly

in summer uniforms with one blanket per man—
and bivouacking that night at 4,500 meters (15,000
feet) ... they moved next day to Yamato La, a 4,000
meter (13,000 foot) pass a mile west and higher. ...
[The commanders in Delhi] pointed out that the
troops could not survive at this altitude without
winter clothing. ... Brigadier Kaul spent a restless
night ... . Like so many of his troops he was suffering from a pulmonary disorder consequent on his
exertions at altitudes to which he was not accustomed. ... [H]e had to be carried over the pass. A
helicopter was waiting ... to lift him to Delhi.[42(p20)]

This conflict, extending the length of the Sino–
Indian frontier, was the first large-scale confrontation between armies at altitudes that can be—and
in this case often were—fatal. Among the Indian
troops, morbidity from mountain sickness ranged
from 4% to 20% in different companies; a third of
the casualties are said to have died. From experience in this theater, many studies of acute mountain sickness and of high-altitude pulmonary and
cerebral edema have been published. There is no
doubt that the Indian troops suffered far more casualties from altitude and cold than from enemy action,
although the numbers still remain classified.[43] The
conflict continues today, occasionally flaring up and
endangering the stability of the subcontinent.

After 18 months of indecisive action, the Chinese
unexpectedly withdrew, although minor skirmishes
persist today as they have for many decades. Hundreds of casualties and deaths among the Indian
troops on the northwestern front, but only a few on
the southeastern, were due to altitude illnesses.

In retrospect, the lessons are clear: at the outbreak
of hostilities the Indian command was forced to
move troops very rapidly to a dangerous altitude,
but they failed to appreciate the importance of acclimatization, which the Chinese understood. It is
not likely that staging troops gradually to higher
from lower elevations would have altered the outcome, but it would have prevented many casualties from cold and altitude. The most important result of the Sino–Indian conflict was not conquest
but major medical contributions to understanding
the pathophysiology of mountain sickness and acclimatization.[42]

India and Pakistan

Kashmir has been fought over for a thousand
years, and it has been a theater for the Great Game

between Britain and Russia since the 17th century;
the territory has been even more bitterly disputed
since the partition of the subcontinent into Pakistan
and India in 1947. Although Kashmir was and still
is predominantly Muslim, the Hindu government
of India immediately sent troops to occupy the state
despite ragged opposition along the always-mili-
tant northwest frontier. Several small, desperately
brave military operations by Pakistani troops took
place in the winter of 1948 at 4,500 m (15,000 ft),
resulting in little gain but great suffering from frostbite and later amputation for those who survived.

As an adjunct to the Kashmir dispute, India and
Pakistan have been fighting a difficult and undeclared
war in the Karakoram Range of the Himalayas since
1985. The arena is the watershed of the Siachen Glacier, comprising about 1,000 square miles of the
highest, least accessible mountains in the world.
This small war is a case study of the problems of
operations in very high mountainous terrain. The
campaign is immobile and consists of holding positions on very high points, raids by both sides, and
daily artillery duels. No large-scale engagements
have been fought. Details are classified but apparently only a few hundred troops on each side are
engaged at any time.

At the beginning of 2002, both India and Pakistan are in full alert across the disputed Kashmir
border, both armed with nuclear weapons. This confrontation threatens to destabilize the smaller-scale
fighting, which has been in progress for 10 years in
the Siachen area as high as 7,000 m (23,000 ft). Personnel rotate through these positions every 6 to 8
weeks, since they are at or above the altitude where
deterioration outstrips acclimatization. Replacements
are taken by truck and airlifted to points from which
they must climb up the remaining few thousand
feet. Supplies follow the same route and are often
air-dropped. Casualties are alleged to be 20% or
higher owing to cold and altitude, because the
troops are exposed without adequate acclimatization.

The same syndrome of right ventricular failure
described in Han Chinese infants in Tibet has been
reported in Indian (and presumably has also appeared in Pakistani) troops who have been stationed
for long periods at great height. The syndrome is
different from the well-studied chronic mountain
sickness (Monge's disease) seen in long-time residents in the high Andes Mountains.[39] Cold injuries
are said to be less important. The medical experience gained has been of great interest to science.

SUMMARY

Throughout history many battles have been fought in mountainous terrain because the high ground can benefit either defense or offense. Small hills offer tactical advantage with few risks or obstacles. On higher mountains, however, the rigors of cold, altitude, difficult and dangerous terrain, and wildly variable weather often exact a heavy price. Even a brief review of military history reveals that these factors are often decisive in mountain warfare. Repeatedly, although not surprisingly, leadership emerges as the most critical factor. Faced with the hazards of high mountains, the courage, genius, and panache of leaders like Xenophon, Alexander, and Hannibal have often brought victory despite great obstacles. Conversely, if the leader falters, or if leadership is divided or uncertain, defeat is more likely. Preparedness has also been a major factor. More often than not soldiers have been led to fight in an environment for which they had inadequate clothing, food, or information—as was the case for Russian troops in the Caucasus. Cold has taken a heavy toll when troops have had inadequate footwear, clothing, or shelter—as happened in the disastrous retreat from the Chosin Reservoir in Korea.

During a few campaigns in the mountains, the oxygen lack at great altitude has caused many casualties among troops required to ascend too rapidly to dangerous altitude; this was especially true among Indian troops in Ladakh. Together, cold and altitude have been devastating, as Alexander found in the Hindu Kush Mountains, and as the Chinese Communist army experienced when crossing the Snowy Mountains. The combatants in the Karakoram Range of the Himalayas today are badly handicapped by the extreme altitude. By contrast, even on high mountains, well-clothed and -acclimatized men have usually prevailed over the enemy, whether defending or attacking. Continuing supplies of food, water, weapons, and clothing are crucial but are often interrupted by terrain and weather. Lack of food, as Xenophon noted, can greatly weaken even the best soldiers. In very cold weather, ice and snow can be changed to water only when fuel for fire is available; lack of water causes weakness from dehydration.

It is ironic that despite sophisticated weapons, clothing, and food; despite airpower and advanced transport; repeated failure to learn such basic lessons from the past has continued to cause avoidable casualties and has too often led to defeat. Mountainous terrain is a special circumstance, one greatly complicating the other hazards of war.

REFERENCES

1. Xenophon; Warner R, trans. *The Persian Expedition.* London, England: Penguin Books; 1949.

2. Arrian; Sélincourt A, trans. *The Campaigns of Alexander.* London, England: Penguin Books; 1971.

3. Dodge TA. *Great Captains: Alexander.* Boston, Mass: Houghton Mifflin; 1891. Reprinted (facsimile) Mechanicsburgh, Pa: Stackpole Books; 1994.

4. Green P. *Alexander of Macedon: 356–323 BC.* Berkeley, Calif: University of California Press; 1991.

5. Quintus Curtius Rufus; Rolfe JC, trans. *History of Alexander.* London, England: Heineman; 1946.

6. De Beer G. *Alps and Elephants.* New York, NY: Dutton; 1956.

7. Lucas JS. *Alpine Elite: German Mountain Troops of World War II.* London, England: Jane's; 1980.

8. Chandler DG. *Atlas of Military Strategy.* New York, NY: Macmillan; 1980.

9. Monelli P. *Toes Up.* London, England: Duckworth; 1930.

10. Buchan JA. *History of the Great War.* Boston, Mass: Houghton Mifflin; 1922.

11. Werth A. *Russia at War 1941–1945.* New York, NY: Dutton; 1964.

12. Ellis J. *Cassino: The Hollow Victory.* New York, NY: McGraw Hill; 1984.

13. Strawson J. *The Italian Campaign.* New York, NY: Carroll and Graf; 1988.

14. Meinke AH. *Mountain Troops and Medics.* Keewaydin, Mich: Rucksack; 1993.

15. Gilbert DL. The first documented report of mountain sickness: The China or Headache story. *Respir Physiol.* 1983;52:10.

16. Fa Hsien. *The Travels of Fa-Hsien (399–414 AD), or Record of the Buddhist Kingdoms.* Westport, Conn: Greenwood Press; 1981.

17. de Acosta J. *Of Some Mervellous Effects of the Windes Which are in Some Parts of the Indies.* Quoted by: West JB, ed. *High Altitude Physiology.* Stroudsburg, Pa: Hutchinson Ross; 1981: 10.

18. de Ovalle A. Quoted by: Pinkerton J, ed. *A General Collection of the Best and Most Interesting Voyages and Travels in all Parts of the World.* London, England: Longman, Hurst, Reese, Orme, and Brown; 1813: 46–47.

19. Gruber. Cited by: Gilbert DL. *Oxygen and Living Processes.* New York, NY: Springer-Verlag; 1981.

20. Morgan D. *The Mongols.* New York, NY: Blackwell; 1986.

21. Dupuy RE, Dupuy TN. *The Encyclopedia of Military History.* New York, NY: Harper & Row; 1970: 277.

22. Mirza Muhammad Haider. *The Tarikh-i-Rashid: History of the Mongols in Central Asia.* Lahore, Pakistan: Book Traders; 1894: 412–413.

23. Hopkirk P. *The Great Game: The Struggle for Empire in Central Asia.* New York, NY: Kodansha; 1994.

24. Keay J. *The Gilgit Game.* Hamden, Conn: Archon; 1979.

25. Forbes A. *The Afghan Wars.* London, England: Seeley; 1906.

26. Urban M. *War in Afghanistan.* New York, NY: St Martin's Press; 1988.

27. Landon P. *The Opening of Tibet.* New York, NY: Doubleday Page; 1905; 52–54.

28. Mehra P. *The Younghusband Expedition.* New York, NY: Asia Publishing House; 1968.

29. Wilson D. *The Long March: The Epic of Chinese Communists' Survival.* New York, NY: Viking; 1971.

30. Salisbury HE. *The Long March: The Untold Story.* New York, NY: Harper & Row; 1985.

31. Hastings M. *The Korean War.* New York, NY: Simon & Schuster; 1987.

32. Pandolf K, Burr RE, Wenger CB, Pozos RS, eds. *Medical Aspects of Harsh Environments, Volume 1.* In: Zajtchuk R, Bellamy RF, eds. *Textbook of Military Medicine.* Washington, DC: Department of the Army, Office of The Surgeon General, and Borden Institute; 2001. Also available at www.armymedicine.army.mil/history.

33. Diamond J. Collision at Cajamarca. In: *Guns, Germs, and Steel: The Fates of Human Societies.* New York, NY: W. W. Norton & Co; 1997: 67–81.

34. Adams JR. José de San Martín. In: *Latin American Heroes.* New York, NY: Ballantine Books; 1991: 57–73.

35. Adams JR. Bernardo O'Higgins. In: *Latin American Heroes.* New York, NY: Ballantine Books; 1991: 74–91.

36. Adams JR. Simón Bolívar. In: *Latin American Heroes*. New York, NY: Ballantine Books; 1991: 28–39.

37. Adams JR. Manuela Sáenz. In: *Latin American Heroes*. New York, NY: Ballantine Books; 1991: 40–56.

38. del Campo J. The Breña Campaign, 1881–1883. Great Military Campaigns of the Peruvian Army and Navy website. Available at http://members.lycos.co.uk/Juan39/THE_BRENA_CAMPAIGN.html. Accessed 12 March 2002.

39. Anand IS. Subacute mountain sickness syndromes: Role of pulmonary hypertension. In: Sutton JR, Houston CS, Coates G, eds. *Hypoxia and Mountain Medicine.* Burlington, Vt: Queen City Press; 1992: 241–251.

40. Fisher WW, Rose LE, Huttenback RA. *Himalayan Battleground: Sino–Indian Rivalry in Ladakh.* New York, NY: Praeger; 1964.

41. Johri SR. *Chinese Invasion of Ladakh.* Lucknow, India: Himalaya Publications; 1969: 20.

42. Houston CS. *Going Higher: Oxygen, Man and Mountains.* Seattle, Wash: Mountaineers; 1998.

43. Singh I, Khanna PK, Srivastava MC, Lal M, Roy SB, Subramanyan CSV. Acute mountain sickness. *N Engl J Med.* 1969;280:175–179, 183–184.

Chapter 21

HUMAN ADAPTATION TO HIGH TERRESTRIAL ALTITUDE

ANDREW J. YOUNG, PhD*; AND JOHN T. REEVES, MD†

*Thermal & Mountain Medicine Division, US Army Research Institute of Environmental Medicine, Natick, Massachusetts 01760-5007
†Department of Medicine, Pediatrics, and Family Medicine, University of Colorado Health Science Center, Denver, Colorado 80262

INTRODUCTION

Soldiers who deploy from sea-level bases for operations in the mountains or high plateaus will experience multiple environmental stressors, but the stress unique to high altitudes is the oxygen-deficient atmosphere. This chapter will focus on the physiological effects of acute and chronic exposure to that stressor. The emphasis will be on the effects experienced during altitude sojourns of the type that military units might conduct (ie, ascent to moderate altitudes [2,500–5,000 m] for a few days to several weeks), although effects of longer and more extreme ascents will also be considered. The mechanisms for these effects will be discussed with a view to explaining functional changes experienced by *lowlanders* (natives or acclimatized inhabitants of low-altitude regions) who are sojourning at altitude.

On arriving at high altitude, lowlanders will be incapable of as much physical exertion as they were at sea level. Further, they may not feel well, and may have impaired mentation. These effects are ultimately due to hypoxia. However, a series of physiological adjustments ensue that are directed at compensating for the reduction in ambient oxygen. These adjustments, which include increases in ventilation, hemodynamic and hematologic changes, altered hormone secretion, and metabolic and body water changes, to name a few, relieve some but not all of the physiological strain of continued residence at high altitude. The time required for altitude adaptations to become manifest varies with the different processes, with the altitude ascended, and with the speed of ascent. The progressive development of these adjustments, usually termed *acclimatization,* alleviates, to varying degrees, the symptoms and physical and mental limitations inflicted by hypoxia. The adjustments to hypoxia that begin immediately with acute hypoxic exposure, together with the continuing processes of acclimatization, collectively comprise the altitude adaptations that will be examined in this chapter.

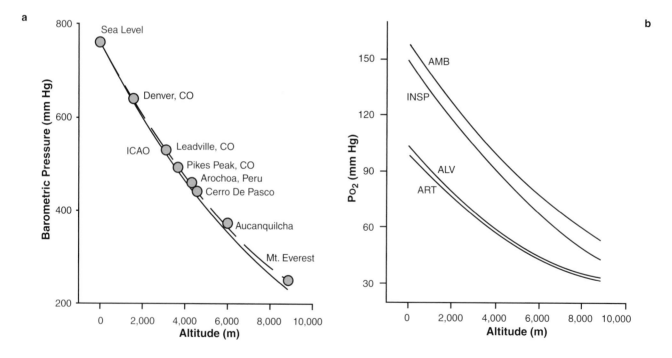

Fig. 21-1. Both atmospheric pressure and the partial pressure of oxygen decrease as functions of altitude. (**a**) The barometric pressure measured at various sites located at different elevations (closed circles and dashed line)[1,2] and the global average (solid line) reported[3] by the International Civil Aviation Organization (ICAO). (**b**) Partial pressures of oxygen (Po_2) at increasing altitude are shown in ambient air (AMB), in the airways after inspired air has been warmed and humidified (INSP), in the alveolus after CO_2 has been added (ALV), and in the arterial blood (ART). Data sources: (1) West JB. Prediction of barometric pressures at high altitudes with the use of model atmospheres. *J Appl Physiol.* 1996;81:1850–1854. (2) Authors' personal unpublished observations. (3) Ward MP, Milledge JS, West JB. *High Altitude Medicine and Physiology.* New York, NY: Oxford University Press; 2000: 26, Table 2.1.

THE HYPOXIC ENVIRONMENT

Elevation, Barometric Pressure, and Inspired Oxygen

The surface of Earth's oceans, which we call sea level, is also the bottom of an ocean of air. Air, unlike water, is compressible. Therefore air is denser at sea level than at higher terrestrial elevations, and barometric pressure (P_B) is not directly proportional to elevation but is logarithmic. Thus, from sea level (P_B = 760 mm Hg) to the summit of Mount Everest (P_B = 253 mm Hg), the highest point on Earth, the relationship of pressure to elevation is a curved, and not a straight, line (Figure 21-1). Also, where P_B has actually been measured at various terrestrial elevations within the temperate zone, it is slightly higher than the "standard barometric pressure" indicated in the table published by the International Civil Aviation Organization (ICAO) to reflect mean conditions over the entire earth's surface.[1] In addition, the ambient barometric pressure is lower in winter than in summer, a decrease that over the years averages 8 mm Hg in Colorado.

Air is a mixture of gases, the summated partial pressures of which equal the P_B. The principal gases in air are oxygen and nitrogen. Their concentrations are essentially constant over Earth's terrestrial elevations. For example, when water vapor is absent, oxygen comprises 20.93% of the air at all elevations. The partial pressure of oxygen (P_{O_2}, in mm Hg) in the atmosphere falls as barometric pressure (P_B, in mm Hg) falls, as defined by Equation 1:

$$(1) \qquad P_{O_2} = P_B \bullet 0.2093$$

Thus, ambient P_{O_2} also depends on the terrestrial elevation, falling with P_B as elevation above sea level increases, as indicated in Figure 21-1b. The atmospheric P_{O_2} (in dry air) is 159 mm Hg at sea level (760 • 0.2093) and 53 mm Hg on the summit of Mount Everest (253 • 0.2093).

When air is inspired, it is warmed to body temperature and saturated with water vapor by the time it reaches the bifurcation of the trachea. The water vapor has a partial pressure, which is also a component of total pressure. At all altitudes, the partial pressure of water vapor (P_{H_2O}) in fully humidified air depends only on temperature, ranging (in mm Hg) from approximately 0.5 at 0°C and 760 at 100°C. At body temperature of 37°C, P_{H_2O} is 47 mm Hg. The dilution of inspired air by water vapor reduces the inspired oxygen pressure (P_{IO_2}) below the ambient P_{O_2}, as illustrated by Equation 2, where the P_{H_2O} is taken to be 47 mm Hg:

$$(2) \qquad P_{IO_2} = (P_B - 47) \bullet 0.2093$$

Thus, P_{IO_2} also falls with increasing elevation. As Figure 21-1(b) shows, P_{IO_2} is 149 mm Hg ([760 – 47] • 0.2093) at sea level and 43 mm Hg ([253 – 47] • 0.2093) on the summit of Mount Everest. Although the major determining factor of P_{IO_2} is P_B, body temperature can affect the P_{IO_2} somewhat. If body temperature falls, P_{H_2O} of saturated inspired air would also fall and P_{IO_2} would rise; conversely, if body temperature were to rise, P_{IO_2} would fall. At a given P_B, the oxygen pressure in the inspired air is therefore independent of ventilation and depends only on body temperature. (Alveolar temperature equals body temperature, but a detailed discussion of this point is beyond the scope of this chapter.)

Overview of the Oxygen-Transport Cascade at High Altitude

For health and even for life itself, oxygen must constantly be transported from the atmosphere to the mitochondria in sufficient quantities to meet tissue demands. Transport can be regarded as a series of steps in a cascade, because the P_{O_2} falls sequentially and progressively, much as cascading water flowing over steps must fall to each new level. The cascade has four steps (Figure 21-2a):

1. oxygen transport by the bellows action of the respiratory system, which brings oxygen from ambient air to the alveolus, from which
2. oxygen passively diffuses across the alveolar–capillary membrane into the blood, which then
3. convectively transports the oxygen via cardiac action to the systemic capillaries, where
4. the oxygen passively diffuses through the tissues to the cells' mitochondria.

Figure 21-2b illustrates the P_{O_2} fall for each step in the cascade during near maximal exercise. At sea level, where the P_{IO_2} is near 150 mm Hg, ventilation normally limits the P_{O_2} pressure fall during the first step in the cascade to approximately 40 mm Hg, resulting in an alveolar P_{O_2} of 110 mm Hg. During the second step in the cascade, the P_{O_2} falls as oxygen diffuses across the pulmonary–capillary membrane from air in the alveolus to pulmonary capillary blood. During heavy exercise, where large amounts of oxygen are to be transported, the diffusion gradient may be large. This is because blood entering the pulmonary capillaries during heavy exercise has relatively little oxygen content to begin with, and the high circulatory flow rate ensures that oxygen is removed quickly after crossing the pulmonary–capillary membrane. In addition, venous shunts allow deoxygenated blood to bypass the lung capillaries and contribute to the P_{O_2} pressure gradient from alveolus to arterial blood. Fig-

ure 21-2b shows the cascade from alveolus to artery as a P_{O_2} pressure fall of about 30 mm Hg during near-maximal exercise at sea level. The third step, convective transport by the circulation, representing cardiac action, normally limits the P_{O_2} pressure fall to about 60 mm Hg (ie, from 80 mm Hg in arterial blood to 20 mm Hg in venous blood). In Figure 21-2b, venous P_{O_2} is assumed to reflect that in the systemic capillaries. The P_{O_2} in the mitochondria is considered to be near zero, so the fourth step in the cascade represents a P_{O_2} fall of about 20 mm Hg.

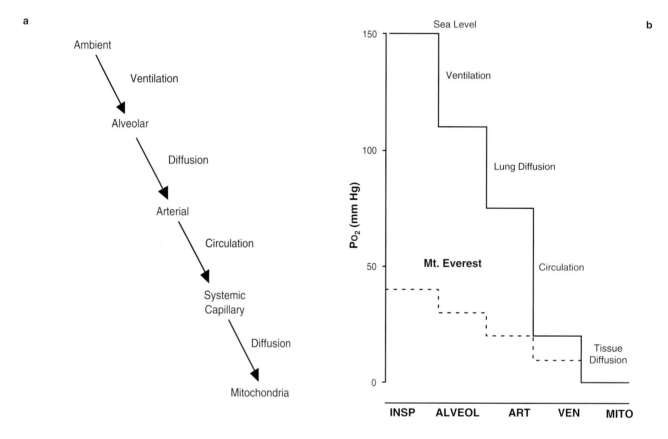

Fig. 21-2. In the oxygen transport cascade, oxygen moves from the atmosphere to the tissues down a decreasing pressure gradient. (**a**) The four steps in the oxygen transport cascade from ambient air to tissue mitochondria use either active (ventilation, circulation) or passive (diffusion) processes. (**b**) The average fall in the partial pressure of oxygen (P_{O_2}) was observed[1–4] at each step in the oxygen transport cascade during near-maximal exercise at sea level (solid line) and at the simulated summit of Mount Everest (dotted line).
INSP: inspired air, warmed and humidified; ALVEOL: in the alveoli, after CO_2 has been added; ART: in the arterial blood, convectively transporting oxygen to metabolically active tissue; VEN: in the venous blood draining from capillaries perfusing metabolically active tissue; MITO: in the mitochondria while oxygen is used in the regeneration of adenosophine triphosphate.
Data sources: (1) Sutton JR, Reeves JT, Wagner PD, et al. Operation Everest II: Oxygen transport during exercise at extreme simulated altitude. *J Appl Physiol.* 1988;64:1309–1321. (2) Wagner PD, Sutton JR, Reeves JT, Cymerman A, Groves BM, Malconian MK. Operation Everest II: Pulmonary gas exchange during a simulated ascent of Mt Everest. *J Appl Physiol.* 1987;63:2348–2359. (3) Cymerman A, Reeves JT, Sutton JR, et al. Operation Everest II: Maximal oxygen uptake at extreme altitude. *J Appl Physiol.* 1989;66:2446–2453. (4) Houston CS, Sutton JR, Cymerman A, Reeves JT. Operation Everest II: Man at extreme altitude. *J Appl Physiol.* 1987;63:877–882.

The overall P_{O_2} pressure gradient that drives oxygen down the transport chain during heavy exercise at sea level is approximately 150 mm Hg from inspired air to the mitochondria. The overall P_{O_2} gradient driving oxygen transport at the highest point on Earth, the summit of Mount Everest, is considerably less than at sea level, about 43 mm Hg from inspired air to the mitochondria, because the atmospheric P_{O_2} is so low at the top of Mount Everest. Nevertheless, men recently ascended Mount Everest successfully without using supplemental breathing oxygen.[2] As shown in Figure 21-2b, the P_{O_2} fall at each successive step in the oxygen-transport cascade is less on Mount Everest than at sea level. Clearly, humans must have a great capacity for physiological adjustments to compensate for the reduced pressure gradient that drives oxygen transport at high altitude. Not surprisingly, the most profound adjustments involve the active transport steps in the cascade, ventilation and circulation, but there are also adjustments affecting the passive transport steps. In the subsequent sections of this chapter, we will use experimental data reported from a variety of studies at high altitudes to focus on the physiology and implications involved in the altitude-related changes in each step in the oxygen-transport cascade, to better understand the normal responses to the combined stresses of exercise and hypoxia.

PULMONARY GAS EXCHANGE AT HIGH ALTITUDE

The Role of Increasing Ventilation

As we will discuss next in detail, one of the principal physiological responses to hypoxia is an increase in ventilation. However, in the preceding section it was pointed out that P_{IO_2} was independent of alterations in ventilation. Therefore, we need to consider what role increasing ventilation plays in adjusting oxygen transport in response to hypoxia.

The alveolus always contains carbon dioxide. Because ambient inspired air contains relatively little carbon dioxide, alveolar carbon dioxide (P_{ACO_2}) reflects the net balance between carbon dioxide diffusion into the alveolus from the capillary blood and removal of carbon dioxide from the alveolus by expiration. When the inspired air reaches the alveolus, it is diluted by the alveolar carbon dioxide, which causes the alveolar P_{O_2} (P_{AO_2}) to fall below the P_{IO_2} (see Figure 21-1b). For practical purposes one may consider that the alveolus contains essentially four gases: nitrogen (including the other inert gases), water vapor, oxygen, and carbon dioxide. When the glottis is open at the end of inspiration and expiration, the total pressure in the alveolus must equal the P_B, which is the sum of the partial pressures of the alveolar gases, as indicated in Equation 3:

(3) $\qquad P_B = (P_{AN_2} + P_{AH_2O} + P_{ACO_2} + P_{AO_2})$

Therefore, by rearranging Equation 3, an expression of the partial pressure of oxygen in the alveolus, Equation 4, is obtained:

(4) $\qquad P_{AO_2} = P_B - (P_{AN_2} + P_{ACO_2} + P_{AH_2O})$

So how can increasing ventilation at any altitude increase the partial pressure of oxygen in the alveolus? The P_B is determined by the altitude and the P_{AH_2O} is determined by body temperature (47 mm Hg at 37°C, as described above). Physiologically, nitrogen is an inert gas, being neither produced nor consumed by the body. Assuming that body temperature is 37°C and that equal volumes of oxygen leave and carbon dioxide enter the alveolus over time (ie, the respiratory exchange ratio, R, equals 1), the alveolar partial pressure of nitrogen (P_{AN_2}) may be expressed as follows in Equation 5:

(5) $\qquad P_{AN_2} = (P_B - 47) \bullet 0.7907$

where 0.7907 is the fraction of nitrogen in dry atmospheric air. Physiological variations in body temperature or R have only small effects on P_{AN_2}, which is relatively high, compared with pressures of other atmospheric gases. Thus, hyperventilation has little or no effect on the P_B, P_{AH_2O}, or P_{AN_2} components of Equation 4 but does have a profound effect on the two remaining components. Hyperventilation increases the rate of removal of carbon dioxide from the alveolus relative to the rate that it diffuses in from the blood. As hyperventilation lowers the P_{ACO_2}, the P_{AO_2} must rise.

Another expression of the steady state relation of P_{AO_2} and P_{ACO_2} is given by the alveolar air equation in Equation 6:

(6) $\qquad P_{AO_2} = P_{IO_2} - P_{ACO_2} (F_{IO_2} + [1 - F_{IO_2}] / R)$

where F_{IO_2} represents the fraction of oxygen in the inspired air (0.2093 during air breathing) and R, the respiratory exchange ratio, represents carbon dioxide production divided by oxygen uptake. As R varies within its usual physiological range of 0.8 to

1.2, P_{ACO_2} will be modified by a factor ranging, respectively, from approximately 1.20 to 0.87. Equation 7 illustrates the special case when R = 1:

$$(7) \qquad P_{AO_2} = P_{IO_2} - P_{ACO_2}$$

It is clear from Equations 6 and 7 that if P_{IO_2} is constant, then P_{AO_2} must rise as P_{ACO_2} falls. Further, when R = 1, there is an equal exchange of O_2 for CO_2. Each mm Hg fall in P_{CO_2} is accompanied by a mm Hg rise in P_{O_2}. Thus, ventilation raises P_{O_2} to the extent that it lowers P_{CO_2}.

It is important to understand that although the relationship between the ventilation expired (V_E) and P_{CO_2} depends on the volume of carbon dioxide to be expired, the expired volumes of ventilation and of carbon dioxide are reported differently. The ventilation expired is usually reported in liters per minute, measured at *body temperature, ambient pressure*, and *saturated* with water vapor (BTPS, designated V_E BTPS). These measurements reflect the volume of gas expired under the conditions within the alveolus, and therefore the actual movement of the diaphragm and chest wall (ie, the bellows function of the respiratory system). But the volumes of carbon dioxide ($\dot{V}_{CO_2}$) are always reported under *standard* conditions of *temperature* (0°C), *pressure* (760 mm Hg), and *dry* ($P_{H_2O} = 0$ mm Hg) (known as STPD) to reflect the number of molecules of gas. (Occasionally, ventilation is reported as V_E STPD to designate the number of molecules transported into and out of the lungs, as will be discussed later in this chapter).

Equation 8 shows that the P_{ACO_2} falls as alveolar ventilation (V_A, total ventilation minus dead space ventilation) rises for any given volume of CO_2 produced ($\dot{V}_{CO_2}$):

$$(8) \qquad P_{ACO_2} = (F \bullet \dot{V}_{CO_2}\ STPD) / V_A\ BTPS$$

where *F* is the factor that converts CO_2 from STPD to BTPS conditions, multiplied by the barometric pressure to allow the alveolar CO_2 to be expressed as a partial pressure rather than a fractional concentration.[3] Because F is nearly constant from sea level (1.21 • 760 mm Hg = 920 mm Hg) to the summit of Mount Everest (4.19 • 253 mm Hg = 1,060 mm Hg), the P_{ACO_2} for a given $\dot{V}_{CO_2}$ depends almost entirely on the V_A measured under BTPS conditions. Further, in normal subjects resting quietly at sea level, P_{ACO_2} and the ratio of $\dot{V}_{CO_2} / V_A$ remain stable over long periods,[4] demonstrating that even at rest, ventilation is tightly coupled to meta-

bolic rate. The tight coupling of resting metabolic rate and ventilation also occurs at altitude, and decreases in P_{ACO_2} reflect altitude-related hyperventilation independent of changes in metabolic rate.[5] Also, carbon dioxide, being a water-soluble molecule, crosses the alveolar–capillary membrane with much greater facility than does oxygen. The result is that the resting alveolar–capillary P_{CO_2} gradient is so small that alveolar and arterial P_{CO_2} values are often used interchangeably. By convention, respiratory physiologists use the carbon dioxide partial pressure in either the alveolus (P_{ACO_2}) or the arterial blood (P_{aCO_2}) as convenient approximations of effective (alveolar) resting ventilation for the various altitudes.

Ventilatory Responses to Acute Hypoxia

Mechanism for Increasing Ventilation With Hypoxia

An increase in ventilation begins within seconds of exposure to hypoxia, but the subsequent time-dependent changes are complex. Figure 21-3 schematically depicts these sequential changes in stages that include a stimulation of ventilation known as the acute hypoxic ventilatory response, hypoxic ventilatory depression, ventilatory acclimatization, and finally hypoxic desensitization. The first two stages occur within minutes of hypoxic exposure, whereas ventilatory acclimatization is developed over the ensuing days to weeks that hypoxia continues and persists for many years of residence in a hypoxic environment. The final stage, hypoxic desensitization, is not usually observed until after decades of chronic hypoxic exposure.

The key sensors that initiate and sustain the increase in ventilation in response to hypoxia appear to be the peripheral chemoreceptor cells in the carotid bodies. The carotid bodies are about the size of the head of a pin and are located bilaterally in the wall of the internal carotid artery at its origin from the common carotid. Decreasing arterial oxygenation increases carotid body neural discharge. The carotid body neural discharge increases hyperbolically with decreasing P_{O_2}, and in inverse proportion to decreasing oxygen saturation below 96%.[6–8] With acute hypoxia, the carotid body neural discharge is tightly coupled with elevated phrenic nerve activity and increased ventilation.[8] Carotid bodies sense oxygen pressure rather than content, as they do not respond to carbon monoxide–induced reductions in arterial oxygen content

(Ca_{O_2}) where the arterial P_{O_2} remains high.[8] Carotid bodies have an extremely high blood flow relative to their size and metabolism (only a 5- to 15-mm Hg P_{O_2} gradient from arterial blood to the chemoreceptor cell), so small changes in arterial oxygenation can be rapidly sensed. Experiments with animals indicate that removal of the carotid bodies prevents ventilatory acclimatization to hypoxia.[9] Animals without carotid body function that are taken to high altitude do poorly and may die. Further, selective carotid body hypoxia induces acclimatization even when the rest of the body, including the brain, is normoxic. Thus, the acute and chronic ventilatory response to hypoxia resides in the carotid bodies.

When the arterial oxygen pressure (Pa_{O_2}) falls, nervelike cells (chemoreceptor cells, also called glomus type I cells) in the carotid body increase afferent

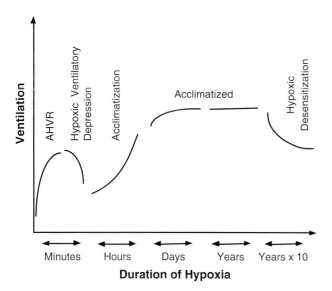

Fig. 21-3. Ventilation responses to hypoxia change as the exposure increases in duration. The acute hypoxic ventilatory response (AHVR) increases ventilation over the first 5 to 8 minutes. After about 10 minutes of hypoxia, some of the initial increase abates during hypoxic ventilatory depression. Over the next hours and days, ventilation increases as the ventilatory depression disappears, and ventilatory acclimatization occurs. Fully developed ventilatory acclimatization is characterized by hyperventilation, which is sustained for years at high altitude. A fall in ventilation that sometimes occurs after decades of altitude residence has been called hypoxic desentization. Adapted with permission from Weil JV. Ventilatory control at high altitude. In: Fishman AP, Cherniak NS, Widdicombe JG, Geiger SR, eds. *Handbook of Physiology. Section 3: The Respiratory System. Vol 2: Control of Breathing, Part 2.* Bethesda, Md: American Physiological Society; 1986: 704.

impulses along the ninth cranial nerve to the respiratory system in the brainstem, resulting in increased respiratory effort. If a subject breathes oxygen-enriched mixtures, the reverse happens (ie, decreased nerve traffic and respiratory effort). Thus, an important mechanism controlling breathing is the Pa_{O_2}, where a decrease in P_{O_2} increases breathing, and an increase in P_{O_2} decreases breathing. In each case, the result is, in effect, the body's effort to maintain constant blood oxygen levels. This concept is fully developed in subsequent sections of this chapter.

How the carotid body senses oxygen levels has been intensively investigated. Following the initial report from Lopez-Barneo,[10] there is increasing evidence that the glomus type I cells have voltage-gated K^+ channels that are altered by oxygen pressure over the physiological range (see review by Benot[11]). When the P_{O_2} is high, the channels are open, allowing the egress of K^+ to maintain the negative transmembrane potential in the interior of the cell, which under these conditions is quiescent. As the P_{O_2} falls, the outward K^+ current is progressively inhibited, causing the interior of the cell to become less negative and thereby inducing membrane depolarization. A reduction in P_{O_2} thus induces electrical discharge of the glomus type I cells, which send afferent impulses up the ninth cranial nerve to the respiratory center in the medulla, resulting in an increase in ventilation within seconds. Whether changing P_{O_2} directly affects the K^+ channels by changing the configuration of key proteins, or whether it alters mitochondrial activity, or works through some other mechanism is not clear.

Many complex factors act on this basic control mechanism to modulate the resultant level of ventilation. For one thing, hypercapnia augments and hypocapnia inhibits the hypoxic response. Changes in Pco_2 exert direct effects on the respiratory center as well as acting indirectly by affecting chemoreceptor function.[12] Although changing Pco_2 levels appear to be foremost, other factors also modulate the hypoxic ventilatory response. Dopamine is thought to profoundly inhibit carotid body chemoreceptor activity, probably via effects on the Na^+ and Ca^{++} channels and the levels of cyclic adenosine monophosphate (AMP) in the glomus type I cells, which modulate the firing rate.[13] Somatic neural impulses to the central nervous system, including those from the lungs, also contribute to regulation of ventilation. With so many influences, ventilation is both highly regulated and variable from one individual to another. The interplay of these various influences within an individual account for changes in ventilation over time at altitude (see Figure 21-3).

The Acute Hypoxic Ventilatory Response

When sea-level residents are made progressively more hypoxemic over 10 minutes, the stimulus–response curve of P_{O_2} to ventilation is hyperbolic (Figure 21-4a). That the curve indeed reflects a stimulus-response relationship is theoretically likely, because P_{O_2} may be considered the actual stimulus for the carotid body, as already discussed. The acute ventilatory response can be described by Equation 9[8,14]:

$$(9) \qquad \dot{V}_E = V_o + A / (P_{O_2} - B)$$

where $\dot{V}_E$ represents minute ventilation (in L/min),

and V_o, the asymptote along the abscissa, represents the minute ventilation (in L/min) when the P_{O_2} is high (ie, when there is no hypoxic stimulation of ventilation). The constant B, empirically determined to equal 32 mm Hg,[8,14] represents the P_{O_2} below which there is no further increase in carotid body neural discharge, and ventilation is assumed to become asymptotic along the ordinate.[6,7] P_{O_2}, by convenience, usually represents the alveolar oxygen pressure (P_{AO_2}, in mm Hg), and A represents the shape parameter for the curve. Figure 21-4a shows clearly that a higher A value corresponds with a greater "drive" to breathe, whereas a lower A value characterizes individuals with a less-sen-

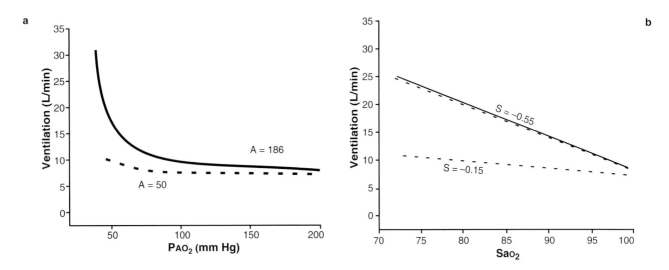

Fig. 21-4. The acute hypoxic ventilatory response is quantified by the increase in ventilation measured as alveolar oxygen pressure (P_{AO_2}) is decreased. (**a**) The stimulus-response curve is generated by plotting minute ventilation as P_{AO_2} is progressively lowered over 5–8 minutes from a high value to about 45 mm Hg. The shape parameter, A, from the response curve's equation, quantifies an individual's "drive" to ventilate ($\dot{V}_E = V_o + A / P_{O_2} - B$), where $\dot{V}_E$ represents minute ventilation (in L/min), and V_o, the asymptote along the abscissa, represents the minute ventilation (in L/min) when the P_{O_2} is high (ie, when there is no hypoxic stimulation of ventilation). The constant B, empirically determined to equal 32 mm Hg, represents the P_{O_2} below which there is no further increase in carotid body neural discharge, and ventilation is assumed to become asymptotic along the ordinate.[1,2] P_{O_2}, by convenience, usually represents the alveolar oxygen pressure (P_{AO_2}, in mm Hg).

The average response (solid line) for 44 normal men and women has a shape parameter equal to 186 (the shape parameter's units are generally ignored), whereas in a subgroup of individuals whose response to hypoxia was at the low end of the normal range (broken line), the value of A is 50.[3,4] (**b**) For the tests plotted in panel (a), the corresponding relationship between minute ventilation and the arterial oxygen saturation (S_{AO_2}) is linear with a negative slope. References for the figure legend: (1) Hornbein TF. The relation between stimulus to chemoreceptors and their response. In: Torrance RW, ed. *Arterial Chemoreceptors*. Oxford, Edinburgh, Scotland: Blackwell Scientific Publications; 1968: 65–78. (2) von Euler US, Liljestrand G, Zotterman Y. The excitation mechanism of the chemoreceptor in the carotid body. *Scand Arch Physiol*. 1939;83:132–152. (3) Weil JV, Byrne-Quinn E, Sodal IE, Filley GF, Grover RF. Hypoxic ventilatory drive in normal man. *J Clin Invest*. 1971;50:186–195. (4) Hirschman CA, McCullough RE, Weil JV. Normal values for hypoxic and hypercapnic ventilatory drives in man. *J Appl Physiol*. 1975;38:1095–1098.
Data sources for the graphs: (1) Weil JV, Byrne-Quinn E, Sodal IE, Filley GF, Grover RF. Hypoxic ventilatory drive in normal man. *J Clin Invest*. 1971;50:186–195. (2) Hirschman CA, McCullough RE, Weil JV. Normal values for hypoxic and hypercapnic ventilatory drives in man. *J Appl Physiol*. 1975;38:1095–1098.

sitive response to falling P_{AO_2}. In a group of 44 normal Denver residents, V_o and A were measured and found to be (mean ± 1 SD) 6.9 ± 2.4 L/min, and 186 ± 85 L • mm Hg/min, respectively.[8,14] The large standard deviation for A indicates the large variability among individuals observed in the normal population.

The strength of an individual's acute ventilatory response during the 10-minute progressive hypoxia test can also be quantified using the relationship between $\dot{V}_E$ and the arterial oxygen saturation (Sa_{O_2}) (Figure 21-4b). As Sa_{O_2} falls, $\dot{V}_E$ rises linearly, such that the slope, S, is negative, as calculated in Equation 10:

$$(10) \qquad S = \Delta\dot{V}_E / \Delta Sa_{O_2}$$

Sa_{O_2} is frequently and conveniently measured using commercial oximeters. Thus, the negative slope of the relation of $\dot{V}_E$ to Sa_{O_2} is a measure of the strength of the hypoxic ventilatory response, where the strength of an individual's hypoxic ventilatory response increases as the slope becomes more negative. The curvilinear relation of $\dot{V}_E$ (and carotid body neural discharge) to P_{AO_2}, as shown in Equation 9 and Figure 21-4a, have been thought to reflect the shape of the oxyhemoglobin dissociation curve (ODC). Therefore, using Sa_{O_2} rather than P_{AO_2} to describe ventilatory responsiveness linearizes the relationship between stimulus and response, although the stimulus to the carotid body is thought to be oxygen pressure rather than hemoglobin saturation. Another advantage of using Sa_{O_2} rather than P_{AO_2} is that arterial blood (and not alveolar air) bathes the carotid chemoreceptor.

Regardless of whether the hypoxic ventilatory response is quantified using oxygen pressure to measure A, or hemoglobin saturation to measure S, it is an inherent characteristic of an individual that provides an accurate index of the strength of the ventilatory response to acute hypoxia. Because there is greater concurrence between identical than fraternal twins, the response may have a familial component.[15] When P_{CO_2} is maintained at normal values during the hypoxic breathing (isocapnia), the response is greater than when P_{CO_2} is allowed to fall.[6,16] The hypoxic ventilatory response correlates with P_{CO_2} at sea level and may be a determinant of ventilation in subjects acclimatized to 4,300 m.[17] The response is increased when the metabolic rate is increased, as with eating, exercise, and hyperthyroidism. The strength of the ventilatory response to hypoxia correlates with the strength of the ventilatory response to hypercapnia,[14] suggesting that the ventilatory responses to low oxygen and high carbon dioxide are linked.

Hypoxic Ventilatory Depression

The strength of the initial hypoxic response is not sustained (Figure 21-5). For example, at P_{AO_2} of approximately 45 mm Hg, the ventilatory response during acute hypoxia rises to a maximum between 5 and 10 minutes, and then over the next 20 minutes partially declines toward the normoxic, control value. This ventilatory depression is not a response to hypocapnia, because it occurs both when P_{CO_2} is held constant (isocapnia) and when it is allowed to vary (poikilocapnia).

This hypoxic ventilatory depression may not originate from the carotid body. Studies using anesthetized cats have demonstrated that when the ventilation falls, the carotid body neural traffic does not decrease.[9] In other studies using cats, selective hypoxia of the brain stem produced the ventilatory depression, indicating that the depression is central in origin.[18] Recent research has focused on the possibility that hypoxic ventilatory depression is mediated by γ-aminobutyric acid (GABA). GABA is a central neurotransmitter released by inhibitory interneurons within the brain and spinal cord during hypoxia and is implicated in the hypoventilation of hibernating and diving animals.[19] Further, GABA administration depresses ventilation, and administration of antagonists to GABA prevents the hypoxic ventilatory depression.[20] Possibly, GABA release is a vestigial remnant of a central mechanism that was active in the aquatically adapted fetus.[21] However, anesthetized animals may not provide an appropriate model of ventilatory control in awake humans, in whom the carotid body may still regulate the ventilatory depression.[22]

Ventilation on Arrival at High Altitude

Thus, in subjects rapidly transported to high altitude, opposing factors alter ventilation on arrival. On the one hand, hypoxia stimulates ventilation; on the other, the ventilatory response is limited by the development of both hypocapnia and hypoxic depression.[16] When all three factors—hypoxic stimulation, hypocapnia, and hypoxic depression—were measured over 30 minutes in a group of individuals at low altitude, these factors largely accounted for the level of ventilation observed on arrival (day 1) at high altitude (see Figure 21-5a). Approximately half of the ventilatory inhibition that occurred on arrival could be attributed to hypoxic depression, and half to the development of hypocapnia. Both inhibitory factors abated over the

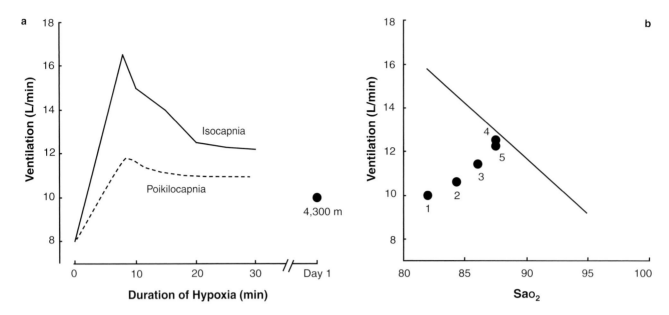

Fig. 21-5. When hypoxia is sustained for more than a few minutes, the increase in ventilation observed with acute hypoxia abates owing to ventilatory depression. (**a**) The acute ventilatory response to hypoxia (partial pressure of alveolar oxygen [P_{AO_2}] ~ 45 mm Hg) and the ventilatory response to hypoxia sustained over the next 30 minutes were measured in 11 male residents of 1,600 m. Ventilation is greater when the partial pressure of alveolar carbon dioxide (P_{ACO_2}) is held constant (isocapnia, solid line) than when it is allowed to fall (poikiolcapnia, dotted line) during the hypoxia. However, ventilatory depression begins after about 10 minutes of hypoxia, regardless of whether the partial pressure of carbon dioxide (P_{CO_2}) is maintained or allowed to fall. Resting ventilation in these subjects on arrival at 4,300 m was near that observed during sustained poikilocapnic hypoxia at 1,600 m. (**b**) For the same 11 subjects at 1,600 m (solid line), the mean values of resting ventilation and the corresponding arterial oxygen saturation (SaO_2) were measured on each of the first 5 days during acclimatization at 4,300 m (closed circles, days 1–5). These observations suggest that ventilation on arrival at altitude could be predicted from low altitude hypoxic tests when there was hypocapnia and hypoxic depression, whereas the acclimatized ventilation could be predicted from the acute isocapnic hypoxic ventilatory response at low altitude. Adapted with permission from Huang SY, Alexander JK, Grover RF, et al. Hypocapnia and sustained hypoxia blunt ventilation on arrival at high altitude. *J Appl Physiol.* 1984;56:604.

next several days at altitude, and the ventilation observed was that predicted by the acute ventilatory response to isocapnic hypoxia at low altitude (see Figure 21-5b). The loss, over several days, of the factors inhibiting ventilation at altitude may contribute to the process of ventilatory acclimatization, as will be discussed in the next section of this chapter.

The increase in ventilation at altitude is a true hyperventilation, in that ventilation increases out of proportion to metabolic requirements. However, resting metabolic rate increases on arrival at altitude,[5,23] and this increased metabolic rate is another contributing factor signaling for an increase in ventilation. This is demonstrated by the findings that propranolol treatment to induce dense β-adrenergic blockade prevented the increase in metabolic rate and lowered ventilation at altitude compared to placebo treatment.[5] However, ventilation rose progressively and Pa_{CO_2} fell progressively in both

propranolol- and placebo-treated subjects.[5] Thus, these data were interpreted to indicate that the increase in metabolic rate on arrival at altitude does stimulate ventilation; however, this effect was separate from the process of ventilatory acclimatization.

Ventilatory Acclimatization to High Altitude

Ventilation increases during the first days after arrival at high altitude through a poorly understood process termed "ventilatory acclimatization." As ventilation increases, P_{CO_2} falls and arterial pH and Sa_{O_2} rise (Figure 21-6). More time is required for full development of ventilatory acclimatization (evidenced by plateauing of these responses) when the altitude ascended increases (Figure 21-7). The rise in ventilation develops progressively over several days following arrival at altitude, even though hypoxemia—a ventilatory stimulus—progressively decreases, and hypocapnic alkalosis—usually considered a ventilatory inhibitor—increases. Concomitantly, the hypoxic ventilatory response increases.[4,24] Paradoxically therefore, both ventilation and the acute ventilatory response to hypoxia increase under conditions not usually considered conducive to such an increase.

Simultaneously defending both arterial Pa_{O_2} and acid–base balance presents a physiological dilemma for the lowlander on arrival at altitude. The dilemma is that a large increase in ventilation to raise Pa_{O_2} would cause severe alkalosis, whereas constraining ventilation at altitude to maintain normal sea-level Pa_{CO_2} and pH would result in severe hypoxemia. The dilemma arises because the ventilatory response to hypoxia occurs immediately, but the renal compensation to respiratory alkalosis requires several days. The body resolves the dilemma with a compromise where the initial increase in ventilation is incomplete on arrival at altitude, thus the acid–base derangement is minimal. The passage

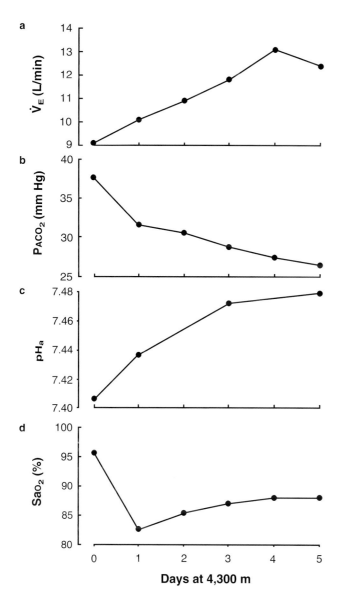

Fig. 21-6. Ventilatory acclimatization at altitude is characterized by time-dependent changes in ventilation. The four panels in this figure show (**a**) ventilation ($\dot{V}_E$), (**b**) the partial pressure of alveolar carbon dioxide (Pa_{CO_2}), (**c**) arterial pH (pHa), and (**d**) oxygen saturation of arterial blood (Sa_{O_2}) measured in 11 normal men at their residence altitude of 1,600 m and on days 1 through 5 after arriving at 4,300 m. Adapted with permission from Huang SY, Alexander JK, Grover RF, et al. Hypocapnia and sustained hypoxia blunt ventilation on arrival at high altitude. *J Appl Physiol.* 1984;56:603.

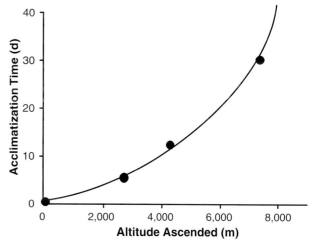

Fig. 21-7. The time required for ventilatory acclimatization varies with elevation ascended above residence altitude. The curve was drawn from three points reflecting altitude gains of 2,700 m (Denver to Pikes Peak[1]), 4,300 m (sea level to Pikes Peak[2]), and 7,380 m (sea level to simulated altitude[3]). The time indicated for ventilatory acclimatization to an ascent of 8,100 m (30 d) should be considered hypothetical because the data at this point were derived from a progressively staged ascent (as opposed to a continuous ascent as in the other data points), and a continous ascent to that elevation is not physiologically tolerable.

Data sources: (1) Huang SY, Alexander JK, Grover RF, et al. Hypocapnia and sustained hypoxia blunt ventilation on arrival at high altitude. *J Appl Physiol.* 1984;56:602–606. (2) Green HJ, Sutton JR, Wolfel EE, Reeves JT, Butterfield GE, Brooks GA. Altitude acclimatization and energy metabolic adaptations in skeletal muscle during exercise. *J Appl Physiol.* 1992;73:2701–2708. (3) Reeves JT, Groves, BM, Sutton R, et al. Adaptations to hypoxia: Lessons from Operation Everest II. In: Simmons DH, ed. *Current Pulmonology.* St Louis, Mo: Mosby–Year Book; 1991: 23–50.

of time for development of the large increase in ventilation that is characteristic of full acclimatization provides time for renal compensation by bicarbonate excretion to limit alkalosis. Although other factors may play a role, the principal mechanisms mediating this ventilatory acclimatization involve the central chemoreceptors (pH receptors in the medulla) and the peripheral chemoreceptors (P_{O_2} receptors in the carotid body).

Central (Medullary) Chemoreceptor Mechanisms

Ventilation is sensitive to small changes in medullary pH, increasing with increased concentration of hydrogen ions [H^+], and decreasing with decreased [H^+]. An early view considered that ventilatory acclimatization reflected a progressive withdrawal of the inhibitory effects exerted by the central chemoreceptor in response to hypocapnic alkalosis. As acclimatization proceeds, the concentration of bicarbonate [HCO_3^-] in the blood and cerebral spinal fluid falls due to renal compensation concomitant with the decline in P_{CO_2}, thus limiting the fall in [H^+]. In addition, hypoxia may increase metabolic production of lactate in the brain, which could increase [H^+] concentration near the medullary chemoreceptor. Either mechanism would tend to restore normal pH in or near the medullary chemoreceptor, despite decreased arterial P_{CO_2}. The ventilatory response to carbon dioxide is shifted to lower P_{CO_2} values, and the slope of the response becomes somewhat steeper. While this early view implicating the central chemoreceptor in the acclimatization process is attractive and may be correct, there is little direct evidence to support it.[12,25]

Peripheral (Carotid) Chemoreceptor Mechanisms

An alternative view attributes ventilatory acclimatization to an increase in hypoxic sensitivity of the carotid (ie, peripheral) chemoreceptor. Studies with animals show neural activity from the carotid body progressively increasing over time at altitude.[26] In goats, acclimatization occurs within hours when the hypoxia is limited to the carotid bodies, but does not occur when the hypoxia is limited to the central nervous system.[9] Further, acclimatization occurs with carotid body hypoxia whether or not there is accompanying hypocapnia.[12,25] The studies have suggested that acclimatization occurs within the carotid body, possibly independent of the changes within the central nervous system.

Experiments involving human subjects appear to confirm the conclusions from those with animals.

In one study, maintaining normocapnia reportedly prevented ventilatory acclimatization in humans who were exposed for 100 hours to hypobaric hypoxia[27]; however, these experiments appeared flawed[4,9,25] in that there was poor control of carbon dioxide, particularly during the first 24 hours of altitude exposure, during which time only one measurement was made. In more-recent and better-controlled human studies, ventilation and the ventilatory response to acute hypoxia were observed to increase progressively during the first 8 hours of hypoxia—even though P_{CO_2} was tightly maintained at sea-level values.[4,24] These results indicate that in man, as in the goat, ventilatory acclimatization to hypoxia can develop in the absence of hypocapnia and, therefore, is not merely a matter of overcoming central hypocapnic alkalosis. Still, ventilation appears to rise more rapidly during hypoxia with normocapnia than with hypocapnia,[4,27] so the possibility of some role for the central chemoreceptor in the process of ventilatory acclimatization cannot be entirely ruled out.[4,24] Nevertheless, the weight of current evidence suggests that acclimatization results primarily from a progressive effect of hypoxia on the carotid body.

Acclimatization to Altitude: Rest

The reduction in P_{aCO_2} and the increase in P_{AO_2} with ventilatory acclimatization at altitude becomes more pronounced with increasing altitude (Figure 21-8). For ethical reasons, unacclimatized subjects are not studied at altitudes above approximately 4,500 m. In unacclimatized subjects, P_{aCO_2} values observed at 4,300 to 4,500 m were approximately 10 mm Hg higher than in acclimatized subjects at the same altitudes. The higher P_{aCO_2} values maintained in the unacclimatized subjects dictate lower P_{AO_2} values than in acclimatized subjects, thus limiting the altitude to which the unacclimatized are able to ascend. Inspection of Figure 21-8b indicates that the unacclimatized subjects at 4,300 to 4,500 m had P_{AO_2} values similar to the values in acclimatized subjects above 7,000 m.

The increasing importance of ventilatory acclimatization with increasing altitude was first noted by Fitzgerald,[28] and later by Rahn and Otis,[29] who illustrated this relationship by plotting their observations on a $P_{aCO_2} - P_{AO_2}$ diagram. This classical representation of the effects of ventilatory acclimatization is depicted in Figure 21-9, in which the early observations by Rahn and Otis[29] are displayed along with more-recent data that were obtained during the American Medical Research Expedition to Everest (AMREE)[1]

Fig. 21-8. The importance of ventilatory acclimatization becomes greater with increasing altitude. This is demonstrated by extrapolating the relationship between (**a**) the partial pressure of alveolar carbon dioxide (P_{ACO_2}) and (**b**) the partial pressure of alveolar oxygen (P_{AO_2}) in subjects unacclimatized to the high elevations (open circles, dotted lines[1-5]) and then comparing the extrapolated values with those observed in acclimatized subjects (closed circles, solid lines[6-12]).

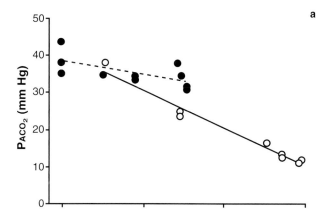

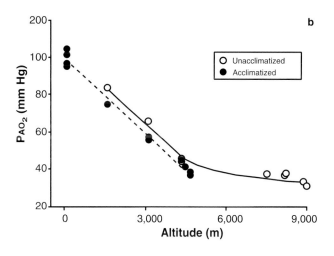

Data sources for a: (1) Sutton JR, Reeves JT, Wagner PD, et al. Operation Everest II: Oxygen transport during exercise at extreme simulated altitude. *J Appl Physiol.* 1988;64:1309–1321. (2) Wagner PD, Gale GE, Moon R.E, Torre-Bueno JR, Stolp BW, Saltzman HA. Pulmonary gas exchange in humans exercising at sea level and simulated altitude. *J Appl Physiol.* 1986;61:260–270. (3) Bender PR, Groves BM, McCullough RE, et al. Oxygen transport to exercising leg in chronic hypoxia. *J Appl Physiol.* 1988;65:2592–2597. (4) Bender PR, McCullough RE, McCullough RG, et al. Increased exercise SaO_2 independent of ventilatory acclimatization at 4300 m. *J Appl Physiol.* 1989;66:2733–2738. (5) Dempsey JA, Reddan WG, Birnbaum ML, et al. Effects of acute through life-long hypoxic exposure on exercise, pulmonary gas exchange. *Resp Physiol.* 1971;13:62–89.

Data sources for b: (6) Huang SY, Alexander JK, Grover RF, et al. Hypocapnia and sustained hypoxia blunt ventilation on arrival at high altitude. *J Appl Physiol.* 1984;56:602–606. (7) Malconian MK, Rock PB, Reeves JT, Cymerman A, Houston CS. Operation Everest II: Gas tensions in expired air and arterial blood at extreme altitude. *Aviat Space and Environ Med.* 1993;64:37–42. (8) Sutton JR, Reeves JT, Wagner PD, et al. Operation Everest II: Oxygen transport during exercise at extreme simulated altitude. *J Appl Physiol.* 1988;64:1309–1321. (9) West JB, Hackett PH, Maret KH, et al. Pulmonary gas exchange on the summit of Mount Everest. *J Appl Physiol.* 1983;55:678–687. (10) Bender PR, Groves BM, McCullough RE, et al. Oxygen transport to exercising leg in chronic hypoxia. *J Appl Physiol.* 1988;65:2592–2597. (11) Dempsey JA, Reddan WG, Birnbaum ML, et al. Effects of acute through life-long hypoxic exposure on exercise, pulmonary gas exchange. *Resp Physiol.* 1971;13:62–89. (12) Authors' unpublished observations.

and Operation Everest II,[30] which are shown for comparison. Despite being obtained at higher altitudes, the more-recent data show good agreement with the earlier findings from lower elevations.

The crucial importance of ventilatory acclimatization for ascent to extreme altitudes is demonstrated in Figure 21-9. Without an increase in ventilation at altitude, human beings breathing air might not be able to climb Mont Blanc, and certainly could not scale Mount Everest. At the summit of Mount Everest, the inspired P_{O_2} is only 43 mm Hg. If there were no increase in ventilation, then the P_{IO_2}-to-P_{AO_2} gradient would remain the same as at sea level, at 40 mm Hg. In that case, the P_{AO_2} would fall to 3 mm Hg, and life would not be possible. However, the increased ventilation with acclimatization enables the resting alveolar P_{AO_2} to be main-

tained at 33 to 35 mm Hg on the summit of Mount Everest, only 8 to 10 mm Hg less than that in the inspired air, values that are compatible with life.[30] Thus the ventilation-mediated reduction in P_{ACO_2} reduces the P_{O_2} gradient from the inspired to the alveolar air, resulting in an alveolar oxygen concentration higher than would otherwise be possible.

Acclimatization to Altitude: Exercise

Exercise and hypoxia act synergistically to increase ventilation.[31] The synergism may be seen by comparing ventilatory changes during progressive hypoxia at rest (ie, the standard hypoxic ventilatory response) with the analogous ventilatory response to progressive hypoxia measured in exercising subjects. At rest, the increase in ventilation

Fig. 21-9. The relationship between the partial pressure of alveolar carbon dioxide (P_{ACO_2}) and oxygen (P_{AO_2}) shifts with ventilatory acclimatization, as indicated by the diagram, which is drawn from data from unacclimatized subjects[1–5] (open symbols) and acclimatized subjects[6–12] (closed symbols). Also shown (solid line) for comparison is the curve redrawn from older data reported by Rahn and Otis.[13]

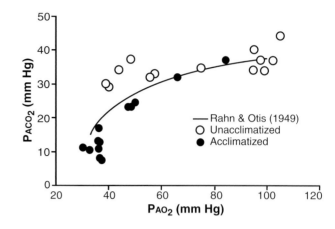

Data sources for unacclimatized subjects: (1) Sutton JR, Reeves JT, Wagner PD, et al. Operation Everest II: Oxygen transport during exercise at extreme simulated altitude. *J Appl Physiol.* 1988;64:1309–1321. (2) Wagner PD, Gale GE, Moon R.E, Torre-Bueno JR, Stolp BW, Saltzman HA. Pulmonary gas exchange in humans exercising at sea level and simulated altitude. *J Appl Physiol.* 1986;61:260–270. (3) Bender PR, Groves BM, McCullough RE, et al. Oxygen transport to exercising leg in chronic hypoxia. *J Appl Physiol.* 1988;65:2592–2597. (4) Bender RR, McCullough RE, McCullough RG, et al. Increased exercise Sa_{O_2} independent of ventilatory acclimatization at 4300 m. *J Appl Physiol.* 1989;66:2733–2738. (5) Torre-Bueno JR, Wagner PD, Saltzman HA, Gale GE, Moon RE. Diffusion limitation in normal humans during exercise at sea level and simulated altitude. *J Appl Physiol.* 1985;58:989–995.

Data sources for acclimatized subjects: (6) Huang SY, Alexander JK, Grover RF, et al. Hypocapnia and sustained hypoxia blunt ventilation on arrival at high altitude. *J Appl Physiol.* 1984;56:602–606. (7) Malconian MK, Rock PB, Reeves JT, Cymerman A, Houston CS. Operation Everest II: Gas tensions in expired air and arterial blood at extreme altitude. *Aviat Space and Environ Med.* 1993;64:37–42. (8) Sutton JR, Reeves JT, Wagner PD, et al. Operation Everest II: Oxygen transport during exercise at extreme simulated altitude. *J Appl Physiol.* 1988;64:1309–1321. (9) West JB, Hackett PH, Maret KH, et al. Pulmonary gas exchange on the summit of Mount Everest. *J Appl Physiol.* 1983;55:678–687. (10) Bender PR, Groves BM, McCullough RE, et al. Oxygen transport to exercising leg in chronic hypoxia. *J Appl Physiol.* 1988;65:2592–2597. (11) Dempsey JA, Reddan WG, Birnbaum ML, et al. Effects of acute through life-long hypoxic exposure on exercise, pulmonary gas exchange. *Resp Physiol.* 1971;13:62–89. (12) Authors' unpublished observations
Data source for comparison curve: (13) Rahn H, Otis AB. Man's respiratory response during and after acclimatization to high altitude. *Am J Physiol.* 1949;157:445–462.

with a falling P_{O_2} is curvilinear, being greater the more severe the hypoxia (Figure 21-10). During exercise, however, the whole curve is shifted to higher values of ventilation for any value of P_{O_2}. The shift to higher ventilation values is more pronounced at low than at high P_{O_2}, and the hypoxic ventilatory response curves at low P_{O_2} values become very much steeper during exercise than at rest. The synergistic effects of exercise and hypoxia on ventilation, which are more than a simple additive effect, are likely to be of great importance at altitude but not at sea level, where, in normal persons, other mechanisms of ventilatory control predominate.[32] The locus of the synergism remains unclear, but exercise may in some way increase the "gain" of the carotid chemoreceptor. For example, as depicted in Figure 21-10a, during exercise, ventilation increases in response to even small decrements in P_{O_2} within what is generally considered the normoxic range. Thus, while the hypoxic ventilatory response curve appears relatively flat in the range of 100 mm Hg in resting subjects, a pronounced slope is apparent in this range in exercising subjects. Figure 21-10b shows that a similar exercise-associated in-

crease in chemoreceptor gain is apparent in the ventilatory response to increasing P_{CO_2}.

At issue is the application of these effects on the exercise ventilation of persons ascending to and remaining at high altitude. The report of Dempsey and colleagues[33] provides insight regarding the time course and magnitude for acclimatization of exercise ventilation during sojourns at high altitude. In that study,[33] ventilation of normal sea-level residents was measured both at rest and during exercise at sea level, before and after they were switched from breathing normoxic gas to a P_{IO_2} of 100 mm Hg, simulating ambient air at Leadville, Colorado (3,100 m). Ventilation was measured again during rest and exercise and while breathing ambient air on days 4, 21, and 45 of residence at Leadville. Figure 21-10c shows that, as panel (a) predicts, resting ventilation remained little changed (8.6–8.7 L/min) with acute hypoxia, even though P_{AO_2} in these subjects fell to 56 mm Hg. In contrast, Figure 21-10d shows that ventilation during exercise increased dramatically when the breathing mixture was acutely switched from normoxic to a P_{IO_2} of 100 mm Hg, even though P_{AO_2} fell similarly (to 55 mm Hg)

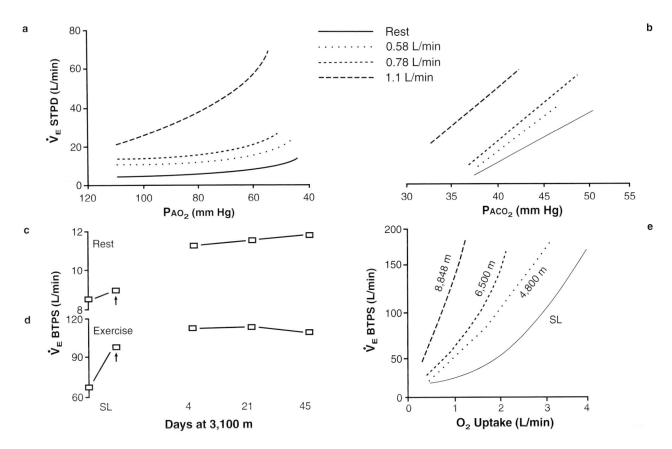

Fig. 21-10. The effect of exercise on ventilation is synergistic with those of hypoxia and hypercapnia. (**a**) Ventilation at standard temperature, pressure, and dry ($P_{H_2O} = 0$) ($\dot{V}_E$ STPD), is measured during acute progressive hypoxia in subjects resting (solid line) or exercising at three different intensities (broken lines) on a supine cycle ergometer. As indicated, increasing metabolism results in increasing ventilation at all partial pressures of alveolar oxygen (P_{AO_2}), but the increments in ventilation with increasing metabolism are greatest at the lowest P_{AO_2}. (**b**) A similar synergism on ventilation of the effects of increasing metabolism is seen with increasing partial pressure of alveolar carbon dioxide (P_{ACO_2}).

The duration of exposure to altitude affects the ventilatory response to exercise. (**c**) Resting ventilation and (**d**) exercise ($\dot{V}_{O_2}$ = 2.29 L/min) ventilation at body temperature, pressure, and saturated ($\dot{V}_E$ BTPS) are shown in subjects at sea level breathing normoxic air and hypoxic air (indicated by the arrow) simulating 3,100 m, and breathing ambient air at Leadville, Colorado (3,100 m), on days 4, 21, and 45. The stimulating effect of acute hypoxia on ventilation at sea level is more pronounced during exercise (seen in **d**) than at rest (seen in **c**), whereas the effect of ventilatory acclimatization appears more pronounced when measured during rest than during exercise. The relation between oxygen uptake ($\dot{V}_{O_2}$) and ventilatory response ($\dot{V}_E$ BTPS) at different altitudes is shown in (**e**). As elevation increases, so does the increment in ventilation for a given $\dot{V}_{O_2}$, but ventilation during maximal effort is only slightly increased at altitude.

Graphs a and b: Adapted with permission from Weil JV, Bryne-Quinn E, Sodal IE, Kline JS, McCullough RE, Filley GF. Augmentation of chemosensitivity during mild exercise in normal man. *J Appl Physiol*. 1972;33:813–819. Graphs c and d: Adapted with permission from Dempsey JA, Forster HV, Birnbaum ML, et al. Control of exercise hyperpnea under varying durations of exposure to moderate hypoxia. *Respir Physiol*. 1972;16:213–231. Graph e: Adapted with permission from Sutton JR, Reeves JT, Wagner PD, et al. Operation Everest II: Oxygen transport during exercise at extreme simulated altitude. *J Appl Physiol*. 1988;64:1309–1321.

during hypoxic exercise and during hypoxic rest. The exercise increased $\dot{V}_{O_2}$ 8-fold above the resting rate, to 2.3 L/min. Ventilation during normoxic exercise was 70 L/min, also 8-fold higher than the resting level; however, during hypoxic exercise, ventilation was almost 12-fold greater than the resting level. After 4 days' residence at Leadville, the effects of ventilatory acclimatization increased resting ventilation by 38% (to 3.7 L/min), whereas exercise ventilation increased only an additional 9% (6 L/min). There were no further changes in resting or exercise ventilation over the remainder of the 45-day stay at Leadville, indicating that, at least for altitudes around 3,100 m, ventilatory acclimatization was complete in 4 days.

Why ventilatory acclimatization appears to have a lesser effect on exercise ventilation than on resting ventilation remains unclear, because mechanisms linking ventilation to metabolism are not fully understood. One possibility is that during exercise when the metabolic rate is high, chemoreceptor sensitivity is augmented so that stimulation of ventilation is very near the maximal levels in response acute hypoxia, with little further potential increase possible following acclimatization. Further, during rest, ventilation rates are low and respiratory muscle fatigue would not be expected to develop or limit ventilatory increases with acclimatization; but during exercise at high altitude, high ventilation rates may well lead to respiratory muscle fatigue, precluding manifestation of ventilatory acclimatization during exercise. Another potential modulating mechanism involves (*a*) the accumulation of metabolic acid (primarily lactic) during exercise and (*b*) the buffering capacity of blood plasma (ie, plasma [HCO_3^-]), both of which change with acute hypoxic exposure and altitude acclimatization. Thus during ventilatory acclimatization, ventilatory stimulation due to changes in blood pH and acid concentration during exercise will be varying. Clearly, mechanisms regulating exercise ventilation during ventilatory acclimatization require further study.

Therefore, subjects acclimatized to high altitude have higher ventilations for a given $\dot{V}O_2$ at altitude than sea level, although maximal ventilation is similar for all altitudes. Further, as the elevation increases, so does the increment in ventilation for a given $\dot{V}O_2$, as depicted in Figure 21-10e. This increase in exercise ventilation at high altitude should be viewed in perspective, however. For many years it has been recognized that when ventilation is expressed under standard (STPD) rather than body (BTPS) conditions, the ventilation during rest and exercise at different intensities is relatively independent of altitude.[34] This suggests that for a given $\dot{V}O_2$, the same number of oxygen molecules is respired at all altitudes, including sea level. The respiratory system seems to function in a remarkably well-regulated manner, regardless of the individual's elevation, acclimatization status, or severity of effort, such that ventilation brings to the lung approximately $1.7 \cdot 10^{23}$ molecules of oxygen for each liter of oxygen consumed.[3]

Blood Acid–Base Balance Following Ventilatory Acclimatization

The bicarbonate buffer system is the body's most important regulator of body fluid pH because of the

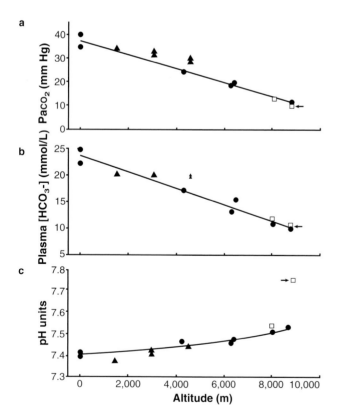

Fig. 21-11. The bicarbonate buffer system minimizes pH changes in persons ascending to high altitudes. (**a**) The closed circles indicate resting partial pressure of arterial carbon dioxide (PaCO_2), (**b**) plasma bicarbonate concentration ([HCO_3^-]), and (**c**) arterial pH (pHa) of acclimatized subjects during a simulated ascent to the summit of Mount Everest.[1] The open squares indicate values reported[2] from an actual climb of Mount Everest, where pHa and [HCO_3^-] at the summit were estimated from alveolar air samples collected at the summit (arrow), and from a venous blood sample taken the next day at a lower altitude. The closed triangles indicate measurements from arterial blood samples obtained during acute altitude exposure.[3,4]

Data sources: (1) Sutton JR, Reeves JT, Wagner PD, et al. Operation Everest II: Oxygen transport during exercise at extreme simulated altitude. *J Appl Physiol.* 1988;64:1309–1321. (2) Sorensen SC, Severinghaus JW. Irreversible respiratory insensitvity to acute hypoxia in man born at high altitude. *J Appl Physiol.* 1968;25:217–220. (3) Gale GE, Torre-Bueno JR, Moon RE, Saltzman HA, Wagner PD. Ventilation perfusion inequality in normal humans during exercise at sea level and simulated altitude. *J Appl Physiol.* 1985;58:978–988. (4) Wagner PD, Gale GE, Moon R.E, Torre-Bueno JR, Stolp BW, Saltzman HA. Pulmonary gas exchange in humans exercising at sea level and simulated altitude. *J Appl Physiol.* 1986;61:260–270.

large body stores of bicarbonate and the link between ventilation and $P_{a_{CO_2}}$. Changes in blood pH, $P_{a_{CO_2}}$, and bicarbonate concentration $[HCO_3^-]$ influence each other, as described by Equation 11, also known as the Henderson-Hasslebach Equation:

$$(11) \quad pH = pK + \log ([HCO_3^-] \div 0.03 \bullet P_{CO_2})$$

where *$[HCO_3^-]$* represents plasma bicarbonate concentration (in mmol/L), P_{CO_2} is expressed in mm Hg, and *pK* represents the equilibrium constant for the formation of carbonic acid from CO_2 and H_2O, which is about 6.1 at body temperature. The equation shows that if a fall in $P_{a_{CO_2}}$ is not accompanied by an offsetting fall in plasma $[HCO_3^-]$, then blood pH will rise. The decline in $P_{a_{CO_2}}$ that occurs with ventilatory acclimatization during ascent to moderate elevations (< 5,000 m) is accompanied by a fall in plasma $[HCO_3^-]$, which maintains higher blood pH values in acclimatized[2,35] compared with unacclimatized[36,37] subjects (Figure 21-11). Over time, HCO_3^- is eliminated from the body in the urine; however, the body stores of HCO_3^- are quite large. For example, a 70-kg person living at sea level with plasma $[HCO_3^-]$ of 25 mEq/L, has approximately 90 mEq $[HCO_3^-]$ in the blood, 260 mEq in the interstitial fluid, and 700 mEq in the intracellular fluid. Elimination of approximately 400 mEq of HCO_3^- to allow blood concentration to fall to 15 mEq/L, the value normally seen after acclimatization at 4,300 m, requires 10 to 14 days.

In well-acclimatized subjects, the $P_{a_{CO_2}}$ and plasma $[HCO_3^-]$ continue to decrease with ascent to higher altitudes, but not sufficiently to prevent a rise in pH. In fact, findings reported from AMREE suggest that pH may rise extraordinarily high in persons ascending to the summit of Mount Everest.[2] During AMREE, a pH of 7.78 was calculated indirectly from $P_{a_{CO_2}}$, which was determined by measuring (*a*) P_{CO_2} in a subject's alveolar air sample, obtained shortly after he reached the summit (8,848 m), and (*b*) plasma $[HCO_3^-]$, which was determined from a blood sample obtained at a lower altitude the following day.[38] In contrast, direct measurements of resting arterial pH in subjects participating in the Operation Everest II altitude chamber study[35] averaged 7.56 at the barometric pressure equivalent of the summit of Mount Everest (P_B = 253 mm Hg). The extreme exertion required to actually reach the summit of Everest, the nonsimultaneous sampling of blood and alveolar air, and the substantially lower pH values in Operation Everest II subjects at the simulated summit raise questions about the validity of extreme alkalotic arterial pH estimated from the

AMREE measurements. Figure 21-11 shows that the calculated pH values reported from AMREE at the slightly lower elevation of 8,050 m, where the blood and alveolar air were sampled at the same altitude and time, fell close to the arterial pH values measured directly at the equivalent pressure during the Operation Everest II study. However, a chamber study does not reproduce all the conditions of a climb, so the issue of how high arterial pH can rise at high altitude remains open, pending direct measurements of arterial pH in subjects actually ascending Everest.

Exercise alters the acid–base balance. The interactions between (*a*) effects of altitude and exercise on acid–base balance and (*b*) the three variables of interest ($[HCO_3^-]$, pH, and P_{CO_2}) may be examined in Figure 21-12. At sea level, release of fixed acids (primarily lactic acid) during exercise of increasing

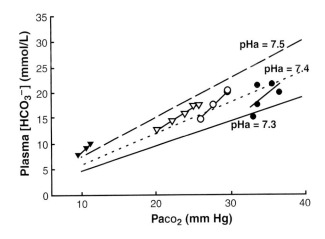

Fig. 21-12. Acute exposure to high altitude and altitude acclimatization affect the components of the Henderson-Hasslebach Equation such that acid–base balance during exercise is altered. At sea level (closed circles), the partial pressure of arterial carbon dioxide ($P_{a_{CO_2}}$), plasma bicarbonate concentration ($[HCO_3^-]$) and arterial ph (pHa) progressively decrease from resting levels (on the right of the graph) as intensity increases to maximal (toward the left). The decrease also occurs at high altitude, but the relationship among $P_{a_{CO_2}}$, plasma $[HCO_3^-]$, and pHa is shifted with acute (unacclimatized at 4,570 m, open circles) and chronic (acclimatized at 4,500 m, open triangles) exposure to altitude, and at the pressure equivalent of the summit of Mount Everest (closed triangles).
Data sources: (1) Sutton JR, Reeves JT, Wagner PD, et al. Operation Everest II: Oxygen transport during exercise at extreme simulated altitude. *J Appl Physiol.* 1988;64:1309–1321. (2) Wagner PD, Gale GE, Moon R.E, Torre-Bueno JR, Stolp BW, Saltzman HA. Pulmonary gas exchange in humans exercising at sea level and simulated altitude. *J Appl Physiol.* 1986;61:260–270.

intensity up to maximal effort causes pH to fall progressively below the resting value with an accompanying slight decrease in P_{aCO_2} and plasma $[HCO_3^-]$. At altitude, the release of fixed acids during exercise also results in acidosis. However, the changes in pH during exercise at altitude are modulated by the respiratory hypocapnic alkalosis, lactate production and disposal, and the buffering capacity of the blood, all of which begin changing on arrival at high altitude. With acute altitude exposure, the exercise-related metabolic acidosis is superimposed over the initial altitude-related respiratory alkalosis that slightly elevates resting pH. For acclimatized subjects at altitude, the hypocapnic alkalosis is fully developed, as evidenced by the more marked fall in resting P_{aCO_2} and plasma $[HCO_3^-]$, and the rise in resting pH. As at sea level, pH falls with progressively increasing exercise intensity up to maximal, accompanied by slight decreases in P_{CO_2} and $[HCO_3^-]$. The important point is that the lactic acid concentration in arterial blood correlates closely with developing acidosis during progressively increasing exercise intensity to maximal both at sea level and at high altitude (Figure 21-13).

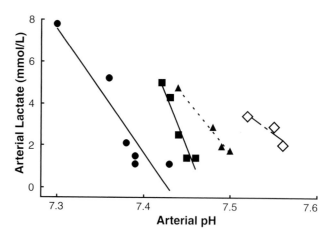

Fig. 21-13. Changes in arterial lactate concentration and arterial pH are closely related during progressive intensity exercise from rest to maximal, both at sea level and at high altitudes, even in acclimatized lowlanders exercising at extreme altitudes, when lactate concentrations do not increase much. The circles, squares, triangles, and diamonds represent measurements that were made at sea level and at simulated altitudes of 4,900, 6,100, and 7,620 m. Data source: Sutton JR, Reeves JT, Wagner PD, et al. Operation Everest II: Oxygen transport during exercise at extreme simulated altitude. *J Appl Physiol.* 1988;64:Tables 2–5.

Summary of Ventilation at High Altitude

The ventilatory changes experienced by lowlanders who ascend to high altitudes and remain can be summarized as follows. As barometric pressure falls, ventilation (the first step in the oxygen cascade) increases, raising alveolar oxygen tension and limiting the fall in the P_{O_2} pressure gradient from the inspired air to the alveolus. The increased ventilation at altitude is driven primarily by the increased carotid chemoreceptor activity. The increased ventilation also increases the removal of carbon dioxide from the blood. The resulting hypocapnic alkalosis, which accompanies the in-

creased ventilation, may be partially responsible for delaying the full increase in ventilation (ie, ventilatory acclimatization), which can require a week or more to develop at moderately high altitudes. Ventilation ($\dot{V}_E$ BTPS) during maximal exercise appears to be similar at all altitudes, but the number of oxygen molecules that can be transported $\dot{V}_E$ STPD decreases with altitude. Given the close relationship of the number of oxygen molecules ventilated and those taken up, then at low barometric pressure, ventilation is particularly important in limiting the fall in maximum exercise capacity.

ALVEOLAR–ARTERIAL OXYGEN PRESSURE GRADIENT

The P_{O_2} gradient from alveolus (P_{AO_2}) to artery (P_{aO_2}) has two components: (1) venous admixture of arterial blood and (2) the oxygen diffusion gradient from alveolus to the lung capillary blood. Although under normal circumstances, systemic arterial P_{O_2} is only slightly less than the P_{O_2} of blood leaving a pulmonary capillary, certain physiological states create a rapid capillary transfer that may not allow for anywhere near normal diffusion time. This effect becomes increasingly apparent during exercise at altitude and can be quantitated by measuring the difference between alveolar P_{O_2} and systemic artery P_{O_2} ($P_{AO_2} – P_{aO_2}$), by convention this being

taken as pressure that drives diffusion. Systemic P_{aO_2}, which can easily be measured, is taken as a surrogate for P_{O_2} at the end of a capillary, which cannot be measured. One characteristic of the $P_{AO_2} – P_{aO_2}$ shown in Figure 21-14 is that it increases with increasing oxygen uptake at all altitudes. However, the relative contribution to the $P_{AO_2} – P_{aO_2}$ by venous admixture versus diffusion changes with increasing altitude.

The ODC is not, strictly speaking, a component of the $P_{AO_2} – P_{aO_2}$ gradient. However, the ODC defines the relationship between changes in P_{aO_2}, S_{aO_2}, and C_{aO_2}. The ODC is determined by the affinity of hemoglobin for oxygen, which varies with Pa_{O_2} as shown in Figure 21-15. The Ca_{O_2} is determined by Equation 12:

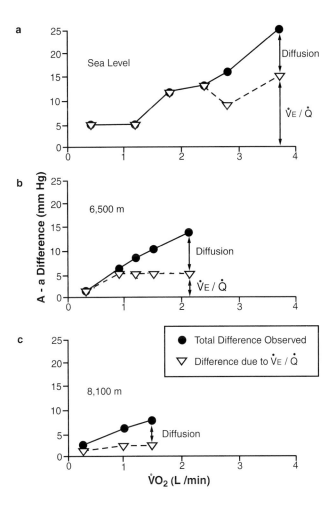

(12) $$Ca_{O_2} = Sa_{O_2} \bullet [Hb] \bullet A$$

where Ca_{O_2} represents arterial oxygen content, Sa_{O_2} represents the oxygen saturation of arterial blood, *[Hb]* represents arterial hemoglobin concentration, and the constant *A* defines the maximal amount of oxygen that can bind to a unit of hemoglobin (the value of which varies among individuals from 1.34 to 1.36 mL of oxygen per gram of hemoglobin). The shape of the ODC allows Sa_{O_2} and Ca_{O_2} to fall minimally with the changes in Pa_{O_2} that occur during the initial ascent from sea level to altitudes around 1,000 m. The changes in Pa_{O_2} that occur when ascending higher, however, occur on the steeper portion of the ODC, and thus cause a disproportionately greater decline in Sa_{O_2} and Ca_{O_2}. Thus, as we discuss next, the shape of the ODC causes more pronounced pulmonary diffusion limitations and ventilation–perfusion inequities during exercise at altitude than at sea level.

Pulmonary Venous Admixture

Venous admixture (the mixing of non-reoxygenated venous blood with oxygenated blood) reduces the Ca_{O_2} and increases the $Pa_{O_2} - Pa_{O_2}$ by two primary mechanisms. First, oxygen-depleted blood draining

Fig. 21-14. The alveolar – arterial difference in the partial pressure of oxygen ($Pa_{O_2} - Pa_{O_2}$) widens with increasing exercise intensity and oxygen consumption per unit time ($\dot{V}_{O_2}$), both at (**a**) sea level and (**b** and **c**) high altitude (6,100 m and 8,100 m, respectively). The $Pa_{O_2} - Pa_{O_2}$ can be partitioned into components of diffusion and venous admixture. Venous admixture results from shunting and ventilation–perfusion mismatch ($\dot{V}_E/\dot{Q}$), with the latter predominating during exercise or at high altitude. When the $\dot{V}_E/\dot{Q}$ component (open symbols) of the $Pa_{O_2} - Pa_{O_2}$ accounts for less than the total $Pa_{O_2} - Pa_{O_2}$ measured (closed symbols), the difference represents the diffusion component. As exercise intensity increases, the diffusion accounts for increasingly more of the total $Pa_{O_2} - Pa_{O_2}$. As elevation increases, the diffusion component becomes significant at lower exercise intensities than at sea level. Adapted with permission from Wagner PD, Sutton JR, Reeves JT, Cymerman A, Groves BM, Malconian MK. Operation Everest II: Pulmonary gas exchange during a simulated ascent of Mt Everest. *J Appl Physiol.* 1987;63:2354.

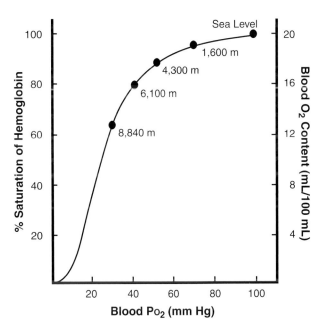

Fig. 21-15. The percentage of hemoglobin that is bound and combined with oxygen, and thus the amount of oxygen in the blood, is not linear over the physiological range of oxygen tension in the blood (blood P_{O_2}), as depicted in the classic oxygen–hemoglobin dissociation curve.

from the intrapulmonary bronchi veins into the pulmonary veins, a process referred to as *shunt*, mixes with the oxygenated blood draining the pulmonary capillaries. Second, blood flow and ventilation are not uniformly distributed over even the normal lung at sea level, nor is the distribution of flow perfectly matched to the distribution of ventilation. The ratio of the rates of ventilation and perfusion ($\dot{V}_E/\dot{Q}$) quantifies this inequality. Capillary blood perfusing poorly ventilated lung (ie, lung units having a low $\dot{V}_E/\dot{Q}$) is inadequately oxygenated, which lowers P_{aO_2} and contributes to the $P_{AO_2} - P_{aO_2}$ at all altitudes.

At sea level, bronchial venous flow is normally less than 1% of resting pulmonary capillary flow. Nevertheless, this small flow of poorly oxygenated blood entering the pulmonary veins measurably decreases the P_{O_2} before the blood reaches the systemic arteries and is the major component of the approximately 10-mm Hg $P_{AO_2} - P_{aO_2}$ gradient at sea level. This is because pulmonary capillary blood P_{O_2} is on the flat part of the ODC, where small reductions in arterial content correspond to relatively large changes in P_{O_2}. In contrast, the lung capillary P_{O_2} at high altitude is on the steep part of the ODC, so while shunt from intrapulmonary bronchi may reduce oxygen content similarly to the reduction at sea level, the corresponding reduction in P_{O_2} is smaller, and it contributes relatively less to the $P_{AO_2} - P_{aO_2}$.[37,39] Furthermore, during exercise, the increase in pulmonary capillary blood flow is much greater than the increase in shunt, so the relative contribution of shunt to the venous admixture component of the $P_{AO_2} - P_{aO_2}$ declines with exercise, both at sea level and at altitude.[37,39] Thus, shunt contributes to the $P_{AO_2} - P_{aO_2}$ during rest at sea level, but during exercise or at high altitude, the venous admixture component of the $P_{AO_2} - P_{aO_2}$ is predominately due to $\dot{V}_E/\dot{Q}$ mismatch.

It is possible to estimate the contribution of $\dot{V}_E/\dot{Q}$ mismatch to the $P_{AO_2} - P_{aO_2}$ using a complex method, the multiple inert gas elimination technique, which involves inhalation of a mixture of gases having different solubilities and measuring these gases in exhaled air and arterial blood.[40] The $\dot{V}_E/\dot{Q}$ mismatch and the resulting $P_{AO_2} - P_{aO_2}$ increase during exercise (see Figure 21-14). Even in normal healthy subjects at sea level, the contribution of low $\dot{V}_E/\dot{Q}$ areas to the $P_{AO_2} - P_{aO_2}$ increased with increasing exertion, and at high altitude, the low $\dot{V}_E/\dot{Q}$ areas still contribute to the $P_{AO_2} - P_{aO_2}$ with exercise. Note in Figure 21-14 that with increasing $\dot{V}_{O_2}$, the observed $P_{AO_2} - P_{aO_2}$ exceeds that which is accounted for by $\dot{V}_E/\dot{Q}$ mismatch, and that the exercise intensity $\dot{V}_{O_2}$ at which this becomes ap-

parent decreases with increasing altitude. The difference between the observed $P_{AO_2} - P_{aO_2}$ and that which can be accounted for by $\dot{V}_E/\dot{Q}$ mismatch is assumed to represent a component of the $P_{AO_2} - P_{aO_2}$ due to the diffusion limitation.[39]

Diffusing Capacity

Having reached the alveolus, the oxygen molecule must diffuse across the alveolar–capillary membrane and into the red blood cells in the pulmonary capillary blood. This diffusion occurs along the oxygen pressure gradient from alveolus to blood. Moving from upright to a supine posture, increasing ventilation, initiating exercise, and exposure to hypoxia all increase distension and recruitment of pulmonary microcirculation (arterioles, capillaries, and venules), increasing the lung surface area for gas exchange, as does an exercise-induced increased microvascular pressure. During maximal effort, lung diffusion capacity for oxygen is maximal ($D_{LO_2}max$). The $D_{LO_2}max$ is proportional to the maximal oxygen uptake ($\dot{V}_{O_2}max$) divided by the oxygen pressure gradient from alveolus (P_{AO_2}) to pulmonary capillary blood (Pc'_{O_2}), as shown in Equation 13:

$$(13) \quad D_{LO_2}max = k \cdot [\dot{V}_{O_2}max \div (P_{AO_2} - Pc'_{O_2})]$$

where the constant *k* represents the oxygen conductivity of the alveolar capillary and the red blood cell membrane. However, membrane thickness, membrane surface area, and reaction of oxygen in the red blood cell are unlikely to be changed by moving to high altitude. Therefore, during maximal exercise in health, microvascular surface area and diffusing membrane thickness are likely to be similar at sea level and at altitude.

In humans, Pc'_{O_2} cannot be measured directly. However, if we assume that during exercise at sea level and during rest and exercise at high altitude, the reduction in arterial content resulting from venous admixture causes but little fall in the P_{aO_2}, then the Pc'_{O_2} can be taken to be approximately equal to P_{aO_2} under those conditions. Therefore, subtracting the contribution of $\dot{V}_E/\dot{Q}$ from the total $P_{AO_2} - P_{aO_2}$ allows us to estimate the contribution of diffusion, as described above and shown in Figure 21-14. As altitude increases, the relative contributions of shunt and $\dot{V}_E/\dot{Q}$ to the $P_{AO_2} - P_{aO_2}$ decrease, while the contribution of diffusion increases. Further, Figure 21-14 shows that at sea level the diffusion limitation of the lung for oxygen transfer does not become apparent until oxygen uptakes exceeds 2.5 L/min, whereas at altitude,

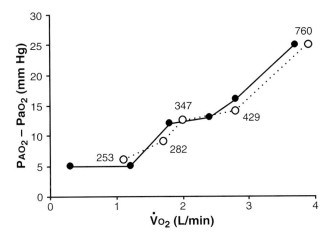

Fig. 21-16. The alveolar – arterial difference in partial pressure of oxygen (P$_{AO_2}$ – Pa$_{O_2}$) widens with increasing oxygen uptake (V̇$_{O_2}$) during exercise. The closed circles show the gradient at sea level during rest and at different incremental stages during progressive intensity exercise up to maximal oxygen uptake. The open circles represent the gradient measured during exercise at maximal oxygen uptake at each barometric pressure shown. Adapted with permission from Sutton JR, Reeves JT, Wagner PD, et al. Operation Everest II: Oxygen transport during exercise at extreme simulated altitude. *J Appl Physiol.* 1988;64:1317.

diffusion limitation becomes apparent at oxygen uptakes of less than 1 L/min.

At sea level, the P$_{AO_2}$ – Pa$_{O_2}$ during exercise widens as exercise intensity increases. Although the P$_{AO_2}$ – Pa$_{O_2}$ results from complex interactions among pulmonary shunting, V̇$_E$/Q̇ mismatch, and pulmonary diffusion (Figure 21-16), the size of the gradient increases in a nearly linear fashion, with increasing oxygen uptakes between 1 and 4 L/min. Even during maximal exercise, Pa$_{O_2}$ is maintained at 80 mm or higher in most normal healthy persons, because arterial oxygenation is occurring on the flat portion of the ODC. Elite, highly conditioned athletes might be an exception to this, in that their cardiovascular systems have the capacity to transport such large amounts of oxygen that the membrane diffusion capacity of the lung may be insufficient to allow arterial oxygen levels to be maintained

constant during maximal exercise, even at sea level.

At altitude, however, Pa$_{O_2}$ is reduced to the range where the limitations inherent in the diffusing capacity of lung membrane become significant relative to the total oxygen pressure gradient, and Pa$_{O_2}$ and saturation fall below resting levels during exercise. As depicted in Figure 21-14, the P$_{AO_2}$ – Pa$_{O_2}$ during maximal exercise at high altitude is largely the result of limitations in pulmonary diffusion. At the summit of Mount Everest, where the inspired P$_{O_2}$ is only 43 mm Hg, the resting P$_{AO_2}$ is severely hypoxic. Exercise, by increasing the oxygen uptake, also increases the alveolar-to-arterial P$_{O_2}$ gradient. Because the P$_{AO_2}$ is little changed, the P$_{O_2}$ must fall. Even at rest, the arterial oxygen saturation is on the steep part of the ODC (resting Sa$_{O_2}$ = 58%), and increasing oxygen uptake required for maximal exercise causes the arterial oxygen saturation to fall to approximately 50%.

The fall in arterial saturation, P$_{AO_2}$ – Pa$_{O_2}$, and the diffusion component of the P$_{AO_2}$ – Pa$_{O_2}$ during rest and near maximal exercise with increasing terrestrial elevation are shown in Figure 21-17a. The exercise saturations are less than those at rest largely because pulmonary diffusing capacity for oxygen is more limiting with increasing altitude.[39] As shown in Figure 21-16 and discussed above, the decrease in total P$_{AO_2}$ – Pa$_{O_2}$ with increasing altitude is linked to the decline in V̇$_{O_2}$max. However, the diffusion component of that difference during maximal exercise remains nearly unchanged (Figure 21-17b). As a result, the diffusion component becomes progressively more significant with increasing altitude (Figure 21-17c).

It is clear that the low environmental oxygen at altitude is associated with reduced Pa$_{O_2}$ at rest. With exercise, diffusion limitation inherent in the normal lung reduces Pa$_{O_2}$ even further. At modest altitudes, diffusion limitation is only apparent during heavy exercise and high oxygen uptake, but with increasing altitude and decreasing Pa$_{O_2}$, the diffusion limitation becomes apparent at progressively lower exercise intensities and oxygen uptakes. In the extreme circumstance, namely, at the summit of Mount Everest, diffusion limitation is apparent, with oxygen uptakes of less than 1 L/min.

SYSTEMIC OXYGEN TRANSPORT AT HIGH ALTITUDE

Unacclimatized Lowlanders on Arrival at High Altitude

The decline in Sa$_{O_2}$ and Ca$_{O_2}$ that lowlanders experience with ascent to high altitude necessitates

adjustments in systemic oxygen transport to maintain sufficient oxygen delivery to meet the metabolic needs of the body. Equation 14, the Fick Equation, defines the relationship between systemic oxygen transport and oxygen uptake:

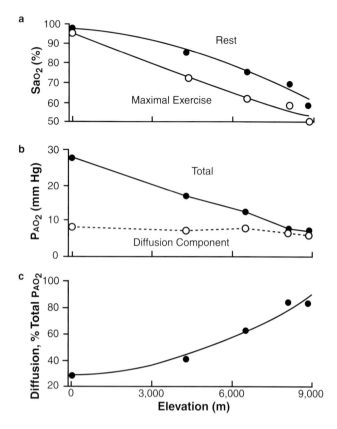

Fig. 21-17. The reduction in ambient and alveolar oxygen pressure with increasing altitude causes (**a**) the decrease in arterial oxgyen saturation (Sao$_2$) during rest (closed circles), and the development of pulmonary diffusing limitations causes the additional decrease during maximal exercise (open circles). (**b**) The total alveolar – arterial difference in partial pressure of oxygen (Pao$_2$ – Pao$_2$, closed circles) decreases with increasing altitude because maximal oxygen uptake declines, but the diffusion component (open circles) remains unchanged in magnitude. Thus, diffusion accounts for (**c**) an increasing proportion of the total Pao$_2$ – Pao$_2$ as altitude increases (closed circles).
Data source: Wagner PD, Sutton JR, Reeves JT, Cymerman A, Groves BM, Malconian MK. Operation Everest II: Pulmonary gas exchange during a simulated ascent of Mt Everest. *J Appl Physiol.* 1987;63:2348–2359.

(14) $\dot{V}o_2 = Qc \bullet (Cao_2 - C\bar{v}o_2),$

where $\dot{V}o_2$ represents oxygen uptake, Qc represents cardiac output, Cao_2 represents arterial oxygen content, and $C\bar{v}o_2$ represents mixed venous oxygen content. The steady state $\dot{V}o_2$ elicited during submaximal exercise at a given absolute exercise intensity or power output is the same at high altitude as at sea level.[41–44] The Fick Equation shows that to sustain a given $\dot{V}o_2$, the reduction in Cao$_2$ at

high altitude could be compensated for by a higher Qc, a lower $C\bar{v}o_2$, or both.

Increased Cardiac Output

Experimental observations indicate that both adjustments are invoked. Oxygen tensions in venous blood that drains contracting muscle fall lower during submaximal exercise at high altitude than at sea level—not low enough, however, to fully compensate for the decrease in Cao$_2$; thus, the arteriovenous oxygen difference narrows (Figure 21-18).[45] Many studies have confirmed that unacclimatized lowlanders exhibit a higher cardiac output for any given $\dot{V}o_2$ during steady state submaximal exercise at high altitude than at sea level.[43,46,47] This increased cardiac output is achieved by an increased heart rate, while stroke volume during exercise tends to be lower on arrival at altitude than at sea level.[43] However, maximal cardiac output remains unchanged from sea-level values in unacclimatized lowlanders, as does the $C\bar{v}o_2$ during maximal exercise.[43] Hence these physiological limits are achieved at lower absolute exercise intensities at high altitude than sea level, and $\dot{V}o_2$max is reduced.

Decrement in Maximal Oxygen Uptake

The decline in $\dot{V}o_2$max at high altitude varies. The primary factor that modulates the decline is the actual elevation ascended above sea level. Lowlanders

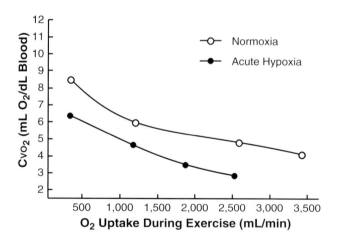

Fig. 21-18. During both rest (left of graph) and exercise (right of graph), venous oxygen content (Cvo$_2$) falls lower under hypoxic than normoxic conditions.
Data source: Bender PR, Groves BM, McCullough RE, et al. Oxygen transport to exercising leg in chronic hypoxia. *J Appl Physiol.* 1988;65:2592–2597.

experience no measurable decline in V̇o₂max until they ascend above about 900 to 1,000 m, and only a small decrement between 1,000 and 2,000 m above sea level.[48] Above 2,000 m elevation, the decrement averages about 10% for every 1,000 meters ascended.[49,50] Although the average decrement in V̇o₂max at any given altitude is predictable for a group of subjects, the decrement varies considerably between individuals.[51] For example, in a group of 51 male sea-level residents, the decrement in V̇o₂max at 4,300 m altitude compared with the decrement at sea level was normally distributed in a range from 9% to 54%, and averaged 27%.[51]

The physiological factors that account for the variability in the decrement in V̇o₂max experienced at a given altitude are not fully understood. Intraindividual variability in hypoxic ventilatory responsiveness, hemoglobin affinity for oxygen, and body fluid movements are a few factors that might play a role. However, one factor in particular, the individual's level of aerobic physical fitness, has received considerable attention.[50–53] As Fulco and Cymerman point out in Chapter 22, Physical Performance at Varying Terrestrial Altitudes, the decrement in V̇o₂max with ascent to high altitude is more pronounced in aerobically fit, compared with less fit, persons. In fact, variability in aerobic fitness may account for as much as one third of the variability in the altitude-induced decrement in V̇o₂max.[51] One explanation that has been postulated for this, although it is unproven, is that highly aerobically fit persons exhibit relative hypoventilation during maximal exercise,[54] and their maximal cardiac outputs, hence maximal pulmonary capillary blood flows, are higher and pulmonary capillary transit times shorter than in less fit persons.[55] Both factors could exaggerate pulmonary diffusion limitations and ventilation perfusion inequalities at high altitude in fit compared with less-fit persons.

Acclimatization Effects on Systemic Oxygen Transport

The initial physiological adjustments in the components of systemic oxygen transport (increased cardiac output, tachycardia, etc) elicited when lowlanders first ascend to high altitude occur at the expense of increases in cardiac work, myocardial oxygen uptake, and coronary blood flow.[56–58] These responses increase cardiovascular strain and probably contribute to the decreased endurance that most lowlanders experience when they arrive at high altitude. However, in lowlanders who remain at high altitude and acclimatize, the acute responses

are progressively replaced by physiological adjustments that alleviate the increased demand on the heart while still allowing systemic oxygen transport requirements of activity to be sustained.

Cardiac Output Declines

One of the more pronounced effects of altitude acclimatization at moderate altitudes is a reduction in cardiac output. The acclimatization-induced reduction in cardiac output is observable during rest[59–61] as well as during both submaximal[59,61] and maximal[41,59,62] exercise. Most studies indicate that this reduction in cardiac output is more pronounced than the initial increase observed on arrival at high altitude. Thus, for any given V̇o₂, cardiac output is not only lower after acclimatization than on arrival at altitude but it is also lower than it was at sea level before ascent (Figure 21-19). At altitudes between 3,000 and 5,000 m, this adjustment first becomes observable in as few as 2 days of acclimatization[61,62] and continues to develop over the following 8 to 10 days.[41,59,61,62] Staging (ie, gradual ascent with stops at intermediate altitudes) appears to blunt both the initial increase in cardiac output and the subsequent decline,[47] and persons who continue ascending to very extreme altitudes (> 6,000 m) do not appear to exhibit a decline in cardiac output below sea-level values.[63]

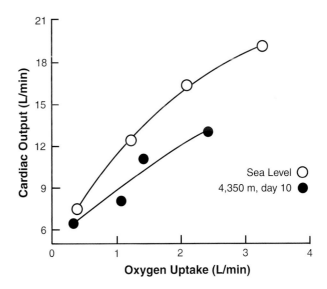

Fig. 21-19. Following altitude acclimatization (closed symbols), cardiac output during exercise is lower than it is at sea level (open symbols).
Data source: Vogel JA, Hartley LH, Cruz JC, Hogan RP. Cardiac output during exercise in sea-level residents at sea level and high altitude. *J Appl Physiol.* 1974;36:169–172.

The reduction in cardiac output with altitude acclimatization results primarily from reduced stroke volume and, to a lesser extent, alleviation of the exercise tachycardia exhibited on arrival at high altitude.[64] Stroke volume, both at rest and during submaximal and maximal exercise, clearly declines with altitude acclimatization, and the time course for this adjustment parallels the decline in cardiac output.[59,61,62] On the other hand, as a comprehensive review[64] details, some reports indicate no effect of acclimatization on heart rate responses, while others indicate that the initial altitude-induced tachycardia abates. Differences in altitude, exposure duration, ascent profile, and individual variability contribute to the disparate observations.[64] Acclimatization effects on heart rate may also vary with exercise intensity. Altitude-induced tachycardia has been reported[65] to be attenuated at high, near-maximal intensities, but not at low intensities.

Conceivably, a depression in myocardial contractility, decreased cardiac filling, or both could cause the decline in stroke volume. The possibility that a hypoxia-related decline in myocardial contractility and function contributed to the decline in stroke volume that was postulated earlier by some investigators[60,61] is not consistent with the most recent experimental observations. Lowlanders who are chronically exposed to very high altitudes exhibit no change in the cardiac filling pressure–stroke volume relationship,[63] and their ejection fraction increases despite reduced ventricular volumes[66] when breathing either hypoxic or normoxic air. Thus, a reduction in cardiac filling is probably the principal mechanism mediating the decrease in stroke volume with altitude acclimatization. The hematological and hemodynamic adjustments experienced as the lowlander acclimatizes to high altitude may act to limit cardiac filling.

Development of Hemoconcentration

The lowlanders' hematocrit and hemoglobin concentration increase during the first 7 to 14 days of altitude acclimatization, concomitant with the decline in stroke volume. The increases in the hematocrit and the hemoglobin concentration during the first 2 to 3 weeks at high altitude are sometimes mistakenly attributed to an increase in circulating red blood cells, but that response does not develop until later in the acclimatization process. The early rise in hematocrit and hemoglobin, in fact, results from a hemoconcentration in which plasma volume is lost[61,67–69] while erythrocyte volume remains unchanged[69]; thus blood volume decreases.[61,67–69] At moderate elevations (3,000–4,300 m), the magnitude of this effect is modest, with plasma volume losses reported averaging 250 to 500 mL[61,67,69]; but at higher altitudes the loss of plasma volume is more pronounced.[70] At face value, this hemoconcentration appears to be the mechanism responsible for the decline in stroke volume that is experienced as lowlanders acclimatize at altitude, because experimental manipulations that prevent the altitude-induced hemoconcentration also prevent the reduction in stroke volume.[71]

Exactly how hemoconcentration exerts this effect remains unresolved, but several mechanisms could be acting to limit cardiac output and stroke volume in acclimatized lowlanders. A reduction in blood volume might reduce stroke volume, according to the Frank-Starling curve, in which cardiac output or stroke volume can be plotted in relation to end diastolic volume. However, infusing 500 mL of dextran into two lowlanders acclimatized 10 days at 3,100 m expanded blood and plasma volume to preacclimatization levels without restoring stroke volume during exercise.[61] In contrast, when 450 mL of whole blood was removed from five lowlanders acclimatized at 4,300 m and replaced with Ringers lactate, hematocrit and viscosity returned to preacclimation levels without a change in blood volume, and stroke volume during exercise increased back to preacclimatization levels.[72] Horstman, Weiskopf, and Jackson suggested that the findings they reported were consistent with the development of a viscosity-related limitation to cardiac filling and stroke volume.[72] However, erythrocyte infusion (also known as blood doping) experiments at sea level demonstrate that hematocrit and viscosity increases that are comparable to changes that occur during acclimatization at moderate altitude do not produce a viscosity impairment of stroke volume and cardiac output.[73] The most plausible explanation for the changes in cardiac output and stroke volume during the first 2 weeks of altitude acclimatization is that the reduced Cao_2 and partial pressure of venous oxygen (Pvo_2) on arrival at high altitude cause a dilation of peripheral vasculature with concomitant elevation in cardiac output (metaboreflex), which is then reversed when the acclimatization-induced hemoconcentration raises Cao_2 and Pvo_2.

Arterial Oxygen Content Increases

Regardless of the precise mechanism for the reduction in stroke volume and cardiac output in lowlanders remaining at altitude, the lower cardiac output for a given oxygen uptake necessitates compensatory adjustments in systemic oxygen transport and delivery. The Fick Equation (see Equation 14 above) indicates that an increased tissue oxygen extraction must accompany the reduction in cardiac output at a given oxygen uptake. This has been experimentally demonstrated.[45,60,74] Figure 21-20 shows that during rest and submaximal exercise, the difference between arterial and venous oxygen contents, which narrowed with ascent to altitude, widens after about 10 days of acclimatization. Following acclimatization, the oxygen content of venous blood draining active muscle during exercise at altitude is the same[45] or only slightly lower[74,75] than it was before. Therefore, the key factor that enables systemic oxygen transport requirements to be achieved with lower cardiac output than before, for a given oxygen uptake after altitude acclimatization, is an increased oxygen extraction that is primarily due to an increased CaO_2.

After 7 to 10 days of acclimatization, lowlanders sojourning at high altitude exhibit higher CaO_2 during both rest and exercise. For example, Hannon and Vogel[76] observed that the average resting CaO_2 of six lowlanders sojourning at 4,300 m increased by 2.6 milliliters of oxygen per 100 milliliters of blood between the 2nd and 14th day of altitude acclimatization. Several physiological adjustments contribute to this increase in CaO_2 with acclimatization. As described before and illustrated in Figure 21-21, a hemoconcentration develops over this same time, increasing hematocrit and owing to a decrease in plasma volume, while erythrocyte volume remains unchanged.[61,69] This hemoconcentration increased hemoglobin concentration by 0.7 grams per 100 milliliters of blood, accounting for about 25% of the increase in CaO_2 over that same time. The remainder of the increase in CaO_2 observed in Hannon and Vogel's study[76] was attributable to an increase in SaO_2.

During the first week or so of acclimatization, lowlanders sojourning at high altitude experience an increase in SaO_2 measured during both rest and exercise. For example, in lowlanders ascending from sea level to the summit of Pikes Peak (4,300 m), resting SaO_2 generally falls to 78% to 80% on arrival, after which it rises, reaching about 84% after 3 to 4 days and 87% after 9 to 10 days.[16,77,78] It has been generally accepted that the increase in saturation reflects the effects of the increase in ventilation that develops progressively over the first few days after arriving at high altitude (ventilatory acclimatization). However, while resting SaO_2

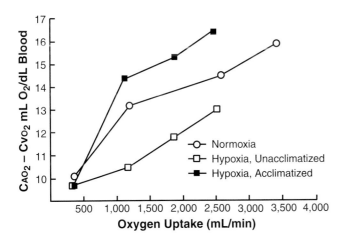

Fig. 21-20. For a given intensity of exercise and oxgyen uptake, extraction of oxgyen (the alveolar – venous oxygen contents, as measured in milliliters of oxygen per deciliters of blood, or $CaO_2 - CvO_2$) decreases on arrival at high altitude compared with at sea level, but with acclimatization extraction increases above sea level values.
Data source: Bender PR, Groves BM, McCullough RE, et al. Oxygen transport to exercising leg in chronic hypoxia. *J Appl Physiol*. 1988;65:2592–2597.

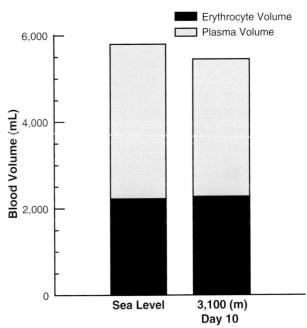

Fig. 21-21. During the first 2 weeks of high-altitude acclimatization, the mass of red blood cells does not change, but a modest decrease in the volume of plasma increases the hematocrit.
Data source: Alexander JK, Hartley LH, Modelski M, Grover RF. Reduction of stroke volume during exercise in man following ascent to 3,100 m altitude. *J Appl Physiol*. 1967;23:849–858.

reaches a plateau after about 8 days of acclimatization, SaO_2 maintained during exercise continues to rise between the 8th and 22nd day of acclimatization, despite the fact ventilation during exercise remains the same over this period.[77] Thus, the rise in SaO_2 that lowlanders experience as they acclimatize to high altitude is only partially explained by the effects of ventilatory acclimatization. A decreased pulmonary capillary transit time secondary to the decline in cardiac output with acclimatization (discussed above) also contributes to an increase in SaO_2 in the acclimatizing lowlander, along with other adjustments that may develop, such as a decreased pulmonary diffusion limitation (increased diffusing capacity), improved $\dot{V}E/\dot{Q}$, and, as will be discussed below, a left shift in the ODC.

While increased erythrocyte volume does not account for the initial rise in hematocrit, hemoglobin concentration, and CaO_2 that lowlanders experience during their first 2 weeks at high altitude,[69] an increased erythrocyte volume is manifested later during acclimatization.[70,79] The time course for the increase in erythrocyte volume has not been adequately investigated and remains unclear, although this appears to be one of the slower adjustments elicited during altitude acclimatization.[70,79] No changes in erythrocyte volume are apparent in lowlanders after 8 days' residence at 1,600 m,[80] 10 days at 3,100 m,[61] or 13 days at 4,300 m.[69] However, Pugh[81] observed a 33% increase in erythrocyte volume in two lowlanders who had remained above 5,800 m for at about 8 weeks and about a 17% increase in three other lowlanders who had resided between 4,650 and 5,800 m for 14 weeks. Pugh's data also indicate that after 3 to 4 months at high altitude, some of the plasma volume lost during the initial phase of acclimatization has been recovered.[81] This blunts further increases in blood hemoglobin concentration despite the expanding erythrocyte volume, and lowlanders who become well acclimatized to altitude (4–6 mo, 4,000–5,800 m elevation) exhibit hemoglobin concentrations (17–20 mg/100 mL blood) that are similar to those of healthy, native-born, high-altitude residents.[70] Thus, while short-term acclimatization brings about a relatively rapid increase in arterial oxygen content by hemoconcentration, in long-term acclimatization, increased arterial oxygen content is sustained by expansion of erythrocyte volume.

Oxyhemoglobin Dissociation Curve Shifts

In lowlanders who ascend to altitudes between 1,800 and 4,500 m and remain, blood samples obtained during rest demonstrate a decrease in hemoglobin's affinity for oxygen. Blood P_{50} (the PO_2 when SaO_2 is 50%) increases due to a rightward shift in the ODC.[82–84] This adjustment occurs within hours after arriving at high altitude[83,84] and persists even in lifelong high-altitude residents.[82,83] The rightward shift in the ODC at these moderately high altitudes represents the net effect of opposing factors. A rise in the erythrocyte concentration of the glycolytic intermediate 2,3 diphosphoglycerate (2,3 DPG) mediates a rightward shift[84] in the ODC. This effect more than compensates for the tendency of blood alkalosis and decreased PCO_2 to shift the curve leftward (the Bohr effect). Interestingly, it is the blood alkalosis associated with increased ventilation that appears to be the factor that stimulates 2,3 DPG to increase at high altitude. Pharmacological intervention to maintain experimental subjects at an acidotic pH during altitude sojourns prevents the rise in 2,3 DPG and the right shift in the ODC.[84] Above about 4,500 m, the Bohr effect becomes sufficient to overcome the 2,3 DPG effect on hemoglobin affinity for oxygen, and the ODC is shifted to the left.

Right shifts in the ODC facilitate oxygen unloading in capillaries of active tissue, because decreased hemoglobin–oxygen affinity allows greater desaturation at a given blood PO_2; whereas left shifts facilitate oxygen loading in the pulmonary capillaries, because increased hemoglobin–oxygen affinity allows higher saturation to be attained at given blood PO_2. Whether a left or a right shift in the ODC confers an advantage or disadvantage to lowlanders sojourning at high altitude appears to depend on the elevation ascended and the intensity of activity. A theoretical analysis of optimal P_{50} suggests that up to moderate altitudes ($PaO_2 > \sim 75$ mm Hg), a high P_{50} (ie, right-shifted ODC) allows a higher partial pressure of venous oxygen (PvO_2) to be sustained, which facilitates oxygen unloading in the tissues without compromising oxygen loading in the pulmonary capillaries, as the ODC at PaO_2 higher than 75 mm Hg is relatively flat.[83,85] As altitude increases and PaO_2 decreases, the advantage of a high P_{50} for maintaining high PvO_2 diminishes, and at altitudes where PaO_2 is lower than 40 mm Hg, a lower P_{50} (left-shifted ODC) maintains the PvO_2 at a higher level. Thus, the right shift in the ODC that is experienced when lowlanders sojourn at low altitudes, followed by the left shift as they ascend higher, both serve to optimize oxygen transport under the conditions in which the shifts occur.

Exercise-induced acidosis would increase the P_{50} and shift the ODC rightward. During exercise, which increases oxygen extraction, the advantage of a left-shifted ODC becomes apparent at either higher Pa_{O_2} or lower elevations, rather than during rest.[85] As is discussed below, exercise-induced shifts due to acidosis are exacerbated in unacclimatized lowlanders on arrival at high altitude compared with sea level, and this effect abates after a few weeks of acclimatization. Thus, the rightward shifts in the ODC may be pronounced when unacclimatized persons exercise at altitude, but the shifts will be less pronounced after acclimatization.

Net Effects of Systemic Oxygen Transport Adjustments

During the first month or so at high altitude, the decline in cardiac output and the increase in Ca_{O_2} with acclimatization appear to offset each other with respect to the net effects on systemic oxygen transport during exercise. Whole-body $\dot{V}_{O_2}$ during steady state submaximal exercise at a given absolute intensity or power output at altitude is unchanged with acclimatization.[78,86–88] The lowlander's $\dot{V}_{O_2}$max remains reduced to the same degree after up to 3 weeks of acclimatization as it was on arrival at altitude,[65,78,86,88,89] perhaps because the hypovolemia and elevated viscosity that result from hemoconcentration limit maximal cardiac output.

However, the hemoconcentration that rapidly increases Ca_{O_2} at the expense of decreased blood volume and increased viscosity during short-term acclimatization is eventually replaced by expansion of erythrocyte volume, which sustains the increased Ca_{O_2} with long-term acclimatization. The expanded erythrocyte volume, in combination with a partial recovery of lost plasma volume, restores normovolemia or may even expand blood volume, and the increase in blood viscosity is to some degree alleviated. If the hypovolemia and elevated viscosity associated with hemoconcentration are indeed the factors limiting stroke volume and cardiac output during maximal exercise for the first month or so that lowlanders live at altitude, as some have suggested,[72,73] then this secondary adaptation with long-term (> 4 mo) sustaining of Ca_{O_2} with a more normal blood volume and viscosity could ameliorate that limitation, perhaps ultimately leading to some recovery of $\dot{V}_{O_2}$max. The reductions in $\dot{V}_{O_2}$max and maximal cardiac output at 4,350 m compared with sea level are smaller for high-altitude natives,[90] who are presumably fully acclimatized, than they are for lowlanders acclimatized for 10 days at 4,350 m,[59] tending to support this suggestion, but confirmatory studies of maximal exercise responses in persons acclimatizing for sufficient time (ie, > 4 mo) to fully develop the expansion of erythrocyte volume are required.

METABOLISM AT HIGH ALTITUDE

High-Altitude Weight Loss

Lowlanders who ascend to high altitude and remain for more than a few days typically lose weight. The magnitude of weight loss observed varies considerably, with values reported in different investigations ranging from 80 to nearly 500 g/d.[91] The large range of weight losses observed undoubtedly relates to discrepancies among the studies with respect to such factors as hydration and dietary control, rate of ascent, altitude attained, duration of exposure, and the activity level of subjects under investigation. Both hypohydration and negative energy balance contribute to the body weight loss experienced by lowlanders sojourning at high altitude.[91–94]

Body Water Changes

Lowlanders usually experience an apparent progressive reduction in total body water when they ascend to high altitude and remain.[67,92,95] At moderate altitudes (eg, 3,500–5,000 m), the reduction in body water is measurable after as few as 3 days and persists for at least 12 days.[67,92,95] Some[92,95] have suggested that this hypohydration causes the decrease in plasma volume described above, as well as decreases in intracellular and extracellular fluid volumes. However, in other studies, lowlanders sojourning at altitude reportedly experienced a decrease in plasma volume or extracellular fluid volume[69,80,96] without a change in total body water. These observations have been interpreted as suggesting that acclimatization causes a redistribution of fluid from extracellular to intracellular compartments, rather than just dehydration. Longitudinal studies have not documented how intracellular and extracellular fluid volumes and total body water respond during altitude sojourns longer than 2 weeks, but cross-sectional studies suggest that total body water is not reduced in either lowlanders who have been acclimatized at altitude for at least 10 weeks[97] or native-born, high-altitude residents.[98]

Both decreased water intake and increased water loss can affect water balance in lowlanders acclimatizing to high altitude. The primary mechanisms for water loss include respiratory and cutaneous evaporation and urine formation. It is widely believed that increased pulmonary ventilation exacerbates respiratory water loss in lowlanders so-journing at high altitude. However, Hoyt and Honig[92] reported that respiratory water losses in soldiers working hard outdoors in winter were similar at moderate altitudes (eg, 2,200–3,100 m) and at sea level, ranging from 400 to 800 mL/d, depending on energy expenditure. This suggests that with the increased ventilation during exertion at moderate elevations in cold weather, inspired air may not become fully saturated. The decreased expired air temperature and lower water vapor pressure at altitude (compared with sea level) reduces maximum water content of saturated expired air, apparently counterbalancing the tendency of elevated ventilation to facilitate respiratory water loss, at least at moderate altitude. On the other hand, prediction modeling indicates that ventilation increases sufficiently at higher altitudes (4,300 m) to outweigh the decreased water content, such that respiratory water loss increases by 200 mL/d or more.[92]

Cutaneous evaporative water loss may be greater at altitude than at sea level. Lowlanders usually engage in more vigorous physical activity at high altitude than they do at sea level, which could increase the requirement for sweating. Unacclimatized lowlanders exposed to hypoxia exhibit suppressed sweating during the onset of exercise. A given change in core temperature produces a smaller rise in sweating rate under hypoxic than under normoxic conditions (Figure 21-22).[99,100] This leads to greater heat storage during the transition from rest to steady state exercise in hypoxic conditions. Thus, core temperature rises higher during prolonged submaximal exercise of a given absolute intensity and duration under hypoxic than it does under normoxic conditions, with a correspondingly higher sweat loss.[101]

Unacclimatized lowlanders also experience diuresis when they breathe moderately hypoxic gas mixtures,[102,103] or during the first few days following arrival at moderate (< 5,000 m) altitudes.[91,92,95,104] As will be discussed later in this chapter, this diuresis is at least partially mediated by hormonal mechanisms. To some degree, diuresis at altitude is probably beneficial because (*a*) individuals who do not exhibit diuresis are more likely to experience the signs and symptoms of altitude illnesses, and (*b*) diuresis may not occur at extreme altitudes, where most persons experience some altitude illness.[104] Some diuresis during altitude sojourn can be attributable to the release of water during catabolism of fat and lean body mass secondary to negative energy balance.[91] However, even when

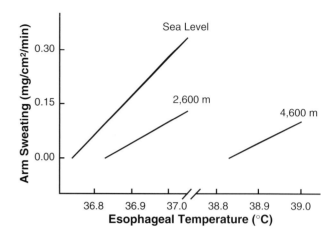

Fig. 21-22. Sweating responses appear to be suppressed in unacclimatized lowlanders exercising at high altitude, compared with acclimatized people, although sweating responses in the latter have not been well characterized. A given change in core temperature causes a smaller increase in sweat rate under hypoxic (altitude: 4,600 m) than normoxic (altitude: 2,600 m) conditions.
Data source: Kolka MA, Stephenson LA, Gonzalez RR. Depressed sweating during exercise at altitude. *J Therm Biol.* 1989;14:167–170.

nutrition is adequate to maintain energy balance and prevent cachexia at altitude, some diuresis still occurs.[91]

Thirst and appetite are diminished at altitude,[91,92,104] which could contribute to negative water balance when drinking is ad libitum. However, water intake can be controlled and standardized such that total body water remains unchanged during altitude sojourns.[69] Thus, while an increase in the rate that body water is lost may be inevitable and perhaps beneficial at altitude, aggressive steps to encouraging drinking can sustain proper hydration in lowlanders ascending to high altitude.

Energy Balance at Altitude

Obviously, individuals who maintain a negative energy balance (caloric intake less than caloric expenditure) will experience cachexia and weight loss over time during altitude sojourns, just as would be expected at sea level.[91,94] Under experimental conditions, a controlled nutritional regimen accurately matching energy intake with energy expenditure can prevent cachexia in lowlanders sojourning at altitudes up to 4,300 m.[91] However, this degree of control over energy balance is not usually maintained by lowlanders trekking and climbing in mountainous regions under expedition conditions.

Several factors may disrupt energy balance in lowlanders sojourning at altitude. Anorexia is common among newcomers at altitude, especially those experiencing symptoms of acute mountain sickness (AMS).[91] Furthermore, appetite suppression can persist even after acclimatization alleviates AMS symptoms.[94] Anecdotal observations[105] and one limited experimental study[106] suggest that in lowlanders sojourning at altitudes above 6,000 m, gastrointestinal fat absorption may deteriorate, which could limit effective energy intake. However, extensive controlled evaluations failed to confirm this observation or demonstrate any evidence that gastrointestinal fat, protein, or carbohydrate absorption is impaired in lowlanders sojourning at more-moderate altitudes up to 5,500 m.[91]

An increase in energy expenditure may shift overall energy balance to negative in lowlanders sojourning at altitude. Energy expenditure required to sustain a given activity (at a given absolute intensity or power output) for a given duration is the same at both altitude and sea level.[107] However, lowlanders typically engage in strenuous activities when they ascend to high altitudes, which increases their energy expenditure. Furthermore, the basal metabolic rate (BMR) increases 7% to 17% over the first 2 to 3 days after arrival at high altitude, declining thereafter.[4,91,106,108,109] Some investigators report that the BMR returns to sea-level values by 7 to 20 days,[106,108] while others report a sustained elevation.[109] Butterfield[91,109] reviewed these discrepant observations and suggested that in those studies in which the BMR fell completely back to sea-level values, negative energy balance and loss of metabolically active tissue had suppressed the subjects' BMRs, whereas when positive energy balance was maintained, the subjects' BMRs remained somewhat elevated throughout the duration of the altitude sojourn.

Thus, a decrease in fluid and energy intake, an increase in energy expenditure, or both can contribute to the inability of lowlanders sojourning at high altitude to maintain proper hydration and energy balance in situations where diet is ad libitum and uncontrolled. The magnitude and composition (ie, water, fat, lean tissue) of the weight loss at altitude will depend on the severity and duration of periods of negative water and energy balance. It is, however, possible to institute countermeasures (eg, nutritional supplementation, enforced eating and drinking regimens) that can ameliorate these effects, minimize dehydration and cachexia, and sustain

body mass during altitude sojourns, at least at moderate elevations below 5,000 m.

Energy Metabolism During Exercise at High Altitude: The Lactate Paradox

The energy demands of contracting skeletal muscle are supplied by the breakdown of biochemical compounds containing high-energy phosphate bonds. The metabolic processes involved in the breakdown and regeneration of these high-energy phosphate compounds during exercise under normoxic conditions are reviewed in detail elsewhere.[110-117] This section of the chapter will consider (1) the pronounced effects that hypoxia and altitude acclimatization have on energy metabolism during exercise, and (2) how these effects contribute to changes in physical work capacity and performance of lowlanders sojourning at high altitude.

The collective manifestation of the effects of hypoxia and subsequent altitude acclimatization on energy metabolism during exercise is a phenomenon referred to as the "lactate paradox." This phenomenon, first reported by Dill[118] and subsequently confirmed by Edwards,[119] is characterized by higher blood lactate concentrations during exercise at altitude than at sea level in unacclimatized persons, but lower blood lactate levels—sometimes even lower than at sea level—in acclimatized persons exercising at altitude. If it is assumed that the hypoxia accelerates blood lactate accumulation in unacclimatized persons exercising at altitude, via Pasteur's effect, then a paradox arises in explaining the decline that acclimatized persons exhibit in lactate accumulation during exercise at high altitude since hypoxia continues unrelieved.

Accelerated Glycolytic Metabolism Before Acclimatization

In one of the earliest studies of altitude effects on blood lactate, Edwards[119] observed that resting concentrations of unacclimatized lowlanders were the same on their first day at high altitude (2,810 m) as at sea level, whereas postexercise concentrations were higher at altitude, despite the fact that the metabolic rate during exercise was the same as at sea level for a given power output. Many subsequent studies have repeated these observations. Hypoxia (rather than hypobaria or other stresses associated with the mountainous environment) causes the higher blood lactate accumulation at altitude, because the same effects can be produced in hypobaric decompression chambers[120–123] or by breathing hypoxic gas mixtures under normobaric conditions.[124,125]

The elevation ascended (ie, the magnitude of hypoxia) and the metabolic rate modulate the altitude effect on blood lactate responses to exercise. In general, the increment in lactate accumulation during exercise becomes greater at a given altitude with increasing exercise intensity,[122,126] and the altitude-induced increment in lactate accumulation at any particular exercise intensity becomes greater as the elevation increases and P_{IO_2} falls.[123,125–127] Thus, elevations in resting lactate concentrations are not observed unless unacclimatized persons are acutely exposed to altitudes above 4,600 m,[120,121] which is fairly rare outside of experimental circumstances. At moderate elevations (2,000 to 4,500 m), blood lactates of unacclimatized lowlanders are similar to sea-level values during rest or low intensity exercise, but when $\dot{V}o_2$ exceeds about 1.5 L/min, an elevation in lactate concentration becomes apparent.[122,126,127] Lactate concentration in unacclimatized persons following maximal exercise is the same at high altitude as at sea level, but because of the reduction in maximal work capacity at altitude, maximal lactate concentrations are achieved at lower power outputs.[78,124,126,128–131]

Interestingly, the altitude effect just described is not observed when lactate concentrations are compared at the same relative intensity (ie, at the same percentage of $\dot{V}o_2$max) (Figure 21-23). Hermansen and Saltin[126] first observed this phenomenon, but others[78,122] have subsequently confirmed that although blood lactate concentrations in unacclimatized lowlanders exercising on arrival at high altitude or during acute hypoxic exposure were higher than during normoxic exercise for a given absolute intensity, lactate concentrations are similar when exercise of the same relative intensity is compared. A similar relationship has been observed for the effect of hypoxia on muscle lactate concentrations during short exercise bouts[122] and during longer (10–30 min) steady state exercise.[89,132] Further, the so-called "lactate threshold" during progressive-intensity exercise occurs at a lower power output and $\dot{V}o_2$ in unacclimatized lowlanders at 4,200 m simulated altitude than in normoxia; however, this threshold, expressed as relative exercise intensity, occurred at about 50% $\dot{V}o_2$max at both simulated high altitude and sea level.[131]

The increased blood lactate accumulation during hypoxic exercise reflects increased lactate release

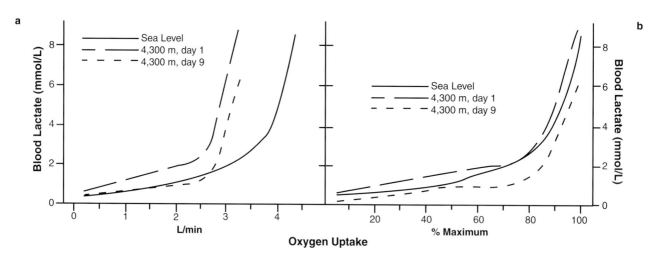

Fig. 21-23. The effects of high altitude on blood lactate accumulation during exercise differ, depending on whether comparisons are made at a given absolute or at a relative exercise intensity. (**a**) For a given absolute exercise intensity, lactate accumulation is accelerated in lowlanders on arrival at high altitude, as compared with sea level. (**b**) In contrast, lactate accumulation in unacclimatized lowlanders exercising at a given percentage of maximum oxygen uptake ($\dot{V}o_2$max) is the same at sea level and on arrival at high altitude. Regardless of whether comparisons are made of similar absolute or relative intensities, following 1 to 3 weeks of altitude acclimatization, a reduction in lactate accumulation during exercise is apparent. Because the lactate accumulation is blunted with altitude acclimatization while the hypoxia persists, this adaptation is referred to as the "lactate paradox" by many altitude researchers.
Data source: Young AJ, Sawka MN, Boushel R, et al. Erythrocyte reinfusion alters systemic O_2 transport during exercise at high altitude. *Med Sci Sports Exerc.* 1995;27:S109.

from active muscle rather than a decrease in lactate clearance. Rowell and colleagues[133] showed that hepatic blood flow increased approximately 10% and hepatic lactate extraction (ie, arterial–hepatic venous lactate difference) increased 5-fold when subjects performing steady state submaximal exercise were switched from a normoxic to a hypoxic ($F_{IO_2} \sim 0.11$) breathing mixture. Thus, lactate uptake by the liver (and probably also by inactive skeletal muscle) is greater during exercise under acute hypoxic conditions than during normoxia. Bender and colleagues[134] observed, on the other hand, an 80% increase in leg muscle lactate release (femoral arterial–femoral venous difference multiplied by femoral blood flow) during steady state exercise while breathing hypoxic ($P_{IO_2} = 83$ mm Hg), as compared with normoxic, air mixtures. More recently, Brooks and colleagues[135] measured simultaneous rates of appearance and removal of blood lactate during exercise at sea level and high altitude, and concluded that both were exaggerated on arrival at high altitude.

Muscle lactate efflux during exercise is increased by acute hypoxia.[134] Muscle lactate efflux increases during exercise because the rate that lactate appears in muscle exceeds the capacity of the muscle to oxidize the lactate. The accelerated muscle lactate efflux in unacclimatized lowlanders exercising under hypoxic conditions could reflect an increase in muscle lactate production, a decrease in lactate oxidation within the muscle, or both. The effects of acute hypoxic exposure on muscle lactate production and oxidation have not been directly measured independent of one another. However, lactic acid formation during exercise is probably accelerated under conditions of acute hypoxia. Lactate dehydrogenase activity is stimulated by increasing cytosolic nicotinamide adenine dinucleotide (reduced form, NADH) availability, and total muscle NADH concentration increases more during exercise with respiratory hypoxia than with normoxia.[136] Whether mitochondrial hypoxia per se is directly responsible for the accelerated muscle NADH accumulation remains controversial.[137] Further, the rate of lactate formation is closely linked to the overall rate of glycolysis due to the mass-action effect of pyruvate accumulation, and there is evidence that muscle glycolysis is accelerated during exercise with acute hypoxic exposure compared with normoxic exercise.

Uptake and clearance of blood glucose by active muscle were observed to increase more on the day of arrival at high altitude than during the same exercise at sea level[138]; however, the investigators questioned whether the increase was sufficient to entirely account for the concomitant increase in blood lactate.[135] Other studies have investigated the effects of hypoxia or acute high-altitude exposure on muscle glycogenolysis during exercise in unacclimatized lowlanders. Young and colleagues[89] observed no difference in muscle glycogen utilization when unacclimatized lowlanders exercised at the same relative intensity (85% $\dot{V}_{O_2}$max) for 30 minutes at sea level and at 4,300 m simulated altitude. In those experiments, however, absolute power output was lower in the hypoxic than in the normoxic experiment to offset the reduction in $\dot{V}_{O_2}$max and to maintain relative intensity constant for both trials.[89] This led to the suggestion that muscle glycogenolysis would have been greater under acute hypoxic conditions than normoxia if the exercise had been done at the same absolute power output,[49] but in subsequent experiments, muscle glycogenolysis was found to be the same or even slightly less during 45 minutes of exercise at given absolute exercise intensity on the first day at high altitude as at sea level.[139] Thus, the accelerated lactate accumulation exhibited by unacclimatized lowlanders exercising at high altitude may reflect an accelerated muscle glycolytic rate fueled by enhanced uptake of glucose by active muscle.

The accelerated muscle glycolysis and lactate accumulation in unacclimatized lowlanders exercising on arrival at high altitude is usually attributed to Pasteur's effect. That is, the decreased Ca_{O_2} at high altitude is thought to cause muscle hypoxia, which, in turn, limits oxidative energy production and necessitates an increase in glycolytic metabolism to satisfy the adenosine 5'-triphosphate (ATP) requirements of muscle contraction.[140] However, experimental findings suggest that this may not be the actual mechanism for the increased lactate accumulation. For one thing, compensatory mechanisms increase blood flow to active muscle when Ca_{O_2} is reduced, allowing the same oxygen delivery and uptake by the muscle to be maintained during exercise at a given absolute intensity under both acute hypoxic conditions and at sea level.[45,127,141] Furthermore, if oxygen availability limited aerobic muscle metabolism during exercise in hypoxic environments, then $\dot{V}_{O_2}$ during steady state submaximal exercise at a given power output should be reduced at high altitude compared with sea level, which it is not. Lastly, as depicted in Figure 21-24, net lactate release by the muscle at a given level of oxygen delivery was greater under acute hypoxic than normoxic conditions.[134]

Muscle glycogen breakdown and lactate accumulation during exercise could be accelerated during

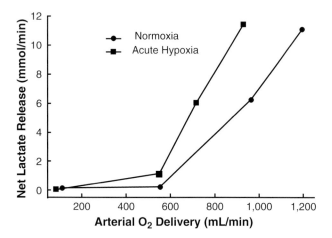

Fig. 21-24. Net lactate release from muscle during exercise (ie, the product of the muscle blood flow rate and the arterial – venous lactate concentration difference) is greater during hypoxia (squares) than normoxia (circles) for any given rate of arterial oxygen delivery to the muscle. This indicates that the mechanism for the accleration in lactate accumulation during exercise at high altitude is not a simple Pasteur effect.
Data sources: (1) Bender PR, Groves BM, McCullough RE, et al. Oxygen transport to exercising leg in chronic hypoxia. *J Appl Physiol.* 1988;65:2592–2597. (2) Bender PR, Groves BM, McCullough RE, et al. Decreased exercise muscle lactate release after high altitude acclimatization. *J Appl Physiol.* 1989;67:1556–1462.

acute hypoxic exposure by mechanisms other than tissue oxygen lack. Experiments with animals indicate that epinephrine stimulates glycolysis in contracting fast-twitch muscle fibers, even at exercise intensities that are otherwise too low to elicit glycogenolysis in the absence of epinephrine.[142] Circulating epinephrine levels of unacclimatized lowlanders exercising under acute hypoxic conditions are elevated, compared with the levels in normoxic conditions, and the elevation in epinephrine concentrations is correlated with the elevation in lactate accumulation.[143] Thus, elevated epinephrine levels in unacclimatized lowlanders exercising at altitude may stimulate muscle glycogenolysis, particularly in fast-twitch (type II) fibers, which have a greater capacity for glycolysis and lactic acid production than slow-twitch (type I) fibers.

Glycogen Sparing With Altitude Acclimatization

Changes in blood lactate responses to exercise were the first reported indication that altitude acclimatization affected muscle metabolism. As mentioned, Edwards[119] reported that acclimatized (6 wk) subjects exercising at 2,810 m exhibited the same or smaller increments in blood lactate as during sea-level exercise at the same power output. Shortly thereafter, Dill and colleagues[118] reported similar observations, and many subsequent investigators have confirmed and extended these findings.

The observation that blood lactate concentrations are lower at altitude than at sea level when acclimatized lowlanders exercise maximally[78,128,144–146] has generated some controversy. Because the reduction in $\dot{V}O_2max$ at altitude persists even after acclimatization, those lower blood lactate values may simply reflect the lower maximal power outputs achieved and reduced exercise durations rather than a metabolic adaptation.[49] This explanation is consistent with observations that the reduction in lactate accumulation during maximal exercise at altitude after acclimatization is associated with a reduced glycolytic flux unrelated to any metabolic impairment due to substrate (ie, glycogen, glucose) availability[146] or inhibition of maximal glycolytic or glycogenolytic enzyme activity.[147] That acclimatized subjects achieve the same maximal lactate concentrations 48 hours after returning to sea level as before ascent is thought to confirm the absence of any metabolic adaptation.[147] One suggestion[146] is that the contractile apparatus does not become as fully activated during maximal exercise at altitude after acclimatization as during maximal exercise at sea level. However, Grassi and colleagues[145] found that in acclimatized lowlanders performing maximal exercise at 5,050 m, acute restoration of normoxia enabled the subjects to attain higher power outputs than while breathing ambient air, but maximal lactate levels did not increase. Collectively, these findings suggest that in acclimatized persons exercising at high altitude, a central fatigue mechanism may limit maximal muscle contractile activity, while another mechanism may limit maximal rates of glycogenolytic/glycolytic metabolism.

The lactate responses to steady state submaximal exercise also change with acclimatization. Maher, Jones, and Hartley[132] observed that plasma lactate concentrations of sea-level residents did not increase as much during 20 minutes of exercise at 75% $\dot{V}O_2max$ on day 12 of residence at 4,300 m as on the second day at high altitude, or at sea level. That blood lactate accumulation during prolonged steady state submaximal exercise decreases with altitude acclimation has been confirmed in many subsequent studies.[89,131,134,135,148,149]

The effect of altitude acclimatization on lactate accumulation during exercise probably reflects a decrease in lactate production and release into the blood rather than an increase in metabolic clearance. Studies involving infusion of radioactively labeled metabolites demonstrate decreases in both lactate removal from the blood and metabolic clearance following altitude acclimatization, secondary to a decrease in the rate of lactate appearance in the blood. This observation (combined with earlier findings that net lactate release from muscle,[134] muscle lactate accumulation,[148] and the decrease in muscle pH[139,149] during submaximal exercise at altitude are all less pronounced after acclimatization, whereas pyruvate oxidation appears unchanged[139]) indicates that the lower lactate concentrations reflect a decreased glycolytic production of lactate in contracting muscle.

Indeed, experimental evidence confirms that altitude acclimatization enables a decreased muscle glycogenolysis during exercise. Young and colleagues[89] measured muscle glycogen utilization of sea-level residents during 30 minutes of exercise at 85% $\dot{V}O_2$max at sea level, during the first 2 hours at a simulated altitude of 4,300 m, and again after 18 days of acclimatization at 4,300 m; the two altitude trials were at the same absolute intensity. Muscle glycogen utilization and blood lactate accumulation during exercise at high altitude before acclimatization were the same as at sea level, but were both reduced after 18 days of altitude acclimatization.[89] Green and colleagues[139] confirmed and extended those findings using a similar altitude protocol but employing the same absolute exercise intensity for all three trials.

The mechanism enabling the glycogen-sparing effect of altitude acclimatization is not fully understood. Young and colleagues[89] originally suggested that an increase in fat oxidation during exercise might provide the energy to enable a decreased muscle glycogenolysis. This speculation was based on differences observed in blood–free fatty acid and -glycerol concentrations during exercise at sea level and at altitude. However, while subsequent studies employing strict dietary control and more-precise approaches to measuring fat metabolism have confirmed the glycogen-sparing effect of altitude acclimatization,[139] the most current findings demonstrate that muscles, in fact, decrease utilization of fat as an energy substrate following altitude acclimatization.[150] On the other hand, uptake and clearance of blood glucose by muscle during exercise at altitude is greater following acclimatization, indicating that increased availability of glucose may permit sparing of glycogen stores within the muscle.[131]

The glycogen-sparing adaptation appears to be due to different mechanisms than the metabolic adaptation resulting from chronic aerobic endurance-type training. In the case of endurance training, increased oxidative enzyme activity in skeletal muscle appears to account, at least in part, for metabolic adaptations to physical training at sea level. However, humans acclimatized for 3 weeks at 4,300 m exhibited no change in hexokinase, glycogen phosphorylase, lactate dehydrogenase, malate dehydrogenase,[149] or citrate synthetase (unpublished observations from this laboratory—AJY) activities in the vastus lateralis muscle. Similarly, during a 40-day altitude exposure simulating a progressive ascent to the summit of Mount Everest (282 mm Hg), eight male subjects exhibited no change in vastus lateralis enzyme activities of 3-hydroxyacyl CoA dehydrogenase, pyruvate kinase, or alpha-glycerophosphate dehydrogenase, decreases in succinic dehydrogenase, and citrate synthetase.[147] Thus, the changes in metabolic responses to exercise observed after 2 to 3 weeks of altitude acclimatization do not appear to be due to changes in muscle glycolytic or oxidative enzyme activities.

A progressive rise in resting plasma norepinephrine with unchanged epinephrine occurs during the same time frame that the aforementioned metabolic adaptations to high altitude take place.[148,151] This prompted Young and colleagues[89] to speculate that increased sympathetic nervous activity mediated those adaptations, based on their conclusion that the glycogen-sparing effect of altitude acclimatization had resulted from increased fatty acid mobilization and subsequent oxidation by muscle, because at sea level, increased sympathetic activity stimulates lipolysis. More-recent observations, however, demonstrate that an increased utilization of fatty acids does not necessarily accompany the reduction in glycogen utilization and lactate accumulation that occur with altitude acclimatization.[148,150] Another possibility is that chronically elevated circulating norepinephrine levels during altitude acclimatization induces a decrease in the number or sensitivity, or both, of muscle β_2-adrenergic receptors. Cardiac β_2-adrenergic receptor density and sensitivity in lowlanders declines during altitude acclimatization.[152,153] Stimulation of β_2-adrenergic receptors in muscle activates glycogenolysis, so down-regulation of these receptors could blunt glycogenolysis and lactate accumulation during exercise. However, β_2-adrenergic blockade with propranolol during altitude acclimatization does not prevent the glycogen-sparing adaptation.[148]

These findings suggest that chronic β_2-adrenergic stimulation during altitude acclimatization may not cause the reduction in glycogen utilization and lactate accumulation during exercise. However, this is not to say that changes in β_2-adrenergic stimulation play no role in the changes in muscle energy metabolism induced by altitude acclimatization. Epinephrine release into the blood during exercise, which is greatly exaggerated on arrival at high altitude compared with that at sea level, is blunted following 2 to 3 weeks of acclimatization.[143,148] As described above, the increase in lactate accumulation during exercise that unacclimatized lowlanders exhibit on arrival at high altitude is closely correlated with the more pronounced increment in epinephrine levels. Thus, a blunting of epinephrine release into the blood appears to be the most likely mechanism by which muscle glycogenolysis and lactate accumulation during exercise at high altitude could be diminished following acclimatization, but this requires experimental verification.

Endocrine Responses at High Altitude

The preceding section described how epinephrine, and perhaps norepinephrine, appeared to mediate the effects of altitude acclimatization on glycogenolysis and lactate accumulation during exercise. While the catecholamines appear to play a principal role in the mechanism by which adjustments in energy metabolism occur during altitude acclimatization, other hormones involved in metabolic regulation may also be affected by sojourn to high altitude. In addition, other hormonal responses to ascent to high altitude and subsequent acclimatization may also modulate the body water adjustments discussed at the beginning of this section.

Insulin and glucagon act to regulate the relative contribution of carbohydrate and fat metabolism to the overall metabolic energy requirements. Glucagon levels appear unchanged in lowlanders sojourning at high altitude, during either rest or exercise.[154] However, changes in the insulin response to exercise, or in the insulin sensitivity of muscle tissue, may contribute to the changes in muscle energy metabolism during exercise at high altitude. Acute hypoxic exposure does not affect resting insulin concentrations in unacclimatized lowlanders up to about 3,000 m.[155] In unacclimatized lowlanders ascending to 4,300 m and higher, resting insulin levels at altitude appear to be elevated, compared with those at sea level.[131,156,157] During exercise at altitude, insulin remains constant at these elevated levels[131,154,156] or increases if the exercise intensity is maximal.[155] Insulin levels, both at rest and during exercise, decrease back to sea-level values with 2 or more weeks of acclimatization,[131,156] unless the sojourner continues ascending to more extreme altitudes.[154]

Thus, on arrival at high altitude, an increase in insulin levels may facilitate glucose uptake by muscle to sustain the accelerated glycolysis and increased lactate accumulation that are apparently stimulated by an exaggerated epinephrine release during exercise. This is consistent with the apparent increase in the uptake and utilization of blood glucose by muscle when unacclimatized lowlanders exercise at high altitude. However, the subsequent decline in insulin levels back to sea-level values that occurs during altitude acclimatization is not consistent with the finding that glucose uptake and utilization by muscle remain elevated. Insulin sensitivity of muscle tissue might increase during acclimatization, but this possibility remains to be investigated. Alternatively, the increased uptake of blood glucose during exercise in acclimatized lowlanders may reflect the actions of growth hormone. Acutely, changes in growth hormone concentrations exert effects on glucose uptake that are similar to those of insulin. Although circulating growth hormone levels during rest are unaffected by sojourn at altitude, growth hormone levels increase more rapidly during exercise at altitude after acclimatization.[87]

The transient elevation in BMR during the first few days after lowlanders arrive at high altitude, which was discussed earlier in this section, appears to be mediated by the thyroid hormones. Within 24 hours after lowlanders arrive at high altitude, plasma thyroxine (T_4) and triiodothyronine (T_3) concentrations both begin to increase.[158] The T_4 and T_3 levels appear to peak between the third and eighth day at altitude,[106,159] and thereafter levels decline.[158,159] This time course parallels that of changes in the BMR.[5,91,106,108,109] When the elevation ascended is extreme (> 5,400 m), thyroid stimulating hormone (TSH) increases along with T_4 and T_3.[160] However, it is interesting to note that at lower altitudes, an increase in TSH has not always been observed to accompany the increase in T_4 and T_3.[158,159] This might suggest that the elevated T_4 and T_3 levels may not be mediated by altitude effects on the hypothalamic-pituitary-thyroid axis activity. Because T_4 and T_3 are transported bound to plasma proteins, changes in these hormone levels may simply reflect the reduction in volume of distribution for the plasma proteins, owing to hemoconcentration during the first week at altitude.

Hormonal responses are thought to be involved in mediating adjustments on body fluid homeostasis experienced by lowlanders during sojourns at high altitude; however, the exact mechanisms are unclear. Arginine vasopressin (AVP), or antidiuretic hormone, regulates water loss in urine by increasing the permeability of the collecting duct to water, thus promoting water resorption. Unacclimatized lowlanders exposed to moderate hypoxia (at elevations of about 11,000 ft [3,385 m]) exhibit a decrease in AVP over the first 2 hours.[161] Exposure to more extreme elevations appears to have no effect or cause no increase in AVP levels.[161] Furthermore, after 24 hours of hypoxic exposure, and thereafter at altitude, AVP levels are similar to those at sea level.[161] Thus, AVP might play a role in initiating the decrease in body water and plasma volume that lowlanders experience during altitude sojourns, but other mechanisms are involved in sustaining that response.

It is generally agreed that on arrival at high altitude, aldosterone levels in lowlanders are decreased, both at rest and during exercise.[161,162] Aldosterone normally functions to defend normal fluid volume. Aldosterone acts on the kidney to increase sodium and water resorption; thus, a decrease in aldosterone levels would contribute to the increased urine formation and decrease in plasma volume that unacclimatized lowlanders experience on arrival at altitude. With several weeks of altitude acclimatization, aldosterone returns to preascent levels, although the reduction in plasma volume appears to persist longer.[162]

At sea level, aldosterone secretion is controlled by the renin–angiotensin mechanism, in which reduced blood volume or pressure stimulates the kidney to secrete renin, which catalyzes conversion of blood angiotensinogin to angiotensin I, which in turn is converted to angiotensin II by the action of angiotensin-converting enzyme (ACE) in the vascular endothelium. Angiotensin II stimulates release of aldosterone, and exerts a vasoconstrictor effect as well. One frequently cited investigation reported that the acute altitude exposure disrupted the control mechanism at the conversion from angiotensin I to II, based on observations that plasma ACE levels decreased in unacclimatized lowlanders newly arrived at high altitude.[38,163] However, the authors repeatedly failed to confirm their observations, either in subsequent follow-up studies or even when archived blood samples from the original study were reanalyzed, which ultimately led them to retract their conclusion. Thus, Maher and colleagues'[162] observations that renin, both at rest and during exercise, decreases along with aldosterone after 14 hours at 4,300 m, and that resting levels of angiotensin II were also decreased (although exercise levels were not), indicate that the fall in aldosterone secretion on arrival at altitude is appropri-

ate and normally regulated by the renin–angiotensin system.

The decrease in aldosterone synthesis may be a response to what is sensed as, but is not, a progressive increase in blood volume. Within several hours after arrival at high altitude, lowlanders exhibit a sustained peripheral venoconstriction, which progressively increases over the first week of acclimatization.[164,165] Peripheral venoconstriction decreases venous vascular capacity, translocating blood to the central circulation (possibly signaling an increase in blood volume to the kidney, which then decreases renin secretion), and ultimately effecting a decrease in aldosterone levels. Alternatively, the decline in aldosterone levels may reflect a decrease in aldosterone synthesis mediated by a hypoxia-induced decrease in expression of genes for enzymes required in the metabolic synthesis of aldosterone.[166]

Another hormonally mediated process altered in lowlanders sojourning at altitude is erythropoieses, which at sea level is stimulated by an increase in circulating erythropoietin levels. Erythropoietin is released mainly by the kidney (and to a lesser degree by the liver and other extrarenal sites) in response to hypoxemia or blood loss. The expansion of erythrocyte volume that lowlanders experience after several months' acclimatization at high altitude is usually attributed to this hormonal mechanism.[70,167] However, the time course for the changes in erythropoietin in lowlanders sojourning at high altitude is difficult to reconcile with the time course of the expansion of erythrocyte volume.

In contrast to the expansion of erythrocyte volume, which is not manifested until the lowlander has spent several months at high altitude, erythropoietin begins increasing within several hours after ascent.[69,70,167] In one study,[69] erythropoietin levels were elevated 3-fold over sea-level values within 10 to 14 hours after rapid ascent from sea level to 4,300 m. Yet, this increase is short lived. Peak erythropoietin levels are achieved between 24 and 48 hours after arrival at 4,300 m,[168] but decline thereafter, reaching preascent values by the ninth day at this altitude.[69,168] A similar response pattern and time course have been reported at lower[169,170] and higher[171] elevations, but a more pronounced increase in circulating erythropoietin is observed[171] with ascent above 5,000 m. Given that the acclimatizing lowlander's hormone levels return to sea-level values well before the expansion of erythrocytes is manifested and without alleviation of hypoxemia, the role of this response in the mechanism of erythrocyte volume expansion is unclear and remains to be fully investigated.

CONCLUDING THOUGHTS

At sea level, circulation is thought to be the dominant factor limiting maximal exercise performance.[172] Indeed, maximum oxygen uptake at sea level varies markedly among subjects, and that variability is closely linked to the variability in maximum cardiac output.[173] However, this variability among subjects in their maximum oxygen uptake is markedly reduced as elevation is increased.[174] Considering the limitation imposed on the number of oxygen molecules that can be ventilated at high altitude, and the limitation of lung diffusing capacity at altitude, one might conclude that the respiratory rather than circulatory system limits maximal oxygen uptake at high altitude. If oxygen does not reach the arterial blood, then increasing cardiac output might not greatly facilitate oxygen transport to the tissues. Wagner's analysis[172] indicates that at the summit of Mount Everest, a doubling of maximal cardiac output will increase maximum oxygen uptake by less than 10%. The altitude limitations in total body oxygen transport begin to appear above 2,000 m, where these respiratory limitations might be expected. Thus, the respiratory system imposes greater limitations on overall exercise performance at altitude than at sea level.

Even if respiratory factors limit maximal oxygen uptake at high altitude more than circulatory factors, this is not to say that the systemic oxygen transport and muscle energy metabolism adjustments that occur at high altitude do not affect physical performance. Most physical activities elicit oxygen uptakes well below the maximal, and thus are not limited by $\dot{V}o_2$max, either at sea level or at high altitude. While ascent to high altitude does causes $\dot{V}o_2$max to de-

crease, it is not until extreme altitudes are reached that the reduction is sufficient that the oxygen uptake required for activities such as walking approaches maximal. In unacclimatized lowlanders arriving at high altitude, steady state submaximal exercise is sustained by an increase in cardiac output and an accelerated glycolysis and lactate accumulation. Both factors could limit endurance for a given activity at high altitude more than at sea level, the first by increased cardiac work and the second by an increased rate of energy substrate depletion.

With as few as 12 to 16 days of acclimatization, submaximal exercise endurance increases 40% to 60% compared with exercise endurance on arrival at altitude, even though maximal oxygen uptake remains lower.[132,175] After altitude acclimatization, systemic oxygen transport requirements during exercise at altitude can be satisfied with a lower cardiac output, and thus reduced cardiac work, than on arrival.[56] In large part, this adaptation is enabled by the higher Sao_2 resulting from ventilatory acclimatization, which, along with hemoconcentration due to high-altitude diuresis during the initial weeks at altitude and expanded erythrocyte volume after several months, raises Cao_2.

The development of a glycogen-sparing adaptation further contributes to the improvement in exercise performance. Thus, in lowlanders ascending to high altitude, maximal performance appears to be limited by respiratory factors and submaximal performance by nonrespiratory factors, but both respiratory and nonrespiratory factors appear to contribute importantly to performance improvements with acclimatization.

REFERENCES

1. Ward MP, Milledge JS, West JB. *High Altitude Medicine and Physiology*. New York, NY: Oxford University Press; 2000.

2. West JB, Hackett PH, Maret KH, et al. Pulmonary gas exchange on the summit of Mount Everest. *J Appl Physiol*. 1983;55:678–687.

3. Reeves JT, Groves BM, Sutton JR, et al. Adaptations to hypoxia: Lessons from Operation Everest II. In: Simmons DH, ed. *Current Pulmonology*. St. Louis, Mo: Mosby–Year Book; 1991: 23–50.

4. Howard LSGE, Robbins PA. Ventilatory response to 8 h of isocapnic and poikilocapnic hypoxia in humans. *J Appl Physiol*. 1995;78:1092–1097.

5. Moore JM, Cymerman A, Huang SY, et al. Propranolol blocks metabolic rate increase but not ventilatory acclimatization to 4300 m. *Respir Physiol*. 1987;70:195–204.

6. Hornbein TF. The relation between stimulus to chemoreceptors and their response. In: Torrance RW, ed. *Arterial Chemoreceptors*. Edinburgh, Scotland: Blackwell Scientific Publications; 1968: 65–78.

7. von Euler US, Liljestrand G, Zotterman Y. The excitation mechanism of the chemoreceptor in the carotid body. *Scand Arch Physiol*. 1939;83:132–152.

8. Weil JV, Byrne-Quinn E, Sodal IE, Filley GF, Grover RF. Hypoxic ventilatory drive in normal man. *J Clin Invest*. 1971;50:186–195.

9. Bisgard GE. The role of arterial chemoreceptors in ventilatory acclimatization to hypoxia. *Adv Exp Med Biol*. 1994;360:109–122.

10. Lopez-Barneo J, Lopez-Lopez JR, Urena J, Gonzales C. Chemotransduction in the carotid body: K+ modulated by Po_2 in type 1 chemoreceptor cells. *Science*. 1988;242:580–582.

11. Benot AR, Ganfornia MD, Lopez-Barneo J. Potassium channel modulated by hypoxia and the redox status in glomus cells of the carotid body. In: Weir EK, Hume JR, Reeves JT, eds. *Ion Flux in Pulmonary Vascular Control*. New York, NY: Plenum Press; 1992: 177–188.

12. Weil JV. Ventilatory control at high altitude. In: Fishman AP, Cherniak NS, Widdicombe JG, Geiger SR, eds. *Handbook of Physiology: The Respiratory System. Control of Breathing, Vol 2* Bethesda, Md: American Physiological Society; 1986: 703–728.

13. Stea A, Jackson L, Macintyre L, Nurse CA. Long-term modulation of inward currents in O_2 chemoreceptors in chronic hypoxia and cyclic AMP in vitro. *J Neurosci*. 1995;15:2192–2202.

14. Hirschman CA, McCullough RE, Weil JV. Normal values for hypoxic and hypercapnic ventilatory drives in man. *J Appl Physiol*. 1975;38:1095–1098.

15. Collins DD, Scoggin CH, Zwillich CW, Weil JV. Hereditary aspects of decreased hypoxic response. *J Clin Invest*. 1978;62(1):105–110.

16. Huang SY, Alexander JK, Grover RF, et al. Hypocapnia and sustained hypoxia blunt ventilation on arrival at high altitude. *J Appl Physiol*. 1984;56:602–606.

17. Reeves JT, McCullough RE, Moore LG, Cymerman A, Weil JV. Sea-level Pco_2 relates to ventilatory acclimatization at 4300 m. *J Appl Physiol*. 1993;75:1117–1122.

18. Van Beek JHGM, Berkenbosch A, Degoode J, Olievier CN. Effects of brainstem hypoxemia on the regulation of breathing. *Respir Physiol*. 1984;57:171–188.

19. Nilsson GE, Lutz PL. Role of GABA in hypoxia tolerance, metabolic depression, and hibernation: Possible links to neurotransmitter evolution. *Comp Biochem Physiol Comp Pharmacol*. 1993;105:329–336.

20. Kazemi H, Hoop B. Glutamic acid and gamma-aminobutyric acid neurotransmitters in central control of breathing. *J Appl Physiol*. 1991;70:1–7.

21. Weil JV. Ventilatory responses to CO_2 and hypoxia after sustained hypoxia in awake cats. *J Appl Physiol*. 1994;76:2251–2252.

22. Robbins PA. Commentary: Hypoxic ventilatory decline. *J Appl Physiol*. 1995;79:373–374.

23. Butterfield GE, Gates J, Fleming S, Brooks GA, Sutton JR, Reeves JT. Increased energy intake minimizes weight loss in men at high altitude. *J Appl Physiol*. 1992;72:1741–1748.

24. Howard LSGE, Robbins PA. Alterations in respiratory control during 8 h of isocapnic and poikilocapnic hypoxia in humans. *J Appl Physiol*. 1995;78:1098–1107.

25. Dempsey JA, Forster HV. Mediation of ventilatory adaptations. *Physiol Rev*. 1982;62:262–331.

26. Visek M, Pickett CK, Weil JV. Increased carotid body sensitivity during acclimatization to hypobaric hypoxia. *J Appl Physiol*. 1987;63:2403–2410.

27. Cruz JC, Reeves JT, Grover RF, et al. Ventilatory acclimatization to high altitude is prevented by CO_2 breathing. *Respiration*. 1980;39(3):121–130.

28. Fitzgerald MP. Further observations on the changes in the breathing and the blood at various high altitudes. *Proc Royal Soc*. 1914;88:248–258.

29. Rahn H, Otis AB. Man's respiratory response during and after acclimatization to high altitude. *Am J Physiol*. 1949;157:445–462.

30. Malconian MK, Rock PB, Reeves JT, Cymerman A, Houston CS. Operation Everest II: Gas tensions in expired air and arterial blood at extreme altitude. *Aviat Space and Environ Med*. 1993;64:37–42.

31. Weil JV, Bryne-Quinn E, Sodal IE, Kline JS, McCullough RE, Filley GF. Augmentation of chemosensitivity during mild exercise in normal man. *J Appl Physiol*. 1972;33:813–819.

32. Waldrop TG, Eldrige FL, Iwamoto GA, Mitchell JH. Central neural control of respiration and circulation during exercise. In: Rowell LB, Sheperd JT, eds. *Handbook of Physiology*. Section 12: *Exercise: Regulation and Integration of Multiple Systems*. New York, NY: Oxford University Press; 1996: 333–380.

33. Dempsey JA, Forster HV, Birnbaum ML, et al. Control of exercise hyperpnea under varying durations of exposure to moderate hypoxia. *Resp. Physiol*. 1972;16:213–231.

34. Christensen EH. Sauerstoff aufnahme and repiratorische functionen in gross hohen [in German]. *Skand Arch Physiol*. 1937;76:88–100.

35. Sutton JR, Reeves JT, Wagner PD, et al. Operation Everest II: Oxygen transport during exercise at extreme simulated altitude. *J Appl Physiol*. 1988;64:1309–1321.

36. Gale GE, Torre-Bueno JR, Moon RE, Saltzman HA, Wagner PD. Ventilation perfusion inequality in normal humans during exercise at sea level and simulated altitude. *J Appl Physiol*. 1985;58:978–988.

37. Wagner PD, Gale GE, Moon RE, Torre-Bueno JR, Stolp BW, Saltzman HA. Pulmonary gas exchange in humans exercising at sea level and simulated altitude. *J Appl Physiol*. 1986;61:260–270.

38. Milledge JS, Catley DM, Ward MP, Williams ES, Clarke CRA. Renin-aldosterone and angiotensin–converting enzyme during prolonged altitude exposure. *J Appl Physiol*. 1983;55:699–702.

39. Wagner PD, Sutton JR, Reeves JT, Cymerman A, Groves BM, Malconian MK. Operation Everest II: Pulmonary gas exchange during a simulated ascent of Mt Everest. *J Appl Physiol*. 1987;63:2348–2359.

40. Evans JW, Wagner PD. $\dot{V}/\dot{Q}$ distributions from analysis of experimental inert gas elimination. *J Appl Physiol*. 1977;42:889–898.

41. Saltin B, Grover RF, Blomqvist CG, Hartley LH, Johnson RL. Maximal oxygen uptake and cardiac output after 2 weeks at 4300 m. *J Appl Physiol*. 1968;25:400–409.

42. Valeri CR, Pivacek LE, Gray AD, et al. The safety and therapeutic effectiveness of human red cells stored at −80°C for as long as 21 years. *Transfusion*. 1989;29:429–437.

43. Stenberg J, Ekblom B, Messin R. Hemodynamic response to work at simulated altitude, 4000 m. *J Appl Physiol*. 1966;21:1589–1594.

44. Pugh LGCE, Gill MB, Lahiri S, Milledge JS, Ward MP, West JB. Muscular exercise at great altitudes. *J Appl Physiol*. 1964;19:431–440.

45. Bender PR, Groves BM, McCullough RE, et al. Oxygen transport to exercising leg in chronic hypoxia. *J Appl Physiol*. 1988;65:2592–2597.

46. Hartley LH, Vogel JA, Landowne M. Central, femoral, and brachial circulation during exercise in hypoxia. *J Appl Physiol*. 1973;34:87–90.

47. Vogel JA, Hansen JE, Harris CW. Cardiovascular responses in man during exhaustive work at sea level and high altitude. *J Appl Physiol*. 1967;23:531–539.

48. Squires RW, Buskirk ER. Aerobic capacity during acute exposure to simulated altitude, 914 to 2286 meters. *Med Sci Sports Exerc*. 1986;14:36–40.

49. Young AJ. Energy substrate utilization during exercise in extreme environments. In: Pandolf KB, Holloszy JO, eds. *Exercise and Sport Sciences Reviews*. Baltimore, Md: Williams & Wilkins; 1990: 65–117.

50. Buskirk ER. Decrease in physical working capacity at high altitude. In: Hegnaurer AH, ed. *Biomedicine Problems of High Terrestrial Elevations*. Natick, Mass: US Army Research Institute of Environmental Medicine; 1969: 204–222.

51. Young AJ, Cymerman A, Burse RL. The influence of cardiorespiratory fitness on the decrement in maximal aerobic power at high altitude. *Eur J Appl Physiol*. 1985;54:12–15.

52. Grover RF, Reeves JT, Grover EB, Leathers JE. Muscular exercise in young men native to 3100 m altitude. *J Appl Physiol*. 1967;22:555–564.

53. Saltin B. Aerobic and anaerobic work capacity at an altitude of 2250 meters. In: Goddard RF, ed. *The Effects of Altitude on Physical Performance*. Albuquerque, NM: The Athletic Institute; 1967: 97–102.

54. Powers SK, Lawler J, Dempsey JA, Dodd S, Landry G. Effects of incomplete pulmonary gas exchange on $\dot{V}o_2$max. *J Appl Physiol*. 1989;66:2491–2495.

55. Astrand PO, Cuddy TE, Saltin B, Stenberg J. Cardiac output during submaximal and maximal work. *J Appl Physiol*. 1964;19:268–274.

56. Grover RF, Lufschanowski R, Alexander JK. Alterations in the coronary circulation of man following ascent to 3100 m altitude. *J Appl Physiol*. 1976;41:832–838.

57. Hultgren HN. Coronary heart disease and trekking. *J Wild Med*. 1990;1:154–161.

58. Grover RF, Tucker CE, McGroaty SR, Travis RR. The coronary stress of skiing at high altitude. *Arch Intern Med*. 1990;150:1205–1208.

59. Vogel JA, Hartley LH, Cruz JC, Hogan RP. Cardiac output during exercise in sea-level residents at sea level and high altitude. *J Appl Physiol*. 1974;36:169–172.

60. Hartley LH, Alexander JK, Modelski M, Grover RF. Subnormal cardiac output at rest and during exercise in residents at 3,100 m altitude. *J Appl Physiol*. 1967;23:839–848.

61. Alexander JK, Hartley LH, Modelski M, Grover RF. Reduction of stroke volume during exercise in man following ascent to 3,100 m altitude. *J Appl Physiol*. 1967;23:849–858.

62. Klausen K. Cardiac output in man in rest and work during and after acclimatization to 3,800 m. *J Appl Physiol*. 1966;21:609–616.

63. Reeves JT, Groves BM, Sutton JR, et al. Operation Everest II: Preservation of cardiac function at extreme altitude. *J Appl Physiol*. 1987;63:531–539.

64. Grover RF, Weil JV, Reeves JT. Cardiovascular adaptation to exercise and high altitude. In: Pandolf KB, ed. *Exercise and Sport Sciences Reviews*. New York, NY: Macmillan; 1986: 269–302.

65. Moore LG, Cymerman A, Shao-Yung H, et al. Propranolol does not impair exercise oxygen uptake in normal men at high altitude. *J. Appl Physiol*. 1986;61:1935–1941.

66. Suarez J, Alexander JK, Houston CS. Enhanced left ventricular performance at high altitude during Operation Everest II. *Am J Cardiol*. 1987;60:137–142.

67. Jain SC, Bardhan J, Swamy YV, Krishina B, Nayar HS. Body fluid compartments in humans during acute high-altitude exposure. *Aviat Space Environ Med*. 1980;51:234–236.

68. Jung RC, Dill DB, Horton R, Horvath SM. Effects of age on plasma aldosterone levels and hemoconcentration at altitude. *J Appl Physiol*. 1971;31:593–597.

69. Sawka MN, Young AJ, Rock PB, et al. Altitude acclimatization and blood volume: Effects of erythrocyte volume expansion. *J Appl Physiol*. 1996;81:636–642.

70. Ward MP, Milledge JS, West JB. *Haematological Changes and Plasma Volume*. London, England: Chapman & Hall; 1989: Chap 9.

71. Grover RF, Reeves JT, Maher JT, et al. Maintained stroke volume but impaired arterial oxygenation in man at high altitude with supplemental CO_2. *Circ Res*. 1976;38:391–396.

72. Horstman D, Weiskopf R, Jackson RE. Work capacity during 3–wk sojourn at 4,300 m: Effects of relative polycythemia. *J Appl Physiol*. 1980;49(2):311–318.

73. Ekblom B, Wilson G, Astrand PO. Central circulation during exercise after venesection and reinfusion of red blood cells. *J Appl Physiol*. 1976;40:379–383.

74. Young AJ, Sawka MN, Boushel R, et al. Erythrocyte reinfusion alters systemic O_2 transport during exercise at high altitude. *Med Sci Sports Exerc*. 1995;27:S109.

75. Dempsey JA, Thomson JM, Forster HV, Cerny FC, Chosy LW. HbO_2 dissociation in man during prolonged work in chronic hypoxia. *J Appl Physiol*. 1975;38:1022–1029.

76. Hannon JP, Vogel JA. Oxygen transport during early altitude acclimatization: A perspective study. *Eur J Appl Physiol*. 1977;36:285–297.

77. Bender PR, McCullough RE, McCullough RG, et al. Increased exercise Sao_2 independent of ventilatory acclimatization at 4300 m. *J Appl Physiol*. 1989;66:2733–2738.

78. Young AJ, Sawka MN, Muza SR, et al. Effects of erythrocyte infusion on $\dot{V}o_2$max at high altitude. *J Appl Physiol*. 1996;81:252–259.

79. Heath D, Williams DR. The blood. In: *Man at High Altitude*. Edinburgh, Scotland: Churchill Livingston; 1977: 39–53.

80. Surks MI, Chinn KSK, Matoush LO. Alterations in body composition in man after acute exposure to high altitude. *J Appl Physiol*. 1966;21:1741–1746.

81. Pugh LGCE. Blood volume and haemoglobin concentration at altitudes above 18,000 ft (5500 m). *J Physiol*. 1964;170:344–354.

82. Torrance JD, Lenfant C, Cruz J, Marticorena E. Oxygen transport mechanisms in residents at high altitude. *Resp Physiol*. 1970;11:1–15.

83. Mairbaurl H. Red blood cell function in hypoxia at altitude and exercise. *Int J Sports Med*. 1994;15:51–63.

84. Goldberg SV, Schoene RB, Haynor D, et al. Brain tissue pH and ventilatory acclimatization to high altitude. *J Appl Physiol*. 1992;72:58–63.

85. Willford DC, Hill EP, Moores WY. Theoretical analysis of optimal P_{50}. *J Appl Physiol*. 1982;52:1043–1048.

86. Reeves JT, Grover RF, Cohn JE. Regulation of ventilation during exercise at 10,200 ft in athletes born at low altitude. *J Appl Physiol*. 1967;22:546–554.

87. Raynaud J, Drouet L, Martineaud JP, Bordacha J, Coudert J, Durand J. Time course of plasma growth hormone during exercise in humans at altitude. *J Appl Physiol*. 1981;50:229–233.

88. Brotherhood J, Brozavic B, Pugh LGC. Haematological status of middle- and long-distance runners. *Clin Sci and Mol Med*. 1975;48:139–145.

89. Young AJ, Evans WJ, Cymerman A, Pandolf KB, Knapik JJ, Maher JT. Sparing effect of chronic high-altitude exposure on muscle glycogen utilization. *J Appl Physiol*. 1982;52:857–862.

90. Vogel JA, Hartley LH, Cruz JC. Cardiac output during exercise in altitude natives at sea level and high altitude. *J Appl Physiol*. 1974;36:173–176.

91. Butterfield GE. Maintenance of body weight at altitude: In search of 500 kcal/day. In: Marriot BM, Carlson SJ, eds. *Nutritional Needs in Cold and in High-Altitude Environments*. Washington, DC: National Academy Press; 1996: 357–378.

92. Hoyt RW, Honig A. Environmental influences on body fluid balance during exercise: Altitude. In: Buskirk, ER, Puhl SM, eds. *Body Fluid Balance: Exercise and Sport*. New York, NY: CRC Press; 1996: 183–196.

93. Fulco CS, Cymerman A, Pimental NA, Young AJ, Maher JT. Anthropometric changes at high altitude. *Aviat Space Environ Med*. 1985;56:220–224.

94. Sutton JR. Effect of acute hypoxia on the hormonal response to exercise. *J Appl Physiol*. 1977;42:587–592.

95. Hoyt RW, Honig A. Body fluid and energy metabolism at high altitude. In: Fregley ML, Blatteis CM, eds. *Handbook of Physiology*. Section 4. *Environmental Physiology, Vol 2*. New York, NY: Oxford University Press; 1995: 1277–1289.

96. Hannon JP, Chinn KSK, Shields JL. Effects of acute high altitude exposure on body fluids. *Fed Proc*. 1969;38:1178–1184.

97. Anand IS, Chandrashekhar Y, Rao SK, et al. Body fluid compartments, renal blood flow and hormones at 6,000 m in normal subjects. *J Appl Physiol*. 1993;74:1234–1239.

98. Picon-Reategui E, Lozano R, Valdivieso J. Body composition at sea level and high altitudes. *J Appl Physiol*. 1961;16:589–592.

99. Kolka MA, Stephenson LA, Rock PB, Gonazlez RR. Local sweating and cutaneous blood flow during exercise in hypobaric environments. *J Appl Physiol*. 1987;62:2224–2229.

100. Kolka MA, Stephenson LA, Gonzalez RR. Depressed sweating during exercise at altitude. *J Therm Biol*. 1989;14:167–170.

101. Greenleaf JE, Greenleaf CJ, Card DH, Saltin B. Exercise-temperature regulation in man during acute exposure to simulated altitude. *J Appl Physiol*. 1969;26:290–296.

102. Tucker A, Reeves JT, Robertshaw D, Grover RF. Cardiopulmonary response to acute altitude exposure: Water loading and denitrogenation. *Respir Physiol.* 1983;54:363–380.

103. Ashack R, Farber MO, Weinberger M, Robertson G, Fineberg N, Manfredi F. Renal and hormonal responses to acute hypoxia in normal individuals. *J Lab Clin Med.* 1985;106:12–16.

104. Anand IS, Chandrashekhar Y. Fluid metabolism at high altitudes. In: Marriott BM, Carlson SJ, eds. *Nutritional Needs in Cold and High-Altitude Environments.* Washington, DC: National Academy Press; 1996: 331–356.

105. Pugh LGCE. Physiological and medical aspects of the Himalayan Scientific and Mountaineering Expedition, 1960–61. *Br Med J.* 1962;2:621–627.

106. Surks MI, Beckwitt HJ, Chidsey CA. Changes in plasma thyroxine concentration and metabolism, catecholamine excretion and basal oxygen consumption in man during acute exposure to high altitude. *J Clin Endocrinol.* 1967;27:789–799.

107. Cymerman A, Pandolf KB, Young AJ, Maher JT. Energy expenditure during load carriage at high altitudes. *J Appl Physiol.* 1981;51:14–18.

108. Grover RF. Basal oxygen uptake in man at high altitude. *J Appl Physiol.* 1963;18:909–912.

109. Butterfield GE, Gates J, Fleming S, Brooks GA, Sutton JR, Reeves JT. Increase energy intake minimizes weight loss in men at high altitude. *J Appl Physiol.* 1992;72:1741–1748.

110. Holloszy JO, Coyle EF. Adaptations of skeletal muscle to endurance exercise and their metabolic consequences. *J Appl Physiol.* 1984;56:831–838.

111. Arner P. Impact of exercise on adipose tissue metabolism in humans. *Int J Obes Relat Metab Disord.* 1995;19:S18–S21.

112. Sherman WM. Metabolism of sugars and physical performance. *Am J Clin Nutr.* 1995;62:228S–241S.

113. Wasserman DH. Regulation of glucose fluxes during exercise in the postabsorptive state. *Annu Rev Physiol.* 1995;57:191–218.

114. Coyle EF. Substrate utilization during exercise in active people. *Am J Clin Nutr.* 1995;61:968S–979S.

115. Brooks GA. Balance of carbohydrate and lipid utilization during exercise: The "crossover" concept. *J Appl Physiol.* 1994;76:2253–2261.

116. Conlee RK. Muscle glycogen and exercise endurance: A twenty-year perspective. In: Pandolf KB, ed. *Exercise and Sport Sciences Reviews.* New York, NY: Macmillan; 1987;15:1–28.

117. Aragon JJ, Lowenstein JM. The purine nucleotide cycle: Comparison of the levels of citric acid cycle intermediates with the operation of the purine nucleotide cycle in rat skeletal muscle during exercise and recovery from exercise. *Eur J Biochem.* 1980;110:371–377.

118. Dill DB, Edwards HT, Folling A, Oberg SA, Pappenheimer AM, Talbot JH. Adaptations of the organism to changes in oxygen pressure. *J Physiol.* 1931;71:47–63.

119. Edwards HT. Lactic acid in rest and work at high altitude. *Am J Physiol.* 1936;116:367–375.

120. Friedemann TE, Haugen GE, Kmieciak TC. The level of pyruvic and lactic acids and lactic pyruvic ratio in the blood of human subjects: The effect of food, light muscular activity, and anoxia at high altitude. *J Biol Chem.* 1945;157:673–689.

121. Harboe M. Lactic acid content in human venous blood during hypoxia at high altitude. *Acta Physiol Scand.* 1957;40:248–253.

122. Knuttgen HG, Saltin B. Oxygen uptake, muscle high-energy phosphates, and lactate in exercise under acute, hypoxic conditions in man. *Acta Physiol Scand*. 1973;87:368–376.

123. Lorentzen FV. Lactic acid in blood after various combinations of exercise and hypoxia. *J Appl Physiol*. 1962;17:661–664.

124. Hogan MC, Cox RH, Welch HG. Lactate accumulation during incremental exercise with varied inspired oxygen fractions. *J Appl Physiol*. 1983;55:1134–1140.

125. Naimark A, Jones NL, Lal S. The effect of hypoxia on gas exchange and arterial lactate and pyruvate concentration during moderate exercise in man. *Clin Sci*. 1965;28:1–13.

126. Hermansen L, Saltin B. Blood lactate concentration during exercise at acute exposure to altitude. In: Margaria R, ed. *Exercise at Altitude*. New York, NY: Excerpta Medica Foundation; 1967: 48–53.

127. Linnarsson D, Karlsson J, Fagraeus L, Saltin B. Muscle metabolites and oxygen deficit with exercise in hypoxia and hyperoxia. *J Appl Physiol*. 1974;36:399–402.

128. Dill DB, Myhre LG, Phillips EE, Brown DK. Work capacity in acute exposures to altitude. *J Appl Physiol*. 1966;21:1168–1176.

129. Boouissou P, Guezennec CY, Defer G, Pesquies P. Oxygen consumption, lactate accumulation, and sympathetic response during prolonged exercise under hypoxia. *Int J Sports Med*. 1987;8:266–269.

130. Fagraeus L, Karlsson J, Linnarsson D, Saltin B. Oxygen uptake during maximal work at lowered and raised ambient air pressures. *Acta Physiol Scand*. 1973;87:411–421.

131. McLellan T, Jacobs I, Lewis W. Acute altitude exposure and altered acid–base states, I: Effects on the exercise ventilation and blood lactate responses. *Eur J Appl Physiol*. 1988;57:435–444.

132. Maher JT, Jones LG, Hartley LH. Effects of high-altitude exposure on submaximal endurance capacity of men. *J Appl Physiol*. 1974;37:895–898.

133. Rowell LB, Blackmon JR, Kenny MA, Escourrou P. Splanchnic vasomotor and metabolic adjustments to hypoxia and exercise in humans. *Am J Physiol*. 1984;247:H251–H258.

134. Bender PR, Groves BM, McCullough RE, et al. Decreased exercise muscle lactate release after high altitude acclimatization. *J Appl Physiol*. 1989;67:1556–1462.

135. Brooks GA, Butterfield GE, Wolfe RR, et al. Decreased reliance on lactate during exercise after acclimatization to 4,300 m. *J Appl Physiol*. 1991;71:333–341.

136. Katz A, Sahlin K. Role of oxygen in regulation of glycolysis and lactate production in human skeletal muscle. In: Pandolf KB, Holloszy JO, eds. *Exercise and Sport Sciences Reviews*. Baltimore, Md: Williams & Wilkins; 1990: 1–28.

137. Stainsby WN, Brooks GA. Control of lactic acid metabolism in contracting muscles and during exercise. In: Pandolf KB, Holloszy JO, eds. *Exercise and Sport Sciences Reviews*. Baltimore, Md: Williams & Wilkins; 1990: 29–63.

138. Brooks GA, Butterfield GE, Wolfe RR, et al. Increased dependence on blood glucose after acclimatization to 4300 m. *J Appl Physiol*. 1991;70:919–927.

139. Green HJ, Sutton JR, Wolfel EE, Reeves JT, Butterfield GE, Brooks GA. Altitude acclimatization and energy metabolic adaptations in skeletal muscle during exercise. *J Appl Physiol*. 1992;73:2701–2708.

140. Hill AV, Lupton H. Muscular exercise, lactic acid and the supply and utilization of oxygen. *Q J Med*. 1923;16:135–171.

141. Horstman DH, Gleser M, Delehunt J. Effects of altering O_2 delivery on $\dot{V}O_2$ of isolated, working muscle. *Am J Physiol*. 1976;230:327–334.

142. Richter EA, Ruderman NB, Gavras H, Belur ER, Galbo H. Muscle glycogenolysis during exercise: Dual control by epinephrine and contractions. *Am J Physiol.* 1982;242:E25–E32.

143. Mazzeo RS, Bender PR, Brooks GA, et al. Arterial catecholamine responses during exercise with acute and chronic high-altitude exposure. *Am J Physiol.* 1991;261:E419–E424.

144. Cerretelli P, di Prampero PE. Aerobic and anaerobic metabolism during exercise at altitude. *Med Sports Sci.* 1985;19:1–19.

145. Grassi B, Marzorati M, Kayser B, et al. Peak blood lactate and blood lactate vs workload during acclimatization to 5050 m and in deacclimatization. *J Appl Physiol.* 1996;80:685–692.

146. Green HJ, Sutton J, Young P, Cymerman A, Houston CS. Operation Everest II: Muscle energetics during maximal exhaustive exercise. *J Appl Physiol.* 1989;66:142–150.

147. Green HJ, Sutton JR, Cymerman A, Young PM, Houston CS. Operation Everest II: Adaptations in human skeletal muscle. *J Appl Physiol.* 1989;66:2454–2461.

148. Young AJ, Young PM, McCullough RE, Moore LG, Cymerman A, Reeves JT. Effect of beta-adrenergic blockade on plasma lactate concentration during exercise at high altitude. *Eur J Appl Physiol.* 1991;63:315–322.

149. Young AJ, Evans WJ, Fisher EC, Sharp RL, Costill DL, Maher JT. Skeletal muscle metabolism of sea level natives following short-term high altitude residence. *Eur J Appl Physiol.* 1984;52:463–466.

150. Roberts AC, Butterfield GE, Cymerman A, Reeves JT, Wolfel EE, Brooks GA. Acclimatization to 4,300-m altitude decreases reliance on fat as a substrate. *J Appl Physiol.* 1996;81:1762–1771.

151. Cunningham WL, Becker EJ, Kreuzer F. Catecholamines in plasma and urine at high altitude. *J Appl Physiol.* 1965;20:607–610.

152. Richalet JP, Le-Trong JL, Rathat C, et al. Reversal of hypoxia-induced decrease in human cardiac response to isoproterenol infusion. *J Appl Physiol.* 1989;67:523–527.

153. Richalet JP, Larmignat P, Rathat C, Keromes A, Baud P, Lhoste F. Decreased cardiac response to isoproterenol infusion in acute and chronic hypoxia. *J Appl Physiol.* 1988;65:1957–1961.

154. Young PM, Sutton JR, Green HJ, et al. Operation Everest II: Metabolic and hormonal responses to incremental exercise to exhaustion. *J Appl Physiol.* 1992;73:2574–2579.

155. Kullmer T, Gabriel H, Jungmann E, et al. Increase of serum insulin and stable c-peptide concentrations with exhaustive incremental graded exercise during acute hypoxia in sedentary subjects. *Exp Clin Endocrinol Diabetes.* 1995;103:156–161.

156. Young PM, Rock PB, Fulco CS, Trad LA, Forte VA, Cymerman A. Altitude acclimatization attenuates plasma ammonia accumulation during submaximal exercise. *J Appl Physiol.* 1987;63:758–764.

157. Young PM, Rose MS, Sutton JR, Green HJ, Cymerman A, Houston CS. Operation Everest II: Plasma lipid and hormonal responses during a simulated ascent of Mt Everest. *J Appl Physiol.* 1989;66:1430–1435.

158. Rastogi GK, Malhotra MS, Srivastava MC, et al. Study of the pituitary-thyroid functions at high altitude in man. *J Clin Endocrinol Metab.* 1977;44:447–452.

159. Stock MJ, Chapman C, Stirling JL, Campbell IT. Effects of exercise, altitude, and food on blood hormone and metabolite levels. *J Appl Physiol.* 1978;45:350–354.

160. Mordes JP, Blume FD, Boyer S, Zheng MR, Braverman LE. High-altitude pituitary-thyroid function on Mount Everest. *N Engl J Med.* 1983;308:1135–1138.

161. Claybaugh JR, Wade CE, Cucinell SA. Fluid and electrolyte balance and hormonal response to the hypoxic environment. In: Claybaugh JR, Wade CE, eds. *Hormonal Regulation of Fluid and Electrolytes*. New York, NY: Plenum; 1989: 187–214.

162. Maher JT, Jones LG, Hartley LH, Williams GH, Rose LI. Aldosterone dynamics during graded exercise at sea level and high altitude. *J Appl Physiol*. 1975;39:18–22.

163. Milledge JS, Catley DM, Williams ES, Withey WR, Minty BD. Effect of prolonged exercise at altitude on the renin–aldosterone system. *J Appl Physiol*. 1983;55:413–418.

164. Weil JV, Byrne-Quinn E, Battock DJ, Grover RF, Chidsey CA. Forearm circulation in man at high altitude. *Clin Sci*. 1971;40:235–246.

165. Wiel JV, Battock DJ, Grover RF, Chidsey CA. Venoconstriction in man upon ascent to high altitude: Studies on potential mechanisms. *Fed Proc*. 1969;28:1160–1162.

166. Raff H, Janowski BM, Engeland WC, Oaks MK. Hypoxia in vivo inhibits aldosterone synthesis and aldosterone synthase mRNA in rats. *J Appl Physiol*. 1996;81:604–610.

167. Winslow RM. High-altitude polycythemia. In: West JB, Lahiri S, eds. *High Altitude and Man*. Bethesda, Md: American Physiological Society; 1984: 163–172.

168. Abbrecht PH, Littell JK. Plasma erythropoietin in men and mice during acclimatization to different altitudes. *J Appl Physiol*. 1972;32:54–58.

169. Gunga HC, Kirsch K, Rocker L, Schobersberger W. Time course of erythropoietin, triiodothyronine, thyroxine and thyroid-stimulating hormone at 2,315 m. *J Appl Physiol*. 1994;76:1068–1072.

170. Gunga HC, Rocker L, Behn C, et al. Shift working in the Chilean Andes (> 3,600 m) and its influence on erythropoietin and the low-pressure system. *J Appl Physiol*. 1996;81:846–852.

171. Richalet JP, Souberbielle JC, Antezana AM, et al. Control of erythropoiesis in humans during prolonged exposure to the altitude of 6,542 m. *Am J Physiol*. 1994;266:R756–R764.

172. Wagner PD. An integrated view of the determinants of maximum oxygen uptake. In: Gonzales NC, Fedde MR, eds. *Oxygen Transfer From Atmosphere to Tissues*. New York, NY: Plenum Press; 1988: 245–256.

173. Reeves JT, Groves BM, Cymerman A, et al. Cardiac filling pressures during cycle exercise at sea level. *Respir Physiol*. 1990;80:147–154.

174. Cymerman A, Reeves JT, Sutton JR, et al. Operation Everest II: Maximal oxygen uptake at extreme altitude. *J Appl Physiol*. 1989;66:2446–2453.

175. Khanna PK, Dham SK, Hoon RS. Exercise in an hypoxic environment as a screening test for ischaemic heart disease. *Aviat Space Environ Med*. 1976;47:1114–1117.

Chapter 22

PHYSICAL PERFORMANCE AT VARYING TERRESTRIAL ALTITUDES

CHARLES S. FULCO, ScD[*]; AND ALLEN CYMERMAN, PhD[†]

INTRODUCTION

PHYSICAL PERFORMANCE
    The Effects of Altitude on Maximal Aerobic Power
    Submaximal Exercise Performance
    Muscle Strength and Power

PRACTICAL ASPECTS OF HUMAN PERFORMANCE AT ALTITUDE
    The Effects of Altitude on Military Occupational Tasks
    Practical Guidelines for Military Operational Planning at Altitude
    Training Strategies for Improving Exercise Performance at Altitude

SUMMARY

ATTACHMENT: DATA SOURCES FOR GRAPHS

[*]*Research Physiologist*
[†]*Team Leader, Research Physiologist, Thermal and Mountain Medicine Division, US Army Research Institute of Environmental Medicine, 42 Kansas Street, Natick, Massachusetts 01760-5007*

INTRODUCTION

The study of physical performance has long been of interest to the military. Scientific studies of military members performing a variety of tasks were among the earliest nonclinical investigations in the area of applied physiological research.[1,2] For example, numerous reports have described the energy cost of marching at various speeds with and without loads under controlled conditions.[1,3–8] It is well accepted that external stresses such as increased load carriage and rugged terrain features can lead to decreases in functional capacities. Yet, despite the considerable mechanization of the modern military, service members still have the burdensome task of carrying essential, often heavy equipment. In mountainous regions, the load carried will almost certainly increase—owing to the additional weight of protective clothing and technical equipment. Other factors that have profound negative influence on military operations in the mountains include steep, rugged, and constantly changing terrain; unpredictable weather conditions; snow-covered ground; and mountain sickness.[9,10] Military physical performance in the mountains may also be adversely affected by sleep deprivation; increased physical or emotional stress, or both; caloric and fluid restrictions; reduced visibility; equipment failures; inadequate communications; and lack of specialized medical equipment.[11]

The hypoxia (ie, low inspired oxygen pressure) associated with mountain (ie, actual) or altitude (ie, experimental) exposures reduces sustained physical performance capabilities to a degree directly proportional to the elevation, with the magnitude of the reduction associated with initial exposure usually greater than that associated with continued exposure. Because of hypoxia-induced physical performance decrements, military personnel rapidly transported from low to high terrestrial elevations should not be committed immediately to patrolling operations, entrenchment, combat, or other physically demanding duties, nor should they be expected to perform as well as they did at sea level.[9] Although it is generally accepted that more-frequent rest breaks, increased time for task completion, and a reduction in the number of daily tasks will be required for proper recovery and should be included in operational planning, the combination of all the above factors makes it difficult or impossible to precisely predict the extent of the negative impact on unit effectiveness that an operation will encounter, or to provide exact guidelines to improve mission success. Mountaineering training (provided by sites such as the Northern Warfare Training Center at Fort Greely, Alaska; the Marine Mountain Warfare Training Center, Bridgeport, California; and the Mountain Warfare Training Site, Jericho, Vermont) is essential to fully appreciate the complexity of the problems to be encountered in mountain environments.

Initially, interest in the human capacity to do physical work at altitude was primarily stimulated by early mountaineering experiences.[12,13] Although mountain climbing is strenuous and can require high levels of skill, the focus of a noncompetitive climb is often related more to successfully completing mountaineering tasks and enjoying the scenery than in climbing the greatest distance in the shortest time. Conversely, military service members are deployed to mountain areas on the basis of their units' mission, and not for recreation or personal challenge. Tactical operations dictate the timing, duration, and location of the mission, often exposing service members to terrain and environmental conditions that would usually not be considered recreational.[11]

Occupational requirements for military operations, mining, aviation, and space science stimulated research that focused on functional limitations, adjustments, and processes of acclimatization at altitudes greater than 3,000 m during rest and low-to-moderate intensity activities.[14,15] Even though in the first half of the 20th century one third of the world's population lived above an altitude of 2,000 m,[16] few early physiological investigations had been conducted in the low-to-moderate altitude range between 2,000 and 3,000 m. [Other experts in epidemiology use a different estimate—a number considerably lower but still enormous—of the world's population living at high altitude: for example, by the 1990s nearly 140 million people resided above 2,500 m (8,000 ft).[17,18]—RFB, ed.] Not until reports of subnormal athletic performances in the longer-lasting events in the 1955 Pan American Games and the 1962 World Pentathlon World Championships in Mexico City (2,300 m), and the 1959 National Amateur Athletic Union at Boulder, Colorado (1,630 m),[19–21] did scientific investigations include the effects of hypoxic stress of more moderate altitudes.

The choice of Mexico City in 1963 as the site for the 19th Olympiad in 1968 stimulated much research on the effects of altitude.[22] International symposia in Switzerland (1965), the United States (1966) and Italy (1967) summarized findings from research and competitive athletic sources and made recommendations to the International Olympic Committee for the 1968 Olympics. Many,[19,23–26] although not all,[27–30] reports from this period indicated that acute altitude exposure impaired exercise performance, while residing or training (or both) at altitude greatly improved altitude maximal or submaximal exercise performances. At this time, it also became apparent that during altitude training and competition, the exercise performance of some but not all athletes was adversely affected, for reasons not well understood.[24,26] Not surprisingly, coaches and representatives of sea-level countries were concerned that

- residence and exercise training at altitude would confer an unfair advantage over those who resided and trained at sea level;
- it was not appropriate to conduct the Olympic trials at lower altitudes to choose individuals for competitions at higher elevations; and
- the moderate elevation of Mexico City would be deleterious to the health of elite athletes coming from sea level.

Although previous competitions at moderate altitudes had provided a general knowledge of what was to be expected from a low-altitude athlete competing at a higher altitude, much of the available information was incomplete or contradictory. For example, recommendations made to the International Olympic Committee for the length of time an endurance athlete should train at altitude prior to competition ranged from less than 48 hours[16] to a minimum of 4 to 6 weeks.[31] Resolution of many of these issues was seen as having important implications for potential military deployment and conflict at altitude.[5]

Since the 1968 Olympics, interest in the effects of altitude residence and exercise training on physical performance at altitude or sea level for civilians and military has not waned.[32] Intensive study by many research, sport, and military organizations has provided some answers to questions regarding the effects of altitude exposure on physical performance. While there appears to be a consensus in the scientific literature that endurance exercise training at altitude improves exercise performance at altitude,[33] controversy still exists whether endurance training or residence at altitude improves subsequent sea-level endurance performance.[34–37]

PHYSICAL PERFORMANCE

The Effects of Altitude on Maximal Aerobic Power

The ability to perform sustained aerobic muscular exercise is assessed using the maximal rate of oxygen uptake ($\dot{V}o_2max$). This widely used performance index is reproducible[38,39] and generally accepted as the single best measure of the functional limit of the respiratory and circulatory systems to deliver oxygen to active muscles and the ability of the active muscles to utilize the oxygen delivered.[40] Maximal aerobic power can be affected by factors that alter any of the processes involved in oxygen transport or utilization. At altitude, a person is exposed to a progressive decrease in atmospheric pressure, with resultant declines in inspired, alveolar, and arterial oxygen pressures. As a consequence of the progressive hypoxia associated with increasing altitude, $\dot{V}o_2max$ declines at a rate inversely proportional to the elevation.[41]

Figure 22-1 illustrates the relationship of the measured percentage of decline in $\dot{V}o_2max$ with increasing actual or simulated elevations (ie, hypobaric chambers or breathing hypoxic gas). The wide range of the mean percentage of decline in $\dot{V}o_2max$ at nearly all altitudes reflects variability owing to differences in experimental design and procedures and physiological differences among subjects (Exhibit 22-1).

The relative contributions of these sources of variation to $\dot{V}o_2max$ decrement differences at a given altitude have yet to be quantified. It is important to note that even under ideal experimental conditions at sea level, owing to measurement error and individual biological variation, 68% of the time values of $\dot{V}o_2max$ for repeat tests can vary by as much as $\pm 5.6\%$; and 98% of the time can vary by as much as $\pm 11.2\%$.[39]

The mean data points in Figure 22-1 represent a database derived from literature sources. The regression line generated from these data provides a visual reference. Systematically isolating and grouping an adequate number of studies with similar experimental designs or subject characteristics from within this database, and then comparing the relative positions of the subgroupings to the entire database, allows a qualitative assessment of the relative importance of various factors in accounting for the total variation.

Fig. 22-1. Maximum oxygen consumption ($\dot{V}O_2$max) decreases with increasing elevation. Each of the 146 points (unfilled circles) on the graph represents a mean value derived from 65 different civilian and military investigations[*] conducted at altitudes from 580 m[1] to 8,848 m.[2,3] Multiple mean data points for a study were included if the study entailed more than one of the following: (1) elevation, (2) group of test subjects, or (3) exposure duration. For studies using hypoxic gas mixtures, inspired oxygen values were converted to altitude equivalents. Mean values are reported because they were the only values common to all investigations. A database regression line (thick curvilinear line) was drawn using the 146 points. Because each of these data points is a mean value of many intrainvestigation individual determinations of $\dot{V}O_2$max, the regression line represents possibly thousands of $\dot{V}O_2$max test values and therefore provides a truer approximation for the expected average decrement at each elevation. Also included are the regression lines of Buskirk and colleagues[4] (dashed line) and Grover and colleagues[5] (dotted line), which represent two of the most-often-quoted relationships of the decrement in

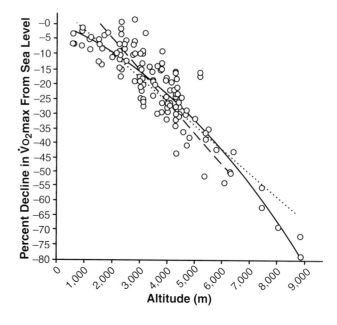

$\dot{V}O_2$max to an increase in elevation. Reproduced with permission from Fulco CS, Rock PB, Cymerman A. Maximal and submaximal exercise performance at altitude. *Aviat Space Environ Med.* 1998;67(8):794.
Sources for the figure legend: (1) Gore CJ, Hahn AG, Scroop GS, et al. Increased arterial desaturation in trained cyclists during maximal exercise at 580 m altitude. *J Appl Physiol.* 1996;80:2204–2210. (2) Cymerman A, Reeves JT, Sutton JR, et al. Operation Everest II: Maximal oxygen uptake at extreme altitude. *J Appl Physiol.* 1989;66(5):2446–2453. (3) West JB, Boyer SJ, Graber DJ, et al. Maximal exercise at extreme altitudes on Mount Everest. *J Appl Physiol.* 1983;55:688–698. (4) Buskirk ER, Kollias J, Picon-Reategui E, Akers R, Prokop E, Baker P. Physiology and performance of track athletes at various altitudes in the United States and Peru. In: Goddard RF, ed. *The Effects of Altitude on Physical Performance.* Albuquerque, NM: The Athletic Institute; 1967: 65–72. (5) Grover RF, Weil JV, Reeves JT. Cardiovascular adaptation to exercise at high altitude. In: Pandolf KB, ed. *Exercise and Sport Science Reviews.* 14th ed. New York, NY: Macmillian; 1986: 269–302.
[*]Sources for the data points are contained in the Attachment at the end of this chapter.

Minimal Altitude for Decrement of, and the Rate of Decline in, Maximal Aerobic Power

Figure 22-1 shows the minimal altitude at which a decrease in $\dot{V}O_2$max has been detected and the rate at which it declines with increasing elevation. Three regression lines have been drawn: one representing data of the current database and the other two representing the more commonly cited relationships in the scientific literature.[42,43] The largest differences between the three lines occur at the lowest and the highest altitudes but the data points at all three lines are at similar locations at the intermediate altitudes. Buskirk and colleagues[42] suggested that there is minimal decrement in $\dot{V}O_2$max until approximately 1,524 m, with an average linear decline of 3.2% for every additional 305 m of altitude (dashed line). When this relationship was first proposed in 1966, the altitude at which $\dot{V}O_2$max began to decline and whether the $\dot{V}O_2$max decline remained linear at the

higher altitudes were not apparent, because there was a paucity of data at altitudes less than 2,500 m and greater than 6,000 m. In more recent years, $\dot{V}O_2$max has been determined in subjects of varying fitness levels at lower[44–59] and higher[60,61] altitudes. Using information from some of these studies,[57,61] Grover, Weil, and Reeves[43] suggested in 1986 that the decline in $\dot{V}O_2$max begins at about 700 m, with a linear reduction of 8% for every additional 1,000 m of altitude up to approximately 6,300 m. In support of their contention, Jackson and Sharkey[34] reported in 1988 that athletes who reside at sea level and train at the Olympic Training Center in Colorado Springs, Colorado (altitude 1,881 m), exhibit a loss in $\dot{V}O_2$max of approximately 1% for every 305 m of ascent above sea level (this line is not shown in Figure 22-1). Consistent with these reports,[34,43] Gore and colleagues[62] reported in 1996 that at 580 m, $\dot{V}O_2$max declines 3.6% in fit, untrained individuals (statistically not significant) and 7% in elite ath-

EXHIBIT 22-1

POTENTIAL SOURCES OF VARIATION OF THE MEAN PERCENTAGE OF DECLINE IN $\dot{V}O_2MAX$ IN COMPETITION AT ALTITUDE

- Subjects' fitness levels
- Residence at altitude prior to a study
- Subjects' gender
- Changes in conditioning level resulting from increased activity during the exposure
- Subjects' smoking status
- Subjects' motivation
- Subjects' age
- Hypoxic ventilatory response
- Altitude sickness (acute mountain sickness, high-altitude pulmonary edema, and high-altitude cerebral edema)
- Sample size
- Rate of ascent to altitude
- Duration of exposure (eg, acute vs chronic)
- Timing of $\dot{V}O_2$max measurements (eg, preacclimatazation and postacclimatization)
- Differences between training and exercise testing modes
- Use of inappropriate exercise mode (eg, elite runners tested with bicycle ergometers)
- Altitude-induced muscle wasting

Sources: (1) Dill DB, Adams WC. Maximal oxygen uptake at sea level and at 3,090-m altitude in high school champion runners. *J Appl Physiol.* 1971;30:854–859. (2) Faulkner JA, Kollias J, Favour CB, Buskirk ER, Balke B. Maximum aerobic capacity and running performance at altitude. *J Appl Physiol.* 1968;24:685–691. (3) Hansen JE, Vogel JA, Stelter GP, Consolazio CF. Oxygen uptake in man during exhaustive work at sea level and high altitude. *J Appl Physiol.* 1967;23:511–522. (4) Jackson CG, Sharkey BJ. Altitude, training and human performance. *Sports Med.* 1988;6:279–284. (5) Kollias J, Buskirk ER. Exercise and altitude. In: Johnson WR; Buskirk ER, eds. *Science and Medicine of Exercise and Sport.* 2nd ed. New York: Harper and Row; 1974: 211–227. (6) Howley ET, Bassett DR Jr, Welch HG. Criteria for maximal oxygen uptake: Review and commentary. *Med Sci Sports Exerc.* 1995;27:1292–1301. (7) Berglund B. High-altitude training: Aspects of haematological adaptation. *Sports Med.* 1992;14:289–303. (8) Boutellier U, Marconi C, Di Prampero PE, Cerretelli P. Effects of chronic hypoxia on maximal performance. *Bull Europ Physiopath Resp.* 1982;18:39–44. (9) Buskirk ER, Kollias J, Picon-Reategui E, Akers R, Prokop E, Baker P. Physiology and performance of track athletes at various altitudes in the United States and Peru. In: Goddard RF, ed. *The Effects of Altitude on Physical Performance.* Albuquerque, NM: The Athletic Institute; 1967: 65–72. (10) Dill DB, Hillyard SD, Miller J. Vital capacity, exercise performance, and blood gases at altitude as related to age. *J Appl Physiol.* 1980;48:6–9. (11) Dill DB, Robinson S, Balke B, Newton JL. Work tolerance: Age and altitude. *J Appl Physiol.* 1964;19:483–488. (12) Lawler J, Powers SK, Thompson D. Linear relationship between $\dot{V}O_2$ and $\dot{V}O_2$max decrement during exposure to acute altitude. *J Appl Physiol.* 1988;64:1486–1492. (13) Schoene RB, Lahiri S, Hackett PH, et al. Relationship of hypoxic ventilatory response to exercise performance on Mount Everest. *J Appl Physiol.* 1984;56:1478–1483. (14) Shephard RJ, Bouhlel E, Vandewalle H, Monod H. Peak oxygen uptake and hypoxia. *Int J Sports Med.* 1988;9:279–283. (15) Terrados N, Melichna J, Sylven C, Jansson E, Kaijser L. Effects of training at simulated altitude on performance and muscle metabolic capacity in competitive road cyclists. *Eur J Appl Physiol Med.* 1988;57:203–209. (16) Young AJ, Cymerman A, Burse RL. The influence of cardiorespiratory fitness on the decrement in maximal aerobic power at high altitude. *Eur J Appl Physiol Med.* 1985;54:12–15.

letes. Even acknowledging the problems with accuracy and sensitivity of $\dot{V}O_2$max measurement techniques,[39] these and other data presented in Figure 22-1 suggest that small declines in $\dot{V}O_2$max begin at a much lower altitude than had been previously assumed by Buskirk and colleagues[42] and by Grover, Weil, and Reeves.[43] In addition, it would appear from Figure 22-1 that there is a more rapid, nonlinear decline in $\dot{V}O_2$max at altitudes in excess of approximately 6,300 m. This more rapid decline may be linked with reduced blood flow, reduction of muscle mass, or metabolic deterioration, conditions that in any combination are often associated with chronic hypoxic exposure.[60,63–66]

Fitness Level and Maximal Aerobic Power Variability

The subgroupings in Figure 22-2 to Figure 22-5, separate discussions of which follow, were limited to the factors of fitness level, prealtitude exposure elevation, gender, and altitude duration, respectively. Other factors such as age or smoking status could not likewise be assessed because of a paucity of published reports at altitude on such topics. The intent is not to present a broad statistical relation-

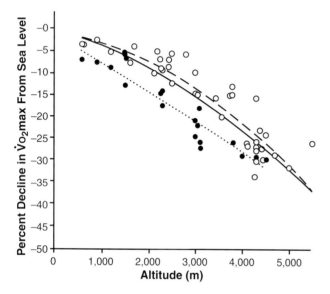

Fig. 22-2. The effect of fitness level on the variability of the decrement of $\dot{V}O_2$max is depicted in studies of highly conditioned (baseline altitude $\dot{V}O_2$max was ≥ 63 mL/kg/min, closed circles)[*] and less-well-conditioned ($\dot{V}O_2$max was ≤ 51 mL/kg/min, open circles)[†] individuals. Only mean data points based on objective fitness criteria (ie, $\dot{V}O_2$max normalized to body weight and measured at the preexposure, resident altitude) are included. Studies that used only descriptive terms such as "highly fit," "well-conditioned," or "trained" to characterize subjects were not included. To minimize possible confounding effects of altitude acclimatization and/or physical conditioning changes due to training while at altitude, data collected beyond the first 3 days of altitude exposure were also excluded. Regression lines for the highly conditioned (dotted line) and less-well-conditioned (dashed line) individuals, as well as the database regression line (solid line), which is redrawn from Figure 22-1 but truncated at 5,500 m altitude, are included. Reproduced with permission from Fulco CS, Rock PB, Cymerman A. Maximal and submaximal exercise performance at altitude. *Aviat Space Environ Med*. 1998;67(8):794.
Sources for the data points for highly conditioned[*] and less-well-conditioned[†] individuals are found in the Attachment at the end of this chapter.

ship but rather to provide an appreciation and perspective of the wide range of factors that modify the decrement in $\dot{V}O_2$max that occurs with altitude exposure.

Figure 22-2 indicates that highly fit (≥ 63 mL/kg/min) individuals (represented in the graph by closed circles) generally have a larger decrement in $\dot{V}O_2$max at altitude than less fit (≤ 51 mL/kg/min) individuals (open circles). Although the data presented were dichotomized to compare widely differing fitness levels, the amount of decline in $\dot{V}O_2$max at a given altitude is inversely related to the degree of fitness, but within a much narrower range than is apparent in Figure 22-2, and seems to exist on a continuum.[67–69] For example, Young, Cymerman, and Burse[68] compiled data from several studies that used a relatively homogeneous group of subjects (51 young, male soldiers) whose values for sea-level $\dot{V}O_2$max were normally distributed from 36 to 60 mL/kg/min. In those studies, the $\dot{V}O_2$max decrement at 4,300 m altitude was greater for the more highly fit subjects ($\dot{V}O_2$max decrement = $\dot{V}O_2$max decrement = $0.52 - 11.39 \cdot \dot{V}O_2$max [sea level], r = 0.56, $P < .05$). At extreme altitudes ($> 7,000$ m), however, there is some evidence suggesting that the difference in $\dot{V}O_2$max decrement owing to fitness levels diminishes.[60] Nevertheless, the collective results indicate that much of the variability in $\dot{V}O_2$max decrement at altitudes up to at least 5,500 m is closely associated with prealtitude exposure fitness levels. Of the studies used to prepare Figure 22-2 that directly compared high with moderate-to-low fitness levels,[49,58,67,70] the greater $\dot{V}O_2$max decrement in the more-fit subjects was associated with pulmonary gas–exchange limitations, evidenced by lower arterial blood saturations that were exacerbated during hypoxic exercise (see Chapter 21, Human Adaptation to High Terrestrial Altitude).

Prealtitude Exposure Elevation and Maximal Aerobic Power Variability

Figure 22-3 demonstrates that the regression lines of the prealtitude exposure elevation—the elevation where experimental, prealtitude exposure baseline data were collected—lower than 100 m do not differ meaningfully from the database regression line. However, mean values for prealtitude exposure elevations higher than 400 m tend to fall above the low baseline altitude and the database regression lines, especially in the range of 2,200 m to 4,300 m altitude. Therefore, the potential $\dot{V}O_2$max decrement measured at any altitude would be lessened if experimental, prealtitude exposure baseline data are

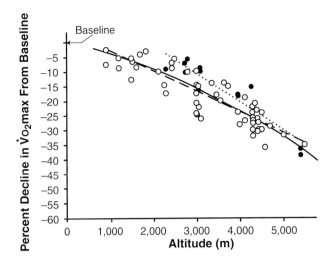

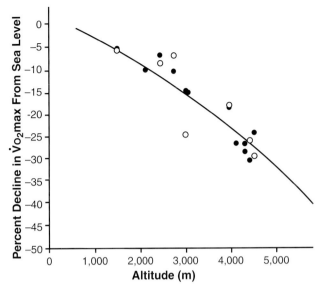

Fig. 22-3. The effects of a difference in prealtitude expo-sure elevations on $\dot{V}O_2$max decrement variability are shown from two subgroupings of studies: those whose baseline resident altitudes were lower than 100 m (open circles)[*] and those whose baseline resident altitudes were higher than 400 m (closed circles).[†] Regression lines were cal-culated for the lower baseline-resident elevations (dashed line) and higher baseline-resident elevations (dotted line) and compared with the database regression line (solid line), which is redrawn from Figure 22-1 but truncated at 5,500 m altitude. To minimize possible confounding effects of changes due to altitude acclimatization and/or physical conditioning while residing at the experimen-tal altitude, only data collected within the first 3 days of hypobaric hypoxia or during hypoxic gas breathing were included. Reproduced with permission from Fulco CS, Rock PB, Cymerman A. Maximal and submaximal exer-cise performance at altitude. *Aviat Space Environ Med.* 1998;67(8):795.
Sources for the data points for baseline resident altitudes < 100 m[*] and > 400 m[†] are found in the Attachment at the end of this chapter.

Fig. 22-4. Gender comparison of the $\dot{V}O_2$max decrement at altitude. Data were derived from seven studies[*] in which $\dot{V}O_2$max decline was reported for women (closed circles) during altitude exposure or during hypoxic gas mixture breathing. Also included are the mean results for men (open circles) from the four of these studies[†] in which direct gender comparisons were made. Data are plotted against the database regression line of Figure 22-1, truncated at 5,500 m. For all seven studies, $\dot{V}O_2$max was measured within an hour of altitude exposure or hypoxic gas mixture breathing. Reproduced with permission from Fulco CS, Rock PB, Cymerman A. Maximal and submax-imal exercise performance at altitude. *Aviat Space Environ Med.* 1998;67(8):796.
Sources for the data points for women[*] and men[†] dur-ing altitude exposure or breathing hypoxic gas mixtures are found in the Attachment at the end of this chapter.

collected at elevations of 400 m or higher. These data indicate that some of the interstudy variability ob-served in $\dot{V}O_2$max decrements at a given higher al-titude is likely due to differences in the elevation where the prealtitude exposure baseline values were obtained.

Gender and Maximal Aerobic Power Variability

Data presented in Figure 22-4 suggest there is no difference between men and women in the percent-age of $\dot{V}O_2$max decrement at altitude; both genders had similar decrements compared with the database regression line of Figure 22-1. In addition, the only reported altitude study controlling for menstrual cycle phase[71] indicated that the $\dot{V}O_2$max decline from sea

level to 4,300 m was not significantly different be-tween early follicular and midluteal cycle phases or different from the database regression line, indi-cating little, if any, effect of cycle menstrual cycle phase.

Altitude Exposure Duration and Maximal Aerobic Power Variability

In Figure 22-5, data from chronic (> 10 d) alti-tude studies or exercise training studies and acute (< 2 h) hypoxic-exposure studies were compared, in an effort to provide a means to assess increases in variation due to changes in physical condition-ing at altitude, altitude acclimatization, or both. The mean decline in the acute altitude-exposure stud-ies lies within two standard deviations of the re-gression line of the database (see Figure 22-1), while

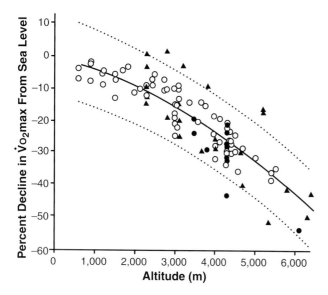

Fig. 22-5. Athletic training, trekking expeditions, and altitude acclimatization all affect the variability of $\dot{V}O_2$max decrement. The studies illustrated represent mean declines in $\dot{V}O_2$max during acute hypobaric hypoxia or hypoxic gas breathing (< 2 h, open circles),[*] altitude acclimatization (± 10 days, closed circles),[†] long-term altitude training,[‡] and trekking[§] (closed triangles). Also shown are the database regression line (——) and ± 2 SD lines (⋯). Reproduced with permission from Fulco CS, Rock PB, Cymerman A. Maximal and submaximal exercise performance at altitude. *Aviat Space Environ Med.* 1998;67(8):796. [*]Sources for the data points for acute hypobaric hypoxia or hypoxic gas breathing,[*] altitude acclimatization,[†] long-term altitude training,[‡] and trekking[§] are found in the Attachment at the end of this chapter.

the mean decline of some of the chronic altitude-exposure studies falls within, and some outside, this range. The studies showing the least decline in mean $\dot{V}O_2$max during chronic exposures to altitudes of 5,200 m or lower were composed of subjects who were neither endurance athletes nor highly conditioned. It is likely that the subjects in these studies improved their fitness level while at altitude.[19,25,63]

The variability of the mean decrements in $\dot{V}O_2$max for exercise training studies involving chronic exposures and using highly conditioned subjects ($\dot{V}O_2$max was > 63 mL/kg/min)[24,27,28,45,72] was indistinguishable from that of the acute altitude-exposure studies (ie, the subjects maintained their fitness levels). Three other studies[60,66,73] of chronic altitude exposure had mean $\dot{V}O_2$max declines at or below the lower standard deviation range line. Two were nonexercise training studies[60,66] in which subjects became detrained owing to reduced activity levels at altitude; in one,[60] a re-

duced muscle mass was documented,[65] which may have reduced maximal exercise capabilities. The third study comprised members of a trekking expedition,[73] whose relatively poor performance during maximal testing likely also resulted from factors such as a reduced muscle mass.

The data presented in Figure 22-5 suggest that if the level of physical condition is not altered significantly by increases in activity or exercise training or by physical deterioration, the magnitude of decline in $\dot{V}O_2$max and the amount of variability at each altitude stays relatively constant during chronic compared with acute altitude exposure. In addition, the data from studies in which daily physical activity was light to moderate (and thus did not provide a sufficient training stimulus that resulted in a $\dot{V}O_2$max increase) do not support the concept that simply residing at altitude improves oxygen transport to an extent that improves $\dot{V}O_2$max.

Submaximal Exercise Performance

Oxygen uptake, or the "metabolic cost" for a particular exercise activity performed at a specified rate (ie, power output), is similar at sea level and altitude.[74–76] But because $\dot{V}O_2$max progressively declines with increasing elevation, a fixed power output represents a progressively greater *relative* exercise intensity (ie, a higher percentage of $\dot{V}O_2$max) as the elevation increases. The practical implication is that it is more difficult to perform submaximal exercise (or work) at a fixed power output at altitude than at sea level. The impairment will be most conspicuous in those activities in which a given distance must be traversed in the least amount of time (eg, a 5-km competitive race), or which involve sustained, arduous exercise that utilizes many muscle groups.[4,10,21,22,77,78] However, it is difficult to predict accurately both (a) the magnitude of an individual's submaximal exercise impairment from the $\dot{V}O_2$max decrement at altitude, and (b) an individual's likely success in exercise events or work activities relative to a similar group of individuals at altitude.[19,79,80]

One reason submaximal exercise performance decrements are hard to predict from the decline in $\dot{V}O_2$max is that $\dot{V}O_2$max measures only the maximal aerobic contribution, whereas exercise episodes of various intensities and durations involve differing proportions of aerobic and anaerobic processes.[26,40] A 400-m, 50-second lap for champion runners at sea level, for example, might require approximately 20% aerobic and 80% anaerobic processes; for a

1,500 m, 4-minute run, the proportion may be 60% to 40%; and for a 5-km, 14-minute run, 90% to 10%.[26,40] Moreover, at altitude, compared with at sea level, there is a reduction in the rate of reaching steady-state oxygen uptake[74,81] that effectively increases the anaerobic component for all distances, and further decreases the accuracy of predicting some submaximal exercise performance impairments. In addition, unlike the objectivity of the $\dot{V}O_2$max "plateau" that indicates high motivation and assures maximal short-term effort,[38] there are no similar criteria for assuring submaximal exercise performance. Therefore, submaximal exercise performance differences due to changes in motivation levels or other factors (eg, such as lack of skill and experience; inability to tolerate pain[29]) are unaccounted for and may significantly but unquantifiably alter the final outcome. All these reasons are likely to induce at least as much variability in submaximal exercise performance at altitude as that associated with the $\dot{V}O_2$max decrement (see Figure 22-1).

One factor that may benefit exercise performance in some athletic events at altitude is the lessened air resistance due to the reduced air density. At a typical exercise training altitude of 2,300 m, the 24% reduction in air density[80] increases the distances for field events such as the shot put by 6 cm, the hammer throw by 53 cm, the javelin by 69 cm, and the discus by 162 cm.[82] For running very short distances, in which there is a small aerobic component and high velocity, the advantage of a reduction in air resistance can result in faster times at altitude than at sea level.[20,22,83] For longer duration events such as 5-and 10-km runs, the small advantage afforded by the reduced air resistance is lessened in comparison with the larger impairment linked to the $\dot{V}O_2$max reduction, and run times are slower than at sea level.[22,45,83] But for events such as speed skating and track cycling, in which velocities are much greater than in running, the reduced air resistance at altitude allows an improved performance compared with sea level.

Measuring submaximal exercise performance using laboratory testing paradigms (such as pedaling a cycle ergometer at a specific exercise intensity until volitional exhaustion) can reduce or eliminate variability due to the influences of wind resistance, skill, and experience (Figure 22-6). However, interindividual and intraindividual differences in motivation and pain tolerance still remain, especially for untrained individuals. One way to minimize such variability is to focus primarily on athletic performances during competitions. By using athletes, who represent a homogeneous group of people who are presumed to be healthy and highly

motivated and who are performing at an "all-out" effort in precisely timed events for which they are trained, the effects of altitude exposure per se on submaximal exercise performance should be more readily apparent.

As can be seen in Figure 22-7, performances in maximal-effort events lasting less than 2 minutes at sea level are not adversely affected by altitude exposure. For events lasting 2 minutes or longer, however, the times to complete events (relative to sea-level performances) tend to increase with elevation. For events lasting 2 to 5 minutes, a mean performance decrement threshold occurs at approximately 1,600 m. For events lasting longer than 20 minutes, the threshold occurs at about 600 m to 700

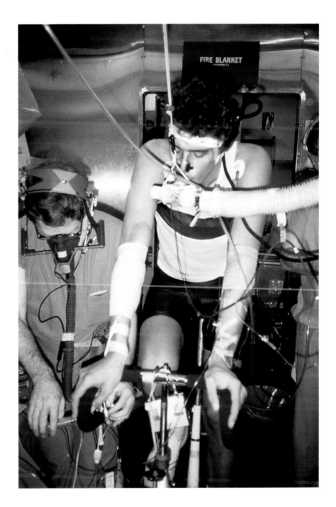

Fig. 22-6. Exercise performance is being measured at a simulated altitude of 5,500 m. The subject is acclimatized and performing heavy exercise on a bicycle ergometer in the Hypobaric Chamber at the US Army Research Institute of Environmental Medicine, Natick, Mass. Note that the unacclimatized investigators must wear oxygen masks to enable them to work at this altitude.

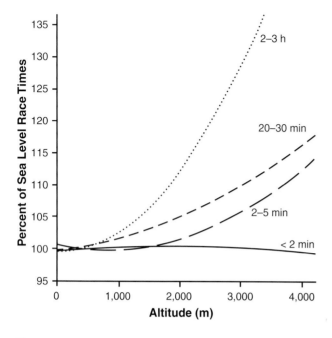

Fig. 22-7. Decrements in athletes' performance (as functions of event duration and altitude) are seen after 10 days of altitude training. The data are derived from several studies that reported results of highly conditioned athletes, primarily during running and swimming competitions,[*] who had lived and trained at altitude for at least 10 days immediately prior to competition. Altitude exposures lasting longer than 10 days were used in the analyses to minimize potentially confounding factors such as mountain sicknesses and nonfamiliarity with the altitude environment. The four regression lines were created using both individual and group data (not shown). They illustrate how sea-level performance would change for events lasting from less than 2 minutes to over 2 hours. For example, at 2,000 m altitude, events lasting less than 5 minutes at sea level would be minimally affected, while events lasting 20 to 30 minutes at sea level would be impaired by about 5%, and events lasting 2 to 3 hours would be impaired by 10% to 15%. Reproduced with permission from Fulco CS, Rock PB, Cymerman A. Maximal and submaximal exercise performance at altitude. *Aviat Space Environ Med.* 1998;67(8):797.
[*]Sources for the data points are found in the Attachment at the end of this chapter.

m, an altitude consistent with significant declines in $\dot{V}O_2$max for similar groups of highly trained subjects.[49,62] These data are consistent with the concept that the magnitude of impairment will be more closely linked to the $\dot{V}O_2$max decrement as the aerobic contribution of an event increases towards 100%. For example, events lasting 2 to 5 minutes at sea level will average about 2% longer at an altitude of

2,300 m; those lasting 20 to 30 minutes, 7% longer; and 2 to 3 hours, 17% longer (see Figure 22-2). At 2,300 m elevation, the mean percentage decline in $\dot{V}O_2$max would be expected to be approximately 15% for a similar group of highly conditioned athletes (see Figure 22-2). The approach used for this analysis can also be used for many military applications. For instance, the average 2-mile physical fitness test in personnel stationed at Fitzsimons Army Medical Center, Denver, Colorado (1,609 m), is increased by 5% (from about 16 to 17 min),[4] a value similar to the decrement that could be estimated from Figure 22-7.

Muscle Strength and Power

Muscle strength and maximal muscle power, determined by the force generated during a single, brief (1–5 sec), maximal muscle contraction (static or dynamic), are generally not adversely affected by acute or chronic altitude exposure[64,76,84–89] as long as muscle mass is maintained.[64,90,91] In addition, alpha-motoneuron excitability, nerve- and muscle-conduction velocity, and neuromuscular transmission are not impaired, even at altitudes exceeding 4,300 m.[76,88,92]

Unchanged maximal force and maximal power generation at altitude may relate to one or both of the following factors:

- maintenance of low resting levels of metabolites[74,91,94] that, if higher (as during more prolonged exercise), could potentially impair function of the contractile machinery[95,96]; and
- preservation of normal resting levels of high energy phosphates sufficient to support the rate of adenosine 5'-triphosphate (ATP) turnover (1–2 mmol/s) for brief maximal muscle performance.[97]

The amounts of ATP and phosphocreatine available at rest in humans prior to a maximal contraction are approximately 26 and 75 mmol/kg dry muscle, respectively.[93,98] Anaerobic performance[99,100] during very intense, maximal or supramaximal exercise (eg, the Wingate test) lasting 30 seconds are generally also not adversely affected at altitude.[90,101,102] For anaerobic performance assessments lasting longer than 30 seconds, there are conflicting results[90]; measurement inconsistencies of the delay and/or the rate of rise of $\dot{V}O_2$ may be contributory factors.[74,81]

PRACTICAL ASPECTS OF HUMAN PERFORMANCE AT ALTITUDE

The Effects of Altitude on Military Occupational Tasks

It is obvious that military personnel are involved in many physical activities other than athletic events (eg, running). Such activities are typically work- or mission-specific and can encompass extremely light to very demanding efforts that use different muscle groups for varying periods of time. In a sense, many work-related tasks have similarities to exercise performance in terms of effort intensity, volumes of active muscle involved, and activity duration. Therefore, the principles discussed above for exercise performance decrements at altitude also relate to decrements in work performance at altitude.

To illustrate the effects of altitude exposure on work performance, 42 tasks[78] were chosen from both the *Soldier's Manual of Common Tasks*, Skill Level 1, STP 21-1-SMCT, Department of the Army,[103] and the Military Occupational Specialty (MOS) Physical Task List, US Army Infantry School, Fort Benning, Georgia[104] (Exhibit 22-2 and Figure 22-8). The tasks are ranked by ascending order of metabolic cost ($\dot{V}O_2$, in mL/kg/min) and the percentage of $\dot{V}O_2$max required to perform the task as determined at sea level and estimated for 2,000 m to 6,000 m (estimates made from the database regression line in Figure 22-1) (Table 22-1). The altitude percentages were calculated with the assumptions that sea-level task intensity and duration were not altered and additional rest breaks were not provided. As can be seen, the percentage of $\dot{V}O_2$max required to complete each task increases progressively with ascending elevation. Note that some tasks (tasks 37 to 42) that are of submaximal intensity at sea level (60% to 70% of $\dot{V}O_2$max) require nearly maximal or greater than maximal oxygen uptakes at higher terrestrial elevations.

Practical Guidelines for Military Operational Planning at Altitude

Although Table 22-1 illustrates how an increase in elevation affects the relative intensity of specific military tasks, it provides little guidance as to modifications that could be made to increase the probability of successfully completing the tasks. Such modifications at altitude, compared with sea level, would include at least one of the following:

- an increase in task duration,

- a reduction in task intensity, or
- more-frequent rest breaks.

The specific amount and type of modification will depend on factors such as type of task involved, task difficulty, elevation, time at altitude, urgency, weather, terrain, and involved muscle mass (eg, arm or leg work). At present, precise adjustments for particular tasks for specific altitudes have not yet been established. Nevertheless, estimates for additional time to complete a task during initial altitude exposure can be made by using information provided by the National Institute for Occupational Safety and Health for lifting tasks, predominantly,[105] and Figure 22-7 for walking and carrying tasks, predominantly. Industrial recommendations stipulate that tasks requiring mostly lifting and less than 30% of $\dot{V}O_2$max can be performed for 2 to 8 hours; those requiring 40% of $\dot{V}O_2$max, 1 to 2 hours; and those requiring 50% or more of $\dot{V}O_2$max, 1 hour or less.[105] Using this information, the data in Table 22-1, task 24, for example, can be performed for 2 to 8 hours at sea level, 1 to 2 hours at 4,000 m, and less than an hour at 6,000 m. Similarly, data illustrated in Figure 22-7 indicate that if task 35 can be performed for 3 hours at sea level, then 30% additional time (about an hour) may have to be allowed at 3,000 m.

Time modifications such as those suggested above are an important means to compensate for impaired physical performance associated with the hypoxia of altitude exposure—especially during the first few days of exposure. With continued exposure, altitude acclimatization occurs and the additional difficulty of exercising and working are lessened. Numerous physiological changes associated with altitude acclimatization that occur to minimize the impact of hypoxia are discussed in Young and Young's chapter in *Human Performance Physiology and Environmental Medicine at Terrestrial Extremes.*[75] Briefly, with initial altitude exposure, arterial oxygen content (CaO_2) is reduced. But for any specified submaximal exercise or work intensity, oxygen transport to the working muscles is maintained because of a compensatory increase in cardiac output. In other words, cardiac output at a given submaximal exercise or work intensity will be greater during initial altitude exposure than at sea level. For maximal levels of exercise or work, maximal cardiac output cannot increase to levels greater than those at sea level, and thus can not compen-

EXHIBIT 22-2

FORTY-TWO SOLDIER TASKS, RANKED IN ORDER OF METABOLIC COST

1. Prolonged standing on a circulation control point: Task #3, MOS 95B (Military Police), Skill Level 1-3. Wearing combat equipment (LBE), stand in place for 15 min.

2. Lift 105-mm projectiles: Task #4, MOS 55D (Missiles/Munitions), Skill level 1-5. Carry 25-kg projectiles 15 m and lift to the height of a 2.5-ton truck (1.32 m), once every 2 min for 15 min.

3. Relocate/establish operations: Task #1, MOS 33S (Intelligence), Skill Level 1-5. Lower/lift 25-kg box to/from ground level from/to the height of a 2.5-ton truck (1.32 m), once every 4 min for 15 min (lift every 2 min/lower every 2 min).

4. Perform emergency destruction operations: Task #24, MOS 16B (Air Defense Artillery), Skill level 1-4. Lift a 6.8-kg shape charge, carry 15 m, and hold at fullest upward reach for 1 min; repeat every 2 min for 15 min.

5. Relocate/establish operations: Task #2, MOS 33S (Intelligence), Skill level 1-5. Lift 22-kg box to the height of a 2.5-ton truck (1.32 m), once per minute for 15 min.

6. Lift 105-mm projectiles: Task #4, MOS 55D (Missiles/Munitions), Skill level 1-5. Carry 25-kg projectiles 15 m and lift to the height of a 2.5-ton truck (1.32 m), once per minute for 15 min.

7. Receive nonperishable subsistence; unload 40-ft container: Task #1, MOS 76X (Quartermaster), Skill Level 1-4. Lift 18-kg ration containers from the floor to 0.9 m and carry 6.1 m, once per minute for 15 min.

8. Relocate/establish operations: Task #1, MOS 33S (Intelligence), Skill Level 1-5. Lower/lift 25-kg box to/from ground level from/to a 2.5-ton truck, once per minute for 15 min (lift every 30 s, then lower every 30 s).

9. Load crates of explosives onto truck: Task #5, MOS 12B (Engineers), Skill level 1-2. Lift a 27.3-kg crate, carry it 4 m, and load it onto a 2.5-ton truck (1.32 m), once per minute for 15 min.

10. Relocate/establish operations: Task #2, MOS 33S (Intelligence), Skill Level 1-5. Lift a 22.7-kg box to the height of a 2.5-ton truck (1.32 m), twice per minute for 15 min.

11. Maintain an M16A1 Rifle: Common Task #071-311-2025. Assemble/disassemble the weapon three to five times for a duration of 5-10 min.

12. Rig a supply load on a modular platform for airdrop: Task #1, MOS 43E (Quartermaster), Skill Level 1-5. Lift a 36-kg ammunition box from ground level to a height of 0.9 m and carry it 6.1 m, once per minute for 15 min.

13. Load artillery pieces in preparation for firing: Task #8, MOS 13B (Field Artillery), Skill Level 1-2. Lift 45-kg projectiles to 1.7 m and carry 5 m, twice per minute for 15 min.

14. Move by foot: Task #1, MOS 11B (Infantry), Skill Level 1-5. Wearing combat equipment (LBE) without a rucksack, march on a level, hard surface at 1.11 m/s for 15 min.

15. Lift, carry, and move patients: Task #7, MOS 91B (Medical), Skill Level 1-2. Given a two-person litter team, move a patient weighing 68 kg over level terrain a distance of 500 m in 20 min.

16. Move by foot: Task #1, MOS 11B (Infantry), Skill Level 1-5. Wearing combat equipment with a 20-kg rucksack, march on a level, hard surface at 1.11 m/s for 15 min.

17. Lift 105 mm Projectiles: Task #2, MOS 55D (Missile/Munitions), Skill Level 1-5. Lift a 25-kg projectile and carry it 15 m at the height of 2.5-ton truck (1.32 m), twice per minute for 15 min.

18. Unload and stack paper stock: Task #2, 74B (Administration), Skill Level 1-2. Lift an 18.2-kg box and carry it 9 m, to include up stairs 2.5 m high, once per minute for 15 min.

19. Move by foot: Task #1, MOS 11B (Infantry), Skill Level 1-5. Wearing combat equipment (LBE) with a 30-kg rucksack, march on a level, hard surface at 1.11 m/s for 15 min.

20. Load artillery pieces in preparation for firing: Task #8, MOS 13B (Field Artillery), Skill Level 1-2. Lift 45-kg projectiles to 1.7 m and carry 5 m, three times per minute for 10 min.

21. Move by foot: Task #1, MOS 11B (Infantry), Skill Level 1-5. Wearing combat equipment (LBE) without a rucksack, march on a level, hard surface at 1.48 m/s for 15 min.

22. Move by foot: Task #1, MOS 11B (Infantry), Skill Level 1-5. Wearing combat equipment (wt: 7 kg), carrying an M-16 (wt: 3 kg), and a 30-kg rucksack, march on a level, hard surface at 1.11 m/s for 15 min.

*(**Exhibit 22-2** continues)*

Exhibit 22-2 *continued*

23. Relocate/establish operations: Task #1, MOS 33S (Intelligence), Skill Level 1-5. Lift 22.7-kg box to height of a 2.5-ton truck (1.32 m), four times per minute for 15 min.

24. Relocate/establish operations: Task #2, MOS 33S (Intelligence), Skill Level 1-5. Lift/lower 22.7-kg box to/from 2.5-ton truck (1.32 m), 6x/min for 10 min (lift in 10 s; then lower in 10 s).

25. Dig individual defensive position: Task #11, MOS 11 B (Infantry), Skill Level 1-5. Using entrenching tool, dig a foxhole 0.45-m deep, approximately 0.6 m wide x 1.8 m long, in sandy soil in 30 min.

26. Load artillery pieces in preparation for firing: Task #8, MOS 13B (Field Artillery), Skill Level 1-2. Lift 45-kg projectiles to 1.7 m and carry 5 m, four times per minute for 10 min.

27. Move by foot: Task #1, MOS 11B (Infantry), Skill Level 1-5. Wearing combat equipment with a 20-kg rucksack, march on a level, hard surface at 1.48 m/s for 15 min.

28. Move by foot: Task #1, MOS 11B (Infantry), Skill Level 1-5. Wearing combat equipment (LBE) with a 20-kg rucksack, march in loose sand at 0.98 m/s for 15 min.

29. Employ hand grenades: Common Task #071-325-4407. Using dummy grenades, engage a 5-m–radius target, 40 m from a covered position, three times per minute for 10 min.

30. Move by foot: Task #1, MOS 11B (Infantry), Skill Level 1-5. Wearing combat equipment (LBE) with 30-kg rucksack, march on a level, hard surface at 1.48 m/s for 15 min.

31. Lift 105-mm projectiles: Task #4, MOS 55D (Missiles/Munitions), Skill Level 1-5. Lift a 25-kg projectile and carry it 15 m to the height of a 2.5-ton truck (1.32 m), four times per minute for 15 min.

32. Carry TOW equipment: Task #1, MOS 11H (Infantry), Skill level 1-4. Wearing combat equipment (LBE), carry a 24.5-kg traversing unit up a grade (10%), at 0.89 m/s for 15 min.

33. Lift, carry, and move patients: Task #7, MOS 91B (Medical), Skill Level 1-2. Given a four-person litter team, move a patient weighing 81.8 kg over level terrain a distance of 1,000 m in 30 min.

34. Lift, carry, and move patients: Task #7, MOS 91B (Medical), Skill Level 1-2. Given a two-person litter team, move a patient weighing 68.2 kg, 100 m every 90 s for 10 min.

35. Move by foot: Task #1, MOS 11B (Infantry), Skill Level 1-5. Wearing combat equipment (wt: 7 kg) and carrying a weapon (wt: 3 kg) with a 30-kg rucksack, march on a level, hard surface at 1.48 m/s for 15 min.

36. Lift, carry, and move patients: Task #7, MOS 91B (Medical), Skill Level 1-2. Given a two-person litter team, carry a patient weighing 68.2 kg for 27.5 m, lift to the height of a 2.5-ton truck (1.32 m), then return 27.5-m to retrieve the next patient; complete 10 cycles in 10 min.

37. Move over, through, and around obstacles: Common Task #071 326-0503. Wearing combat equipment (LBE), traverse a 150-m obstacle course in 2 min at a constant rate; complete 5 cycles in 10 min.

38. Move by foot: Task #1, MOS 11B (Infantry), Skill Level 1-5. Wearing combat equipment (LBE) with a 20-kg rucksack, march in sand at 1.31 m/s for 15 min.

39. Move under direct fire (rush and crawl): Common Task #071-326 0502. Wearing combat equipment (LBE) and carrying a weapon, conduct high crawl and rush maneuvers over wooded terrain; complete 136.5-m course in 90 s; repeat five times.

40. Move by foot: Task #1, MOS 11B (Infantry), Skill Level 1-5. Wearing combat equipment (LBE) without a rucksack, move on a level, hard surface at 2.24 m/s for 10 min.

41. Carry TOW equipment: Task #1, MOS 11B (Infantry), Skill Level 1-4. Wearing full combat equipment, carry a 24.5-kg traversing unit up a grade (20%), at 0.89 m/s for 15 min.

42. Carry an M5 smoke pot in preparation of a smoke line: Task #1, MOS 54C (Chemical), Skill Level 1-2. Lift two 13.6 kg smoke pots, carry 30 m, and then lower the smoke pots, four times per minute for 10 min.

LBE: load-bearing equipment
TOW: tube-launched, optically tracked, wire-guided (missile system)
Adapted from Patton JF, Murphy MM, Bidwell TR, Mello RP, Harp ME. *Metabolic Cost of Military Physical Tasks in MOPP 0 and MOPP 4*. Natick, Mass: US Army Research Institute of Environmental Medicine; 1996. USARIEM Technical Report T95-9: 5–9.

sate for the reduced CaO_2. The result is a reduction in maximal oxygen transport and $\dot{V}O_2$max. With sustained exposures of 2 to 3 weeks, CaO_2 increases toward sea-level values, owing to both hemoconcentration due to the loss of plasma volume and an increase in arterial oxygen saturation (SaO_2).

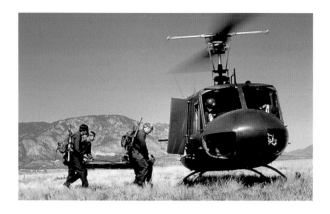

Fig. 22-8. Lift, carry, and move patients (MOS 91B, task 33; see Exhibit 22-2). A four-person litter team is moving an 81.8-kg patient over level terrain at a rate of 305 m/ 30 min. The energy cost of this task would require approximately 46%, 53%, and 66% of $\dot{V}O_2$max at sea level, 3,000 m, and 5,000 m, respectively.

As a consequence of the decreased plasma volume, however, stroke volume and cardiac output are both reduced. During submaximal levels of exercise or work, the restored CaO_2 compensates for the reduced cardiac output such that oxygen transport to the working muscles is maintained. But during maximal levels of exercise or work, the restored CaO_2 cannot compensate for the altitude-induced decline in maximal cardiac output, and maximal oxygen transport and $\dot{V}O_2$max do not improve.[43,106] Additionally, many other ventilatory, hematological, and metabolic adaptations may aid oxygen transport and improve exercise capabilities or military task performance. Some of these may include increases in 2,3-diphosphoglycerate (2,3-DPG) concentration,[54] muscle capillary proliferation,[107] oxidative enzymes,[108] myoglobin,[108] usage of free fatty acids,[109] buffering capacity,[107] oxygen deficit,[107] and decreased ammonia accumulation[66] and dependence on muscle glycogen.[109] These hypoxia-produced changes in oxygen delivery and metabolic profile have been suggested by many within the scientific and athletic communities as a potential means of inducing an additive or potentiating effect on exercise performance—not only at altitude but also on return to sea level. Before we review and summarize the results of such information, it is important that we describe exercise training fundamentals and experimental study considerations. Doing so will allow a more accurate appraisal of the postulate that exercise training or living, or both, under hypoxic conditions enhances $\dot{V}O_2$max and other measures of exercise performance, compared with both living and training at sea level.

Training Strategies for Improving Exercise Performance at Altitude

A plethora of information exists about how various combinations of exercise stimuli—intensity, duration, and frequency—can improve both $\dot{V}O_2$max and submaximal exercise performance at sea level.[110–114] In general, that information suggests that the higher the exercise intensity, the longer the exercise duration, the more frequent the training sessions, and the lower the initial fitness level, the greater will be the performance improvements.[114,115] The exercise training stimuli required to continue producing salutary effects increases as physical conditioning improves.[40,114,115] Therefore, the training stimuli for newly conditioned or highly conditioned individuals must necessarily be greater than for those less conditioned. For this reason, the same absolute training stimuli should not be used for all participants in an exercise training program but should be adjusted to accommodate each individual's current level of conditioning. Not maintaining exercise intensity, duration, and/or frequency of training can result in declines in $\dot{V}O_2$max and submaximal exercise performance.[111–114] Exercise training intensity, however, appears to be the principal stimulus.[111]

As stated above in the discussion of submaximal exercise, exercise at altitude, performed at the same power output as at sea level, represents a higher relative exercise intensity. During training at altitude, a higher exercise intensity may not be desirable because of issues such as not being able to sustain a given task for a required duration. Therefore, to maintain a comparable relative exercise intensity at altitude as at sea level, power outputs must be reduced during exercise training at altitude. However, reducing power output may result in relative deconditioning[23,36] that may offset any potential altitude-induced physiological benefits. Whether an altitude exercise training regimen will be successful in improving exercise performance more at altitude than at sea level would seem, then, to be the net result of a complex interaction of conditioning level, training stimuli, deconditioning, altitude acclimatization, and level of hypoxia.

For research purposes, it is also important to note that unless a matched group of individuals (ie, control group) train similarly while residing at sea level, it is difficult to assess the relative contributions of exercise training or detraining from the effects of hypoxia or altitude acclimatization. In addition, research studies may report only the assessment of $\dot{V}O_2$max in evaluating exercise training or hypoxia-induced results. If a subject's $\dot{V}O_2$max does not im-

TABLE 22-1

PERCENTAGE OF MAXIMAL AEROBIC POWER FOR 42 MILITARY OCCUPATIONAL TASKS AT INCREASING ALTITUDES

Task	$\dot{V}O_2$ (mL/kg/min)	%$\dot{V}O_2$max					
		SL[1]	2,000 m altitude[2]	3,000 m altitude[2]	4,000 m altitude[2]	5,000 m altitude[2]	6,000 m altitude[2]
1	4.9	9	10	11	12	13	16
2	6.7	13	14	15	16	18	22
3	6.7	12	14	15	16	18	22
4	7.4	14	15	16	18	20	24
5	7.5	15	15	17	18	21	24
6	8.5	16	17	19	21	23	27
7	9.1	18	19	20	22	25	29
8	9.5	18	19	21	23	26	31
9	9.6	18	20	21	23	26	31
10	9.8	19	20	22	24	27	32
11	11.0	20	22	24	27	30	35
12	11.0	21	22	24	27	30	35
13	11.0	21	22	24	27	30	35
14	11.8	21	24	26	29	33	38
15	12.0	22	24	27	29	33	39
16	12.2	24	25	27	30	34	39
17	12.4	23	25	28	30	34	40
18	13.7	25	28	31	33	38	44
19	13.9	27	28	31	34	38	45
20	14.0	27	29	31	34	39	45
21	14.4	28	29	32	35	40	46
22	15.2	29	31	34	37	42	49
23	15.4	29	31	34	37	42	50
24	16.5	30	34	37	40	45	53
25	17.1	33	35	38	42	47	55
26	17.4	34	35	39	42	48	56
27	18.1	33	37	40	44	50	58
28	19.1	37	39	43	46	53	62
29	19.7	36	40	44	48	54	64
30	21.1	41	43	47	51	58	68
31	22.9	45	47	51	56	63	74
32	23.2	44	47	52	56	64	75
33	23.9	46	49	53	58	66	77
34	24.6	47	50	55	60	68	79
35	25.7	48	52	57	63	71	83
36	27.0	52	55	60	66	74	87
37	29.5	58	60	66	72	81	95
38	29.7	59	60	66	72	82	96
39	30.3	59	62	67	74	83	98
40	33.5	62	68	75	82	92	108
41	39.0	75	79	87	95	107	126
42	41.4	76	84	92	101	114	134

SL: sea level
Data sources: (1) Patton JF, Murphy MM, Bidwell TR, Mello RP, Harp ME. *Metabolic Cost of Military Physical Tasks in MOPP 0 and MOPP 4*. Natick, Mass: US Army Research Institute of Environmental Medicine; 1996. USARIEM Technical Report T95-9. (2) Estimated from the database regression line in Figure 22-1.

prove, some of these studies may conclude that the altitude exposure and/or the exercise training regimen had no effect. This interpretation is questionable because significant improvements may occur in the response to standard submaximal endurance tests and during athletic performances with or without an increase in $\dot{V}O_2$max.[33,40,47,114,116,117]

Given the above considerations, findings based on appropriately controlled studies[30,45,118] support a beneficial effect of altitude training for altitude, but not subsequent sea-level performances (to be discussed below). In contrast, many anecdotal reports based on the practical experiences of coaches and athletes indicate that altitude exercise training—especially for elite endurance athletes—is not only beneficial but may be required for optimal performance at sea level.[47,119–123] This belief is so strong that it has stimulated a proliferation of moderate altitude (1,500–2,800 m) training sites and facilities around the world.[119,121]

The reasons for the dissimilar conclusions between the research and athletic communities with regard to the efficacy of altitude training for subsequent sea-level exercise performance are not readily apparent. Perhaps laboratory studies that assess changes in exercise performance do not provide an adequate basis for the assessment of specific athletes in competitive athletic events.[19,28,79,80,124] Exercise performance based solely on changes on laboratory estimates of $\dot{V}O_2$max, for example, may miss improvements in anaerobic capacity[107] that could result in improved track and field performances. Also, the level of athletic skill and judgment necessary for athletic success may not be adequately accounted for in the laboratory.[29] Or perhaps altitude training may be beneficial for some athletes but not others.[26,42,124] If so, then small individual improvements in athletic performance—enough to achieve competitive success—may be undetectable by the usual scientific statistical analyses that tend to assess only overall group changes.[125] It may also be that better results could result from

- a strong commitment to train harder at altitude than at sea level,
- training with the best athletes and coaches available,
- an athletic event's being perceived as easier on return to sea level, and
- the belief of athletes and coaches that altitude (or hypoxia) exercise training *does* provide an advantage.

Given these considerations, the following four sections assess the efficacy of residence or exercise training, or both, at altitude or sea level for the enhancement of exercise performance. In each section, a table presents studies from the literature that test the hypothesis that training or living or both under hypoxic conditions enhances $\dot{V}O_2$max, submaximal endurance exercise performance, and other measures of exercise performance compared to both living and training at sea level. Taken together, these studies also provide an appreciation of the complex interaction of the numerous factors that contribute to the lack of consensus about the efficacy of using hypoxia as a exercise performance enhancing aid. The studies selected represent a large sampling of the available exercise training studies that were conducted at different altitudes (1,300 m to 5,700 m), different training and residence durations (12 d–19 wk), and using civilian and military volunteer subjects with a range of fitness levels (mean sea-level $\dot{V}O_2$max values ranging from 37 to 74 mL/kg/min).

Hypoxic Exercise Training During Altitude Acclimatization

Table 22-2 presents studies that evaluated exercise performance of subjects who trained while residing at altitude. Of the 13 studies that lack control groups, seven reported a significant increase in $\dot{V}O_2$max either at altitude or on return to sea level. Of the four studies that included an exercise control group, none reported an improvement in $\dot{V}O_2$max—during or after altitude training—that could not be accounted for by the sea-level control group. The reason for the difference in findings between the studies with and without control groups cannot be attributed to differences in training altitudes, training durations, or subject fitness levels. Collectively, the results of these studies indicate that improvements in $\dot{V}O_2$max may occur during training while residing at altitude and that the higher $\dot{V}O_2$max may be retained on return to sea level. However, the improvement in $\dot{V}O_2$max likely results from exercise training alone and not to physiological changes associated with altitude acclimatization.

Conversely, maximal effort exercise performance at altitude for events lasting longer than 2 minutes can improve during altitude acclimatization independently of an increase in either training intensity or $\dot{V}O_2$max. Figure 22-9 shows data from elite athletes who were highly trained prior to altitude exposure and whose race times were recorded in the conduct of their primary event at the beginning and the end of their altitude exposure. Because of their high fitness levels and relatively short evaluation–reevaluation intervals, the improvement in athletic performance at altitude was not likely due to an increase in training. This conclusion is consistent with other controlled studies that show that altitude exposure with only maintenance training improves endurance performance, with[116] or without[33] an increase in $\dot{V}O_2$max.

Studies that have specifically assessed whether altitude exercise training during residence at altitude improves subsequent sea-level $\dot{V}O_2$max and maximal effort endurance exercise performance in the same subjects have produced conflicting or inconclusive results, however. On return to sea level, either both $\dot{V}O_2$max and athletic performance did not improve,[27,45] or both $\dot{V}O_2$max and athletic performance improved,[19,47] or $\dot{V}O_2$max did not improve but athletic performance did.[107,126] The reason or reasons for these conflicting results is not clear, but it probably is not related to differences in the level of prealtitude exposure fitness levels because the subjects in these studies were all highly conditioned. Differences in results may be related to a complex interaction of factors that include interstudy differences in exercise intensity, altitude duration, or types of exercise performance evaluations used, in any combination, and also to interindividual differences in training responsiveness. In addition, it should be noted that a small, statistically nonsignificant, training-induced improvement in mean $\dot{V}O_2$max (often reported as "no change") can result in a significant increase in submaximal exercise performance. For example, a 1% to 3% rise in $\dot{V}O_2$max results in a 12% to 45% improvement in endurance time to exhaustion.[33,48,117] These studies emphasize the importance of (1) not using $\dot{V}O_2$max as the sole criteria to judge the efficacy of an altitude training program, and (2) reporting individual rather than only group data for *both* $\dot{V}O_2$max and other measures of submaximal exercise performance, as some individuals may benefit from altitude training while others may not.

Hypoxic Exercise Training Without Altitude Residence

Short-duration hypobaric chamber studies or studies utilizing hypoxic gas mixtures during exercise training address the effects of training under repeated acute hypoxic conditions without inducing some of the physiological changes associated with altitude acclimatization such as increased hemoglobin and hematocrit concentrations,[56,127,128] and a reduction in maximal cardiac output.[43,75] Submaximal endurance exercise training during repeated short-duration hypoxic exposures may also enhance peripheral changes such muscle fiber size,[129] capillary density,[129,130] myoglobin concentration,[108] muscle oxidative capacity,[108] glycolytic activity,[108] and interfibrillar mitochondrial volume density[129]—but it has been difficult to determine from the reported data if the magnitude of these potentially salutary changes are greater during hypoxia training than during similar sea-level training.

The collective findings of the studies in which subjects trained daily for short periods at altitude or in hypoxia, but lived at sea level, are presented in Table 22-3. Improvements in $\dot{V}O_2$max were reported for some studies during testing in hypoxia[56,128–132] or normoxia,[66,128,131,132] whether or not control groups were used. In another study,[130] work capacity (ie, the total amount of aerobic work performed during an exhaustive incremental test) but not $\dot{V}O_2$max improved more for the experimental group than for the control group—but in hypoxia

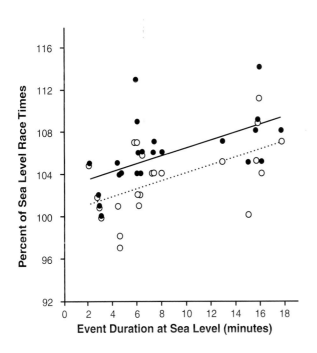

Fig. 22-9. The effect of training at altitude on performance at altitude (2,240 m to 2,800 m). The X axis is the event duration at sea level and the Y axis is the percentage change from the sea-level performance. Data* are from eight of the studies used to develop Figure 22-5. The data used in the graph above are for the same individuals and events but for two different altitude durations: acute exposures (< 5 d, closed circles) and chronic exposures (> 10 days, open circles). The regression lines depict the acute (solid line) and chronic (dashed line) exposure. Reprinted with permission from Fulco CS, Rock PB, Cymerman A. Maximal and submaximal exercise performance at altitude. *Aviat Space Environ Med.* 1998;67(8):798. *Sources for the data points are found in the Attachment at the end of this chapter.

TABLE 22-2

HYPOXIC EXERCISE WITH ALTITUDE ACCLIMATIZATION

Data Source	Training Altitude	Duration	Fitness (mL/kg/min)	Control Group?	$\dot{V}O_2$max Improvement at Altitude	on Return	Comments
1	2,300 m	10 d	?	No	+6%	+8%	Anaerobic capacity and 400-m run time not affected.
2	3,800 m	5 wk	37	No	+4%	+14%	—
3	3,475 m	20 d	44	No	0%	0%	Training not specified; no advantage of residing at 1,610 m altitude on 3,475-m performance.
4	2,300 m	23 d	?	No	+2%	+9%	Pre- to postaltitude 275-m, 1,609-m, and 3,218-m run times, but not swim times, improved.
5	4,300 m	12 d	48	No	0% (assumed)	n/a	45% increase in endurance time to exhaustion.
6	4,300 m	16 d	51	No	+10%	n/a	60% increase in endurance time to exhaustion.
7	4,000 m	55 d	63	No	+3%	0%	Greatly reduced exercise intensity at altitude. Altitude endurance performance equaled sea level control time after 20 d. No pre-to-post altitude difference in 400-m, 800-m, 1,609-m, and 3,218-m run times. Detraining effect was postulated.
8	2,270 m	4 wk	65	No	+5%	n/a	Improved $\dot{V}O_2$max, and 1,609 m and 4,828 m run times at altitude.
9	2,250 m	19 d	> 60 ?	No	+5%	n/a	4 weeks minimum altitude adaptation.
10	2,300 m–4,300 m	Varying durations	≥ 60	No	0%	0%	Some 1,609-m and 4,828-m run times improved at altitude.
11	2,300 m	Alternate training (1–2 wk) at sea level with training at altitude	74	No	+4%	+4%	Rigorous altitude training. 1,609-m and 3,218-m time trials improved at altitude and at return to sea level. Many personal best times.
12	3,090 m		72	No	+2%	+4%	—
13	2,700 m	17 d; 2 wk	72	No	0%	0%	17% increase in short-term running performance; increases in O$_2$ deficit and muscle buffering capacity.
14	4,300 m	4 wk	38	Yes	n/a	+10%	$\dot{V}O_2$max increase not greater than that of control group.
15	3,100 m	17 d	66–68	Yes	0%	0%	Significant reductions in $\dot{V}O_2$max for some runners pre-to-postaltitude exposure; 220-m and 440-m run times reduced at altitude. Laboratory tests not predictive of track performances.
16	2,300 m	3 wk	73	Yes	0%	0%	3,218-m run times improved at altitude, but not pre-to-postaltitude exposure; altitude training was at 6.5% less absolute power output.
17	2,100 m	2 wk	74	Yes	n/a	0%	Increase in O$_2$ deficit.

Data sources: (1) Balke B, Nagle FJ, Daniels J. Altitude and maximal performance in work and sport activity. *JAMA*. 1965;194:646–649. (2) Klausen K, Robinson S, Micahel ED, Myhre LG. Effect of high altitude on maximal working capacity. *J Appl Physiol*. 1966;21:1191–1194. (3) Consolazio CF, Nelson RA, Matoush LO, Hansen JE. Energy metabolism at high altitude (3,475 m). *J Appl Physiol*. 1966;21:1732–1740. (4) Faulkner JA, Daniels JT, Balke B. Effects of training at moderate altitude on physical performance capacity. *J Appl Physiol*. 1967;23:85–89. (5) Maher JT, Jones LG, Hartley LH. Effects of high-altitude exposure on submaximal endurance capacity of men. *J Appl Physiol*. 1974;37:895–898. (6) Horstman D, Weiskopf R, Jackson RE. Work capacity during 3-week sojourn at 4,300 m: Effects of relative polycythemia. *J Appl Physiol*. 1980;49:311–318. (7) Buskirk ER, Kollias J, Akers RF, Prokop EK, Reategui P. Maximal performance at altitude and on return from altitude in conditioned runners. *J Appl Physiol*. 1967;23:259–266. (8) Pugh LGCE. Athletes at altitude. *J Physiol (Lond)*. 1967;192:619–646. (9) Saltin B. Aerobic and anaerobic work capacity at an altitude of 2,250 meters. In: Goddard RF, ed. *The Effects of Altitude on Physical Performance*. Albuquerque, NM: The Athletic Institute; 1967: 97–102. (10) Faulkner JA, Kollias J, Favour CB, Buskirk ER, Balke B. Maximum aerobic capacity and running performance at altitude. *J Appl Physiol*. 1968;24:685–691. (11) Daniels J, Oldridge N. The effects of alternate exposure to altitude and sea level on world-class middle-distance runners. *Med Sci Sports*. 1970;2:107–112. (12) Dill DB, Adams WC. Maximal oxygen uptake at sea level and at 3,090-m altitude in high school champion runners. *J Appl Physiol*. 1971;30:854–859. (13) Mizuno M, Juel C, Bro Rasmussen T, et al. Limb skeletal muscle adaptation in athletes after training at altitude. *J Appl Physiol*. 1990;68:496–502. (14) Hansen JE, Vogel JA, Stelter GP, Consolazio CF. Oxygen uptake in man during exhaustive work at sea level and high altitude. *J Appl Physiol*. 1967;23:511–522. (15) Grover RF, Reeves JT. Exercise performance of athletes at sea level and 3,100 meters altitude. *Med Thorac*. 1966;23:129–143. (16) Adams WC, Bernauer EM, Dill DB, Bomar JB Jr. Effects of equivalent sea-level and altitude training on V̇o₂max and running performance. *J Appl Physiol*. 1975;39:262–266. (17) Svedenhag J, Saltin B, Johansson C, Kaijser L. Aerobic and anaerobic exercise capacities of elite middle-distance runners after two weeks of training at moderate altitude. *Scan J Med Sci Sports*. 1991;1:205–214.
Adapted with permission from Fulco CS, Rock PB, Cymerman A. Improving athletic performance: Is altitude residence or altitude training helpful? *Aviat Space Environ Med*. 2000;71(2):165.

TABLE 22-3

HYPOXIC EXERCISE WITH ALTITUDE ACCLIMATIZATION

Data Source	Training Altitude	Duration	Fitness (mL/kg/min)	Control Group?	V̇o₂max Improvement at Altitude	V̇o₂max Improvement on Return	Comments
1	4,200 m	19 wk	45	No	+14%	+36%	Interval training in normoxia and hypoxia during alternating weeks. Endurance time to exhaustion increased > 100% in both normoxia and hypoxia.
2	3,050–4,268 m	3 wk	54	Yes	+10%	+10%	Because of small n, pre-to-postchange in normoxia and hypoxia V̇o₂max not significantly different from controls (0% and 4%, respectively). Endurance performance improved for hypoxia training group in normoxia but not in hypoxia.
3	2,250 m	4 wk	46	Yes	+8%	+18%	Control group increased V̇o₂max by 6% in normoxia, 4% at 2,250 m, and 0% at 3,450 m.
	3,450 m	4 wk	46	Yes	+14%	+10%	
4	2,500 m	5 wk	43	Yes	+12% to +18%	+11% to +15%	V̇o₂max increases not greater than that of control group; endurance performance improvement specific to training altitude.
5	4,100–5,700 m	3 wk	56	Yes	+11	0%	Training for the control normoxic groups was at the same relative and absolute workloads as in hypoxia. No performance difference compared with controls. Training in hypoxia increased mitochondrial density, muscle fiber area, and capillary-to-fiber ratio.
6	2,300 m	4 wk	71	Yes	0%	0%	No V̇o₂max increase for either group; work capacity increased more for the hypoxia-trained group, but only in hypoxia.

Data sources: (1) Bannister EW, Woo W. Effects of simulated altitude training on aerobic and anaerobic power. *Eur J Appl Physiol Med*. 1978;38:55–69. (2) Loeppky JA, Bynum WA. Effects of periodic exposure to hypobaria and exercise on physical work capacity. *J Sports Med Phys Fitness*. 1970;10:238–247. (3) Roskamm H, Landry F, Samek L, Schlager M, Weidemann H, Reindell H. Effects of a standardized ergometer training program at three different altitudes. *J Appl Physiol*. 1969;27:840–847. (4) Levine BD, Engfred K, Friedman DB, Kjaer M, Saltin B. High altitude endurance training; Effect on aerobic capacity and work performance. *Med Sci Sports Exerc*. 1990;22:S35. Abstract. (5) Desplanches D, Hoppeler H, Linossier MT, et al. Effects of training in normoxia and normobaric hypoxia on human muscle ultrastructure. *Pflugers Arch*. 1993;425:263–267. (6) Terrados N, Melichna J, Sylven C, Jansson E, Kaijser L. Effects of training at simulated altitude on performance and muscle metabolic capacity in competitive road cyclists. *Eur J Appl Physiol Med*. 1988;57:203–209.
Adapted with permission from Fulco CS, Rock PB, Cymerman A. Improving athletic performance: Is altitude residence or altitude training helpful? *Aviat Space Environ Med*. 2000;71(2):167.

TABLE 22-4

ALTITUDE ACCLIMATIZATION WITH NORMOXIC EXERCISE

Data Source	Training Altitude	Duration	Fitness (mL/kg/min)	Control Group?	$\dot{V}O_2$max Improvement at Lower Altitude	Comments
1	1,300 m	4 wk	65	Yes	5%	Experimental and control groups trained together at 1,300 m, but the experimental group lived at 2,500 m ("living high, training low"). Blood volume increased 500 mL and 5-km run time decreased 30 sec in experimental group. No changes in $\dot{V}O_2$max, blood volume, or run time for control group.

Data source: (1) Levine BD, Stray-Gundersen J, Duhaime G, Snell PG, Friedman DB. "Living High—Training Low": The effect of altitude acclimatization/normoxic training in trained runners. *Med Sci Sports Exerc.* 1991;23:S25. Abstract.

TABLE 22-5

NORMOXIC AND HYPOXIC EXERCISE AFTER ALTITUDE ACCLIMATIZATION

Data Source	Training Altitude	Breathing	Duration	Fitness (mL/kg/min)	Work Load	$\dot{V}O_2$max Improvement in Hypoxia	in Normoxia	Comments
1	3,600 m	Ambient‡	6 wk	42	Control	15%	14%	Training for the two experimental groups was at the same relative or absolute work load as the control hypoxia group, but while training, the experimental groups breathed only high concentrations of O_2 gas (eg, "living high, training low").
	0 m†	0.314%			Same relative	17%	20%	
	0 m†	0.314%			Same absolute	8%	10%	

*Control hypoxia group: altitude natives breathing ambient altitude air
†Experimental group
‡O_2 content of ambient air: 0.2093%

Data source: (1) Levine BD, Stray-Gundersen J, Duhaime G, Snell PG, Friedman DB. "Living High—Training Low": The effect of altitude acclimatization/normoxic training in trained runners. *Med Sci Sports Exerc.* 1991;23:S25.

Adapted with permission from Fulco CS, Rock PB, Cymerman A. Improving athletic performance: Is altitude residence or altitude training helpful? *Aviat Space Environ Med.* 2000;71(2):168.

only. It is interesting that most studies of this design report results that are consistent with an additive or potentiating role of hypoxic exercise training for subsequent hypoxic or normoxic performance evaluations.[56,128–131]

Why living at sea level and training at altitude may be more beneficial for improving exercise performance than both living and training at altitude is not well understood. Possible differences in success rates between these two experimental approaches do not seem to be related to differences in absolute exercise intensity, training altitude, training program duration, subject fitness levels, and peripheral muscle changes. The only consistent differences are increases in hematocrit and hemoglobin in subjects who both trained and resided at altitude, compared with studies in which subjects trained in hypoxia but lived at sea level. Of course, during a typical 2- to 5-week period of living and training at altitude (a typical length of time for most of these studies), increases in hematocrit and hemoglobin concentrations primarily reflect hemoconcentration that, as was mentioned above, is due to decreases in plasma and blood volume—changes that may attenuate the effects of hypoxia per se[43,75] but may not provide an additional benefit for altitude or sea-level physical performance.

When results of the physiological and exercise performance changes of the two experimental approaches are compared, the data suggest that, for both sea-level and altitude exercise performance, training but not living under hypoxic conditions may be more beneficial than training and living at altitude, and that the benefit may be related to a maintained blood volume. It is unfortunate that studies in which subjects live at sea level and train under hypoxic conditions have not typically reported timed track trials and other athletic-event evaluations. Doing so would likely allow a more accurate appraisal of the potential benefits of training, but not living, in hypoxia. Thus, the limited data from studies using widely differing experimental designs preclude forming firm conclusions regarding the efficacy of periodic hypoxic training for subsequent sea-level exercise performance.

Normoxic Exercise Training During Altitude Acclimatization

It is documented that inability to maintain exercise intensity during exercise training at sea level can result in a decline in $\dot{V}O_2max$.[111] It is possible, therefore, that the necessary reduction in exercise intensity while training at altitude may lead to "relative deconditioning" and offset potential beneficial changes resulting from altitude acclimatization.[26] Living at altitude but training at a lower altitude ("living high and training low") theoretically allows both the advantageous changes of acclimatization to develop and the opportunity to train without reducing exercise intensity.

Using this approach, Levine and colleagues[133] trained nine highly conditioned runners ($\dot{V}O_2max$ [sea level] = 64.9 mL/kg/min) for 4 weeks at 1,300 m. All subjects trained together at the same exercise intensity. Three of the subjects lived at 1,300 m (the "sea-level" group) and six lived at 2,500 m (the "altitude" group). Before training, there were no differences between groups in $\dot{V}O_2max$, 5-km run time, or blood volume. For the sea-level group, there were no significant changes in any of the measures after training. For the altitude group, however, both $\dot{V}O_2max$ and blood volume increased and the time to run 5 km decreased (Table 22-4). The investigators concluded that altitude acclimatization with sea-level training improved exercise performance at sea level.

Because of these findings, Levine and Stray-Gundersen[36] and Levine, Roach, and Houston[37] hypothesized 1 year later that altitude acclimatization rather than hypoxic exercise per se was the key to altitude training because the natural form of "blood doping" (increased blood volume and hemoglobin) enhanced oxygen transport. In contrast, as discussed above, hypoxic exercise training has been reported to increase $\dot{V}O_2max$ without inducing changes in hemoglobin concentration or blood volume.[56,133] Perhaps hypoxic exercise training increases the "training effect," as evidenced by greater increase in aerobic enzyme activities and other peripheral changes.[108,129,130] Additional studies with the experimental design of "living high and training low" are still needed to confirm or refute these results.

Normoxic and Hypoxic Exercise Training After Altitude Acclimatization

The studies reviewed above were conducted using sea-level residents who lived or trained, or both, under hypoxic conditions. Some[19,24,25,47,56,128,131,133,134] reported that hypoxic exercise training enhances maximal performance compared to normoxic training on return to sea level, while others[27–30,45,52,107,126,129,130,132] report no such enhancement. The discrepancies have been ascribed to[135]

1. differences in the level and duration of altitude exposure
2. differences in the degree of prealtitude exposure fitness levels,
3. differences in the interindividual rate of early altitude acclimatization, and
4. variable intensity training programs between or within studies.

Some altitude exercise training studies were conducted during the early altitude exposure period and ended long before altitude acclimatization was complete. Other altitude exercise training studies were accomplished during repeated acute hypoxic exposures where some indices of acclimatization were purposefully avoided. Having individuals train at altitude after "complete" acclimatization should both minimize the confounding variability due to changes associated with altitude acclimatization and allow assessment of hypoxic exercise training only.

To test this hypothesis, Favier and colleagues[135] trained 30 native-born, high-altitude residents, (sea-level $\dot{V}O_2$max ~ 42 mL/kg/min), at 3,600 m on a cycle ergometer 30 min/d, five times per week, for 6 weeks (Table 22-5). Subjects were randomly assigned to one of three groups of ten. One group trained at altitude at 70% of $\dot{V}O_2$max breathing ambient air (the control group). The other two groups trained at altitude but inhaled a normoxic gas mix-ture (FIO_2 = 0.314 at 500 mmHg, sea-level equivalent) and exercised at the same relative work load (70% of normoxic $\dot{V}O_2$max) or at the same absolute work load (70% of hypoxic $\dot{V}O_2$max) as the control group. The normoxic training groups were, in essence, living at high altitude and training at low. As the fitness levels of the subjects improved, the work loads were increased to maintain exercise intensities at the desired levels. All three groups demonstrated an improvement in $\dot{V}O_2$max in response to training (the magnitude of which was similar to that of the same conditioning program used for an earlier sea-level training study conducted by the research team).[136] The results suggest that the documented increase in hemoglobin concentration induced by altitude acclimatization does not provide additional benefits in terms of increasing $\dot{V}O_2$max with training. The results also indicate that the combination of altitude acclimatization and oxygen supplementation during exercise training (to allow training at an increased power output and training intensity) does not produce an increase in $\dot{V}O_2$max greater than training in hypoxia. These results do not support the belief that the potential beneficial effect of hypoxia is lessened by the inability to exercise at a high intensity at altitude.[28,37,42] The reason or reasons for the diverging results and conclusions of this study[135] and those of Levine and colleagues[133] are not readily apparent. More studies with these experimental approaches are warranted.

SUMMARY

The ability to perform muscular exercise is usually evaluated by measuring maximal aerobic power ($\dot{V}O_2$max) during increasingly severe exercise that leads to exhaustion within minutes. In ascending to altitude, an individual is exposed to a progressive decrease in atmospheric pressure that is associated with reductions in inspired, alveolar, and arterial oxygen pressures. As a consequence, $\dot{V}O_2$max also declines. A comprehensive review of the literature indicates that the minimal elevation at which a decrease in $\dot{V}O_2$max is detectable is approximately 580 m. It is possible that the minimal altitude is even lower, especially for highly conditioned individuals. Sixteen experimental and physiological factors have been implicated in the wide variation in percentage $\dot{V}O_2$max decrement at altitudes from 580 m to 6,000 m. Fitness level, preexposure elevation, gender, and duration of exposure were all qualitatively assessed to determine their contribution to the overall variability. Of these, fitness-level differences caused the most variability and gender differences contributed the least.

Submaximal oxygen uptake is similar for a given activity at sea level and at altitude. But because $\dot{V}O_2$max declines, the relative exercise intensity is increased and therefore submaximal exercise performance is adversely affected. To maintain the same level of perceived difficulty at altitude for training or working on civilian or military tasks, the exercise or work loads must necessarily be reduced. Long-duration activities will be impaired more than shorter-duration activities at a given altitude. Muscle strength, maximal muscle power, and, likely, anaerobic performance are not affected at altitude as long as muscle mass is maintained. Physical performance may be improved at altitude compared with sea level in activities that have a minimal aerobic component and can be performed at high velocity (eg, sprinting).

Altitude acclimatization is associated with a

multitude of ventilatory, hematological, and metabolic adaptations that have been thought to induce a beneficial effect on exercise performance. Training or living, or both, at altitude can improve altitude exercise performance in athletic events or military activities lasting longer than about 2 minutes. In contrast, findings based on controlled studies do not support a beneficial effect of altitude training on subsequent sea-level performance. Any potential benefit induced by altitude acclimatization for subsequent sea-level performance may be offset by the inability to maintain exercise intensity. Living at altitude but training at a lower altitude permits the theoretical advantage of both acclimatization and training without reducing exercise intensity. This paradigm appears promising but is still open to question, since native-born, high-altitude residents who trained at altitude with oxygen supplementation (in essence, living high but training low) did not improve $\dot{V}O_2max$ more than native-born, high-altitude residents who trained at altitude without supplementation. More research is clearly warranted to determine the most advantageous strategy, if any, for improving sea-level exercise performance.

REFERENCES

1. Goldman RF. Energy expenditure of soldiers performing combat type activities. *Ergonomics*. 1965;8:321–327.

2. Brezina E, Kolmer W. Uber den energieverbrauch beider geharbeit unter dem einflussverschiedener geschwindigheiten und verschiedener belastungen [in German]. *Biochem Ztschr*. 1912;38:129–153.

3. Cymerman A, Pandolf KB, Young AJ, Maher JT. Energy expenditure during load carriage at high altitude. *J Appl Physiol*. 1981;51:14–18.

4. Perry ME, Browning RJ, Jackson R, Meyer J. The effect of intermediate altitude on the Army Physical Fitness Test. *Mil Med*. 1992;157:523–526.

5. Evans WO, Hansen JE. Troop performance in high altitudes. *Army*. 1966;16:54–57.

6. Goldman RF, Iampietro PF. Energy cost of load carriage. *J Appl Physiol*. 1962;17:675–676.

7. Pandolf KB, Haisman MF, Goldman RF. Metabolic energy expenditure and terrain coefficients for walking on snow. *Ergonomics*. 1976;19:683–690.

8. Givoni B, Goldman RF. Predicting metabolic energy cost. *J Appl Physiol*. 1971;30:429–433.

9. US Department of the Army. *Medical Problems of Man at High Terrestrial Elevations*. Washington, DC: DA; 1975. Technical Bulletin Medical (TB MED) 288.

10. US Department of the Army. *Mountain Operations*. Washington, DC: DA; 1980. Field Manual 90–6.

11. Cymerman A, Rock PB. *Medical Problems in High Mountain Environments: A Handbook for Medical Officers*. Natick, Mass: USARIEM; 1994.

12. Balke B. Work capacity at altitude. In: Johnson WR, ed. *Science and Medicine of Exercise and Sports*. New York, NY: Harper & Brothers; 1960: 339–347.

13. Houston CS. *Going Higher*. Boston, Mass: Little, Brown & Company; 1987.

14. Balke B, Faulkner JA, Daniels JT. Maximum performance capacity at sea level and at moderate altitude before and after training at altitude. *Schweizerische Zeitschrift Fur Sportmedizin*. 1966;14:106–116.

15. Faulkner JA. Maximum exercise at medium altitude. In: Shephard RJ, ed. *Frontiers of Fitness*. Springfield, Ill: Charles C Thomas; 1971: 360–375.

16. Goddard RF, ed. *The Effects of Altitude on Physical Performance*. Albuquerque, NM: The Athletic Institute; 1967.

17. Moore L. *Yearbook of Physical Anthropology*. Vol 41. New York, NY: Wenner-Gren Foundation for Anthropological Research; 1998: Table 1, p28.

18. West JB. Personal communication (letter) to RF Bellamy, Colonel, Medical Corps, US Army (Ret); Military Medical Editor, *Textbook of Military Medicine*, Borden Institute; Walter Reed Army Medical Center, Washington, DC; July 2001.

19. Faulkner JA, Daniels JT, Balke B. Effects of training at moderate altitude on physical performance capacity. *J Appl Physiol.* 1967;23:85–89.

20. Jokl E, Jokl P. The effect of altitude on athletic performance. In: Jokl E, Jokl P, eds. *Exercise and Altitude.* New York, NY: Karger; 1968: 29–34.

21. Reeves JT, Jokl P, Cohn JE. Performance of olympic runners at altitudes of 7,350 and 5,350 feet. In: Jokl E, Jokl P, eds. *Exercise and Altitude.* New York, NY: Karger; 1968: 49–54.

22. Craig AB. Olympics 1968: A post-mortem. *Med Sci Sports.* 1969;1:177–180.

23. Balke B. Work capacity and its limiting factors at high altitude. In: Weihe WH, ed. *The Physiological Effects of High Altitude.* New York, NY: Pergamon Press; 1964: 233–247.

24. Dill DB, Adams WC. Maximal oxygen uptake at sea level and at 3,090-m altitude in high school champion runners. *J Appl Physiol.* 1971;30:854–859.

25. Klausen K, Robinson S, Micahel ED, Myhre LG. Effect of high altitude on maximal working capacity. *J Appl Physiol.* 1966;21:1191–1194.

26. Saltin B. Aerobic and anaerobic work capacity at an altitude of 2,250 meters. In: Goddard RF, ed. *The Effects of Altitude on Physical Performance.* Albuquerque, NM: The Athletic Institute; 1967: 17, 97–102.

27. Buskirk ER, Kollias J, Akers RF, Prokop EK, Reategui P. Maximal performance at altitude and on return from altitude in conditioned runners. *J Appl Physiol.* 1967;23:259–266.

28. Faulkner JA, Kollias J, Favour CB, Buskirk ER, Balke B. Maximum aerobic capacity and running performance at altitude. *J Appl Physiol.* 1968;24:685–691.

29. Grover RF, Reeves JT. Exercise performance of athletes at sea level and 3,100 meters altitude. *Med Thorac.* 1966;23:129–143.

30. Hansen JE, Vogel JA, Stelter GP, Consolazio CF. Oxygen uptake in man during exhaustive work at sea level and high altitude. *J Appl Physiol.* 1967;23:511–522.

31. Heath D, Williams DR. Athletic performance at moderate altitude. In: Heath D; Williams DR, eds. *Man at High Altitude: The Pathophysiology of Acclimatization and Adaptation.* Edinburgh, Scotland: Churchill Livingstone; 1977: 240–246.

32. Richalet J-P, Brouns F, Guezennec Y, Bittel J, eds. Proceedings of the International Congress on Mountain Sports. *Int J Sports Med.* 1992;13(suppl):entire issue.

33. Maher JT, Jones LG, Hartley LH. Effects of high-altitude exposure on submaximal endurance capacity of men. *J Appl Physiol.* 1974;37(6):895–898.

34. Jackson CG, Sharkey BJ. Altitude, training and human performance. *Sports Med.* 1988;6:279–284.

35. Kollias J, Buskirk ER. Exercise and altitude. In: Johnson WR, Buskirk ER, eds. *Science and Medicine of Exercise and Sport.* 2nd ed. New York, NY: Harper & Row; 1974: 211–227.

36. Levine BD, Stray-Gundersen J. A practical approach to altitude training: Where to live and train for optimal performance enhancement. *Int J Sports Med.* 1992;13(suppl 1):S209–S212.

37. Levine BD, Roach RC, Houston CS. Work and training at altitude. In: Sutton JR, Coates G, Houston CS, eds. *Hypoxia and Mountain Medicine.* Burlington, Vt: Queen City Printers; 1992: 192–201.

38. Howley ET, Bassett DR Jr, Welch HG. Criteria for maximal oxygen uptake: Review and commentary. *Med Sci Sports Exerc.* 1995;27:1292–1301.

39. Katch VL, Sady SS, Freedson P. Biological variability in maximum aerobic power. *Med Sci Sports Exerc.* 1982;14:21–24.

40. Åstrand P-O, Rodahl K. *Textbook of Work Physiology: Physiological Bases of Exercise.* 3rd ed. New York, NY: McGraw-Hill Book Co; 1986.

41. Ferretti G, Moia C, Thomet JM, Kayser B. The decrease of maximal oxygen consumption during hypoxia in man: A mirror image of the oxygen equilibrium curve. *J Physiol (Lond).* 1997;498(1):231–237.

42. Buskirk ER, Kollias J, Picon-Reategui E, Akers R, Prokop E, Baker P. Physiology and performance of track athletes at various altitudes in the United States and Peru. In: Goddard RF, ed. *The Effects of Altitude on Physical Performance.* Albuquerque, NM: The Athletic Institute; 1967: 65–72.

43. Grover RF, Weil JV, Reeves JT. Cardiovascular adaptation to exercise at high altitude. In: Pandolf KB, ed. *Exercise and Sport Science Reviews.* 14th ed. New York, NY: Macmillan; 1986: 269–302.

44. Adams RP, Welch HG. Oxygen uptake, acid–base status, and performance with varied inspired oxygen fractions. *J Appl Physiol.* 1980;49:863–868.

45. Adams WC, Bernauer EM, Dill DB, Bomar JB Jr. Effects of equivalent sea-level and altitude training on Vo_2max and running performance. *J Appl Physiol.* 1975;39:262–266.

46. Andersen HT, Smeland EB, Owe JO, Myhre K. Analyses of maximum cardiopulmonary performance during exposure to acute hypoxia at simulated altitude: Sea level to 5,000 meters (760–404 mm Hg). *Aviat Space Environ Med.* 1985;56:1192–1195.

47. Daniels J, Oldridge N. The effects of alternate exposure to altitude and sea level on world-class middle-distance runners. *Med Sci Sports.* 1970;2:107–112.

48. Gleser MA, Vogel JA. Effects of acute alterations of Vo_2max on endurance capacity of men. *J Appl Physiol.* 1973;34:443–447.

49. Gore CJ, Hahn AG, Watson DB, et al. Vo_2max and arterial O_2 saturation at sea level and 610 m. *Med Sci Sports Exerc.* 1995;27:S7.

50. Greenleaf JE, Greenleaf CJ, Card DH, Saltin B. Exercise-temperature regulation in man during acute exposure to simulated altitude. *J Appl Physiol.* 1969;26:290–296.

51. Hogan MC, Cox RH, Welch HG. Lactate accumulation during incremental exercise with varied inspired oxygen fractions. *J Appl Physiol.* 1983;55:1134–1140.

52. Levine BD, Friedman DB, Engfred K, et al. The effect of normoxic or hypobaric hypoxic endurance training on the hypoxic ventilatory response. *Med Sci Sports Exerc.* 1992;24:769–775.

53. Levitan BM, Bungo MW. Measurement of cardiopulmonary performance during acute exposure to a 2,440-m equivalent atmosphere. *Aviat Space Environ Med.* 1982;53:639–642.

54. Mairbaurl H, Schobersberger W, Humpeler E, Hasibeder W, Fischer W, Raas E. Beneficial effects of exercising at moderate altitude on red cell oxygen transport and on exercise performance. *Pflugers Arch.* 1986;406:594–599.

55. Paterson DJ, Pinnington H, Pearce AR, Morton AR. Maximal exercise cardiorespiratory responses of men and women during acute exposure to hypoxia. *Aviat Space Environ Med.* 1987;58:243–247.

56. Roskamm H, Landry F, Samek L, Schlager M, Weidemann H, Reindell H. Effects of a standardized ergometer training program at three different altitudes. *J Appl Physiol.* 1969;27:840–847.

57. Squires RW, Buskirk ER. Aerobic capacity during acute exposure to simulated altitude, 914 to 2,286 meters. *Med Sci Sports Exerc*. 1982;14:36–40.

58. Terrados N, Mizuno M, Andersen H. Reduction in maximal oxygen uptake at low altitudes: Role of training status and lung function. *Clin Physiol*. 1985;5(suppl 3):75–79.

59. Tucker A, Stager JM, Cordain L. Arterial O_2 saturation and maximum O_2 consumption in moderate-altitude runners exposed to sea level and 3,050 m. *JAMA*. 1995;252:2867–2871.

60. Cymerman A, Reeves JT, Sutton JR, et al. Operation Everest II: Maximal oxygen uptake at extreme altitude. *J Appl Physiol*. 1989;66(5):2446–2453.

61. West JB, Boyer SJ, Graber DJ, et al. Maximal exercise at extreme altitudes on Mount Everest. *J Appl Physiol*. 1983;55:688–698.

62. Gore CJ, Hahn AG, Scroop GS, et al. Increased arterial desaturation in trained cyclists during maximal exercise at 580 m altitude. *J Appl Physiol*. 1996;80:2204–2210.

63. Boutellier U, Marconi C, Di Prampero PE, Cerretelli P. Effects of chronic hypoxia on maximal performance. *Bull Eur Physiopathol Respir*. 1982;18:39–44.

64. Ferretti G, Hauser H, Di Prampero PE. Maximal muscular power before and after exposure to chronic hypoxia. *Int J Sports Med*. 1990;11:S31–S34.

65. Rose MS, Houston CS, Fulco CS, Coates G, Sutton JR, Cymerman A. Operation Everest II: nutrition and body composition. *J Appl Physiol*. 1988;65(6):2545–2551.

66. Young PM, Rock PB, Fulco CS, Trad LA, Forte VA Jr, Cymerman A. Altitude acclimatization attenuates plasma ammonia accumulation during submaximal exercise. *J Appl Physiol*. 1987;63(2):758–764.

67. Lawler J, Powers SK, Thompson D. Linear relationship between $\dot{V}o_2$max and $\dot{V}o_2$max decrement during exposure to acute altitude. *J Appl Physiol*. 1988;64:1486–1492.

68. Young AJ, Cymerman A, Burse RL. The influence of cardiorespiratory fitness on the decrement in maximal aerobic power at high altitude. *Eur J Appl Physiol Med*. 1985;54:12–15.

69. Koistinen P, Takala T, Martikkala V, Leppaluoto J. Aerobic fitness influences the response of maximal oxygen uptake and lactate threshold in acute hypobaric hypoxia. *Int J Sports Med*. 1995;26:78–81.

70. Martin D, O'Kroy J. Effects of acute hypoxia on the $\dot{V}o_2$max of trained and untrained subjects. *J Sports Sci*. 1993;11:37–42.

71. Beidleman BA, Rock PB, Muza SR, et al. Menstrual cycle phase does not affect work performance at sea level and 4,300 m. In: Sutton JR, Houston CS, Coates G, eds. In: *Hypoxia and the Brain: 9th International Hypoxia Symposium, 14–18 Feb 1995*. Lake Louise, Alberta, Canada: Queen City Printers; 1995.

72. Reeves JT, Grover RF, Cohn JE. Regulation of ventilation during exercise at 10,200 ft in athletes born at low altitude. *J Appl Physiol*. 1967;22(3):546–554.

73. Christensen EH, Forbes WH. Der Kreislauf in grossen Hohen. *Skand Arch Physiol*. 1937;76:75–89.

74. Knuttgen HG, Saltin B. Oxygen uptake, muscle high-energy phosphates, and lactate in exercise under acute hypoxic conditions in man. *Acta Physiol Scand*. 1973;87:368–376.

75. Young AJ, Young PM. Human acclimatization to high terrestrial altitude. In: Pandolf KB, Sawka MN, Gonzalez RR, eds. *Human Performance Physiology and Environmental Medicine at Terrestrial Extremes*. Indianapolis, Ind: Benchmark Press (now Traverse City, Michigan: Cooper Publishing Group); 1988: 497–543.

76. Fulco CS, Lewis SF, Frykman PN, et al. Muscle fatigue and exhaustion during dynamic leg exercise in normobaria and hypobaria. *J Appl Physiol.* 1996; 81:1891–1900.

77. Hackney AC, Kelleher DL, Coyne JT, Hodgdon JA. Military operations at moderate altitude: Effects on physical performance. *Mil Med.* 1992;157:625–629.

78. Patton JF, Murphy MM, Bidwell TR, Mello RP, Harp ME. *Metabolic Cost of Military Physical Tasks in MOPP 0 and MOPP 4.* Natick, Mass: US Army Research Institute of Environmental Medicine; 1996. USARIEM Technical Report T95-9.

79. Buskirk ER. Decrease in physical working capacity at high altitude. In: Hegnauer AH, ed. *Biomedicine of High Terrestrial Elevations.* Natick, Mass: US Army Research Institute of Environmental Medicine; 1969: 204–222.

80. Pugh LGCE. Athletes at altitude. *J Physiol (Lond).* 1967;192:619–646.

81. Linnarsson D, Karlsson J, Fagraeus L, Saltin B. Muscle metabolites and oxygen deficit with exercise and hypoxia and hyperoxia. *J Appl Physiol.* 1974;36:399–402.

82. Dickinson ER, Piddington MJ, Brain T. Project Olympics. *Schweizerische Zeitschrift Fur Sportmedizin.* 1966;14:305–313.

83. Stiles MH. Athletic performance at Mexico City. In: First Conference on Cardiovascular Disease, ed. *Hypoxia, High Altitude and the Heart.* 5th ed. New York, NY: Karger; 1970: 17–23.

84. Bowie W, Cumming GR. Sustained handgrip-reproducibility: Effects of hypoxia. *Med Sci Sports.* 1971;3:24–31.

85. Burse RL, Cymerman A, Young AJ. Respiratory response and muscle function during isometric handgrip exercise at high altitude. *Aviat Space Environ Med.* 1987;58:39–46.

86. Eiken O, Tesch PA. Effects of hyperoxia and hypoxia on dynamic and sustained static performance of the human quadriceps muscle. *Acta Physiol Scand.* 1984;122:629–633.

87. Fulco CS, Cymerman A, Muza SR, Rock PB, Pandolf KB, Lewis SF. Adductor pollicis muscle fatigue during acute and chronic altitude exposure and return to sea level. *J Appl Physiol.* 1994;77:179–183.

88. Garner SH, Sutton JR, Burse RL, McComas AJ, Cymerman A, Houston CS. Operation Everest II: Neuromuscular performance under conditions of extreme simulated altitude. *J Appl Physiol.* 1990;68:1167–1172.

89. Young A, Wright J, Knapik J, Cymerman A. Skeletal muscle strength during exposure to hypobaric hypoxia. *Med Sci Sports Exerc.* 1980;12:330–335.

90. Coudert J. Anaerobic performance at altitude. *Int J Sports Med.* 1992;13(suppl 1):S82–S85.

91. Kayser B, Narici M, Milesi S, Grassi B, Cerretelli P. Body composition and maximum alactic anaerobic performance during a one month stay at high altitude. *Int J Sports Med.* 1993;14:244–247.

92. Kayser B, Bokenkamp R, Binzoni T. Alpha-motoneuron excitability at high altitude. *Eur J Appl Physiol Med.* 1993;66:1–4.

93. Sahlin K. Metabolic changes limiting muscle performance. In: Saltin B, ed. *Biochemistry of Exercise VI.* 16th ed. Champaign, Ill: Human Kinetics; 1986: 323–343.

94. Sutton JR. Effect of acute hypoxia on the hormonal response to exercise. *J Appl Physiol.* 1977;42:587–592.

95. Maclaren DPM, Gibson H, Parry-Billings M, Edwards RHT. A review of metabolic and physiological factors in fatigue. In: Pandolf KB, ed. *Exercise and Sport Sciences Reviews.* 17th annual ed. Baltimore, Md: American College of Sports Medicine, Williams & Wilkins; 1989: 29–66.

96. Fitts RH. Cellular mechanisms of muscle fatigue. *Physiol Rev.* 1994;74:49–94.

97. Edwards RHT. Metabolic changes during isometric contractions of the quadriceps muscle. In: Jokl E, ed. *Medicine and Sport: Advances in Exercise Physiology.* 9th ed. New York, NY: Karger; 1976: 114–131.

98. Chasiotis D, Bergstrom M, Hultman E. ATP utilization and force during intermittent and continuous muscle contractions. *J Appl Physiol.* 1987;63:167–174.

99. Green S. Measurement of anaerobic work capacities in humans. *Sports Med.* 1995;19:32–42.

100. Vanderwalle H, Peres G, Monod H. Standard anaerobic exercise tests. *Sports Med.* 1987;4:268–289.

101. Bedu M, Fellmann N, Spielvogel H, Falgairette G, Van Praagh E, Coudert J. Force-velocity and 30-s Wingate tests in boys at high and low altitudes. *J Appl Physiol.* 1991;70:1031–1037.

102. McLellan TM, Kavanagh MF, Jacobs I. The effect of hypoxia on performance during 30 s or 45 s of supramaximal exercise. *Eur J Appl Physiol Med.* 1990;60:155–161.

103. Department of the Army. *Soldier's Manual of Common Tasks.* Washington, DC: DA; Oct 1990. Cited in: Patton JF, Murphy MM, Bidwell TR, Mello RP, Harp ME. *Metabolic Cost of Military Physical Tasks in MOPP 0 and MOPP 4.* Natick, Mass: US Army Research Institute of Environmental Medicine; 1996. USARIEM Technical Report T95-9.

104. US Army Infantry School. *Military Occupational Specialty (MOS) Physical Task List.* DA; US Army Infantry School, Ft Benning, Ga; Oct 1978. Cited in: Patton JF, Murphy MM, Bidwell TR, Mello RP, Harp ME. *Metabolic Cost of Military Physical Tasks in MOPP 0 and MOPP 4.* Natick, Mass: US Army Research Institute of Environmental Medicine; 1996. USARIEM Technical Report T95-9.

105. Waters TR, Putz-Anderson V, Garg A, Fine LJ. Revised NIOSH equation for the design and evaluation of manual lifting tasks. *Ergonomics.* 1993;36:749–776.

106. Grover RF, Reeves JT, Maher JT, et al. Maintained stroke volume but impaired arterial oxygenation in man at high altitude with supplemental CO_2. *Circ Res.* 1976;38:391–396.

107. Mizuno M, Juel C, Bro Rasmussen T, et al. Limb skeletal muscle adaptation in athletes after training at altitude. *J Appl Physiol.* 1990;68:496–502.

108. Terrados N, Jansson E, Sylvén C, Kaijser L. Is hypoxia a stimulus for synthesis of oxidative enzymes and myoglobin? *J Appl Physiol.* 1990;68:2369–2372.

109. Young AJ, Evans WJ, Cymerman A, Pandolf KB, Knapik JJ, Maher JT. Sparing effect of chronic high-altitude exposure on muscle glycogen utilization. *J Appl Physiol.* 1982;52:857–862.

110. Blomqvist CG, Saltin B. Cardiovascular adaptations to physical training. In: Annual Reviews Inc, ed. *Annual Review of Physiology.* 45th annual ed. 1983: 169–189.

111. Hickson RC, Foster C, Pollock ML, Galassi TM, Rich S. Reduced training intensities and loss of aerobic power, endurance, and cardiac growth. *J Appl Physiol.* 1985;58:492–499.

112. Hickson RC, Kanakis C, Davis JR, Moore AM, Rich S. Reduced training duration effects on aerobic power, endurance, and cardiac growth. *J Appl Physiol.* 1982;53:225–229.

113. Hickson RC, Rosenkoetter MA. Reduced training frequencies and maintenance of increased aerobic power. *Med Sci Sports Exerc.* 1981;13:13–16.

114. Pollock ML. The quantification of endurance training programs. In: Wilmore JH, ed. *Exercise and Sport Science Reviews.* New York, NY: Academic Press; 1973: 155–188.

115. Hickson RC, Bomze HA, Holloszy JO. Linear increase in aerobic power induced by a strenuous program of endurance exercise. *J Appl Physiol.* 1977;42:372–376.

116. Horstman D, Weiskopf R, Jackson RE. Work capacity during 3-week sojourn at 4,300 m: Effects of relative polycythemia. *J Appl Physiol.* 1980;49:311–318.

117. Gleser MA, Vogel JA. Endurance capacity for prolonged exercise on the bicycle ergometer. *J Appl Physiol.* 1973;34:438–442.

118. Davies CT, Sargeant AJ. Effects of hypoxic training on normoxic maximal aerobic power output. *Eur J Appl Physiol Med.* 1974;33:227–236.

119. Crothers T. The secret of their success? *Sports Illustrated.* 1990;72:1–12.

120. Daniels J. Training where the air is rare. *Runner's World.* 1980;Jun:50–52.

121. Dick FW. Training at altitude in practice. *Int J Sports Med.* 1992;13(suppl 1):S203–S206.

122. Longman J. 13,800 feet up, runners toil to excel below. *The New York Times.* 1995;40.

123. Potts F. Running at high altitudes. In: Goddard RF, ed. *The Effects of Altitude on Physical Performance.* Albuquerque, NM: The Athletic Institute; 1967: 73–75.

124. Daniels J. Altitude and athletic training and performance. *Am J Sports Med.* 1979;7:371–373.

125. Smith MH, Sharkey BJ. Altitude training: Who benefits? *The Physician and Sportsmedicine.* 1984;12:48–62.

126. Svedenhag J, Saltin B, Johansson C, Kaijser L. Aerobic and anaerobic exercise capacities of elite middle-distance runners after two weeks of training at moderate altitude. *Scan J Med Sci Sports.* 1991;1:205–214.

127. Berglund B. High-altitude training: Aspects of haematological adaptation. *Sports Med.* 1992;14:289–303.

128. Loeppky JA, Bynum WA. Effects of periodic exposure to hypobaria and exercise on physical work capacity. *J Sports Med Phys Fitness.* 1970;10:238–247.

129. Desplanches D, Hoppeler H, Linossier MT, et al. Effects of training in normoxia and normobaric hypoxia on human muscle ultrastructure. *Pflugers Arch.* 1993;425:263–267.

130. Terrados N, Melichna J, Sylven C, Jansson E, Kaijser L. Effects of training at simulated altitude on performance and muscle metabolic capacity in competitive road cyclists. *Eur J Appl Physiol Med.* 1988;57:203–209.

131. Bannister EW, Woo W. Effects of simulated altitude training on aerobic and anaerobic power. *Eur J Appl Physiol Med.* 1978;38:55–69.

132. Levine BD, Engfred K, Friedman DB, Kjaer M, Saltin B. High altitude endurance training: Effect on aerobic capacity and work performance. *Med Sci Sports Exerc.* 1990;22:S35. Abstract.

133. Levine BD, Stray-Gundersen J, Duhaime G, Snell PG, Friedman DB. "Living High—Training Low": The effect of altitude acclimatization/normoxic training in trained runners. *Med Sci Sports Exerc.* 1991;23:S25

134. Balke B, Nagle FJ, Daniels J. Altitude and maximal performance in work and sport activity. *JAMA.* 1965;194:646–649.

135. Favier R, Spielvogel H, Desplanches D, et al. Training in hypoxia vs training in normoxia in high-altitude natives. *J Appl Physiol.* 1995;78:2286–2293.

136. Hoppeler H, Howald H, Conley K, et al. Endurance training in humans: Aerobic capacity and structure of skeletal muscle. *J Appl Physiol.* 1985;59:320–327.

Chapter 22: ATTACHMENT

DATA SOURCES FOR GRAPHS IN CHAPTER 22

Fig. 22-1. Civilian and military investigations: (1) Cymerman A, Pandolf KB, Young AJ, Maher JT. Energy expenditure during load carriage at high altitude. *J Appl Physiol.* 1981;51:14–18. (2) Faulkner JA, Daniels JT, Balke B. Effects of training at moderate altitude on physical performance capacity. *J Appl Physiol.* 1967;23:85–89. (3) Dill DB, Adams WC. Maximal oxygen uptake at sea level and at 3,090-m altitude in high school champion runners. *J Appl Physiol.* 1971;30:854–859. (4) Klausen K, Robinson S, Micahel ED, Myhre LG. Effect of high altitude on maximal working capacity. *J Appl Physiol.* 1966;21:1191–1194. (5) Buskirk ER, Kollias J, Akers RF, Prokop EK, Reategui P. Maximal performance at altitude and on return from altitude in conditioned runners. *J Appl Physiol.* 1967;23:259–266. (6) Faulkner JA, Kollias J, Favour CB, Buskirk ER, Balke B. Maximum aerobic capacity and running performance at altitude. *J Appl Physiol.* 1968;24:685–691. (7) Grover RF, Reeves JT. Exercise performance of athletes at sea level and 3,100 meters altitude. *Med Thorac.* 1966;23:129–143. (8) Maher JT, Jones LG, Hartley LH. Effects of high-altitude exposure on submaximal endurance capacity of men. *J Appl Physiol.* 1974;37(6):895–898. (9) Boutellier U, Marconi C, Di Prampero PE, Cerretelli P. Effects of chronic hypoxia on maximal performance. *Bull Europ Physiopath Resp.* 1982;18:39–44. (10) Lawler J, Powers SK, Thompson D. Linear relationship between $\dot{V}o_2$max and $\dot{V}o_2$max decrement during exposure to acute altitude. *J Appl Physiol.* 1988;64:1486–1492. (11) Shephard RJ, Bouhlel E, Vandewalle H, Monod H. Peak oxygen uptake and hypoxia. *Int J Sports Med.* 1988;9:279–283. (12) Adams RP, Welch HG. Oxygen uptake, acid–base status, and performance with varied inspired oxygen fractions. *J Appl Physiol.* 1980;49:863–868. (13) Adams WC, Bernauer EM, Dill DB, Bomar JB Jr. Effects of equivalent sea-level and altitude training on $\dot{V}o_2$max and running performance. *J Appl Physiol.* 1975;39:262–266. (14) Andersen HT, Smeland EB, Owe JO, Myhre K. Analyses of maximum cardiopulmonary performance during exposure to acute hypoxia at simulated altitude—Sea level to 5,000 meters (760–404 mm Hg). *Aviat Space Environ Med.* 1985;56:1192–1195. (15) Daniels J, Oldridge N. The effects of alternate exposure to altitude and sea level on world-class middle-distance runners. *Med Sci Sports.* 1970;2:107–112. (16) Gleser MA, Vogel JA. Effects of acute alterations of $\dot{V}o_2$max on endurance capacity of men. *J Appl Physiol.* 1973;34:443–447. (17) Gore CJ, Hahn AG, Watson DB, et al. $\dot{V}o_2$max and arterial O_2 saturation at sea level and 610 m. *Med Sci Sports Exerc.* 1995;27:S7. (18) Greenleaf JE, Greenleaf CJ, Card DH, Saltin B. Exercise-temperature regulation in man during acute exposure to simulated altitude. *J Appl Physiol.* 1969;26:290–296. (19) Hogan MC, Cox RH, Welch HG. Lactate accumulation during incremental exercise with varied inspired oxygen fractions. *J Appl Physiol.* 1983;55:1134–1140. (20) Levine BD, Friedman DB, Engfred K, et al. The effect of normoxic or hypobaric hypoxic endurance training on the hypoxic ventilatory response. *Med Sci Sports Exerc.* 1992;24:769–775. (21) Levitan BM, Bungo MW. Measurement of cardiopulmonary performance during acute exposure to a 2,440-m equivalent atmosphere. *Aviat Space Environ Med.* 1982;53:639–642. (22) Mairbaurl H, Schobersberger W, Humpeler E, Hasibeder W, Fischer W, Raas E. Beneficial effects of exercising at moderate altitude on red cell oxygen transport and on exercise performance. *Pflugers Arch.* 1986;406:594–599. (23) Paterson DJ, Pinnington H, Pearce AR, Morton AR. Maximal exercise cardiorespiratory responses of men and women during acute exposure to hypoxia. *Aviat Space Environ Med.* 1987;58:243–247. (24) Roskamm H, Landry F, Samek L, Schlager M, Weidemann H, Reindell H. Effects of a standardized ergometer training program at three different altitudes. *J Appl Physiol.* 1969;27:840–847. (25) Squires RW, Buskirk ER. Aerobic capacity during acute exposure to simulated altitude, 914 to 2,286 meters. *Med Sci Sports Exerc.* 1982;14:36–40. (26) Tucker A, Stager JM, Cordain L. Arterial O_2 saturation and maximum O_2 consumption in moderate-altitude runners exposed to sea level and 3,050 m. *JAMA.* 1995;252:2867–2871. (27) Cymerman A, Reeves JT, Sutton JR, et al. Operation Everest II: Maximal oxygen uptake at extreme altitude. *J Appl Physiol.* 1989;66(5):2446–2453. (28) West JB, Boyer SJ, Graber DJ, et al. Maximal exercise at extreme altitudes on Mount Everest. *J Appl Physiol.* 1983;55:688–698. (29) Gore CJ, Hahn AG, Scroop GS, et al. Increased arterial desaturation in trained cyclists during maximal exercise at 580 m altitude. *J Appl Physiol.* 1996;80:2204–2210. (30) Young PM, Rock PB, Fulco CS, Trad LA, Forte VA Jr, Cymerman A. Altitude acclimatization attenuates plasma ammonia accumulation during submaximal exercise. *J Appl Physiol.* 1987;63(2):758–764. (31) Koistinen P, Takala T, Martikkala V, Leppaluoto J. Aerobic fitness influences the response of maximal oxygen uptake and lactate threshold in acute hypobaric hypoxia. *Int J Sports Med.* 1995;26:78–81. (32) Martin D, O'Kroy J. Effects of acute hypoxia on the $\dot{V}o_2$max of trained and untrained subjects. *J Sports Sci.* 1993;11:37–42. (33) Beidleman BA, Rock PB, Muza SR, et al. Menstrual cycle phase does not affect work performance at sea level and 4,300 m. In: Sutton JR, Houston CS, Coates G, eds. *Hypoxia and the Brain: 9th International Hypoxia Symposium, 14–18 Feb 1995.* Lake Louise, Alberta, Canada: Queen City Printers; 1995. (34) Reeves JT, Grover RF, Cohn JE. Regulation of ventilation during exercise at 10,200 ft in athletes born at low altitude. *J Appl Physiol.* 1967;22(3):546–554. (35) Christensen EH, Forbes WH. Der Kreislauf in grossen Hohen. *Skand Arch Physiol.* 1937;76:75–89. (36) Pugh LGCE. Athletes at altitude. *J Physiol (Lond).* 1967;192:619–646. (37) Linnarsson D, Karlsson J, Fagraeus L, Saltin B. Muscle metabolites and oxygen deficit with exercise and hypoxia and hyperoxia. *J Appl Physiol.* 1974;36:399–402. (38) Terrados N, Jansson E, Sylvén C, Kaijser L. Is hypoxia a stimulus for synthesis of oxidative enzymes and myoglobin? *J Appl Physiol.* 1990;68:2369–2372. (39) Young AJ, Evans WJ, Cymerman A, Pandolf KB, Knapik JJ, Maher JT. Sparing effect of chronic high-altitude exposure on muscle glycogen utilization. *J Appl Physiol.* 1982;52:857–862. (40) Horstman D, Weiskopf R, Jackson RE. Work capacity during 3-week sojourn at 4,300 m: Effects of relative polycythemia. *J Appl Physiol.* 1980;49:311–318. (41) Loeppky JA, Bynum WA. Effects of periodic exposure to hypobaria and exercise on physical work capacity. *J Sports Med Phys Fitness.* 1970;10:238–247. (42) Desplanches D, Hoppeler H, Linossier MT, et al. Effects of training in normoxia and normobaric hypoxia on human muscle ultrastructure. *Pflugers Arch.* 1993;425:263–267. (43) Balke B, Nagle FJ, Daniels J. Altitude and maximal performance in work and sport activity. *JAMA.* 1965;194:646–649. (44) Fulco CS, Rock PB, Trad L, Forte V Jr, Cymerman A. Maximal cardiorespiratory responses to one- and two-legged cycling during acute and long-term exposure to 4,300 meters altitude. *Eur J Appl Physiol.* 1988;57:761–766. (45) Dua GL, Sen Gupta J. A study of physical work capacity of sea level residents on prolonged stay at high altitude and comparison with high altitude native residents. *Ind J Physiol Pharmac.* 1980;24:15–24. (46) Bouissou PF, Peronnet F, Brisson G, Helie R, Ledoux M. Metabolic and endocrine responses to graded exercise under acute hypoxia. *Eur J Appl Physiol.* 1986;55:290–294. (47) Drinkwater BL, Folinsbee LJ, Bedi JF, Plowman SA, Loucks AB, Horvath SM. Response of women mountaineers to maximal exercise during hypoxia. *Aviat Space Environ Med.* 1979;50:657–662. (48) Elliot PR, Atterbom HA. Comparison of exercise responses of males and females during acute exposure to hypobaria. *Aviat Space Environ Med.* 1978;49:415–418. (49) Consolazio CF, Nelson RA, Matoush LO, Hansen JE. Energy metabolism at high altitude (3,475 m). *J Appl Physiol.* 1966;21:1732–1740. (50) Maresh CM, Noble BJ, Robertson KL, Sime WE. Maximal exercise during hypobaric hypoxia (447 torr) in moderate-altitude natives. *J Appl Physiol.* 1983;15:360–365. (51) Pugh LGCE, Gill MB, Lahiri S, Milledge JS, Ward MP, West JB. Muscular exercise at great altitudes. *J Appl Physiol.* 1964;19:431–440. (52) Saltin B, Grover RF, Blomqvist CG, Hartley LH, Johnson RLJ. Maximal oxygen uptake and cardiac output after 2 weeks at 4,300 m. *J Appl Physiol.* 1968;25:400–409. (53) Hughes RL, Clode M, Edwards RHT, Goodwin TJ, Jones NL. Effect of inspired O_2 on cardiopulmonary and metabolic responses to exercise in man. *J Appl Physiol.* 1968;24:336–347. (54) Shephard RJ, Bouhlel E, Vandewalle H, Monod H. Muscle mass as a factor limiting physical work. *J Appl Physiol.* 1988;64:1472–1479. (55) Dill DB, Myhre LG, Phillips J Jr, Brown DK. Work capacity in acute exposures to altitude. *J Appl Physiol.* 1966;21:1168–1176. (56) Vogel JA, Hartley LH, Cruz JC, Hogan RP. Cardiac output during exercise in sea-level residents at sea level and high altitude. *J Appl Physiol.* 1974;36:169–172. (57) Wagner JA, Miles DS, Horvath SM, Reyburn JA. Maximal work capacity of women during acute hypoxia. *J Appl Physiol.* 1979;47:1223–1227. (58) Benoit H, Germain M, Barthelemy JC, Denis C, Castells J, Dormois D, Lacour JR, Geyssant A. Pre-acclimatization to high altitude using exercise with normobaric hypoxic gas mixtures. *Int J Sports Med.* 1992;13(suppl 1):S213–S215. (59) Fagraeus L, Karlsson J, Linnarsson D, Saltin B. Oxygen uptake during maximal work at lowered and raised ambient air pressures. *Acta Physiol Scand.* 1973;87:411–421. (60) Schoene RB, Bates PW, Larson EB, Pierson DJ. Effect of acetazolamide on normoxic and hypoxic exercise in humans at sea level. *J Appl Physiol.* 1983;55:1772–1776. (61) Robertson RJ, Gilcher R, Metz KF, et al. Effect of induced erythrocythemia on hypoxia tolerance during exercise. *J Appl Physiol.* 1982;53:490–495. (62) Forte VA Jr, Muza SR, Fulco CS, et al. Smoking accentuates the maximal oxygen uptake decrement at high altitude. *FASEB J.* 1996;10:A418. Abstract. (63) Stenberg J, Ekblom B, Messin R. Hemodynamic response to work at simulated altitude: 4,000 m. *J Appl Physiol.* 1966;21:1589–1594. (64) Hartley LH. Adjustments of the oxygen transport system during residence at high altitude. In: Brewer GJ, ed. *Hemoglobin and Red Cell Structure and Function.* New York, NY: Plenum Publishing Corp; 1972: 349–360. (65) Hartley LH, Vogel JA, Landowne M. Central, femoral, and brachial circulation during exercise in hypoxia. *J Appl Physiol.* 1973;34:87–90.

Fig. 22-2. *Highly conditioned individuals: (1) Faulkner JA, Daniels JT, Balke B. Effects of training at moderate altitude on physical performance capacity. *J Appl Physiol.* 1967;23:85–89. (2) Dill DB, Adams WC. Maximal oxygen uptake at sea level and at 3,090-m altitude in high school champion runners. *J Appl Physiol.* 1971;30:854–859. (3) Buskirk ER, Kollias J, Akers RF, Prokop EK, Reategui P. Maximal performance at altitude and on return from altitude in conditioned runners. *J Appl Physiol.* 1967;23:259–266. (4) Grover RF, Reeves JT. Exercise performance of athletes at sea level and 3,100 meters altitude. *Med Thorac.* 1966;23:129–143. (5) Lawler J, Powers SK, Thompson D. Linear relationship between $\dot{V}O_2$max and $\dot{V}O_2$max decrement during exposure to acute altitude. *J Appl Physiol.* 1988;64:1486–1492. (6) Adams WC, Bernauer EM, Dill DB, Bomar JB Jr. Effects of equivalent sea-level and altitude training on $\dot{V}O_2$max and running performance. *J Appl Physiol.* 1975;39:262–266. (7) Daniels J, Oldridge N. The effects of alternate exposure to altitude and sea level on world-class middle-distance runners. *Med Sci Sports.* 1970;2:107–112. (8) Gore CJ, Hahn AG, Watson DB, et al. $\dot{V}O_2$max and arterial O_2 saturation at sea level and 610 m. *Med Sci Sports Exerc.* 1995;27:S7. (9) Paterson DJ, Pinnington H, Pearce AR, Morton AR. Maximal exercise cardiorespiratory responses of men and women during acute exposure to hypoxia. *Aviat Space Environ Med.* 1987;58:243–247. (10) Terrados N, Mizuno M, Andersen H. Reduction in maximal oxygen uptake at low altitudes: Role of training status and lung function. *Clin Physiol.* 1985;5(suppl 3):75–79. (11) Tucker A, Stager JM, Cordain L. Arterial O_2 saturation and maximum O_2 consumption in moderate-altitude runners exposed to sea level and 3,050 m. *JAMA.* 1995;252:2867–2871. (12) Gore CJ, Hahn AG, Scroop GS, et al. Increased arterial desaturation in trained cyclists during maximal exercise at 580 m altitude. *J Appl Physiol.* 1996;80:2204–2210. (13) Martin D, O'Kroy J. Effects of acute hypoxia on the $\dot{V}O_2$max of trained and untrained subjects. *J Sports Sci.* 1993;11:37–42. (14) Reeves JT, Grover RF, Cohn JE. Regulation of ventilation during exercise at 10,200 ft in athletes born at low altitude. *J Appl Physiol.* 1967;22(3):546–554. (15) Pugh LGCE. Athletes at altitude. *J Physiol (Lond).* 1967;192:619–646. (16) Terrados N, Jansson E, Sylvén C, Kaijser L. Is hypoxia a stimulus for synthesis of oxidative enzymes and myoglobin? *J Appl Physiol.* 1990;68:2369–2372.

†Less-well-conditioned individuals: (1) Cymerman A, Pandolf KB, Young AJ, Maher JT. Energy expenditure during load carriage at high altitude. *J Appl Physiol.* 1981;51:14–18. (2) Klausen K, Robinson S, Micahel ED, Myhre LG. Effect of high altitude on maximal working capacity. *J Appl Physiol.* 1966;21:1191–1194. (3) Lawler J, Powers SK, Thompson D. Linear relationship between $\dot{V}o_2$max and $\dot{V}o_2$max decrement during exposure to acute altitude. *J Appl Physiol.* 1988;64:1486–1492. (4) Andersen HT, Smeland EB, Owe JO, Myhre K. Analyses of maximum cardiopulmonary performance during exposure to acute hypoxia at simulated altitude: Sea level to 5,000 meters (760–404 mm Hg). *Aviat Space Environ Med.* 1985;56:1192–1195. (5) Gleser MA, Vogel JA. Effects of acute alterations of $\dot{V}o_2$max on endurance capacity of men. *J Appl Physiol.* 1973;34:443–447. (6) Gore CJ, Hahn AG, Watson DB, et al. $\dot{V}o_2$max and arterial O_2 saturation at sea level and 610 m. *Med Sci Sports Exerc.* 1995;27:S7. (7) Hogan MC, Cox RH, Welch HG. Lactate accumulation during incremental exercise with varied inspired oxygen fractions. *J Appl Physiol.* 1983;55:1134–1140. (8) Levine BD, Friedman DB, Engfred K, et al. The effect of normoxic or hypobaric hypoxic endurance training on the hypoxic ventilatory response. *Med Sci Sports Exerc.* 1992;24:769–775. (9) Levitan BM, Bungo MW. Measurement of cardiopulmonary performance during acute exposure to a 2,440-m equivalent atmosphere. *Aviat Space Environ Med.* 1982;53:639–642. (10) Mairbaurl H, Schobersberger W, Humpeler E, Hasibeder W, Fischer W, Raas E. Beneficial effects of exercising at moderate altitude on red cell oxygen transport and on exercise performance. *Pflugers Arch.* 1986;406:594–599. (11) Paterson DJ, Pinnington H, Pearce AR, Morton AR. Maximal exercise cardiorespiratory responses of men and women during acute exposure to hypoxia. *Aviat Space Environ Med.* 1987;58:243–247. (12) Roskamm H, Landry F, Samek L, Schlager M, Weidemann H, Reindell H. Effects of a standardized ergometer training program at three different altitudes. *J Appl Physiol.* 1969;27:840–847. (13) Terrados N, Mizuno M, Andersen H. Reduction in maximal oxygen uptake at low altitudes: Role of training status and lung function. *Clin Physiol.* 1985;5(suppl 3):75–79. (14) Gore CJ, Hahn AG, Scroop GS, et al. Increased arterial desaturation in trained cyclists during maximal exercise at 580 m altitude. *J Appl Physiol.* 1996;80:2204–2210. (15) Martin D, O'Kroy J. Effects of acute hypoxia on the $\dot{V}o_2$max of trained and untrained subjects. *J Sports Sci.* 1993;11:37–42. (16) Beidleman BA, Rock PB, Muza SR, et al. Menstrual cycle phase does not affect work performance at sea level and 4,300 m. In: Sutton JR, Houston CS, Coates G, eds. *Hypoxia and the Brain: 9th International Hypoxia Symposium, 14–18 Feb 1995.* Lake Louise, Alberta, Canada: Queen City Printers; 1995. (17) Terrados N, Jansson E, Sylvén C, Kaijser L. Is hypoxia a stimulus for synthesis of oxidative enzymes and myoglobin? *J Appl Physiol.* 1990;68:2369–2372. (18) Young AJ, Evans WJ, Cymerman A, Pandolf KB, Knapik JJ, Maher JT. Sparing effect of chronic high-altitude exposure on muscle glycogen utilization. *J Appl Physiol.* 1982;52:857–862. (19) Horstman D, Weiskopf R, Jackson RE. Work capacity during 3-week sojourn at 4,300 m: Effects of relative polycythemia. *J Appl Physiol.* 1980;49:311–318. (20) Balke B, Nagle FJ, Daniels J. Altitude and maximal performance in work and sport activity. *JAMA.* 1965;194:646–649. (21) Fulco CS, Rock PB, Trad L, Forte V Jr, Cymerman A. Maximal cardiorespiratory responses to one- and two-legged cycling during acute and long-term exposure to 4,300 meters altitude. *Eur J Appl Physiol.* 1988;57:761–766. (22) Dua GL, Sen Gupta J. A study of physical work capacity of sea level residents on prolonged stay at high altitude and comparison with high altitude native residents. *Ind J Physiol Pharmacol.* 1980;24:15–24. (23) Drinkwater BL, Folinsbee LJ, Bedi JF, Plowman SA, Loucks AB, Horvath SM. Response of women mountaineers to maximal exercise during hypoxia. *Aviat Space Environ Med.* 1979;50:657–662. (24) Consolazio CF, Nelson RA, Matoush LO, Hansen JE. Energy metabolism at high altitude (3,475 m). *J Appl Physiol.* 1966;21:1732–1740. (25) Maresh CM, Noble BJ, Robertson KL, Sime WE. Maximal exercise during hypobaric hypoxia (447 torr) in moderate-altitude natives. *J Appl Physiol.* 1983;15:360–365. (26) Pugh LGCE, Gill MB, Lahiri S, Milledge JS, Ward MP, West JB. Muscular exercise at great altitudes. *J Appl Physiol.* 1964;19:431–440. (27) Hughes RL, Clode M, Edwards RHT, Goodwin TJ, Jones NL. Effect of inspired O_2 on cardiopulmonary and metabolic responses to exercise in man. *J Appl Physiol.* 1968;24:336–347. (28) Shephard RJ, Bouhlel E, Vandewalle H, Monod H. Muscle mass as a factor limiting physical work. *J Appl Physiol.* 1988;64:1472–1479. (29) Wagner JA, Miles DS, Horvath SM, Reyburn JA. Maximal work capacity of women during acute hypoxia. *J Appl Physiol.* 1979;47:1223–1227. (30) Robertson RJ, Gilcher R, Metz KF, et al. Effect of induced erythrocythemia on hypoxia tolerance during exercise. *J Appl Physiol.* 1982;53:490–495.

Fig. 22-3. *Baseline resident altitudes < 100 m: (1) Grover RF, Reeves JT. Exercise performance of athletes at sea level and 3,100 meters altitude. *Med Thorac.* 1966;23:129–143. (2) Lawler J, Powers SK, Thompson D. Linear relationship between $\dot{V}o_2$max and $\dot{V}o_2$max decrement during exposure to acute altitude. *J Appl Physiol.* 1988;64:1486–1492. (3) Shephard RJ, Bouhlel E, Vandewalle H, Monod H. Peak oxygen uptake and hypoxia. *Int J Sports Med.* 1988;9:279–283. (4) Adams RP, Welch HG. Oxygen uptake, acid–base status, and performance with varied inspired oxygen fractions. *J Appl Physiol.* 1980;49:863–868. (5) Adams WC, Bernauer EM, Dill DB, Bomar JB Jr. Effects of equivalent sea-level and altitude training on $\dot{V}o_2$max and running performance. *J Appl Physiol.* 1975;39:262–266. (6) Andersen HT, Smeland EB, Owe JO, Myhre K. Analyses of maximum cardiopulmonary performance during exposure to acute hypoxia at simulated altitude: Sea level to 5,000 meters (760–404 mm Hg). *Aviat Space Environ Med.* 1985;56:1192–1195. (7) Gleser MA, Vogel JA. Effects of acute alterations of $\dot{V}o_2$max on endurance capacity of men. *J Appl Physiol.* 1973;34:443–447. (8) Hogan MC, Cox RH, Welch HG. Lactate accumulation during incremental exercise with varied inspired oxygen fractions. *J Appl Physiol.* 1983;55:1134–1140. (9) Levitan BM, Bungo MW. Measurement of cardiopulmonary performance during acute exposure to a 2,440-m equivalent atmosphere. *Aviat Space Environ Med.* 1982;53:639–642. (10) Paterson DJ, Pinnington H, Pearce AR, Morton AR. Maximal exercise cardiorespiratory responses of men and women during acute exposure to hypoxia. *Aviat Space Environ Med.* 1987;58:243–247. (11) Tucker A, Stager JM, Cordain L. Arterial O_2 saturation and maximum O_2 consumption in moderate-altitude runners exposed to sea level and 3,050 m. *JAMA.* 1995;252:2867–2871. (12) Young PM, Rock PB, Fulco CS, Trad LA, Forte VA Jr, Cymerman A. Altitude acclimatization attenuates plasma ammonia accumulation during submaximal exercise. *J Appl Physiol.* 1987;63(2):758–764. (13) Beidleman BA, Rock PB, Muza SR, et al. Menstrual cycle phase does not affect work performance at sea level and 4,300 m. In: Sutton JR, Houston CS, Coates G, eds. *Hypoxia and the Brain: 9th International Hypoxia Symposium, 14–18 Feb 1995.* Lake Louise, Alberta, Canada: Queen City Printers; 1995. (14) Christensen EH, Forbes WH. Der Kreislauf in grossen Hohe. *Skand Arch Physiol.* 1937;76:75–89. (15) Pugh LGCE. Athletes at altitude. *J Physiol (Lond).* 1967;192:619–646. (16) Linnarsson D, Karlsson J, Fagraeus L, Saltin B. Muscle metabolites and oxygen deficit with exercise and hypoxia and hyperoxia. *J Appl Physiol.* 1974;36:399–402. (17) Terrados N, Jansson E, Sylvén C, Kaijser L. Is hypoxia a stimulus for synthesis of oxidative enzymes and myoglobin? *J Appl Physiol.* 1990;68:2369–2372. (18) Young AJ, Evans WJ, Cymerman A, Pandolf KB, Knapik JJ, Maher JT. Sparing effect of chronic high-altitude exposure on muscle glycogen utilization. *J Appl Physiol.* 1982;52:857–862. (19) Horstman D, Weiskopf R, Jackson RE. Work capacity during 3-week sojourn at 4,300 m: Effects of relative polycythemia. *J Appl Physiol.* 1980;49:311–318. (20) Fulco CS, Rock PB, Trad L, Forte V Jr, Cymerman A. Maximal cardiorespiratory responses to one- and two-legged cycling during acute and long-term exposure to 4,300 meters altitude. *Eur J Appl Physiol.* 1988;57:761–766. (21) Bouissou PF, Peronnet F, Brisson G, Helie R, Ledoux M. Metabolic and endocrine responses to graded exercise under acute hypoxia. *Eur J Appl Physiol.* 1986;55:290–294. (22) Drinkwater BL, Folinsbee LJ, Bedi JF, Plowman SA, Loucks AB, Horvath SM. Response of women mountaineers to maximal exercise during hypoxia. *Aviat Space Environ Med.* 1979;50:657–662. (23) Consolazio CF, Nelson RA, Matoush LO, Hansen JE. Energy metabolism at high altitude (3,475 m). *J Appl Physiol.* 1966;21:1732–1740. (24) Hughes RL, Clode M, Edwards RHT, Goodwin TJ, Jones NL. Effect of inspired O_2 on cardiopulmonary and metabolic responses to exercise in man. *J Appl Physiol.* 1968;24:336–347. (25) Shephard RJ, Bouhlel E, Vandewalle H, Monod H. Muscle mass as a factor limiting physical work. *J Appl Physiol.* 1988;64:1472–1479. (26) Dill DB, Myhre LG, Phillips J Jr, Brown DK. Work capacity in acute exposures to altitude. *J Appl Physiol.* 1966;21:1168–1176. (27) Vogel JA, Hartley LH, Cruz JC, Hogan RP. Cardiac output during exercise in sea-level residents at sea level and high altitude. *J Appl Physiol.* 1974;36:169–172. (28) Wagner JA, Miles DS, Horvath SM, Reyburn JA. Maximal work capacity of women during acute hypoxia. *J Appl Physiol.* 1979;47:1223–1227. (29) Schoene RB, Bates PW, Larson EB, Pierson DJ. Effect of acetazolamide on normoxic and hypoxic exercise in humans at sea level. *J Appl Physiol.* 1983; 55: 1772–1776. (30) Robertson RJ, Gilcher R, Metz KF, et al. Effect of induced erythrocythemia on hypoxia tolerance during exercise. *J Appl Physiol.* 1982;53:490–495. (31) Forte VA Jr, Muza SR, Fulco CS, et al. Smoking accentuates the maximal oxygen uptake decrement at high altitude. *FASEB J.* 1996;10:A418. Abstract. (32) Stenberg J, Ekblom B, Messin R. Hemodynamic response to work at simulated altitude: 4,000 m. *J Appl Physiol.* 1966;21:1589–1594. (33) Hartley LH. Adjustments of the oxygen transport system during residence at high altitude. In: Brewer GJ, ed. *Hemoglobin and Red Cell Structure and Function.* New York, NY: Plenum Publishing Corp; 1972: 349-360. (34) Hartley LH, Vogel JA, Landowne M. Central, femoral, and brachial circulation during exercise in hypoxia. *J Appl Physiol.* 1973;34:87–90.

†Baseline resident altitudes > 400 m: (1) Mairbaurl H, Schobersberger W, Humpeler E, Hasibeder W, Fischer W, Raas E. Beneficial effects of exercising at moderate altitude on red cell oxygen transport and on exercise performance. *Pflugers Arch.* 1986;406:594–599. (2) Tucker A, Stager JM, Cordain L. Arterial O_2 saturation and maximum O_2 consumption in moderate-altitude runners exposed to sea level and 3,050 m. *JAMA.* 1995;252:2867–2871. (3) Loeppky JA, Bynum WA. Effects of periodic exposure to hypobaria and exercise on physical work capacity. *J Sports Med Phys Fitness.* 1970;10:238–247. (4) Balke B, Nagle FJ, Daniels J. Altitude and maximal performance in work and sport activity. *JAMA.* 1965;194:646–649. (5) Elliot PR, Atterbom HA. Comparison of exercise responses of males and females during acute exposure to hypobaria. *Aviat Space Environ Med.* 1978;49:415–418. (6) Maresh CM, Noble BJ, Robertson KL, Sime WE. Maximal exercise during hypobaric hypoxia (447 torr) in moderate-altitude natives. *J Appl Physiol.* 1983;15:360–365. (7) Benoit H, Germain M, Barthelemy JC, Denis C, Castells J, Dormois D, Lacour JR, Geyssant A. Pre-acclimatization to high altitude using exercise with normobaric hypoxic gas mixtures. *Int J Sports Med.* 1992;13(suppl 1):S213–S215.

Fig. 22-4. *Women: (1) Shephard RJ, Bouhlel E, Vandewalle H, Monod H. Peak oxygen uptake and hypoxia. *Int J Sports Med.* 1988;9:279–283. (2) Levitan BM, Bungo MW. Measurement of cardiopulmonary performance during acute exposure to a 2,440-m equivalent atmosphere. *Aviat Space Environ Med.* 1982;53:639–642. (3) Paterson DJ, Pinnington H, Pearce AR, Morton AR. Maximal exercise cardiorespiratory responses of men and women during acute exposure to hypoxia. *Aviat Space Environ Med.* 1987;58:243–247. (4) Beidleman BA, Rock PB, Muza SR, et al. Menstrual cycle phase does not affect work performance at sea level and 4,300 m. In: Sutton JR, Houston CS, Coates G, eds. *Hypoxia and the Brain: 9th International Hypoxia Symposium, 14–18 Feb 1995.* Lake Louise, Alberta, Canada: Queen City Printers; 1995. (5) Drinkwater BL, Folinsbee LJ, Bedi JF, Plowman SA, Loucks AB, Horvath SM. Response of women mountaineers to maximal exercise during hypoxia. *Aviat Space Environ Med.* 1979;50:657–662. (6) Elliot PR, Atterbom HA. Comparison of exercise responses of males and females during acute exposure to hypobaria. *Aviat Space Environ Med.* 1978;49:415–418. (7) Wagner JA, Miles DS, Horvath SM, Reyburn JA. Maximal work capacity of women during acute hypoxia. *J Appl Physiol.* 1979;47:1223–1227.

†Men: (1) Shephard RJ, Bouhlel E, Vandewalle H, Monod H. Peak oxygen uptake and hypoxia. *Int J Sports Med.* 1988;9:279–283. (2) Levitan BM, Bungo MW. Measurement of cardiopulmonary performance during acute exposure to a 2,440-m equivalent atmosphere. *Aviat Space Environ Med.* 1982;53:639–642. (3) Paterson DJ, Pinnington H, Pearce AR, Morton AR. Maximal exercise cardiorespiratory responses of men and women during acute exposure to hypoxia. *Aviat Space Environ Med.* 1987;58:243–247. (4) Elliot PR, Atterbom HA. Comparison of exercise responses of males and females during acute exposure to hypobaria. *Aviat Space Environ Med.* 1978;49:415–418.

Fig. 22-5. *Acute hypobaric hypoxia or hypoxic gas breathing: (1) Cymerman A, Pandolf KB, Young AJ, Maher JT. Energy expenditure during load carriage at high altitude. *J Appl Physiol.* 1981;51:14–18. (2) Lawler J, Powers SK, Thompson D. Linear relationship between $\dot{V}O_2$max and $\dot{V}O_2$max decrement during exposure to acute altitude. *J Appl Physiol.* 1988;64:1486–1492. (3) Shephard RJ, Bouhlel E, Vandewalle H, Monod H. Peak oxygen uptake and hypoxia. *Int J Sports Med.* 1988;9:279–283. (4) Adams RP, Welch HG. Oxygen uptake, acid–base status, and performance with varied inspired oxygen fractions. *J Appl Physiol.* 1980;49:863–868. (5) Andersen HT, Smeland EB, Owe JO, Myhre K. Analyses of maximum cardiopulmonary performance during exposure to acute hypoxia at simulated altitude: Sea level to 5,000 meters (760–404 mm Hg). *Aviat Space Environ Med.* 1985;56:1192–1195. (6) Gleser MA, Vogel JA. Effects of acute alterations of $\dot{V}O_2$max on endurance capacity of men. *J Appl Physiol.* 1973;34:443–447. (7) Gore CJ, Hahn AG, Watson DB, et al. $\dot{V}O_2$max and arterial O_2 saturation at sea level and 610 m. *Med Sci Sports Exerc.* 1995;27:S7. (8) Greenleaf JE, Greenleaf CJ, Card DH, Saltin B. Exercise-temperature regulation in man during acute exposure to simulated altitude. *J Appl Physiol.* 1969;26:290–296. (9) Hogan MC, Cox RH, Welch HG. Lactate accumulation during incremental exercise with varied inspired oxygen fractions. *J Appl Physiol.* 1983;55:1134–1140. (10) Levitan BM, Bungo MW. Measurement of cardiopulmonary performance during acute exposure to a 2,440-m equivalent atmosphere. *Aviat Space Environ Med.* 1982;53:639–642. (11) Paterson DJ, Pinnington H, Pearce AR, Morton AR. Maximal exercise cardiorespiratory responses of men and women during acute exposure to hypoxia. *Aviat Space Environ Med.* 1987;58:243–247. (12) Squires RW, Buskirk ER. Aerobic capacity during acute exposure to simulated altitude, 914 to 2,286 meters. *Med Sci Sports Exerc.* 1982;14:36–40. (13) Tucker A, Stager JM, Cordain L. Arterial O_2 saturation and maximum O_2 consumption in moderate-altitude runners exposed to sea level and 3,050 m. *JAMA.* 1995;252:2867–2871. (14) Gore CJ, Hahn AG, Scroop GS, et al. Increased arterial desaturation in trained cyclists during maximal exercise at 580 m altitude. *J Appl Physiol.* 1996;80:2204–2210. (15) Young PM, Rock PB, Fulco CS, Trad LA, Forte VA Jr, Cymerman A. Altitude acclimatization attenuates plasma ammonia accumulation during submaximal exercise. *J Appl Physiol.* 1987;63(2):758–764. (16) Koistinen P, Takala T, Martikkala V, Leppaluoto J. Aerobic fitness influences the response of maximal oxygen uptake and lactate threshold in acute hypobaric hypoxia. *Int J Sports Med.* 1995;26:78–81. (17) Beidleman BA, Rock PB, Muza SR, et al. Menstrual cycle phase does not affect work performance at sea level and 4,300 m. In: Sutton JR, Houston CS, Coates G, eds. *Hypoxia and the Brain: 9th International Hypoxia Symposium, 14–18 Feb 1995.* Lake Louise, Alberta, Canada: Queen City Printers; 1995. (18) Christensen EH, Forbes WH. Der Kreislauf in grossen Hohen. *Skand Arch Physiol.* 1937;76:75–89. (19) Linnarsson D, Karlsson J, Fagraeus L, Saltin B. Muscle metabolites and oxygen deficit with exercise and hypoxia and hyperoxia. *J Appl Physiol.* 1974;36:399–402. (20) Terrados N, Jansson E, Sylvén C, Kaijser L. Is hypoxia a stimulus for synthesis of oxidative enzymes and myoglobin? *J Appl Physiol.* 1990;68:2369–2372. (21) Young AJ, Evans WJ, Cymerman A, Pandolf KB, Knapik JJ, Maher JT. Sparing effect of chronic high-altitude exposure on muscle glycogen utilization. *J Appl Physiol.* 1982;52:857–862. (22) Loeppky JA, Bynum WA. Effects of periodic exposure to hypobaria and exercise on physical work capacity. *J Sports Med Phys Fitness.* 1970;10:238–247. (23) Fulco CS, Rock PB, Trad L, Forte V Jr, Cymerman A. Maximal cardiorespiratory responses to one- and two-legged cycling during acute and long-term exposure to 4,300 meters altitude. *Eur J Appl Physiol.* 1988;57:761–766. (24) Bouissou PF, Peronnet F, Brisson G, Helie R, Ledoux M. Metabolic and endocrine responses to graded exercise under acute hypoxia. *Eur J Appl Physiol.* 1986;55:290–294. (25) Drinkwater BL, Folinsbee LJ, Bedi JF, Plowman SA, Loucks AB, Horvath SM. Response of women mountaineers to maximal exercise during hypoxia. *Aviat Space Environ Med.* 1979;50:657–662. (26) Elliot PR, Atterbom HA. Comparison of exercise responses of males and females during acute exposure to hypobaria. *Aviat Space Environ Med.* 1978;49:415–418. (27) Maresh CM, Noble BJ, Robertson KL, Sime WE. Maximal exercise during hypobaric hypoxia (447 torr) in moderate-altitude natives. *J Appl Physiol.* 1983;15:360–365. (28) Shephard RJ, Bouhlel E, Vandewalle H, Monod H. Muscle mass as a factor limiting physical work. *J Appl Physiol.* 1988;64:1472–1479. (29) Dill DB, Myhre LG, Phillips J Jr, Brown DK. Work capacity in acute exposures to altitude. *J Appl Physiol.* 1966;21:1168–1176. (30) Wagner JA, Miles DS, Horvath SM, Reyburn JA. Maximal work capacity of women during acute hypoxia. *J Appl Physiol.* 1979;47:1223–1227. (31) Benoit H, Germain M, Barthelemy JC, Denis C, Castells J, Dormois D, Lacour JR, Geyssant A. Pre-acclimatization to high altitude using exercise with normobaric hypoxic gas mixtures. *Int J Sports Med.* 1992;13(suppl 1):S213–S215. (32) Fagraeus L, Karlsson J, Linnarsson D, Saltin B. Oxygen uptake during maximal work at lowered and raised ambient air pressures. *Acta Physiol Scand.* 1973;87:411–421. (33) Schoene RB, Bates PW, Larson EB, Pierson DJ. Effect of acetazolamide on normoxic and hypoxic exercise in humans at sea level. *J Appl Physiol.* 1983;55:1772–1776. (34) Robertson RJ, Gilcher R, Metz KF, et al. Effect of induced erythrocythemia on hypoxia tolerance during exercise. *J Appl Physiol.* 1982;53:490–495. (35) Forte VA Jr, Muza SR, Fulco CS, et al. Smoking accentuates the maximal oxygen uptake decrement at high altitude. *FASEB J.* 1996;10:A418. Abstract. (36) Stenberg J, Ekblom B, Messin R. Hemodynamic response to work at simulated altitude: 4,000 m. *J Appl Physiol.* 1966;21:1589–1594. (37) Hartley LH. Adjustments of the oxygen transport system during residence at high altitude. In: Brewer GJ, ed. *Hemoglobin and Red Cell Structure and Function.* New York, NY: Plenum; 1972: 349–360. (38) Hartley LH, Vogel JA, Landowne M. Central, femoral, and brachial circulation during exercise in hypoxia. *J Appl Physiol.* 1973;34:87–90.

†Altitude acclimatization: (1) Maher JT, Jones LG, Hartley LH. Effects of high-altitude exposure on submaximal endurance capacity of men. *J Appl Physiol.* 1974;37(6):895–898. (2) Cymerman A, Reeves JT, Sutton JR, et al. Operation Everest II: Maximal oxygen uptake at extreme altitude. *J Appl Physiol.* 1989;66(5):2446–2453. (3) Young PM, Rock PB, Fulco CS, Trad LA, Forte VA Jr, Cymerman A. Altitude acclimatization attenuates plasma ammonia accumulation during submaximal exercise. *J Appl Physiol.* 1987;63(2):758–764. (4) Young AJ, Evans WJ, Cymerman A, Pandolf KB, Knapik JJ, Maher JT. Sparing effect of chronic high-altitude exposure on muscle glycogen utilization. *J Appl Physiol.* 1982;52:857–862. (5) Horstman D, Weiskopf R, Jackson RE. Work capacity during 3-week sojourn at 4,300 m: Effects of relative polycythemia. *J Appl Physiol.* 1980;49:311–318. (6) Fulco CS, Rock PB, Trad L, Forte V Jr, Cymerman A. Maximal cardiorespiratory responses to one- and two-legged cycling during acute and long-term exposure to 4,300 meters altitude. *Eur J Appl Physiol.* 1988;57:761–766. (7) Consolazio CF, Nelson RA, Matoush LO, Hansen JE. Energy metabolism at high altitude (3,475 m). *J Appl Physiol.* 1966;21:1732–1740. (8) Saltin B, Grover RF, Blomqvist CG, Hartley LH, Johnson RLJ. Maximal oxygen uptake and cardiac output after 2 weeks at 4,300 m. *J Appl Physiol.* 1968;25:400–409. (9) Vogel JA, Hartley LH, Cruz JC, Hogan RP. Cardiac output during exercise in sea-level residents at sea level and high altitude. *J Appl Physiol.* 1974;36:169–172.

‡Long-term altitude training: (1) Balke B, Faulkner JA, Daniels JT. Maximum performance capacity at sea level and at moderate altitude before and after training at altitude. *Schweizerische Zeitschrift Fur Sportmedizin.* 1966;14:106–116. (2) Faulkner JA, Daniels JT, Balke B. Effects of training at moderate altitude on physical performance capacity. *J Appl Physiol.* 1967;23:85–89. (3) Dill DB, Adams WC. Maximal oxygen uptake at sea level and at 3,090-m altitude in high school champion runners. *J Appl Physiol.* 1971;30:854–859. (4) Klausen K, Robinson S, Micahel ED, Myhre LG. Effect of high altitude on maximal working capacity. *J Appl Physiol.* 1966;21:1191–1194. (5) Buskirk ER, Kollias J, Akers RF, Prokop EK, Reategui P. Maximal performance at altitude and on return from altitude in conditioned runners. *J Appl Physiol.* 1967;23:259–266. (6) Faulkner JA, Kollias J, Favour CB, Buskirk ER, Balke B. Maximum aerobic capacity and running performance at altitude. *J Appl Physiol.* 1968;24:685–691. (7) Adams WC, Bernauer EM, Dill DB, Bomar JB Jr. Effects of equivalent sea-level and altitude training on $\dot{V}O_2$max and running performance. *J Appl Physiol.* 1975;39:262–266. (8) Daniels J, Oldridge N. The effects of alternate exposure to altitude and sea level on world-class middle-distance runners. *Med Sci Sports.* 1970;2:107–112. (9) Reeves JT, Grover RF, Cohn JE. Regulation of ventilation during exercise at 10,200 ft in athletes born at low altitude. *J Appl Physiol.* 1967;22(3):546–554. (10) Pugh LGCE. Athletes at altitude. *J Physiol (Lond).* 1967;192:619–646. (11) Balke B, Nagle FJ, Daniels J. Altitude and maximal performance in work and sport activity. *JAMA.* 1965;194:646–649. (12) Counsilman JE. The effect of altitude upon swimming performance. In: Goddard RF, ed. *The Effects of Altitude on Physical Performance.* Albuquerque, NM: The Athletic Institute; 1967: 126–131.

§Trekking: (1) Boutellier U, Marconi C, Di Prampero PE, Cerretelli P. Effects of chronic hypoxia on maximal performance. *Bull Europ Physiopath Resp.* 1982;18:39–44. (2) West JB, Boyer SJ, Graber DJ, et al. Maximal exercise at extreme altitudes on Mount Everest. *J Appl Physiol.* 1983;55:688–698. (3) Christensen EH, Forbes WH. Der Kreislauf in grossen Hohen. *Skand Arch Physiol.* 1937;76:75–89. (4) Pugh LGCE, Gill MB, Lahiri S, Milledge JS, Ward MP, West JB. Muscular exercise at great altitudes. *J Appl Physiol.* 1964;19:431–440.

Fig. 22-7. *Highly conditioned athletes during running and swimming competitions: (1) Balke B, Faulkner JA, Daniels JT. Maximum performance capacity at sea level and at moderate altitude before and after training at altitude. *Schweizerische Zeitschrift Fur Sportmedizin.* 1966;14:106–116. (2) Faulkner JA, Daniels JT, Balke B. Effects of training at moderate altitude on physical performance capacity. *J Appl Physiol.* 1967;23:85–89. (3) Reeves JT, Jokl P, Cohn JE. Performance of Olympic Runners at Altitudes of 7,350 and 5,350 feet. In: Jokl E; Jokl P, eds. *Exercise and Altitude.* New York, NY: Karger; 1968: 49–54. (4) Buskirk ER, Kollias J, Akers RF, Prokop EK, Reategui P. Maximal performance at altitude and on return from altitude in conditioned runners. *J Appl Physiol.* 1967;23:259–266. (5) Daniels J, Oldridge N. The effects of alternate exposure to altitude and sea level on world-class middle-distance runners. *Med Sci Sports.* 1970;2:107–112. (6) Pugh LGCE. Athletes at altitude. *J Physiol (Lond).* 1967;192:619–646. (7) Daniels J. Altitude and athletic training and performance. *Am J Sports Med.* 1979;7:371–373. (8) Balke B, Nagle FJ, Daniels J. Altitude and maximal performance in work and sport activity. *JAMA.* 1965;194:646–649. (9) Counsilman JE. The effect of altitude upon swimming performance. In: Goddard RF, ed. *The Effects of Altitude on Physical Performance.* Albuquerque, NM:

The Athletic Institute; 1967: 126–131. (10) Goddard RF, Favour CB. United States Olympic Committee Swimming Team performance in International Sports Week, Mexico City, October, 1965. In: Goddard RF, ed. *The Effects of Altitude on Physical Performance.* Albuquerque, NM: The Athletic Institute; 1967: 135–150. (11) Grover RF, Reeves JT. Exercise performance of athletes at sea level and 3,100 meters altitude. In: Goddard RF, ed. *The Effects of Altitude on Physical Performance.* Albuquerque, NM: The Athletic Institute; 1967: 80–87.

Fig. 22-9. The effect of training at altitude on performance at altitude: (1) Balke B, Faulkner JA, Daniels JT. Maximum performance capacity at sea level and at moderate altitude before and after training at altitude. *Schweizerische Zeitschrift Fur Sportmedizin.* 1966;14:106–116. (2) Faulkner JA, Daniels JT, Balke B. Effects of training at moderate altitude on physical performance capacity. *J Appl Physiol.* 1967;23:85–89. (3) Faulkner JA, Kollias J, Favour CB, Buskirk ER, Balke B. Maximum aerobic capacity and running performance at altitude. *J Appl Physiol.* 1968;24:685–691. (4) Adams WC, Bernauer EM, Dill DB, Bomar JB Jr. Effects of equivalent sea-level and altitude training on $\dot{V}o_2$max and running performance. *J Appl Physiol.* 1975;39:262–266. (5) Daniels J, Oldridge N. The effects of alternate exposure to altitude and sea level on world-class middle-distance runners. *Med Sci Sports.* 1970;2:107–112. (6) Pugh LGCE. Athletes at altitude. *J Physiol (Lond).* 1967;192:619–646. (7) Balke B, Nagle FJ, Daniels J. Altitude and maximal performance in work and sport activity. *JAMA.* 1965;194:646–649. (8) Counsilman JE. The effect of altitude upon swimming performance. In: Goddard RF, ed. *The Effects of Altitude on Physical Performance.* Albuquerque, NM: The Athletic Institute; 1967: 126–131.

Chapter 23

COGNITIVE PERFORMANCE, MOOD, AND NEUROLOGICAL STATUS AT HIGH TERRESTRIAL ELEVATION

LOUIS E. BANDERET, PhD[*]; AND BARBARA SHUKITT-HALE, PhD[†]

INTRODUCTION

SELECTED SYSTEMS OR PROCESSES AFFECTED BY EXPOSURE TO HIGH
TERRESTRIAL ELEVATION
Mobility and Mission Accomplishment
Mood States
Personality
Cognitive and Psychomotor Performance
Vision, Hearing, and Taste
Speech
Sleep
Neuronal Cells
Neurochemical Mechanisms
Changes in the P300 Waveform

VARIABLES THAT INFLUENCE EFFECTS AT HIGH TERRESTRIAL ELEVATION
Threshold Altitude for Effects
Time Course of Effects
Temporary Versus Long-Term Effects
Cognitive Task Complexity and Practice
Individual Differences
Performance Tradeoffs of Speed Versus Accuracy
Correlations Between Measured Effects

COPING WITH HIGH TERRESTRIAL ELEVATION AND MINIMIZING
ADVERSE EFFECTS
Psychological Strategies
Operational Strategies
Medical Strategies

SUMMARY

[*]US Army Research Institute of Environmental Medicine, Military Performance Division, Natick, Massachusetts 01760-5007
[†]US Department of Agriculture, The Human Nutrition Research Center on Aging, Tufts University, 711 Washington Street, Room 919, Boston, Massachusetts 02111

INTRODUCTION

Many military, recreational, and industrial settings expose people to the effects of high terrestrial elevation (HTE). Such high-altitude environments (ie, 3,000–8,848 m) often involve risk; moreover, the consequences of faulty judgment or a cognitive error can be deadly or costly. Some of the earliest information about the psychological effects of HTE came from people working or living in high mountainous regions or people exploring conditions involving hypoxia.[1,2] Regions at high elevations are often important for military, economic, geopolitical, and other reasons.

High ground is usually sought during military operations.[3,4] High terrestrial elevations offer advantageous sites for observation and grant the holder the strategic advantage in that area. Hence the military was interested in balloons and explored their feasibility for observation and scouting in the late 1700s.[1,2,5] In the late 1960s, analyses of military history were published that showed that combat units that resided at altitudes higher than 3,000 m for a few days before engaging in warfare at even higher altitude (eg, 4,000 m) gained a dramatic advantage.[6,7] In contrast, unacclimatized troops coming immediately from positions near sea level experienced the rigors of the terrain, the liabilities of acute mountain sickness (AMS), and an adversary who was already emplaced.

Such effects, and others to be described in this chapter, result because above 3,000 m the substantially reduced atmospheric pressure associated with HTE causes hypoxemia (inadequate oxygenation of the blood), because the lungs cannot extract sufficient oxygen. The importance of oxygen for normal functioning and survival is emphasized by the fact that even at sea level the brain requires a disproportionately large amount of blood (enriched with oxygen) to function normally. Specifically, an adult human brain receives about 15% of the total volume of blood pumped by the heart, whereas the brain is only 2% of the body's weight. Normally, a healthy adult brain consumes 3.3 mL of oxygen per 100 g of brain tissue per minute,[8] which is approximately 20% of the oxygen consumed by the human body under resting conditions.

Hypoxemia results when individuals are exposed to HTE. Hypoxemia also results from procedures that are used to simulate the effects of HTE (eg, exposure to gas mixtures with ~ 13% oxygen, or special environments with atmospheric pressure ~ 70% that at sea level). This chapter will therefore describe findings resulting from exposure to HTE and the use of methods to simulate the effects of HTE.

In the last 100 years, technology has created microenvironments that are of special interest because some make people hypoxemic. Early airplanes, which did not have supplemental oxygen or internal compartment pressurization, made pilots, crews, and passengers hypoxemic.[9–12] Stowaways traveling infrequently in wheel compartments or nonpressurized areas of newer commercial aircraft experienced even more extreme conditions.[13] Surprisingly, sometimes stowaways survived extreme hypoxemia and cold (11,000 m and −65°C) during such flights. Today, another microenvironment that sometimes causes hypoxemia is astronomical observatories at HTE with large telescopes for viewing the galaxies, planets, comets, and stars. Observatories, constructed at altitudes of 4,000 to 5,000 m, provide better views of the solar system because they are above most of the low-altitude haze and pollutants.[14,15] Although observatories at HTE enhance the optics of the telescope, such work sites create new problems for the employees because their bodies and brains are hypoxemic. An important military microenvironment that can cause hypoxemia is the submarine. In some modern submarines, the atmospheric pressure is deliberately reduced so that the risk and destructiveness of fires on board are greatly decreased.[16] Selection of appropriate, reduced atmospheric pressures inside submarines was heavily guided by choosing those that would provide an optimal compromise between the adverse impact on personnel aboard (hypoxemia) while providing reasonable protection against fires.

Today, many land masses at HTE are especially important for military and recreational purposes.[4] Military personnel train for varied high-altitude missions, because mountain passes and flat expanses at high altitude (altiplano) are of great strategic and military importance.[3,4] Phenomena at HTE are also of interest to many civilians because, since 1970, many more have climbed to altitudes above 5,000 m.[17–21] Also, recent trends in climbing dictate that it is fashionable and desirable to climb the highest mountains in the world, often without oxygen, such as Mount Everest (8,848 m). Today, sites at HTE are more accessible than ever before, the climbing equipment and clothing are matchless, and people with minimal experience are attempting Mount Everest and other high mountains.[17,19–21]

This chapter will examine some of the psychological consequences that result from exposure to HTE, such as its effects on our senses, sleep, mood, judgment, memory, and ability to perform cognitive and psychomotor tasks. We will review the minimum altitude for threshold effects and evaluate data that suggest that long-term effects may result from exposure to extreme elevations. Lastly, we will look at some of the strategies used to reduce the adverse effects of high altitude so that people can function better and experience a greater sense of well-being at HTE.

SELECTED SYSTEMS OR PROCESSES AFFECTED BY EXPOSURE TO HIGH TERRESTRIAL ELEVATION

Exposure to high altitude affects many bodily processes and functions. Moreover, the onset of effects varies from immediate to several days or weeks. In planning military operations at HTE it is important to be able to predict the types, magnitudes, and time courses of impairments that will be experienced. This section describes adverse changes that usually occur after exposure to HTE higher than 4,000 m, such as those in mobility and mission accomplishment, mood states, cognitive and psychomotor performances, the senses, and sleep.

Mobility and Mission Accomplishment

The strenuous demands of a military training exercise in an intermediate high altitude (2,100–3,050 m) and a cold environment have been described aptly by Davis and colleagues[22]:

> The high-altitude, snow-covered environment is unique in the demands imposed on marines. Failure to recognize and consider the implications of this environment can drastically distort operational requirements. It is difficult to convey all the encumbrances associated with maintenance of basal tasks in this environment.[22(p37)]

Even at lesser altitudes of 2,065 to 2,620 m, 9 of 638 Marines (1.4%) in a US Marine Corps Battalion Landing Team that was conducting mountainous warfare training experienced incapacitating symptoms (eg, headache, nausea, malaise) of AMS.[23] Considering the exceptional motivation and discipline that is typical of Marine units, it is likely that although some individuals were uncomfortable and affected by the effects of high altitude, they did not seek medical help. The fact that this incidence occurred at altitudes only slightly higher than that of Denver, Colorado, suggests the generality and relevance of this information, because intermediate altitudes such as these are experienced by many military personnel, skiers, novice climbers, and hikers.

Historical data from civilian climbing expeditions have shown that conditions associated with climbing, high altitude, and cold can be life-threatening and sometimes fatal. Even lesser mountains such as Mount McKinley (6,194 m) in Alaska, with its highly unpredictable and extreme weather, is a foreboding challenge. In 1992, 13 climbers died (a 2- to 6-fold increase over most prior years) while attempting to climb the mountain. Of those who tried to climb Mount McKinley in the first 6 months that year, only 39% succeeded, a percentage much lower than usual. By the end of June 1992, 11 climbers had died; this 6-month total surpassed any previous 12-month total. By contrast, from 1980 to 1992 the median percentage of successful attempts was 51%, and the number of deaths per year averaged 2.5.[20] Although military personnel will be required to go where their mission demands, it is likely that they will be better-trained and -supervised than expeditions undertaken by many civilian climbers, especially those who are novices. The challenges and reputation of Mount Everest are even more fateful. Since the first Western Expedition in 1922, only 600 people have reached the summit, while more than 140 have died in the attempt; in terms of the mission objective, 1 of 7 climbers have reached the summit.[17]

Mood States

Observed behaviors and personal anecdotes suggest that the initial mood state experienced at altitude is euphoria, followed by depression. Euphoria can lead to dangerous consequences because its effects are usually not recognized by the affected person.[1] With time, individuals may also become quarrelsome, irritable, anxious, and apathetic.[24] At higher altitudes, irritability, not elation, is the more consistent manifestation. Sensitivity to criticism or instruction, aggressiveness, and a free-floating impatience are also more common at higher than at lower altitudes.[25] Overconfidence, often a problem at HTE, occurs frequently with elation and also with an irritable, aggressive mood.[25] Although disturbances in emotional control have been noticed at HTE for decades, until recently there have been few systematic and quantitative studies assessing mood at altitude.

In 1977, Banderet[26] conducted one of the first systematic studies of mood changes at HTE using the Clyde Mood Scale to determine the self-rated moods of volunteers. His effort was part of a larger study

designed to evaluate the efficacy of staging plus acetazolamide (treatment) for the prevention of
AMS.[27] Staging involves ascending to one (or more)
intermediate altitudes and allowing time for some
physiological acclimatization; then, the climber ascends to the summit (or the desired site) at HTE.[1,27,28]
Mood states were assessed at 200 m (baseline), 1,600
m (the staging site), and 4,300 m (Pikes Peak,
Colo).[26] Mood changes were not observed at 1,600
m, but four of the six mood factors were sensitive
to 4,300 m altitude. At 4,300 m, all volunteers (treatment and control groups) rated themselves as less
friendly and clear thinking and more sleepy and dizzy
than at 200 m. At 4,300 m, the treatment strategy
(acetazolamide and staging) resulted in improved
mood on the friendly, sleepy, and dizzy factors, but
not on the clear-thinking factor. (The characteristics of AMS, its pathophysiology, and its treatment

are described in Chapter 24, Altitude Illness: Acute
Mountain Sickness and High-Altitude Cerebral
Edema.)

In 1988, Shukitt and Banderet,[29] using the original database of Banderet,[26] compared moods measured with the Clyde Mood Scale at three different
altitudes and two times of day (morning and
evening) (Figure 23-1). Baseline values were determined at 200 m; moods were then assessed for 2
days at 1,600 m in one group, or for 4 days at 4,300
m with a second group. Only sleepiness changed
at 1,600 m; volunteers were sleepier at this altitude
compared with sea level. At 4,300 m, moods differed from baseline (200 m) after 1 to 4 hours and
differed even more after 18 to 28 hours; volunteers
became less friendly, less clear thinking, and diz-
zier.[29] They also became sleepier and happier, with
effects being greatest after 1 to 4 hours. Aggressive-

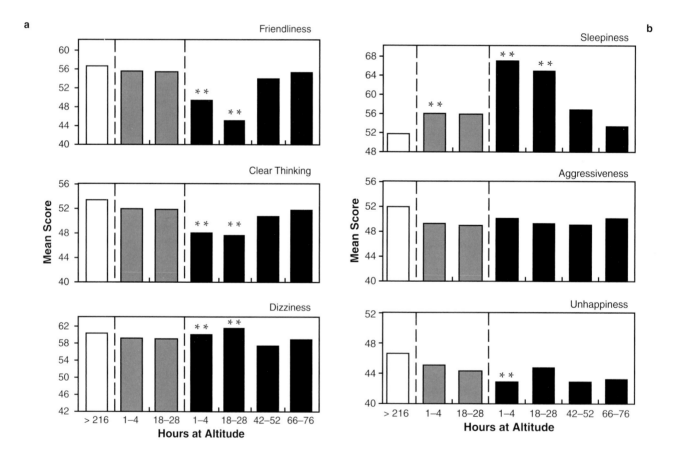

Fig. 23-1. Time courses of varied mood states: (**a**) friendliness, clear thinking, and dizziness, and (**b**) sleepiness, aggressiveness, and unhappiness at simulated altitude conditions of 200 m (no shading), 1,600 m (light shading), and
4,300 m (dark shading). Two asterisks atop a bar indicate that the mood state was significantly different (*P* ≤ .01) at
4,300 m than at 200 m. Reprinted with permission from Shukitt-Hale B, Lieberman HR. The effect of altitude on
cognitive performance and mood states. In: Marriott B, Carlson SJ eds. *Nutritional Needs in Cold and in High-Altitude
Environments.* Washington, DC: National Academy Press; 1996: 437.

ness did not change.[29] However, by 42 to 52 hours after ascent to 4,300 m, all moods returned to baseline levels. Mood states each morning and evening were similar at each altitude (1,600 and 4,300 m). Therefore, at 4,300 m, five moods differed from baseline 1 to 4 hours after arrival, three differed even more after 18 to 28 hours, and after 42 to 52 hours all previously affected moods returned to baseline values. Mood states were adversely affected by both duration of exposure and level of altitude (1,600 and 4,300 m); changes in mood states at altitude had a distinct and measurable time course.[29]

In another study, mood states were evaluated using the Profile of Mood States and the Clyde Mood Scale during a 4.5-hour exposure to a simulated altitude of 4,200 or 4,700 m to examine changes as a function of altitude level and duration of exposure.[30] Effects of 4,700 m altitude were seen for 75% of mood factors (friendliness, sleepiness, dizziness, hostility, depression, anxiety, confusion, fatigue, tension, anger, and vigor), while the effects of 4,200 m altitude were seen for only 25% of mood factors (sleepiness, dizziness, tension, and confusion). More adverse changes were noted with longer durations after ascent, especially for 4,700 m simulated altitude. This study, like Banderet's earlier study,[26] demonstrated that moods are significantly altered after only a few hours of exposure to simulated altitude; effects increase (incidence and magnitude) when testing is conducted at 4,700 compared with 4,200 m.[30]

In still another study, Shukitt-Hale, Rauch, and Foutch[31] evaluated self-rated symptoms and mood states during a climb of Mount Sanford in Alaska. Self-rated moods and symptoms were determined with the Profile of Mood States and the Environmental Symptoms Questionnaire.[32–35] In their 1990 study, Shukitt-Hale and colleagues[31] studied seven males for 7 days during a climb to 3,630 m. The volunteers were tested at four increasing altitudes: they were tested twice at 2,225 m and once at 2,530 m, 3,080 m, and 3,630 m. Seven symptom factors and two mood factors were adversely affected by changes in altitude. The volunteers experienced more respiratory AMS, exertion stress, and muscular discomfort, and they were colder, less alert, less vigorous, and more fatigued at the higher altitudes. Fewer adverse effects on day 2 at 2,225 m suggest that some acclimatization may have taken place from day 1 to day 2 at this altitude. It is interesting to note that even though the climb to the moderate altitude of 3,630 m in this study was relatively slow (< 300 m/d), adverse changes at this and lower altitudes were evident. These data demonstrate that a climb to 3,630 m produces adverse changes in symptomatology and mood states, and that other variables associated with a climb (eg, physical exertion or exercise) can affect these parameters.[15]

Personality

Changes in personality associated with exposure to high altitude were reported by several investigators, including Hertzman, Seitz, and Orlansky,[36] who in 1955 examined the relationship between personality and hypoxia. When their subjects spent 47 to 49 minutes at a simulated altitude of 5,638 m, they showed some loss of emotional control, with a tendency toward emotional disorganization and increased anxiety, followed by a counteracting tendency to become more constrictive.

In a different investigation, three standard personality questionnaires and a Mountain Sickness Anticipation Questionnaire were completed prior to departure to the Himalayas to assess the role of personality and expectations in the development of AMS.[37] The symptomatology of AMS was assessed by clinical interview and by peer review. The severity of AMS and its occurrence were not predicted with these methods and bore no significant relationship to personality. For comparison, daily self-assessment of the signs and symptoms of AMS were also conducted throughout the expedition, using graduated and graphic rating scales. Ratings from these graphical rating scales were found to be unreliable and dependent on personality factors. Therefore, the authors concluded that personality is of no significance in the development of AMS, but that it is important in influencing self-ratings of symptom severity.

Intellectual functioning and changes in personality were examined during a 35-day mountaineering expedition to Mount McKinley.[38] At 3,800 m, these indices varied minimally. However, at 5,000 m, undesirable changes were evident; that is, there was a marked deterioration in cognitive ability, a sharp increase in paranoia and obsessive-compulsiveness, and smaller increases in depression and hostility. While these psychological changes may have resulted from high altitude, the heavy physical demands, enforced intragroup dependence required of mountain climbing, close living quarters, extremely cold temperatures, sensory deprivation, and frequent periods of reduced visual fields may also have affected them.

The effects of chronic hypoxemia on cognition and behavior have been studied in women exposed to high-altitude mountaineering.[39] Neuropsychological tests, psychosocial questionnaires, and physiological questionnaires were given to women before, during, and after a Himalayan climb to 6,248 m. Cognitive functioning remained relatively intact with only two significant decrements, complex abstract reasoning and word-finding ability. Significant changes were found on all psychosocial and physiological questionnaires. High positive affect toward others and anxiety, both high before the climb, declined significantly after the expedition. In contrast to this decreased acceptance of others, subjects' self-ratings of their abilities improved after the expedition (ie, increased self-esteem). Self-perception of cognitive and affective functioning was more related to emotional states and physical symptoms than to actual ability to perform. Anxiety, depression, fatigue, and altitude eroded self-confidence, emphasizing the presence of psychological as well as physiological demands of high-altitude mountaineering.

Ryn[40] also described mental disturbances in climbers that he claims are related to duration of stay and level of altitude. The neurasthenic syndrome was common at 3,000 to 4,000 m and is characterized by fatigability, lack of motivation, feelings of inadequacy, and psychosomatic symptoms. The cyclothymic syndrome occurred at 4,000 to 5,000 m and involved alternating depressed and elevated moods. Acute organic brain syndromes occurred above 7,000 m and resulted from structural or functional defects in the central nervous system (CNS). The climber's personality, the emotional atmosphere associated with climbing, the high degree of risk, and other biological and psychological factors were important in the etiology of such mental disturbances.

Cognitive and Psychomotor Performance

In a review of research literature on high-altitude physiology and medicine, Cudaback[14] included some anecdotal reports of astronomers working at high altitude; he reported that the effects of high altitude on performance are often larger than those recognized either by its victims or their colleagues at the same altitude. He suggested that at 4,000 m most unacclimatized people will lose approximately 20% of their sea level abilities, and some loss may persist even after moderate acclimatization. At least half the people with no acclimatization will suffer some sickness starting a few hours after ascent and lasting a few days. Between 0.1% and 1% of individuals going to 4,000 m HTE will suffer serious illness at some time, and that illness may become

life-threatening if the victim does not descend. Mental performance in unacclimatized people on simple, well-learned tasks was impaired 12% to 28%, and impairments on complex tasks were expected to be larger.

High altitude produces substantial impairments in a number of cognitive performances. Impairments in psychomotor performance, mental skills, reaction time, vigilance, memory, and logical reasoning have been demonstrated at altitudes above 3,000 m.[41,42] Performance changes do not follow the same time course at altitude as do symptoms of AMS or moods; therefore, with time, performance will often be affected differently than symptoms or many moods.[43–45] Cognitive performance is usually more vulnerable to altitude than psychomotor performance,[14,28,46] and complex tasks are typically affected before simple tasks.[14] Additionally, activities requiring decisions and strategies are more vulnerable than automatic processes.[47] Deficits of learning and retention of information in perceptual and memory tasks were measured in climbers; climbers also performed more slowly on most tasks than did a control group.[48] (See Exhibit 19-1 in Chapter 19, Mountains and Military Medicine: An Overview, for definitions of climbers and other categories of people who visit mountains.) Motivation and training may compensate for the degradation in performance imposed by high altitude.[49]

In 1937, McFarland,[50] in a classic study of the behavioral effects of exposure to HTE conditions, found decrements on several measures of cognitive performance. In 1948, Russell[51] exposed 244 volunteers to simulated altitude (5,486 m) for 35 minutes and measured finger dexterity, arm–hand coordination, and simple addition. Decrements in performance appeared immediately after the introduction to hypoxia, rapid adjustment occurred as the duration of hypoxia increased, and continued practice under hypoxic conditions resulted in improvement. Other investigations have found decrements above 3,000 m in psychomotor performance,[52] problem solving,[53] symbol substitution,[54] card sorting,[55] reaction time,[56,57] vigilance performance,[58] and rifle marksmanship.[59,60]

In 1989, Kennedy and colleagues[61] investigated cognitive function at simulated altitude in a repeated-measures study of performance of seven volunteers; the atmospheric pressure in their chamber was systematically reduced for 40 days to a final altitude equivalent of 8,848 m, the height of Mount Everest (Operation Everest II). Significant impairments in cognitive function were seen for three of the five tests in the computerized test battery (Sternberg, pattern comparison, grammatical reasoning), and on two paper-and-pencil tests (grammatical reasoning and pattern comparison), every volunteer showed a substantial decrement at 7,625 m. Another study,[62] actually conducted on Mount Everest at altitudes above 6,400 m, showed no reliable effect on the retrieval of general information from memory, and this robustness of retrieval occurred for both recall and forced-choice recognition. However, extreme altitude did affect metacognition (ie, the monitoring and control of one's own cognitive processes); climbers showed a decline in their feeling of knowing, both while at altitude and 1 week after returning from altitude. This study demonstrated that exposures to extreme altitudes produced a decline in feelings of knowing, although there was no change in retrieval as assessed by accuracy of recall, latency of recall, and accuracy of recognition.

In 1985, Forster[63] studied two groups of sea-level residents at the summit of Mauna Kea (4,200 m) in Hawaii to examine the effect of different ascent profiles on performance. People in both groups ascended the mountain in a vehicle. "Commuters" spent 6 hours at the summit, while "shift workers" resided on the mountain for 5 days. Commuters experienced fewer symptoms of altitude sickness than shift workers on the first day at 4,200 m. After 5 days, shift workers reported fewer symptoms and performed better at tests of numerate memory and psychomotor ability than commuters. Therefore, the impairments in cognition at altitudes of 4,200 m are moderate but short-lived when individuals stay at HTE continuously.

In 1991, Koller and colleagues[64] found a 20% increase in errors on a test of mental arithmetic in 7 nonacclimatized subjects during stepwise, acute ascent to 6,000 m, compared with an error rate of about 7% in 10 acclimatized subjects. Because human cognitive function is sensitive to changes in oxygen availability, exposure to hypoxia should produce a continuum of effects as either the level of HTE or the duration of exposure is increased. In a laboratory study, Shukitt-Hale and colleagues[30] evaluated the behavioral effects of hypoxia as a function of duration of exposure and altitude level with various standardized tests of cognitive performance. Each test was administered from one to three times to participants in an altitude chamber during 4.5-hour–exposures to three levels of simulated altitude: 500 m (the baseline); 4,200 m; and 4,700 m. A number of measures were affected during the first administration of the tests (after 90 min of exposure). Cognitive performance was signifi-

cantly impaired on 7 of 10 performance measures at 4,700 m; whereas only 4 of 10 measures were affected at 4,200 m. When the results for 4,200 m and 4,700 m were compared, even relatively simple performance tasks (simple and choice reaction time), as well as complex tests of cognition (addition test), resulted in graded impairments. The number of hits on the Bakan vigilance task decreased with increasing altitude, simple reaction time increased as a function of increased altitude, and percentage errors increased on the four-choice reaction time test. The number of correct responses (a measure reflecting both the speed and accuracy of performance) decreased on the addition, coding, number comparison, and pattern recognition with increasing altitude and duration at altitude. Therefore, adverse changes in cognitive performance appeared within 90 minutes of exposure to altitude and were greater with higher altitudes and longer durations (< 4.5 h).

Therefore, it is generally accepted that hypoxia has few effects on human performance at altitudes lower than 3,000 m. Higher than 3,000 m, however, substantial impairments occur in cognitive performance, such as mental skills, reaction time, vigilance, memory, and logical reasoning.

Vision, Hearing, and Taste

Himalayan climbers often report visual and auditory hallucinations.[65] Usually, the senses are affected by altitude before cognitive and psychomotor performances.[42] Temporary visual changes are uncommon but can include blurred vision, flashing lights, blindness, or double vision.[66] Retinal hemorrhages can also occur above 3,600 m; they rarely cause symptoms and heal rapidly.[66] McFarland[12] gives estimates for the loss of function for visual parameters at 4,300 m: 10% in central field extent, 30% in central brightness contrast, 34% in dark adaptation, and 36% in central acuity. Adverse effects on vision may be partially responsible for some of the cognitive performance decrements seen at altitude.[12] As examples, the latencies to read briefly displayed visual stimuli increased with hypoxia,[67] latencies to detect visual stimuli increased with hypoxia,[68] and the detection of signals decreased as the perceptual sensitivity of the visual system changed.[58]

Vision is the first sense affected by hypoxia, with some effects seen at altitudes as low as 1,220 to 1,520 m.[12] Sensitivity to light, visual acuity, and color discrimination decreased at altitudes higher than 3,000 m. Night vision and dark adaptation are particularly sensitive to the effects of hypoxia, because retinal rods and cones are impaired in their ability to adapt to the dark.[69] Kobrick and colleagues[70] found a continued impairment of night vision (dark adaptation) that prevailed during sustained hypoxia (16 d at 4,300 m) but that recovered substantially when hypoxia was reduced (but not eliminated). They demonstrated that such visual impairments may persist after recovery from symptoms, adverse moods, and impaired performances.[70] Another study[71] found that visual acuity in 11 male and 6 female pilots using the Aviator Night Vision Imaging System (ANVIS) was degraded slightly after 30 minutes of exposure to 4,300 m, although less than what would be expected with unaided night vision under these conditions. There were no visual effects attributable to gender.[71] Therefore, ANVIS might limit degradation of visual performance resulting from hypoxia under low illumination conditions.

Auditory thresholds for different frequencies of sound were relatively insensitive to hypoxia, with few or no changes at HTE as high as 4,600 m.[24,72] Recently, this belief has been challenged by several investigators[73–75] who believe that audition may be more sensitive to hypoxia than previously believed. Although there was a drop in speech discrimination under hypoxia, no significant deterioration in hearing for pure tones was found for 4,600- and 6,100-m conditions in a chamber.[76] The changes in speech discrimination were thought to be due to either lack of oxygen in the cochlea or inattention caused by hypoxia.[76]

The four basic tastes of salt, sour, bitter, and sweet become less pronounced after ascent to moderate altitude, although the appetite for sweet foods is said to increase.[28] This change in taste sensation may be a factor in high-altitude anorexia, a self-induced starvation.[42] Animals[77] and humans[78] lose body weight when exposed to high-altitude conditions, due to reduced daily food intake and perhaps other factors. One study[78] found that hypoxia was associated with an 8.9% reduction in initial body weight, with appetite suppression and decreased caloric intake lasting for several weeks (during the study), particularly due to a decrease in carbohydrate preference, despite access to ample varieties and quantities of highly palatable foods.

Speech

Some nonperceptible characteristics of speech appear to change after exposure to HTE. Lieberman and colleagues[79,80] reported an innovative and promising methodology that they used to measure small but important changes in speech from five male climbers during the 1993 Sagarmatha Expedition of Mount Everest. They measured a time interval associated with selective speech sounds, which they called the "voice onset time" (VOT). In normal communications, separation intervals for VOT for "voiced" and "unvoiced" consonants differ by 20 milliseconds or more, so that the sounds from the two types of consonants are distinctive and discernible to a human listener.

Values of the VOT were determined at different altitudes from each climber's speech utterances when he read a list of monosyllabic words. The list contained words like "bat" and "kid," which had voiced and unvoiced consonants at the beginning and end of each word, respectively. These measurements were determined at 5,300 m (the base camp), 6,300 m, 7,150 m, 8,000 m, and on return to 5,300 m. As the climbers ascended to each test altitude, they communicated the standard words on the list to the experimenters (at the base camp). During each test session, the experimenter recorded the climbers' verbalizations for subsequent analysis.

Exposure to high altitude changed the VOTs. The separation interval between voiced and unvoiced consonants changed from 24.0 to 5.4 milliseconds.[79,80] This suggests that it would be more difficult to understand and process verbal communications at high altitude because stop consonants may not be readily perceived. Lieberman and colleagues[79,80] inferred that this change in speech results from the effects of hypoxia on subcortical pathways to the prefrontal cortex.

A second test used by these investigators measured the time required for each climber to process simple and complex sentences; the sentences that were used could be processed easily by a 10-year-old, fluent in the English language.[79,80] Each climber looked at a small booklet with three illustrations per page that reflected various interpretations of a simple or a complex sentence. Before each sentence, the climber announced the number of the page he was viewing; this provided a start event for each reaction time and ensured that the pages in the booklets were synchronized for the climber on the mountain and the experimenter at the base camp. The experimenter read the sentence and the climber verbalized the letter of the alternative he thought was correct. As with the investigation of the VOTs, the climber's verbalization was transmitted over the radio to the experimenter at the base camp and recorded.

The duration required to process sentences was influenced directly by degree of both high altitude and sentence complexity.[79,80] Interestingly, VOT separation width (in milliseconds) and the latency to process sentences were correlated –0.77.[79,80] This correlation coefficient implies that 60% of the impaired processing of sentences under these conditions was predicted by the VOT index. Fortunately, these changes in speech and in processing of language were transient; they recovered after descent to the base camp (5,300 m).

This methodology, which is based on changes in speech, may be useful in other stressful situations that involve hypoxia, such as flying in aircraft (without cabin pressurization or supplemental oxygen); high-altitude parachuting; and aspects of mountain climbing. Because speech (real-time or recorded) is the basic datum for this technique, this methodology can be employed unobtrusively, at a distance, and (perhaps eventually) with automated equipment to aid analysis.

Sleep

Mountain climbers, soldiers, hikers, tourists, and workers at high altitude have reported disturbed and fitful sleep.[1,3,14] People are seldom rested or refreshed even after a full night's sleep at HTE; respiratory periodicity with apnea (eg, actual pauses in breathing for 5–10 s during sleep) and sleep disruption occur.[28,81–84] Self-ratings of sleepiness increased after acute ascent to 1,600 to 4,700 m[26,29] or gradual ascent to 7,000 to 7,600 m.[85]

Scientific studies of sleep have been conducted under conditions of high altitude since the 1970s. Many studies were conducted in laboratory hypobaric chambers; others were conducted in tents or shelters at high altitude. In 1972, sleep was studied at high altitude for the first time with electroencephalography (EEG).[86] The investigation, carried out at 4,300 m at the US Army Pikes Peak Laboratory Facility, a part of the US Army Research Institute of Environmental Medicine (USARIEM), Natick, Massachusetts, found that sleep stages 3 and 4 decreased and periodic breathing occurred; however, total time asleep did not change. During days 1 through 12 at 4,300 m, EEG characteristics, the number of awakenings during sleep, and subjective ratings of sleep quality returned to sea-level values. In other investigations during acclimatization, changes in ventilatory and blood–gas measures were described for various sleep stages and wakefulness.[84] At higher altitudes (eg, 5,000 m), disturbances of sleep may last for many days or weeks.[28]

In 1975, Reite and colleagues[86] noted a disparity between objective and subjective measures of sleep quality at high altitude. These investigators suggested that the difference was related to the frequency of arousals during sleep and concluded that the subjects' intense complaints were disproportionate for the situation. Reite and colleagues did not recognize that such brief arousals might disrupt sleep and dramatically influence subjective appraisals of sleep quality.

In 1985, EEG was used to study brain wave characteristics during sleeping, walking, and climbing in 12 males on an expedition to Mount Api (7,130 m) in the Himalayas.[87] This was the first study of sleep at high altitude that also included ambulatory EEG with free-roving climbers. Each climber wore a small portable medical (physiological) recorder to record EEG signals. Recordings were made during acclimatization from 4,115 m to 6,220 m. Collection of these data was a remarkable scientific and technological feat, especially under such challenging and extreme environmental conditions. Stage 4 sleep was reduced 65% to 74% at 4,115 m (compared with values at sea level); stage 4 did not change with altitudes higher than 4,115 m. Rapid eye movement sleep was also reduced at high altitude. During sleep, EEG records showed no gross abnormalities or epilepsy-like phenomena, nor did records during ambulation and climbing. These investigators were reassured that such abnormalities were not observed, because it was suspected (in 1985) that extreme altitude conditions might cause prolonged damage to the CNS in some climbers; the investigators thought that their climbers may have been "protected" by being well-acclimatized and by practicing good hydration discipline. However, this study provided evidence that sleep quality at high altitude was impaired even in well-maintained, healthy, and acclimatized climbers.

In 1985, during Operation Everest II, the male volunteers frequently reported that they slept poorly at night at high altitude. Their complaints included difficulties in falling asleep, frequent nighttime awakenings, and feeling less refreshed than expected on awakening. In 1992, Anholm and colleagues[81] modified procedures to score sleep EEG records and noted episodes of marked hypoxemia at night and several 3- to 4-second arousals during sleep (eg, they measured 22, 63, and 161 arousals per hour at 180, 4,572, and 7,620 m, respectively). Earlier efforts of these investigators established that traditional scoring of EEG records would not detect brief arousals of 3 to 4 seconds observed during sleep at high altitude, because brief arousals are not predominant phenomena in a 20- to 30-second scoring epoch.[88] Brief arousals were not observed in all apnea cycles; however, all volunteers experienced them.[81] These objective sleep data suggested many reasons for the complaints of poor sleep at high altitude. Compared with sea level, volunteers at 7,620 m experienced more frequent awakenings (37.2 vs 14.8), total sleep time was reduced (167 vs 337 min), rapid eye movement sleep was a smaller portion of total sleep time (4.0% vs 17.9%), and, as noted, brief arousals during sleep were more frequent.[81]

Looking closely at brief events in the EEG records from high altitude (ie, 4,572, 6,100, and 7,200 m), these researchers[81,88] found a relationship between the number of arousals during nighttime sleep and deficits in daytime performance. The number of arousals and the degree of apnea-induced hypoxemia during sleep were better predictors of daytime cognitive impairments than alterations in sleep stages. During nighttime sleep at altitude ($\geq$ 4572 m), values for arterial oxygen tension (PaO_2) were lower than those observed in the daytime[28,81,84,88]; such acutely decreased PaO_2 values in the daytime while awake would probably be lethal in an unacclimatized volunteer.[28,81] Sleep efficiency and number of awakenings during sleep did not change at altitudes higher than 4,572 m; higher than 6,100 m, however, volunteers were less active behaviorally and spent more time napping.[81] Rapid eye movement sleep was decreased by 70% during hypoxemia, but slow-wave sleep did not change.[81]

At 6,100 m, different sleep stages had minimal effects on the oxygen saturation of arterial blood (SaO_2); however, SaO_2 was negatively correlated (–0.72) with the number of brief arousals during sleep.[81] The lowest values of SaO_2 in all five volunteers during the study were measured during sleep. The difference between daytime and nighttime SaO_2 values increased as altitude increased. All volunteers exhibited periodic breathing with apnea during much of the night at 6,100 and 7,620 m. Periodic breathing in all volunteers was central in origin, not obstructive. These data suggest that the use of supplemental oxygen during the evening (the equivalent of sleeping at a lower altitude) may improve sleep and, therefore, subsequent daytime performance.

Climbers and other team members often experience poor-quality sleep at high altitude and are tempted to take different medications to improve sleep.[14,89] Acetazolamide appears to be the best sleep-enhancing drug at high altitude because it reduces periodic breathing, improves oxygenation, and is a safe medication to improve sleep.[89] Sleep quality, quantity, and self-ratings of sleep characteristics are improved by the use of acetazolamide.[82,83] Other sleep-improving drugs at high altitude, such as diphenhydramine, triazolam, or temazepam, can be used; however, they are potentially dangerous because they depress ventilation, relax the muscles of respiration, and further complicate conditions associated with hypoxemia at high altitude.[82,83,89,90] Therefore, the choice of an inappropriate sleep aid may increase hypoxemia, complicate sleep apnea at high altitude, and impair daytime cognitive performance in some individuals at high altitude. (Strategies for improving sleep at HTE and decreasing the adverse effects of exposure to altitude are also reviewed in Chapter 24, Acute Mountain Sickness and High-Altitude Cerebral Edema, and Chapter 25, High-Altitude Pulmonary Edema.)

A review by Heath and Williams[28] in 1989 examined the phenomena of nocturnal periodic breathing at high altitudes. Paradoxically, people with the greatest ventilatory drive in response to hypoxia in the daytime (an adaptive response) have the most pronounced periodic breathing at night.[28,84] The greatest effect of periodic breathing during *sleep* is that SaO_2 is reduced during sleep to less than what one would expect for that level of altitude during the daytime. This significant reduction during the nighttime affects both sleep quality and subsequent cognitive capabilities during waking hours. Several investigators reported that people at altitude whose arterial blood became the most desaturated at night also performed more poorly on daytime tests of cognitive performance.[81,91] Hence, subjects best able to adapt to hypoxemia and perform *physical* work during waking hours were most impaired in their daytime *cognitive* performances because of their ventilatory responses during sleep. This finding is also consistent with an experimental study[92] of sleep apneics at sea level that demonstrated that sleep apneics also experience daytime cognitive performance decrements resulting from their hypoxemia during sleep.

Currently, there is controversy as to whether daytime performance impairments in individuals with sleep apnea (at sea level) result from severe hypoxic episodes induced by apnea during sleep or from disrupted EEG sleep stages and associated fragmented sleep.[93] In a correlational study of patients with sleep apnea, the best predictor of the hypoxic aspects of apnea episodes was the number of episodes during sleep when SaO_2 fell by 4% or more.[46] This criterion of hypoxemia correlated with several of the patients' daytime performance measures but did not predict changes in sleep stages. Also, in the experimental study of patients with sleep apnea, daytime cognitive impairments were found to result from hypoxemic episodes during the evening and to a lesser extent from sleep fragmentation.[92]

Thus, in patients with sleep apnea, the degree of hypoxemia during sleep, rather than changes in sleep architecture, is correlated with impairments in daytime performance.

Neuronal Cells

Severe, chronic hypoxia can produce permanent damage to neurons, depending on the severity of the exposure.[94] Evidence gathered from magnetic resonance imaging (MRI) during the 1990s supports the idea that some hypoxic CNS damage induced by HTE may be long-term.[18,95] Calcium appears to play an integral role in the production of ischemic and hypoxic cell damage. Ischemic damage to the plasma membrane of the cell disrupts its relative impermeability to calcium and results in an influx of calcium. Large accumulations of free calcium disrupt metabolic function and eventually cause neuronal death.[96] This massive increase in intracellular free calcium occurs preferentially in the cells that appear to be selectively vulnerable to ischemia.[97,98] Neuronal injury from hypoxia can be prevented if calcium accumulation is blocked.[99]

Histological studies with small laboratory animals showed that some cortical layers (III, V, and VI) and the hippocampus, striatum, thalamus, and amygdala are especially vulnerable to hypoxic damage.[94] Pyramidal cells in the hippocampus are vulnerable to ischemically induced damage; morphological degeneration of these cells occurs 2 to 4 days after the ischemic insult.[98,100] Severe ischemia (10–15 min in duration) extended neuronal death to other regions, such as the hippocampal CA3 and CA4 subfield, cerebral cortex, striatum, and thalamus.[101] Additionally, there is evidence that transient hypoxia (4.5% oxygen for 30 min) can induce irreversible neuronal damage in the CA1 subfield; such hippocampal lesions can result in deterioration of cognitive memory function.[102]

Repeated exposures to extreme altitude can cause mild but persistent cognitive impairment because the brain areas most vulnerable to chronic hypoxia seem to be the hippocampal structures.[103] The hippocampus, an area thought to be involved in learning and memory processes, is rich in cholinergic innervation; as shown by studies with rats, the central cholinergic system is particularly vulnerable to hypoxia.[104] Rats subjected to forebrain ischemia developed severe damage to the CA1 region of the hippocampus, which led to impaired behavioral performance on memory tasks.[105] Other investigators suggested that cognitive deficits correlated more with cell losses observed in the CA2 and CA3 sectors than with damage to the CA1 region of the hippocampus.[106]

In yet another study with rats, morphological changes were observed with light microscopy in rats' brains following a 4-day exposure to altitude.[77] Damage was observed in some rats exposed to altitudes of 5,500 or 6,400 m, with cell degeneration and death increasing as altitude increased. Also, the longer the time following exposure before sacrifice, the more noticeable the damage, which suggests delayed neurotoxicity. These data suggest how exposure to extreme high altitude may result in permanent brain damage, but the conditions that cause such damage and the consequences of such damage on subsequent behavioral performance are only beginning to be determined.

Neurochemical Mechanisms

The central mechanisms responsible for the effects of hypoxia on behavior and cognitive processes are not known. Additionally, none of the drugs currently employed to treat the effects of hypoxia, such as acetazolamide or dexamethasone, have specific mechanisms of action that act centrally.[107] Numerous studies[69,104,108–111] have sought to determine the effects of hypoxia on central neurotransmitters and their metabolites. The direct effects of mild transient hypoxia on the brain are likely to be variations in the level of specific neurotransmitters, transient morphological changes, or both. Because the synthesis of several neurotransmitters is oxygen-dependent, abnormalities of neurotransmitter metabolism may mediate the early functional changes due to acute hypoxia.[104] Some of the behavioral decrements caused by hypoxia may be attributable to changes in neurotransmitter utilization and concentration.[108]

The central cholinergic system is particularly vulnerable to hypoxia, and it appears that acetylcholine (ACh), which is involved in the regulation of learning and memory processes,[108] is the neurotransmitter primarily affected.[104] The rates of synthesis of other neurotransmitters (eg, dopamine, serotonin, and the amino acids), are also sensitive to hypoxia, but perhaps less so than the rate of ACh synthesis.[109] A decrease in ACh synthesis has been documented following mild hypoxia without any reduction in neuronal ACh concentration; this is consistent with the hypothesis that hypoxia acts through inhibition of ACh release.[107,110] Hypobaric hypoxia (equivalent to 5,500 m simulated altitude) reduced extracellular hippocampal ACh release,[111] lending support to the hypothesis that decreases in ACh metabolism and release are caused by altitude exposure. Impaired ACh synthesis and release could account for many of the behavioral symptoms of hypoxia.[104]

Changes in the P300 Waveform

The P300 waveform, a positive, endogenous, event-related brain potential, provides a new tool for investigating cognitive performance impairments. This measure reflects the processes of evaluation rather than those involved with selecting or executing a response. Decreasing the PaO_2 increased P300 latencies and reaction times in an experimental study; hypoxemia had no effect on P300 amplitudes.[112] Measures of P300 latencies and reaction times to the stimuli were highly correlated, whereas P300 amplitudes and reaction times were not. Increased P300 latencies are thought to indicate that hypoxemia slows stimulus evaluation processes. Another study[113] demonstrated that both the reaction time and movement components of a reaction time task were affected by hypoxemia.

In 1993, Kida and Imai[114] investigated 38 male volunteers at successive levels of simulated altitude in a hypobaric chamber (0 m; 3,000 m; 4,000 m; 5,000 m; 6,000 m; and 0 m) with an auditory oddball reaction time paradigm. All altitude conditions were tested the same day; testing was for 45 minutes at each altitude. The volunteers were classified into three groups based on their auditory reaction times for the different altitudes. This post-hoc classification yielded a group with increased reaction times at altitudes of 4,000 m; a second group with increased reaction times at 5,000 m; and a third group with no increases, not even at 6,000 m. Using this classification of responses to altitude, these investigators believed that they found several distinctive waveforms in event-related potentials that may be predictive of whether a person's cognitive performance will be vulnerable to hypoxia.

In 1995, Fowler and Prlic[75] investigated 6 volunteers to determine the influence of stimulus modality (vision or audition) on the slowing of the P300 waveform produced by hypoxia. Thresholds were estimated from measures of reaction time and the event-related brain potential P300. Volunteers responded to oddball light flashes or tone pips while breathing low-oxygen mixtures manipulated to produce SaO_2 of 77% to 86%. Both reaction time and P300 slowed in a dose-dependent manner with hypoxia, suggesting that the role of the stimulus-evaluation processes may be important in slowing. The threshold altitude for slowing was similar for both modalities (ie, 81%–82% SaO_2). The P300 amplitude exhibited an inverted-U dose-response function and was different from the response time measures. These investigators inferred that the slowing of reaction times and the P300 duration result from perceptual, rather than central, processes and that the inverted-U function for increasing hypoxia and P300 amplitude may reflect the activity of physiological compensatory mechanisms.

VARIABLES THAT INFLUENCE EFFECTS AT HIGH TERRESTRIAL ELEVATION

A number of other variables besides the level of HTE contribute to the type and magnitude of the adverse psychological impairments observed after exposure to altitude. Some adverse effects are more sensitive to high altitude (eg, visual changes result at lower levels of HTE than the symptoms of AMS). The time courses of various adverse effects are often dissimilar; effects may begin, be maximal, or end at different times. The late 1980s also brought the recognition that very extreme altitudes may cause long-term, if not permanent, impairments in some cognitive and psychomotor performances. Characteristics of military, survival, or psychological assessment tasks, such as task complexity and the amount and distribution of practice on them, also influence adverse effects. Likewise, some characteristics of the soldier or the climber are also important. They include his or her strategy for optimizing speed versus accuracy of his or her performance on a task, sensitivity to hypoxia, and individual differences that affect adverse psychological effects.

Threshold Altitude for Effects

Knowing and predicting the effects of varying degrees of high altitude are of critical importance for many military and civilian enterprises and activities. This section is concerned with the altitude (threshold) at which illness and other adverse effects occur.[3,115] In planning for military operations at high altitude, commanders must consider how much illness and impaired performance must be anticipated at a given altitude.[4,6,7] Likewise, other personnel specialists also make similar judgments (eg, astronomers determine if supplemental oxygen is required in their observatories above 3,800 m[14,15]; and regulatory specialists in commercial aviation specify minimum altitudes [eg, 1,800–2,438 m] above which supplemental oxygen or pressurization in the aircraft is required) based on high-altitude research and experience. Such guidelines are reevaluated periodically to ensure that human capabilities are sustained in especially demanding environments and that safety guidelines produce specifications that are not excessive (structural specifications, weight, and safety systems of aircraft or requirements for observatories).[10] Individual responses to high altitude, supplemental oxygen, or pressurization of an aircraft will vary greatly; other factors such as physical activity, smoking, heart and lung disease, and alcohol consumption will degrade a person's adaptation to a given level of altitude.[10,15]

Sensation, symptoms, moods, and physiological functions are more sensitive to the effects of high altitude than is cognitive performance.[11] Changes in cognitive functioning are usually reported for altitudes in excess of 3,048 m, whereas changes in sensation, symptoms, moods, and physiological functioning are often observed at lower altitudes. McFarland[11] reported the incidence for varied complaints in 200 volunteers at 3,048 m altitude as headache (10%), altered respiration (> 15% after 10 min), dizziness during locomotion (~ 4%), and sensory impairments (~ 5%). Thresholds for the dark-adaptation function were increased at 1,524 and 2,255 m; such increases were evident 2 minutes after the start of dark adaptation at 2,255 m.[11] Shukitt and Banderet[29] found increased sleepiness in volunteers at 1,600 m. Fraser and colleagues[116] reported increased postural sway at 1,521, 2,438, and 3,048 m; however, their statistical analyses and interpretations were challenged.[117]

Other variables than the degree of high altitude influence the threshold for effects, such as the dependent measure of interest. For example, the duration until one loses consciousness after exposure to HTE, such as during special altitude training in a hypobaric chamber, does not change until higher than 5,000 m,[118] whereas many other dependent measures of effects such as mood states would change after exposure to 3,000 m or 4,000 m. Other critical variables are the duration of exposure before measurements are assessed, the rate of ascent, the choice of dependent measures within a class of phenomena (eg, mood state of sleepiness vs dizziness),[29] and the statistical power of the study design.

Studies of psychological effects at altitudes of approximately 3,000 m or lower often have equivocal outcomes. Performance (rate of problem solving) on Baddeley's Grammatical Reasoning Test was not significantly impaired at 2,440 m or 3,050 m of altitude in four groups of 30 civilians[119]; interestingly, the authors of the study attributed the greater error rate at 3,050 m to apprehension rather than to the effects of

altitude per se. In a clinical study, seven subjects were exposed to 3,048 m for 6.5 hours.[120] When the effects of only responsive subjects were emphasized, subjects' cognitive performances appeared affected; inferential statistics were not used because of large individual differences.[120] At altitudes higher than 3,048 m, incremental changes were demonstrated with progressively higher altitudes for pattern perception, alertness, memory, computation, decision making, and attention.[11]

Tune's[121] 1964 literature review suggested that an altitude of 3,048 m or higher will cause perceptual–motor impairments. However in 1966, Denison, Ledwith, and Poulton[122] found increased reaction times on a spatial task while subjects exercised at 2,438 m, an altitude 650 m lower than that specified by Tune.[121] They suggested that task novelty, resulting from new learning of task information, made performance more vulnerable at these low altitudes. Guided by these data, the recommendation was made that cabin altitudes in aircraft (cabin pressures) be maintained below the equivalent of 2,438 m to ensure the performance of aircrews.[9] A more-recent investigation (1995) evaluated 12 male volunteers at simulated altitudes of 30 m, 2,134 m, and 3,658 m with a signal-detection approach and found that response times were slower at the two high altitudes.[123] These investigators suggested 2,134 m as a threshold for effects in this study—an unexpectedly low threshold value. Another explanation for this lower threshold is that it is an artifact, since the variability of Sao_2 from person to person can be great (eg, 82%–98%, with a mean of 91.2%) when ambient pressure is manipulated to simulate a specific altitude condition. Hence, the variability of Sao_2 values (which can result from manipulating ambient pressure) or the greater sensitivity of the signal-detection paradigm that was used may account for these apparent effects at 2,134 m.

Many performances appear more robust to the effects of hypoxemia than was suggested by the two investigations just described.[122,123] In 1963, Tichauer[124] studied machine shop operators producing bicycle axles at 2,740 m and observed that their performance at that altitude was not different from sea-level performance; such tasks were affected in shops at 4,120 m. It is likely that some of the conflicting work on the minimum threshold for altitude effects may depend on whether the researcher controlled Sao_2 or ambient pressure. In 1985, Fowler and colleagues[125] attempted to replicate the 1966 study of Denison and colleagues,[122] and found that altitudes higher than 2,134 to 2,438 m were required to produce the effects that had been suggested by Denison and colleagues. The Fowler investigation also showed the importance of controlling PaO_2 (a measure highly correlated with SaO_2), rather than atmospheric pressure or gas mixtures, to ensure comparable hypoxemia. They concluded that the findings of Denison and colleagues[122] probably resulted from unusually low arterial PaO_2, caused by the resistance of breathing through a facial mask, which became more significant during hypoxia, exercise, and hypoventilation. Hence, Fowler and colleagues[125] concluded that 2,438 m was substantially lower than the actual altitude threshold that affects performance. Their investigation also suggested that new learning is no more vulnerable than prior learning to the effects of hypoxemia.

To determine the minimum altitude that causes changes on perceptual motor performance, in 1987 Fowler and colleagues[126] established altitude-response curves for the serial choice reaction time task for two levels of stimulus brightness. PaO_2 was manipulated in small increments by having six subjects breathe low-oxygen gas mixtures so that varied levels of hypoxemia (simulating altitudes of 2,712–3,475 m) were produced. Response times slowed in an altitude-dependent manner; the minimum altitude (ie, the threshold) for effects was estimated at 2,972 m. These data from a choice reaction time task are strong support for Tune's assertion in 1964 that the minimum

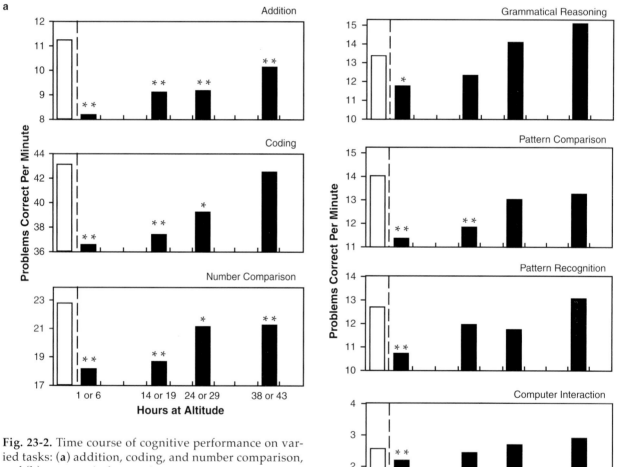

Fig. 23-2. Time course of cognitive performance on varied tasks: (**a**) addition, coding, and number comparison, and (**b**) grammatical reasoning, pattern comparison, pattern recognition, and computer interaction, all at 4,600 m simulated altitude. The measure of performance—problems correct per minute—incorporates both accuracy and speed of performance in the index. At each data collection interval, some of the volunteers were evaluated at one time and the remainder at a different time (eg, 1 h or 6 h). Asterisks above a bar indicate a statistically significant difference ($P \le .05 = *$; $P \le .01 = **$) from the baseline (200 m) value. Data source: Banderet LE, Shukitt B, Crohn EA, Burse RL, Roberts DE, Cymerman A. Effects of various environmental stressors on cognitive performance. *Proceedings of the 28th Annual Meeting of the Military Testing Association.* Mystic, Conn: US Coast Guard Academy; 1986: 594. DTIC No. AD 188762.

threshold for altitude effects on most performance tasks is approximately 3,050 m.[121] Hence, an earlier estimate of the minimum altitude that produces performance impairments (ie, 2,438 m), and its implied requirements for greater aircraft pressurization, was unnecessarily cautious.[125,126]

Time Course of Effects

Because adverse changes in mood and cognitive performance occur after exposure to high altitude, two interesting questions are "What is the time course of these effects?" and "Are adverse changes in mood and cognitive performances related to increases in AMS?" The number, severity, rapidity of onset, and the duration of symptom, mood, and performance changes vary from person to person and are related to both level of altitude and rate of ascent.[42,44] The faster one ascends and the higher one climbs, the more likely the chances of being affected.[3,42] It is usually assumed that individuals afflicted with AMS will be more susceptible to changes in mood, cognitive and psychomotor performance, and the like; however, their time courses are sometimes different and may reflect different mechanisms.[42]

Symptoms of AMS start to appear after 6 hours, increase from 6 to 24 hours, and reach maximum severity during 30 to 40 hours of exposure.[3,127,128] The time courses of other factors measured by the Environmental Symptoms Questionnaire[32–35] (eg, cold, alert, exertion, muscular discomfort, fatigue) and some mood states appear similar to that of the symptomatology of AMS (AMS-C, the "cerebral" factor on the Environmental Symptoms Questionnaire), although these trends are not as well documented.[29,44] At 4,300 m, moods (friendliness, clear thinking, dizziness, sleepiness, and happiness) were adversely affected after 1 to 4 hours on the day of arrival and differed most after 18 to 28 hours.[29] By 42 to 52 hours after ascent, all moods returned to baseline levels. Adverse changes in mood states were also measured 90 minutes after ascent to a 4.5-hour exposure to 4,200 or 4,700 m during the first administration of the cognitive tests and mood questionnaires.[30,129]

The time course of performance impairments, however, appears somewhat different than that for AMS and some moods. Decrements on all seven tasks administered 1 or 6 hours after ascent to 4,600 m have been found.[43,45,130] At 14 hours or 19 hours, only four tasks were still impaired, and by 38 hours or 42 hours, only two were still impaired (Figure 23-2). Therefore, changes in performance were greatest at 1 hour or 6 hours (ie, soon after ascent), a time when the symptoms of AMS are only starting

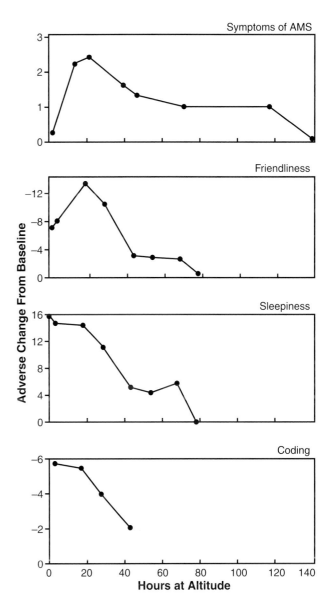

Fig. 23-3. Adverse changes at 4,300 m simulated altitude for selected measures of symptoms of acute mountain sickness (AMS), moods, and cognitive performance. The units for each dependent measure were retained but transformed so that baseline for each measure equals 0. The first three measures (symptoms of AMS, friendliness, and sleepiness) are based on subjective ratings; the fourth, coding, is a measure of cognitive performance and is scored as the number of problems correct per minute. Symptoms of AMS and the mood state friendliness have similar time courses. The time courses of sleepiness and coding are analogous but different from those for AMS and sleepiness. The time courses of coding performance and the symptoms of AMS, however, are dissociated and dissimilar.

to appear. Figure 23-3 emphasizes the dissociation between performance impairments while doing coding, the cognitive task, and the symptoms of AMS; performance on the coding task was somewhat improved when the symptoms of AMS were most severe (after 20–30 h). It also shows that the mood state of friendliness had a time course like that of AMS, whereas sleepiness had a time course like that of coding performance.

A study by Cahoon[131] in 1972 exposed volunteers to 4,570 m for 48 hours, during which they performed four card-sorting tasks after 3 hours, 20 hours, 24 hours, and 45 hours of exposure. The greatest decrement on all tasks occurred during the test at 3 hours; after that, performance improved. Other studies[16,30,43,129] have confirmed that adverse changes in cognitive performance were measured at 90 minutes of exposure to 4,200 or 4,700 m simulated altitude, which was the earliest that performance tasks were administered at altitude.[30]

Temporary Versus Long-Term Effects

There is growing concern, heightened dramatically in the past 10 years, that some undesirable consequences of extreme high-altitude exposure may be long-term or even permanent. Mountain climbers, balloonists, and pilots who did not use supplemental oxygen have known that high altitude produces changes in affective behavior, judgment, and cognitive performance.[1,2] Long-term residents at even moderate altitudes of 4,328 m had 3- to 4-fold more migraine headaches than residents at sea level; tension headaches, however, were not affected.[132] Peter Habeler—who climbed Mount Everest in 1978 with the mountaineer Reinhold Messner, together making the first ascent without supplemental oxygen—suffered nightmares and memory lapses even a few years after the climb.[72] A case study described the fate of a man who was briefly subjected to 7,620 m during a malfunction in a hypobaric chamber.[133] Although the man was revived and quickly returned to sea level, 15 years later he still experiences loss of taste and throbbing headaches in both temples three or four times weekly. Some medical professionals (some of whom are also climbers) express concerns that extreme climbs (almost resulting in death or completed without supplemental oxygen) may produce long-term behavioral and cognitive changes.[18,134]

Practices that put climbers at unnecessary risk for CNS damage also raise another concern: some neurological effects of extreme exposures to high altitude may be latent and have minimal impact until the brain is subsequently traumatized by another injury or stressor.[135] If so, an earlier impairment from climbing could combine with and magnify the degradation from a new trauma.

In a review prepared in 1989, Banderet and Burse[42] concluded that long-term effects caused by ascent to extreme high altitude were a reliable and important phenomenon. At that time, there were many older studies with no adverse findings; only a few new studies supported the idea of extreme high altitude causing long-term effects to the CNS. In that review, they said:

> New trends in climbing increase the risk of damage to the nervous system, since some climbers choose special procedures to deliberately increase the challenge of climbing high mountains.[40,134,136] Climbers may ascend without time scheduled for staging, without supplemental oxygen, during the winter, or without securing ropes.[42(p240)]

Since then, it has become clear that many factors are putting greater numbers of climbers at risk for long-term, perhaps permanent, CNS effects. Climbing without supplemental oxygen has become fashionable in the last few years, since a small group of elite climbers has scaled all 14 of the peaks above 8,000 m in the world without supplemental oxygen.[18] (Some mountain climbers, from Russia, for example, choose not to use supplemental oxygen during a climb because they feel it is unethical and wrong to use it.[137]) In addition, blatant commercialism and promotion of climbing expeditions to extremely high altitudes expose inexperienced and unseasoned climbers to perilous conditions.

What data support the idea that climbs to very high altitudes engender long-term changes to the CNS? Studies demonstrating such effects were rare before and during the 1980s. More than 100 climbers who spent time above 5,500 m in the mid 1970s indicated by survey that they did not feel that they or their peers were permanently impaired by altitude.[1] More than 20 individuals who climbed higher than 5,300 m were carefully studied by means of several psychological tests; these data, published in 1983, supported the earlier findings of no long-term effects.[138] Climbers who spent at least 4 days above 7,200 m, and two who reached the summit of Mount Everest, were assessed in 1989.[139] Temporary impairments were observed during the climb at altitudes higher than 5,200 m; after descent, there was no evidence of impairment.

Recent studies provide much stronger evidence for long-term effects by documenting both behavioral and structural phenomena. Personality and mental effects were documented in 80 Polish Alpinists from 1960 through 1985. In some climbers, permanent injury to the CNS was inferred because of the persistence of mental changes long after the climb.[40] In 1985, Townes, Hornbein, and Schoene[140] studied 51 climbers from five expeditions to Mount Everest. Various neuropsychological tests suggested transient changes in verbal expression and possibly memory. Most remarkable and persistent was a bilateral motor impairment even 1 year after the climb. Such changes at high altitude and immediately after descent were replicated in Operation Everest II.[91]

Impairments after high-altitude exposure have also been demonstrated for HTE less extreme than Mount Everest. Long-term effects from climbing to 5,947 m were demonstrated in 1993.[141] Also in 1993, Kramer, Coyne, and Strayer[48] published their comparison of 18 men and 2 women who climbed Mount Denali (6,194 m) in Alaska with their matched controls. After descent, the climbers showed deficits of learning and retention in perceptual and memory tasks. With each administration of the memory search and choice reaction time tasks, the climbers responded more slowly on these tasks than the control group, demonstrated less transfer from practice on the tasks, and were more disrupted by the time intervals between practice sessions.[48]

Memory studies in seven people who climbed without supplemental oxygen to 7,100 m were published in 1987; even 75 days after the climb, memory impairments persisted.[95] A subsequent study with 10 climbers (9 men and 1 woman) who spent 14 days at 5,300 to 7,000 m without supplementary oxygen confirmed memory deficits even 75 days after the climb.[142] The investigators speculated in 1990 that the impairments were created by the effect of extreme hypoxia on the temporal lobes.[142] They were surprised to find the impairments in this study, as this climb was made during the summer so that atmospheric pressure and weather conditions would be less severe than during the other seasons. Still another study,[141] published in 1993 by this same team of investigators, studied 11 male climbers from two separate expeditions who ascended to 5,947 or 7,439 m without supplemental oxygen; all climbers spent at least 14 days above 5,200 m. Seventy-five days after the climbers returned to sea level, testing showed that measures of associative memory, reaction times, and concentration were impaired, compared with their performances before the climb. The investigators suggested that one climb may have been sufficient to produce these effects because (1) none of these climbers had climbed before outside the Alps and (2) none were professional climbers.[141]

In 1989, Regard and colleagues[103] measured small impairments in concentration, short-term memory, and ability to shift concepts and control errors in five of the eight world-class climbers that they studied who had scaled mountains approximately 350 m lower than Mount Everest. Some 2 to 11 months earlier, all climbers had been at altitudes above 8,500 m for 2 to 15 days.[103] More-detailed analyses of these climbers' performances published the next year[65] indicated that although all climbers were highly motivated and achievement oriented, the performance of five of the eight climbers showed significant decrements of concentration, short-term memory, and cognitive flexibility. Their perceptual abilities, language, and spatial-constructive abilities were intact so the measured impairments in the five climbers affected probably reflected mild, but permanent, malfunctioning of fronto-temporo-basal brain areas. Conventional EEG recordings, evaluated by two independent experts, showed pathological findings in the two climbers with the greatest cognitive impairments. After their ascent, seven of the eight climbers underwent evaluation of their brains and spinal cords with MRI. The two climbers who showed abnormal MRI findings were among the most cognitively impaired.[65]

Hornbein and colleagues[91,143] tested 35 mountaineers before and 1 to 30 days after ascent to 5,488 and 8,848 m, and 6 volunteers before and after a 40-day ascent to a simulated altitude of 8,848 m. Impairments were manifested by deficits in memory phenomena (storage and recall), aphasia, concentration, and finger-tapping speed.[143] Visual long-term memory was impaired in both groups after descent; however, the mountaineers made twice as many aphasic errors after, compared with before, the climb.[91] Each person's cognitive impairment was positively correlated with his or her ventilatory response to hypoxia.[91,143] Verbal long-term memory was also affected, but only in the volunteers experiencing altitude in a hypobaric chamber.[91] This finding from the laboratory study is of special interest because it suggests that even when the hardships and extreme conditions (eg, cold and storms) associated with climbing a mountain are minimized, cognitive impairments may still persist several days after descent.

Further support for long-term effects was provided by a study[144] of 26 male and female climbers who did not use supplemental oxygen during ascents to extreme HTE. After descent from 7,000 m or higher (7,000–8,848 m), 46% of the climbers had abnormalities detected by MRI, and 58% had significant neurobehavioral impairments. The MRI images for the climbers and matched personnel were scored blind by experts; no MRI abnormalities were observed in any of the 21 matched age and gender controls. The MRI abnormalities suggested cortical atrophy (19% of climbers) and hyperintensity lesions (19% of climbers); two climbers (8%) exhibited both of these MRI abnormalities. The MRI abnormalities that were observed were not associated with age, gender, clinical symptoms, maximal altitude climbed, or duration of exposure to HTE.

Some[1,137] believe that the physical trauma, dehydration, and weight loss at HTE (such as Ryn[40] and others) are responsible for such long-term changes. In contrast, others[48] suggest that the experimental design and assessment methodology are critical, or such effects may be missed. The latter emphasize that they would not have found such effects in their climbers without the use of matched controls. The study of Kramer, Coyne, and Strayer[48] also demonstrates that cognitive impairments after descent may result from a failure to profit fully from practice or the continued performance of a cognitive task. This insight may be a critical new dimension for evaluating the impact of such impairments induced by exposure to extreme HTE.

Others accept the data and conclude that such studies demonstrate long-term impairments. J. B. West, a researcher, physician, and climber, was the first to recognize such long-term effects (in 1986) and called early for an increased awareness of these phenomena, because unless they are informed, climbers, physicians, and educators cannot appraise the risks and choose conditions appropriate for long-term well-being.[134] In a review article[18] that also supports the idea that long-term effects are associated with extreme exposure to high altitude, these concerns were reinforced by the work of others. For example, Cavaletti and colleagues[18] are strongly convinced that climbing to extreme altitudes without supplemental oxygen may create long-term changes in the CNS that affect cognitive and memory processes. They assert that researchers, physicians, and climbers have an ethical responsibility to be aware of these data and to inform relevant others.

Cognitive Task Complexity and Practice

Complex performances are usually affected before simpler performances,[59,145] so activities requiring decisions and strategies are more vulnerable than automatic processes.[47] Cognitive performance is more vulnerable to hypoxemia than is psychomotor performance.[46] Performances involving visual processing of shapes, patterns, and contours are thought to be more vulnerable to impairments at altitude than those involving numbers, words, or characters.

The trends for complexity of the task were nicely illustrated by various displays of the Manikin Task. The effects of staging for 5 successive days at 4,500 m to 7,000 m were investigated (8 h/d) in an altitude chamber.[146] Measures of cognitive performance were determined from four male climbers with a mental rotation task (eg, a Manikin Task), during the acclimation procedure. The latency to mentally rotate simpler manikin displays was not affected by any altitude, not even 7,000 m (eg, rear view requires rotation about one axis only). At 6,500 and 7,000 m, responses to more complex displays of the manikin required longer latencies and climbers also made more errors than at lower altitudes. It is significant that these were experienced climbers; unacclimatized personnel probably would not have tolerated these altitudes.

Two vigilance tasks that varied in difficulty were investigated at a simulated altitude of either 610 or 2,438 m.[147] In this experiment, large numbers of volunteers were tested in both conditions of task complexity. The easier task was investigated with 44 volunteers; the more difficult, with 36. With the easier task, there was no significant difference between performance at either altitude. With the more difficult task, the volunteers' initial performance was significantly worse for the high-altitude group compared with the control group's. The impairment in performance observed initially at high altitude did not occur during the last half of the test trials.

The amount of practice on a cognitive task indirectly affects its sensitivity to the effects of high altitude. Thirty-six medical students performed a vigilance task at a simulated altitude of 2,438 m, and their performance was compared with that of a control group at 610 m.[148] If the students were not familiar with the test before assessment, the hypoxic participants performed poorer on the first half of the test than did the control group; there was no significant difference between groups on performance of the last half of the test. When the students become familiar with the test before exposure to high altitude, the performance of hypoxic and control participants was not statistically different.

In another study,[62] during a gradual mountain ascent (> 6,500 m) climbers served as data collectors by encoding responses and recording audio information for subsequent analysis. Reliability and validity checks of the data-collector climbers indicated that 36% of all errors happened during the first test session at 1,200 m. Overall accuracy for the entire study was 99.6%. It is clear that additional practice and familiarization during the first data-collection session greatly improved subsequent performance, even when it was at high altitude.

Individual Differences

Studies conducted at altitude frequently show large individual variations in dependent measures among volunteers; there appears to be wide individual response to the effects of altitude. Carson and colleagues,[127] describing the effects of 4,300 m high altitude, reported:

> Variability in the degree of symptomatology of AMS is the rule rather than the exception. In our experience with placebo or untreated subjects on Pikes Peak, 10–20%, on the average, appear almost unaffected and 40–50% are temporarily incapacitated.[127(p1085)]

Others assert that the effects of altitude vary greatly from person to person, and some people show great variations from time to time. Such individual differences result from genetic, experimental, and psychological factors.[14]

Individual differences in response to altitude may explain why some studies have shown more pronounced effects of altitude than others. Barach[25] alluded to the difference in behavior that is produced by the environment in which the individual is tested for the effects of hypoxia. In a study with male volunteers, when the experimenter was an attractive female physician, the manifestations of impairment of emotional control differed greatly from those previously observed when the experimenter was a man. When a series of medical students and a group of patients were exposed to an atmosphere of 13% oxygen (simulating approximately 3,660 m altitude) for a 3-hour period, about 60% of the subjects registered euphoria, elation, and boisterous excitement, whereas 40% showed depression, mental dullness, and drowsiness from the start. In the male volunteers who manifested the euphoric tendency, exaggerated self-esteem and frank sexual advances toward the female experimenter were frequently encountered.[25]

The impairment in emotional control that is the result of hypoxia is also determined by the personality and behavior of the individual.[25] Mental efficiency and performance of discrete motor movements were affected at altitudes of 3,660 m,[11] and some individuals experienced altitude-related symptoms such as sleepiness, fatigue, and euphoria. Limited physical exertion at high altitude appeared to minimize symptoms[149]; however, individuals with superb physical conditioning were just as likely to experience the effects of high altitude and the symptoms of AMS.[150] Athletes, however, generally tolerate discomfort well; although symptomatic, they may appear less affected by the illness than nonathletes.[151]

Some individuals believe that altitude will have a great effect on themselves, their performance, or both, while others believe that altitude will have little or no effect. Perhaps this could explain why some individuals' performance and moods are greatly affected at higher elevations, but not others'. Previous exposure to altitude may also influence an individual's psychological response to altitude. In other words, prior exposure might help to remove psychological barriers.[151] Additionally, motivation and training can effectively compensate for the stress imposed by a high-altitude atmosphere, with motivation a more important factor than training in maintaining performance at high altitude.[49]

In 1957, Greene[152] described several effects of chronic hypoxia. For example, chronic hypoxia affects people differently. It influences what system or process is affected and how greatly it is affected. Typically, memory is seriously affected, although the degree of impairment varies from person to person. The capacity to perform mental work accurately is usually degraded. Lastly, Green observed that an afflicted person's emotional instability may be severe, usually taking the form of irritability.

Sensitivity to hypoxia is an individual difference that affects one's responses to high altitude. Hypoxia normally causes an increase in breathing rate, breathing depth, or both; this increase is normally an adaptive response to hypoxia because it results in greater oxygen availability for delivery to the brain, tissues, and bodily organs. Surprisingly, researchers[81,91] found that climbers with the greatest sensitivity to hypoxia were the most hypoxic during sleep; these climbers also had some of the largest daytime cognitive performance deficits. Hornbein and colleagues[91] found that a greater ventilatory response to hypoxia correlated with a reduction in verbal learning and poor long-term verbal memory after ascent. A greater ventilatory response to hypoxia also correlated with an increase in the number of aphasic errors on the aphasic screening test in both the simulated-ascent group and a subgroup of 11 mountaineers. They concluded that persons with a more vigorous ventilatory response to hypoxia have more residual neurobehavioral impairment after returning to lower elevations. According to Hornbein and colleagues, this finding may be explained by poorer oxygenation of the brain despite greater ventilation, perhaps because of a decrease in cerebral blood flow caused by hypocapnia that more than offsets the increase in arterial oxygen saturation.

Hornbein and colleagues[90] state that increased oxygen delivery to muscle during exercise is responsible for the finding that people with greater hypoxic ventilatory responses (who appear more impaired cognitively after exposure to extremely high altitude) are the ones who seem to perform best physically at great heights. On the other hand, Herr[153] suggests that the cognitive impairment demonstrated by Hornbein and colleagues[91] may be the link between a greater ventilatory response to hypoxia and better physical performance. The impairments may be associated with a mild decline in neurobehavioral function that blunts pain, leading to both better physical performance and the recollection of having performed better.[153]

Performance Tradeoffs of Speed Versus Accuracy

Performance impairments at high altitude can reflect increased errors, slowing of performance, or a combination of these effects. Banderet and colleagues[130] studied cognitive tasks requiring processing of numbers, words, and patterns under conditions of cold, dehydration, and simulated altitude (4,300–7,600 m). Before the experiment, subjects practiced the tasks extensively, received performance feedback, and maintained low error rates. During exposure to each stressful environment, the rate of problem solving decreased; a few errors resulted but contributed little to the impairments. Such trends for varied high altitudes are shown in Figure 23-4.[130] Data were not collected for each altitude for all cognitive tasks. The average change in performance (from baseline) for the volunteers tested in each high altitude condition is shown for the contribution from increased errors or the contribution from decreased rates of performance. Although some errors occurred, it is clear that the strategy observed in these studies at varied high altitudes was a slowing of performance while maintaining accuracy. This strategy is consistent with that observed by us for other stressful, nonaltitude conditions.[130] These findings illustrate a common functional strategy observed in several studies where the volunteer sets the pace of the task: the rate of performance is often sacrificed for accuracy.[46,145] With time, performance at 4,600 m recovered to rates observed previously at low altitude; there was also a slight decrease in the number of

errors.[43,130] Other analyses suggested that the rate of each person's performance at low altitude (baseline) does not predict performance impairments resulting from altitude or other environmental stressors.[43,130]

Cahoon[131] studied eight participants with cognitive and psychomotor tasks at 4,570 m for 48 hours or less and found that cognitive tasks showed a greater decrement in speed and accuracy than simple tasks. Moreover, speed was generally sacrificed to maintain accuracy. Cognitive data, collected at altitudes from 5,500 to 7,600 m from six or seven volunteers in the Operation Everest II study, also exhibited a slowing of the rate of response for tasks administered by computer[61] and paper-and-pencil tasks.[130] Tapping keys on a computer keyboard with fingers on the preferred or nonpreferred hands was not affected.[61] These studies are consistent with the notion that hypoxemia affects cognitive functioning more than motor functioning.[61,131]

Investigators[123] used a signal detection approach to evaluate responses in 12 male volunteers to altitudes of 30 m, 2,134 m, and 3,658 m, simulated in an altitude chamber. On each trial, volunteers indicated if one of four symbols (rectangle, ellipse, the letter "A," or the numeral "1") was upright or rotated up to 90° counterclockwise by pressing one of two keys. Response times were slower at 2,134 m and 3,658 m than at 30 m. Also, a signal-detection analysis showed that at 2,134 m the accuracy of the volunteers' judgments about the orientation of the symbols decreased; their response criterion did not change.[123]

Twenty climbers from the Birmingham Medical Research Expeditionary Society were investigated during two separate climbs to 5,000 m. Climbers who were ill with AMS had increased reaction times. Increased errors also occurred, but they were not related to altitude or symptomatology.[57]

Tharion and colleagues[60] investigated the effects of acute and chronic hypoxia on marksmanship (days 2–4 and days 15–17 after ascent) resulting from residence at 3,700 to 4,300 m. Volunteers fired a laser-equipped training rifle at a 2.3-cm target 5 m away. Performance when firing a rifle during days 2 through 4 at high altitude was 9% less accurate than that at sea level, but the time taken for sighting was briefer at altitude. The change in performance strategy during acute exposure to altitude suggests a different speed–accuracy tradeoff or shift than that described previously: volunteers fired more quickly but less accurately at altitude than at sea level. During days 15 through 17 at high altitude, both measures of performance (timeliness and

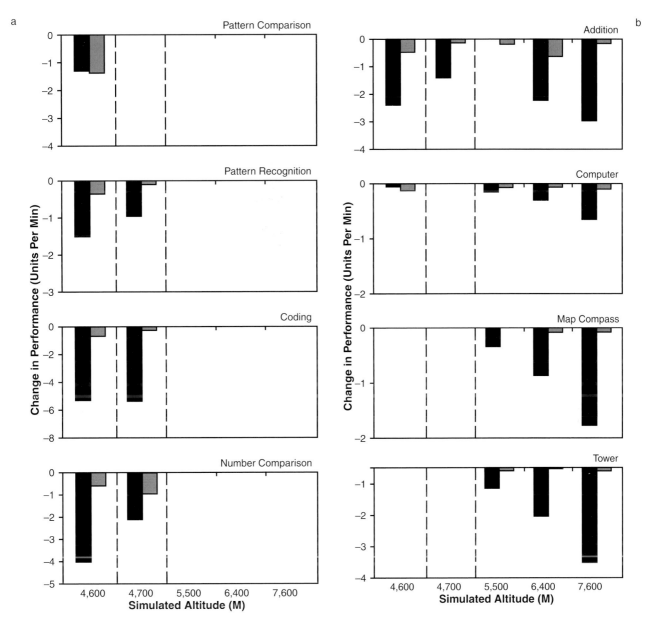

Fig. 23-4. Contributions of increased errors (shaded bars) or slowing of performance (solid bars) to performance impairments observed at varied simulated high attitudes. These graphs show data for (**a**) the pattern comparison, pattern recognition, coding, and number comparison tasks at altitudes of 4,600 m and 4,700 m (except for the pattern comparison task, which was done only at 4,600 m), and (**b**) the addition, computer (computer interaction), map compass, and tower tasks (which, except for the addition task, were not collected for all altitudes). These data suggest that the performance impairments at high altitude on these cognitive tasks result primarily from a slowing of performance rather than decreased accuracy (ie, increased errors). Adapted with permission from Banderet LE, Shukitt B, Crohn EA, Burse RL, Roberts DE, Cymerman A. Characteristics of cognitive performance in stressful environments. *Proceedings of the 28th Annual Meeting of the Military Testing Association.* Mystic, Conn: US Coast Guard Academy; 1986: 427.

accuracy) were similar to those at sea level[60]; this suggests that after 15 to 17 days, performance at altitude had recovered to that observed earlier at sea level. Evans[59] studied eight men on a pistol-fir-

ing task at sea level and at 4,300 m. His results show a different speed–accuracy tradeoff than that of Tharion and colleagues[60] or the ones shown previously in Figure 23-4.[130] In Evans's[59] study at high altitude, volunteers both took longer to fire and were less accurate at altitude than at sea level. These studies illustrate the importance of using measures that include both the speed and the accuracy of performance; otherwise, shifts or tradeoffs in performance criteria will not be evident and interpretations of the data may be misleading.

Schlaepfer, Bartsch, and Fisch[67] evaluated the effects of 3,450 m by transporting 10 volunteers to the Jungfraujoch (in the Swiss Bernese Alps) by helicopter, and by evaluating 10 other volunteers with gas mixtures equivalent to altitudes of either 3,450 m or sea level. All volunteers exposed to hypoxic conditions were assessed 15 minutes after exposure. The dependent variable involved systematically increasing the duration that letters were presented tachistoscopically each time a letter was identified incorrectly, until eight successive letters were recognized correctly. This study suggested that visual perception was improved by hypoxemia, because a briefer presentation was required for both the mountainous and the hypoxic gas-mixture conditions. Unfortunately, accuracies for the different conditions were not specified. Assessment 15 minutes after exposure may have changed the volunteers' response criteria (factors unrelated to the stimulus properties, eg, experience with the task) without any changes in stimulus discriminability occurring. Without more information, it cannot be determined if the reported trend reflected a shift in the volunteers' speed–accuracy tradeoffs.

Another study[154] investigated six physicians (three women and three men) at the Vallot Mont Blanc Observatory at an altitude of 4,382 m for 60 hours. Six control volunteers were also studied and tested at sea level at the same times of day as the altitude group. All 12 volunteers were evaluated on a task that involved entering letter sequences with a 9-number keypad like that on a computer keyboard. The pairing of letters with the keys was defined for each trial and indicated with a diagram, spatially analogous to the keypad, that showed a letter on each key. A five-letter sequence that was to be entered on the keypad was also indicated on the diagram. Character-entry performance under these conditions was scored with a derived index that incorporated both the speed and the accuracy of performance. After 8 to 20 hours at high altitude, a measure of performance on the data-entry task that combined both speed and accuracy was less than control values; after 48 to 60 hours at high altitude, performance recovered to sea-level values.

Fine and Kobrick[155] reported that they found increased errors during exposure to hypoxia on tasks such as receiving information from radio transmissions. Tichauer[124] found that even fully acclimatized personnel working in machine shops at 4,120 m committed more errors and required more time to produce bicycle axles than personnel at lower altitudes. Varied performance outcomes are common, since the characteristics of the task influence the quality of performance and number and types of errors.[145] For example, errors are more likely to occur when tasks are paced by external conditions such as an assembly line or receiving radio transmissions that cannot be "said again." When the pace of the task is set by the subject under stressful conditions (eg, cognitive tasks administered via paper and pencil), response rates are likely to be sacrificed for low error rates. A slowed-processing model in the scientific literature incorporates conditions such as altitude exposure, aging,[156] and nitrogen narcosis.[157]

Correlations Between Measured Effects

Shukitt-Hale, Banderet, and Lieberman[44] conducted a study to determine whether individuals afflicted with initial symptoms of AMS would be more susceptible to adverse changes in other symptoms, mood states, and performance. The AMS-Cerebral (AMS-C) factor of the Environmental Symptoms Questionnaire was chosen as a measure of altitude sickness because it is a commonly used standard index of the degree of illness. Thirty-eight other measures were chosen to assess various symptoms, moods, and performance. Volunteers were evaluated after exposure to 4,700 m for 5 to 7 hours on 11 symptom, 13 mood, and 14 cognitive–motor performance measures.[44,45] The AMS-C scores were significantly correlated with composite measures of symptoms ($r = 0.90$), moods ($r = 0.77$), and performance ($r = 0.59$). After 5 to 7 hours at 4,700 m, the measure of mountain sickness (AMS-C) was most like (ie, most associated with) other symptoms seen at altitude. This measure of mountain sickness was less like adverse mood changes and least like measures of impaired cognitive performances. One reason why the different magnitudes of correlations with composite measures of symptoms, moods, and performance result is because the time courses of these measures are different. Therefore, it is important to measure a variety of parameters during altitude studies so that the varied changes can be characterized.

In a study by Crowley and colleagues,[158] soldiers ascended to a simulated altitude of 4,300 m and remained there for 2.5 days. A test battery consisting of nine cognitive tests, a mood scale, and an AMS questionnaire was administered four times daily.

Transient deficits in cognitive performance occurred on day 1 (code substitution, Stroop test, and logical reasoning). Moods of volunteers who were ill with AMS were more negative and their performance improved less than volunteers with lesser illness. The researchers concluded that after rapid ascent (10 min) to 4,300 m, performance is most affected during the first 8 hours; the performance of individuals affected by AMS improves more slowly; and these afflicted individuals have more negative moods than those who feel well.

Regard and colleagues[159] showed that rapid ascent to 4,559 m within 24 hours had small, but different, effects on cognitive performance, depending on the later development of AMS. Climbers who developed AMS within a 24- to 48-hour stay at high altitude were mildly impaired in short-term memory but improved in conceptual tasks. Climbers who remained healthy had better short-term memory performance but no improvement in cognitive flexibility.

The relationship between psychological factors and AMS was explored in another study.[160] Individuals susceptible to AMS were significantly more anxious (both in trait anxiety and state anxiety before final ascent) than those who were not. Therefore, anxiety appears to be a good psychological predictor of AMS, although it is unknown if it is the cause or a correlate. Anxiety-reducing methods such as relaxation training and self-hypnosis may be used to prepare susceptible climbers before expeditions.

COPING WITH HIGH TERRESTRIAL ELEVATION AND MINIMIZING ADVERSE EFFECTS

Earlier in this chapter, we emphasized that most adverse changes occur in symptoms, moods, and cognitive and psychomotor performances after ascent to altitudes higher than 3,000 m. Treatments to minimize these adverse effects include psychological, operational, and medical strategies. Psychological strategies often involve training and familiarization with the adverse effects that will be experienced at HTE. Learned compensatory practices and behaviors, together with greater tolerance of unpleasant situations, help military personnel cope better with adverse effects.[161,162] Much military training is designed with such objectives and outcomes in mind. Operational strategies include staging at intermediate altitudes, acclimatizing, and using supplemental oxygen from tanks or oxygen generators. Lastly, medical strategies often involve use of medications.

In addition, new strategies need to be developed that are more effective and better suited to varied deployment requirements for HTE. Laboratory work with small animals suggests that a neurochemical approach may be promising for reducing adverse behavioral changes at HTE; in the future, adverse performance and mood changes in humans may be controlled by altering neurochemistry.

This section describes the characteristics, limitations, and potential benefits of these strategies for minimizing the adverse effects of HTE, as well as some of the medical contraindications and complicating factors. In many situations in the field, the beneficial strategies discussed are employed together.

Psychological Strategies

The fact that we can live, work, and play in adverse environments testifies to our adaptive capabilities.[163] Physiological compensations greatly facilitate coping with adverse conditions and are the most important. For example, the body changes the amount of blood flowing to the brain to compensate for the availability of oxygen and the brain's requirements for oxygen. Cerebral blood flow during rest is 700 to 750 mL/min at sea level; at 5,800 m, it may be almost doubled; and at 7,600 m, it may be increased 4-fold.[8] But psychological adaptations and strategies are also critical,[15,42] as they can facilitate coping and functioning in high-altitude environments.[72,164] In a hiking or climbing party, reassurance to the afflicted person can have a beneficial effect on reducing the symptoms of AMS and the discomforts at high altitude.[15] This observation suggests the importance of social and interpersonal variables in influencing reactions to symptoms and discomfort.[161] Reassurance and time can do much to hasten acclimatization to a more challenging, high-altitude environment.

A study[165] of Army personnel showed that the more the soldiers expected to dislike the environmental conditions, the more tense, depressed, angry, fatigued, and physically uncomfortable they were during cold weather training at moderate altitudes. Experience in stressful environments makes cognitive performance more robust because of adaptive changes in behavioral arousal, attentional capacity, or controlled versus automatic processing of the task.[157,163,166] Involvement in a performance task during high-altitude exposure apparently decreases the types and intensities of discomforts reported.[167] Experiencing the symptoms and discomforts of a stressful environment will facilitate subsequent coping in similar situations.[157,161–163,168] If people are aware of the nature and time course of altitude effects, they can devote extra attention to tasks, create checks for errors, manage personnel to ensure redundancy of procedures during critical times, and develop other compensatory strategies.[47,167,169]

Operational Strategies

Prolonged stay at HTE results in physiological acclimatization, which produces adaptive effects on oxygen delivery and regulation of metabolites.[72,150,170,171] Beneficial effects occur within days to weeks, depending on the altitude, rate of ascent, and the dependent measures chosen for evaluation. With enough time at altitude, there is usually a dramatic reduction in symptoms, adverse moods, and behavioral impairments. Lyons and colleagues[172] demonstrated that after acclimation (16 d continuously at 4,300 m altitude), six male volunteers experienced few symptoms of AMS when they were exposed again to 4,300 m, even after living at sea level for 8 days.

Acclimatization can be induced in many ways. Mountain climbers and others use the strategy of slow ascent to high altitude, providing time for acclimatization and symptoms to subside.[1,3,4,6,7,150,173,174] A leaflet by the Himalayan Rescue Association emphasized this strategy for trekkers proceeding above 3,658 m: "The golden rule: Don't go 'too fast too high.'"[15(p153)] Others try staging, where people stay at one altitude for a few days before ascending farther.[27,85,150] However, wearing a rebreathing device at sea level that produced hypoxic breathing at altitude was not found to be beneficial.[175]

As described above, another strategy was evaluated in personnel who worked in observatories at 4,200 m.[63] Some lived and slept at low altitude but drove to the top to work. Personnel with intermittent exposures to high altitude experienced AMS symptoms for more days than personnel who stayed on the mountain continuously.

Supplemental oxygen reduces or defers most effects of high altitude. Pilots in high-performance fighter aircraft use it, as do some mountain climbers.[1,3,134] Its main limitations are logistical (ie, the weight, bulk, and difficulty of transporting it) but the Gamow Bag (US distributor: Chinook Medical Gear, Inc, Durango, Colo), a large 6.6-kg, inflatable nylon bag with an air-tight zipper, and the Certec (a French product) offer promise to individuals who are severely afflicted with altitude disorders.[15,176–179] An important feature of these inventions is that, by encapsulating an individual and introducing ambient air under modest pressure into the bag, lower altitudes and greater barometric pressures are created, thereby obviating the necessity of transporting heavy, bulky oxy-

gen tanks up the mountain and usually making the transporting down of stricken climbers less urgent.

In some work situations, it may be advantageous to add supplemental oxygen to the ambient environment or administer it through a nasal clip or facial mask.[14,180] For example, a telescope technician who arrives from sea level by car to provide repairs to an inoperative telescope may well provide the highly critical and necessary support on the observatory in less than an hour and then return to sea level. Daily shift workers at an observatory often drive to work, work their shift, and then return to low altitude.[63] If supplemental oxygen was provided at the observatory, the well-being and functioning of personnel could be sustained as it is at sea level.[14] West[180] demonstrated that increasing the oxygen concentration from 21% to 25% at high altitudes of 4,000 to 5,500 m reduced the effective altitude by 1,500 m. An increased hazard of fire was not a real concern because under these conditions of reduced atmospheric pressure, items burned less readily than they would have at sea level.[180]

Medical Strategies

Some medications improve functioning at high altitude; others do not. Acetazolamide, the current medication of choice,[3,15,149,150,174,181–183] enables most personnel to work and function at high altitude with less time devoted to acclimatization.[15] Acetazolamide is a carbonic anhydrase inhibitor; it stimulates ventilation and partially corrects acid–base and gas-exchange imbalances in the blood without impairing cognitive performance.[184] It increases Pao_2 at high altitude,[83] improves sleep and reduces symptoms of hypoxia,[185] and ameliorates adverse moods.[26] Acetazolamide reduces symptoms best when combined with staging.[27]

Dexamethasone, a powerful anabolic steroid, is even more effective than acetazolamide.[15,174,186–188] It reduces performance impairments and adverse moods without significant psychological effects.[189] The drug is best used with caution, however, because it may have physical side effects.[3,190,191]

Tyrosine, a precursor of the neurotransmitter norepinephrine, reduces some of the adverse effects of high altitude and cold.[129,192–194] Tyrosine improved symptoms, moods, and various performances in volunteers who showed average or greater than average adverse effects during an environmental challenge in which they had been treated with a placebo.[129,192,193]

The drugs furosemide,[150] phenytoin,[195,196] and naproxen,[197] are ineffective or possibly harmful. Sleep preparations, alcohol, and sedatives should be avoided.[15] Stimulants may increase the symptoms of AMS and impair performances that require subtle discriminations or judgments. Common antacid tablets did not reduce altitude effects[198]; this finding is consistent with earlier data from others.[150] Supplemental intake of potassium is contraindicated.[72]

Climbing or driving to high altitudes, and even flying in aircraft (pressurized or nonpressurized), can result in decompression sickness if a person experiences reduced atmospheric pressures too soon after he or she has scuba dived. In addition to Navy divers or SEALS, such concerns may be relevant for other military personnel who perform parachute and free-fall jumps from high altitudes. The article "Medical Guidelines for Air Travel"[199] specifies the minimum interval between diving and flying in pressurized commercial aircraft (pressure equivalent to ~ 3,000 m). Twelve hours is considered sufficient after one dive per day. If diving occurred more than once per day or was performed over several days, then more than 12 hours should

elapse between the last dive and flying.

"Medical Guidelines for Air Travel"[199] also describes medical disorders (eg, cardiovascular and pulmonary disease) that may complicate flight in an aircraft or balloon. These diseases may also compromise climbing and functioning at high altitude. Such concerns are supported by empirical data. For example, 24 patients with known ischemic heart disease were evacuated with military aircraft; cabin pressure was maintained at 2,100 m; during flight, the average saturation of oxygen in the blood was 94.5%.[200] Although these data do not indicate a life-threatening or critical level of oxygen desaturation, they suggest that people with such medical conditions may be at greater risk in commercial aircraft or at high altitude because hypoxemia even in a partially pressurized aircraft can be potentiated by their preexisting disorders. Military personnel and civilians planning to climb or work at high altitude should be medically evaluated to ensure that they are healthy enough to deal with the specific challenges of exposure to HTE.

SUMMARY

Cognitive and psychomotor performance and mood states, including many critical behavioral functions such as sleep, memory, reasoning, and vigilance, are significantly impaired by ascent to HTE higher than 3,000 m. Impairments in behavior caused by HTE can degrade military operations because the judgment and rate and accuracy of performance of military personnel can be affected. Such adverse effects have distinct and measurable time courses; onset of some effects is immediate (cognitive performance), whereas the onset of others is delayed (symptoms of AMS or adverse moods). The behavioral consequences of HTE are primarily dependent on the level of altitude, the duration of exposure, the rate of ascent, an individual's state of physiological acclimation or acclimatization, characteristics of the task performed, and characteristics of the individual such as hypoxic sensitivity.

Military history documents that the adverse effects induced by HTE need to be considered when military operations at altitude are planned and un-

dertaken. Current research indicates that some performance decrements induced by ascent to extremely high mountains (eg, Mount Everest, 8,848 m) may persist for a year or longer after return to lower elevations.

Psychological, operational, and medical strategies have been employed to minimize these adverse effects. Psychological strategies often involve training and familiarization with the adverse effects that will be experienced at high altitude. Operational strategies include staging at intermediate altitudes, acclimatizing, and using supplemental oxygen from tanks or oxygen generators. Medical strategies often involve the use of medications to improve functioning at altitude and techniques to avoid complications.

In most situations, multiple strategies are employed. The strategies now available and new developments to come will ensure that high-altitude military operations in the future will be less affected by adverse changes in cognitive and psychomotor performance and mood.

ACKNOWLEDGMENT

We thank Allyson Nolan, Patricia Bremner, and Pam Dotter from the Natick Soldier Center Technical Library, Natick, Massachusetts, for their dedication in providing expert information for this manuscript. Marilyn Banderet's linguistic and grammar skills improved our writing. We also recognize the commitment, diligence, and continued resourcefulness of Sergeant Sabrina Carson, Specialist Michelle Worrell, and Jennifer Collins to this effort. Specialist Eliseo DeJesus created the figures in this chapter.

REFERENCES

1. Houston CS. *Going Higher: The Story of Man and Altitude.* Boston, Mass: Little, Brown; 1987.

2. Ward MP, Milledge JS, West JB. *High Altitude Medicine and Physiology.* Philadelphia, Pa: University of Pennsylvania Press; 1989.

3. Cymerman A, Rock PB. *Medical Problems in High Mountain Environments.* Natick, Mass: US Army Research Institute of Environmental Medicine; 1994. Report TN94-2.

4. Desmond EW. War at the top of the world. *Time.* 1989:(31 Jul)26–27, 29.

5. Bert P. Balloon ascensions. In: Hitchcock M, Hitchcock F, trans-eds. *Barometric Pressure: Researches in Experimental Physiology.* Columbus, Ohio: College Book Company; 1943: 171–194.

6. Roy S. Acute mountain sickness. In: Hegnauer AH, ed. *Biomedicine Problems of High Terrestrial Elevations.* Natick, Mass: US Army Research Institute of Environmental Medicine; 1969.

7. Singh GI, Roy SB. High altitude pulmonary edema: Clinical, hemodynamic, and pathologic studies. In: Hegnauer AH, ed. *Biomedicine Problems of High Terrestrial Elevations.* Natick, Mass: US Army Research Institute of Environmental Medicine; 1969.

8. Milnor WR. Circulation in special districts. In: Mountcastle VB, ed. *Medical Physiology.* St Louis, Mo: Mosby; 1968: 221–227.

9. Ernsting J. Prevention of hypoxia—Acceptable compromises. *Aviat Space Environ Med.* 1978;49(3):495–502.

10. Ernsting J. Mild hypoxia and the use of oxygen in flight. *Aviat Space Environ Med.* 1984;55(5):407–410.

11. McFarland RA. Human factors in relation to the development of pressurized cabins. *Aerospace Med.* 1971;12:1303–1318.

12. McFarland RA. Psychophysiological implications of life at high altitude and including the role of oxygen in the process of aging. In: Yousef MK, Horvath SM, Bullard RW, eds. *Physiological Adaptations, Desert and Mountain.* New York, NY: Academic Press; 1972.

13. Veronneau SJH, Mohler SR, Pennybaker AL, Wilcox BC, Sahiar F. Survival at high altitudes: Wheel-well passengers. *Aviat Space Environ Med.* 1996;67(8):784–786.

14. Cudaback DD. Effects of altitude on performance and health at 4 km high telescopes. *Publications of the Astronomical Society of the Pacific.* 1984;96:463–477.

15. Heath D, Williams DR. *High-Altitude Medicine and Pathology.* 4th ed. New York, NY: Oxford University Press; 1995.

16. Shukitt-Hale B, Burse RL, Banderet LE, Knight DR, Cymerman A. *Cognitive Performance, Mood States, and Altitude Symptomatology in 13–21% Oxygen Environments.* Natick, Mass: US Army Research Institute of Environmental Medicine; 1988. Technical Report 18/88.

17. Adler J, Nordland R. High risk. *Newsweek.* 1996;27 May:50–57.

18. Cavaletti G, Tredici G. Effects of exposure to low oxygen pressure on the central nervous system. *Sports Med.* 1992;13(1):1–7.

19. Gates D, Miller S. A case of altitude chicness? *Newsweek.* 1996;27 May:58.

20. Taylor LA, Lee C. Brutal year for climbers on Alaska's Mt. *USA Today.* 1992;29 June:4A.

21. Nordland R. The gods must be angry. *Newsweek.* 1997;26 May:44–45.

22. Davis PO, Curtis AV, Bachinski T. *Physical Performance Tasks Required of US Marines Operating in a High-Altitude Cold Weather Environment.* Langley Park, Md: Institute of Human Performance; 1982.

23. Pigman EC, Karakla DW. Acute mountain sickness at intermediate altitude: Military mountainous training. *Am J Emerg Med.* 1990;8(1):7–10.

24. Van Liere EJ, Stickney JC. *Hypoxia.* Chicago, Ill: University of Chicago Press; 1963.

25. Barach AL. Impairment in emotional control produced both by lowering and raising the oxygen pressure in the atmosphere. *Med Clin North Am.* 1944;28:704–718.

26. Banderet LE. Self rated moods of humans at 4300 meters pretreated with placebo or acetazolamide plus staging. *Aviat Space Environ Med.* 1977;48(1):19–22.

27. Evans WO, Robinson SM, Horstman DH, Jackson RE, Weiskopf RB. Amelioration of the symptoms of acute mountain sickness by staging and acetazolamide. *Aviat Space Environ Med.* 1976;47(5):512–516.

28. Heath D, Williams DR. *High-Altitude Medicine and Pathology.* 3rd ed. New York, NY: Butterworths; 1989.

29. Shukitt B, Banderet LE. Mood states at 1600 and 4300 meters terrestrial altitude. *Aviat Space Environ Med.* 1988;59(6):530–532.

30. Shukitt-Hale B, Banderet LE, Lieberman HR. Elevation-dependent symptom, mood, and performance changes produced by exposure to hypobaric hypoxia. *Int J Aviat Psychol.* 1998;8:319–334.

31. Shukitt-Hale B, Rauch TM, Foutch R. Altitude symptomatology and mood states during a climb to 3630 meters. *Aviat Space Environ Med.* 1990;61(3):225–228.

32. Sampson JB, Kobrick JL. The Environmental Symptoms Questionnaire: Revisions and new field data. *Aviat Space Environ Med.* 1980;51(9):872–877.

33. Sampson JB, Cymerman A, Burse RL, Maher JT, Rock PB. Procedures for the measurement of acute mountain sickness. *Aviat Space Environ Med.* 1983;54(12):1063–1073.

34. Shukitt BL, Banderet LE, Sampson JB. The Environmental Symptoms Questionnaire: Corrected computational procedures for the alertness factor. *Aviat Space Environ Med.* 1990;61(1):77–78.

35. Sampson JB, Kobrick, JL, Johnson RF. Measurement of subjective reactions to extreme environments: The Environment Symptoms Questionnaire. *Mil Psych.* 1994;6(4):215.

36. Hertzman M, Seitz CP, Orlansky J. Stability of personality under anoxia. *J Gen Psychol.* 1955;52:65–73.

37. Olive JE, Waterhouse N. Birmingham Medical Research Expeditionary Society 1977 Expedition: Psychological aspects of acute mountain sickness. *Postgrad Med J.* 1979;55:464–466.

38. Nelson M. Psychological testing at high altitudes. *Aviat Space Environ Med.* 1982;53(2):122–126.

39. Petiet CA, Townes BD, Brooks RJ, Kramer JH. Neurobehavioral and psychosocial functioning of women exposed to high altitude in mountaineering. *Percept Mot Skills.* 1988;67(2):443–452.

40. Ryn Z. Psychopathology in mountaineering: Mental disturbances under high-altitude stress. *Int J Sports Med.* 1988;9:163–169.

41. Bahrke MS, Shukitt-Hale B. Effects of altitude on mood, behavior, and cognitive functioning: A review. *Sports Med.* 1993;16(2):97–125.

42. Banderet LE, Burse RL. Effects of high terrestrial altitude on military performance. In: Gal R, Mangelsdorff D, eds. *Handbook of Military Psychology.* Vol 1. New York, NY: Wiley; 1991: 233–254.

43. Banderet LE, Shukitt B, Crohn EA, Burse RL, Roberts DE, Cymerman A. Effects of various environmental stressors on cognitive performance. *Proceedings of the 28th Annual Meeting of the Military Testing Association.* Mystic, Conn: US Coast Guard Academy; 1986: 592–597. DTIC No. AD 188762.

44. Shukitt-Hale B, Banderet LE, Lieberman HR. Relationships between symptoms, moods, performance, and acute mountain sickness at 4,700 meters. *Aviat Space Environ Med.* 1991;62:865–869.

45. Shukitt-Hale B, Lieberman HR. The effect of altitude on cognitive performance and mood states. In: Marriott B, Carlson SJ, eds. *Nutritional Needs in Cold and in High-Altitude Environments.* Washington, DC: National Academy Press; 1996: 435–451.

46. Berry DTR, Webb WB, Block AJ, Bauer RM, Switzer DA. Nocturnal hypoxia and neuropsychological variables. *J Clin Exp Neuropsychol.* 1986;8(3):229–238.

47. Defayolle M. Deterioration of mental performances. *Med Sport Sci.* 1985;19:122–131.

48. Kramer AF, Coyne JT, Strayer DL. Cognitive function at high altitude. *Hum Factors.* 1993;35(2):329–344.

49. Cahoon RL. Monitoring army radio-communications networks at high altitude. *Percept Mot Skills.* 1973;37:471.

50. McFarland RA. Sensory and motor responses during acclimatization. *Comp Psychol.* 1937;23(1):227–258.

51. Russell RW. The effects of mild anoxia on simple psychomotor and mental skills. *J Exp Psychol.* 1948;38:178–187.

52. Shephard RJ. Physiological changes and psychomotor performance during acute hypoxia. *J Appl Physiol.* 1956;9:343–351.

53. Phillips LW, Griswold RL, Pace N. Cognitive changes at high altitude. *Psychol Rep.* 1963;13:423–430.

54. Evans WO, Witt NF. The interaction of high altitude and psychotropic drug action. *Psychopharmacologia.* 1966;10:184–188.

55. Gill MB, Poulton EC, Carpenter A, Woodhead MM, Gregory MHP. Falling efficiency at sorting cards during acclimatization at 19,000 feet. *Nature.* 1964;203:436.

56. Ledwith F. The effects of hypoxia on choice reaction time and movement time. *Ergonomics.* 1970;13(4):465–482.

57. Mackintosh JH, Thomas DJ, Olive JE, Chesner IM, Knight RJE. The effect of altitude on tests of reaction time and alertness. *Aviat Space Environ Med.* 1988;59:246–248.

58. Cahoon RL. Vigilance performance under hypoxia. *J Appl Psychol.* 1970;54:479–483.

59. Evans WO. Performance on a skilled task after physical work or in a high altitude environment. *Percept Mot Skills.* 1966;22:371–380.

60. Tharion WJ, Hoyt RW, Marlowe BE, Cymerman A. Effects of high altitude and exercise on marksmanship. *Aviat Space Environ Med.* 1992;63:114–117.

61. Kennedy RS, Dunlap WP, Banderet LE, Smith MG, Houston CS. Cognitive performance deficits in a simulated climb of Mount Everest: Operation Everest II. *Aviat Space Environ Med.* 1989;60(2):99–104.

62. Nelson TO, Dunlosky J, White DM, Steinberg J, Townes BD, Anderson D. Cognition and metacognition at extreme altitudes on Mount Everest. *J Exp Psychol Gen.* 1990;119(4):367–374.

63. Forster PJG. Effect of different ascent profiles on performance at 4200 m elevation. *Aviat Space Environ Med.* 1985;56(8):758–764.

64. Koller EA, Bischoff M, Buhrer A, Felder L, Schopen M. Respiratory, circulatory, and neuropsychological responses to acute hypoxia in acclimatized and non-acclimatized subjects. *Eur J Appl Physiol*. 1991;62:67–72.

65. Oelz O, Regard M, Wichmann W, et al. Cognitive impairment, neurological performance, and MRI after repeat exposure to extreme altitude. In: Sutton JR, Coates G, Remmers JE, eds. *Hypoxia: The Adaptations*. Toronto, Ontario, Canada: BC Decker Inc; 1990: 206–209.

66. Houston CS. The lowdown on altitude. *Backpacker*. 1995:22–25.

67. Schlaepfer TE, Bartsch P, Fisch HU. Paradoxical effects of mild hypoxia and moderate altitude on human visual perception. *Clin Sci (Colch)*. 1992;83(5):633–636.

68. Fowler B, White PL, Wright GR, Ackles KN. The effects of hypoxia on serial response time. *Ergonomics*. 1982;25(3):189–201.

69. Gibson GE, Pulsinelli W, Blass JP, Duffy T. Brain dysfunction in mild to moderate hypoxia. *Am J Med*. 1981;70:1247–1254.

70. Kobrick JL, Zwick H, Witt CE, Devine JA. Effects of extended hypoxia on night vision. *Aviat Space Environ Med*. 1984;55(3):191–195.

71. Davis HQ, Kamimori GH, Kulesh DA, et al. Visual performance with the aviator night vision imaging system (ANVIS) at a simulated altitude of 4300 meters. *Aviat Space Environ Med*. 1995;66:430–434.

72. Heath D, Williams DR, Harris P. *Man at High Altitude: The Pathophysiology of Acclimatization and Adaptation*. London, England: Churchill Livingstone; 1981.

73. Carlile S, Bascom DA, Paterson DJ. The effect of acute hypoxia on the latency of the human auditory brainstem evoked response. *Acta Otolaryngol (Stockh)*. 1992;112:939–945.

74. Carlile S, Paterson DJ. The effects of chronic hypoxia on human auditory system sensitivity. *Aviat Space Environ Med*. 1992;63:1093–1097.

75. Fowler B, Prlic H. A comparison of visual and auditory reaction time and P300 latency thresholds to acute hypoxia. *Aviat Space Environ Med*. 1995;66:645–650.

76. Burkett PR, Perrin WF. Hypoxia and auditory thresholds. *Aviat Space Environ Med*. 1976;47(6):649–651.

77. Shukitt-Hale B, Kadar T, Marlowe BE, et al. Morphological alterations in the hippocampus following hypobaric hypoxia. *Hum Exp Toxicol*. 1996;15:312–319.

78. Rose MS, Houston CS, Fulco CS, Coates G, Sutton JR, Cymerman A. Operation Everest II: Nutrition and body composition. *J App Physiol*. 1988;65:2545–2551.

79. Lieberman P, Protopapas A, Reed E, Youngs JW, Kanki BG. Cognitive defects at altitude [letter]. *Nature*. 1994;372(6504):325.

80. Lieberman P, Protopapas A, Kanki BG. Speech production and cognitive deficits on Mt Everest. *Aviat Space Environ Med*. 1995;66(9):857–864.

81. Anholm JD, Powles AC, Downey R III, et al. Operation Everest II: Arterial oxygen saturation and sleep at extreme simulated altitude. *Am Rev Respir Dis*. 1992;145(4 pt 1):817–826.

82. Sutton JR, Houston CS, Mansell AL, et al. Effect of acetazolamide on hypoxemia during sleep at high altitude. *N Engl J Med*. 1979;301(24):1329–1331.

83. Sutton JR. Sleep disturbances at high altitude. *Physician Sportsmed*. 1982;10(6):79–84.

84. White DP, Gleeson K, Pickett CK, Rannels A, Cymerman A, Weil J. Altitude acclimatization: Influence on periodic breathing and chemo-responsiveness during sleep. *J Appl Physiol*. 1987;63(1):401–412.

85. Houston CS, Sutton JR, Cymerman A, Reeves J. Operation Everest II: Man at extreme altitude. *J App Physiol*. 1987;63(2):877–882.

86. Reite M, Jackson D, Cahoon RL, Weil JV. Sleep physiology at high altitude. *Electroenceph Clin Neurophysiol*. 1975;38;463–471.

87. Finnegan TP, Abraham P, Docherty TB. Ambulatory monitoring of the electroencephalogram in high altitude mountaineers. *Electroenceph Clin Neurophysiol*. 1985;60(3):220–224.

88. Powles ACP, Anholm JD, Houston CS, Sutton JR. Sleep and breathing at simulated extreme altitude. In: Sutton JR, Coates G, Houston CS, eds. *Hypoxia: The Tolerable Limits*. Indianapolis, Ind: Benchmark Press; 1988: 161–168.

89. Hackett PH, Roach RC. High-altitude medicine. In: Auerbach PS, ed. *Wilderness Medicine*. St Louis, Mo: Mosby; 1995: 1-37.

90. Harper RM. Obstructive sleep apnea. In: Sutton J, Houston C, Jones N, eds. *Hypoxia, Exercise, and Altitude*. New York, NY: Alan Liss; 1983: 97–105.

91. Hornbein TF, Townes BD, Schoene RB, Sutton JR, Houston CS. The cost to the central nervous system of climbing to extremely high altitude. *N Engl J Med*. 1989;321(25):1714–1719.

92. Potolicchio SJ, Hu EH, Kay GG. Effects of hypoxia on neuropsychological tests in patients with obstructive sleep apnea. *Neurology*. 1988;38(suppl 1):247.

93. Bonnet MH. Effects of sleep disruption on sleep, performance, and mood. *Sleep*. 1985;8(1):11–19.

94. Brierley JB. Cerebral hypoxia. In: Blackwood W, Corsellis JAN, eds. *Greenfield's Neuropathology*. London, England: Edward Arnold; 1976: 43–85.

95. Cavaletti G, Moroni R, Garavaglia P, Tredici G. Brain damage after high-altitude climbs without oxygen. *Lancet*. 1987;1(8524):101.

96. Mitani A, Kadoya F, Kataoka K. Distribution of hypoxia-induced calcium accumulation in gerbil hippocampal slice. *Neurosci Lett*. 1990;120:42–45.

97. Gibson GE, Freeman GB, Mykytyn V. Selective damage in striatum and hippocampus with in vitro anoxia. *Neurochem Res*. 1988;13:329–335.

98. Jensen MS, Lambert JDC, Johansen FF. Electrophysiological recordings from rat hippocampus slices following in vivo brain ischemia. *Brain Res Bull*. 1991;554:166–175.

99. Marcoux FW, Probert AW, Weber ML. Hypoxic neuronal injury in tissue culture is associated with delayed calcium accumulation. *Stroke*. 1990;21(suppl 3):3-71–3-74.

100. Kirino T. Delayed neuronal death in the gerbil hippocampus following ischemia. *Brain Res*. 1982;239:57–69.

101. Katoh A, Ishibashi C, Shiomi T, Takahara Y, Eigyo M. Ischemia-induced irreversible deficit of memory function in gerbils. *Brain Res*. 1992;577:57–63.

102. Ando S, Kametani H, Osada H, Iwamoto M, Kimura N. Delayed memory dysfunction by transient hypoxia, and its prevention with forskolin. *Brain Res*. 1987;405:371–374.

103. Regard M, Oelz O, Brugger P, Biol D, Landis T. Persistent cognitive impairments in climbers after repeated exposure to extreme altitude. *Neurology*. 1989;39:210–213.

104. Gibson GE, Duffy TE. Impaired synthesis of acetylcholine by mild hypoxic hypoxia or nitrous oxide. *J Neurochem.* 1981;36:28–33.

105. Voll CL, Whishaw IQ, Auer RN. Postischemic insulin reduces spatial learning deficit following transient forebrain ischemia in rats. *Stroke.* 1989;20:646–651.

106. Wiard RP, Carroll MS, Beek O, Cooper BR. Assessment of the effects of various durations of cerebral ischemia followed by reperfusion on performance in the Morris water maze in gerbils. *Soc Neurosci Abstr.* 1992;18:1581.

107. Peterson C, Gibson GE. 3,4-Diaminopyridine alters acetylcholine metabolism and behavior during hypoxia. *J Pharmacol Exp Therapeut.* 1982;222:576–582.

108. Freeman GB, Gibson GE. Dopamine, acetylcholine, and glutamate interactions in aging: Behavioral and neurochemical correlates. *Ann N Y Acad Sci.* 1988;515:191–202.

109. Freeman GB, Nielsen P, Gibson GE. Monoamine neurotransmitter metabolism and locomotor activity during chemical hypoxia. *J Neurochem.* 1986;46:733–738.

110. Gibson GE, Peterson C, Sansone J. Decreases in amino acid and acetylcholine metabolism during hypoxia. *J Neurochem.* 1981;37:192–201.

111. Shukitt-Hale B, Stillman MJ, Levy A, Devine JA, Lieberman HR. Nimodipine prevents the in vivo decrease in hippocampal extracellular acetylcholine produced by hypobaric hypoxia. *Brain Res Bull.* 1993;621:291–295.

112. Fowler B, Kelso B, Landolt JP, Porlier G. The effects of hypoxia on P300 and reaction time. *AGARD Conference Proceedings.* Loughton, Essex, UK: Specialized Printing Services Ltd; 1988: 16-1–16-6. No. 432.

113. Fowler B, Taylor M, Porlier G. The effects of hypoxia on reaction time and movement time components of a perceptual–motor task. *Ergonomics.* 1987;30(10):1475–1485.

114. Kida M, Imai D. Cognitive performance and event-related brain potentials under simulated high altitudes. *J Appl Physiol.* 1993;74(4):1735–1741.

115. US Department of the Army. *US Army Medical Problems of Man at High Terrestrial Elevations.* Washington, DC: DA; 1975. Technical Bulletin Medical 288.

116. Fraser WD, Eastman DE, Paul MA, Porlier JA. Decrement in postural control during mild hypobaric hypoxia. *Aviat Space Environ Med.* 1987;58:768–772.

117. Hamilton AJ. Untitled [letter]. *Aviat Space Environ Med.* 1988;59(10):996.

118. Beatty JK. Breathing lessons. *Air and Space.* 1986;Oct–Nov:12–13.

119. Green RG, Morgan DR. The effects of mild hypoxia on a logical reasoning task. *Aviat Space Environ Med.* 1985;56:1004–1008.

120. Vaernes RJ, Owe JO, Myking O. Central nervous reactions to a 6.5 hour altitude exposure at 3048 meters. *Aviat Space Environ Med.* 1984;55:921–926.

121. Tune GS. Psychological effects of hypoxia: Review of certain literature from 1950–1963. *Percept Mot Skills.* 1964;19:551–562.

122. Denison DM, Ledwith LF, Poulton EC. Complex reaction times at simulated cabin altitudes of 5000 feet and 8000 feet. *Aviat Space Environ Med.* 1966;37:1010–1013.

123. McCarthy D, Corban R, Legg S, Faris J. Effects of mild hypoxia on perceptual–motor performance: A signal-detection approach. *Ergonomics.* 1995;38(10):1979–1992.

124. Tichauer ER. Operation of machine tools at high altitudes. *Ergonomics*. 1963;6(1):51–73.

125. Fowler B, Paul M, Porlier G, Elcombe DD, Taylor M. A re-evaluation of the minimum altitude at which hypoxic performance decrements can be detected. *Ergonomics*. 1985;28(5):781–791.

126. Fowler B, Elcombe DD, Kelso B, Porlier G. The threshold for hypoxia effects on perceptual–motor performance. *Hum Factors*. 1987;29:61–66.

127. Carson RP, Evans WO, Shields JL, Hannon JP. Symptomatology, pathophysiology, and treatment of acute mountain sickness. *Fed Proc*. 1969;28(3):1085–1091.

128. Hackett PH. *Mountain Sickness: Prevention, Recognition and Treatment*. New York, NY: American Alpine Club; 1980.

129. Banderet LE, Lieberman HR. Treatment with tyrosine, a neurotransmitter precursor, reduces environmental stress in humans. *Brain Res Bull*. 1989;22(4):759–762.

130. Banderet LE, Shukitt B, Crohn EA, Burse RL, Roberts DE, Cymerman A. Characteristics of cognitive performance in stressful environments. *Proceedings of the 28th Annual Meeting of the Military Testing Association*. Mystic, Conn: US Coast Guard Academy; 1986: 425–430.

131. Cahoon RL. Simple decision making at high altitude. *Ergonomics*. 1972;15(2):157–164.

132. Arregui A, Cabrera J, Leon-Velarde F, Paredes S, Viscarra D, Arbaiza D. High prevalence of migraine in a high altitude population. *Neurology*. 1991;41:1668–1670

133. Kassirer MR, Von Pelejo Such R. Persistent high-altitude headache and ageusia without anosmia. *Arch Neurol*. 1989;46:340–341.

134. West JB. Do climbs to extreme altitude cause brain damage? *Lancet*. 1986;2(8503):387–388.

135. Ewing R, McCarthy D, Gronwall D, Wrightson P. Persisting effects of minor head injury observable during hypoxic stress. *J Clin Neuropsychol*. 1980;2(2):147–155.

136. Rennie D. See Nuptse and die [editorial]. *Lancet*. 1976;2(7996):1177–1179.

137. Sutton JR, Coates G, Remmers JE, eds. Discussion: The brain at altitude. In: *Hypoxia: The Adaptations*. Toronto, Ontario, Canada: BC Decker; 1990: 215–217.

138. Clark CF, Heaton RK, Wiens AN. Neuropsychological functioning after prolonged high-altitude exposure in mountaineering. *Aviat Space Environ Med*. 1983;54(3):202–207.

139. Jason GW, Pajurkova EM, Lee RG. High-altitude mountaineering and brain function: Neuropsychological testing of members of a Mount Everest expedition. *Aviat Space Environ Med*. 1989;60:170–173.

140. Townes BD, Hornbein TF, Schoene RB. *Human Cerebral Function at High Altitude: Final Report*. Seattle, Wash: University of Washington; 1985. DTIC No. AD A165 851. (DTIC authors: Hornbein TF, Townes BD, Schoene RB.)

141. Cavaletti G, Tredici G. Long-lasting neuropsychological changes after a single high altitude climb. *Acta Neurol Scand*. 1993;87(2):103–105.

142. Cavaletti G, Garavaglia P, Arrigoni G, Tredici G. Persistent memory impairment after high altitude climbing. *Int J Sports Med*. 1990;11(3):176–178.

143. Hornbein TF. Long term effects of high altitude on brain function. *Int J Sports Med*. 1992;13(suppl 1):S43–S45.

144. Garrido E, Castello A, Ventura JL, Capdevila A, Rodriguez FA. Cortical atrophy and other brain magnetic resonance imaging (MRI) changes after extremely high-altitude climbs without oxygen. *Int J Sports Med.* 1993;14(4):232–234.

145. Woodward DP, Nelson PA. *A User Oriented Review of the Literature on the Effects of Sleep Loss, Work–Rest Schedules, and Recovery on Performance.* Arlington, Va: Office of Naval Research; 1974. Technical Report ONR-ACR-206.

146. Leifflen D, Poquin D, Savourey G, Raphel C, Bittel J. High altitude and cognitive performance: Effects of acute hypobaric hypoxia on mental imagery processes. *Travaux Scientifiques des Chercheurs du Service de Sante des Armees.* 1994;15:269–270.

147. Kelman GR, Crow TJ. Impairment of mental performance at a simulated altitude of 8,000 feet. *Aerosp Med.* 1969;40(9):981–982.

148. Crow TJ, Kelman GR. Psychological effects of mild hypoxia. *J Physiol.* 1969;204:24P–25P.

149. Mountain RD. High-altitude medical problems. *Clin Orthop.* 1987;216:50–54.

150. Hultgren HN. High-altitude medical problems. *West J Med.* 1979;131:8–23.

151. Smith MH, Sharkey BJ. Altitude training: Who benefits? *Physician Sportsmed.* 1984;12(4):48–62.

152. Greene R. Mental performance in chronic anoxia. *Br Med J.* 1957;1(5026):1028–1031.

153. Herr RD. High altitude and the central nervous system. *N Engl J Med.* 1990;322(25):1821–1822.

154. Bonnon M, Noel-Joraznd MC, Therme P. Psychological changes during altitude hypoxia. *Aviat Space Environ Med.* 1995;66(4):330–335.

155. Fine BJ, Kobrick JL. Effects of altitude and heat on complex cognitive tasks. *Hum Factors.* 1978;20(1):115–122.

156. Hale S, Myerson J, Wagstaff D. General slowing of nonverbal information processing: Evidence for a power law. *J Gerontol.* 1987;42(2):131–136.

157. Fowler B, Ackles KN, Porlier G. Effects of inert gas narcosis on behavior: A critical review. *Undersea Biomedical Research.* 1985;12(4):369–402.

158. Crowley JS, Wesensten N, Kamimori G, Devine J, Iwanyk E, Balkin T. Effect of high terrestrial altitude and supplemental oxygen on human performance and mood. *Aviat Space Environ Med.* 1992;63(8):696–701.

159. Regard M, Landis T, Casey J, et al. Cognitive changes at high altitude in healthy climbers and in climbers developing acute mountain sickness. *Aviat Space Environ Med.* 1991;62(4):291–295.

160. Missoum G, Rosnet E, Richalet J-P. Control of anxiety and acute mountain sickness in Himalayan mountaineers. *Int J Sports Med.* 1992;13(suppl 1):S37–S39.

161. Stokes JW, Banderet LE. Psychological aspects of chemical defense and warfare. *Mil Psych.* 1997;9(4):395-415.

162. Krueger GP, Banderet LE. Effects of chemical protective clothing on military performance: A review of the issues. *Mil Psych.* 1997;9(4):255-286.

163. Bachrach A. *The Human in Extreme Environments.* Bethesda, Md: US Naval Medical Research Institute; 1982. Technical Report 82-88. DTIC No. AD A133204.

164. Hornbein TF. Everest without oxygen. In: Sutton JR, Houston CS, Jones NL, eds. *Hypoxia, Exercise, and Altitude.* New York, NY: Alan R. Liss; 1983: 409–414.

165. Johnson RF, Branch LG, McMenemy DJ. Influence of attitude and expectation on moods and symptoms during cold weather military training. *Aviat Space Environ Med*. 1989;60:1157–1162.

166. Hancock PA. The effect of skill on performance under an environmental stressor. *Aviat Space Environ Med*. 1985;57:59–64.

167. Nesthus TE, Bomar JB Jr, Holden RD, O'Connor RB. Cognitive workload and symptoms of hypoxia. *Proceedings of the Survival and Flight Equipment Association 25th Annual Symposium*. Newhall, Calif: Survival and Flight Equipment Association; 1987: 45–47.

168. Stretch RH, Heslegrave RS, Angus RG. Cognitive impairment during sustained operations: Implications for selection and training. *Proceedings of the 29th Annual Meeting of the Military Testing Association*. Ottawa, Ontario, Canada: National Defence Headquarters; 1987: 368–373.

169. Druckman D, Kraman JA. *Enhancing Human Performance: Issues, Theories, and Techniques*. Washington, DC: National Academy Press; 1988.

170. West JB. High living: Lessons from extreme altitude. *Am Rev Respir Dis*. 1984;130:917–923.

171. Young AJ, Young PM. Human acclimatization to high terrestrial altitude. In: Pandolf KB, Sawka MN, Gonzalez RR, eds. *Human Performance Physiology and Environmental Medicine at Terrestrial Extremes*. Indianapolis, Ind: Benchmark Press (now Traverse City, Mich: Cooper Publishing Group); 1988: 497–543.

172. Lyons TP, Muza SR, Rock PB, Cymerman A. The effect of altitude pre-acclimatization on acute mountain sickness during reexposure. *Aviat Space Environ Med*. 1995;66(10):957–962.

173. Krueger GP. Environmental medicine research to sustain health and performance during military deployment: Desert, arctic, high altitude stressors. *J Therm Biol*. 1993;18(5–6):687–690.

174. Foulke GE. Altitude-related illness. *Am J Emerg Med*. 1985;3(3):217–226.

175. Burse RL, Forte VA Jr. Acute mountain sickness at 4500 m is not altered by repeated eight-hour exposures to 3200–3500 m normobaric hypoxic equivalent. *Aviat Space Environ Med*. 1988;59(3):942–949.

176. Bohnn CR, Jean D, Robertson JA. Correspondence: Field experience with two commercially available portable pressure bags. *Journal of Wilderness Medicine*. 1991;2:151–152.

177. Caughey P. Pumped up. *Summit Magazine*. 1989;Spring:6–7.

178. Gamow RI, Geer AD, Kasic JF, Smith HM. Methods of gas-balance control to be used with a portable hyperbaric chamber in the treatment of high-altitude illness. *Journal of Wilderness Medicine*. 1990;1:165–180.

179. Sandrock M, Gamov I. Reinventing the running shoe—Among other things. *Running Times*. 1993;68–71.

180. West JB. Fire hazard in oxygen-enriched atmospheres at low barometric pressures. *Aviat Space Environ Med*. 1997;68:159.

181. Birmingham Medical Research Expeditionary Society Mountain Sickness Study Group. Acetazolamide in control of acute mountain sickness. *Lancet*. 1981;1(8213):180–183.

182. Lassen NA, Severinghaus JW. Acute mountain sickness and acetazolamide. In: Sutton JR, Houston CS, Coates G, eds. *Hypoxia and Cold*. New York, NY: Praeger; 1987: 493–504.

183. McIntosh IB, Prescott RJ. Acetazolamide in prevention of acute mountain sickness. *J Int Med Res*. 1986;14:285–287.

184. White AJ. Cognitive impairment of acute mountain sickness and acetazolamide. *Aviat Space Environ Med*. 1984;55(7):598–603.

185. Fulco CS, Cymerman A. Human performance and acute hypoxia. In: Pandolf KB, Sawka MN, Gonzalez RR, eds. *Human Performance Physiology and Environmental Medicine at Terrestrial Extremes.* Indianapolis, Ind: Benchmark Press (now Traverse City, Mich: Cooper Publishing Group); 1988: 467–496.

186. Johnson TS, Rock PB, Fulco CS, Trad LA, Spark RF, Maher JT. Prevention of acute mountain sickness by dexamethasone. *N Engl J Med.* 1984:310(11):683–686.

187. Johnson TS, Rock PB. Current concepts: Acute mountain sickness. *N Engl J Med.* 1988;319(13):841–845.

188. Rock PB, Johnson TS, Cymerman A, Burse RL, Falk LJ, Fulco CS. Effect of dexamethasone on symptoms of acute mountain sickness at Pikes Peak, Colorado (4300 m). *Aviat Space Environ Med.* 1987;58(7):668–672.

189. Jobe JB, Shukitt-Hale BS, Banderet LE, Rock PB. Effects of dexamethasone and high terrestrial altitude on cognitive performance and affect. *Aviat Space Environ Med.* 1991;62(8):727–732.

190. Ellsworth AJ, Larson EB, Strickland D. A randomized trial of dexamethasone and acetazolamide for acute mountain sickness prophylaxis. *Am J Med.* 1987;83:1024–1030.

191. Zell SC, Goodman P. Acetazolamide and dexamethasone in the prevention of acute mountain sickness. *West J Med.* 1988;148(5):541–545.

192. Lieberman HR. Tyrosine and stress: Human and animal studies. In: Marriot BM, ed. *Food Components to Enhance Performance.* Washington, DC: National Academy Press; 1994: 277–299.

193. Lieberman HR, Shukitt-Hale B. Food components and other treatments that may enhance mental performance at high altitudes and in the cold. In: Marriott B, Carlson SJ, eds. *Nutritional Needs in Cold and in High-Altitude Environments.* Washington, DC: National Academy Press; 1996: 453–465.

194. Shukitt-Hale B, Stillman MJ, Lieberman HR. Tyrosine administration prevents hypoxia-induced decrements in learning and memory. *Physiol Behav.* 1996;59(4–5):867–871.

195. Burse RL, Landowne M, Young AJ, Maher JT. Phenytoin: Ineffective against acute mountain sickness. *Aviat Space Environ Med.* 1982;53(3):221–225.

196. Wohns RNW, Colpitts M, Clement T, et al. Phenytoin and acute mountain sickness on Mount Everest. *Am J Med.* 1986;80(1):32–36.

197. Meehan RT, Cymerman A, Rock P, et al. The effect of naproxen on acute mountain sickness and vascular responses to hypoxia. *Am J Med Sci.* 1986;292(1):15–20.

198. Roach RC, Larson EB, Hornbein TF, et al. Acute mountain sickness, antacids and ventilation during rapid, active ascent of Mount Rainier. *Aviat Space Environ Med.* 1983;54(5):397–401.

199. Aerospace Medical Association. Medical guidelines for air travel. *Aviat Space Environ Med.* 1996;67(sec 2, suppl):B1–B16.

200. Bendrick GA, Nicolas DK, Krause BA, Castillo CY. Inflight oxygen saturation decrements in aeromedical evacuation patients. *Aviat Space Environ Med.* 1995;66(1):40–44.

Chapter 24

ACUTE MOUNTAIN SICKNESS AND HIGH-ALTITUDE CEREBRAL EDEMA

ROBERT ROACH, PhD[*]; JAN STEPANEK, MD[†]; AND PETER HACKETT, MD[‡]

*Scientist, New Mexico Resonance, PO Box 343, Montezuma, New Mexico 87731; Adjunct Assistant Professor, Department of Medicine, University of New Mexico School of Medicine, Albuquerque, New Mexico 87131, and Adjunct Assistant Professor, Department of Surgery, University of Colorado School of Medicine, Denver, Colorado 80220
†Senior Associate Consultant, Section of Aerospace Medicine, Department of Preventive and Occupational Medicine, Mayo Clinic, Rochester, Minnesota 55905
‡Affiliate Associate Professor of Medicine, Department of Medicine, University of Washington School of Medicine, Seattle, Washington 98195

INTRODUCTION

Acute mountain sickness (AMS) and high-altitude cerebral edema (HACE) are syndromes that probably occur along a continuum of severity from mild, benign AMS to severe, life-threatening HACE. They strike people who travel too fast beyond altitudes to which they are adjusted. AMS and HACE can destroy the effectiveness of even the fittest mountain troops on ascent to high altitude. In this chapter, we describe the clinical features of AMS and HACE, including what is known of their pathophysiology, and the best available approaches to prevention and treatment.

The scope of the chapter is limited to a critical appraisal of the scientific literature concerning AMS and HACE to provide an up-to-date perspective focused on pathophysiology. Further exhaustive information on history, incidence, treatment, and prevention are available,[1–11] and only the essence of that material is covered here. This chapter provides the information needed by military medical personnel deploying to the mountain regions of the world by (*a*) providing a thorough description of the clinical syndromes of AMS and HACE, including symptoms, signs, and diagnosis; (*b*) using the latest advances in research into the causes of AMS and HACE to thoroughly describe what is known (and hint at what is not yet known) about their pathophysiology; and (*c*) giving practical advice for the prevention and treatment of AMS and HACE based on an explanation of the underlying physiology.

The major importance of AMS to the readers of this volume is that

- AMS can sharply reduce a military unit's effectiveness in the field, especially in the first few days following insertion to high altitude, and
- if AMS worsens and HACE develops, the risk of fatality is significant and the disruption of planned activities to arrange rescue or temporizing measures can be considerable.

Fortunately, most cases of AMS and HACE can be prevented, personnel can be trained to identify the syndromes early and reliably in the field without sophisticated instruments, and if AMS and HACE are recognized early, most cases respond rapidly with complete recovery in a few hours (in the case of AMS) to days (for HACE).

Enduring descriptions in English of AMS and HACE come from observations of European travelers to the Andes Mountains in South America at or just before the turn of the 20th century. Edward Whymper[12] described the symptoms of AMS at about 3,500 m thus:

> I found myself lying on my back, incapable of making the least exertion. We...had intense headaches, and were unable to satisfy our desire for air, except by breathing with open mouths. Headache with all three of us was intense, and rendered us almost frantic or crazy. ... Of course there was no inclination to eat.[12(pp26–28)]

An early and important description of HACE comes from T. H. Ravenhill's experiences as a mining camp physician in the Andes Mountains during the early part of the 20th century.[13,14] He frequently observed AMS, called "puna" in the local dialect, and wrote a classic description of "nervous puna" as a type of AMS characterized by predominant neurological features, known today as HACE:

> The most marked case I had was a young Chileno, aged 19. He arrived at the neighboring mine in the usual way; three days later I was called to see him. He was then unable to speak, there were violent spasmodic movements of the limbs, and he resisted examination. The face was blanched, the lips almost white, the pupils slightly dilated. Temperature and respiration were normal; the pulse 140. He was unable to stand or to walk. I was told that he had been in this condition almost since his arrival, and that he had been delirious, talking all sorts of nonsense. I could find nothing organically wrong on physical examination. He was sent down the same day; three days later, ie, by the time he had just reached the coast, he had quite recovered.[13(p315)]

HACE remains rare and largely confined to altitudes over 4,000 m, although recent evidence[15] from magnetic resonance imaging (MRI) scans suggests that HACE may also occur at lower altitudes (3,000–3,500 m). In one survey of 1,925 soldiers at altitudes ranging from 3,350 to 5,000 m, only 23 men (1.2%) developed the severe neurological signs of HACE[16]; similarly, only 5 (1.8%) of 278 trekkers were diagnosed with HACE at 4,243 m.[17] (Please see Exhibit 19-1 in Chapter 19, Mountains and Military Medicine: An Overview, for definitions of climbers, trekkers, and other categories of people who visit mountains.) Increasingly, data from clinical studies support the notion that AMS is caused by cerebral edema.[15,16,18] When the degree of cerebral edema passes a critical threshold, the neurological signs are increasingly observed and diagnosis of HACE becomes clear.

MODERN MILESTONES IN UNDERSTANDING THE SYNDROMES

Paul Bert's[19] identification in late-19th-century France of hypoxia as the main environmental challenge for balloonists (and mountaineers) was the beginning of scientific investigation into the human responses to the stress of high altitude. By the late 1950s, AMS and HACE had been described clinically, and acclimatization to high altitude was understood to be a process not to be rushed. The India–China–Pakistan border conflicts during the late 1960s focused medical attention on practical problems of military troops abruptly deployed to very high altitudes without time for acclimatization. The classic study by Singh and colleagues[16] (Figure 24-1) described the Indian Army's experience in the conflict and laid the groundwork for future research into the pathogenesis of AMS and HACE.

Who is at risk for developing AMS is a question that has only recently been explored in detail with a large study population. Investigators in Colorado completed the largest epidemiological survey to date on 3,158 travelers visiting resorts in the Rocky Mountains of Colorado.[20] Of those, 790 (about 25%) developed AMS, and most decreased their daily activity because of their symptoms. Tourists whose permanent residence was below 3,000 m had a risk for AMS that was 3.5-fold greater than those who permanently resided above 3,000 m. Women, obese persons, and those with underlying lung disease also had a slightly higher occurrence of AMS.[20] The next step in this type of research is to couple large-scale epidemiological surveys with noninvasive physiological measurements at sea level and at altitude to better describe physiological characteristics that predispose to high-altitude illness.

Singh and colleagues[16] mentioned results of several autopsies from HACE victims, but it was several more years before detailed postmortem reports and case histories of HACE were published.[20–25] Only recently have significant advances been made in the understanding of HACE. Numerous groups have attempted to use noninvasive scanning technologies (MRI and computed tomography [CT] scans) to investigate cerebral edema in mountaineers, and to follow their recoveries.[15,18,26] The recent MRI work of Hackett and colleagues[15] shows that

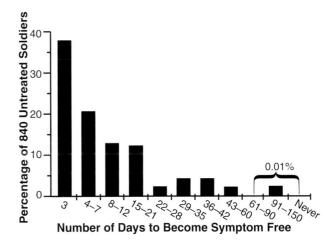

Fig. 24-1. The natural course of acute mountain sickness in 840 soldiers who received no treatment for their symptoms at altitudes ranging from 3,350 to 5,000 m. Note that about one third were free of symptoms after only 3 days, whereas the next third took as long as 12 days to be symptom free. Data source: Singh I, Khanna PK, Srivastava MC, Lal M, Roy SB, Subramanyam CS. Acute mountain sickness. *N Engl J Med.* 1969;280:177.

the edema is characterized by reversible white-matter edema, which has important implications for understanding the underlying pathophysiology.

Most major problems of prevention and treatment of AMS were solved within 2 decades after Singh's seminal paper[16] had been published (ie, by 1990). Acetazolamide was identified as effective prophylaxis[17,27,28] and treatment for AMS[29] and is now considered the drug of choice for prevention of AMS.[30,31] The study of Singh and colleagues[16] also suggested that the steroid betamethasone was an effective treatment of severe AMS. Researchers have confirmed and extended these original observations with dexamethasone. Dexamethasone effectively treats severe AMS and HACE,[27,32,33] and in persons intolerant of acetazolamide, it can also be used for prophylaxis of AMS.[34] Its exact mechanism is unclear. The next advances in AMS and HACE research will likely incorporate sophisticated imaging studies, pharmacological interventions, and perhaps biochemical and molecular markers of the onset or the resolution of brain edema.

DESCRIPTION

AMS is a syndrome that occurs in susceptible individuals when ascent to high altitude outpaces the ability to acclimatize. The symptoms, although often incapacitating, are usually self-limited. The incidence and severity of AMS depend on the rate of ascent and the altitude attained, the length of time at altitude, the degree of physical exertion, and the individual's physiological susceptibility.[35] The chief significance of AMS for the military is that large numbers of troops rapidly deployed to high altitude may be completely incapacitated in the first few days at a new altitude. Additionally, in a few individuals, AMS may progress to life-threatening HACE or to high-altitude pulmonary edema (HAPE), which is the subject of Chapter 25, High-Altitude Pulmonary Edema.

Symptoms and Signs

Headache is the cardinal symptom of AMS and is usually accompanied by insomnia, unusual fatigue (beyond that expected from the day's activities), dizziness, anorexia, and nausea (Table 24-1).[36] As Ravenhill[13] noted in 1913 and King and Robinson[37] confirmed in 1972, the headache is often frontal (bitemporal) and worsens during the night and with exertion. Insomnia is the next most frequent complaint (70% in Nepal trekkers at 4,243 m). The physi-

ology of sleep at high altitude has been extensively investigated,[38–41] with general support for the view that, independent of AMS, disturbed sleep is prevalent.[42] Poor sleep can occur secondary to periodic breathing, severe headache, dizziness, and shortness of breath, among other causes. Anorexia,[43,44] nausea, and dizziness complete the list of most common symptoms.[16,17,20] Anorexia and nausea are common (~ 35%), with vomiting reported less frequently (14%) in trekkers to 4,243 m.[17]

Surprising to many sea-level residents on their first encounter with AMS is the debilitating lassitude that strikes—so severe in some cases that victims are unable to look after the most basic daily tasks.[35] Afflicted persons commonly complain of a deep inner chill, unlike mere exposure to cold temperature.[5,13] Other symptoms may include irritability and marked dyspnea on exertion.[16,17,20] The incidence and severity of AMS can be measured with a variety of tools; two (the Environmental Symptoms Questionnaire and the Lake Louise AMS symptom score) are described in detail later in this chapter.

Decreased urinary output,[45–47] independent of fluid intake,[47–49] is commonly observed. In 67% of 1,925 soldiers ill with AMS, Singh and colleagues[16] noted bradycardia (average pulse rate of 66 beats per min). Localized rales are common.[50] Fever is absent unless HAPE is present.[16]

The following case history (from our [RR, PH] clinical experience in 1988) illustrates a typical clinical presentation and setting for AMS with particular reference to armed forces personnel rapidly transported to high altitudes:

TABLE 24-1

FREQUENCY OF SYMPTOMS OF ACUTE MOUNTAIN SICKNESS IN MOUNTAIN TREKKERS AND TOURISTS

Frequency of Symptom	Trekker*,1 (%)	Tourists†,2 (%)
Headache	96	62
Insomnia	70	31
Anorexia	38	11
Nausea	35	—
Dizziness	27	21
Dyspnea on exertion	25	21
Reduced urinary output	20	—
Marked lassitude	13	—
Vomiting	14	3
Incoordination	11	—

*Data from 146 mountain trekkers ill with acute mountain sickness (AMS) at 4,243 m in the Himalayas at Pheriche, Nepal
†Data from 3,158 tourists (total tourists, not only those with AMS) studied at 1,900–3,000 m in the Rocky Mountains of the western United States.
—: Question not asked
Data sources: (1) Hackett PH, Rennie ID, Levine HD. The incidence, importance, and prophylaxis of acute mountain sickness. *Lancet.* 1976;2:1149–1154. (2) Honigman B, Theis MK, McLain J, et al. Acute mountain sickness in a general tourist population at moderate altitudes. *Ann Intern Med.* 1993;118:587–592.

Case History 1. C. A., a 26-year-old Special Forces unit commander, was airlifted in 1 hour with 12 other soldiers from S. L. to 4,200 m. They immediately erected camp, consisting of mountaineering tents surrounded by hand-cut ice blocks. The labor was strenuous and time consuming. After 6 hours of heavy labor, C. A. developed a throbbing bilateral frontal headache and nausea. He had maintained fluid intake but was oliguric. His headache was so severe that he ceased work and rested. His symptoms worsened until he developed an intense, migrainelike headache, where any movement was painful. Over a few hours he became disoriented and confused, and severe nausea and occasional vomiting were also noted. At this point he transferred command of his unit to the fittest senior soldier in his unit.

Diagnostic physical findings in AMS only become apparent when the syndrome progresses to HACE. Prior to such progression, AMS is distinguished only by symptoms, absent any objective signs. The progression of AMS to HACE is marked by development of truncal ataxia; severe lassitude; and altered mental status, including impaired mental capacity, drowsiness, and stupor.[5,21,24] Coma may develop as soon as 24 hours after the onset of ataxia or change in mental status.

The following case report describes the typical development of HACE in the field setting:

Case History 2. H. E. was a 26-year-old German lumberjack with extensive mountaineering experience. He ascended to 5,200 m from 2,000 m in 4 days, and attempted the summit (6,194 m) on the fifth day. At 5,800 m he turned around owing to severe fatigue, headache, and malaise. He returned alone to 5,200 m, stumbling on the way because of loss of coordination. He had no appetite and crawled into his sleeping bag too weak, tired, and disoriented to undress. He recalled no pulmonary symptoms. In the morning, H. E. was unarousable, slightly cyanotic, and noted to have Cheyne–Stokes respirations. After 10 minutes on high-flow oxygen, H. E. began to regain consciousness although he was completely disoriented and unable to move. A rescue team lowered him down a steep slope, and on arrival at 4,400 m 4 hours later, H. E. was conscious but still disoriented, able to move his extremities but unable to stand. Respiratory rate was 60 breaths per minute and heart rate was 112 beats per minute. Papilledema and a few rales were present. The oxygen saturation of arterial blood (Sao_2) was 54% on room air (normal is 85% to 90%). On a non-rebreather oxygen mask with 14 L/min oxygen, the Sao_2 increased to 88% and his respiratory rate decreased to 40. Eight mg of dexamethasone was administered intramuscularly at 1620 hours, and continued orally, 4 mg every 6 hours. At 1720 hours, H. E. began to respond to commands. The next morning H. E. was still ataxic, although able to stand, take fluids, and eat heartily. He was evacuated by air to Anchorage, Alaska (sea level), at 1200 hours, where he recovered fully within several days.[5]

This climber was fortunate to become ill on a high mountain where a sophisticated medical research laboratory was on site. Without the medical care provided by the researchers there, HACE and HAPE would have almost certainly been fatal. The rationale for his treatment and strategies for preventing the syndromes are discussed later in the chapter.

Incidence, Severity, and Natural Course

The incidence of AMS in visitors to the western United States, with a sleeping altitude of 2,000 to 3,000 m, is 18% to 40%,[20] and in climbers of Mount Rainier, with a sleeping altitude of 3,000 m and a summit of 4,300 m, the incidence was 67% (Figure 24-2).[27] The subgroup of patients developing HACE is much smaller and ranges from 0.01% in visitors to western states with a sleeping altitude of 2,000 m[20,51] to 1.2%

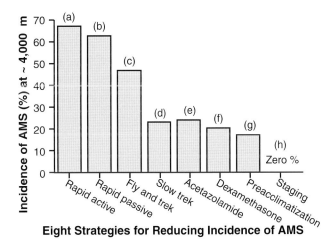

Fig. 24-2. The incidence of acute mountain sickness (AMS) is reduced with slower ascents. For clarity, only one or two studies are referenced in a particular category (a–h), although all done within each category support the trend illustrated here. (**a**) Climbers ascending Mount Rainier from sea level in less than 48 hours.[1] (**b**) Rapid, passive ascent from sea level by subjects in the field[2,3] or from chamber studies.[4,5] (**c**) Trekkers who flew to 2,800 m, then, over 1 to 2 days, hiked to 4,243 m.[6] (**d**) From the same study[6] as (c), but in this case the trekkers hiked for 10 to 13 days to reach 4,243 m. (**e**) Acetazolamide[1] and (**f**) dexamethasone[2,4] each reduced AMS incidence to about 20% to 25%. After acclimatizing to 4,300 m, (**g**) six men went to sea level for 8 days before being reexposed to altitude in a hypobaric chamber when their incidence of AMS was only 17%,[7] in the same range as for dexamethasone or acetazolamide. Only long and slow staging (**h**) at intermediate altitudes results in no symptoms of AMS at approximately 4,000 m. The volunteers in this study spent 1 week at 1,584 m, then 1 week at 3,500 m, before finally going up to 4,300 m.[3]

Data sources: (1) Larson EB, Roach RC, Schoene RB, Hornbein TF. Acute mountain sickness and acetazolamide: Clinical efficacy and effect on ventilation. *JAMA.* 1982;288:328–332. (2) Hackett PH, Roach RC, Wood RA, et al. Dexamethasone for prevention and treatment of acute mountain sickness. *Aviat Space Environ Med.* 1988;59:950–954. (3) Hansen JE, Harris CW, Evans WO. Influence of elevation of origin, rate of ascent and a physical conditioning program on symptoms of AMS. *Mil Med.* 1967;132:585–592. (4) Johnson TS, Rock PB, Fulco CS, Trad LA, Spark RF, Maher JT. Prevention of acute mountain sickness by dexamethasone. *N Engl J Med.* 1984;310:683–686. (5) Roach RC, Loeppky JA, Icenogle MV. Acute mountain sickness: Increased severity during simulated altitude compared with normobaric hypoxia. *J Appl Physiol.* 1996;81(5):1908–1910. (6) Hackett PH, Rennie ID, Levine HD. The incidence, importance, and prophylaxis of acute mountain sickness. *Lancet.* 1976;2:1149–1154. (7) Lyons TP, Muza SR, Rock PB, Cymerman A. The effect of altitude pre-acclimatization on acute mountain sickness during reexposure. *Aviat Space Environ Med.* 1995;66:957–962.

in the Indian armed forces, where the sleeping altitude is up to 5,500 m,[52,53] to 1.8% in trekkers at 4,300 m on their way to Mount Everest base camp.[17] Controlled studies have not yet determined whether men and women differ in their susceptibility to AMS. Limited epidemiological studies suggest that women have the same or slightly greater incidence of AMS but may be less susceptible to HAPE. Honigman and colleagues[20] studied 3,158 adults visiting moderate altitude (1,900–3,000 m). Of 1,255 women included in that study, 28% developed AMS, compared with 24% of the men ($P < 0.01$). In another survey conducted at a higher altitude (4,243 m), Hackett and colleagues[17] studied 278 unacclimatized trekkers in Nepal and noted no gender differences in AMS susceptibility.

Prior physical condition has little influence on incidence.[54] Older adults consistently report less AMS than younger people with similar altitude exposure. Whether this difference results from behavioral adjustments or has a basis in physiological differences is not known. It is important to note that older age, by itself, does not preclude travel to moderate high altitude. In one study of 97 elderly (average age = 69.8 y) visitors to 2,500 m, only 16% reported AMS,[55] compared with 20% to 25% persons aged about 44 years at a similar altitude.[20]

The natural course of AMS varies with the initial altitude, rate of ascent, clinical severity, and individual susceptibility. Of 840 soldiers not treated with any drugs for their AMS symptoms at 3,300 to 5,500 m, only 40% were symptom-free after 3 days[16] (see Figure 24-1). After 3 weeks, 80% were symptom-free. The remaining 20% coped with symptoms for up to 6 months; indeed, 9 soldiers were never free of AMS symptoms during the 6-month study. At lower altitudes more frequently visited by tourists, 99% of symptoms resolved within the first 36 hours at altitude, and most individuals resumed normal activities shortly thereafter.[20] Previous experience is the best predictor of an individual's response to altitude and of the natural course of AMS.

Predisposing and Contributing Factors

An understanding of predisposing and contributing factors to the development of AMS and HACE is important to aid preventive action and early recognition. Because HACE is on a continuum with AMS,[5] risk factors for the development of AMS may be viewed as risk factors for the development of HACE in susceptible individuals. The lack of proper acclimatization (ie, too rapid ascent), or any factors that impede acclimatization, clearly increases the risk of AMS and HACE.[21] In their series of 1,925

soldiers exposed to high altitude, Singh and colleagues[16] reported that the exposure to cold environmental conditions and physical exertion seemed to aggravate the condition of individuals already having symptoms of AMS or precipitate the condition in persons who initially were well.

Ross[56] hypothesized that the person who will tolerate hypoxic brain-swelling least well is the one with small intracranial and intraspinal capacity and thus limited compliance. He based his deductions on pressure volume index measurements carried out by Shapiro and colleagues,[57] which indicate that in a person under the age of 30, the intracranial space not occupied by the brain is less than 1% and that this value increases up to 5.9% by 70 to 80 years of age. More research is necessary to fit this interesting work to the known minimal effect of age (up to 60 y) on susceptibility to AMS.

Lack of acclimatization can certainly predispose climbers, hikers, and others to AMS. Mentioned earlier (see Case History 2) was the effect on Sao_2 during exercise, as affected by the degree of acclimatization: the better the acclimatization, the higher the Sao_2 during exercise. For example, among 104 climbers studied at 4,200 m before attempting to climb to the summit of Mount McKinley (6,200 m),[58] those whose Sao_2 fell the furthest during exercise were the most likely to develop AMS during their climb.

In another attempt to predict subsequent AMS, Savourey and colleagues[59] completed a number of tests at sea level in both normoxia and hypoxia. On a subsequent high-altitude trek, the AMS score did not relate to body size, pulmonary function, hypoxic or hypercapnic ventilatory responses, or the cold pressor test. The end-tidal partial pressure of oxygen ($Peto_2$) during submaximal exercise at sea level was highly correlated ($r = 0.92$, $P < 0.001$) with the subsequent AMS score. Reeves and colleagues[60] had earlier reported that Sao_2 at altitude was best predicted by the sea-level resting end-tidal partial pressure of carbon dioxide ($Petco_2$), such that the lower the sea-level $Petco_2$, the higher was the Sao_2 on ascent to altitude. Further investigations into breathing pattern, hypoxia, oxygen and carbon dioxide chemosensitivity, and AMS are necessary to clarify these relationships.

Scoring Systems

Awareness of the scoring systems is of practical importance to the military medical officer to allow identification and rapid quantification of the severity of AMS and HACE. In the context of mountaineering, the rule of thumb is that a severe headache with nausea, vomiting, dizziness, or undue fatigue is probably AMS. The lack of objective criteria to identify AMS has put an emphasis on techniques to score AMS symptoms. Questionnaires have been developed based on survey or clinical approaches and yield similar results. The Environmental Symptoms Questionnaire (ESQ) contains 67 questions and was developed to survey large groups of US armed forces personnel exposed to a variety of harsh environments.[61–63] Twenty-one of the 67 questions are necessary to derive the two subscores used for AMS research: the AMS-Respiratory and the AMS-Cerebral scores (Exhibit 24-1). These 21 questions com-

---

EXHIBIT 24-1

THE ENVIRONMENTAL SYMPTOMS QUESTIONNAIRE ITEMS AND THE DERIVATIVE AMS-CEREBRAL AND AMS-RESPIRATORY SCORES

The 21 Environmental Symptoms Questionnaire (ESQ) items necessary to derive the Acute Mountain Sickness-Cerebral (AMS-C) and -Respiratory (AMS-R) scores are listed below, followed by the equations for using the questionnaire. Subjects are instructed to complete the questionnaire regarding how they feel *at that moment* and to score each item from 0 to 5. ESQ score weight: zero = none at all; 1 = slight; 2 = somewhat; 3 = moderate; 4 = quite a bit; 5 = extreme or severe.

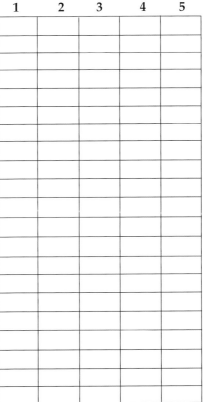

ESQ Items	Word Association Score
	1 2 3 4 5
I feel lightheaded	
I have a headache	
I feel dizzy	
I feel faint	
My vision is dim	
My coordination is off	
I am short of breath	
It is hard to breathe	
It hurts to breathe	
I have stomach cramps	
I feel weak	
My back aches	
My stomach aches	
I feel sick to my stomach	
My nose feels stuffed up	
I've been having nose bleeds	
I've lost my appetite	
I feel sick	
I feel hungover	
I couldn't sleep	
I feel depressed	

AMS-C score equation: (lightheaded • 0.489 + headache • 0.312 + dizzy • 0.446 + faint • 0.346 + vision • 0.501 + coordination off • 0.519 + feel weak • 0.387 + sick to stomach • 0.347 + lost appetite • 0.413 + feel sick • 0.692 + feel hungover • 0.584) / 25.95

AMS-R score equation: (headache • 0.312 + short of breath • 0.745 + hard to breathe • 0.763 + hurts to breathe • 0.734 + stomach cramps • 0.516 + back aches • 0.686 + stomach aches • 0.744 + sick to stomach • 0.691 + nose stuffy • 0.534 + nose bleeds • 0.578 + could not sleep • 0.355 + depressed • 0.48) / 35.69

Adapted with permission from Sampson JB, Cymerman A, Burse RL, Maher JT, Rock PB. Procedures for the measurement of acute mountain sickness. *Aviat Space Environ Med.* 1983;54(12):1065.

prise a questionnaire of reasonable length and proven reliability, and a lengthy literature is available for comparison. The major shortcoming of the ESQ is that the entire system is based on the statistical agreement between artificial clusters of symptoms used for the AMS-Cerebral and AMS-Respiratory

scores and the single response of "I feel sick."

Clinicians, favoring a more direct approach, have developed a number of scoring systems that recently have evolved into an international standard, known as the Lake Louise AMS scoring system (Exhibit 24-2).[64] This system has two parts, a symptom score section

---

EXHIBIT 24-2

LAKE LOUISE ACUTE MOUNTAIN SICKNESS SCORING SYSTEM

The Lake Louise Acute Mountain Sickness (AMS) score provides a system for both self-assessment and clinical assessment of the symptoms and signs of AMS. The self-assessment score can also be administered by a healthcare provider or researcher. A person is considered to have AMS *only* if he or she has a headache score of at least mild severity and one additional symptom. The person's total points (maximum 15) are summed to become his or her AMS score.

1. Self-Assessment

    a. Headache

        0 No headache
        1 Mild headache
        2 Moderate headache
        3 Severe headache (incapacitating)

    b. Gastrointestinal symptoms

        0 No gastrointestinal symptoms
        1 Poor appetite or nausea
        2 Moderate nausea or vomiting
        3 Severe nausea or vomiting (incapacitating)

    c. Fatigue, weakness, or both

        0 Not tired or weak
        1 Mild fatigue or weakness
        2 Moderate fatigue or weakness
        3 Severe fatigue or weakness (incapacitating)

    d. Dizziness or Lightheadedness

        0 Not dizzy or lightheaded
        1 Mild dizziness or lightheadedness
        2 Moderate dizziness or lightheadedness
        3 Severe dizziness or lightheadedness (incapacitating)

    e. Difficulty Sleeping

        0 Slept as well as usual
        1 Did not sleep as well as usual
        2 Woke many times, poor night's sleep
        3 Could not sleep at all

2. Clinical Assessment

    a. Change in mental status

        0 No change in mental status
        1 Lethargy or lassitude
        2 Disoriented or confused
        3 Stupor or unconsciousness

    b. Ataxia (heel to toe walking)

        0 No ataxia
        1 Maneuvers to maintain balance
        2 Falls down
        3 Can't stand

    c. Peripheral edema

        1 No peripheral edema
        2 Peripheral edema at one location
        3 Peripheral edema at two or more locations

3. Functional Score

    Overall, if you had any symptoms, how did they affect your activity?

        0 No reduction in activity
        1 Mild reduction in activity
        2 Moderate reduction in activity
        3 Severe reduction in activity

Adapted with permission from Roach RC, Bärtsch P, Hackett PH, Oelz O, and the Lake Louise AMS Scoring Consensus committee. The Lake Louise Acute Mountain Sickness scoring system. In: Sutton JR, Houston CS, Coates G, eds. *Hypoxia and Molecular Medicine*. Burlington, Vt: Queen City Press; 1993: 273–274.

and a clinical examination section. The symptom score may be completed by clinical interview or it can be self-administered, like the ESQ can. An important feature of this scoring system is that it emphasizes the importance of headache in the definition of AMS. To have AMS in this scoring system, the respondent must have a headache of at least mild severity. The second part of the questionnaire is useful for identifying the progression of AMS to HACE because it asks about mental status, ataxia, and peripheral edema, and it includes a functional score that assesses the impact of any symptoms on normal daily activity. An added advantage of the Lake Louise AMS symptom score is that the score can be derived in a few seconds by hand (even at 4,000 m!), whereas the ESQ requires considerably more time for manual calculation.

In summary, both systems adequately quantify subjective AMS symptom responses and are appropriate for use in field or laboratory studies of AMS.

The scores could also be used by field medics for triage or in making initial management decisions (eg, should the casualty be evacuated?)

Differential Diagnosis

Symptoms suggestive of AMS in a setting of recent ascent to a new altitude are probably due to altitude sickness and should be treated as such until proven otherwise.[35] It is common to misdiagnose AMS as a viral flulike illness; and alcohol hangover, exhaustion, and dehydration are also invoked. All misdiagnoses must be eliminated by physical exam, history, or treatment. As noted previously, fever is usually absent in AMS, and alcohol or other drug use can be excluded by the history. Rest and rehydration can eliminate fatigue and dehydration in the differential diagnosis of AMS. Mental confusion and ataxia, the hallmarks of HACE, are also present with hypothermia.

PATHOPHYSIOLOGY

Despite dozens of investigations, the basic mechanisms of AMS (and HACE) remain elusive. The extremely low incidence of HACE limits research into its pathophysiology largely to conclusions drawn from the similarity in the pathophysiology of AMS and HACE. Available evidence suggests that the pathophysiology of AMS is brain swelling. This is aggravated by poor ventilatory response, fluid retention or overhydration, and cerebral vasodilation and leakage of the blood–brain barrier.

The pathophysiology of AMS and HACE includes many common features, some well-understood and others that remain obscure despite intense scientific scrutiny. Singh and colleagues[16] proposed in 1969 that the high-altitude syndromes are secondary to the body's responses to hypobaric hypoxia, not due simply to hypoxemia. They based this conclusion on two observations: (1) there is a delay between the onset of hypoxia and the onset of symptoms after ascent (from hours to days) and (2) not all symptoms are immediately reversed with oxygen. Scientists have long assumed that AMS and HACE are due solely to the hypoxia of high altitude, based largely on two reports: the pioneering experiments of Paul Bert[19] and the Glass House experiment of Barcroft.[65] Until recently, no studies have challenged the assumption that hypoxia *alone* was responsible for the symptoms of AMS. A comparison of symptom responses to simulated altitude, hypoxia alone, and hypobaric normoxia revealed more AMS with simulated altitude, compared with

either normobaric hypoxia or normoxic hypobaria[66] (Figure 24-3).

The pathophysiology of AMS that has been described

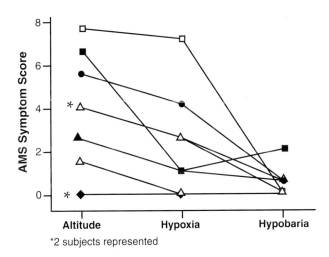

*2 subjects represented

Fig. 24-3. Acute mountain sickness (AMS) symptom scores (averages for hours 6 and 9) from nine subjects exposed to simulated altitude, normobaric hypoxia, and normoxic hypobaria. Overall, symptoms were worse during the altitude exposure, although some illness was present with normobaric hypoxia. See Exhibit 24-2 for AMS scoring. Reproduced with permission from Roach RC, Loeppky JA, Icenogle MV. Acute mountain sickness: Increased severity during simulated altitude compared with normobaric hypoxia. *J Appl Physiol.* 1996;81(5):1909.

includes relative hypoventilation,[46,67] a widened alveolar–arterial oxygen tension difference ($P_{AO_2} - P_{aO_2}$),[29,68] and decreased vital capacity and peak expiratory flow[16,27,69]; subclinical pulmonary edema may be common.[70] Fluid retention,[46,47,71–73] proteinuria,[74,75] weight gain,[46] increased cerebrospinal fluid (CSF) pressure,[16,76,77] and cerebral edema are also noted.[16,18,26] We quickly recognize pulmonary, fluid-balance, and cerebral components in the pathophysiology of AMS. What determines how AMS will progress is not presently known. The findings documented in HACE related to pathophysiology include elevated CSF pressures,[16] evidence of cerebral edema on CT scan[18] and MRI,[15] and gross cerebral edema on postmortem examination.[23–25] Well-documented cases of HACE often include pulmonary edema.

Writing in 1924, Barcroft[65] elegantly argued that the brain's response to hypoxia was central to understanding the pathophysiology of mountain sickness. He wrote:

> Taking it, therefore, as settled that mountain sickness is due to oxygen want, the question arises, "oxygen want of what?" And the answer is, "of the brain." Such evidence as is at our disposal goes to show that the brain wants but little oxygen; that little, however, it wants very badly indeed.[65(p91)]

By 1970, enough had been learned of the basic pathophysiology of AMS and HACE to allow Hansen and Evans[78] to develop an elegant hypothesis of the pathogenesis of these illnesses. Their theory is that compression of the brain, either by increased cerebral venous volume, reduced absorption of CSF, or increased brain-tissue hydration, initiates the development of the symptoms and signs of AMS and HACE. This approach is increasingly supported by studies of brain edema in the syndromes (Figure 24-4). That the pulmonary and fluid-balance abnormalities of AMS and HACE are secondary to central nervous system (CNS) responses to sustained hypoxia may help explain the varied results from the large number of studies done on these topics since about 1950. Consequently, the following discussion of the pathophysiology of AMS and HACE primarily deals with the response of the brain to sustained hypoxia. But first we shall briefly review the known factors associated with AMS and HACE.

Ventilation and Gas Exchange

Relative hypoventilation is an inappropriately low ventilation for the level of hypoxemia encountered at high altitude. Reports of low ventilatory response and increased symptoms of AMS led to intensive investigation of a link between the chemical control of ventilation and the pathogenesis of AMS.[46,79,80] By and large, the results of these investigations indicate that for most people, the ventilatory response to hypoxia has little predictive value. If the extremes of ventilatory responsiveness are contrasted, those with low ventilatory drives are more likely to suffer AMS than those with high. Ventilatory responses of eight men with known AMS susceptibility and from four men without a history of AMS—and free of AMS on this occasion—are shown in Figure 24-5. The "sick" subjects had a low hypoxic ventilatory response at sea level and breathed less and had disproportionately lower S_{aO_2} values at altitude, although the difference in oxygenation between the "sick" and "well" groups was small.[80] The protective role of the hypoxic ventilatory response may be due to increased oxygen transport and decreased arterial carbon dioxide levels, with less cerebral hypoxia and vasodilation.

Pulmonary dysfunction in AMS includes decreased vital capacity and peak expiratory flow,[27,69,70] increased $P_{AO_2} - P_{aO_2}$,[29,68] decreased transthoracic impedance,[81,82] and a high incidence of rales.[50,70] These findings are compatible with interstitial edema (ie, increased extravascular lung water). Careful measurements of ventilation–perfusion ratios ($\dot{V}/\dot{Q}$) in the lung at various altitudes (4,300–8,848 m) confirmed gross inequalities consistent with increased lung water in subjects without clinical evidence of pulmonary edema or even AMS.[83] Accumulation of interstitial fluid is most likely minor or low-grade pulmonary edema, with a mechanism perhaps similar to that of HAPE (see Chapter 25, High-Altitude Pulmonary Edema). Interstitial fluid will impair gas exchange and worsen hypoxemia.

Fluid Homeostasis and Permeability Abnormalities

As persons become ill with AMS, the handling of renal water switches from net loss or no change to net gain of water. Singh and colleagues[16] noted less of a diuresis (fluid intake minus urinary output: –1,100 to +437 mL) in 118 soldiers with known susceptibility to AMS, compared with that seen in 46 "absolutely immune" (+930 to +4,700 mL) soldiers. They also noted that clinical improvement was preceded by diuresis. Subsequent investigations[46,47,84–89] have failed to elucidate the exact mechanism of the fluid retention. It is likely to be multifactorial and capable of dynamically adjusting to oxygenation, neural input and hormonal action.

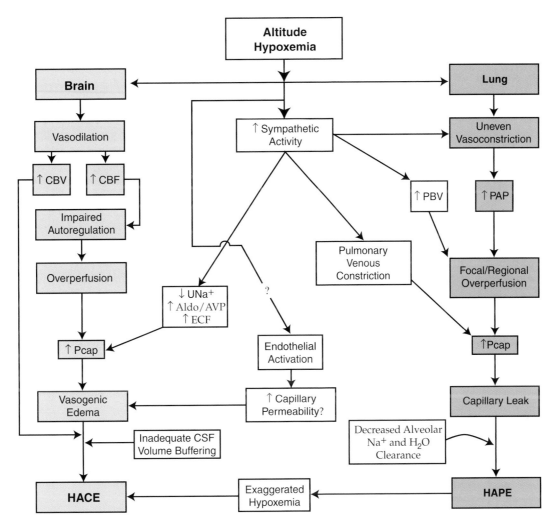

Fig. 24-4. Proposed pathophysiology of acute mountain sickness (AMS), high-altitude cerebral edema (HACE), and high-altitude pulmonary edema (HAPE). At high altitudes, hypoxemia can lead to overperfusion, elevated capillary pressure, and leakage from the cerebral and pulmonary microcirculation.[1-3] Increased sympathetic activity has a central role in this process, and increased permeability of capillaries, as a result of endothelial activation (inflammation), may also have a role. Reproduced with permission from Hackett PH, Roach RC. High-altitude illness. *N Engl J Med.* 2001;345:109.
Aldo: aldosterone; AVP: arginine vasopressin; CBF: cerebral blood flow; CBV: cerebral blood volume; CSF: cerebral spinal fluid; ECF: extracellular fluid; PAP: pulmonary artery pressure; PBV: pulmonary blood volume; Pcap: capillary pressure; UNa+: urinary sodium
(1) Hackett PH, Roach RC. High-altitude medicine. In: Auerbach PA, ed. *Wilderness Medicine.* St Louis, Mo: Mosby; 2001: 2–43. (2) Hackett PH. High altitude cerebral edema and acute mountain sickness: A pathophysiology update. In: Roach RC, Wagner PD, Hackett PH, eds. *Hypoxia: Into the Next Millennium.* New York, NY: Plenum/Kluwer Academic Publishing; 1999: 23–46. (3) Bartsch P, Roach RC. Acute mountain sickness and high-altitude cerebral edema. In: Hornbein TF, Schoene RB, eds. *High Altitude: An Exploration of Human Adaptation.* New York, NY: Marcel Dekker; 2001: 731–776.

Renal responses to hypoxia are variable and depend in part on the hypothalamic arginine vasopressin (AVP) response. Increases in urinary AVP excretion with increasing hypoxia have been demonstrated,[90-93] but caution in interpreting these results is called for because nausea, independent of AMS, stimulates AVP,[94] as does exercise.[95] Aldosterone increases or does not change in persons ill with AMS, compared

with those free of illness.[90] Plasma renin activity increases with AMS.[86] Atrial natriuretic peptide is also increased in AMS,[90] and although the rise is likely compensatory, increases in this cardiac-secreted amino acid compound may significantly worsen AMS by increasing microvascular permeability.[96,97]

An important link has been described among hypoxia, ventilation, and fluid balance. In a study of 15

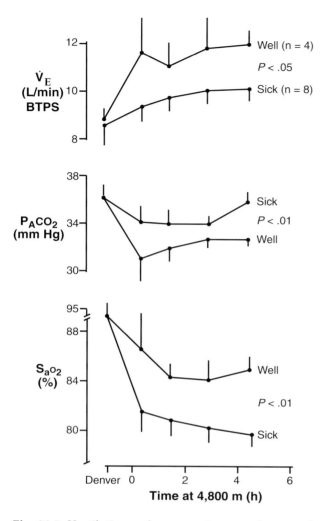

Fig. 24-5. Ventilation and oxygenation were lower and P_{ACO_2} greater in subjects who had a prior history of acute mountain sickness (AMS) (sick) , compared with subjects who were immune to AMS on previous visits (well), suggesting that the sick subjects have a low hypoxic sensitivity. Reproduced with permission from Moore LG, Harrison GL, McCullough RE, et al. Low acute hypoxic ventilatory response and hypoxic depression in acute altitude sickness. *J Appl Physiol.* 1986;60:1407–1412. $\dot{V}_E$ BTPS: expiratory ventilation at *b*ody *t*emperature, (ambient) *p*ressure, *s*aturated (with H_2O vapor); P_{ACO_2}: end-tidal CO_2 tension; Sa_{O_2}: O_2 saturation of arterial blood

volunteers breathing hypoxic gas mixtures for 6 hours, Swenson and colleagues[98] found a positive relationship between increased ventilatory sensitivity to hypoxia and hypoxic diuresis (Figure 24-6). In other words, individuals who breathed more when hypoxic also had a greater urinary output. This phenomenon had previously been well described in animals,[99] but Swenson's[98] was the first careful study in humans. It could be that the hypoxic ventilatory response varies

widely in its relationship to AMS because the ventilatory response exerts its influence on AMS through fluid balance, which is ultimately influenced by other, perhaps overriding, factors.

The hypothesis that CNS responses to hypoxia cause AMS and HACE may explain the observed fluid abnormalities via increased activation of the sympathetic nervous system. Krasney[100] postulated that cerebral edema causes brain compression and that this will lead to an increase in peripheral sympathetic nervous system activity. Increased sympathetic stimulation causes vasoconstriction of the renal circulation and subsequent renal hypoperfusion, increased aldosterone and antidiuretic hormone levels, and reduces glomerular filtration rate and urinary output.

Increased sympathetic activity is consistent with the increased norepinephrine levels in AMS victims, which has been noted in some studies.[90,101] During 8 hours of normobaric hypoxia, Kamimori and colleagues[101] noted that epinephrine was increased in all subjects with AMS, but arterial norepinephrine values did not discriminate between those with and those without AMS, suggesting that adrenal medullary responses may play an important role in the pathophysiology of AMS. In men exposed to a simulated altitude of 4,500 m, muscle sympathetic nerve

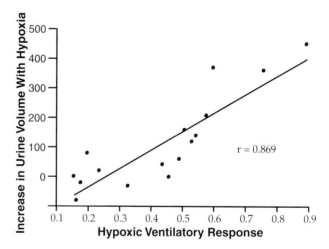

Fig. 24-6. The hypoxic ventilatory response (HVR) of 16 subjects was measured before they breathed hypoxic (F_{IO_2} = 0.12) gas for 6 hours. Here, the HVR is plotted against the subsequent increase in urinary volume that occurs with hypoxia. Those with a strong HVR had the greatest hypoxic diuresis. Reproduced with permission from Swenson ER, Duncan TB, Goldberg SV, Ramirez G, Ahmad S, Schoene RB. Diuretic effect of acute hypoxia in humans: Relationship to hypoxic ventilatory responsiveness and renal hormones. *J Appl Physiol.* 1995;78:380.

activity increased 2-fold after 1 hour at simulated altitude and remained elevated after 24 hours.[102] Too few subjects experienced AMS in this study to draw conclusions about a relationship between elevated sympathetic tone and AMS; the important point is that direct measurements of sympathetic activity indicate a high degree of activation by hypoxia that is maintained during at least the first 24 hours of altitude exposure. Whether differences in the intensity of this response may be related to who gets sick and who remains free of AMS remains to be determined. Additionally, α-adrenergic blockade has been shown to be effective for the treatment of HAPE,[103] acting presumably by decreasing sympathetically mediated pulmonary hypertension (see Chapter 25, High-Altitude Pulmonary Edema).

Additional support for a role of sympathetic activation in the pathogenesis of AMS comes from the work by Fulco and colleagues,[104] showing that subjects with β-adrenergic blockade had less AMS than subjects taking placebo. More complete adrenergic blockade may result in even greater decrease in AMS responses if the hypothesis is correct that sympathetic activation plays a central role in the pathogenesis of AMS. Taken together, the evidence points to the possibility that the sympathetic nervous system has a role in the early development of AMS and HACE.

A generalized permeability defect has been hypothesized as an early defect common to the edemas of altitude.[105] With the discovery of many vasoactive mediators of endothelial permeability, several studies briefly explored this important area. Urinary leukotriene E_4 levels were measured in 8 healthy men at sea level and after 36 hours at 4,300 m.[106] Leukotriene E_4 levels were nearly doubled at altitude, and the concentration was related to the severity of AMS symptoms. In another study in 10 subjects exposed to 4,350 m for 8 days, leukotriene B_4 levels mirrored the increase in AMS symptom score from sea level to high altitude, and decreased as symptoms resolved over time at altitude.[107] Further studies are needed to establish cause and effect for these modulators of endothelial permeability in the pathogenesis of AMS and HACE.

The Brain

Factors that determine the brain's responses to sustained hypoxia include changes in cerebral blood flow (CBF) and metabolism, CSF pressure, and cerebrovascular hemodynamics. Each response is now considered and examined for how they comprise the brain's responses to sustained hypoxia.

Cerebral Blood Flow and Metabolism

For a better understanding of the concepts that will be discussed in this and the following section, it is useful to recall a few physiological principles regarding CBF. The three variables on which CBF depends are systemic blood pressure, vascular resistance, and intracranial pressure; their relationship can adequately be described by Equation 1:

$$(1) \qquad CBF = \frac{CPP}{CVR} = \frac{BP - IP}{CVR}$$

where *CBF* represents cerebral blood flow; *CPP*, cerebral perfusion pressure; *BP*, systemic blood pressure; *IP*, intracranial pressure; and *CVR*, cerebrovascular resistance.

Various factors influence regulation of the cerebral vasculature, acting especially on the arterioles. Chemoregulation, autoregulation, and possibly neuromodulation[108–111] are distinguished by sympathetic nerves that innervate the cerebral vessels as principal mechanisms that affect CBF. Cerebral vessels vasodilate with a decrease in extracellular pH, increase in P_{CO_2}, and marked decrease of P_{O_2} (< 50 mm Hg). Cerebral vasoconstriction is seen as a reaction to decreases in P_{CO_2} and increases in extracellular pH. Autoregulation is the term given to the ability of the cerebral vasculature to maintain a constant CBF despite fluctuations of cerebral perfusion pressure (CPP) within certain limits. This means that a drop in CPP will produce a vasodilatory response, and an increase in CPP, a vasoconstriction. The capability for autoregulation fails if CPP is less than 60 mm Hg or is greater than 160 mm Hg. It is not known if these cerebrovascular autoregulatory mechanisms remain intact during periods of prolonged hypoxia or if they are reset to a higher level of CBF in an attempt to adapt to the persistent hypoxic stimulus.[100] Data gathered by Curran-Everett, Meredith, and Krasney[112] in an experimental sheep model for HACE showed powerful cerebrovascular vasodilation during hypoxia and hypercapnia. After ventilatory acclimatization, the same stimuli induced paradoxical cerebral vasoconstriction. Krasney[100] hypothesized that this response may be due to increased activation, by the arterial chemoreceptors, of sympathetic vasoconstrictor nerves innervating the cerebral vasculature and concluded that this physiological mechanism may protect the blood–brain barrier from cerebral autoregulatory breakthrough.

In a person ascending to high altitude, two physiological alterations occur:

1. the reduced partial pressure of inspired oxygen (P_{IO_2}) leads to progressive hypoxia, and
2. the ventilatory acclimatization induces hyperventilation with subsequent hypocapnia.

The former (reduced P_{IO_2}) leads to a decrease in CVR; the latter usually induces cerebrovascular constriction, but its effects are offset by the hypoxic stimulus. The net effect is an increase in CBF; this fact has been documented in animal models[113–115] and in human subjects[116–118] exposed to high altitude. The magnitude of the increase of CBF reaches up to 40%.[116–118] The increased CBF correlates nicely with increased middle cerebral artery flow-velocities measured with transcranial doppler.[76,119,120] Interestingly, in a study performed by Jensen and colleagues[121] in 12 subjects, the increase in CBF (up to +24% at an altitude of 3,475 m, measured by the radioactive xenon technique) did not correlate with symptoms of AMS. In a study by Baumgartner and colleagues[120] (Figure 24-7), CBF was measured by transcranial doppler and found to be higher in subjects with AMS than in healthy climbers, with a direct correlation between CBF and symptom severity. A follow-up study[122] did not support these early results, however, and a similar study by Otis and colleagues[119] also did not find such a correlation.

The key question in this context is, To what, if any, extent, is increased CBF responsible for symptoms of AMS? Judging from available evidence it appears doubtful that increased CBF is a primary factor. The rise in CBF is virtually instantaneous, as opposed to the symptoms of AMS and HACE, which arise only after several hours to days. Another important issue in this context is whether the cerebrovascular bed is homogeneous in its reactivity and susceptibility to hypoxia-induced changes. Hackett and colleagues[15] found in 1998 that edema appears to form preferentially in the corpus callosum (especially in its splenium) of subjects with HACE, as seen on examination with MRI scans. In part, this particular distribution could be explained by the fact that the posterior cerebral arteries receive less adrenergic innervation[108–111] than the other CNS arteries, rendering them more susceptible for breakthrough of autoregulation. Experimental work in conscious, hypoxic rats showed a greater increase in CBF in the brainstem and posterior circulation than in the cerebral cortex.[123] Studies by Cutler and Barlow[124] in guinea pigs subjected to severe hypercapnia (25% CO_2) showed that transcapillary fluid leakage in the CNS was nonuniform, with distinct predilection to leakage in the thalamus, hypothalamus, mesencephalon, and medulla. The CBF re-

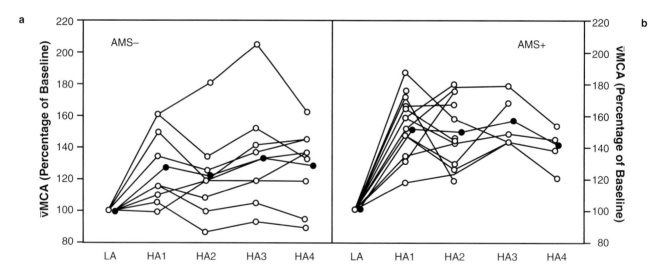

Fig. 24-7. In 24 healthy men (open circles) exposed to 4,559 m altitude for 4 days (HA1–HA4), mean blood flow velocity of the middle cerebral arteries ($\overline{v}$MCA) was significantly higher in (**b**) the 14 men with AMS (AMS+) after day 1, compared with (**a**) the 9 men who remained free of AMS (AMS–). $\overline{v}$MCA remained higher on day 2, but by day 3, symptoms of AMS and $\overline{v}$MCA were similar in the two groups. Closed circles represent mean values ± 95% confidence intervals. Difference of mean values between AMS+ and AMS– subjects were statistically significant ($P < .025$) on HA1 and HA2. Reproduced with permission from Baumgartner RW, Bärtsch P, Maggiorini M, Waber U, Oelz O. Enhanced cerebral blood flow in acute mountain sickness. *Aviat Space Environ Med.* 1994;65:726–729.
LA: low altitude (490 m); HA: high altitude (4,559 m)

mained constant or even decreased in these areas, as opposed to in the cerebral hemispheres, which experienced the most significant increase in CBF without any edema formation. Certainly, many questions remain open in this regard.

Early hypotheses of the pathogenesis of HACE postulated that hypoxia may cause a dysfunction in cellular Na^+/K^+ adenosine triphosphatase (ATPase), producing an influx of sodium into cells and thus causing cytotoxic CNS edema.[125] Metabolic studies focusing on cerebral oxygen and glucose uptake revealed that these parameters are maintained even during prolonged hypoxic exposure of 5 days.[112] In fact, the CNS optimizes oxygen uptake during hypoxemia, resulting in increased oxygen extraction. Interestingly, there appears to be a relationship between oxygen extraction capacity and the propensity to develop the AMS–HACE continuum in sheep, as described by Curran-Everett and colleagues.[126] They found that animals susceptible to AMS and HACE showed a lower oxygen extraction and higher CBF during normoxic conditions, and hypothesized that this predisposed the animals to high cerebral capillary pressures during hypoxia, leading to a transcapillary fluid shift. A similar investigation needs to be done in humans.

Changes in Cerebrospinal Fluid Pressure and Cerebral and Intracranial Hemodynamics

In the following section, hemodynamic and CSF pressure changes observed during the development of AMS and HACE are discussed. To that end, it is useful to recall a few pertinent physiological concepts and classifications.

The blood–brain barrier is the physiological mechanism that prevents free transition of substances from the bloodstream into the extracellular CNS compartment. The anatomical structure responsible for the barrier function is at the tight junctions between adjacent endothelial cells, and in the CNS parenchyma astrocytic foot-processes that are closely associated with the endothelial cells and their basement membrane. The blood–brain barrier is not uniform, and in select areas of the CNS it is virtually absent. In other areas (eg, eminentia mediana hypothalami, glandula pinealis), it is diminished by the presence of fenestrated capillaries.

Classification of Central Nervous System Edema

In his classic description in 1967, Klatzo[127] divided the pathological entity of brain edema into two distinct categories:

1. *Vasogenic* edema: protein-rich fluid spreads into the extracellular space through a compromised blood–brain barrier. The preferential site for this type of edema is the white matter.
2. *Cytotoxic* edema: intracellular fluid accumulation in neurons and neuroglia occurs after a severe insult (eg, toxins, ischemia). This type of edema is preferentially located in the gray matter.

A third type of brain edema was later added to the classification to include the edema associated with derangements of CSF[125] (Figure 24-8):

3. *Interstitial* edema: block of CSF absorption results in increased cerebral fluid located in the cellular interstitium. This type of cerebral edema is preferentially located in the periventricular white matter.

Clear distinctions among these subtypes are often not possible, because a mixed picture may be seen with the progression of the causative pathology. For example, severe anoxia may compromise cellular metabolism and lead to cytotoxic edema, but the concomitant vascular damage will produce progressive vasogenic edema as well. In his original description, Klatzo[127] commented on the particular predilection of white matter in the setting of vasogenic edema and hypothesized that the regular arrangement of extracellular channels offers less resistance to the invasion of edema fluid than does the dense meshwork of the cerebral gray matter. The following overview synopsizes the events that occur:

- During the initial stages of AMS and HACE, responses related to decreased P_{IO_2} and the hypobaric environment predispose to, or act as risk factors for the development of, the ensuing pathophysiological cascade.
- Next, hypobaric hypoxia generates a compensatory increase in CBF and ventilation. The concomitant hypocapnia (caused by the increased ventilation) causes a respiratory alkalosis, which in turn acts as a slowing mechanism on the central respiratory center, preventing excessive increases in ventilation.[5] The kidneys excrete bicarbonate to compensate for the respiratory alkalosis. The cerebrum also compensates for the respiratory alkalosis by reducing the bicarbonate content of the CSF. A progressive, mild, increase in CSF pressure is seen with in-

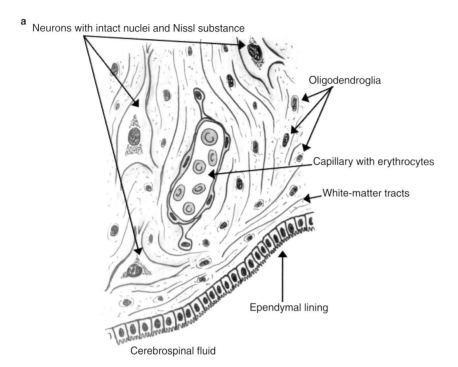

a Neurons with intact nuclei and Nissl substance

Oligodendroglia

Capillary with erythrocytes

White-matter tracts

Ependymal lining

Cerebrospinal fluid

Fig. 24-8. A schematic illustration of the distinctive features of vasogenic, cytotoxic, and interstitial edema. (**a**) Normal anatomy, labeled for reference. (**b**) Vasogenic cerebral edema (with special predilection to white matter). (**c**) Cytotoxic cerebral edema, preferentially located in the gray matter. (**d**) Interstitial cerebral edema, preferentially located in the periventricular white matter. The red arrows on views b and d indicate the direction of fluid movement; gray areas in views b, c, and d indicate edema.

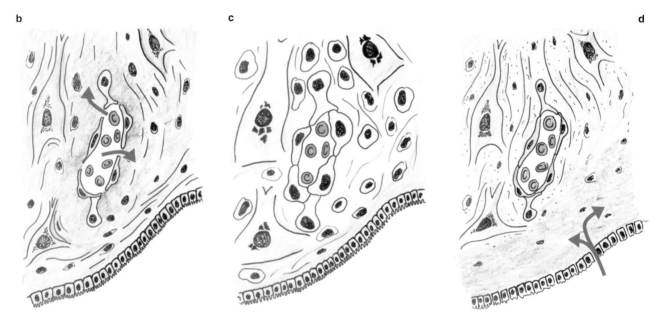

b   **c**   **d**

creasing hypoxia.[76] In the sheep model[128] for HACE, the choroid plexus blood flow clearly declines during progressive hypocapnic hypoxia, leading to a decrease in CSF production. In HACE and severe AMS, compensation for edema formation may begin with increases in CSF absorption, and CSF may finally shift caudally.

- Finally, progressive edema formation and accompanying anatomical changes occur. At this stage, CSF pressure increases mark-

edly (as does intracranial pressure) and anatomical shifts start to occur, leading to severe neurological symptoms. These changes may range from focal neurological deficits to coma and potentially to death if vital centers of the medulla oblongata are compressed during caudal herniation of brain parenchyma.

The pathogenesis of AMS and HACE has been and is still being studied intensely, and although many advances have been made in the understanding of the pathophysiology, many questions still remain open and require further study. With a focus on the blood–brain barrier and the role of the cus on the blood–brain barrier and the role of the endothelium and its mediators, as well as the role of the neuroglial component, and with the use of the available animal models, further advances should be forthcoming.

PROPHYLAXIS

The fundamentals of prevention are similar for AMS and HACE. They are based on slow ascent, time for acclimatization, a low sleeping altitude, and avoidance of any factors that increase hypoxemia, such as sedative hypnotics and alcohol.

Acclimatization and Staging

Gradual ascent with appropriate time to adjust to new altitudes above 2,500 m is the safest prophylaxis for AMS. How slow is best determined by previous experience. A general guideline is to avoid rapid ascent from sea level to a sleeping altitude above 3,000 m, and to spend 2 to 3 days at this altitude for initial acclimatization. As Heber and Bristol wrote in 1921, the "altitude of happiness" varies for each individual, noting that they felt good at 3,300 m but "a good deal less so" at 4,100 m.[129(p1148)] The concept of "sleeping altitude" is important to understanding the practical aspects of the acclimatization process. As is mentioned in Chapter 25, High-Altitude Pulmonary Edema, respiration can vary widely among individuals at high altitude, with the two extreme conditions being respiration during exercise and during sleep. By sleeping at too high an altitude too soon after arrival, severe periodic breathing during sleep can occur, causing marked arterial oxygen desaturation and poor sleep and thus hindering acclimatization. After acclimatization to approximately 3,000 m, stopping for an extra night is recommend every time the sleeping altitude increases 500 to 1,000 m. Above 3,000 m, climbing or hiking to higher altitudes during the day aids acclimatization. Abrupt increases of more than 500 to 1,000 m in sleeping altitudes should be avoided without prior daytime exposures to the higher sleeping altitudes. Spending several nights at 3,000 m and climbing to 4,000 m in the intervening days will allow the sleeping altitude to be increased to 4,000 m with few problems; in contrast, the increase to 4,000 m after several days and nights spent at only at 3,000 m would likely result in difficult acclimatization and perhaps AMS. Staged acclimatization is time consuming but very effective (see Figure 24-1). By having subjects spend 1 week at 1,584 m followed by 1 week at 3,500 m before driving them to 4,300 m, Hansen, Harris, and Evans[54] were able to completely prevent AMS in their volunteers.

Overexertion should be avoided while ascending.[130] Early in their altitude exposure, six of seven volunteers experienced significantly worse AMS when they exercised compared with when they were resting. During exercise, Sao_2 levels dropped 8%, but at rest after exercise, ventilation and fluid balance were not significantly different than the same variables measured during rest without exercise.[130]

After acclimatization, in contrast, Sao_2 is better defended during exercise than on sudden exposure to high altitude.[58,131] Diets high in carbohydrate content (> 70% of caloric intake as carbohydrate) may influence acclimatization by increasing Sao_2 levels.[132] High-carbohydrate diets decreased AMS symptoms 30%,[133] presumably by increasing the respiratory quotient ($\dot{V}co_2/\dot{V}o_2$) and thereby stimulating ventilation and increasing oxygenation.[134,135] These findings were not confirmed in subjects who breathed hypoxic gas at sea-level pressure for 12 hours.[135]

Climbers maintain that recent acclimatization is protective. Scientific support for this argument comes from Lyons and colleagues[136] who took six young, healthy men to the US Army Pikes Peak Laboratory Facility (a part of the US Army Research Institute of Environmental Medicine, Natick, Mass), located at 4,300 m, for 16 days, and measured AMS symptoms and Sao_2. On day 1, four of the six (67%) had AMS, and their average Sao_2 was 77%. After 14 days at 4,300 m, as expected, their AMS scores had decreased to near zero and their Sao_2 levels had increased about 10%. The new finding from this study came a week later when the same subjects, who had been at sea level for the intervening week, were reexposed to altitude in a hypobaric chamber. Their symptoms were much less pronounced than they had been during their initial exposure (only one subject of six was ill with AMS) and their Sao_2 levels were 83%—higher than on day 1 on Pikes Peak (77%) but somewhat lower than on day 14 (87%). This suggests that factors that protect against AMS are activated during acclimatization, and they continue to function after 1 week (or more?) at sea level.

Drugs

When rapid ascent is unavoidable, or known susceptibility to AMS and HACE exists, several drugs are helpful for prevention of the conditions (Exhibit 24-3; also see Figure 24-1). Acetazolamide is the drug of choice for prophylaxis of AMS.[6,30] As a carbonic anhydrase inhibitor, acetazolamide reduces reabsorption of bicarbonate and sodium in the kidney, thus causing a bicarbonate diuresis and a metabolic acidosis. These effects start within 1 hour after oral ingestion and rapidly enhance ventilatory and renal acclimatization to high altitude. Arterial oxygenation is improved. Acetazolamide's diuretic action counteracts the fluid retention characteristic of AMS, and perhaps more importantly, decreases CSF production and volume and possibly CSF pressure.[93]

Indications for acetazolamide prophylaxis include rapid ascent (≤ 1 d) to altitudes higher than 3,000 m, a rapid gain in sleeping altitude, a history of recurrent AMS, and troublesome periodic breathing. Doses of 125 to 250 mg twice daily, starting 24 hours prior to ascent, are as effective as higher doses

started earlier.[5,6,30] A 500-mg sustained-action capsule of acetazolamide given once every 24 hours is probably equally effective.[5,137] Once acclimatization is established, acetazolamide can be safely discontinued or reserved solely for prevention of persistent periodic breathing during sleep.[6,138] Spironolactone and other diuretics have shown equivocal results for AMS prevention.[139–141]

Another drug, dexamethasone, has also proven effective for AMS prophylaxis. In eight healthy, young men rapidly exposed to 4,570 m in a hypobaric chamber, 4 mg every 6 hours decreased AMS symptoms 75%, compared with placebo treatment.[34] A field study on Pikes Peak (4,300 m) reported a 21% reduction in AMS symptoms.[142] Various dexamethasone dose regimens have been tested, from 4 mg every 6 hours to 0.25 mg every 12 hours. Based on the findings of Rock and colleagues,[143] the lowest effective dose for AMS prophylaxis is 4 mg given every 12 hours, which reduced symptoms by 52%. In one study, combined acetazolamide and dexamethasone proved superior to the use of either agent alone.[144] Unlike acetazolamide, however, dexamethasone does not aid acclimatization. Once dexamethasone is discontinued, rebound of AMS is likely.[32,143] Dexamethasone, therefore, should

---

EXHIBIT 24-3

FIELD TREATMENT OF ACUTE MOUNTAIN SICKNESS AND HIGH-ALTITUDE CEREBRAL EDEMA

Mild Acute Mountain Sickness
  Stop ascent; rest and acclimatize at the same altitude
  Administer acetazolamide, 125 to 250 mg twice daily, to speed acclimatization
  Treat symptoms as necessary with analgesics and antiemetics
  Or, descend 500 m or more

Moderate Acute Mountain Sickness
  Administer low-flow oxygen, if available
  Administer acetazolamide, 125 to 250 mg twice daily, with or without dexamethasone, 4 mg every 6
    hours, by mouth, intramuscularly, or intravenously
  Administer hyperbaric therapy
  Or, immediately descend 500 m or more

High-Altitude Cerebral Edema
  Descend immediately until symptoms resolve
  Administer oxygen, 2 to 4 L/min
  Administer dexamethasone, 4 mg every 6 hours, by mouth, intramuscularly, or intravenously
  Hyperbaric therapy (simulated descent)
  Consider administering furosemide 80 mg orally every 12 hours for a total of 2 doses

Sources: (1) Hackett PH, Roach RC. High-altitude medicine. In: Auerbach PA, ed. *Wilderness Medicine.* St Louis, Mo: Mosby; 2001: 2–43. (2) Hackett PH, Roach RC. High-altitude illness. *N Engl J Med.* 2001;345:107–114.

be reserved for *treatment* of AMS and HACE, rather than *prevention*, except when necessary in persons intolerant of acetazolamide.

Two studies have found that a herbal remedy made from the plant *Ginkgo biloba* (a) prevented AMS during a gradual ascent to 5,000 m[145] and (b) reduced both the symptoms and the incidence of AMS by 50% during an abrupt ascent to 4,100 m.[146] Extracts from the plant *G biloba* are potent antioxidants, and it may be this property that is responsible for the herbal remedy's effectiveness in AMS.[147]

With respect to high-altitude headache, prophylactic aspirin (325 mg every 4 hours for a total of three doses) reduced the incidence from 50% to 7%.[148]

TREATMENT

Treatment of mild AMS can include additional time to acclimatize at the present altitude, symptomatic therapy for headache and nausea, or both. Symptoms often resolve in 1 to 2 days (see Figure 24-2). Moderate-to-severe AMS and HACE should be treated with immediate descent when possible. In a patient with mild AMS, any deterioration of neurological status or signs of pulmonary edema demand immediate descent. In the following descriptions of simulated descent, oxygen therapy and pharmacological approaches to the treatment of AMS and HACE are expected, in moderate-to-severe illness, to serve only as temporizing measures until real descent can be accomplished. Treatment options are summarized in Exhibit 24-3.

Descent, Both Real and Simulated

"When in doubt, DESCEND," is the mantra of altitude medicine. Mountaineering physicians have noted that descent of as little as 500 m yields striking clinical improvement in AMS and HACE victims. Descent is not always practical, however, and with the advent of pressure chambers in the late 1970s and early 1980s, simulated descent is now an option widely available to expeditions and trekking groups. The first portable chamber for treating altitude illness was assembled and tested at the Himalayan Rescue Association clinic in Pheriche, Nepal, in 1975 (Figure 24-9). Results from 15 patients with AMS, HACE, and HAPE confirmed previous clinical observations that descent was a safe, effective means of reversing altitude illness. Subsequent controlled studies verified and extended these findings.[149–151]

In summary, hyperbaria is as effective as oxygen breathing for the treatment of AMS and HACE. Real descent is the safest form of treatment for all the high-altitude illnesses because neither equipment failure (eg, pumps, chambers) nor supply limitation (eg, of oxygen) can interfere with recovery once descent is accomplished.

Oxygen and Pharmacological Treatment

Oxygen does not immediately relieve all the symptoms of AMS and HACE, although it provides

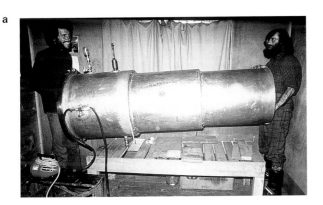
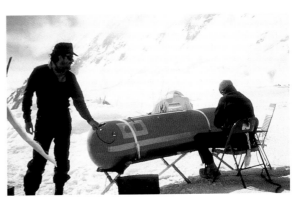

Fig. 24-9. Increasing pressure by descent or by putting a patient in a hyperbaric chamber effectively treats acute mountain sickness (AMS) and high-altitude cerebral edema (HACE). Hyperbaric pressurization, descent, and oxygen therapy are of equivalent effectiveness for treating AMS and HACE. (**a**) This pressure chamber was first used in Pheriche, Nepal, in 1975 for recompression of patients ill with AMS or HACE. (**b**) A fabric hyperbaric chamber has the advantage over portable oxygen cylinders of being lightweight, being easy to transport, and offering simulated descent for as long as the operator can pressurize the chamber by manual pump.

significant symptomatic relief in mild-to-moderate cases. Oxygen can be a life-saving temporizing measure in cases of severe AMS and HACE.

In mild AMS, acetazolamide (125–250 mg, administered orally twice daily) will speed acclimatization and alleviate illness. Headache can be treated with analgesics[6] such as aspirin (650 mg), acetaminophen (650–1,000 mg),[148,152] or ibuprofen (≥ 200 mg).[153] Nausea and vomiting respond well to prochlorperazine (5–10 mg, administered intramuscularly). Alcohol and sedative hypnotics should be avoided because of their depressive effect on respiration, especially during sleep. In moderate AMS, acetazolamide (250 mg, given three times daily) was effective in relieving symptoms and improving pulmonary gas exchange and $SaO_2\%$.[29] Dexamethasone is effective for treatment of moderate AMS. Using a dose of either 4 mg every 6 hours[32] or an 8-mg initial dose followed by 4 mg every 6 hours,[33] symptoms were notably minimized, with no significant side effects. However, dexamethasone does not aid acclimatization, and symptom rebound has repeatedly been observed.[32,33,142] Therefore, dexamethasone could be used to relieve symptoms and acetazolamide to speed acclimatization.

Successful treatment of HACE requires early recognition. At the first sign of ataxia or change in consciousness, descent should be started, dexamethasone (initially 4–8 mg intravenously, intramuscularly, or by mouth, followed by 4 mg every 6 h) administered, and oxygen (2–4 L/min by mask or nasal cannula) applied, if available. Oxygen can be titrated to maintain SaO_2 at or higher than 90% if oximetry is available. Comatose patients require additional airway management and bladder drainage. Attempting to decrease intracranial pressure by intubation and hyperventilation is a reasonable approach, although these patients are already alkalotic and over-hyperventilation could result in cerebral ischemia. Loop diuretics such as furosemide (40–80 mg) or bumetanide (1–2 mg) may help reduce brain hydration, but an adequate intravascular volume to maintain perfusion pressure is critical. Hypertonic solutions of saline, mannitol, and urea have been suggested[7] but are used rarely in the field. Controlled studies are lacking, but empirically, the response to steroids and oxygen seems to be excellent if given early in the course of the illness and disappointing if not started until the patient is unconscious. Coma may persist for days, even after evacuation to low altitude, in which case other causes of coma must be considered and ruled out by appropriate evaluation. Sequelae lasting weeks are common; longer-term follow-up has been limited.

MILITARY OPERATIONS AT ALTITUDE

The rapid deployment of troops to high altitude (ie, > 2,500 m) may pose significant logistical, technical, environmental, tactical, and medical problems.[16,154,155] The routes for supply in difficult mountainous terrain may be restricted to air-drop and may be hampered by unfavorable weather conditions—necessitating autonomy in regard to food, clothing, and equipment. The environment may require special attention to dangers of rockfall; high ultraviolet light exposures; difficult technical ascents requiring special gear; avalanches; and severe, prolonged periods of cold weather in the winter season. The human factors that have to be taken into consideration are more likely to be crucial in this setting. The lack of experience in a new environment and insufficient physical and psychological preparedness are factors that can be overcome by careful planning and training for the specific operation. The environmental conditions (eg, low temperatures, difficult ascents) can produce a state of physical and psychological exhaustion that may affect decision making and result in faulty assessments of terrain and the feasibility of tasks at hand. The medical issues that arise during a military operation at high altitude are multiple and complex; the following discussion will focus on the potential dangers of AMS and HACE.

The symptomatology of the two syndromes is unfortunately not specific in its initial presentation and thus requires constant attention from the medical officer for early detection. Headache, lassitude, and mild ataxia are early warning signs that should be carefully watched and acted on as necessary. The observations by Singh and colleagues[16] are the most comprehensive series of published observations made in troops exposed to a high-altitude environment. Singh studied 1,925 soldiers, aged 18 to 53 years, air-lifted to the Indian Himalaya at altitudes of 3,350 to 5,500 m. A variety of neurological manifestations were observed, including headaches (the most prevalent and most persistent symptom), decreased ability to concentrate, blurred vision, and, in 24 soldiers, more-severe signs and symptoms including papilledema, stupor, coma, seizures, and focal neurological deficits. In Singh's series, three patients died from neurological complications and two had marked cerebral edema on postmortem examination.

The neurological changes seen in AMS after rapid exposure to high altitude may thus have significant impact on the physical and mental functioning of susceptible individuals. These changes in conjunction with the hardships of the environment can make troop leadership difficult. Constant attention to the physical and mental state of the troops is necessary to detect early changes that can be appropriately treated. Lack of attention to these early issues will entail secondary dangers to the military operation, such as misjudgments of tactical situations and mistakes made during the operation of vehicles, weapons, or complex instruments. The capability for rapid deployment is a hallmark of today's modern armies and confers obvious strategic advantages. However, rapid deployment itself exposes the troops to a higher risk of altitude-related illnesses in the mountainous environment. To avoid disability and death of the troops, the fol-lowing actions must be taken by the commanding officer, in collaboration with the medical officer:

1. Allow time for acclimatization through graded ascent to high altitude.
2. Educate troops about signs and symptoms of AMS and HACE to ensure early reporting (make use of the "buddy-system," in which individuals observe each other for occurrence of symptoms).
3. Evaluate the need for pharmacological prophylaxis, in view of the nature of the mission and the available time.
4. Minimize severe exertion and exposure to cold as possible precipitating factors.
5. Plan ahead for rapid evacuation (to lower altitude) for severe cases.
6. Plan for treatment of AMS to keep soldiers functional and to avoid evacuations.

SUMMARY

Altitude-related illnesses such as AMS are usually a nuisance (eg, headaches, anorexia, nausea) rather than a threat to life and are most commonly self-limited. However, they may have a significant impact on an individual's ability to function. Military commanders and medical officers can prevent or reduce altitude-related illnesses by following the six actions enumerated just above.

To avoid fatal outcomes, severe complications such as HACE in susceptible individuals may require rapid recognition and efficient treatment, such as evacuation to lower altitude, simulated descent in a hyperbaric bag, and pharmacological therapy.

If descent is not an option, then acetazolamide and dexamethasone effectively reverse AMS, and HACE is reversed with dexamethasone. Aspirin successfully treats high-altitude headache.

Pharmacological prevention can include acetazolamide, dexamethasone, and a herbal remedy made from the plant *Ginko biloba*. Recent studies support the effectiveness of *G biloba* extract in small study groups; larger trials are underway. Prevention can largely be achieved by slow, staged ascent. All travelers to high altitude should be mindful that awareness of the early symptoms of AMS and HACE can be the most effective strategy for preventing fatal outcomes.

REFERENCES

1. Sutton JR, Lassen NA. Pathophysiology of acute mountain sickness and high altitude pulmonary edema: An hypothesis. In: Brendel W, Link RA, eds. *High Altitude Physiology and Medicine.* New York, NY: Springer-Verlag; 1982: 266–267.

2. Malconian MK, Rock PB. Medical problems related to altitude. In: Pandolf KB, Sawka MN, Gonzalez RR, eds. *Human Performance Physiology and Environmental Medicine at Terrestrial Extremes.* Dubuque, Iowa: Brown & Benchmark; 1986: 545–564.

3. Johnson TS, Rock PB. Acute mountain sickness. *N Engl J Med.* 1988;319:841–845.

4. Houston CS. Mountain sickness. *Sci Am.* 1992;267:58–66.

5. Hackett PH, Roach RC. High-altitude medicine. In: Auerbach PA, ed. *Wilderness Medicine.* St Louis, Mo: Mosby; 2001: 2–43.

6. Hackett PH, Roach RC. Medical therapy of altitude illness. *Ann Emerg Med.* 1987;16:980–986.

7. Hackett PH, Roach RC. High-altitude illness. *N Engl J Med.* 2001;345:107–114.

8. Roach RC, Hackett PH. Frontiers of hypoxia research: Acute mountain sickness. *J Exp Biol.* 2001;204:3161–3170.

9. Hackett PH. High altitude cerebral edema and acute mountain sickness: A pathophysiology update. *Adv Exp Med Biol.* 1999;474:23–45.

10. Hackett PH. The cerebral etiology of high-altitude cerebral edema and acute mountain sickness. *Wilderness Environ Med.* 1999;10:97–109.

11. Bärtsch P, Roach RC. Acute mountain sickness and high-altitude cerebral edema. In: Hornbein TF, Schoene RB, eds. *High Altitude: An Exploration of Human Adaptation.* New York, NY: Marcel Dekker; 2001: 731–776.

12. Whymper E; Shipton E, ed. *Travels Amongst the Great Andes of the Equator.* London, England: Charles Knight; 1972. Republished; originally published in London, England: Murray; 1891–1892.

13. Ravenhill TH. Some experiences of mountain sickness in the Andes. *J Trop Med Hygiene.* 1913;1620:313–320.

14. West JB. T. H. Ravenhill and his contributions to mountain sickness. *J Appl Physiol.* 1996;80:715–724.

15. Hackett PH, Yarnell PR, Hill R, Reynard K, Heit J, McCormick J. High altitude cerebral edema evaluated with magnetic resonance imaging: Clinical correlation and pathophysiology. *JAMA.* 1998;280(22):1920–1925.

16. Singh I, Khanna PK, Srivastava MC, Lal M, Roy SB, Subramanyam CS. Acute mountain sickness. *N Engl J Med.* 1969;280:175–218.

17. Hackett PH, Rennie ID, Levine HD. The incidence, importance, and prophylaxis of acute mountain sickness. *Lancet.* 1976;2:1149–1154.

18. Matsuzawa Y, Kobayashi T, Fujimoto K, Shinozaki S, Yoshikawa S. Cerebral edema in acute mountain sickness. In: Ueda G, Reeves JT, Sekiguchi M, eds. *High Altitude Medicine.* Matsumoto, Japan: Shinshu University Press; 1992: 300–304.

19. Bert P. *La Pression Barométrique: Recherches de Physiologie Expérimentale.* Paris, France: G. Masson; 1878. Reprinted as *Barometric Pressure.* Bethesda, Md: Undersea Medical Society; 1978.

20. Honigman B, Theis MK, McLain J, et al. Acute mountain sickness in a general tourist population at moderate altitudes. *Ann Intern Med.* 1993;118:587–592.

21. Houston CS, Dickinson JG. Cerebral form of high altitude illness. *Lancet.* 1975;2:758–761.

22. Wilson R, Mills WJ Jr, Rogers DR, Propst MT. Death on Denali: Fatalities among climbers in Mount McKinley National Park 1903–1976: Analysis of injuries, illnesses and rescues in 1976. *West J Med.* 1976;128:471–476.

23. Wilson R. Acute high altitude illness in mountaineers and problems of rescue. *Ann Intern Med.* 1973;78:421–427.

24. Dickinson JG. High altitude cerebral edema: Cerebral acute mountain sickness. *Semin Respir Med.* 1983;5:151–158.

25. Dickinson JG, Heath J, Gosney J, Williams D. Altitude related deaths in seven trekkers in the Himalayas. *Thorax.* 1983;38:646–656.

26. Levine BD, Yoshimura K, Kobayashi T, Fukushima M, Shibamoto T, Ueda G. Dexamethasone in the treatment of acute mountain sickness. *N Engl J Med.* 1989;321:1707–1713.

27. Larson EB, Roach RC, Schoene RB, Hornbein TF. Acute mountain sickness and acetazolamide: Clinical efficacy and effect on ventilation. *JAMA.* 1982;288:328–332.

28. Forwand SA, Landowne M, Folansbee IN, Hansen JE. Effect of acetazolamide on acute mountain sickness. *N Engl J Med*. 1968;279:839–845.

29. Grissom CK, Roach RC, Sarnquist FH, Hackett PH. Acetazolamide in the treatment of acute mountain sickness: Clinical efficacy and effect on gas exchange. *Ann Intern Med*. 1992;116:461–465.

30. Editorial. Acetazolamide for acute mountain sickness. *FDA Drug Bull*. 1983;13:27.

31. Editorial. High altitude sickness. *Med Lett Drugs Ther*. 1992;34:84–86.

32. Hackett PH, Roach RC, Wood RA, et al. Dexamethasone for prevention and treatment of acute mountain sickness. *Aviat Space Environ Med*. 1988;59:950–954.

33. Ferrazzini G, Maggiorini M, Kriemler S, Bärtsch P, Oelz O. Successful treatment of acute mountain sickness with dexamethasone. *Br Med J*. 1987;294:1380–1382.

34. Johnson TS, Rock PB, Fulco CS, Trad LA, Spark RF, Maher JT. Prevention of acute mountain sickness by dexamethasone. *N Engl J Med*. 1984;310:683–686.

35. Hackett PH. *Mountain Sickness: Prevention, Recognition and Treatment*. New York, NY: American Alpine Club; 1980.

36. Sanchez del Rio M, Moskowitz MA. High altitude headache: Lessons from headaches at sea level. *Adv Exp Med Biol*. 1999;474:145–153.

37. King AB, Robinson SM. Vascular headache of acute mountain sickness. *Aerospace Med*. 1972;43:849–851.

38. Weil JC, Kryger MH, Scoggin CH. Sleep and breathing at high altitude. In: Guilleminault C, Demant WC, eds. *Sleep Apnea Syndromes*. New York, NY: AR Liss; 1978: 119–136.

39. Reite M, Jackson D, Cahoon RL, Weil JV. Sleep physiology at high altitude. *Electroencephalogr Clin Neurophysiol*. 1975;38:463–471.

40. Powles AP, Sutton JR. Sleep at altitude. *Semin Respir Med*. 1983;5:175–180.

41. Anholm JD, Powles AC, Downey R, et al. Operation Everest II: Arterial oxygen saturation and sleep at extreme simulated altitude. *Am Rev Respir Dis*. 1992;145:817–826.

42. Powles AP, Sutton JR, Gray GW, Mansell AL, McFadden M, Houston CS. Sleep hypoxemia at altitude: Its relationship to acute mountain sickness and ventilatory responsiveness to hypoxia and hypercapnia. In: Folinsbee LJ, Wagner JA, Borgia JF, Drinkwater BL, Gliner JA, Bedi JF, eds. *Environmental Stress: Individual Human Adaptations*. New York, NY: Academic Press; 1978: 317–324.

43. Westerterp-Plantenga MS, Westerterp KR, Rubbens M, Verwegen CR, Richelet JP, Gardette B. Appetite at "high altitude" (Operation Everest III [Comex-'97]): A simulated ascent of Mount Everest. *J Appl Physiol*. 1999;87:391–399.

44. Bailey DM, Davies B, Milledge JS, et al. Elevated plasma cholecystokinin at high altitude: Metabolic implications for the anorexia of acute mountain sickness. *High Alt Med Biol*. 2000;1:9–23.

45. Singh MV, Rawal SB, Tyagi AK. Body fluid status on induction, reinduction and prolonged stay at high altitude of human volunteers. *Int J Biometeorol*. 1990;34:93–97.

46. Hackett PH, Rennie ID, Hofmeister SE, Grover RF, Grover EB, Reeves JT. Fluid retention and relative hypoventilation in acute mountain sickness. *Respiration*. 1982;43:321–329.

47. Bärtsch P, Shaw S, Wiedmann P, Franciolli M, Maggiorini M, Oelz O. Aldosterone, antidiuretic hormone and atrial natriuretic peptide in acute mountain sickness. In: Sutton JR, Coates G, Houston CS, eds. *Hypoxia and Mountain Medicine*. Burlington, Vt: Queen City Press; 1992: Chap 8.

48. Aoki VS, Robinson SM. Body hydration and the incidence and severity of acute mountain sickness. *J Appl Physiol*. 1971;31:363–367.

49. Heyes MP, Sutton JR. High altitude ills: A malady of water, electrolyte, and hormonal imbalance? *Semin Respir Med*. 1983;5:207–212.

50. Hackett PH, Rennie ID. Rales, peripheral edema, retinal hemorrhage and acute mountain sickness. *Am J Med*. 1979;67:214–218.

51. Montgomery AB, Mills J, Luce JM. Incidence of acute mountain sickness at intermediate altitude. *JAMA*. 1989;261:732–734.

52. Singh I, Roy SB. High altitude pulmonary edema: Clinical, hemodynamic, and pathologic studies. In: Hegnauer A, ed. *Biomedical Problems of High Terrestrial Elevations*. Springfield, Va: Federal Science and Technical Information Service; 1962: 108–120.

53. Singh I, Kapila CC, Khanna PK, Nanda RB, Rao BD. High altitude pulmonary oedema. *Lancet*. 1965;1:229–234.

54. Hansen JE, Harris CW, Evans WO. Influence of elevation of origin, rate of ascent and a physical conditioning program on symptoms of AMS. *Mil Med*. 1967;132:585–592.

55. Roach RC, Houston CS, Honigman B, et al. How well do older persons tolerate moderate altitude? *West J Med*. 1995;162:32–36.

56. Ross RT. The random nature of cerebral mountain sickness. *Lancet*. 1985;1:990–991.

57. Shapiro K, Marmarou A, Shulman K. Characterization of clinical CSF dynamics and neural axis compliance using the pressure volume index, I: The normal pressure–volume index. *Ann Neurol*. 1980;7:508–514.

58. Roach RC, Lium D, Hackett PH. Arterial oxygen desaturation may determine subsequent acute mountain sickness [abstract]. *Med Sci Sport Exerc*. 1994;26:S22.

59. Savourey G, Moirant C, Eterradossi J, Bittel J. Acute mountain sickness relates to sea-level partial pressure of oxygen. *Eur J Appl Physiol*. 1995;70:469–476.

60. Reeves JT, Moore LG, Cymerman A, Weil JV. Sea-Level Pco_2 relates to ventilatory acclimatization at 4,300 m. *J Appl Physiol*. 1993;75:1117–1122.

61. Kobrick JL, Sampson JB. New inventory for the assessment of symptom occurrence and severity at high altitude. *Aviat Space Environ Med*. 1979;50:925–929.

62. Sampson JB, Kobrick JL. The environmental symptoms questionnaire: Revisions and new field data. *Aviat Space Environ Med*. 1980;51:872–877.

63. Sampson JB, Cymerman A, Burse RL, Maher JT, Rock PB. Procedures for the measurement of acute mountain sickness. *Aviat Space Environ Med*. 1983;54:1063–1073.

64. Roach RC, Bärtsch P, Oelz O, Hackett PH. The Lake Louise Acute Mountain Sickness scoring system. In: Sutton JR, Houston CS, Coates G, eds. *Hypoxia and Molecular Medicine*. Burlington, Vt: Queen City Press; 1993: Chap 26.

65. Barcroft J. Mountain sickness. *Nature*. 1924;2855:90–92.

66. Roach RC, Loeppky JA, Icenogle MV. Acute mountain sickness: Increased severity during simulated altitude compared with normobaric hypoxia. *J Appl Physiol*. 1996;81(5):1908–1910.

67. Matsuzawa Y, Fujimoto K, Kobayashi T, et al. Blunted hypoxic ventilatory drive in subjects susceptible to high-altitude pulmonary edema. *J Appl Physiol*. 1989;66:1152–1157.

68. Sutton JR, Bryan AC, Gray GW, et al. Pulmonary gas exchange in acute mountain sickness. *Aviat Space Environ Med*. 1976;47:1032–1037.

69. Anholm JD, Houston CS, Hyers TM. The relationship between acute mountain sickness and pulmonary ventilation at 2,835 meters (9,300 feet). *Chest*. 1979;75:33–36.

70. Cremona G, Asnaghi R, Baderna P, et al. Pulmonary extravascular fluid accumulation in recreational climbers: A prospective study. *Lancet*. 2002;359:303–309.

71. Bärtsch P, Pfluger N, Audetat M, et al. Effects of slow ascent to 4559m on fluid homeostasis. *Aviat Space Environ Med*. 1991;62:105–110.

72. Claybaugh JR, Brooks DP, Cymerman A. Hormonal control of fluid and electrolyte balance at high altitude in normal subjects. In: Sutton JR, Coates G, Houston CS, eds. *Hypoxia and Mountain Medicine*. Burlington, Vt: Queen City Press; 1992: Chap 7.

73. Singh MV, Rawal SB, Tyagi AK, Bhagat JK, Parshad R, Divekar HM. Changes in body fluid compartments on re-induction to high altitude and effects of diuretics. *Int J Biometeorol*. 1988;32:36–40.

74. Editorial. Proteinuria at high altitude. *Br Med J*. 1979;1:508–509.

75. Winterborn MH, Bradwell AR, Chesner IM, Jones GT. The origin of proteinuria at high altitude. *Postgrad Med J*. 1987;63:179–181.

76. Hartig GS, Hackett PH. Cerebral spinal fluid pressure and cerebral blood velocity in acute mountain sickness. In: Sutton JR, Coates G, Houston CS, eds. *Hypoxia and Mountain Medicine*. Burlington, Vt: Queen City Press; 1992: Chap 24.

77. Schaltenbrand G. Atmospheric pressure, circulation, respiration and cerebrospinal fluid pressure. *Acta Aerophysiol*. 1933;1:65–78.

78. Hansen JE, Evans WO. A hypothesis regarding the pathophysiology of acute mountain sickness. *Arch Environ Health*. 1970;21:666–669.

79. King AB, Robinson SM. Ventilation response to hypoxia and acute mountain sickness. *Aerospace Med*. 1972; 43:419–421.

80. Moore LG, Harrison GL, McCullough RE, et al. Low acute hypoxic ventilatory response and hypoxic depression in acute altitude sickness. *J Appl Physiol*. 1986;60:1407–1412.

81. Hoon RS, Balasubramanian V, Tiwari SC, Mathew OP, Behl A. Changes in transthoracic electrical impedance at high altitude. *Br Heart J*. 1977;39:61–66.

82. Roy SB, Balasubramanian V, Khan MR, Kaushik VS, Manchanda SC, Guha SK. Transthoracic electrical impedance in cases of high-altitude hypoxia. *Br Med J*. 1974;3:771–775.

83. Wagner PD, Sutton JR, Reeves JT, Cymerman A, Groves BM, Malconian MK. Operation Everest II: Pulmonary gas exchange during a simulated ascent of Mt Everest. *J Appl Physiol*. 1987;63:2348–2359.

84. Bartsch P, Shaw S, Francioli M, Gnadinger MP, Weidmann P. Atrial natriuretic peptide in acute mountain sickness. *J Appl Physiol*. 1988;65:1929–1937.

85. Hannon JP, Chinn KS, Shields JL. Effects of acute high altitude exposure on body fluids. *Fed Proc*. 1969;28:1178–1184.

86. Claybaugh JR, Hansen JE, Wozniak DB. Response of antidiuretic hormone to acute exposure to mild and severe hypoxia in man. *J Endocrinol*. 1978;77:157–160.

87. Claybaugh JR, Sato AK, Eichinger MR. Blood pressure, AVP, ACTH, and PRA responses to IV and IVT angiotensin II during hypoxia [abstract]. In: Sutton JR, Coates G, Houston CS, eds. *Hypoxia and Mountain Medicine.* Burlington, Vt: Queen City Press; 1993: 296.

88. Olsen NV, Kanstrup IL, Richalet JP, Hansen JM, Plazen G, Galen FX. Effects of acute hypoxia on renal and endocrine function at rest and during graded exercise in hydrated subjects. *J Appl Physiol.* 1992;73:2036–2043.

89. Westerterp KR, Robach P, Wouters L, Richalet JP. Water balance and acute mountain sickness before and after arrival at high altitude of 4,350 m. *J Appl Physiol.* 1996;80:1968–1972.

90. Bärtsch P, Maggiorini M, Schobersberger W, et al. Enhanced exercise-induced rise of aldosterone and vasopressin preceding mountain sickness. *J Appl Physiol.* 1991; 711:136–143.

91. Hackett PH, Forsling ML, Milledge JS, Rennie ID. Release of vasopressin in man at altitude. *Horm Metab Res.* 1978;10(6):571.

92. de Souich P, Saunier C, Hartemann D, et al. Effect of moderate hypoxemia on atrial natriuretic factor and arginine vasopressin in normal man. *Biochem Biophys Res Commun.* 1987;148:906–912.

93. Senay LC, Tolbert DL. Effect of arginine vasopressin, acetazolamide and angiotensin II on CSF pressure at simulated altitude. *Aviat Space Environ Med.* 1984;55:370–376.

94. Convertino VA, Brock PJ, Keil LC, Bemauer EM, Greenleaf JE. Exercise training induced hypervolemia: Role of plasma albumin, renin and vasopressin. *J Appl Physiol.* 1980;48:665–669.

95. Robertson GL. Regulation of vasopressin in health and disease. *Recent Progress in Hormone Research.* 1987;33:333–385.

96. Westendorp RG, Roos ANA, Tjiong MY, et al. Atrial natriuretic peptide improves pulmonary gas exchange in subjects exposed to hypoxia. *Am Rev Respir Dis.* 1993;148(2):304–309.

97. Lockette W, Brennaman B. Atrial natriuretic factor increases vascular permeability. *Aviat Space Environ Med.* 1990;61:1121–1124.

98. Swenson ER, Duncan TB, Goldberg SV, Ramirez G, Ahmad S, Schoene RB. Diuretic effect of acute hypoxia in humans: Relationship to hypoxic ventilatory responsiveness and renal hormones. *J Appl Physiol.* 1995;78:377–383.

99. Honig A. Peripheral arterial chemoreceptors and reflex control of sodium and water homeostasis. *Am J Physiol.* 1989;257:R1282–R1302.

100. Krasney JA. A neurogenic basis for acute altitude illness. *Med Sci Sport Exerc.* 1994;26:195–208.

101. Kamimori GH, Davis HO, Ruocco M, Balkin TJ, Lawless N, Robles H. Effects of hypoxia (12% O_2) on cerebral edema and acute mountain sickness in men and women [abstract]. *Med Sci Sport Exerc.* 1995;28:S203.

102. Roach RC, Vissing SF, Calbet JAL, Savard GK, Saltin B. Peak exercise heart rate after 24 hours at high altitude. *FASEB J.* 1996;10:A811.

103. Hackett PH, Roach RC, Hartig GS, Greene ER, Levine BD. The effect of vasodilators on pulmonary hemodynamics in high altitude pulmonary edema: A comparison. *Int J Sports Med.* 1992;13:S68–S70.

104. Fulco CS, Rock PB, Reeves JT, Trad LA, Young PM, Cymerman A. Effects of propranolol on acute mountain sickness (AMS) and well-being at 4,300 meters of altitude. *Aviat Space Environ Med.* 1989;60:679–683.

105. Hackett PH, Rennie ID, Grover RF, Reeves JT. Acute mountain sickness and the edemas of high altitude: A common pathogenesis? *Respir Physiol.* 1981;46:383–390.

106. Roach JM, Muza SR, Rock PB, Lyons TP, Cymerman A. Urinary leukotriene levels are elevated upon exposure to high altitude and correlate with symptoms of acute mountain sickness [abstract]. In: Sutton JR, Coates G, Houston CS, eds. *Hypoxia and Mountain Medicine*. Burlington, Vt: Queen City Press; 1995: 337.

107. Richalet JP, Hornych A, Rathat C, Aumont J, Larmignant P, Remy P. Plasma prostaglandins, leukotrienes and thromboxane in acute high altitude hypoxia. *Respir Physiol.* 1991;85:205–215.

108. Vatner SF, Priano LL, Rutherford JD, Manders WT. Sympathetic regulation of the cerebral circulation by the carotid chemoreceptor reflex. *Am J Physiol.* 1980;238:H594–H598.

109. Busija DW. Sympathetic nerves reduce blood flow during hypoxia in awake rabbits. *Am J Physiol.* 1984;247:H446–H451.

110. Kissen I, Weiss HR. Cervical sympathectomy and cerebral microvascular and blood flow responses to hypocapnic hypoxia. *Am J Physiol.* 1989;256:H460–H467.

111. Kissen I, Weiss HR. Effect of peripheral and central alpha adrenoceptor blockade on cerebral microvascular and blood flow responses to hypoxia. *Life Sci.* 1991;48:1351–1363.

112. Curran-Everett DC, Meredith MP, Krasney JA. Acclimatization to hypoxia alters cerebral convective and diffusive oxygen delivery. *Respir Physiol.* 1992;88:355–371.

113. Krasney J, McDonald BW, Matalon S. Regional circulatory responses to 96 hours of hypoxia in conscious sheep. *Respir Physiol.* 1984;57:73–88.

114. Krasney J, Miki K, McAndrews K, Hajduczok G, Curran-Everett DC. Peripheral circulatory responses to 96 hours of eucapnic hypoxia in conscious sheep. *Respir Physiol.* 1985;59:197–211.

115. Yang Y, Sun B, Yang Z, Wang J, Pong Y. Effects of acute hypoxia on intracranial dynamics in unanesthetized goats. *J Appl Physiol.* 1993;74:2067–2071.

116. Jensen JB, Sperling B, Severinghaus JW, Lassen NA. Augmented hypoxic cerebral vasodilation in men during 5 days at 3,810 m altitude. *J Appl Physiol.* 1996;80:1214–1218.

117. Severinghaus JW, Chiodi H, Eger EI, Brandstater B, Hornbein TF. Cerebral blood flow in man at high altitude: Role of cerebrospinal fluid pH in normalization of flow in chronic hypoxia. *Circ Res.* 1966;19:274–282.

118. Roy SB, Guleria JS, Khanna PK, et al. Immediate circulatory response to high altitude hypoxia in man. *Nature.* 1968;217:1177–1178.

119. Otis SM, Rossman ME, Schneider PA, Rush MP, Ringelstein EB. Relationship of cerebral blood flow regulation to acute mountain sickness. *J Ultrasound Med.* 1989;8:143–148.

120. Baumgartner RW, Bärtsch P, Maggiorini M, Waber U, Oelz O. Enhanced cerebral blood flow in acute mountain sickness. *Aviat Space Environ Med.* 1994;65:726–729.

121. Jensen JB, Wright AD, Lassen NA, et al. Cerebral blood flow in acute mountain sickness. *J Appl Physiol.* 1990;69:430–433.

122. Baumgartner RW, Spyridopoulos I, Bärtsch P, Maggiorini M, Oelz O. Acute mountain sickness is not related to cerebral blood flow: A decompression chamber study. *J Appl Physiol.* 1999;86:1578–1582.

123. Edelman NH, Santiago TV, Neubauer JA. Hypoxia and brain blood flow. In: West JB, Lahiri S, eds. *High Altitude and Man*. Bethesda, Md: American Physiological Society; 1984: 101–114.

124. Cutler RW, Barlow CF. The effect of hypercapnia on brain permeability to protein. *Arch Neurol.* 1966;14:54–63.

125. Fishman RA. Brain edema. *N Engl J Med.* 1975;293:706–711.

126.   Curran-Everett DC, Iwamoto J, Meredith MP, Krasney JA. Intracranial pressures and O_2 extraction in conscious sheep during 72 h of hypoxia. *Am J Physiol.* 1991;261:H103–H109.

127.   Klatzo I. Presidential address: Neuropathological aspects of brain edema. *J Neuropathol Exp Neurol.* 1967;26(1):1–14.

128.   Iwamoto J, Curran-Everett DC, Krasney E, Krasney JA. Cerebral metabolic and pressure-flow responses during sustained hypoxia in awake sheep. *J Appl Physiol.* 1991;71:1447–1453.

129.   Heber AR, Bristol CB. Some effects of altitude on the human body. *Lancet.* 1921;i:1148–1150.

130.   Roach RC, Maes D, Sandoval D, et al. Exercise exacerbates acute mountain sickness at simulated high altitude. *J Appl Physiol.* 2000;88:581–585.

131.   West JB, Lahiri S, Gill MB, Milledge JS, Pugh LG, Ward MP. Arterial oxygen saturation during exercise at high altitude. *J Appl Physiol.* 1962;17:617–621.

132.   Lawless NP, Dillard TA, Torrington KG, Davis Ha, Kamimori G. Improvement in hypoxemia at 4600 meters of simulated altitude with carbohydrate ingestion. *Aviat Space Environ Med.* 1999;70:874–878.

133.   Consolazio CF, Matoush LO, Johnson HL, Krzywicki HJ, Daws TA, Isaac GJ. Effects of a high-carbohydrate diet on performance and clinical symptomology after rapid ascent to high altitude. *Fed Proc.* 1969;28:937–943.

134.   Hansen JE, Hartley LH, Hogan RP. Arterial oxygen increased by high-carbohydrate diet at altitude. *J Appl Physiol.* 1972;33:441–445.

135.   Swenson ER, MacDonald A, Treadwell A, Allen R, Vatheuer M, Schoene RB. Effect of increased dietary carbohydrate on symptoms of acute mountain sickness and circulating cytokines [abstract]. In: Sutton JR, Coates G, Houston CS, eds. *Hypoxia and Mountain Medicine.* Burlington, Vt: Queen City Press; 1995: 341.

136.   Lyons TP, Muza SR, Rock PB, Cymerman A. The effect of altitude pre-acclimatization on acute mountain sickness during reexposure. *Aviat Space Environ Med.* 1995;66:957–962.

137.   Hackett P. Pharmacological prevention of acute mountain sickness: Many climbers and trekkers find acetazolamide 500 mg/day to be useful. *BMJ.* 2001;322:48. Discussion 49.

138.   Sutton JR, Houston CS, Marsell AL, McFadden MD, Hackett PH. Effect of acetazolamide on hypoxemia during sleep at high altitude. *N Engl J Med.* 1979;301:1329–1331.

139.   Larsen RF, Rock PB, Fulco CS, Edelman B, Young AJ, Cymerman A. Effect of spironolactone on acute mountain sickness. *Aviat Space Environ Med.* 1986;57:543–547.

140.   Singh MV, Jain SC, Rawal SB, et al. Comparative study of acetazolamide and spironolactone on body fluid compartments on induction to high altitude. *Int J Biometeorol.* 1986;30:33–41.

141.   Jain SC, Singh MV, Rawal SB. The effects of acetazolamide and spironolactone on the body water distribution of rabbits during acute exposure to simulated altitude. *Int J Biometeorol.* 1984;28:101–107.

142.   Rock PB, Johnson TS, Cymerman A, Burse RL, Falk LJ, Fulco CS. Effect of dexamethasone on symptoms of acute mountain sickness at Pikes Peak, Colorado (4,300 m). *Aviat Space Environ Med.* 1987;58(7):668–672.

143.   Rock PB, Johnson TS, Larsen RF, Fulco CS, Trad LA, Cymerman A. Dexamethasone as prophylaxis for acute mountain sickness: Effect of dose level. *Chest.* 1989;95:568–573.

144.   Zell SC, Goodman PH. Acetazolamide and dexamethasone in the prevention of acute mountain sickness. *West J Med.* 1988;148:541–545.

145.   Roncin JP, Schwartz F, D'Arbigny P. EGb 761 in control of acute mountain sickness and vascular reactivity to cold exposure. *Aviat Space Environ Med.* 1996;67:445–452.

146. Leadbetter G, Maakestad K, Olson S, Hackett PH. *Ginkgo biloba* reduces incidence and severity of acute mountain sickness. *High Altitude Medicine and Biology.* 2001;2(12):110.

147. Bailey DM, Davies B. Acute mountain sickness: Prophylactic benefits of antioxidant vitamin supplementation at high altitude. *High Alt Med Biol.* 2001;2:21–29.

148. Burtscher M, Likar R, Nachbauer W, Philadelphy M. Aspirin for prophylaxis against headache at high altitudes: Randomised, double blind, placebo controlled trial. *BMJ.* 1998;316:1057–1058.

149. Kasic JF, Yaron M, Nicholas RA, Lickteig JA, Roach RC. Treatment of acute mountain sickness: Hyperbaric versus oxygen therapy. *Ann Emerg Med.* 1991;20:1109–1112.

150. Bärtsch P, Merki B, Hofstetter D, Maggiorini M, Kayser B, Oelz O. Treatment of acute mountain sickness by simulated descent: A randomised controlled trial. *Br Med J.* 1993;306:1098–1101.

151. Kayser B, Jean D, Herry JP, Bärtsch P. Pressurization and acute mountain sickness. *Aviat Space Environ Med.* 1993;64:928–931.

152. Burtscher M, Likar R, Nachbauer W, Philadelphy M, Puhringer R, Lammle T. Effects of aspirin during exercise on the incidence of high-altitude headache: A randomized, double-blind, placebo-controlled trial. *Headache.* 2001;41:542–545.

153. Broome JR, Stoneham MD, Beeley JM, Milledge JS, Hughes AS. High altitude headache: Treatment with ibuprofen. *Aviat Space Environ Med.* 1994;65:19–20.

154. Dusek ER, Hansen JE. Biomedical study of military performance at high terrestrial elevation. *Mil Med.* 1969;134:1497–1507.

155. Pigman EC, Karakla DW. Acute mountain sickness at intermediate altitude: Military mountainous training. *Am J Emerg Med.* 1990;8:7–10.

Chapter 25

HIGH-ALTITUDE PULMONARY EDEMA

JAMES M. ROACH, MD[*]; AND ROBERT B. SCHOENE, MD[†]

INTRODUCTION AND HISTORICAL BACKGROUND

CLINICAL PRESENTATION
  Incidence and Setting
  Symptoms and Physical Findings
  Radiographic Findings
  Ancillary Findings
  Autopsy Findings

PATHOPHYSIOLOGY
  Role of Pulmonary Hypertension
  Role of Exercise and Cold Exposure
  Role of Inflammation
  Role of Hypoxic Ventilatory Response
  Role of Fluid Alterations
  Role of Alveolar Fluid Clearance

TREATMENT AND PREVENTION
  Nonpharmacological Modalities
  Pharmacological Modalities

SUMMARY

[*]Executive Medical Director, Medical Affairs, Sepracor, Inc, 111 Locke Drive, Marlborough, Massachusetts 02139; formerly Major, Medical Corps, US Army
[†]Professor of Medicine, University of Washington School of Medicine; and Chief of Medicine, Swedish Providence Medical Center, 500 17th Avenue, Seattle, Washington 98122

INTRODUCTION AND HISTORICAL BACKGROUND

High-altitude pulmonary edema (HAPE) is a noncardiogenic pulmonary edema that develops in susceptible people who ascend quickly from low to high altitude. The incidence of HAPE increases with the rate of ascent and the ultimate altitude attained. HAPE is a cause of significant morbidity in people who sojourn to high altitude, and although it is usually easily treatable, it remains the most common cause of illness-related death. (Please see Exhibit 19-1 in Chapter 19, Mountains and Military Medicine: An Overview, for definitions of sojourners, trekkers, climbers, and other categories of visitors to mountain environments.)

Undoubtedly, HAPE has occurred and existed for as long as people have sojourned into the mountains, although it was not recognized as a distinct clinical entity until the 1950s and 1960s. A description of what would now be regarded as acute mountain sickness (AMS) appeared in Chinese documents dating back to 37 to 32 BC,[1] but not until the year AD 403 did the first "case report" of probable HAPE appear in a written document. Hui Jiao, a Chinese archivist, noted that his traveling companion in the Lesser Snowy Mountains, Hui Jing,

> was in a serious condition, frothing at the mouth, losing his strength rapidly and fainting away now and then. Finally he dropped dead on the snowy ground.[2(p58)]

Altitude illness remained a relatively uncommon and obscure problem for several centuries; largely because people had little interest in venturing into the mountains and as means of rapid transportation were not yet available, the few who did were unable to travel high enough and quickly enough to become symptomatic. Mountaineering became more popular in the mid to late 19th century; consequently, the scientific and medical community became interested in investigating the physiological and pathophysiological effects of exposure to hypobaric hypoxia. In 1891, Dr Etienne Henri Jacottet ascended Mont Blanc (on the common border of France, Italy, and Switzerland) to make scientific measurements on the summit. He became quite ill but refused to descend so that he could "observe the acclimatization process" in himself.[3] He died soon thereafter; autopsy revealed "a suffocative catarrh accompanied by acute edema of the lungs."[3]

It was not uncommon for mountaineers to develop severe dyspnea at high altitude, particularly if they had ascended quickly and were engaged in strenuous activity; however, their symptoms were usually attributed to pneumonia or heart failure.[4,5] Railroads were built into the mountains—particularly in areas of mining such as the Andes of South America—early in the 20th century. For the first time, people could be transported rapidly from low altitude to high altitude. Dr Thomas Ravenhill, a physician working for a mining company in Chile, published the first comprehensive description of altitude illness in the English medical literature in 1913.[5] He depicted three types of *puna* (ie, altitude illness): normal, nervous, and cardiac. These descriptions are consistent with what would now be identified as AMS, high-altitude cerebral edema (HACE), and HAPE, respectively. Symptoms of cardiac puna included severe dyspnea, cough productive of white frothy or sometimes blood-stained sputum, cyanosis, and crepitations.[5,6] In a South American publication in 1937, Hurtado[7] described a case of pulmonary edema occurring in a resident of high altitude who visited sea level briefly and became ill shortly after returning to his native environment. Lizarraga[8] reported several similar cases of HAPE in 1955. Although Hurtado mentioned these cases and speculated on the mechanism of HAPE in the American journal *Military Medicine* in 1955,[9] not until Charles S. Houston, MD, published a case report in the *New England Journal of Medicine* in 1960[10] was HAPE brought to the attention of the English-speaking medical community at large.

The military relevance of HAPE is best illustrated by the experience of the Indian Army during the Sino–Indian border conflict in the 1960s, when the incidence of HAPE was noted to be as high as 15.5% in a group of "fresh inductees" who were rapidly transported to altitudes between 3,355 and 5,490 m (11,000–18,000 ft).[11,12] Morbidity and mortality from HAPE were significant, and a commanding general was one of several who died of the disease.[13] The threat posed by HAPE to military personnel who could be stationed at high altitude was well recognized by military physicians in the United States at that time.[14] Since the mid 1980s, Indian and Pakistani military forces have been engaged in a border conflict in northern Kashmir at altitudes between 5,185 and 5,490 m (17,000–18,000 ft); both sides have acknowledged that about 80% of casualties were caused by the harsh environmental conditions.[15] Mortality from HAPE has been reported to be as high as 44% when descent is not possible and supplemental oxygen is not available[16]—conditions that may be encountered in a combat situation.

The basic altitude physiology and the pathophysiology of altitude illness in general have been extensively reviewed in previous chapters of this textbook. The focus of this chapter is the clinical presentation, pathophysiology, and treatment of HAPE. Many other reviews in the medical literature present HAPE from different perspectives and provide some supplementary material.[4,6,13,17–25]

CLINICAL PRESENTATION

Incidence and Setting

The incidence of HAPE depends on the rate of ascent and the altitude achieved (Table 25-1).[12,13,17] The reported range of incidence is from an estimated 0.01% in people who traveled from low altitude to Vail, Colorado (2,501 m [8,200 ft]),[26] to 15.5% in a group of male Indian soldiers who were transported rapidly to between 3,355 and 5,490 m (11,000–18,000 ft).[11] Children of both genders appear to be more predisposed to HAPE than adults,[27] but the overall incidence of HAPE in adult women is much lower than in men.[26,28] Other factors that are believed to contribute to the development of HAPE include vigorous exertion and exposure to the cold,[11,13] although in one case series HAPE occurred more often in sedentary subjects than in those who had recently exerted themselves.[12] People who have experienced a previous episode of HAPE have a 60% to 70% likelihood of recurrence on reascent to high altitude.[29–31]

HAPE occurs in two common settings:

1. in residents of sea level or relatively low altitude who ascend to high altitude; and
2. in high-altitude natives (or people who reside at high altitude for at least several months) who descend to low altitude, stay for a period of time, and then reascend to high altitude.

These different manifestations of HAPE have been referred to as Type I and Type II but are more commonly called "HAPE" and "reentry HAPE," respectively. It has been suggested that these "variants" are epidemiologically different[26]; however, not enough data are available to substantiate this hypothesis. Singh and colleagues[11] stated that the incidence of HAPE was similar in "fresh inductees and reinductees"[11(p229)] to altitude. The relative incidence and prevalence of HAPE and reentry HAPE reported in the literature are probably more a re-

TABLE 25-1

INCIDENCE OF ALTITUDE ILLNESS IN VARIOUS EXPOSED GROUPS

Study Group*	Number at Risk per Year	Sleeping Altitude (m)	Average Days to Reach Sleeping Altitude From Low Altitude	Maximum Altitude Reached (m)	Percentage with AMS	Percentage with HAPE and/or HACE
Visitors to western US states	30 million	~ 2,000 ~ 2,500 ≥ 3,000	1–2	3,500	18–20, 22 27–42	0.01
Mt Everest trekkers	6,000	3,000–5,200	1–2 (fly in) 10–13 (walk in)	5,500	47 23	1.6 0.05
Mt McKinley climbers	800	3,000–5,300	3–7	6,194	30	2–3
Mt Rainier climbers	6,000	3,000	1–2	4,392	67	‡
Indian army soldiers	Unknown	3,000–5,500	1–2	5,500	†	2.3–15.5

AMS: acute mountain sickness; HACE: high-altitude cerebral edema; HAPE: high-altitude pulmonary edema
*See Exhibit 19-1 in Chapter 19, Mountains and Military Medicine: An Overview, for definitions of groups
†Reliable estimate unavailable
‡No data available
Adapted with permission from Hackett PH, Roach RC. High-altitude medicine. In: Auerbach PS, ed. *Wilderness Medicine*. 4th ed. Philadelphia, Pa: Mosby; 2001: 3.

flection of the demographics and geographical location of the population being studied than a representation of two distinct clinical entities, however.

Most early reports from South America concentrated on native highlanders and, as such, most of their cases were of the reentry HAPE variety.[7,8,31,32] In these cases, the average length of stay at a lower elevation prior to returning to high altitude was about 12 days, although one individual had remained at low altitude for 5 months. HAPE has also been reported to occur after descents as brief as 24 hours. Reentry HAPE usually developed between 3 and 48 hours after arriving at altitudes between 3,660 and 4,575 m (12,000–15,000 ft). Most episodes occurred within the first 24 to 36 hours of reexposure to altitude but can occur several weeks after ascent, particularly at extreme altitude. This time course and altitude profile is also similar for lowlanders who ascend rapidly to high altitude. Although the incidence of HAPE is low below altitudes of 3,050 m (10,000 ft), Maldonado[33] described a number of people who developed Type II HAPE in Bogotá, Colombia, at an altitude of 2,641 m (8,660 ft), illustrating that the diagnosis of HAPE should be considered in the appropriate clinical setting, even at relatively low altitudes. HAPE also occurs occasionally in people who have resided at high altitude for several months and have not recently changed elevation, although this is unusual.[11,12]

Symptoms and Physical Findings

The symptoms and findings of the physical examination in HAPE are similar to those seen in cardiogenic forms of pulmonary edema, although the illness may begin insidiously.[11,13,18] Early manifestations of HAPE include decreased exercise tolerance at altitude and a longer recovery period after exertion. Most victims of HAPE initially experience symptoms consistent with AMS, such as headache, lethargy and fatigue, nausea, and difficulty sleeping.[11,12,34] Then respiratory symptoms such as dyspnea on exertion, chest discomfort, and dry cough develop and begin to predominate the clinical picture. As the disease progresses, dyspnea is noticeable at rest and in severe cases, the cough becomes productive of blood-tinged, frothy sputum. Symptoms often develop and worsen during the night,[35] presumably because of decreased ventilation (and subsequent decrease in arterial oxygen saturation [Sa_{O_2}]), and redistribution of blood flow that occurs when subjects are in a recumbent position.[13] Signs and symptoms of HACE (discussed in Chapter 24, Acute Mountain Sickness and High-Altitude Cerebral Edema) may accompany HAPE, especially at higher altitudes.

Physical examination typically reveals tachypnea and tachycardia, with orthopnea and cyanosis becoming manifest in more severe cases.[12,31,32] A low-grade fever is often present.[12,27] Examination of the lungs reveals rales, often asymmetrical in distribution and initially located in the right midlung field,[13,17,18] but as the disease progresses, the rales spread throughout both lung fields. Of note, there is no accompanying evidence of cardiac failure such as a third heart sound or distention of the neck veins,[31] although the second component of the pulmonic heart sound is often palpable and accentuated.[12] Marticorena and Hultgren[36] developed a scoring system to grade the severity of HAPE based on clinical symptoms, signs, and radiographic findings (Exhibit 25-1). From a clinical and a research standpoint, their scoring system is useful in grading the severity of HAPE.

In 1971, Lenfant speculated that "a diffuse, asymptomatic pulmonary edema"[37(p1303)] was at least partially responsible for the ventilation–perfusion mismatching and gas-exchange abnormality often seen in people who ascend to high altitude. In support of this theory, Jaeger and colleagues[38] demonstrated that in a group of 25 male soldiers, thoracic intravascular fluid volume increased abruptly following rapid ascent to 14,000 ft, although none of these men had findings on physical or radiographic examination suggestive of pulmonary edema. The incidence of rales in trekkers in the Himalayas in another study was noted to be 23% overall; 40% of people with rales had no clinical evidence of AMS or HAPE.[39] These findings suggest that subclinical pulmonary edema occurs frequently in people ascending to high altitude. The true prevalence of subclinical HAPE, and the percentage of people with mild interstitial edema who eventually develop disease severe enough to be recognized clinically, is unknown.

Radiographic Findings

The chest roentgenogram findings in HAPE have been well described.[11,12,30,31,33,34,40,41] Although one study suggests that "[a] peripheral, often patchy or nonhomogeneous distribution of densities is typical,"[30(p665)] others emphasize the wide variety of findings that are seen in patients with HAPE. Infiltrates may be patchy or diffuse, unilateral or bilateral, and distributed primarily in a central or a peripheral location.[31,33,41] This diversity of radiographic abnormalities is most likely related to the stage of disease at which the roentgenogram was taken. It has been hypothesized that the infiltrates start patchy and peripheral, and as the disease

EXHIBIT 25-1

SEVERITY CLASSIFICATION OF HIGH-ALTITUDE PULMONARY EDEMA

Grade	Clinical Symptoms and Signs	Roentgenographic Findings and Example Chest Films
1. Mild	Minor symptoms with dyspnea on moderate exertion. May be able to perform light activity. Heartbeats per minute: < 110 Breaths per minute: < 20	Minor opacities involving < 1/4 of one lung field:
2. Moderate	Symptoms of dyspnea, weakness, fatigue on slight effort. Cannot perform light activity. Headache with cough, dyspnea at rest. Heartbeats per minute: 110–120 Breaths per minute: 20–30	Opacities involving at least 1/2 of one lung field:
3. Serious	Severe dyspnea, headache, weakness, nausea at rest. Loose, recurrent, productive cough. Wheezy, difficult respirations; obvious cyanosis. Heartbeats per minute: 121-140 Breaths per minute: 31–40	Opacities involving at least 1/2 of each lung field, or unilateral exudate involving all of one lung field:
4. Severe	Clouded consciousness, stupor, or coma. Unable to stand or walk. Severe cyanosis. Bubbling rales present with copious sputum, usually bloody. Severe respiratory distress. Heartbeats per minute: > 140 Breaths per minute: > 40	Bilateral opacaties involving > 1/2 of each lung field: 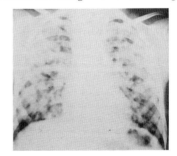

Adapted with permission from Marticorena E, Hulgren HN. Evaluation of therapeutic methods in high altitide pulmonary edema. *Am J Cardiol*. 1979; 43:308, 309.

progresses they become more diffuse, homogenous, and consolidated.[41] When the infiltrates are unilateral, they are more frequently located on the right side.[31,41] The symmetrical "bat-wing" distribution of edema, typically seen in cardiogenic pulmonary edema, is distinctly unusual.[34] Enlargement of the right ventricle has also been reported,[34,40] although other reports describe the heart size as being normal[30,33,42] or normal to minimally elevated.[41] Kerley B lines and pleural effusions are very unusual but may be observed in a minority of patients; when present, effusions usually develop in the recovery period.[41] Peribronchial and perivascular cuffing is almost always present.[41]

Main pulmonary arteries may be prominent and dilated in HAPE.[11,30,31,33,34,40,42] One Japanese study[40] compared the chest radiographs of 16 patients with HAPE, obtained at hospital admission, with those obtained following their recovery and documented a decrease in both the area and the volume of the main pulmonary artery, as calculated from the posteroanterior projection. Vock and colleagues[30] studied 25 male volunteers whose chest radiographs were taken at an altitude of 550 m (1,805 ft) and again at 6, 18, and 42 hours after they were rapidly transported to 4,559 m (14,958 ft). Eight of these subjects subsequently developed HAPE (six had experienced HAPE previously). Within 6 hours after arrival at high altitude, the diameter of the central pulmonary arteries increased by 17% to 30% in all subjects; there was no statistically significant difference in this measurement between the group that developed HAPE and the group that did not.[30] This observation suggests that dilation of the pulmonary arteries is characteristic in individuals acutely exposed to high altitude, and it should not be considered a finding that is unique to HAPE. In addition, this study documented the time course of radiographic evidence of HAPE, and the relationship between the extent of radiographic abnormalities and the presence of rales.

Changes consistent with the diagnosis of HAPE were generally present within 18 hours after arrival, and in all subjects except one, the infiltrates had progressed during the next 24 hours. Rales were absent in half the observations of subjects who simultaneously had radiographic evidence of HAPE, implying that the diagnosis of HAPE should not be excluded on the basis of normal lung sounds with auscultation. Conversely, rales were detected in several subjects with normal chest roentgenograms who later developed radiographic evidence of HAPE, indicating that radiographic changes may be insensitive in detecting early pulmonary edema and may lag behind the physical findings. Radio-graphic abnormalities may be expected to resolve very quickly (ie, within 24–72 h) with appropriate therapy.[11,13,27,32,42]

Ancillary Findings

Laboratory Findings

Several analyses of patients with HAPE that have reported blood test results have demonstrated that hematocrit and hemoglobin levels are normal.[12,26,27,33,34] One of these studies[34] noted that the hematocrit was lower on recovery, suggesting that hemoconcentration occurred during the acute illness, although another investigation[12] showed no change with recovery. Leukocyte counts are usually elevated[12,26,27,31,33,34] and frequently associated with a leftward shift of the granulocyte series.[12,26,33,34] Serum chemistries[33,34] and sedimentation rates[12,31,33] are typically normal; however, one study[34] reported a significant elevation of creatine kinase (CK), presumably secondary to muscle damage. Of five patients on whom CK isoenzyme analysis was performed, two had elevations of the CK-BB component (to about 1% of the total), which the authors of the study believed to be indicative of brain damage. Decreased serum iron levels, mild thrombocytopenia, and a slight increase in prothrombin time have also been reported.[34] Urinalysis results are not consistent, with some investigations reporting normal results[12,33] and others reporting increased specific gravity[31] and a preponderance of albuminuria.[34]

At a given altitude, Sao_2 is significantly lower in people with HAPE, compared with those without.[30,43] At 2,745 to 3,355 m (9,000–11,000 ft), the mean Sao_2 in HAPE subjects was 73.7%, compared with 90.6% in healthy controls[43]; and in another study conducted at 4,559 m (14,958 ft), these values were 59% and 80%, respectively.[30] Arterial blood gases (ABGs) typically reveal severe hypoxemia and respiratory alkalosis.[34,40,44,45] Kobayashi and colleagues[34] evaluated 27 patients who developed HAPE at altitudes ranging from 2,680 to 3,190 m (8,793–10.466 ft); mean ABG values within 3 hours of arrival at the hospital (altitude 610 m [2,001 ft]) were pH, 7.47; $Paco_2$, 30.6; and Pao_2, 46.1.

Electrocardiographic, Hemodynamic, and Echocardiographic Findings

The electrocardiographic (ECG) tracings in patients with HAPE invariably reveal sinus tachycardia.[12,32,33] Findings suggestive of right ventricular strain and hypertrophy, such as right axis deviation, right bundle-branch block, an S_1Q_3 pattern, and tall R waves over the right precordial leads have also been described.[31–33] A variety of changes in T wave morphology, to include diffuse flattening and inversion[12,33] as well as an increase in the size of the T waves in both the precordial and the limb leads,[32] have also been reported. Peaked P waves in leads 2 and V_1 or V_2 (suggestive of right atrial enlargement—thought to be caused by an acute increase in pulmonary artery pressure [PAP]) have also been noted.[31,32,42] Some studies have stated that except for sinus tachycardia, the ECG is usually normal,[12] whereas others noted that at least some of the abnormalities described above are present more often than not.[11,31–33] Q waves[12] or T wave changes in the standard (bipolar) lead I, the augmented limb lead aVL, and the precordial leads[31] are not characteristic of HAPE. On recovery, most patients' ECG abnormalities resolve,[31,33] although despite clinical improvement, T wave changes often persist for several weeks if the individual remains at altitude.[11,12,33] It should be noted that right axis deviation, T wave abnormalities, and P wave abnormalities have also been described in individuals without HAPE who were exposed to hypobaric hypoxia,[46,47] suggesting that these changes may be more closely associated with the degree of elevation of PAP than with the development of HAPE per se.

In 1962, Fred and colleagues[48] published the first report of hemodynamic data in a patient with HAPE. Cardiac catheterization in this patient revealed a markedly elevated PAP (68/39), which decreased substantially while the patient breathed 100% oxygen, and normal left atrial and pulmonary venous pressures. On the basis of these findings, they concluded that left ventricular failure was not the cause of edema formation, and also that the increased resistance to blood flow was largely due to hypoxic pulmonary vasoconstriction (HPV). Hultgren and colleagues[49] in 1964 and Roy and colleagues[44] in 1969 confirmed these findings and also demonstrated that the pulmonary capillary wedge pressure in HAPE was normal or low in all patients, thus providing further evidence that HAPE is not caused by cardiac failure or pulmonary venous constriction. Other, more-recent studies that have compared hemodynamic data during the acute illness and the recovery phase reveal that the resolution of infiltrates on the chest radiograph,[34,40] as well as improvement in Sao_2,[34] are associated temporally with the normalization of PAP.

Obtaining invasive hemodynamic measurements at high altitude is obviously problematic. Echocardiography has been employed in several studies evaluating pulmonary hemodynamic responses to hypoxia in subjects who have previously experienced HAPE (and are therefore HAPE-susceptible, discussed below in this chapter).[50–52] Echocardiography has also been utilized since the early 1990s in evaluating the effects on pulmonary hemodynamics and cardiac function of various pharmacological agents proposed for use in the prophylaxis and treatment of HAPE.[29,53,54] These studies demonstrated a marked increase in PAP in HAPE subjects and HAPE-susceptible subjects, compared with controls.

Bronchoalveolar Lavage Findings

In two separate studies, Schoene and colleagues[55,56] performed bronchoscopy with bronchoalveolar lavage (BAL) in 14 people (6 with HAPE, 4 with AMS,

TABLE 25-2

CONSTITUENTS OF BRONCHOALVEOLAR LAVAGE PERFORMED AT HIGH ALTITUDE

Substance Recovered	Controls (n=4)	Patients AMS (n=4)	HAPE (n=8)
Total WBC ($\bullet\ 10^5$/mL)	0.7 ± 0.6	0.9 ± 0.4	3.5 ± 2.0
Polymorphonuclear Leukocytes (%)	2.8 ± 1.5	2.4 ± 1.7	25.4 ± 20.0
Alveolar Macrophages (%)	93.8 ± 5.2	93.8 ± 3.4	67.4 ± 28.1
Total Protein (mg/dL)	12.0 ± 3.4	10.4 ± 8.3	616 ± 329.1

AMS: acute mountain sickness; HAPE: high-altitude pulmonary edema; WBC: white blood cells
Reproduced with permission from Schoene RB. High altitude pulmonary edema: Pathophysiology and clinical review. *Ann Emerg Med.* 1987;16:988.

and 4 without altitude illness) on Mount McKinley in Alaska, at an altitude of 4,400 m (14,436 ft). The results of these procedures are summarized in Table 25-2. Analysis of the BAL fluid revealed a 60-fold increase in high molecular weight proteins in HAPE subjects, compared with AMS subjects and controls, a finding consistent with increased permeability of the pulmonary vascular endothelium. Other notable findings included detectable levels of several potent chemical mediators in the HAPE fluid, including $C5_a$, leukotriene B_4 (LTB_4), and thromboxane B_2, as well as a substantial increase in total leukocytes (particularly neutrophils and alveolar macrophages). For the sake of comparison, subjects with severe HAPE have much higher protein concentrations and similar numbers of total leukocytes, albeit much lower numbers of neutrophils, than patients with another form of high-permeability pulmonary edema, adult respiratory distress syndrome (ARDS).[57] The implication is that although acute inflammation may not be as important in the pathogenesis of HAPE as it is in ARDS, it probably plays a role, possibly in the perpetuation of the permeability leak.

Several other studies[58–60] have confirmed the findings of protein, inflammatory cells, and various chemical markers of inflammation in BAL fluid of patients with HAPE.

Autopsy Findings

Autopsy results on several victims of HAPE have been published[11,32,34,42,61,62] and have consistently demonstrated (*a*) severe pulmonary edema, with bloody, frothy fluid present in the airways; (*b*) right atrial and ventricular distention and hypertrophy; (*c*) no left-sided cardiac enlargement; and (*d*) patent coronary arteries. In addition to being blood-tinged, the fluid found in the alveoli has been described as "proteinaceous,"[11] or protein-rich.[34] Other common findings include marked congestion and distention of the pulmonary vessels, with evidence of thrombi formation in small pulmonary arteries and septal capillaries. Although it has been speculated that the formation of thrombi may be involved in the pathophysiology of HAPE, research published in the late 1980s by Bärtsch and colleagues[63,64] suggests that in vivo fibrin generation is more likely an epiphenomenon of, rather than the cause of, edema formation.

Hyaline membranes are often[32,61] but not always[42] a characteristic of HAPE. As an aside, electron microscopy performed on the lungs of rats exposed to high altitude (barometric pressure [PB] 265 mm Hg) for only 12 hours revealed the formation of multiple endothelial vesicles that contained a granular material.[65] Heath, Moosavi, and Smith[65] speculated that these "oedema vesicles" could conceivably exert a significant hemodynamic effect by protruding into the pulmonary venous capillaries; however, as no electron microscopy data have been published in humans, the significance of this finding is uncertain. In summary, the pathological findings described in HAPE collectively support the concept that rather than being cardiogenic in origin, the edema is of the "high-permeability" type, similar to the hemodynamic data and BAL studies mentioned above.

PATHOPHYSIOLOGY

Role of Pulmonary Hypertension

Although the exact mechanism of illness is unknown, most investigators believe that HAPE and the other major altitude illnesses, AMS and HACE, are caused by the *consequences* of exposure to acute hypoxia, rather than by hypoxia per se (Figure 25-1).[19,66–69] Perhaps the most important physiological effect of low ambient and arterial oxygen tensions relative to the development of HAPE is pulmonary vasoconstriction. Houston speculated in 1960 that HAPE was caused by elevated PAP secondary to anoxia, leading to failure of the left ventricle.[10] Although subsequent investigations of hemodynamics in patients with HAPE proved him wrong with regard to overt left ventricular failure (there is some reported evidence for ventricular dysfunction during exercise[70,71] and diastolic dysfunction at rest[72]), several lines of evidence suggest that pulmonary hypertension is critical to the development of HAPE.

Altitude Exposure and Pulmonary Arterial Pressure

The hypoxic pulmonary vasoconstriction response (HPVR), which is manifested by an increase in PAP, was initially described in an animal model (cats) in 1946.[73] One year later, Motley and colleagues[74] demonstrated that mean PAP increased from 13 to 23 mm Hg in five normal human volunteers following their exposure to a fraction of inspired oxygen (FIO_2) of 0.1. Rotta and colleagues[75] first described the relationship between PAP and altitude in 1956. Not surprisingly, PAP rises as altitude increases (Figure 25-2) because of the associated decrease in inspired oxygen tension at higher altitudes. It should be emphasized, however, that the degree of this response is highly variable between individuals.[76–78] Those with exaggerated responses to hypoxia appear to be predisposed to developing HAPE.

People who have previously experienced HAPE have been the subject of many investigations, in an attempt to determine whether something unique or remarkable about their physiological response to hypoxia makes them susceptible to the condition. Hultgren, Grover, and Hartley[45] measured PAP in five HAPE-susceptible (HAPE-S) subjects at sea level and also 24 hours following their ascent to 3,100 m (10,171 ft), and demonstrated that their HPVRs were markedly exaggerated both at rest and during exercise, compared with what would be expected in normal individuals at that altitude. None of the subjects developed clinically apparent pulmonary edema, suggesting that elevation of PAP can occur prior to, rather than as a consequence of, the development of edema—a phenomenon that

since then has been explicitly demonstrated.[29,53,78] Viswanathan and colleagues[79] evaluated the effect of breathing a hypoxic gas mixture ($FIO_2 = 10\%$) for 5 minutes in 51 HAPE-S subjects and 44 controls and also found greater HPVRs in the HAPE-S group. Although this finding was questioned by Naeije, Melot, and Lejeune[80] in 1986, more-recent studies[50–52,70,71,81] have repeatedly shown that HAPE-S individuals have a "constitutional abnormality in the pulmonary vascular response to hypoxia,"[51(p801)] which is even more pronounced during exercise.[50,70,71]

As yet, the constitutional abnormality responsible for the increased HPVRs in HAPE-S individuals has not been precisely defined, although research findings have identified several possible contributing mechanisms. One possible mechanism is an increased hypoxia-related sympathetic nervous system stimulation. Thus, Duplain and colleagues[78] found an increased rate of sympathetic nerve discharge that correlated with increased PAP in HAPE-S subjects, compared with control subjects at high altitude. Further, the increase in sympathetic nerve activity and pulmonary pressure preceded the development of HAPE in HAPE-S subjects. Another possible mechanism involves an imbalance in pulmonary endothelial vasoconstrictor and vasodilator mediators. Sartori and colleagues[82] demonstrated an increase of the pulmonary vasoconstrictor endothelin-1 at high altitude in HAPE-S subjects relative to normal control subjects, and the levels correlated with PAP. HAPE-S subjects have been shown to have decreased pulmonary production of

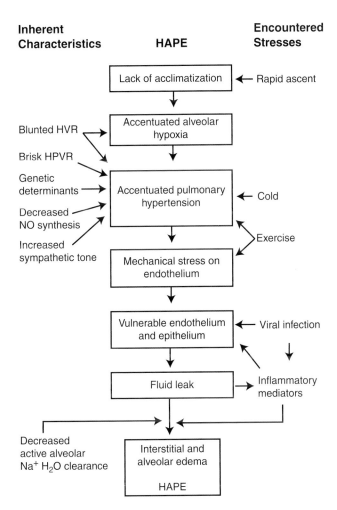

Fig. 25-1. Proposed pathophysiology of high-altitude pulmonary edema (HAPE). Interaction of the magnitude of ascent-induced hypoxia with other stresses and inherent characteristics of the individual cause accentuated pulmonary hypertension. Mechanical stress from the exaggerated increase in pulmonary vascular pressure increases normally low rate of fluid leak into the interstitial space. Increased fluid leak has both a hydrostatic component from pressure gradient and a permeability component from vascular endothelial disruption. Inflammatory mediators generated by hypoxia and tissue damage further exaggerate the permeability fluid leak. Buildup of fluid in the interstitial space and disruption of bronchial-alveolar epithelium causes alveolar flooding. Decreased sodium and fluid clearance by dysfunctional epithelium may also contribute to the abnormal fluid accumulation. Adapted with permission from Schoene RB, Swenson EK, Hultgren HN. High-altitude pulmonary edema. In: Hornbein TF, Schoene RB, eds. *High Altitude, An Exploration of Human Adaptation.* New York, NY: Marcel Dekker; 2001; 779.

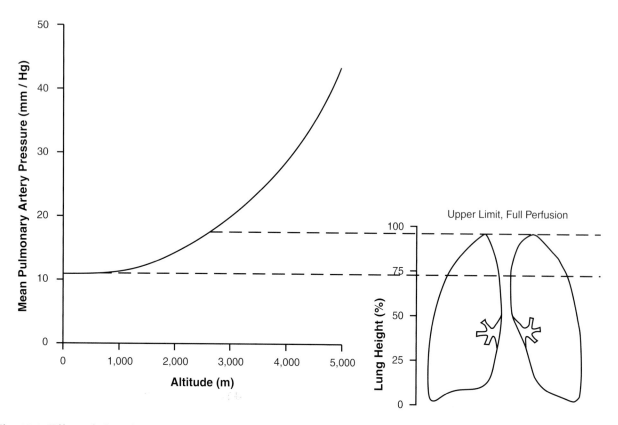

Fig. 25-2. Effect of altitude on mean pulmonary artery pressure measured in relation to lung hilum. Note that from sea level to 1,000 m (3,280 ft) in an erect body position, only the lower 70% of the lungs are continuously perfused (the upper lungs are perfused only during the systolic pulse). At an elevation of about 2,500 m (8,200 ft), the hypoxia-induced increase in mean pulmonary artery pressure allows continuous perfusion of the total lungs. Above 2,500 m, there is progressive pulmonary artery hypertension. Adapted with permission from Lenfant C, Sullivan K. Adaptation to high altitude. *N Engl J Med.* 1971;284:1303.

endothelial-derived nitric oxide when breathing a hypoxic gas mixture,[83] and populations indigenous to high altitude have high levels of exhaled nitric oxide, suggesting high production in their lungs, relative to low-altitude populations.[84] Additionally, inhaled nitric oxide has been shown to significantly reduce increased PAP and improve arterial oxygenation in HAPE-S subjects at high altitude.[85] Finally, the observation that HAPE-S individuals frequently have a smaller lung volumes compared with mountaineers who seem not to experience HAPE[70,79] caused Eldridge and colleagues[70] to speculate that a smaller pulmonary vascular bed in HAPE-S individuals might contribute to their exaggerated HPVRs.

Overperfusion of Pulmonary Vessels

The location of the fluid leak caused by hypoxia-induced pulmonary vasoconstriction is not known. For instance, the pulmonary vasoconstriction in HAPE may initially be heterogeneous and unevenly distributed, as suggested by the asymmetric distri-

bution of rales and infiltrates seen on physical and radiographic examinations performed early in the course of the edema. Vessels that are not constricted are subjected to high pressures and flow and are relatively "overperfused," compared with vessels that are protected by the HPVR,[20,86] and the areas upstream from the constriction may also have very high intravascular pressures. The increase in hydrostatic forces in these overperfused areas can then lead to transudation of fluid into the alveoli, and edema may form in the interstitial spaces around the extraalveolar vessels proximal to the vasoconstriction. By the "classic" definition, if the edema in HAPE were caused only by an increase in hydrostatic forces, then it would be expected to have a low protein content.[87] The protein-rich nature of the lavage fluid and low capillary wedge pressure characteristically found in HAPE suggest that the edema is of the high-permeability variety, which could be secondary to very high pressures and flow that break down the pulmonary capillary endothelium.

Hackett and colleagues[88] reported four cases of

unilateral (left-sided) HAPE occurring at moderate altitudes (2,000–3,000 m [6,562–9,843 ft]) in adult patients whose right pulmonary artery was absent, and Rios and colleagues[89] reported a similar case in a 10-year-old child who also lacked a right pulmonary artery. Unilateral HAPE at moderate altitude has also been reported in a man with a hypoplastic right pulmonary artery[90] and in another with occlusion of the right pulmonary artery by calcified lymph nodes associated with granulomatous mediastinitis.[91] In these settings, all of the cardiac output (C.O.) is directed to one lung. The presumption is that as the individuals became more hypoxic, C.O. (and PAP) increased and led to exceedingly high pressures and flows in the vulnerable lung and the subsequent development of edema. HAPE has also been reported in association with pulmonary thromboembolism[92] and partial anomalous pulmonary venous drainage without an atrial septal defect.[93] (A similar situation is seen in individuals who have had pneumonectomy and develop pulmonary edema during exercise.[94]) These cases provide further indirect evidence of the importance of overperfusion of the pulmonary vascular bed in the pathophysiology of HAPE.

Stress Failure in the Pulmonary Circuit

West and colleagues[95–97] have shown that pulmonary capillaries that are exposed to high pressures may experience damage to the vascular endothelium and widening of the pores between endothelial membranes of adjacent cells, which can lead to high molecular weight proteins and red blood cells leaking into the interstitial and alveolar spaces. This concept, termed "stress failure" of the pulmonary capillaries, could explain the seemingly paradoxical finding of an edema caused by regional overperfusion, which should be transudative in nature, instead being characterized by high protein content in the alveolar fluid, a condition more suggestive of a high-permeability leak (see Figure 25-1). In an animal model, the integrity of the capillary membrane has been shown to be restored within minutes following a reduction in pressure.[98] Although this has yet to be proven in humans, it may explain why patients with HAPE often respond quickly to treatment with oxygen and other treatments aimed at lowering PAP (see the section on Treatment and Prevention, below).

Role of Exercise and Cold Exposure

Several of the early descriptions of HAPE,[10–12,49] as well as more-recent reviews,[13,17,22,77] state that vigorous exercise, exposure to the cold, or both, may be risk factors associated with the development of HAPE or may exacerbate the condition. This suggestion has yet to be demonstrated unequivocally, but there is good reason to believe that exercise and cold exposure may predispose to HAPE because they increase blood flow and pressure in pulmonary circulation.

The earliest evidence that exercise might contribute to increased PAP at altitude came in the 1960s, when Peñaloza and colleagues[99] found a greater increase in PAP during exercise at high altitude in individuals born and reared there than in sea-level residents exercising at sea level. Later, Wagner and colleagues[100,101] measured C.O. and PAP in eight normal subjects at rest and during exercise at sea level and simulated altitudes of 3,048 m (10,000 ft; PB 523 mm Hg) and 4,572 m (15,000 ft; PB 429 mm Hg). Their work demonstrates that (*a*) at all altitudes tested, PAP and C.O. increase with exercise intensity, and (*b*) for a given workload, PAP and C.O. are progressively elevated at higher altitudes, compared with sea level (Figure 25-3). Hultgren and colleagues[45] found a similar rise in the PAP of HAPE-S subjects exercising at altitude. More telling, perhaps, is that HAPE-S subjects have been shown to have a greater rise in PAP during exercise at sea level than normal control subjects,[50,71] and Eldridge and colleagues[70] found that during exercise at high altitude, HAPE-S subjects also have a greater rise in PAP than normal controls. Thus, pulmonary blood pressure and flow increase during exercise, and theoretically can lead to further overperfusion and stress on the pulmonary capillary wall, especially in HAPE-S individuals, predisposing to the development of edema. Although demonstration of a direct connection between the exercise-induced increase in PAP and HAPE has not been reported, Anholm and colleagues[102] have reported a prospective study in which they found radiographic evidence for early pulmonary edema in 33 elite bicycle racers following prolonged intensive exercise at 2,097 to 3,121 m (6,880–10,240 ft) altitude.

As does exercise, cold exposure increases PAP. Exposure to the cold has been shown to cause a significant increase in PAP in cattle,[103] rats,[104] and sheep.[105] The latter study further demonstrated that during exposure to cold ambient temperature (3°C) or hypoxia (F_{IO_2} = 11%), the rise in PAP was 24% and 27%, respectively. When the sheep were exposed to both hypoxia and cold simultaneously, the rise in PAP was greater (61%) than the sum of the two separate conditions, illustrating the independent (and perhaps synergistic) effects of cold exposure and hypoxia on the pulmonary vasculature.

Reeves and colleagues[106] reported epidemiological data that suggest the incidence of HAPE in human visitors to Summit County, Colorado (2,650–2,950 m [8,700–9,700 ft]), may be affected by cold conditions. In the only direct study reported on the effect of cold on PAP in humans, Hasen Nuri, Ali

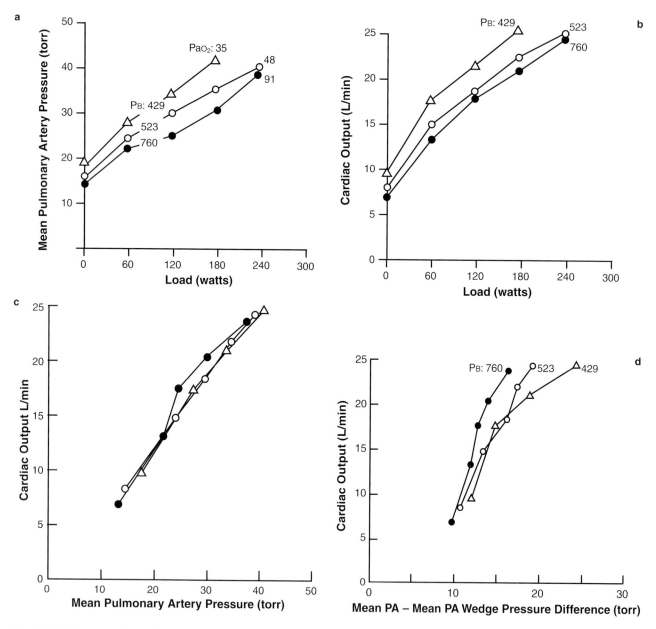

Fig. 25-3. Pulmonary hemodynamics during acute exposure to hypobaric hypoxia. Data represent mean values obtained by pulmonary artery catheter in eight normal volunteer subjects at rest and during three and four exercise (bicycle ergometer) work loads (in watts) at sea level (SL), 523 mm Hg (3,050 m/10,000 ft) and 429 mm Hg (4,574 m/15,000 ft) in a hypobaric chamber. Mean arterial oxygen (PaO$_2$) values at rest and during peak exercise at each simulated altitude were 95 and 91 mm Hg at SL; 56 and 48 mm Hg at P$_B$ = 523 torr; and 39 and 35 mm Hg at P$_B$ = 429 torr. (**a, b, c**) The panels show a parallel increase in mean pulmonary artery pressure (PAP$_{mean}$, mm Hg) and cardiac output (ie, blood flow; L/min) with increasing altitude and work level. (**d**) The panel shows increased pulmonary vascular resistance (PAP$_{mean}$ − mean pulmonary capillary wedge pressure [PCWP$_{mean}$], mm Hg) with both altitude and higher work load. • = 760 mm Hg, ○ = 523 mm Hg, = 429 mm Hg. Repr oduced with permission from Wagner PD. Hypobaric effects on the pulmonary circulation and high altitude pulmonary edema. In: Weir EK, Reeves JT, eds. *Pulmonary Vascular Physiology and Pathophysiology.* Vol 38. In: Lenfant C, ed. *The Lung in Health and Disease.* New York, NY: Marcel Dekker; 1989: 177–178.

Kahn, and Quraishi[107] evaluated the PAP response to a cold pressor test in a group of Indian soldiers and found a greater increase in PAP in HAPE-S subjects, compared with controls.

Role of Inflammation

The pathophysiology of HAPE is generally thought to be related to increased hydrostatic pressure within the pulmonary vasculature *in association with* increased endothelial permeability.[13,19,21,66,68,108,109] This so-called "hydrostatic permeability" hypothesis[21] suggests that the development of edema is accentuated by the simultaneous release of (*a*) vasoactive substances (leading to increased perfusion pressure) and (*b*) mediators that lead to increased endothelial permeability. Because the inflammatory process is mediated by substances that affect both blood flow and endothelial permeability, there has been much speculation as to a possible role of inflammation in HAPE.

Early evidence of an association of inflammation with HAPE came from autopsy findings that showed leukocyte infiltration and hyaline membranes in the alveoli of HAPE fatalities.[11,43,61,62,110] Results of epidemiological studies also support a possible role of inflammation in HAPE. A retrospective study of clinical records from children who developed HAPE at moderate altitudes in Colorado found that a preponderance of children with HAPE had a history of preexisting illness (most often upper respiratory infection), suggesting that the inflammation associated with their illness was a possible predisposing factor to developing HAPE.[111] Similarly, Hanaoka[112] and associates reported a greater number of the major histocompatibility-complex genotypes HLA-DR6 and HLA-DQ4 among adult HAPE-S individuals, compared with a normal population, a finding consistent with a possible genetic inflammatory predisposition.

The strongest evidence for inflammation's playing a role in HAPE stems from the findings of presence of inflammatory mediators in blood and BAL fluid of individuals with established HAPE and in HAPE-S and normal volunteer subjects exposed to high altitude. Richalet and colleagues[21] found an increase, followed by a decrease in the peripheral blood, of a number of eicosanoids, many of which play a role in inflammation, in normal volunteers during exposure to 4,350 m (13,998 ft) altitude. The time course and pattern of blood levels of specific eicosanoids that affect vasodilatation, vasoconstriction, or increasing permeability paralleled the time course of AMS. Elevated levels of urinary leukotriene

E_4, a general marker of inflammation, were found to be increased in patients with HAPE seen in medical clinics in Summit County, Colorado (> 2,727 m [9,000 ft]), compared with patients without HAPE.[113] In addition to blood and urine, evidence for ongoing inflammation has been found on multiple occasions in BAL fluid from patients with HAPE.[34,55,56,58–60] Increased protein content and white blood cells, mostly alveolar macrophages and neutrophils, is a consistent finding in all BAL studies. Other findings include inflammatory eicosanoids,[55,56] cytokines,[58–60] and complement activation products.[55,56]

Although the evidence noted above certainly suggests that HAPE may be accompanied by inflammation, it does not answer the question of whether inflammation contributes to the initial vascular leak, because the data are either retrospective or were obtained from cases after the edema was well established. As such, these data do not provide very strong support for a role for inflammation in the onset of HAPE. Prospective studies have failed to demonstrate increase in inflammatory mediators prior to development of HAPE. For example, in a prospective study of HAPE-S subjects during 50 hours of altitude exposure (4,000 m [13,124 ft]) in a hypobaric chamber with exercise (30 min at 50% maximal oxygen uptake), Pavlicek and colleagues[114] found slight increase in acute-phase proteins C3 and α_1AT in peripheral blood but not in other acute-phase proteins or the vascular endothelial growth factor. None of the volunteer subjects developed HAPE, however. Kleger and colleagues[115] studied normal and HAPE-S subjects in the first 2 to 3 hours after they arrived at a research facility located on a mountain summit in the Swiss Alps at 4,559 m (14,958 ft). The researchers found only a modest increase in systemic albumin escape (a marker of vessel permeability) prior to development of HAPE in four of the volunteer subjects. After the onset of HAPE, proinflammatory cytokines and C-reactive protein increased in the peripheral blood. At the same location in the Swiss Alps, HAPE-S subjects had no increase in urinary leukotriene B_4 prior to developing HAPE but had an increase once HAPE was clinically apparent.[116] Finally, again at the same research location, Swenson and colleagues[117] performed BAL on HAPE-S subjects within hours of ascent and found protein in BAL fluid but no neutrophils or inflammatory cytokines. Considering all the evidence, most authorities believe that inflammation does not play a significant role in the onset of HAPE. This was conclusively demonstrated by Swenson and colleagues in 2002.[117b] That inflammation may play a later role in edema formation has not been excluded.[22]

Role of Hypoxic Ventilatory Response

The role of a reduced ventilatory response to hypoxia in the pathogenesis of altitude illness has previously been discussed. In general, people with a low hypoxic ventilatory response (HVR) are predisposed to developing AMS. This is presumably because the degree of hypoxia that develops at a given altitude in an individual is at least partially dependent on the HVR. If altitude illness is caused by the consequences of hypoxia, it is logical to expect that the incidence and prevalence of illness are proportional to the degree of hypoxia. Several studies have documented a similar relationship between a low HVR and susceptibility to developing HAPE.

In 1975, Lakshminarayan and Pierson[118] had the opportunity to study a young man who developed

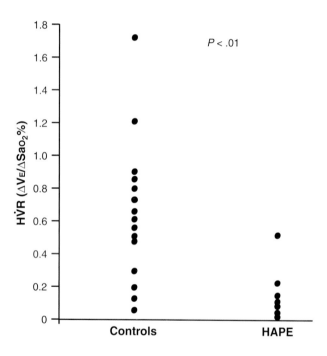

Fig. 25-4. Hypoxic ventilatory response (HVR) in 17 climbers without altitude illness (controls) and 7 climbers with high-altitude pulmonary edema (HAPE) measured at 4,400 m (14,436 ft) on Denali (Mount McKinley, Alaska). The mean value for the HAPE group was statistically significantly lower than that of the controls. The observation that some individuals in the control group had HVR values as low as individuals in the HAPE group yet did not experience HAPE suggests that a low HVR alone is not sufficient to cause HAPE. Adapted with permission from Hackett PH, Roach RC, Schoene RB, Harrison GL, Mills WJ Jr. Abnormal control of ventilation in high-altitude pulmonary edema. *J Appl Physiol.* 1988;64(3):1270.

recurrent HAPE in the absence of any symptoms of respiratory distress and noted that his HVR was blunted. A few years later, Hyers and colleagues[119] exposed a group of HAPE-S subjects and controls to a simulated altitude of 4,150 m (13,616 ft) for 12 hours and found that relative to controls, the HAPE-S group developed more-pronounced hypoxemia associated with relative hypoventilation by 6 hours of exposure. The most convincing studies are those from Hackett and colleagues[120] (Figure 25-4), Matsuzawa and colleagues,[121] and Hohenhaus and colleagues[122]; these studies demonstrate that subjects susceptible to HAPE have a significantly lower HVR, compared with controls. However, these investigations also revealed that HAPE can develop in the presence of a normal HVR, and further that individuals with a low HVR do not necessarily develop HAPE. Cases have been reported in people with a high HVR as well.[123] Hackett and colleagues[120] concluded that a low HVR plays a permissive rather than a causative role in the pathogenesis of HAPE. Individuals with a low HVR and an exaggerated HPVR may be particularly prone to developing HAPE.[18] HAPE has frequently been reported to occur or to progress during the night. HAPE-S subjects have been reported to have irregular nocturnal breathing patterns,[124] but this abnormal breathing appears to be an effect, rather than a cause, of HAPE.[125]

Role of Fluid Alterations

The alterations in fluid homeostasis that occur during ascent to high altitude and the association between these changes and the development of AMS and HACE were reviewed in Chapter 24, Acute Mountain Sickness and High-Altitude Cerebral Edema. Bärtsch and colleagues[126] demonstrated that HAPE-S subjects develop fluid retention even during a relatively slow ascent to high altitude, and also that this alteration in fluid balance was associated with a widening of the right atrium and an increase in atrial natriuretic peptide (ANP).

Several other studies have documented that ANP levels are elevated in HAPE subjects,[127–129] as well as subjects with a history of HAPE who were then subjected to an acute hypoxic stress.[130] ANP levels correlate with the cross-sectional dimension of the right atrium as measured by echocardiography,[126] as well as the degree of elevation of PAP.[130] It has been speculated that ANP levels are elevated in HAPE subjects as a result of right atrial stretching caused by elevated PAP, fluid retention, and centralization of blood volume.[126] But it is unclear whether elevated ANP levels contribute to the development of edema in HAPE, or whether this finding is simply an epiphenomenon.

Role of Alveolar Fluid Clearance

Accumulation of edema fluid in the pulmonary interstitial spaces and alveoli is not only a function of the rate at which fluid leaves the vasculature but is also dependent on how fast the extravasated fluid is cleared.[131] Findings consistent with decreased epithelial handling of sodium in the respiratory epithelium of HAPE-S, compared with HAPE-resistant subjects, suggest that individuals susceptible to HAPE may have a genetic impairment of their ability to clear edema fluid from their lungs.[132] Scherrer and colleagues[133] suggest that the combination of high PAP from an exaggerated HPVR and decreased alveolar fluid clearance may help explain differences between individuals in HAPE susceptibility.

TREATMENT AND PREVENTION

Although the treatment of HAPE depends to some degree on the severity of illness, descent is *always* an effective treatment.[4,13,17,18,66,109,134] Unfortunately, descending may not always be feasible owing to extreme weather conditions, concomitant trauma, or the tactical situation. Descent is not always necessary in cases of mild or moderate HAPE if bed rest, oxygen, and patient observation are available. For example, in many recreation sites (ie, ski areas), patients with HAPE may present with mild-to-moderate disease. If the patients' blood oxygen saturation can be improved with low-flow oxygen to 90% or greater and if they can be observed at night by family or friends, then it is reasonable to send the patients to their accommodations overnight and see them again the next day. Hultgren[23] presented a classification of HAPE severity based on the patient's specific signs and symptoms and electrocardiographic and chest radiographic findings, and suggested that patients with Grades 1 and 2 (mild and moderate, respectively) HAPE could often be treated with bed rest alone. This approach of bed rest and the initiation of oxygen therapy at 4 to 8 L/min by nasal cannula or mask will lead to a dramatic improvement in symptoms within 2 to 6 hours,[11] and complete recovery and resolution of pulmonary edema over the next few days.[31,42]

Mortality has been reported[16] to be as high as 44% in one case series of 166 patients when descent was impossible and supplemental oxygen was unavailable. This situation is not an unusual one for mountaineers to encounter, and so it is obvious that a search for other effective therapeutic options is warranted. Several pharmacological and nonpharmacological modalities directed at improving oxygen tension, lowering PAP, or both have been evaluated in the treatment of HAPE. Given the low incidence of the disease, studying these various modalities in a prospective, randomized, placebo-controlled fashion is very difficult. Despite these limitations, however, several recommendations can be made based on information available in the literature.

Nonpharmacological Modalities

Several nonpharmacological approaches have been evaluated, recommended, or both as potential HAPE therapies when descent is not possible. These include bed rest alone, expiratory positive airway pressure (EPAP), and simulated descent using a portable hyperbaric chamber (see Figure 24-9 [b] in Chapter 24, Acute Mountain Sickness and High-Altitude Cerebral Edema). Marticorena and Hultgren[36] studied 36 children and young adults who developed HAPE of mild-to-moderate severity at an altitude of 3,750 m (12,303 ft). Sixteen subjects were treated with bed rest alone, and 20 subjects received "traditional" treatment including continuous administration of oxygen (6–12 L/min) and bed rest. Although oxygen therapy resulted in quicker resolution of symptoms and greater reductions in heart rate, all subjects treated with bed rest alone fully recovered. Furthermore, the average length of stay in the hospital was similar in both groups. The authors concluded that HAPE of mild-to-moderate severity that develops at relatively low altitude can be treated with bed rest alone, but that this should not be substituted for descent, supplemental oxygen, or both, if feasible and available.

The application of positive expiratory pressure was first proposed as an adjunctive treatment for HAPE in 1977; Feldman and Herndon's[135] rationale was that "positive airway pressure is an effective treatment for pulmonary oedema of any cause."[135(p1037)] The device that they described was cumbersome and untested in the mountainous setting and also impractical to bring on field expeditions; however, the advent of the Downs mask—a lightweight, portable mask developed for use in nonintubated hospital patients—made it possible to study this concept in HAPE. Two uncontrolled studies, with a total of seven patients with HAPE, have demonstrated that the application of EPAP at 5 to 10 cm H_2O pressure for several minutes leads to increased SaO_2.[136,137] The mask was well tolerated and did not lead to any obvious adverse effects; however, in subjects who wore the mask for several hours, symptoms and signs of HAPE returned shortly after the masks were removed. In addition, the application of EPAP at higher levels (> 10–15 cm H_2O) may cause barotrauma or lead to a decreased C.O. A case of HACE believed to be caused by using positive end-expiratory pressure (PEEP) as a treatment for HAPE has also been reported.[138] EPAP may be useful as a temporizing measure until descent is possible, but more experience is needed before it can be widely recommended.

Another nonpharmacological modality that has been employed in the treatment of HAPE is the portable hyperbaric chamber (PHC). The rationale for its use in other forms of altitude illness has been discussed in Chapter 24, Acute Mountain Sickness and High-Altitude Cerebral Edema. The PHC has been used in several patients with HAPE and has been reported to be very effective, but these reports are descriptive in nature and uncontrolled, and often the patients were receiving other concurrent therapies; thus, the independent beneficial contribution of the PHC was difficult to ascertain.[139,140] Theoretically, the PHC should be as useful as supplemental oxygen because both of these interventions work by increasing arterial oxygen tension (Pao_2). It is often impractical to carry heavy metal tanks of oxygen on an expedition; the few groups that bring oxygen usually only carry a single bottle.[141] As a consequence, the supply of oxygen in the field is usually limited. The PHC offers the advantage of being lightweight and more easily transportable, and it can be used repeatedly and for long periods of time.

Hackett[142] compared the effect of supplemental oxygen with the PHC in nine individuals who developed HAPE on Mount McKinley (at an altitude of 4,300 m [14,108 ft]). Alveolar oxygen tensions (Pao_2) were matched during both treatments, and symptomatic improvement was similar in both groups. The authors of another study,[143] the primary focus of which was to compare the effect of the PHC versus supplemental oxygen in AMS, concluded that simulated descent with the PHC and supplemental oxygen were equally effective for relieving symptoms of AMS. This study included six people with coexisting "mild" HAPE; analysis of the data in this subset yielded similar results.

Although patients with HAPE may have difficulty tolerating the recumbent position necessary for optimal use of the PHC,[144] it is an effective temporizing measure for the treatment of HAPE and

may be lifesaving in instances where descent is impossible and oxygen is not available. Additionally, most PHC devices are sufficiently lightweight and portable so that they can be positioned at a sloping angle, with the head of the enclosed patient higher than the feet. Areas of further research should focus on the optimal duration of treatment, the incidence of recurrence of disease after treatment, and the potential synergistic effects of pressurization and supplemental oxygen.

Vigorous coughing in the head-down position accompanied by steady pressure applied to the upper abdomen has been reported to be effective in facilitating drainage of edema fluid and temporarily improving symptoms.[145] Other, more-general, treatment considerations include minimizing exertion and keeping the victims warm (and having them breathe warmed air if possible), as exercise and exposure to cold may lead to an increase in PAP.

Pharmacological Modalities

Historically, a wide variety of drugs such as antibiotics, corticosteroids, digitalis, morphine, atropine, aminophylline, and diuretics have been utilized in the treatment of HAPE[11,12,27,31,42,67]; however, controlled studies evaluating the effectiveness of any of these therapies have not been performed. As more is understood about the pathophysiology of HAPE, it is clear that little rationale exists for the indiscriminate use of antibiotics, digitalis preparations, aminophylline, atropine, or corticosteroids. Given that HAPE is noncardiogenic and that patients are often intravascularly volume-depleted, it is also possible that treatment with diuretics (and perhaps morphine) may have a detrimental effect.

Although comparative investigations have not been performed, Scoggin and colleagues[27] stated that in a group of 39 people with HAPE, "there were no differences in response between oxygen treatment alone (n = 8) and oxygen combined with drugs"[27(p1271)] (ie, some combination of antibiotics, corticosteroids, and diuretics). In another study[26] of 32 patients with HAPE, all of whom were treated with supplemental oxygen, 20 received furosemide; this group had a longer mean hospital stay compared with the group treated only with oxygen. Gray and colleagues,[146] in a study indirectly evaluating the effect of acetazolamide and furosemide on AMS, noted that "subjects started on furosemide on arrival at altitude quickly became medical casualties,"[146(p84)] and concluded that "[p]owerful diuretics such as furosemide … in fact may be dangerous at high altitude."[116(p84)] In 1962, Hultgren, Spickard, and

Lopez[42] were originally in favor of using diuretics; however, in 1975, Hultgren[147] commented on the considerable risks associated with the use of furosemide in HAPE and pointed out that there was insufficient evidence to justify its use.

Recent reviews of HAPE[4,6,13,17,109,134] generally suggest that (*a*) there are no data to substantiate the use of diuretics, morphine, or both in HAPE, and their use remains controversial; (*b*) diuretics and morphine are not useful in treating HAPE in the field because of the potential adverse effects; or (*c*) when used, diuretics and morphine should only be given in situations where blood pressure and fluid status can be closely monitored.

Another medication that has been suggested for use in the prevention and treatment of HAPE is acetazolamide because it has proven efficacy in AMS; however, supportive data from controlled studies are not available. Acetazolamide reduces symptoms and prevents further impairment of pulmonary gas exchange in AMS subjects,[148] improves SaO_2 and reduces periodic breathing during sleep at high altitude,[149,150] and is effective in the prophylaxis of AMS.[151] In the latter study, it was noted that vital capacities were increased in the acetazolamide-treated group at high altitude, and Larson and colleagues[151] surmised that these climbers developed less interstitial edema in the lung. They further speculated that if this was true, "acetazolamide could diminish the incidence and severity of HAPE"[151(p332)] and also "could prove effective in preventing HAPE, as well as improving performance at altitude."[151(p332)] Hackett and colleagues,[35] while participating in the Denali Medical Research Project on Mount McKinley from 1982 to 1985, had the opportunity to treat many HAPE victims. Acetazolamide, in their opinion, "seemed to be beneficial when given early in the course of the illness."[35] They also remarked that HAPE responded so well to supplemental oxygen and descent that no one needed to be evacuated, and except for acetazolamide, no other medications were administered. Because nifedipine, a calcium channel–blocking agent, became the standard pharmacological adjunct to both prevent and treat HAPE during the 1990s and early 2000s[17,24,25] (see below), the long-standing debate on whether diuretics, morphine, and acetazolamide are indicated in the management of this disease may well be obsolete.

A mountaineer who was also a physician and scientist interested in altitude physiology and medicine (Oswald Oelz) developed HAPE in 1986 while ascending Mount Makalu in Nepal. He treated himself with 20 mg of nifedipine sublingually, and

noted that within 15 minutes his dyspnea improved and sputum production decreased.[152,153] He took 20 mg of a slow-release preparation periodically and additional sublingual doses as needed until he had descended safely. His experience prompted further interest in examining the effect of nifedipine in patients with HAPE. Dr Oelz studied 6 male subjects who developed clinical and radiographic evidence of HAPE while ascending Monte Rosa, an Alpine peak between Italy and Switzerland (on which a research laboratory is located at 4,559 m [14,958 ft]). Oelz and colleagues[53] found that treating these subjects with 10 mg of nifedipine sublingually followed by 20 mg of a slow-release preparation every 6 hours led to an improvement in symptoms, usually within 15 to 30 minutes after the first sublingual dose. Nifedipine was postulated to be effective because it reduced PAP (measured by doppler echocardiography) to values approaching that of controls, thereby reducing the hydrostatic forces that lead to the transudation of fluid into the alveoli.

In a prospective, randomized, placebo-controlled, double-blind study, Bärtsch and colleagues[29] proved in 1991, in a group of subjects who had a previous history of HAPE, that nifedipine is effective in decreasing PAP and preventing the development of HAPE. In 1994, these same researchers[154] found that nifedipine was not effective in preventing AMS symptoms in subjects who were not HAPE-susceptible; they believed that its use in high-altitude medicine should be limited to preventing HAPE in susceptible subjects and treating HAPE when immediate descent is not possible and supplemental oxygen is not available.

Hackett and colleagues[54] compared the effects of oxygen, nifedipine, hydralazine, phentolamine, and a combination of oxygen and phentolamine on the pulmonary vasculature in HAPE subjects. All of the vasodilators studied decreased pulmonary vascular resistance and mean PAP to varying degrees and improved gas exchange (Figure 25-5), thus providing more indirect evidence that pulmonary vasoconstriction is associated with edema formation. It is interesting to note that the α-adrenergic blocking agent phentolamine caused the greatest reduction in these parameters and also had an additive effect when combined with oxygen therapy, implying that the sympathetic nervous system may be involved in the pathophysiology of HAPE. Controlled studies evaluating the therapeutic benefit of these other agents are warranted; however, they cannot be recommended for use at this time.

In summary, although some of the pharmacological (particularly nifedipine) and nonpharmacological

Fig. 25-5. The percentage change in mean pulmonary artery pressure (Ppa) and pulmonary vascular resistance (PVR) with five different interventions (see key to graph, below) in a total of 16 patients with high-altitude pulmonary edema (HAPE) and 6 controls. Data are pooled from three data-collection periods, and some individuals must have been included in more than one category (eg, the 10 persons in the first two cagetories apparently received oxygen first and then nifedipine). All changes in Ppa and PVR from baseline were significant ($P < .05$) for all interventions. For Ppa reduction, phentolamine was statistically more effective than either oxygen or hydralazine. Oxygen with phentolamine was more effective than phentolamine alone. For PVR reduction, oxygen and phentolamine were more effective than hydralazine. Phentolamine and phentolamine with oxygen were more effective than nifedipine. Reproduced with permission from Hackett PH, Roach RC, Hartig GS, Greene ER, Levine BD. The effect of vasodilators on pulmonary hemodynamics in high altitude pulmonary edema: A comparison. *Int J Sports Med.* 1992;13 suppl 1:S69.

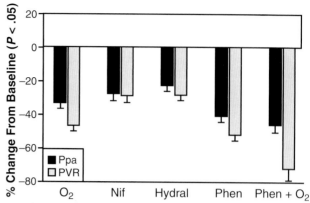

O_2: oxygen (n=10); Nif: nifedipine (n=10); Hydral: hydralazine (n=3); Phen: phentolamine (n=6); Phen+O_2: phentolamine and oxygen (n=6).

modalities (particularly the PHC) discussed may be appropriate as temporizing or prophylactic measures in specific circumstances, they should not be utilized in place of either standard prevention measures (ie, acclimatization and slow ascent) or treatment strategies (ie, descent, supplemental oxygen).

SUMMARY

HAPE is a is a noncardiogenic pulmonary edema that occurs in unacclimatized individuals who ascend rapidly from low altitude to altitudes usually over 2,500 m (8,203 ft) and remain there for more than a few hours. Because HAPE can rapidly be fatal, it is a serious threat to military personnel who may be required to ascend rapidly into high mountains as a contingency of their mission. The pathophysiological mechanisms that cause HAPE are not precisely defined, but they appear to involve an exaggerated hypoxia-induced increase in pulmonary blood pressure, which may cause overperfusion of parts of the pulmonary circuit and stress failure of capillaries with subsequent leak of fluid, protein, and cells into the interstitial tissue and alveoli of the lungs. Hypoxia-induced decrease of alveolar epithelial sodium pump function may limit fluid clearance and contribute to the edema. The leak of fluid and cells may trigger an inflammatory reaction that also contributes to the edema. Some individuals seem much more susceptible to HAPE than others, suggesting that a component of genetic predisposition may be present in the pathophysiology.

HAPE is characterized by a persistent cough that progresses to a production of a pink-tinged or blood-flecked sputum; inappropriate dyspnea with exertion that progresses to dyspnea at rest; and lethargy and fatigue that progresses to confusion, decreased consciousness, and coma.

Untreated HAPE can rapidly be fatal. Descent to a lower altitude is the mainstay of treatment in HAPE, and immediate descent often results in rapid and complete recovery. Descent of as few as 300 m (~1,000 ft) can be lifesaving in some instances. Accepted adjunctive therapies for HAPE include supplemental oxygen and the calcium-channel antagonist nifedipine. HAPE can often be prevented by slow ascent, which allows the body to acclimatize to hypoxia, and by nifedipine taken prophylactically.

REFERENCES

1. Gilbert DL. The first documented report of mountain sickness: The China or Headache Mountain story. *Respir Physiol.* 1983;52:315–326.

2. Houston CS. Mountain sickness. *Sci Am.* 1992;267:58–62, 66.

3.   Mosso A. *Life of Man in the High Alps.* London, England: T. Fisher Unwin; 1898.

4.   Rabold M. High-altitude pulmonary edema: A collective review. *Am J Emerg Med.* 1991;7:426–433.

5.   Ravenhill TH. Some experience of mountain sickness in the Andes. *J Trop Med Hyg.* 1913;20:313–320.

6.   Sutton JR. Mountain sickness. *Neurol Clin.* 1992;10:1015–1030.

7.   Hurtado A. *Aspectos Fisicos y Patologicos de la Vida en Las Alturas* [*Physical and Pathological Aspects of Life at High Altitude*]. Lima, Peru: Imprenta Rimac; 1937.

8.   Lizarraga L. Soroche agudo: Edema agudo del pulmon [Acute mountain sickness: Acute edema of the lungs]. *An Fac Med (Lima).* 1955;38:244.

9.   Hurtado A. Pathological aspects of life at high altitudes. *Mil Med.* 1955;117:272–284.

10.   Houston CS. Acute pulmonary edema of high altitude. *N Engl J Med.* 1960;263:478–480.

11.   Singh I, Kapila CC, Khanna PK, Nanda RB, Rao BDP. High-altitude pulmonary oedema. *Lancet.* 1965;i:229–231.

12.   Menon ND. High-altitude pulmonary edema: A clinical study. *N Engl J Med.* 1965;273:66–73.

13.   Hackett PH, Roach RC. High altitude pulmonary edema. *J Wild Med.* 1990;1:3–26.

14.   Colcolough HL. Pulmonary edema of high altitude: A review of clinical and pathological considerations. *Mil Med.* 1966;131:1504–1509.

15.   Desmond EW. War at the top of the world. *Time.* 1989;31 Jul:26-29.

16.   Lobenhoffer HP, Zink RA, Brendel W. High altitude pulmonary edema: Analysis of 166 cases. In: Brendel W, Zink RA., eds. *High Altitude Physiology and Medicine.* New York, NY: Springer; 1982: 219–231.

17.   Hackett PH, Roach RC. High-altitude medicine. In: Auerbach PS, ed. *Wilderness Medicine.* 4th ed. St Louis, Mo: Mosby; 2001: Chap 1: 2–43.

18.   Schoene RB. Pulmonary edema at high altitude: Review, pathophysiology, and update. *Clin Chest Med.* 1985;6(3):491–507.

19.   Hackett PH, Roach RC, Sutton JR. High altitude medicine. In: Auerbach PS, Geehr EC, eds. *Management of Wilderness and Environmental Emergencies.* St Louis, Mo: C. V. Mosby; 1989: 1–34.

20.   Hultgren HN. High altitude pulmonary edema. In: Staub NC, ed. *Lung Water and Solute Exchange.* New York, NY: Marcel Dekker; 1978: 437–469.

21.   Richalet JP, Hornych A, Rathat C, Aumont J, Larmignat P, Remy P. Plasma prostaglandins, leukotrienes and thromboxane in acute high altitude hypoxia. *Respir Physiol.* 1991;85:205–215.

22.   Schoene RB, Swenson EK, Hultgren HN. High-altitude pulmonary edema. In: Hornbein TF, Schoene RB, eds. *High Altitude: An Exploration of Human Adaptation.* New York, NY: Marcel Dekker; 2001: 777–814.

23.   Hultgren HN. High altitude medical problems. *West J Med.* 1979;131:8–23.

24.   Hackett PH, Roach RC. High-altitude illness. *N Engl J Med.* 2001;345:107–114.

25.   Bärtsch P. High altitude pulmonary edema. *Med Sci Sports Exerc.* 1999;31(suppl):S23–S27.

26.   Sophocles AM Jr. High-altitude pulmonary edema in Vail, Colorado, 1975–1982. *West J Med.* 1986;144:569–573.

27. Scoggin CH, Hyers TM, Reeves JT, Grover RF. High-altitude pulmonary edema in the children and young adults of Leadville, Colorado. *N Engl J Med.* 1977;297:1269–1272.

28. Sophocles AM Jr, Bachman J. High-altitude pulmonary edema among visitors to Summit County, Colorado. *J Fam Pract.* 1983;17:1015–1017.

29. Bärtsch P, Maggiorini M, Ritter M, Noti C, Vock P, Oelz O. Prevention of high-altitude pulmonary edema by nifedipine. *N Engl J Med.* 1991;325:1284–1289.

30. Vock P, Fretz C, Franciolli M, Bärtsch P. High-altitude pulmonary edema: Findings at high-altitude chest radiography and physical examination. *Radiology.* 1989;170:661–666.

31. Hultgren HN, Spickard WB, Hellriegel K, Houston CS. High altitude pulmonary edema. *Medicine.* 1961;40:289–313.

32. Marticorena E, Tapia FA, Dyer J, et al. Pulmonary edema by ascending to high altitudes. *J Dis Chest.* 1964;45:273–283.

33. Maldonado D. High altitude pulmonary edema. *Radiol Clin North Am.* 1978;16:537–549.

34. Kobayashi T, Koyama S, Kubo K, Fukushima M, Kusama S. Clinical features of patients with high-altitude pulmonary edema in Japan. *Chest.* 1987;92:814–821.

35. Hackett PH, Roach RC, Schoene RB, Hollingshead F, Mills WJ Jr. The Denali Medical Research Project, 1982–85. *Am Alpine J.* 1986;28:129–137.

36. Marticorena E, Hultgren HN. Evaluation of therapeutic methods in high altitude pulmonary edema. *Am J Cardiol.* 1979;43:307–312.

37. Lenfant C, Sullivan K. Adaptation to high altitude. *N Engl J Med.* 1971;284:1298–1309.

38. Jaeger JJ, Sylvester JT, Cymerman A, Berberich JJ, Denniston JC, Maher JT. Evidence for increased intrathoracic fluid volume in man at high altitude. *J Appl Physiol: Respirat Environ Exercise Physiol.* 1979;47(4):670–676.

39. Hackett PH, Rennie D. Rales, peripheral edema, retinal hemorrhage and acute mountain sickness. *Am J Med.* 1979;67:214–218.

40. Koizumi T, Kawashima A, Kubo K, Kobayashi T, Sekiguchi M. Radiographic and hemodynamic changes during recovery from high-altitude pulmonary edema. *Intern Med.* 1994;33:525–528.

41. Vock P, Brutsche MH, Nanzer A, Bärtsch P. Variable radiomorphologic data of high altitude pulmonary edema: Features from 60 patients. *Chest.* 1991;100:1306–1311.

42. Hultgren H, Spickard W, Lopez C. Further studies of high altitude pulmonary edema. *British Heart Journal.* 1962;24:95–102.

43. Bachman JJ, Beatty T, Levene DE. Oxygen saturation in high-altitude pulmonary edema. *J Am Board Fam Pract.* 1992;5:429–431.

44. Roy SB, Guleria JS, Khanna PK, Manchanda SC, Pande JN, Subba PS. Haemodynamic studies in high altitude pulmonary oedema. *British Heart Journal.* 1969;31:52–58.

45. Hultgren HN, Grover RF, Hartley LH. Abnormal circulatory responses to high altitude in subjects with a previous history of high-altitude pulmonary edema. *Circulation.* 1971;44:759–770.

46. Malconian M, Rock P, Hultgren H, et al. The electrocardiogram at rest and exercise during a simulated ascent of Mt Everest (Operation Everest II). *Am J Cardiol.* 1990;65:1475–1480.

47. Milledge JS. Electrocardiographic changes at high altitude. *British Heart Journal.* 1962;25:291–298.

48. Fred HL, Schmidt AM, Bates T, Hecht HH. Acute pulmonary edema of altitude: Clinical and physiologic observations. *Circulation.* 1962;25:929–937.

49. Hultgren HN, Lopez CE, Lundberg E, Miller H. Physiologic studies of pulmonary edema at high altitude. *Circulation.* 1964;29:393–408.

50. Kawashima A, Kubo K, Kobayashi T, Sekiguchi M. Hemodynamic responses to acute hypoxia, hypobaria, and exercise in subjects susceptible to high-altitude pulmonary edema. *J Appl Physiol.* 1989;67(5):1982–1989.

51. Yagi H, Yamada H, Kobayashi T, Sekiguchi M. Doppler assessment of pulmonary hypertension induced by hypoxic breathing in subjects susceptible to high altitude pulmonary edema. *Am Rev Respir Dis.* 1990;142:796–801.

52. Vachiery JL, McDonagh T, Moraine JJ, et al. Doppler assessment of hypoxic pulmonary vasoconstriction and susceptibility to high altitude pulmonary oedema. *Thorax.* 1995;50:22–27.

53. Oelz O, Maggiorini M, Ritter M, et al. Nifedapine for high altitude pulmonary oedema. *Lancet.* 1989;2:1241–1244.

54. Hackett PH, Roach RC, Hartig GS, Greene ER, Levine BD. The effect of vasodilators on pulmonary hemodynamics in high altitude pulmonary edema: A comparison. *Int J Sports Med.* 1992;13(suppl 1):S68–S71.

55. Schoene RB, Hackett PH, Henderson WR, et al. High-altitude pulmonary edema: Characteristics of lung lavage fluid. *JAMA.* 1986;256:63–69.

56. Schoene RB, Swenson ER, Pizzo CJ, et al. The lung at high altitude: Bronchoalveolar lavage in acute mountain sickness and pulmonary edema. *J Appl Physiol.* 1988;64(6):2605–2613.

57. Schoene RB. High altitude pulmonary edema: Comparison with other forms of lung injury. *Am Rev Respir Dis.* 1986;133:A269.

58. Kubo K, Hanaoka M, Yamaguchi S, et al. Cytokines in bronchoalveolar lavage fluid in patients with high altitude pulmonary oedema at moderate altitude in Japan. *Thorax.* 1996;51:739–742.

59. Kubo K, Hanaoka M, Hayano, et al. Inflammatory cytokines in BAL fluid and pulmonary hemodynamics in high-altitude pulmonary edema. *Respir Physiol.* 1998;111:301–310.

60. Droma Y, Hayano T, Takabayashi Y, et al. Endothelin-1 and interleukin-8 in high altitude pulmonary oedema. *Eur Respir J.* 1996;9:1947–1949.

61. Arias-Stella J, Kruger H. Pathology of high altitude pulmonary edema. *Arch Pathol Lab Med.* 1963;76:147–157.

62. Hultgren HN, Wilson R, Kosek JC. Lung pathology in high-altitude pulmonary edema. *Wilderness Environ Med.* 1997;8:218–220.

63. Bärtsch P, Haeberli A, Franciolli M, Kruithof EKO, Staub PW. Coagulation and fibrinolysis in acute mountain sickness and beginning pulmonary edema. *J Appl Physiol.* 1989;66(5):2136–2144.

64. Bärtsch P, Waber U, Haeberli A, et al. Enhanced fibrin formation in high-altitude pulmonary edema. *J Appl Physiol.* 1987;63(2):752–757.

65. Heath D, Moosavi H, Smith P. Ultra structure of high altitude pulmonary edema. *Thorax.* 1973;28:694–700.

66. Hackett PH, Roach RC. Medical therapy of altitude illness. *Ann Emerg Med.* 1987;16:980–986.

67. Singh I, Khanna PK, Srivastava MC, Lal M, Roy SB, Subramanyam CVS. Acute mountain sickness. *N Engl J Med.* 1969;280:175–183.

68. Hansen JE, Evans WO. A hypothesis regarding the pathophysiology of acute mountain sickness. *Arch Environ Health.* 1970;21:666–669.

69. Meehan RT, Zavala DC. The pathophysiology of acute high-altitude illness. *Am J Med*. 1982;73:395–403.

70. Eldridge MW, Podolsky A, Richardson RS, et al. Pulmonary hemodynamic response to exercise in subjects with prior pulmonary edema. *J Appl Physiol*. 1996;81:911–921.

71. Grünig E, Mereles D, Hildebrandt W, et al. Stress doppler echocardiography for identification of susceptibility to high altitude pulmonary edema. *J Am Coll Cardiol*. 2000;35:980–987.

72. Ritter M, Jenni R, Maggorini M, et al. Abnormal left ventricular diastolic filling patterns in acute hypoxic pulmonary hypertension at high altitude. *Am J Noninvas Cardiol*. 1993;7:33–38.

73. Euler von US, Liljestrand G. Observations on the pulmonary arterial blood pressure in the cat. *Acta Physiol Scand*. 1946;12:301–320.

74. Motley HL, Cournand A, Werko L, Himmelstein A, Dresdale D. The influence of short periods of induced anoxia upon pulmonary artery pressures in man. *Am J Physiol*. 1947;150:315–320.

75. Rotta A, Canepa A, Hurtado A, Velasquez T, Chavez T. Pulmonary circulation at sea level and at high altitudes. *J Appl Physiol*. 1956;9:328–336.

76. Lockhart A, Saiag B. Altitude and the human pulmonary circulation. *Clin Sci*. 1981;60:599–605.

77. Gibbs JSR. Pulmonary hemodynamics: Implications for high altitude pulmonary edema (HAPE). In: Roach RC, Wagner PD, Hackett PH, eds. *Hypoxia: Into the Next Millennium.* New York, NY: Kluwer Academic/Plenum Pub; 1999: 81–91.

78. Duplain H, Vollenweider L, Delabays A, Nicod P, Bärtsch P, Scherrer U. Augmented sympathetic activation during short-term hypoxia and high-altitude exposure in subjects susceptible to high-altitude pulmonary edema. *Circulation*. 1999;99:1713–1718.

79. Viswanathan R, Jain KS, Subramanian S, Subramanian TAV, Dua L, Giri J. Pulmonary edema of high altitude, II: Clinical, aero-hemodynamic and biochemical studies in a group with a history of pulmonary edema of high altitude. *Am J Respir Dis*. 1969;100:334–341.

80. Naeije R, Melot C, Lejeune P. Hypoxic pulmonary vasoconstriction and high altitude pulmonary edema. *Am Rev Respir Dis*. 1986;134:332–333.

81. Marriorini M, Mélot C, Pierre S, et al. High-altitude pulmonary edema is initially caused by an increase in capillary pressure. *Circulation*. 2001;103:2078–2083.

82. Sartori C, Vollenweider L, Löeffler, et al. Exaggerated endothelin release in high-altitude pulmonary edema. *Circulation*. 1999;99:2665–2668.

83. Busch T, Bärtsch, Pappert D, et al. Hypoxia decreases exhaled nitric oxide in mountaineers susceptible to high-altitude pulmonary edema. *Am J Respir Crit Care Med*. 2001;163:368–373.

84. Beall CM, Laskowski D, Strohl KP, et al. Pulmonary nitric oxide in mountain dwellers. *Nature*. 2001;414:411–412.

85. Scherrer U, Vollenweider L, Delabays A, et al. Inhaled nitric oxide for high-altitude pulmonary edema. *N Engl J Med*. 1996;334:624–629.

86. Kleiner JP, Nelson WP. High altitude pulmonary edema: A rare disease? *JAMA*. 1975;234:491–495.

87. Staub NC. Pulmonary edema—Hypoxia and overperfusion. *N Engl J Med*. 1980;302:1085–1086.

88. Hackett PH, Creagh CE, Grover RF, et al. High-altitude pulmonary edema in persons without the right pulmonary artery. *N Engl J Med*. 1980;302:1070–1073.

89. Rios B, Driscoll DJ, McNamara DG. High-altitude edema with absent right pulmonary artery. *Pediatrics.* 1985;75:314–317.

90. Fiorenzano G, Rastelli V, Greco V, Di Stefano A, Dottorini M. Unilateral high-altitude pulmonary edema in a subject with right pulmonary artery hypoplasia. *Respiration.* 1994;61:51–54.

91. Torrington KG. Recurrent high-altitude illness associated with right pulmonary artery occlusion from granulomatous mediastinitis. *Chest.* 1989;96:1422–1423.

92. Nakagawa S, Kubo K, Koizumi T, Kobayashi T, Sekiguchi M. High-altitude pulmonary edema with pulmonary thromboembolism. *Chest.* 1993;103:948–950.

93. Derks A, Bosch FH. High-altitude pulmonary edema in partial anomalous pulmonary venous connection of drainage with intact atrial septum. *Chest.* 1993;103:973–974.

94. Waller DA, Keavey P, Woodfine L, Dark JH. Pulmonary endothelial permeability changes after major lung resection. *Ann Thorac Surg.* 1996;61(5):1435–1440.

95. West JB, Mathieu-Costello O. High altitude pulmonary edema is caused by stress failure of pulmonary capillaries. *Int J Sports Med.* 1992;13(suppl 1):S54–S58.

96. West JB, Mathieu-Costello O. Pulmonary blood–gas barrier: A physiological dilemma. *News in Physiological Sciences.* 1993;8:249–253.

97. Mathieu-Costello OA, West JB. Are pulmonary capillaries susceptible to mechanical stress? *Chest.* 1994;105(suppl):102S–107S.

98. Elliott AR, Fu Z, Tsukimoto K, Prediletto R, Mathieu-Costello O, West JB. Short-term reversibility of ultrastructural changes in pulmonary capillaries caused by stress failure. *J Appl Physiol.* 1992;73:1150–1158.

99. Peñaloza D, Sime I, Banchero N, Gamboa R. Pulmonary hypertension in healthy men born and living at high altitude. *Am J Cardiol.* 1963;11:150–157.

100. Wagner PD, Gale GE, Moon RE, Torre-Bueno JR, Stolp BW, Saltzman HA. Pulmonary gas exchange in humans exercising at sea level and simulated altitude. *J Appl Physiol.* 1986;61(1):260–270.

101. Wagner PD. Hypobaric effects on the pulmonary circulation and high altitude pulmonary edema. In: Weir EK, Reeves JT, eds. *Pulmonary Vascular Physiology and Pathophysiology.* New York, NY: Marcel Dekker; 1989: 173–198.

102. Anholm JD, Milne ECN, Stark P, Bourne JC, Friedman P. Radiographic evidence of interstitial pulmonary edema after exercise at altitude. *J Appl Physiol.* 1999;86:503–509.

103. Will DH, McMurtry IF, Reeves JT, Grover RF. Cold-induced pulmonary hypertension in cattle. *J Appl Physiol.* 1978;45:469–473.

104. Kashimura O. Effects of acute exposure to cold on pulmonary arterial blood pressure in awake rats. *Nippon Eiseigaku Zasshi.* 1993;48:859–863.

105. Chauca D, Bligh J. An additive effect of cold exposure and hypoxia on pulmonary artery pressure in sheep. *Res Vet Sci.* 1976;21:123–124.

106. Reeves JT, Wagner J, Zafren K, Honigman B, Schoene RB. Seasonal variation in barometric pressure and temperature in Summit County: Effect on altitude illness. In: Sutton JR, Houston CS, Coates G, eds. *Hypoxia and Molecular Medicine.* Burlington, Vt: Queen City Press; 1993: 275–281.

107. Masud ul Hasan Nuri M, Zulfiqar Ali Khan M, Shuaib Quraishi M. High altitude pulmonary oedema: Response to exercise and cold on systemic and pulmonary vascular beds. *Journal of the Pakistan Medical Association.* 1988;38:211–217.

108. Bezruchka S. High altitude medicine. *Med Clin North Am*. 1992;76:1481–1497.

109. Schoene RB. High altitude pulmonary edema: Pathophysiology and clinical review. *Ann Emerg Med*. 1987;16:987–992.

110. Nayak N, Roy S, Narayanan T. Pathologic features of altitude sickness. *Am J Pathol*. 1964;45:381–391.

111. Durmowicz AG, Noordeweir E, Nicholas R, Reeves JT. Inflammatory process may predispose children to high-altitude pulmonary edema. *J Pediat*. 1997;130:838–340.

112. Hanaoka M, Kubo K, Yamazaki Y, et al. Association of high-altitude pulmonary edema with the major histocompatibility complex. *Circulation*. 1998;97:1124–1128.

113. Kaminsky DA, Jones K, Schoene RB, Voelkel NF. Urinary leukotriene E_4 levels in high-altitude pulmonary edema: A possible role for inflammation. *Chest*. 1996;110:939–945.

114. Pavlicek V, Marti HH, Grad S, et al. Effects of hypobaric hypoxia on vascular endothelial growth factor and the acute phase response in subjects who are susceptible to high-altitude pulmonary oedema. *Eur J Appl Physiol*. 2000;81:497–503.

115. Kleger G-R, Bärtsch P, Vock P, Heilig B, Roberts LJ II, Ballmer PE. Evidence against an increase in capillary permeability in subjects exposed to high altitude. *J Appl Physiol*. 1996;81:1917–1923.

116. Bärtsch P, Eichenberger U, Ballmer PE, et al. Urinary leukotriene E_4 levels are not increased prior to high-altitude pulmonary edema. *Chest*. 2000;117:1393–1398.

117. Swenson E, Mogovin S, Gibbs S, et al. Stress failure in high altitude pulmonary edema [abstract]. *Am Rev Respir Crit Care Med*. 2000;161:A418.

117b. Swenson ER, Maggiorini M, Mongovin S, et al. Pathogenesis of high-altitudepulmonary edema: Inflammation is not an etiologic factor. *JAMA*. 2002;287(17):2228–2235.

118. Lakshminarayan S, Pierson DJ. Recurrent high altitude pulmonary edema with blunted chemosensitivity. *Am Rev Respir Dis*. 1975;111:869–872.

119. Hyers TM, Scoggin CH, Will DH, Grover RF, Reeves JT. Accentuated hypoxemia at high altitude in subjects susceptible to high-altitude pulmonary edema. *J Appl Physiol: Respirat Environ Exercise Physiol*. 1979;46:41–46.

120. Hackett PH, Roach RC, Schoene RB, Harrison GL, Mills WJ Jr. Abnormal control of ventilation in high-altitude pulmonary edema. *J Appl Physiol*. 1988;64(3):1268–1272.

121. Matsuzawa Y, Fujimoto K, Kobayashi T, et al. Blunted hypoxic ventilatory drive in subjects susceptible to high-altitude pulmonary edema. *J Appl Physiol*. 1989;66(3)1152–1157.

122. Hohenhaus E, Paul A, McCullough RE, Kücherer, Bärtsch P. Ventilatory and pulmonary vascular response to hypoxia and susceptibility to high altitude pulmonary oedema. *Eur Respir J*. 1995;8:1825–1833.

123. Selland MA, Stelzner TJ, Stevens T, Mazzeo RS, McCullough RE, Reeves JT. Pulmonary function and hypoxic ventilatory response in subjects susceptible to high-altitude pulmonary edema. *Chest*. 1993;103:111–116.

124. Fujimoto K, Matsuzawa Y, Hirai K, et al. Irregular nocturnal breathing patterns at high altitude in subjects susceptible to high-altitude pulmonary edema (HAPE): A preliminary study. *Aviat Space Environ Med*. 1989;60:786–791.

125. Eichenberger U, Weiss E, Riemann D, Oelz O, Bärtsch P. Nocturnal periodic breathing and the development of acute high altitude illness. *Am J Respir Crit Care Med*. 1996;154:1748–1754.

126. Bärtsch P, Pfluger N, Audetat M, et al. Effects of slow ascent to 4559 m on fluid homeostasis. *Aviat Space Environ Med*. 1991;62:105–110.

127. Tianyi W. Atrial natriuretic peptide in high altitude pulmonary edema. *International Society for Mountain Medicine Newsletter*. 1993;3(3):8–10.

128. Cosby RL, Sophocles AM, Durr JA, Perrinjaquet CL, Yee B, Schrier RW. Elevated plasma atrial natriuretic factor and vasopressin in high-altitude pulmonary edema. *Ann Intern Med*. 1988;109:796–799.

129. Bärtsch P, Shaw S, Franciolli M, Gnadinger MP, Weidmann P. Atrial natriuretic peptide in acute mountain sickness. *J Appl Physiol*. 1988;65(5):1929–1937.

130. Kawashima A, Kubo K, Matsuzawa Y, Kobayashi T, Sekiguchi M. Hypoxia-induced ANP secretion in subjects susceptible to high-altitude pulmonary edema. *Respir Physiol*. 1992;89:309–317.

131. Staub NC. Pulmonary edema. *Physiol Rev*. 1974;54;678–811.

132. Sartori C, Lepori M, Maggiorini M, Allerman Y, Nicod P, Scherrer U. Impairment of amiloride-sensitive sodium transport in individuals susceptible to high altitude pulmonary edema [abstract]. *FASEB J*. 1998;12:A231.

133. Scherrer U, Sartori C, Lepori M, et al. High-altitude pulmonary edema: From exaggerated pulmonary hypertension to a defect in transepithelial sodium transport. In: Roach RC, Wagner PD, Hackett PH. *Hypoxia Into the Next Millennium*. New York, NY: Kluwer Academic/Plenum; 1999: Chap 8: 93–107.

134. Tso EL, Wagner TJ Jr. What's up in the management of high-altitude pulmonary edema? *Md Med J*. 1993;42:641–645.

135. Feldman KW, Herndon SP. Positive expiratory pressure for the treatment of high–altitude pulmonary edema. *Lancet*. 1977;1:1036–1037.

136. Schoene RB, Roach RC, Hackett PH, Harrison G, Mills WJ Jr. High altitude pulmonary edema and exercise at 4,400 meters on Mount McKinley: Effect of expiratory positive airway pressure. *Chest*. 1985;87:330–333.

137. Larson EB. Positive airway pressure for high-altitude pulmonary oedema. *Lancet*. 1985;1:371–373.

138. Oelz O. High-altitude cerebral oedema after positive airway pressure breathing at high altitude. *Lancet*. 1983;2:1148.

139. Taber RL. Protocols for the use of a portable hyperbaric chamber for the treatment of high altitude disorders. *J Wild Med*. 1990;1:181–192.

140. King SI, Greenlee RR. Successful use of the Gamow hyperbaric bag in the treatment of altitude illness at Mount Everest. *J Wild Med*. 1990;1:193–202.

141. Robertson JA, Shlim DR. Treatment of moderate acute mountain sickness with pressurization in a portable hyperbaric (Gamow) bag. *J Wild Med*. 1991;2:268–273.

142. Hackett PH. A portable, fabric hypobaric chamber for treatment of high altitude pulmonary edema [abstract]. In: Sutton JR, Coates G, Remmers JE, eds. *Hypoxia: The Adaptations*. Philadelphia, Pa: B. C. Decker; 1995: 291.

143. Kasic JF, Yaron M, Nicholas RA, Lickteig JA, Roach R. Treatment of acute mountain sickness: Hyperbaric versus oxygen therapy. *Ann Emerg Med*. 1991;20:1109–1112.

144. Murdoch D. The portable hyperbaric chamber for the treatment of high altitude illness. *N Z Med J*. 1992;105:361–362.

145. Bock J, Hultgren HN. Emergency maneuver in high-altitude pulmonary edema. *JAMA*. 1986;255:3245–3246.

146. Gray GW, Bryan AC, Frayser R, Houston CS, Rennie IDB. Control of acute mountain sickness. *Aerospace Med*. 1971;42:81–84.

147. Hultgren HN. Furosemide for high altitude pulmonary edema. *JAMA*. 1975;234:589–590.

148. Grissom CK, Roach RC, Sarnquist FH, Hackett PH. Acetazolamide in the treatment of acute mountain sickness: Clinical efficacy and effect on gas exchange. *Ann Intern Med.* 1992;116:461–465.

149. Sutton JR, Houston CS, Mansell AL, et al. Effect of acetazolamide on hypoxemia during sleep at high altitude. *N Engl J Med.* 1979;301(24):1329–1331.

150. Hackett PH, Roach RC, Harrison GL, Schoene RB, Mills WJ. Respiratory stimulants and sleep periodic breathing at high altitude: Almitrine versus acetazolamide. *Am Rev Respir Dis.* 1987;135:896–898.

151. Larson EB, Roach RC, Schoene RB, Hornbein TF. Acute mountain sickness and acetazolamide: Clinical efficacy and effect on ventilation. *JAMA.* 1982;248:328–332.

152. Oelz O. A case of high-altitude pulmonary edema treated with nifedipine. *JAMA.* 1987;257:780.

153. Oelz O, Maggiorini M, Ritter M, et al. Prevention and treatment of high altitude pulmonary edema by a calcium channel blocker. *Int J Sports Med.* 1992;13(suppl 1):S65–S68.

154. Hohenhaus E, Niroomand F, Goerre S, Vock P, Oelz O, Bärtsch P. Nifedipine does not prevent acute mountain sickness. *Am J Respir Crit Care Med.* 1994;150:857–860.

Chapter 26

ADDITIONAL MEDICAL PROBLEMS IN MOUNTAIN ENVIRONMENTS

PAUL B. ROCK, DO, PhD[*]; AND THOMAS H. MADER, MD[†]

[*]Colonel, Medical Corps, US Army (Ret); Associate Professor of Medicine, Center for Aerospace and Hyperbaric Medicine, Oklahoma State University Center for the Health Sciences, Tulsa, Oklahoma 74132; formerly, US Army Research Institute of Environmental Medicine, Natick, Massachusetts 01760
[†]Colonel, Medical Corps, US Army (Ret); formerly, Chief of Ophthalmology, Madigan Army Medical Center, Tacoma, Washington 98431-5000; currently, Alaska Native Medical Center, Anchorage, Alaska 99508

INTRODUCTION

Acute mountain sickness (AMS), high-altitude cerebral edema (HACE), and high-altitude pulmonary edema (HAPE), which were discussed in the two previous chapters of this textbook (Chapter 24, Acute Mountain Sickness and High-Altitude Cerebral Edema, and Chapter 25, High-Altitude Pulmonary Edema), are probably the most familiar and notorious altitude-associated medical problems to mountaineers and medical personnel. These disorders occur only in high mountains, are common, and are potentially life-threatening. From a military standpoint they are important because they increase the rate of disease and nonbattle injuries and degrade performance, both of which can jeopardize a military unit's mission. These well-known altitude illnesses are not the only medical problems that occur in mountain terrain, however, and certainly are not the only ones to have significant potential impact on soldier performance. The complex tableaux of terrain and climatic features of mountains can cause a variety of medical problems in visitors and permanent inhabitants alike. Although many of these problems are not caused by hypoxia and, therefore, are not unique to high altitude (ie, hemorrhoids), the specific *constellation* of problems is characteristic of high mountain environments. Steele's[1] lively description of the medical support of the 1971 International Himalayan Expedition, for instance, provides an example of the scope of injury and illness that can be inflicted by the mountain environment. To be adequately prepared to care for people in the mountains, military and civilian medical personnel should be familiar with the whole range of problems that can occur.

The purpose of this chapter is to describe the types of illness and injury other than AMS, HACE, and HAPE that commonly occur in high mountain environments. The intent is to facilitate an awareness of the characteristic constellation of problems so that medical personnel supporting military units deploying to mountain regions are prepared to treat more than the familiar altitude illnesses. Problems that are unique to mountains (ie, those directly related to hypobaric hypoxia) are described in some detail. These include peripheral edema, altitude-related eye problems, sleep disturbances, thromboembolic disorders, suppression of immune function, wound healing, high-altitude pharyngitis and bronchitis, and exacerbation of preexisting medical conditions. Conditions that occur in mountains but may be more characteristic of other environments (eg, cold injury, carbon monoxide poisoning) are described in less detail. Readers are referred to other chapters in this volume or different volumes in the *Textbook of Military Medicine* series for more-extensive discussion of those problems, and to Exhibit 19-1 in Chapter 19, Mountains and Military Medicine: An Overview, for definitions of the categories of visitors to high mountains.

MEDICAL PROBLEMS CAUSED BY HYPOXIA

The spectrum of hypoxia-related medical problems other than "classic" altitude illness is a potpourri, affecting different body systems and ranging from benign to serious in consequence and from common to rare in occurrence. All of these problems can have a negative impact on military operations by diminishing unit manpower or degrading individual performance. Because they are related to hypoxia, they tend to be increasingly frequent and more severe at higher elevations. Most are rare and mild at altitudes under 3,000 m and quite common at altitudes over 5,000 m. As with AMS, HACE, and HAPE, the most effective treatment for all of these hypoxia-related problems is descent to lower altitude, a treatment option that may not always be available during bad weather or combat.

High-Altitude Peripheral Edema

Given that the progressive hypobaric hypoxia in high mountain environments can cause edema in the brain and lungs, it should not be surprising that edema occurs in other tissues as well. "High-altitude peripheral" or "systemic" edema refers to edema of the face, extremities, or both during altitude exposure in the absence of other causes of edema (eg, congestive heart failure, cirrhosis, kidney failure). Two manifestations of altitude-related peripheral edema are described in the literature, one associated with altitude illness, the other occurring as a seemingly isolated clinical condition. Additionally, "stasis" edema (which is not caused by hypoxia and can be seen in other settings) can occur in the arms and legs due to impeded venous blood return by constriction from climbers' bulky, multilayered clothing or from tight straps on rucksacks and climbing harnesses.

Although the Moguls in central Asia apparently described "swelling of the hands and feet" as a sign of mountain sickness in the 14th century,[2] and climbers have been aware of the condition for many years, the first descriptions of high-altitude peripheral edema in the modern medical literature were in the 1960s and early 1970s. Waterlow and Bunjè[3] recorded "oedema of the hands and face" in a single volunteer test subject whose symptoms were consistent with HACE. Singh and colleagues[4] reported lower-extremity edema occurring in many soldiers who had symptoms of altitude illness. Shortly thereafter, a seemingly benign form of peripheral edema affecting the face and extremities while climbing a mountain in the tropics was reported by Sheridan and Sheridan.[5] Although some literature describes this peripheral edema without accompanying altitude illness as if it were an independent entity,[6] the consensus is that all altitude edemas are manifestations of the same pathological process, a concept first proposed by Hackett and colleagues.[7]

Signs and symptoms of high-altitude peripheral edema include facial edema, often prominent periorbital edema, and/or edema in the upper and lower extremities (Figure 26-1). It is associated with a weight gain of 4 to 6 kg (6–12 lb),[6] or as much as 6% of body weight.[8] Steele[1] described a young woman whose peripheral edema at 5,300 m (17,800 ft) was accompanied by a weight gain of 8.6 kg (19 lb), or approximately 20% of her normal body weight. The weight gain associated with peripheral edema is often apparent as a bloated feeling or uncomfortable tightness of clothing. Facial edema may become apparent as creases left in the skin by sun goggles or headbands. Likewise, edema of the extremities may cause skin indentations left by rings, watch bands, gloves, or socks and boots.

The incidence of high-altitude peripheral edema has not been well delineated but may be substantial even at lower altitudes. Hackett and Rennie[9] documented a 16% to 18% incidence in trekkers at 4,243 m in the Himalayan mountains, while Bärtsch and colleagues[10,11] reported a 40% to 70% incidence in male mountaineers at 4,559 m in the Alps. High-altitude peripheral edema appears to be more common in women than men but is not clearly associated with the fluctuation of menstrual cycle hormones or with ingestion of birth control pills or estrogen replacement therapy.[9,12] It also is much more common in individuals with altitude illness. Bärtsch and colleagues[11] found facial edema in 73% of individuals with AMS, compared with 28% in individuals without. Hackett and Rennie[12] reported some form of peripheral edema in 64% of individuals with AMS and 43% of individuals without.

There is a general consensus that the underlying pathophysiology of all the altitude-related edemas

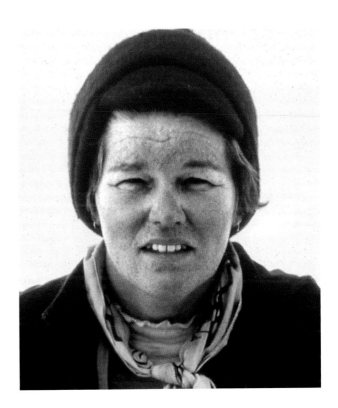

Fig. 26-1. High-altitude peripheral edema manifested by periorbital and facial swelling is seen in a woman at about 4,400 m during a mountain-climbing expedition. Other common signs of this condition include body-weight gain and swelling in the distal portions of the arms and legs. Altitude-related peripheral edema is often associated with altitude illness, and this woman had symptoms of acute mountain sickness. High-altitude peripheral edema may be more common in women than men but is not related to either the menstrual cycle or hormone therapy. Photograph: Courtesy of Peter Hackett, MD, Seattle, Washington.

is similar,[7] and various postulated mechanisms are presented in Chapter 21, Human Adaptation to High Terrestrial Altitude; Chapter 24, Acute Mountain Sickness and High-Altitude Cerebral Edema; and Chapter 25, High-Altitude Pulmonary Edema. Low arterial oxygen saturation (Sa_{O_2}) from relative hypoventilation probably initiates increased capillary and small-vessel leakage[8] through activation of permeability mediators.[13,14] Increased blood flow and blood pressure in specific organs and tissues, mediated through increased sympathetic nervous activity, accelerates edema formation in the brain, lungs, and peripheral tissues.[15] Insufficient peripheral arterial chemoreceptor-mediated diuresis and natriuresis,[16] changes in renal blood flow,[17] and perturbations in the fluid-volume regulatory hormones (renin-angiotensin-aldosterone system, arginine vasopressin, and atrial natriuretic peptide) due to hypoxia,[10] exertion, or both probably also contribute.[11,18] The extent and distribution of edema formation is a function of the complex interaction of all these factors and possibly more.

Diagnosis of high-altitude peripheral edema is based on the presence of signs and symptoms of edema in the face or extremities following ascent to a higher altitude. A history of previous episodes in mountain terrain helps to strengthen the diagnosis. Some individuals seem to develop peripheral edema consistently above a certain "trigger" altitude.[6,12] It is important to rule out other potential causes of peripheral edema, especially edema associated with life-threatening medical conditions. The differential diagnosis includes the usual causes of edema seen at sea level such as congestive heart failure, cirrhosis, renal failure, and so forth, none of which is likely in a relatively young, healthy, military population. Anand and colleagues[19] reported congestive heart failure in young soldiers deployed to extreme altitude for long periods of time, however. Most of the conditions included in the differential diagnosis can be ruled out through clinical history and physical exam. Stasis edema due to pressure of pack straps or constrictive clothing is identified by its resolution after the constriction is removed. Given that most altitude-induced peripheral edema is associated with other forms of altitude illness, its presence should prompt an evaluation for HAPE or HACE.

Recommended treatment of uncomplicated high-altitude peripheral edema is poorly defined because no controlled studies have been reported. The usual treatment is salt restriction and induction of a mild diuresis. Adequate salt restriction can usually be achieved by avoiding foods with high sodium content (eg, meat jerky, junk foods, some ethnic foods, many military rations) and by not adding salt to foods during preparation or consumption. When necessary, appropriate diuresis can be achieved with low-dose furosemide (20 mg/d) or another diuretic. Prophylaxis consists of starting salt restriction several days prior to ascending and starting a diuretic during the ascent. Prophylaxis for AMS using acetazolamide will also prevent peripheral edema and may be the best choice for individuals with a history of AMS accompanied by peripheral edema.[20]

The clinical course of altitude peripheral edema is not well documented, but the prognosis appears relatively good if it is not associated with more menacing forms of altitude illness. Many untreated individuals remain edematous for the entire time

they are above their trigger altitude but diurese rapidly when they return to lower elevations.[6] Others may eventually diurese at high altitude as they acclimatize. Most are uncomfortable enough while edematous that they prefer not to remain at altitude waiting to acclimatize. Treatment and prophylaxis are said to be nearly universally effective, but in susceptible individuals, edema may recur on every ascent if not treated. Given the benign but predictably recurrent nature of this condition, susceptible military personnel do not need to be medically restricted from high altitude but should probably receive prophylactic treatment when the mission takes them into mountain terrain.

Problems in the Eye

Several problems can occur in the eyes during high altitude exposure. Both the retina and the cornea are affected by hypoxia. Snowblindness from exposure to high levels of ultraviolet (UV) radiation is also a potential problem. Although most altitude-related eye problems are temporary, changes in visual acuity can increase the risk for accidents and put a soldier at great risk during combat.

High-Altitude Retinopathy

The term high-altitude retinopathy (HAR) describes a spectrum of retinal changes associated with exposure to prolonged hypobaric hypoxia at high altitude. The changes include retinal hemorrhage, vitreous hemorrhage, cotton wool spots, and optic disc edema. HAR is common during altitude exposure and has been well documented for several decades. In the 1930s, Sedan[21] described retinal hemorrhages in hypertensive subjects at 3,650 m. Singh and colleagues[4] reported papilledema and engorgement of retinal veins and vitreous hemorrhages in Indian troops exposed to high altitude in 1969. In 1970, Frayser and colleagues[22] reported a 37.5% incidence of high-altitude retinal hemorrhages (HARHs) among otherwise healthy climbers at 5,360 m on Mount Logan in Canada. McFadden and colleagues[23] first reported cotton wool spots in the retina at high altitude in 1981. Numerous other reports have described high-altitude retinal changes in studies of climbers,[24–31] at high-altitude laboratories,[22,23] and in a hypobaric chamber.[32]

The first retinal changes associated with altitude exposure are usually disc hyperemia and an increase in retinal vascular diameter and tortuosity (Figure 26-2).[22–26,33–36] These changes are almost universally observed at altitude and probably represent a normal

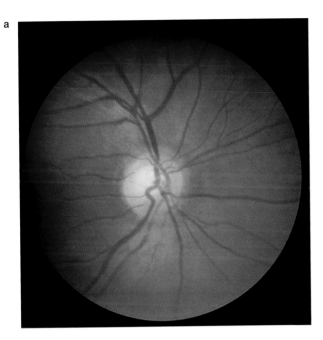
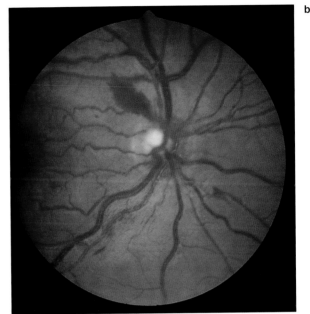

Fig. 26-2. High-altitude retinopathy in the right eye of a 26-year-old male volunteer test subject (**a**) at sea level and (**b**) at 7,620 m altitude-equivalent pressure in a hypobaric chamber following a gradual decompression over 4 weeks.[1] At high altitude, the vessels are engorged and tortuous. There is a large, flame-shaped hemorrhage in the peripapillary region. There are smaller flame-shaped hemorrhages further away from the optic disk and a "dot-blot" hemorrhage near the macula. There is slight papilledema. The retinopathy did not cause symptoms and resolved completely over several weeks following descent. (1) Rock PB, Meehan RT, Malconian MK, et al. Operation Everest II: Incidence of retinal pathology during simulated ascent of Mt Everest [abstract]. *Federation Proceedings.* 1986;45:1030.

response to hypoxia (as opposed to a true pathological condition). Although apparently benign, retinal vascular dilation and tortuosity may be striking on examination, and the mechanism of these changes may provide some insight into the early retinal vascular response to altitude exposure. The overall blood supply to the retina is from the terminal branches of the internal carotid artery. The retina itself has a dual blood supply. The central retinal artery branches from the optic disc to supply the inner layers of the retina, and its diameter is controlled by autoregulation. The choroid, which supplies the outer retina, is a spongy vascular plexus without autoregulation. With increasing altitude, there is a precipitous drop in ocular oxygenation.[37] As the level of oxygenation decreases, autoregulation causes observable dilation of retinal arteries and veins. In conjunction with the increase in retinal vascular diameter, there is a concurrent lengthening of the vessel. Because the vasculature is tethered to the retina and cannot elongate longitudinally, this lengthening results in vascular tortuosity. These changes progress with increasing altitude and may be prominent at extreme altitude. The changes are purely vascular, however, and reverse with decreasing altitude, leaving no residual effects.

The most widely recognized manifestation of HAR is HARH. These retinal hemorrhages have been reported extensively in the medical literature, particularly since the early 1970s. Although one report[32] described HARH in subjects exposed to hypobaric hypoxia in an altitude chamber, all other reports have involved subjects exposed to high altitude in mountain laboratories[22,23] or during mountaineering expeditions.[21,22,24–31]

The exact appearance and position of the hemorrhages varies somewhat but most are flame-shaped, "dot and blot," or splinter hemorrhages and appear in the peripapillary area or near or between the vascular arcades. Fundus photographs suggest that the hemorrhages can be preretinal,[22,23] intraretinal,[29,36] or extend into the vitreous.[4,29] Fluorescein angiography of established hemorrhages has demonstrated blockage of underlying fluorescence with no leakage in the hemorrhagic area.[23]

Hemorrhages occurring outside the macula are usually asymptomatic, self-limited, and resolve without sequelae. HARHs are *not* always transient and innocuous, however. Macular hemorrhages may cause a sudden loss of central vision.[27] Although some degree of recovery can be anticipated, a permanent decrement in central visual acuity or a pericentral scotoma can occur following macular hemorrhage.[22,23,31]

There is no clear threshold altitude for occurrence of HARHs, and they have been reported at altitudes as low as 3,650 m.[21] The reported incidence is extremely variable, probably owing to differences in altitude, rates of ascent, method of documentation, and duration of altitude exposure. In general, however, the higher the ascent, the higher will be the incidence and severity of HARH. HARHs occur in approximately one third to one half of subjects exposed to altitudes in excess of 5,000 m.[23,26,28,30] They occur in nearly 100% of those ascending above 6,500 m.[25]

Although HARH has been observed in both healthy climbers and those with AMS,[22] HARH may be more common in those with AMS. Schumacher and Petajan[28] reported a progressive rise in the incidence of retinal hemorrhages correlated with increased intensity of high-altitude headaches. Hackett and Rennie[9] found that of 13 mountain trekkers with HARH, 11 had AMS, 7 had pulmonary rales, and 4 had HAPE or HACE. Wiedman and Tabin[38] reported a statistically significant correlation between HAR and HACE in climbers who reached altitudes between 4,800 and 8,854 m on Mount Everest; although they reported a high incidence of HACE, however, they did not report the criteria that they used for diagnosing HACE.

There is conflicting information regarding the effect of acclimatization, as reflected by slower ascent rate, on the incidence of HARH. In a study[9] of more than 200 trekkers at 4,243 m in the Himalayan mountains examined for retinal hemorrhage, no difference was found in the incidence of HARH in subjects who flew to an altitude of 2,800 m and then ascended on foot compared with those who walked from 1,300 m and, therefore, were better acclimatized. One other report[22] also suggests no relation between HARH and rate of ascent. This is in contrast with studies that suggest that the incidence of HARH was decreased in subjects who had undergone gradual, as opposed to more rapid, ascent.[23,28,29]

HARH may be exacerbated by exercise. During a study at 5,360 m on Mount Logan in Canada, McFadden and colleagues[23] observed new hemorrhages in 7 of 34 subjects after maximum exertion on a cycle ergometer. Additionally, peripapillary fluorescein leakage associated with exercise-induced hemorrhages was noted in 8 of 20 subjects examined with fluorescein. Whether the retinal vasculature leakage was due to increased mechanical pressure from increased blood flow, exercise-

induced hypoxemia, or a combination of both, was unclear.

The pathogenesis of HARH is a subject of debate but is probably due to the complex interaction of several factors. The hypoxia-induced increase in retinal blood flow at high altitude is accompanied by retinal vascular dilation. With dilation, linear velocity of the blood decreases and lateral pressure increases, causing more mechanical stress on the vessel wall.[24] It is possible that while the vasculature is distended, increases in venous back pressure may cause fragile vessel walls to rupture. Valsalva stress associated with coughing, defecating, and strenuous exercise may cause an elevation in reflex venous pressure in the eye and increase the likelihood of vessel rupture.[24,26,28] The finding of fluorescein leakage following vigorous exercise at 5,360 m reinforces this hypothesis.[23] The hypothesis is also supported by reports of retinal hemorrhages similar in appearance to HARH associated with Valsalva stress in the absence of hypoxia.[39,40]

Hypoxia and hypocapnia may have a direct effect on the vascular endothelium, causing increased vascular permeability.[22–24,41] Microscopic examination of retinal tissue from a climber who died as a result of HACE after an ascent to 5,330 m documented endothelial damage to the retinal vasculature at the nerve fiber layer level in an area of macroscopic retinal hemorrhage.[42] Based on their findings, Lubin, Rennie, and Hackett[42] hypothesized that hypoxia may cause a defect in capillary endothelial integrity, leading to extravasation of blood. They concluded that the hemorrhages were from both retinal capillaries and retinal veins. The fact that HARHs frequently occur away from major vessels also supports a capillary origin. Because most retinal hemorrhages occur in the nerve fiber layer within the distribution of the radial peripapillary capillaries, it is possible that some HARHs may also occur in this vascular net. The radial peripapillary capillaries are a distinct strata of capillaries occupying the superficial portion of the nerve fiber layer in the peripapillary retina.[43–46]

Many other possible causes for HARH have been suggested. Decreased intraocular pressure (IOP) reported in some altitude studies has been hypothesized to set the stage for HARH, presumably due to the decreased tamponade effect of IOP on the retinal vasculature.[31,35,36,47] However, not all studies have found a decrease in IOP at altitude.[29,48] Systemic hypertension has also been implicated as a causative factor.[24] Other possible predisposing factors include hemoconcentration and blood hyperviscosity caused by fluid shifts and dehydration at altitude.[31,42,49] These conditions may lead to increased coagulability and decreased oxygen transport, which could contribute to the pathogenesis of HARH.

Some researchers suggest that high-altitude exposure may lead to low-grade cerebral edema, increased cerebrospinal fluid pressure, mild papilledema, and compression of retinal veins, all of which may predispose a climber to HARH.[31,42] However, in experimentally produced intracranial hypertension in rhesus monkeys, Hayreh and Hayreh[50] documented that venous dilation is a comparatively late phenomenon and should not be used as a criteria for early papilledema. Even eyes with marked optic disc edema showed no capillary dilation or retinal hemorrhages.[50]

The actual contribution of any of the proposed factors predisposing to HARH is open to question. Additionally, a wide spectrum of retinal changes is noted in individuals with nearly identical climbing profiles (ie, altitude exposures). Thus, retinal vascular response to altitude appears to be diverse, suggesting that different factors may be more or less important in different individuals.

Other than avoiding high-altitude exposure, there are few agreed-on measures to prevent HARH. Although anecdotal information suggests some protection from previous exposure to high altitude, there appears to be no significant correlation between preclimb altitude exposure and the incidence of HARH.[29,30] Acetazolamide decreases the symptoms and incidence of AMS but has not been conclusively demonstrated to lessen the incidence of HARH.[22,23] Although evidence is scanty, gender and race probably have no impact on the rate of occurrence or extent of HARH.[23] Since HARH can be associated with AMS, it seems logical to follow the same general guidelines that are used to lessen the symptoms of AMS (see Chapter 24, Acute Mountain Sickness and High-Altitude Cerebral Edema). Avoidance of vigorous exercise and performing Valsalva maneuvers at altitude also may be prudent.

There is no specific treatment for HARH, and the hemorrhages usually resolve in 2 to 3 months.[24,31] Administration of oxygen may alleviate symptoms of AMS, but it does not necessarily prevent or decrease the extent of retinal hemorrhages. Hemodilution, which may decrease blood viscosity and coagulability in dehydrated climbers, has been reported[49] as a treatment for retinal hemorrhages associated with visual decrement. Documentation of the best corrected baseline visual acuity to provide a comparison for any subsequent visual loss is prudent.

Any unexplained visual complaints during altitude exposure should prompt bilateral, dilated fundus examination to search for intraocular pathology. As with all altitude illness, the most effective measure to prevent further hemorrhage is evacuation to a lower altitude, preferably lower than 3,000 m. Asymptomatic HARHs, those not involving the macula, are usually not considered significant enough to dictate descent to a lower altitude.[23] It may be prudent to evacuate individuals with macular or vitreous hemorrhages to a lower altitude, because such changes may interfere with central vision and could worsen with increasing altitude. It is also advisable that individuals with previous symptomatic retinal hemorrhages not return to high altitude because of the possibility that hemorrhage will recur to the same area.

Several authors have hypothesized that owing to similarities in the cerebral and the retinal circulation, changes observed in the retina may also occur simultaneously in the brain.[25,42] Such changes were documented by Lubin, Rennie, and Hackett[42] in autopsy studies. From these studies, Wiedman and Tabin[25] concluded that (1) HARH may be a prognostic indicator for altitude illness and (2) those ascending to high altitude should be monitored by funduscopic exam for HARH as an early warning sign of impending, more-serious altitude illness. Because HARH may occur in healthy individuals or those with minimal symptoms of AMS, it is probably not necessary to do serial dilated exams on all asymptomatic individuals at high altitude. This obviously would be very difficult in a military unit deployed in a tactical situation. However, Wiedman and Tabin[25] recommend that if a person has symptoms or signs of cerebral edema, then careful serial fundus examinations may provide useful additional information.

Edema of the optic disc at high altitude has been well described, and it occurs as a result of HACE. Ocular manifestations include pronounced disc hyperemia and swelling. It should be emphasized that, using direct ophthalmoscopy, it can be difficult to distinguish prominent disc hyperemia and vasodilatation from true early disc edema. Binocular examination by a 78-diopter (D) or 90 D lens at a slitlamp is probably the most reliable method of documentation. Because the facilities for such examinations are rarely available at altitude, serial examinations using a hand-held direct ophthalmoscope are usually the most practical option. Regardless of specific etiology, *true disc edema represents the ocular manifestation of increased intracranial pressure and should be considered a life-threatening condition.*

Immediate evacuation to a lower altitude is mandatory, with treatment as detailed in Chapter 24, Acute Mountain Sickness and High-Altitude Cerebral Edema.

High-altitude exposure may predispose a climber to other sight-threatening conditions. Although not common, cotton wool spots (an area of infarction of the nerve fiber layer[51]) have been observed at high altitude.[23,29] Since systemic hypoxemia would not be expected to cause localized areas of ischemia, it is hypothesized that these may occur as a result of microembolization. Microemboli may be formed by platelet aggregates, which have been reported to develop during hypoxic conditions.[23,52] Cotton wool spots cause scotoma in the visual fields corresponding to the size and location of the lesion. McFadden and associates[23] documented a persistent visual field loss 2 years after a well-documented occurrence of a cotton wool spot during a high-altitude laboratory study. There is no specific treatment for cotton wool spots, but descent to a lower altitude is never inappropriate.

Central retinal vein occlusion with permanent visual loss has also been reported at altitude. Butler and colleagues[29] described a patient whose vision, after what was thought to be a vitreous hemorrhage, deteriorated to "finger counting" following ascent to 5,909 m. Following resolution of the vitreous hemorrhage, a widespread area of capillary nonperfusion was noted by fluorescein angiography, consistent with ischemic central retinal vein occlusion. The patient subsequently underwent panretinal photocoagulation. Although central retinal vein occlusion at high altitude is extremely uncommon, this report underscores the potential for permanent visual loss associated with high-altitude exposure.

In summary, HAR consists of retinal changes ranging in severity from relatively asymptomatic retinal hemorrhages to potentially sight-threatening conditions such as macular hemorrhages and nerve fiber layer infarcts. Life-threatening HACE may be manifest in the eye as papilledema. All of the retinal changes occur as the result of hypobaric hypoxia associated with exposure to increased altitude. Individuals vary widely in their susceptibility to high-altitude retinopathy, and other than avoiding altitude exposure, there are no sure means to prevent it. There is no definitive treatment. Individuals who develop symptoms should be evacuated to lower altitude to avoid worsening of any visual decrement.

High Altitude and Refractive Surgery

Since the mid 1980s, refractive surgery for the correction of myopia has become increasingly popular. In the military it is an attractive alternative to eyeglasses or contact lenses in the field and eliminates the necessity for optical inserts in protective masks. Historically, the most popular procedure for the correction of myopia has been radial keratotomy (RK), which is widely available, heavily advertised, and performed extensively in active young people wishing to rid themselves of glasses. The procedure normally consists of four to eight radial incisions made in the periphery of the cornea at approximately 90% corneal depth, leaving the central 3 to 4 mm of the cornea untouched. These incisions cause the cornea to steepen peripherally and flatten centrally, thus decreasing myopia and improving distance visual acuity. The procedure requires minimal instrumentation to perform, is comparatively inexpensive, causes only mild discomfort, and usually results in excellent, predictable vision almost immediately following surgery.

Evidence suggests that some radial keratotomy patients may experience visual difficulties following exposure to changing oxygen concentration.[48,53–56] In the late 1980s and early 1990s, two case reports described a hyperopic (farsighted) shift in refraction and increased corneal flattening in radial keratotomy patients exposed to altitudes of 2,743 m to 3,048 m.[53,57] At the time, the authors of the 1988 report[57] hypothesized that hypobaria alone was responsible for the observed changes.

In 1994, research confirmed a significant increase in spherical equivalence in four eyes that had undergone RK surgery (ie, four RK eyes) exposed to altitude compared with four "normal" controls.[54] The average increase in spherical equivalent, cycloplegic refraction from sea level to 3,657 m was 1.03 ± 0.16 D and from sea level to 5,182 m was 1.94 ± 0.26 D. A flattening of the cornea that increased with altitude was also noted. The subjects who had undergone RK surgery (ie, RK subjects) did not have a subjective change in visual acuity until after an overnight stay at either altitude. This study also documented a prominent decrease in near and far visual acuity in a 49-year-old RK subject at 5,182 m. The individual was unable to read his watch, operate a combination lock, or even assemble a portable cookstove at this altitude, and his distance visual acuity was reduced from 20/20 at sea level to 20/50 bilaterally at altitude. Fortunately, this severe visual impairment occurred in an indoor research facility rather than in an environment where such visual changes could have proved dangerously debilitating. The same year, Ng and colleagues[56] failed to find a hyperopic shift in nine RK subjects following 6 hours at a simulated altitude of 3,660 m in an altitude chamber. This extended time to produce visual changes suggests a metabolic origin, as opposed to a purely pressure-related phenomenon.

A more-definitive study was performed in 11 eyes of six RK subjects, 12 eyes of six subjects who had undergone photorefractive keratectomy (PRK), and 17 eyes of nine myopic controls during a 72-hour exposure to 4,270 m.[48] Cycloplegic refraction, IOP, keratometry, computerized video keratography, and corneal pachymetry were measured every 24 hours. Although no measurable change occurred on day 1, RK eyes had a significant shift by day 3, with a 3.75 D shift documented in one patient. Keratometry confirmed a 1.29 D corneal flattening by day 3 in the RK group. There was no significant change in cycloplegic refraction or keratometry in the PRK or control groups. No change in IOP was found in any group, but all three groups had a statistically significant increase in peripheral corneal thickness. A myopic shift back to baseline refraction occurred several days after return to sea level. This study firmly established that a progressive increase in hyperopia and corneal thickness occurred in RK eyes during 72 hours of high-altitude exposure. It also established that PRK corneas were stable at high altitude.

In 1996, 20 eyes in 10 subjects who had undergone RK surgery and 20 eyes of 10 myopic controls were studied at sea level to determine whether the changes seen at altitude were due to hypoxia or hypobaria.[55] Subjects were fitted with airtight goggles in which one eye was exposed to anoxic conditions (humidified nitrogen, 0% oxygen), and the other eye was exposed to humidified room air. There was a significant hyperopic shift of 1.24 D and corneal flattening of 1.19 D after only 2 hours in the RK eyes exposed to nitrogen. Radial keratotomy eyes exposed to humidified room air had no refractive change, nor did non-RK eyes exposed to either nitrogen or room air. Both RK and non-RK eyes exposed to nitrogen had a significant increase in corneal thickness. These findings strongly supported the hypothesis that hypoxia causes metabolic alterations within the RK cornea that result in refractive change. Because all the changes occurred at sea level, hypobaria could not be the cause.

The specific physiological mechanism responsible for refractive changes in RK eyes is not proven. However, research suggests that when the normal corneal architecture is weakened by radial incisions, the hypoxic cornea may expand in two dimensions (both thickness and circumference) perpendicular to the keratotomy incisions.[48,54,55,58] Perhaps even a small amount of hypoxia-induced increase in stromal hydration near the RK sites may cause a circumferential expansion and subsequent elevation of the cornea peripheral to the optical zone. This annular band of corneal expansion could lead to central corneal flattening within the optical zone and a resultant hyperopic shift. The cornea of an RK eye appears to adjust constantly to changing environmental oxygen concentration, producing a new refractive error over a period of 24 hours or more. The data suggest that both the hyperopic shift and the corneal flattening in radial keratotomy subjects (1) are progressive with increasing altitude and (2) return to normal after reexposure to sea level.[48,54–56,58]

The hypoxia-induced changes in RK eyes result in delayed visual difficulties at high altitude.[59] All reports have documented that approximately 24 hours of altitude exposure are needed to cause the hyperopic shift and associated visual changes.[48,53,54,58,59] Thus visual changes might not be observed immediately on arrival at a new altitude. A soldier or pilot could arrive at a new elevation with normal vision but awaken the following morning to a prominent change in visual acuity. The additional hypoxic insult of lid closure during sleep may add to the magnitude of the change.

The magnitude of postoperative refractive error is an important factor in predicting visual problems in RK eyes during high-altitude exposure. The starting point of the hyperopic shift is as important a determinant of visual changes as the absolute amount of shift.[58] For example, if an RK subject with 2 D of residual myopia at sea level has a 2-D hyperopic shift at altitude, then he will note an improvement in distant visual acuity. However, an RK emmetrope (no refractive error) may observe a very noticeable decrease in visual acuity associated with a 2-D hyperopic shift. Additionally, older subjects with diminished accommodative amplitude may experience more profound visual changes than younger subjects with greater amplitude.

There is no known practical method to reverse the hyperopic shift that can occur in RK eyes during altitude exposure. However, soldiers who have undergone RK may be aided by plus lenses (reading glasses) at high altitudes for crisp near and far vision. One RK climber has successfully used such lenses during ascents to altitudes in excess of 6,000 m.[58] Unfortunately, it is very difficult to predict the exact lens power needed at a given altitude. Thus, if travel to extreme altitude is planned, multiple spectacles with increasing plus power should be considered.

Since the mid 1990s, two additional methods of refractive surgery (*laser in situ keratomileusis* [LASIK] and photorefractive keratectomy [PRK]) for correcting corneal abnormalities to improve myopia and hyperopia have largely replaced the RK technique. Both LASIK and PRK use laser light to reshape the overall cornea more uniformly than is possible with the few narrow radial incisions made in the cornea during RK. Theoretically, a cornea reshaped with these techniques should swell uniformly when it becomes hypoxic at high altitude and, thus, not change its refractive index as drastically as corneas subjected to RK. LASIK, however, incorporates a circumferential surgical flap in the cornea that might affect hypoxia-induced swelling in a manner similar to RK. Indeed, anecdotal reports and results of initial studies suggest that the vision of individuals who have undergone LASIK is affected by hypoxia, while individuals who have undergone PRK may not experience the vision problems.

A case report[60] of a woman with low myopia 2 years after LASIK stated that she had stable refraction, uncorrected visual acuity, and near-point conversion between 3,300 and 4,800 m altitude for 1 to 10 days. However, when Nelson and colleagues[61] studied 40 eyes in 20 subjects who had undergone LASIK and 40 eyes in 20 myopic control subjects who had not undergone LASIK, using air-tight goggles to expose one eye of each subject to humidified nitrogen to create ocular surface hypoxia and the other eye to humidified air (normoxia) for 2 hours, they found increased central corneal thickness in all eyes, which was associated with a myopic shift in refraction in the post-LASIK subjects. They attributed the changes to a combination of mechanical and metabolic mechanisms.

Unlike RK and LASIK, post-PRK eyes may not be greatly affected by exposure to high altitude. Mader and colleagues[62] studied six subjects (12 eyes) who had undergone PRK at sea level and during 72 hours exposure to 4,300 m and compared them with six subjects (11 eyes) who had undergone RK and nine unoperated myopic control subjects (17 eyes) undergoing the same altitude exposure. They reported significant hypoxia-induced corneal thickening in all individuals, but only the post-RK

individuals demonstrated a shift in refractive error. On the basis of these results of the studies reported to date, it appears that PRK is preferable to both RK and LASIK for correcting acuity related to corneal shape abnormalities in individuals who may spend time at high altitudes.

Sleep Disturbances

"Poor sleep" is a nearly universal experience during a trip to high mountains. Many mountain travelers attribute their sleep problems to travel-related factors such as jet lag, cold temperature, an unfamiliar bed, sleeping on the ground, and other causes of "insomnia" that are common at low altitude and very common during military deployments. While such factors may contribute, the primary cause of sleep disturbances at high altitude is hypobaric hypoxia. The distinction is important, for mistaking the cause of altitude-induced sleep problems may lead to a certain complacency. In the context of civilian recreational mountaineering, poor sleep is more a nuisance than a significant disability. For the military, however, sleep deprivation from any cause during deployment may affect mission success through the performance decrements it causes. In high mountains, where hypoxia generates significant performance deficits by itself (see Chapter 22, Physical Performance at Varying Terrestrial Altitudes, and Chapter 23, Cognitive Performance, Mood, and Neurological Status at High Terrestrial Elevation), the addition of sleep deprivation acts synergistically[63] and could cause disaster for a soldier and his or her unit. Given their prevalence and potential, altitude-related sleep disturbances are not a problem that can be safely ignored during military operations.

The four common manifestations of high-altitude sleep disturbances include

1. periodic breathing with prolonged periods of apnea,
2. sleep "fragmentation" with frequent arousals and alterations of sleep stages,
3. decreased arterial oxygen content, and
4. cardiac rhythm disturbances.

Most unacclimatized individuals experience all of these manifestations to some degree following initial ascent. The symptoms are so frequent that poor sleep often has been considered a part of the AMS syndrome,[64–66] but at present, altitude-related sleep problems are considered to be a separate entity from AMS (see Chapter 24, Acute Mountain Sickness and High-Altitude Cerebral Edema). Many believe that sleep disturbances may play a causal role in altitude illnesses, however. This opinion stems from the observations that AMS symptoms often increase in severity in the early morning after sleeping[64,67–69] and that the onset of HAPE is often after an overnight sleep.[70] The relationship is thought to be due to worsening during sleep of the already low SaO_2.[66,67,71] That concept was called into question during a study by Eichenberger and colleagues,[72] who suggested that the periodic breathing during sleep at altitude in HAPE-susceptible individuals may be caused by their profound hypoxemia rather than a cause of their HAPE.

Periodic Breathing and Apnea

Altitude-induced periodic breathing is probably the most overtly apparent of the altitude-induced sleep disturbances. The most characteristic pattern is cyclic increase and decrease in tidal volume over two to six breaths[73,74] followed by a prolonged period of apnea lasting from 6 to 20 seconds.[65,71,74] Each breathing cycle lasts from 15 to 24 seconds,[64,68] and the cycles get shorter with increasing altitude.[71,75] Another pattern consists of cyclic fluctuations of respiration without periods of apnea. In contrast to these regular cycles, a few individuals have a very disorganized breathing pattern with irregular frequency and tidal volume.[76,77] The percentage of sleep time consumed by altered breathing, especially periodic breathing with apnea, increases with increasing altitude.[71,75,78] Although periodic breathing and prolonged apnea can be alarming to a casual observer, such as someone sharing the tent, it does not seem to cause the sleeper distress unless it is associated with arousal (see below). Sleepers who are awakened during apnea often describe a sensation of suffocation, or dreams of being smothered by a collapsing tent or an avalanche.[65]

Periodic breathing during sleep occurs in nearly everyone above 3,000 m and is universal above 6,000 m.[20,71,79] Periodic breathing has been documented in some awake individuals at rest at 2,440 m,[75] so presumably it might also occur during sleep at that altitude. Individuals vary significantly in their pattern and amount of periodic breathing at altitude.[72,78–81] Some of the variation may be related to differences in respiratory drive among individuals, for several researchers have described a positive association with respiratory drive as measured by hypoxic ventilatory response (HVR)[77,79,81–83] and hypercapnic ventilatory response (HCVR).[79,84] Others have failed to find a strong association with either HVR or HCVR.[65,71] Periodic breathing may be

less frequent in women,[20] but as yet no supporting data exist. Although periodic breathing can occur during all stages of sleep at altitudes greater than 4,600 m,[72,78,85] it is much more common during non–rapid eye movement (REM) sleep.[74,80,86]

Fragmented Sleep

"Sleep fragmentation" in mountain environments refers to hypoxia-induced changes in normal sleep architecture. The overall sleep/wakefulness pattern in mountain expedition settings is often a function of living in the field without electricity or other amenities, and it tends to conform to the seasonal light/dark cycle.[87] This may not be true in a military setting where operations are driven by tactical considerations. However, even if an adequate amount of time is available for sleep in mountain environments, changes in the length of sleep stages and more-frequent awakening and arousals (ie, brief periods of alpha-wave activity on electroencephalographic recordings or changes to a lighter sleep stage) cause more time awake compared with lower altitudes in most,[74,78,88] but not all,[86,89] individuals. Usually REM sleep decreases.[78] "Deep" or "slow-wave" sleep (Stages 3 and 4) may also decrease, although that change has not been consistently observed.[78,89] As a result of the decrease in deep and REM sleep, there are often increases in "transition" and "light" sleep (Stages 1 and 2, respectively)[66,74,89] and/or in wakefulness.[74,78,88] The symptoms caused by changes in sleep stages are vivid dreams or nightmares, a feeling of poor or unrefreshing sleep, or a feeling of not having slept much at all.[66,74,80,90] Daytime fatigue is common. The awakening and arousals are thought to be the most responsible for the subjective symptoms of poor sleep in the mountains.[91]

Like periodic breathing, sleep fragmentation is nearly universal in altitude sojourners,[73] especially at altitudes higher than 5,000 m.[78] Sleep fragmentation may be common at lower altitudes, but there are few data to delineate the lower limit for the effect. One study found little effect at 3,200 m,[89] while another found evidence for sleep disturbance between 1,100 m and 2,750 m.[85]

Decreased Arterial Oxygen Content

Slight hypoxemia due to decrease in ventilation during sleep at low altitude is a well-known and "normal" phenomenon.[92] It also occurs during sleep at high altitude. SaO_2 measured with a peripheral oximeter during sleep at high altitude shows a cyclic pattern that tracks periodic breathing, although the peak and trough levels characteristically lag peak and trough ventilatory excursions.[80,83] Mean saturations are somewhere between 4% and 10% below the awake values.[66,71–73,78] That amount of desaturation from the already low values caused by the hypobaric hypoxia can result in profoundly low blood oxygen levels during sleep.

The absolute amount of SaO_2 during sleep is directly related to altitude,[71,78] as is the amount of desaturation relative to awake values.[78] There is a great deal of individual variability in the amount of desaturation that occurs.[72,78,93,94] Some evidence indicates that individuals with higher HVRs have less desaturation,[77,81] although others have not found a significant relationship.[66,73]

Cardiac Arrhythmias

Cardiac rhythm during sleep in high-altitude sojourners is characterized by an overall relative tachycardia compared with that found at lower altitudes[74,95] and by an almost universal sinus arrhythmia, often with profound periods of bradycardia. The bradycardia at extreme altitude can go as low as 20 to 30 beats per minute with beat-to-beat (R–R) intervals as long as 3.6 seconds.[96,97] The bradycardia may be followed by sudden acceleration of heart rate in the range of 130 to 135 beats per minute.[97,98] Like SaO_2, the sinus arrhythmia tracks periodic breathing with increasing bradycardia during apneic periods and the sudden increase in heart rate with the resumption of respirations.[71,74,81,97] The association is so characteristic that changes in heart rate are sometimes used as surrogate markers for periodic breathing during sleep studies at high altitude, because heart rate measured by continuous electrocardiogram is easier to obtain in extreme field settings than are measures of respiration.[71]

In addition to relative tachycardia and sinus arrhythmia that occur during sleep at high altitude, other arrhythmias have been noted but seem to be fairly rare. Premature atrial and ventricular contractions have been observed,[71,86] as well as atrial bigeminy[98] and sinus arrest with junctional escape.[97] Given that these arrhythmias can also be seen in healthy individuals at low altitude, they are probably not very physiologically significant or medically portentous.

Pathophysiology of Altitude Sleep Disturbances

The pathophysiological mechanisms of hypoxia-related sleep disturbances are not precisely known, nor are the relationships between the various sleep phenomena well defined. A useful approach to understanding sleep at high altitude is to consider periodic breathing to be the primary problem, with the other phenomena (ie, arterial desaturation, sleep fragmentation, and cardiac arrhythmias) related to that abnormal breathing pattern. This approach is useful because it provides a focus for treatment option; in other words, if the concept is correct, then treating periodic breathing would also treat the other problems.

The most prominent theory of the cause of periodic breathing during sleep at high altitude is that it results from an hypoxia-induced instability in the feedback system that controls ventilation.[99,100] Hypoventilation occurs during sleep at both low and high altitude owing to (1) the loss of a suprapontine stimulus associated with the awake state and (2) an increase in upper airway resistance due to reduced phasic stimulation of upper airway musculature. At high altitude, the combination of hypobaric hypoxia and hypoxia due to the relative hypoventilation associated with sleep effectively increases the gain of the peripheral (carotid) chemoreceptors, which respond primarily to arterial oxygen pressure (PaO_2) without altering the apneic threshold of the central (medullary) chemoreceptors to carbon dioxide pressure (PCO_2) or hydrogen ion concentration [H^+]. Hyperventilation driven by the peripheral chemoreceptors lowers the PCO_2 below the central chemoreceptor threshold, causing a centrally mediated apnea in which all respiratory efforts cease. The apnea causes an increase in PCO_2 at the central chemoreceptors and a decrease in PaO_2 at the peripheral chemoreceptors, which stimulates resumption of breathing. Owing to the increased gain of the peripheral chemoreceptors, hyperventilation then occurs, which lowers the arterial carbon dioxide pressure ($PaCO_2$) and the PCO_2 below the apneic threshold again, and the cyclic pattern of alternating hyperventilation and apnea is perpetuated.[99,100] Additional factors that have been postulated to contribute include (1) decreased body stores of oxygen and carbon dioxide, which may change the relative response times of the chemoreceptors, and (2) the loss of a central, chemoreceptor-independent ventilatory drive ("afterdischarge"), which normally functions to dampen ventilatory depression after hyperventilation.[101]

Many people view reduced oxygen content of the arterial blood as the most significant consequence of periodic breathing during sleep at high altitude, because low oxygen levels drive many pathophysiological processes. SaO_2 during sleep at altitude is a function of the following:

1. the underlying level of hypobaric hypoxia associated with the decreased partial pressure of oxygen at a specific altitude (see Chapter 22, Physical Performance at Varying Terrestrial Altitudes), combined with
2. the normal 4% to 6% desaturation associated with sleep-induced hypoventilation,[92] and
3. any desaturation due to the apneic phase of altitude-associated increases in periodic breathing.

The contribution of underlying hypobaric hypoxia to sleep desaturation increases with increasing altitude. Desaturation owing to sleep-associated hypoventilation remains relatively fixed but assumes more and more physiological significance as the underlying hypobaric hypoxia positions the individual further down on the steep portion of the oxyhemoglobin dissociation curve (see Chapter 21, Human Adaptation to High Terrestrial Altitude). The contribution of periodic breathing to the overall level of hypoxia is somewhat controversial, however. It makes sense that recurrent apnea would cause arterial desaturation, and it does. As previously noted, SaO_2 measured during sleep with peripheral oximeters shows a cyclic pattern of decreasing and increasing saturation that tracks cyclic breathing. West and colleagues[71] found that apneas at very high altitudes were associated with the lowest SaO_2 measured during the 24-hour day. The question is whether the *mean* saturation during periodic breathing is low. Some investigators found that it was,[76,93,94] while others found little relationship between SaO_2 and amount of periodic breathing.[72,73] Masuyama and colleagues[77] found a negative correlation between the amount of periodic breathing and the degree of SaO_2 during sleep. On the basis of their findings, they suggested that individuals with high ventilatory drives maintain higher saturation during sleep by means of periodic breathing. The findings of Lahiri and colleagues[102] that acclimatized climbers from low altitudes had higher HVRs, more periodic breathing, and higher SaO_2 during sleep than high-altitude, native-born Sherpas, who had a blunted hyperventilatory response, no periodic breathing, and lower saturation, also suggests that periodic breathing might have an adaptive value for maintaining saturation during sleep in altitude sojourners.

The sleep fragmentation that occurs at high altitude is generally believed to be related to periodic breathing.[65,68,74,78] The mechanism is thought to be the triggering of arousal and awakenings by periods of apnea. The arousals or awakening functions to stimulate respiration and terminate the apnea. Arousal may sometimes occur in the absence of apnea,[78] which suggests that the body may respond more to the level of desaturation than to the absence of feedback from respiratory movements. There is little information in the literature to suggest that altitude-induced hypoxemia has any effect on central mechanisms that control sleep architecture.

As noted previously, the sinus arrhythmias seen during sleep at high altitude are so consistently related to periodic breathing that the recurrent episodes of bradycardia have been used as surrogate markers for periods of sleep apnea.[71] The cyclic variation in heart rate has been suggested to be mediated through alterations in the predominance of the sympathetic versus the parasympathetic influence of the autonomic nervous system.[95,97] The other bradyarrhythmias that have been observed undoubtedly result from parasympathetic activity on the sinoatrial node through the vagus nerves.[97]

Diagnosis and Treatment of Sleep Disturbances at Altitude

The diagnosis of altitude-related sleep disorder is made by noting the signs and symptoms of disordered sleep in an individual who has recently ascended to moderate or high altitude, or at any time in an individual at very high and extreme altitudes. It is useful to try to differentiate altitude-related sleep disturbance from other causes to ensure appropriate treatment. As noted below, inappropriate treatment of altitude-induced sleep problems with hypnotic drugs (ie, sleeping pills) can be dangerous, owing to depression of ventilation. Other possible causes of poor sleep in the setting of a military deployment to mountain terrain include environmental factors other than hypoxia (eg, cold, unfamiliar bedding or sleeping surface, crowded sleeping quarters, etc) and disruption of circadian rhythms by work schedules or moving across time zones (ie, jet lag).

Preexisting pathological sleep disorders should be rare in military populations, which generally consist of relatively young, healthy individuals who have often been medically screened as a condition of entering military service. However, acquired sleep disorders are possible in the command and senior noncommissioned officer populations, which are traditionally older. Preexisting sleep-disordered breathing occurs in 4% to 9% of middle-aged persons[103] and may be a cause of chronic hypertension.[104] Most sleep problems that are not directly related to altitude can be identified on the basis of clinical history. Medical officers should remember, however, that the signs and symptoms of many pre-existing conditions of sleep-disordered breathing, including Cheyne-Stokes respiration in chronic heart failure and obstructive sleep apnea syndrome, are similar to those seen in altitude periodic breathing.

Raising Arterial Oxygen Content During Sleep

Because hypobaric hypoxia is the ultimate cause of altitude-related sleep disturbances, treatment is based on increasing the oxygen content of the blood. This can be accomplished either by raising the inspired oxygen or by increasing ventilation to raise lung alveolar oxygen content. Conversely, anything that decreases respiration will worsen altitude sleep disturbances and is potentially harmful at altitude.[66] Transient or short-term insomnia related to deployment and environmental factors other than hypobaric hypoxia can be treated by changing the sleep environment, sleep schedule, or both. Use of sleeping pills that are routinely used at low altitude is possible at high altitude so long as those treatments do not depress respiration.

Descent. The most reliable method to raise inspired oxygen during sleep is to descend in elevation, which effectively increases the oxygen content of the ambient air. Mountaineers codified this principle many years ago in the axiom "climb high, sleep low." Ideally, one should descend to a level at which the partial pressure of oxygen is sufficient to eliminate periodic breathing during sleep. Given individual variability, this altitude will differ for different individuals, and some individuals exhibit periodic breathing at sea level.[103] However, descent below 2,500 m will significantly reduce altitude-induced sleep problems for the vast majority of people.

Supplemental Oxygen. Sleeping low, or at least at low-enough elevations to decrease sleep problems related to hypoxia, is not always a viable option in mountain environments where severe weather conditions and rugged terrain can significantly limit mobility. Tactical situations may also limit descent during military deployment. When descent is not possible, the inspired oxygen levels can be raised using supplemental oxygen administered by mask or nasal cannula. Supplemental oxygen has been demonstrated to eliminate apnea and eliminate or attenuate periodic breathing depending on the altitude and the amount of oxygen supplied.[71,74,78–81] The mountain climbing community has known about the benefits of low-flow, supplemental oxygen during sleep and has used it for years at high camps and bivouacs.[105]

The biggest problem with the use of supplemental oxygen is obtaining a sufficient supply. Metal oxygen tanks are heavy, cumbersome, and cold in an environment where those characteristics are potential liabilities. The high camps on Mount Everest (and other mountains that are popular to climb) are littered with used and abandoned oxygen tanks, because the difficulty of transporting them down outweighs any perceived utility. Additionally, it would require vast amounts of oxygen and equipment to supply the personnel of any unit bigger than a squad or platoon for any period of time. Bottled oxygen is also an explosive hazard if it is struck by bullets or fragments. In a static situation or a relatively fixed site with adequate power supplies, molecular-sieve oxygen concentrators may be more cost effective than transporting bottled oxygen. The use of portable, cloth, hyperbaric chambers or fixed-facility hyperbaric chambers to sleep in will also allow an increased inspired oxygen level owing to the increase in barometric pressure. Both of these solutions could present a supply problem for larger units, however.

Pharmacological Aids to Sleep. Increasing ventilation during sleep at altitude is accomplished most practically by using pharmacological respiratory stimulants. Drugs that have been evaluated in that role include carbonic anhydrase inhibitors, almitrine, and progestogens. Of these, acetazolamide, a carbonic anhydrase inhibitor, is the best studied and probably the most useful.

Acetazolamide is not generally thought of as a respiratory stimulant, but it is effective in this role during sleep at high altitude at a dose that is also effective for prophylaxis of AMS (ie, 250 mg/8 h).[65,68,83,85,94] It increases the oxygen in arterial blood and decreases periodic breathing, arousals, and awakenings without changing the HVR (Figure 26-3).[65,83] Another carbonic anhydrase inhibitor, benzolamide, has been shown to have similar actions.[106] The drugs probably stimulate respiration by inducing a metabolic acidosis, which counteracts the respiratory depression effect of the altitude-induced respiratory alkalosis (see Chapter 21, Human Adaptation to High Terrestrial Altitude). They may also have a stimulatory effect on the central respiratory chemoreceptor.[106] Regardless of the mechanism of action, acetazolamide is relatively effective and safe for preventing sleep problems at high altitude. Its additional advantage—that of being safe and effective for preventing AMS—make it the drug of choice for both indications.

Other respiratory stimulants that have been evaluated during sleep at high altitude include almitrine and methyl progesterone.[65,76,83] Almitrine increases periodic breathing by raising the HVR and increases SaO_2 about as effectively as acetazolamide.[83] To the extent that periodic breathing contributes to frequent arousals or awakening, almitrine is not as effective as acetazolamide in treating altitude sleep problems. Methyl progesterone, on the other hand, decreases periodic breathing but only moderately increases SaO_2 in altitude sojourners. It increases SaO_2 during sleep more effectively in altitude residents with chronic mountain polycythemia (Monge's disease) and prevents transient episodes of severe desaturation that characterize this group of patients.[65,76] Given its relative ineffectiveness and potential side effects, progesterone is probably not a good option for treating altitude-related sleep disturbances in young, healthy, military personnel.

Use of hypnotic medications such as benzodiazepines to treat sleep problems at high altitude is relatively contraindicated due their ability to depress respiration and worsen sleep hypoxemia. Nonetheless, they have been suggested as appropriate therapy for sleep problems that are not directly related to hypobaric hypoxia.[107] In reality, individuals who are not medically trained tend not to differentiate among various causes of insomnia and treat all sleep problems, including those related to hypoxia, with "sleeping pills." It is well known that mountain climbers often use hypnotic medications to help them sleep at high altitude,[82] sometimes with disastrous results.[108]

Few studies of hypnotic medication use at high altitude have been reported, and all the studies were of benzodiazepines. Diazepam in a 10-mg dose was found to decrease Stage 3 sleep and increase hypoxemia[66]; the authors suggested that this drug might be dangerous to use at high altitude. Triazolam 0.125 mg was used to promote sleep at 7,600 m in a hypobaric chamber without apparent harmful effects, but it was not formally studied.[109] One milligram of loprazolam did not alter sleep architecture or increase periodic breathing at 4,800 m.[82] Likewise, 10 mg of temazepam reduced sleep-onset latencies and increased sleep efficiency without increasing periodic breathing above 4,000 m but was more effective when taken in addition to 500 mg acetazolamide per day.[85] This approach of combining a hypnotic with acetazolamide, which stimulates respiration during sleep, seems to offer a method for avoiding respiratory depression. Diphenhydramine 50 to 75 mg has been recommended as a means to treat insomnia at high altitude without resorting to benzodiazepines,[106] but no studies have been reported.

For most people, the prognosis for untreated hypoxia-induced sleep problems is good at altitudes under 5,000 m because they will improve with acclimatization.[74,94,110] Additionally, the sleep problems can be successfully treated with acetazolamide or supplemental oxygen as described above. At altitudes higher than 5,000 m, periodic breathing and its associated sleep disturbances appear to persist indefinitely; although treatment may improve sleep somewhat at very high and extreme altitudes, sleep is never normal.[71]

The attitude of many civilians who venture into the mountains for recreation is that altitude-induced sleep problems are "a nuisance rather than a disability."[93(p172)] As previously noted, sleep problems cannot be safely ignored in a military deployment because of their detrimental effects on performance. Strong consideration should be given to treating all military personnel deployed to mountain environments above 3,000 m to prevent altitude-related sleep problems during their initial ascent. At altitudes under 5,000 m, treatment can be discontinued for most individuals as they successfully acclimatize. At higher altitudes, treatment

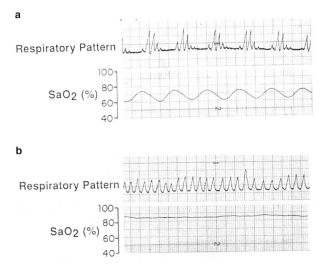

Fig. 26-3. Periodic breathing during sleep in a volunteer test subject at 4,400 m on Mount McKinley in Alaska. Each panel contains a tracing of respiratory excursion and arterial oxygen saturation (SaO_2, %) measured by pulse oximeter. (**a**) During treatment with placebo the subject had periodic breathing and low arterial oxygen saturation. (**b**) Acetazolamide treatment decreased periodic breathing and improved oxygen saturation. Adapted with permission from Hackett PH, Roach RD, Harrison GL, Schoene RB, Mills WJ Jr. Respiratory stimulants and sleep periodic breathing at high altitude: Almitrine versus acetazolamide. *Am Rev Respir Dis.* 1987;135:897.

should be continued indefinitely. At present, the safest and most practical treatment for use in military operations in the mountains is probably acetazolamide in the same dosages that are effective for preventing AMS (ie, 125–250 mg twice daily, or 500 mg slow-release formulation once a day in the evening.)

Blood Clotting Disorders

Exposure to high mountain environments is associated with intravascular blood clot (thromboembolic) problems and minor bleeding phenomena that suggest a possible altitude-induced disruption of normal hemostatic mechanisms. Thromboembolic events include pulmonary embolism and stroke in healthy, young individuals, who do not ordinarily develop such catastrophic problems. Given that most military units are composed largely of relatively young individuals, effective medical support for deployment to high altitude should include some provision to manage thromboembolism.

Case reports and anecdotal descriptions of thromboembolic phenomena are surprisingly frequent in the mountaineering literature. Superficial thrombophlebitis[111] and deep venous thrombosis (DVT) in the lower extremity,[1] DVT with subsequent pulmonary embolus (PE),[112–116] transient ischemic attack (TIA),[117] and thromboembolic stroke[113,115,118,119] have all been reported as occurring in the high mountains. Additionally, blood clots have been observed in the small vessels of the lungs and other organs of persons who died of altitude illness.[113,120,121] Those autopsy findings were the basis of a hypothesis that HACE results from an altitude-induced coagulopathy,[122] a theory that is not widely held at present (see Chapter 24, Acute Mountain Sickness and High-Altitude Cerebral Edema).

Although reports of thromboembolic phenomena in high mountains are surprisingly common, the actual incidence of such events is not known. The number of reports could merely reflect an exaggerated interest in these phenomena; however, the consensus is that thromboembolic phenomena at high altitude are not unusual. The events tend to occur at very high altitudes (> 4,500 m), however. Proposed risk factors include either preexisting or altitude-induced coagulopathy, polycythemia, dehydration, cold, climbing without supplemental oxygen, and long periods of forced inactivity in small tents owing to bad weather.[20]

The clinical signs and symptoms of altitude-related thromboembolic disease are the same as those that occur at low altitude:

- peripheral venous thrombi can cause pain, swelling, and warmth in the affected limb;
- pulmonary emboli can cause chest pain, dyspnea, hypoxemia, cough, and hemoptysis; and
- cerebral thrombi and emboli can cause transient or permanent, focal or global neurological abnormalities; coma; and death.

Diagnosis of thromboembolic disease in a high mountain environment usually relies solely on signs and symptoms because the sophisticated diagnostic equipment that is available in fixed medical facilities is lacking. If the patient can be evacuated to appropriate facilities, an attempt to confirm the diagnosis can be made using standard methods (eg, doppler ultrasound, roentgenography, angiography, various scans). The differential diagnosis must include other altitude-related conditions that can have similar manifestations. HACE, HAPE, and cellulitis resulting from altitude-related suppression of immune function (see below) can cause signs and symptoms similar to those of thromboembolism and should be considered in the differential diagnosis.

The most common type of abnormal bleeding at high altitude is retinal hemorrhage, which was described earlier in this chapter. Other bleeding phenomena that have been reported include "splinter" hemorrhages under the fingernails thought to be caused by hand trauma associated with technical climbing,[123,124] rare instances of unexplained gross gastrointestinal and urinary tract hemorrhage that resolved with descent,[125] and subarachnoid hemorrhage.[113,126] Diagnosis of hemorrhage based on direct observation of retinal or significant gastrointestinal or urinary bleeding is relatively uncomplicated. As with cerebral thromboembolism, the signs and symptoms of subarachnoid hemorrhage may be similar to those of HACE, and the definitive diagnosis will require evacuation and more extensive study.[126]

The pathophysiology of thrombosis and abnormal bleeding at high altitude has not been well established. Because bleeding problems at altitude seem relative minor, most attention has been directed toward explaining the mechanisms responsible for the abnormal clotting. The concept of Virchow's triad suggests that intravascular blood clot formation is due to the interaction of at least two of three factors: stasis of blood flow, injury to the vessel epithelium, and changes in blood coagulability.[127] Stasis of blood due to constrictive clothing, cold temperatures, and forced inactivity in cramped quarters during bad weather are well-recognized risk factors in mountain environments.

Likewise, the possibility of vessel injury due to trauma, including pressure trauma from pack straps, climbing ropes, and harnesses, or due to cold injury are also recognized risk factors. What has been the most intriguing to researchers, however, is the possibility of a hypoxia-induced hypercoagulable state. Results of many early investigations, including the autopsy findings of extensive clotting in individuals who died from altitude illness, seemed to support that possibility.[113] In the aftermath of the Sino–Indian border conflict of the early 1960s, researchers from India did a series of studies of the effects of high altitude on coagulation and platelet function, which suggested that both coagulability and fibrinolysis increased with altitude exposure in normal individuals, but that coagulation was activated without a compensatory increase in fibrinolysis in patients with HAPE.[128,129] Platelet adhesiveness was found to be increased in individuals at high altitude with symptoms of altitude illness and stroke.[130,131] Studies since that time have not provided consistent evidence for a hypercoagulable state or abnormal platelet function induced by altitude (see Cucinell and Pitts[132] for a summary of the work up to 1987).

Bärtsch and colleagues[133–135] did an extensive series of studies of coagulation in individuals with and without AMS and HAPE. They found no significant alteration of coagulation or platelet activity in individuals without AMS, and partial activation of coagulation without fibrin formation in individuals with AMS and individuals who later developed HAPE. Once HAPE was established, there was activation of coagulation with production of fibrin and decreased fibrinolysis. They concluded from these results that the hypercoagulation associated with HAPE is an epiphenomenon *resulting* from, not *causing*, HAPE.[135]

A hypercoagulable state does not have to be induced by hypoxia to cause problems at high altitude. Congenital hypercoagulable states caused by deficiencies of proteins C and S or antithrombin III, or by activated protein C resistance due to the factor V Leiden mutation or the prothrombin G20210A mutation may not result in thrombosis in young adults until middle age, or until they are exposed to the many risk factors for intravascular clot formation found in the mountain environment. The Leiden mutation is prevalent in Caucasian populations[136] and has been hypothesized to contribute to frequent DVT formation in aviators.[137] This and similar undetected hereditary defects in coagulation are likely to play a role in thromboembolic events at high altitude.

Pulmonary embolus arising from a DVT is a well-recognized clinical entity and probably explains most of these cases in high mountains. The origin of cerebral venous thrombosis *at high altitude* has been suggested to occur from the combination of hemoconcentration causing a functional hypercoagulable state combined with stasis of blood in the brain owing to HACE.[118] A preexisting hypercoagulable state could also play a role. Thromboembolic stroke has been suggested to result from emboli traveling through the foramen ovale, which is opened by increased right atrial pressure from hypoxia-induced pulmonary hypertension.[20] The causes of subarachnoid hemorrhage and hemorrhagic stroke at high altitude are not known. An effect of hypoxia-related increase in cerebral blood flow and cerebral blood pressure on preexisting aneurysms or arteriovenous malformations may play a role.[126]

Treatment of thromboembolic disease involves

1. preventing the formation of further blood clots or emboli through anticoagulation and elimination of risk factors, and
2. restoring blood circulation to affected areas using pharmacological thrombolysis, surgical extirpation, or waiting for collateral circulation to develop.

The technical equipment and facilities for adequate treatment are not usually available in mountain field settings, where thromboembolic events may occur. Consequently, treatment virtually always requires descent and evacuation to higher-echelon medical support with the capabilities to provide a more-definitive diagnosis and to monitor anticoagulation and thrombolytic therapy. Unfortunately, evacuation from high mountains can often be difficult. Houston and Bates[112] give a gripping account of the attempted evacuation of an individual with DVT and PE from near the summit of K2, an attempt that led to one of the most famous accidents in mountaineering history.

Supportive treatment in the field prior to and during evacuation includes bed rest and ensuring adequate hydration and oxygenation by whatever means are available. The patient should be kept warm, but care should be taken to ensure that clothing, blankets, or equipment do not constrict blood flow. Anticoagulation with heparin or warfarin at high altitude while awaiting evacuation is generally considered to be dangerous without the ability for monitoring coagulation parameters to guide dose adjustments.[20,107] Subcutaneous low molecular weight heparin, which can be used with relative safety in standard doses without the necessity of monitoring coagulation parameters, provides a means of beginning anticoagulation while awaiting evacuation.[20] Anticoagulation should not be started in cases of possible cerebral thromboembolism without a definitive diagnosis to identify possible subarachnoid hemorrhage or hemorrhagic stroke.

Prophylactic measures to prevent thromboembolic disease consists of eliminating risk factors for abnormal blood clot formation. This includes ensuring adequate hydration, protection from cold temperatures, and avoiding situations that promote restriction of blood flow. Prophylactic use of anticoagulation or antiplatelet therapy runs the risk of exacerbating HARHs or other altitude-related bleeding and is not generally recommended.[107]

The prognosis for thromboembolic events occurring at high altitude is the same as at sea level, assuming that the patient can be evacuated for treatment in a timely fashion. Mortality and morbidity are very high if the patient remains at high altitude without treatment.[20] During military deployment to mountain environments, thromboembolic events other than superficial thrombophlebitis create functional casualties, for the afflicted unit members cannot be returned to duty in the time frame of most military operations. The limitations on return to duty include the necessity for prolonged anticoagulant therapy, neurological deficits from stroke, and decreased lung function from pulmonary emboli. The incidence of recurrent thromboembolic disease during subsequent altitude exposure in individuals who have had a previous event in the mountains is not known. Presumably, individuals with a preexisting coagulopathy would be at increased risk. There are anecdotal reports of mountain climbers returning to high altitude successfully after recovering from an altitude-related thromboembolic event. However, military members with a previous history of thromboembolic phenomenon at high altitude should probably be restricted from deployment to the mountains to limit potential impact of a recurrent event on unit strength.

Suppression of the Immune System

Infectious diseases can be a serious medical problem during any military deployment. Consequently, anything that compromises immune function of personnel in a military unit must be viewed as a medical threat. Hypobaric hypoxia at high altitude has been shown[138] to degrade immune function in experimental conditions, although the clinical significance of that finding has not been determined. Nonetheless, military medical personnel should be alert for possible adverse consequences related to effects of altitude on immune function.

Speculation about a possible effect of high altitude on the immune system was originally generated from reports of apparent differences in the occurrence of specific infectious diseases between Indian soldiers stationed at high and low altitudes,[139] and from accounts of persistent skin infections and cellulitis associated with minor trauma in climbers on Mount Everest.[1,140] Although these specific phenomena could have other causes than immune suppression, subsequent research has documented some degree of hypoxia-related immune system dysfunction.

Exposure to high altitude for prolonged periods can depress cell-mediated immunity but seems to have little effect on humoral immune function. Effects on cell-mediated immunity that have been observed include (1) a decreased ability for in vitro monocyte activation despite an increase in monocyte numbers, and (2) a decrease in measures of natural killer cell cytotoxicity.[140,141] The intraindividual variability in cell-mediated response effects was large.[141] These effects are postulated to be the result of altitude-induced increases in adrenal corticosteroid hormone levels.[141] Measures of humoral immune function, including serum immunoglobulin levels[141,142] and B cell response to vaccination with T cell–independent antigen, remain intact at high altitude.[143] Additionally, there is no depression of mucosal immunity, as measured by lysozyme and immunoglobulin A content in nasopharyngeal washings.[141]

Clinical importance of altitude-induced immune suppression appears limited to an increase in skin infections and cellulitis that may not respond well to treatment while the patient remains at high altitude. Poor personal hygiene in the always-difficult mountain environment may contribute to the incidence of these infections.[140] Nagging minor infections can affect morale and performance and should not be dismissed as insignificant by medical personnel. Additionally, infectious complications of all wounds and burns should be anticipated,[107] although there is little information in literature on the subject. Careful attention to wound care and appropriate antibiotics should be attempted to prevent or resolve infections. When possible, descent to a lower altitude or continuous supplemental oxygen therapy will improve immune function and facilitate resolution of the infections.

Wound Healing

Casual observations during climbing expeditions suggest that superficial wounds heal slowly at altitudes higher than 5,000 m.[1,105] No field studies have been reported to confirm this; however, experimental evidence suggests that very low oxygen levels may slow wound healing.[144] Whether levels of oxygen in tissues reach low-enough levels to slow healing as a result of hypobaric hypoxia alone is hard to say, but it is a theoretical possibility at very high altitudes. Certainly the combination of low tissue saturation and cold temperatures at high altitude might decrease the circulation in the extremities enough to be a factor. Whether wound healing would be a problem with surgical and deep soft-tissue wounds is not known but is also a theoretical possibility. The prudent course is to evacuate wounded patients to low altitude or provide them with supplemental oxygen therapy.

High-Altitude Pharyngitis and Bronchitis

Pharyngitis and bronchitis are very common at altitudes above 4,500 m.[1,107,140] The cause is thought not to be infection but rather irritation of the mucosal lining of the respiratory passages by an increased volume of cold, dry air moving across them from the hypoxia-induced increased ventilation.[107] The condition is characterized by sore throat and a dry, nonproductive, hacking cough that can occur in paroxysms. At extreme altitudes, the coughing spells can be severe enough to fracture ribs.[1,30] Throat lozenges and cough suppressants are the mainstays of treatment. The condition resolves without permanent effects after descent, but it may take days to several weeks to completely resolve. Preventive measures include adequate hydration and breathing through a balaclava or face mask to retain moisture. Chronic cough could cause significant problems in a tactical situation by degrading performance and giving the enemy auditory clues to the location of the individual or the unit.

Exacerbation of Preexisting Medical Conditions

Although most military personnel who deploy to high mountain terrain will be relatively healthy, some could have preexisting medical conditions that would be made worse by the environment. Because physical standards and medical screening prevent individuals with significant medical problems from entering or remaining in active-duty military service, the types of medical problems that could be present in a military unit at deployment do not represent the full spectrum seen in the civilian sector. At worst, most military units could be expected to have some acute illnesses and injuries and few chronic health problems. Officers and noncommissioned officers at higher ranks are selected for their experience and training, however, and are older and more likely to have chronic, age-related medical problems. Often they have received waivers for their medical problems to enable them to be retained in active military service for their skills and leadership.

Few studies have been done of preexisting medical problems at high altitude, but the number of anecdotal reports is growing owing to increasing numbers of civilians with medical problems traveling to mountains for recreational purposes. Even in the absence of good data, the progressive decrease in oxygen content of ambient air at altitude provides a basis for prediction of potential problems. The significance of a preexisting medical problem depends largely on its interaction with hypobaric hypoxia. Hypothetical outcomes to that interaction include (1) the medical condition could increase the degree of hypoxia, (2) hypoxia could worsen the medical condition, and (3) no significant effect of either. (In reality, most preexisting medical conditions both increase the degree of hypoxia at altitude and are worsened by it, but the conceptual framework is probably useful.)

Any condition that interferes with oxygen transport will increase the degree of hypoxia experienced at any altitude. Thus chronic heart and lung diseases could be problems at high altitude. Most active-duty military personnel do not have significant heart and lung disease, however. Conditions involving the heart or lungs that might be found in military populations include mild chronic obstructive pulmonary disease (COPD), elevated carbon monoxide levels, or both, due to smoking tobacco; mild asthma; and mild or moderate sleep apnea.

Individuals with mild COPD or mildly elevated carbon monoxide do have lower Sao_2 at altitude,[145,146] but this might not cause significant clinical problems or greatly impact the individuals' performances except at higher altitudes. If individuals with COPD develop significant problems or performance decrements, they should be redeployed to lower elevations, for it is unlikely that they can be adequately managed at high altitude. Elevated carbon monoxide levels will resolve with cessation of tobacco smoking, and these individuals may be able to remain at high altitude if they discontinue smoking.

Asthmatics are at increased risk for broncho-constriction at high altitude due to inhalation of cold air and airway drying from hypoxia-stimulated ventilation. However, they may also benefit from a decrease in allergen load and lower density of the air. Asthma that is mild and well-enough controlled to allow staying in the military is probably not a major contraindication for deployment to high altitude.

Sleep apnea increases nocturnal hypoxemia and also the risk of pulmonary and systemic hypertension, cardiac arrhythmia, and daytime performance decrements at both high and low altitudes.[104] The effect will be greater at high altitude owing to altitude-induced periodic breathing (see above). *Individuals known to have sleep apnea should not be deployed to high elevations.* Those with occult sleep apnea may do poorly at high altitude, but sleep apnea will be difficult to diagnose in the presence of the typical altitude-induced periodic breathing.

Sedatives and any other medications that depress ventilation will increase hypoxia at high altitude and should be avoided. All medications being taken by deploying unit members should be screened prior to deployment to identify those that could worsen hypoxia. This could be a significant problem if unit members are allowed to bring their own supplies of medications during deployment, especially sleeping pills. Medications that depress ventilation should be discontinued prior to deployment or given only under medical supervision.

Hypobaric hypoxia can worsen many chronic medical conditions through direct or indirect effects. The exacerbation of chronic congestive heart failure at mountain resorts due to hypoxia-stimulated increase in catecholamine levels is the classic example of this phenomenon.[20] Congestive heart failure is not prevalent in active-duty military populations, however. Conditions that can be found in military populations and could be made worse by hypoxia include essential hypertension, sickle cell trait, occult coronary artery disease, pulmonary hypertension, migraine headache, and pregnancy.

Blood pressure increases in almost everyone at high altitude prior to acclimatization, owing to autonomic nervous system activation.[147] In normal individuals, the level of increase is not enough to warrant treatment, but patients being treated for hypertension at low altitude will have to continue or increase their medication at altitude to control their blood pressure.

Individuals with sickle cell trait can have splenic syndrome or vaso-occlusive crisis at high altitude.[20,148] Given that many military members may have sickle cell trait, medical personnel should be prepared to treat that condition. Occasionally, splenic syndrome or a vaso-occlusive crisis during altitude deployment may be the first manifestation of an otherwise occult sickle cell trait condition.[20]

Other occult conditions in military populations that could be worsened by hypobaric hypoxia include coronary artery disease, pulmonary hypertension, and seizure disorders. The evidence that exists on established coronary artery disease at high altitude suggests that there is little increased risk for acute events, possibly because of a protective effect of altitude-related limitations of physical work.[149] Whether this situation would hold during combat at high altitude is questionable.

Pulmonary artery pressure increases with altitude exposure and may contribute to HAPE (see Chapter 25, High-Altitude Pulmonary Edema). Individuals with known pulmonary hypertension should be restricted from altitude exposure, but they normally would not be serving on active duty. Likewise, individuals with known seizure disorders would not be serving on active duty. New onset of seizures at high altitude requires that the individual be evacuated to low altitude for evaluation.

Migraine headaches have been reported at high altitude,[150] but the exact incidence and significance are not well established. Worsening of migraine frequency or severity in the mountains is an obvious indication for redeployment to low altitude and future deployment restrictions.

Women living at high altitude have an increased incidence of hypertension and preeclampsia syndrome during pregnancy, and low-birth-weight babies.[151] Pregnant women visiting high altitude may have increased bleeding complications and preterm labor.[152] Although there is little evidence for other significant problems associated with pregnancy at high altitude, pregnant women in the military probably should not be deployed to altitudes greater than 2,500 m.

MEDICAL PROBLEMS CAUSED BY OTHER ENVIRONMENTAL FACTORS

Although hypobaric hypoxia is unique to the high mountains, it is not the only factor in that environment that can cause medical problems. A significant number of other factors play a role, often in conjunction with hypoxia. Some, like cold injury, may be obvious, because most people associate high mountains with snow and cold. Others, like hemorrhoids, may not be expected, but medical units that deploy to high altitude without provisions to treat hemorrhoids will not be able to provide adequate care for a common problem. In many instances, these hypoxia-*unrelated* problems may be far more clinically significant than those caused by hypoxia itself (eg, a lightning strike will cause more disability than retinal hemorrhages.) Often they will be more frequent than hypoxia-related problems (eg, cold injuries usually outnumber cases of HACE). Although not unique to the high-altitude environment per se, these medical problems are significant contributors to the constellation of environmentally related medical problems that affects military units during deployment to the mountains, and the medical support system must be prepared for them.

Trauma

A substantial amount of trauma occurs in high mountain environments. It is likely that the incidence of nonballistic injury due to accidents in units deploying to mountain terrain could be relatively higher than that in other environments, but few data exist to substantiate that supposition. Certainly, the array of traumatic injuries associated with civilian recreation activities in the mountains suggests that a significant threat exists. (Interested readers can also consult the Pictorial Atlas of Freezing Cold Injury by William J. Mills, Jr, MD, which is appended to *Medical Aspects of Harsh Environments, Volume 1.*[153] In addition to freezing cold injuries per se, the Atlas contains numerous descriptions and photographs of trauma in freezing cold and high terrestrial environments.)

The combination of rugged topography with hypoxia-impaired judgment and reasoning abilities is a major contributing factor to traumatic injury in high mountain regions. Other environmental factors may also play a role. Hypothermia can contribute to decrements in judgment and mental processes, and cold fingers and toes may not have the sensitivity needed for safe technical climbing maneuvers. Snow, rain, and ice make footing and handholds more tenuous than when the weather is dry.[154] Bad weather can also make vehicular travel, which is often precarious in the mountains, treacherous. Mountains can inflict trauma directly through rockslides and avalanches. In military operations, the trauma due to environmental factors is compounded by the well-known, early-entry stresses of traveling and a novelty location's causing more accidents early in any deployment.

The traumatic injuries seen in mountain environments form a pattern that results from the interactions among environment, activity, and equipment (Figure 26-4). The combination of rugged terrain and the effects of hypobaric hypoxia on performance cause falls to be a major contributor to the tally of injuries. The injuries caused by falls are characteristic because of their types. Owing to steep terrain, falls tend to be long and uncontrolled, causing multiple blunt trauma. Abrasions are generally not seen because of the protective effect of heavy clothing worn to protect against cold. In the military setting, the wearing of field uniforms also helps protect against abrasion. Falls in mountain terrain are often complicated by specialized equipment used for technical climbing or skiing. Equipment with sharp points and surfaces, such as ski poles and ice crampons, can cause lacerations and penetrating injuries during a long fall.[155] Climbing harnesses and ropes meant to prevent serious falls can cause specific types of injury if misused or if they fail. Free-falling equipment can also inflict injury on personnel at lower levels who are not directly involved in the fall. Blunt trauma and lacerations caused by runaway skis with sharp edges are well-known injuries in recreational ski areas, for example. Weapons carried by military personnel in tactical operations could add an additional hazard during falls.

Different mountaineering activities are associated with different types and locations of injuries. Downhill skiing generates many lower-extremity injuries, but it also causes serious injuries to the head and upper body due to high-speed impacts. Owing to slower speeds, falls during cross-country skiing are associated with fewer serious head injuries. Cross-country skiers tend to have both upper- and lower-extremity injuries, however, owing to falling with backpacks.

Serious trauma is less-often associated with hiking and backpacking. Whereas the higher speeds associated with skiing tend to break bones and tear muscle tissue, hiking and backpacking are associated with strains and sprains of joints and other soft-tissue injuries. Upper-extremity neuropathy due to brachial plexus injury from pack-strap trauma (a form of Erb palsy) can occur due to shifting of rucksack position during climbs and descents.[156] Overuse injuries are common in the mountains owing to traveling up and down steep slopes. Technical climbing, which relies heavily on the arms and hands, is associated with a characteristic set of upper-extremity soft-tissue injuries, including serious hand trauma.[157]

Avalanches and rockslides cause multiple trauma. They often bury individuals, causing crush injury

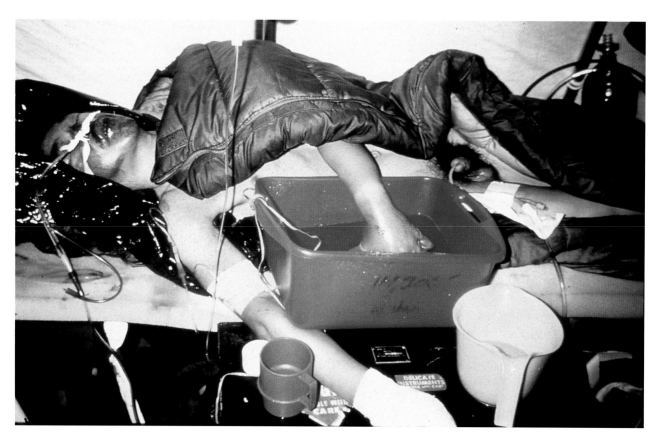

Fig. 26-4. A mountain climber with multiple environmental injuries receives initial treatment in a tent on Mount McKinley, Alaska. The patient had high-altitude pulmonary edema (HAPE), dehydration, multiple trauma from a fall, and severe frostbite injury to his hands. The fall was presumed to be the result of decreased physical and mental functioning caused by hypoxia and altitude illness. Multiple environmental injuries are common in mountain environments. Photograph: Courtesy of Peter Hackett, MD, Seattle, Washington.

and asphyxiation. It is not unusual for whole groups to be caught and injured in a avalanche or rockslide, creating a mass casualty situation.

Diagnosis and treatment of trauma in high mountains is the same as at sea level, with the admonition that transport of the patient may present problems due to rough terrain. Adequate protection of the patient from harsh climatic conditions, especially cold, is also important. Specific treatment of traumatic injuries is not the subject of this chapter but is covered in standard textbooks on orthopedics and sports medicine.

Prevention of trauma in mountain terrain requires appropriate training and equipment. Training should include proper use of equipment such as skis and climbing harnesses. Use of hiking sticks seems to prevent falls during recreational hiking in the mountains even though their use does not ease the strain on the legs and back in most individuals.[158] Unit personnel should also be familiarized with relevant environmental hazards, such as ava-

lanches and rockslides, and know how to avoid being caught in them. Good physical conditioning helps prevent accidents in the mountains by lessening the contributions of fatigue and lack of strength to accidents.

Thermal Injury and Illness

It is no surprise to medical personnel that cold injuries occur in mountain environments, for most people associate mountains with cold and snow. The concept that heat stress can also occur in mountain environments is less obvious but nonetheless true (for an example, see the Preface in *Medical Aspects of Harsh Environments, Volume 1*[153]). Consequently, medical personnel supporting troops deployed to high altitude must anticipate the full spectrum of thermal injuries, although cold injuries are much more frequent. Prevention of thermal injuries through increased awareness and training should be a high priority. Increasing awareness in unit and command personnel has been shown to decrease the incidence of cold injuries in the setting of military deployment to high altitude.[159]

Cold Injuries

Cold injuries are very frequent at high altitude. Mean ambient temperature drops approximately 2°C to 6°C for each 1,000 m increase in elevation, as a function of the inability of the decreased mass of atmospheric gas to absorb or retain significant amounts of heat. Progressively lower temperatures, combined with the high winds and precipitation that are frequent components of mountain weather, create significant cold stress. At the same time, the effects of hypobaric hypoxia on the body and on psychological function increase vulnerability to the cold. Altitude-induced increases in red blood cell mass and peripheral vasoconstriction from decreased plasma volume and dehydration significantly increase the risk of frostbite or freezing injury.[115] Hypoxia-related errors in judgment and blunted reasoning ability hinder the normal behaviors that protect against cold stress. One of the most common scenarios in the mountains is that of climbers taking off their gloves and, owing to hypoxia, forgetting to put them back on, causing severe freezing injuries to their hands.[115]

Diagnosis and treatment of cold injuries in the high-altitude environment is the same as at low altitude and is discussed extensively in *Medical Aspects of Harsh Environments, Volume 1*,[153] particularly Chapter 14, Clinical Aspects of Freezing Cold Injuries; Chapter 15, Nonfreezing Cold Injuries; and Chapter 16, Treatment of Accidental Hypothermia. Evacuation or descent to a lower altitude, or use of supplemental oxygen will help in treating cold injury that occurred at high altitude.

Heat Illness

Heat illness is much less common than cold injury in the mountains, but it does occur in certain situations. It is usually due to a combination of factors that increases an individual's heat load. In high mountain environments, the most common factors are increased solar load due to lack of shade above timberline; increased light reflection off of rock, snow, and ice surfaces (albedo); dehydration; and increased metabolic heat production due to the increased physical effort needed to accomplish work while hypoxic. Heat exhaustion due to these conditions is often referred to as "glacier lassitude" and has been chronicled during climbing expeditions for

many years.[105]

The full spectrum of heat illness is possible at high altitude, but severe forms are not common. Diagnosis and treatment of heat injuries in the mountains is the same as at low altitude and is described in *Medical Aspects of Harsh Environments, Volume 1*,[153] particularly Chapter 8, Clinical Diagnosis, Management, and Surveillance of Exertional Heat Illness. Because hypoxia does not appear to make a significant contribution to the pathophysiology of heat injury, there is no reason to believe that descent or the provision of supplemental oxygen would be of any significant benefit in treating heat injury itself. Increased Sa_{O_2} would certainly not be harmful to a patient with heat injury, however, and might be beneficial for any coexisting altitude illness.

Ultraviolet Radiation Injury

Excessive UV radiation from sunlight (UV-A and UV-B; UV-C is almost entirely filtered out except at the polar regions) is a serious threat to military personnel operating in high mountain regions during daylight hours, because several factors in the environment increase its damaging potential. The decreased UV filtering by the thinner atmosphere at high altitude causes an increased intensity of exposure (~ 4% for every 300 m) and a shift of the UV spectrum to more-harmful short wave lengths.[107] Reflection from snow and ice not only significantly increases the intensity of exposure (~ 75% of the incident radiation is reflected) but also creates different directions for sources of exposure (UV radiation in sunlight usually comes from overhead; reflected UV radiation can come from the side or below). UV exposure can cause significant short-term disability to military personnel through severe sunburn and snow blindness. It can also cause discomfort through mild sunburn and reactivation of cold sores on the lips.

Prevention is the key to lessening the impact of solar radiation injuries on military operations. Prevention is facilitated by threat awareness and the use of sunscreen, protective clothing, and UV protective eyewear. As with most preventive measures, command emphasis may be very successful in ensuring compliance with preventive measures.

(Interested readers may also wish to explore two other volumes in the *Textbook of Military Medicine* series: *Occupational Health: The Soldier and the Industrial Base*,[160] and *Military Dermatology*,[161] in which sunburn, solar keratitis, and other damaging effects of UV exposure are also discussed.)

Sunburn

Sunburn is a well-known hazard of outdoor activity in high mountains. It occurs more rapidly than at lower altitudes, and is often more severe. Because people at high altitude are usually well clothed for protection from the cold temperatures, the sunburn is often confined to the exposed skin of the face, especially the nose and lips. The pattern of the burn can include the underside of the nose, chin, and eyebrows, owing to light's being reflected up from ice, snow fields, and large rock surfaces. This pattern is similar to that seen in people who spend considerable time on large bodies of water, where light is reflected up from the water surface, or in arctic areas, where it is also reflected off the snow and ice. In areas of the mountains where the ambient temperatures are warmer and people hike or work in short pants or take off their shirts, extremities and torsos can be burned in addition to the face. Individuals are often lured into a false sense of security about sunburn because the ambient temperature is still cool, although relatively warmer than at night or at higher altitudes.

The diagnosis and treatment of sunburn at high altitude is the same as that at low altitude. Due to the increased albedo, sunburn may occur in unusual areas such as inside the ears and nostrils, around the eyes, and under the chin. In the setting of military deployment where a decrement in manpower due to sunburn may have an adverse impact on the mission, aggressive treatment with systemic corticosteroids might be considered, to limit the period of disability.

Prevention of sunburn at high altitude relies on covering as much skin as possible with clothing and using sunblocking creams and lotions on exposed skin during the day. At high altitude, special attention should be given to protecting areas of skin that are vulnerable to albedo.

Snow Blindness

In addition to sunburned skin, the increased UV-A and UV-B radiation and reflection off snow and ice in high mountain environments can cause snow blindness (corneal keratitis and uveitis) similar to that seen in arctic regions. This condition is not only very painful, but the effective visual decrement resulting from severe light sensitivity (ie, photophobia) also makes ambulation or vehicle operation by the afflicted individual dangerous, if not impossible, in rugged mountain terrain. It would be similar in a combat situation. Snowblindness, like sunburn, can

easily be prevented and usually occurs as the result of failure to take adequate preventive measures. Consequently, the incidence is quite variable.

Diagnosis and treatment of snow blindness is not different in the high-altitude setting than in the arctic. Signs and symptoms include severe eye pain (due to exposure of corneal nerve endings by sloughing of the damaged outer corneal layer), photophobia with constricted pupil and spasm of swollen and/or sometimes blistered eyelids, profuse tearing, and prominent blood vessels in the sclera and conjunctiva. Symptoms are often maximal 6 to 8 hours after exposure and resolve in 48 to 72 hours.[162] Patching the eye and controlling pain are the mainstays of treatment. Dilating the pupil and using ocular antibiotics are helpful. Pain control may require oral analgesics, sedatives, or both. The prognosis is generally good, although in severe cases permanent damage can occur.[163]

Prevention of UV injury to the eye is achieved by use of protective eyewear that filters UV light (ie, effective sunglasses). To prevent injury from reflected light, protective eyewear should have side shields. Additionally, the eyewear should have a safety cord or strap to prevent its being lost accidentally.

Cold Sores

The occurrence of cold sores on the lips due to reactivation of latent herpes simplex virus infection by UV light exposure is a common and well-known phenomenon at high altitude. Lesions can be treated with local application of an antiviral ointment such as acyclovir. There is probably little utility in treating with an oral antiviral medication in a healthy individual during a military deployment to high altitude. Likewise, there is probably no reason to use oral antiviral medication prophylactically. Prevention of UV exposure by using a sunblock such as zinc oxide is generally effective in preventing cold sores at altitude.

Lightning Strikes

Lightning strikes are a significant seasonal hazard in the mountains, especially in exposed areas above timberline. The thunderstorms that generate lightning are more frequent over high mountains, and many people are killed or injured by lightning in mountain regions.[164] Dusek and Hansen[165] reported a fatality and several injuries in soldiers struck by lightning during maneuvers in the Colorado mountains.

Lightning can strike a person in several ways.[166]

It can strike a person directly or strike an object that the person is touching or holding. These strikes tend to cause the most severe injuries. Lightning can jump from a nearby object that has been struck (ie, splash) or travel through the ground or water (ie, step voltage), types of lightning strikes that are often less severe than direct ones. Military personnel in close proximity to metal vehicles, armament, and communication equipment are at risk for splash strikes. Step voltage can cause injury to large groups with a single strike; military units moving in close formation are at risk for this kind of indirect strike. All strikes can cause blunt trauma if the person struck is thrown by violent muscle contraction or falls while unconscious.[167]

The electrical properties of lightning are those of massive voltage and current applied for a very short time. The current tends to run over the outside of the body (ie, flashover) so that there are fewer deep burns with lightning compared with high-voltage injuries from man-made sources, where the current is long-lasting.[166,168]

Lightning strikes usually cause initial cardiopulmonary arrest due to massive depolarization of muscle tissue and the central nervous system. The heart often resumes its normal beating rapidly, while the respiratory function lags behind due to prolonged paralysis of the diaphragm and the respiratory control areas in the of the brainstem. If victims get cardiopulmonary resuscitation support until the heartbeat and breathing resume, they can often survive. Other injuries include neurological abnormalities, burns, tympanic membrane rupture, ocular injuries, and blunt trauma from falling or being thrown. Neurological problems include confusion, anterograde amnesia, and sometimes transient seizures.[169]

Superficial burns can be linear or in a feathery pattern called Lichtenberg's ferning (also called Lichtenberg's flower). Linear burns are due to the current's following areas of sweat concentration. The mechanism of ferning is not known and it may not cause actual burns, for they fade within hours. Ferning is pathognomonic of lightning injury. Punctate burns through the skin are common with lightning strikes.[168] Second- and third-degree burns occur when metal objects such as rings or coins on the skin are heated by the lightning. Rupture of one or both tympanic membranes due to the blast effect of the lightning strike is common. Ocular injuries are also common, and many individuals will develop cataracts within a few days of being struck.[168] The extent of blunt trauma a victim sustains is a function of the distance that he or she falls or is thrown.

Initial treatment of lightning injury consists of cardiopulmonary resuscitation support. In multiple casualty situations, the apparently dead individuals should be resuscitated *before* medical officers attend those whose breathing and cardiac function are spontaneous,[170] a reversal of usual triage procedure. Once the heart and respiratory function return, treatment of the other injuries is by standard methods. Unlike victims of other high-voltage burns, lightning victims usually do not need massive amounts of fluid because they generally have few internal burns.[167] Tetanus prophylaxis is required in individuals with burns or open wounds.[167]

The prognosis for victims of lightning strikes who survive is good, initially, but after they recover from their acute injuries, victims may experience long-term effects, including posttraumatic stress disorder and other neuropsychological symptoms such as sleep and memory difficulties.[167]

Measures to prevent lightning strikes are essential for military units deployed to mountain terrain, and medical personnel should brief units appropriately. Where the pattern of thunderstorms can be predicted (eg, afternoon storms caused by the adiabatic water cycle), it may be possible to avoid high-risk areas (eg, above timberline). This may not be possible in combat situations. Personal protection includes staying at least 5 m away from tall and large metal objects, and from electrical and communication equipment. The recommended protective position in open terrain is crouching in a low spot with feet and legs pressed together. The interior of fully enclosed metal vehicles offers protection because a strike will flow over the outer surface of the vehicle.

Infectious Disease

It is a basic tenet of military medicine that infectious disease is a serious threat during any deployment. To effectively counter that threat, unit medical personnel must anticipate the general pattern of diseases associated with the environment to which the unit is being deployed.

The pattern of infections seen in high mountain areas appears different from that at low altitude,[139,140,159] and the cause of that difference has been speculated to be hypoxia-induced immune depression (discussed above). However, incidence of infection is a function of both the opportunity for exposure and the susceptibility of the population exposed. Consequently, factors other than immune function alone must be involved in determining the pattern of infectious diseases that occurs in the mountains. Some of those factors that are characteristic of mountain environments are discussed below. A more-extensive discussion of infectious disease in military deployment is presented in another volume in the *Textbook of Military Medicine* series, *Military Preventive Medicine: Mobilization and Deployment*.[171]

Potential exposure to infectious diseases at high altitude is greatly affected by two factors: (1) the absence of many arthropod vectors and (2) the generally low socioeconomic status of many indigenous populations of mountain regions, with concomitant poor sanitation and public health. Additionally, some viral and parasitic infections seem to be found only in specific mountain regions of the world.

Arthropods serve as vectors to transmit a variety of infectious diseases. In mountain regions their populations decrease with increasing elevation,[172] probably as a function of the decrease in humidity and ambient temperature rather than the lower oxygen content of the air. Free-living insect vectors such as mosquitoes are limited to low altitudes except in regions of higher humidity.[173] As a result, the malaria they transmit is not generally seen at higher altitudes. Commensal arthropods such as fleas, lice, and mites, however, range to higher elevations because they inhabit man-made microhabitats. Infrequent bathing owing to harsh, cold conditions probably also contributes to the frequency of these vectors. Diseases spread by these pests, such as louse-borne typhus, can be expected to occur in high mountain regions. At high-enough altitude, even commensal arthropods cannot survive, possibly due to desiccation of their eggs. Eggs and oocysts of arthropod vectors and other parasites (eg, *Toxoplasma gondii*, the organism that transmits toxoplasmosis) are particularly vulnerable to low-humidity cold and increased UV radiation at high altitude. For example, the low prevalence of toxoplasmosis in Colorado is thought to be due to the effects of the mountain environment on the survival of oocysts in the soil.[174]

Poor sanitation and personal hygiene are common in both indigenous populations and sojourners at high altitude owing to cold climate, harsh living conditions, and low socioeconomic conditions (Figure 26-5). Fecal–oral transmission of viruses, such those causing hepatitis and bacterial enteritis, are common.[175,176] Fecal contamination of climbing routes on popular mountains such as Mount Everest and Denali is well known to climbers and trekkers. Given the significant role that these diseases have played in military operations in all environments, fecal contamination would be expected to also be a

problem in deployment to high altitude. Anecdotal reports suggest that it is. Additionally, early in deployment, unit members may manifest diseases that were acquired at low altitude.[159]

Some infectious diseases seem fairly localized to specific mountain regions. Carrion's disease, which is caused by *Bartonella bacilliformis* and includes Oroya fever and characteristic skin lesions called verruga peruana, is the classic example. It is transmitted by a sandfly that is found only in river valleys of the Andes mountains.[177]

Diagnosis and treatment of infectious diseases at high altitude are the same as at low altitude and rely on antibiotics, supportive care, or both. Descent may improve immune function, but whether by relieving hypoxia or improving general health and nutrition status is hard to say.

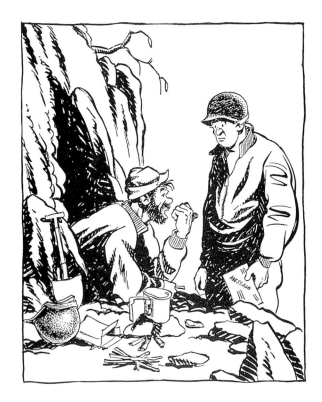

Fig. 26-5. *"Ya must've missed Headquarters on the way up. It's halfway between where the timber stops growin' an' the sojers start shavin'."* There is less concern with personal hygiene in high mountain terrain, as this Bill Mauldin cartoon from World War II illustrates. Causes include inclement weather, limited water supply, and the effects of hypoxia on judgment and motivation. Poor hygiene may contribute to increased infections and the prevalence of disease-carrying arthropod pests. Copyright 1944. By Bill Mauldin. Reprinted with permission by Bill Mauldin.

Poor Hydration and Nutrition

Hypohydration

The poor hydration status of unit personnel is a potential problem in most military deployments, but it is a consistent occurrence during deployments to high mountain environments (interested readers should consult Marriot and Carlson's book[178] on this subject). At high altitude, hypohydration is nearly universal, and it degrades performance and contributes to various environmentally related injuries. Medical personnel in support of units that are deploying to mountain terrain need to be prepared to prevent and to treat problems related to inadequate hydration. The physiological mechanisms involved in altitude-related perturbations of hydration are described in the chapter by Montain in *Medical Aspects of Harsh Environments, Volume 3*.[179]

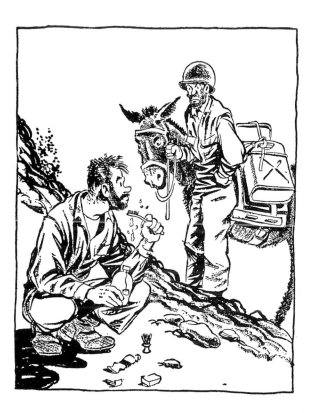

Fig. 26-6. *"I don't haul no water up no crummy mountain fer luxuries."* Cartoonist Bill Mauldin documented the problem of limited water supplies in mountain terrain during World War II. Hypohydration is almost universal in high mountain environments, owing to insufficient fluid intake and increased loss of body water. Limited access to sufficient water supplies is a major factor causing inadequate fluid intake. Copyright 1944. By Bill Mauldin. Reprinted with permission by Bill Mauldin.

Hypohydration in high mountain environments is the result of fluid intake inadequate to compensate for the high rate of fluid loss. Fluid loss is increased over that at low altitude owing to low ambient humidity and the body's response to hypobaric hypoxia and cold. The avenues of fluid loss include increased insensible loss through the skin and respiratory tract and a cold and hypoxia-induced diuresis. Insufficient fluid intake is due to a combination of decreased thirst and volitional behaviors. Thirst is suppressed by both hypoxia and cold. Hypoxia-induced malaise and effects on judgment and reasoning can further limit intake. Obtaining enough fluid to drink in the high mountains requires effort, for it must be either carried on the person and protected from freezing or acquired from melting snow and ice. When an individual is hypoxic, the effort to obtain and consume sufficient water may not seem important (Figure 26-6). Additionally, a conscious decision may be made to limit water intake to avoid having to remove clothing to urinate in cold weather and dangerously rugged terrain (ie, voluntary dehydration).

Diagnosis of hypohydration in a high-altitude setting is somewhat complicated, because many of the common signs and symptoms (eg, malaise, anorexia, dizziness, tachycardia, headache) could be due to hypobaric hypoxia or AMS. Even dry oral mucous membranes could be due to increased ventilation rather than a sign of disordered fluid status. Facilities for laboratory evaluation to support a diagnosis are seldom available during initial deployment or in a field setting. However, because hypohydration is so common at high altitude, it is probably appropriate to consider everyone at altitude to be at least mildly "dry" until proven otherwise. At altitudes below about 5,000 m, many individuals will regain normal hydration status after several weeks. Above that altitude, most will remain chronically hypohydrated.

Hypohydration, while very common at high altitude, is not inevitable. Short of providing continuous supplemental oxygen and adequate protection from cold, little can probably be done to decrease fluid losses. Therefore, prevention of dehydration in mountain environments relies on increasing fluid intake to match losses.

Poor Nutrition

Poor nutrition is a potential problem during deployment to many environments, including high terrestrial altitude. The consistent observation of body weight loss during high-altitude climbing expeditions suggests that inadequate nutrition is an inevitable consequence of altitude exposure, and some research results support that concept. Consequently, unit medical personnel must be prepared to confront nutrition problems during deployment to mountain regions.[178]

Loss of body weight during sojourns to very high altitude (> 5,000 m) is so common it has been labeled "climbers' cachexia" (Figure 26-7). Weight loss at altitude is the result of hypohydration and negative energy balance. Negative energy balance is the result of

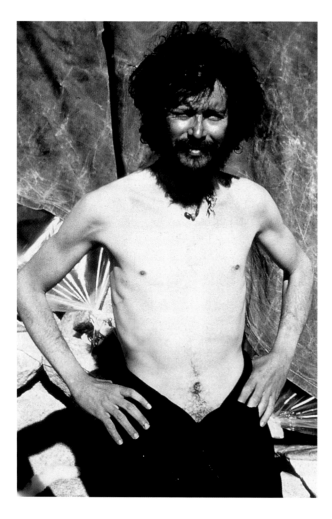

Fig. 26-7. Altitude-induced cachexia in a mountain climber after spending 4 weeks above 6,400 m on Mount Everest. This individual lost approximately 12 kg. Wasting of fat and muscle tissue occurs in everyone at altitudes greater than 5,500 m and is termed "climbers' cachexia." It is caused by the combination of chronic hypoxia, inadequate caloric intake, and hypohydration. Photograph: Courtesy of Peter Hackett, MD, Seattle, Washington.

decreased intake of food due to anorexia and behavioral phenomena combined with a possible increased energy expenditure. Anorexia can be the result of AMS early in deployment but is probably due to hypohydration and the effects of hypoxia later in exposure and at very high altitudes. Hypoxia-induced malaise and effects on judgment and reasoning can limit intake of food and fluid. Additionally, carbohydrates and fat from food that is consumed at very high altitude may be malabsorbed, although this has not been well demonstrated. Increased energy balance is the result of increased metabolic rate and increased energy expenditure to accomplish physical work. Initial weight loss at lower altitudes is largely due to mobilization of fat stores, but both fat and muscle protein are lost at high altitude and during chronic exposure.

Weight loss is the primary sign of inadequate nutrition during deployment to high altitude. Most healthy individuals tolerate the loss fairly well and recover the weight when they redeploy to lower altitude. Although manifestations of poor nutrition other than weight loss are possible, they are not often seen in the time frame of usual climbing expeditions (ie, 6–8 wk). It has been demonstrated that high-altitude weight loss can be prevented at lower altitudes[180,181] and lessened at very high altitudes.[182]

Carbon Monoxide Poisoning

Carbon monoxide poisoning is known to occur in mountain environments. The actual incidence at high altitude is unknown, but anecdotal reports suggest that it is not uncommon.[183] The potential for exposure to hazardous levels of carbon monoxide during deployment to high terrestrial elevations has been recognized by the US Army for many years.[172] Exposure is most often due to increased production in a closed space. Carbon monoxide production by vehicle engines, cook stoves, and the like is increased owing to inefficient combustion caused by the lower oxygen content of the air. Outside of shelters, this increased production does not lead to increased exposure unless a person is in a position to breathe exhaust fumes. Because of the cold conditions at high altitude, people often try to stand close to engines and stoves to find warmth, and in doing so may be exposed to exhaust. Additionally, they may deliberately operate engines and stoves in poorly ventilated, enclosed areas (eg, tents, caves, and vehicles) to create heat. Increased levels of carbon monoxide from cooking stoves have been documented in tents, igloos, and snow caves at altitude,[184,185] and the carbon monoxide levels in snow caves were shown to increase blood levels of carboxyhemoglobin in people inside the cave.[185] Foutch and Henrichs[183] reported that a small, backpacking-type stove caused the deaths of two men by carbon monoxide poisoning in a closed tent during a snowstorm at 4,300 m.

Carbon monoxide binds to hemoglobin in red blood cells much more tightly than does oxygen and thereby decreases the amount of oxygen that the blood can carry. It also shifts the oxyhemoglobin dissociation curve to the left[186] and decreases 2,3-diphosphoglycerate (2,3-DPG) in the red blood cell[187]—changes that decrease oxygen delivery to tissues. At high altitude, where the amount of oxygen in the blood is already limited, it takes less carbon monoxide to cause more significant tissue hypoxia than at lower altitudes. Because low levels of carbon monoxide exposure cause measurable decrements in physical performance at low altitude, they probably have increasingly significant effects at high altitude.[188]

Because the mechanism of injury in carbon monoxide poisoning is hypoxia, the early signs and symptoms are similar to those of AMS and HACE. They include headache, nausea, malaise, and shortness of breath, and they progress to coma. Retinal hemorrhages similar to HARH are also seen in carbon monoxide poisoning.[189] Consequently, it may be difficult at times to distinguish carbon monoxide poisoning from AMS or HACE in unacclimatized individuals during early altitude exposure. A high index of suspicion for carbon monoxide poisoning is appropriate in this setting. Evidence of exposure to possible sources of carbon monoxide should be sought. It is also important to not to rule out carbon monoxide poisoning based on the lack of cherry red skin color, as that is a late and inconsistent clinical sign.

The initial step in treatment is to prevent further exposure by removing the source of carbon monoxide or removing the patient from the source. Treatment then is similar to that at low altitude and consists of administration of 100% oxygen and providing appropriate supportive care. Since descent in elevation increases oxygen pressure, it is helpful to evacuate the patient to lower altitude. Individuals who recover without neurological damage can return to high-altitude duty without limitation.

Prevention of carbon monoxide poisoning in the military setting entails educating people to the danger and identifying the situations and behaviors to avoid.

Constipation and Exacerbation of Hemorrhoids

Constipation and exacerbation of hemorrhoids are so common in the high mountains[1,159] that the problems have achieved the status of medical lore in the climbing community. The common saying is that "the only chronic diseases of climbers are bedsores and hemorrhoids." "Bedsores" refers to a situation that climbers often face, that of being confined to small tents in a recumbent position during prolonged periods (days to a week or more) of inclement weather. Although the climbers find the confinement to be uncomfortable and frustrating, they do not actually develop bed sores. The combination of cold, blood stasis, and elevated hematocrit can cause thromboembolic events, as discussed earlier in this chapter.

Unlike bedsores, however, constipation and hemorrhoids are very real problems at high altitude. Although the phenomenon is well know anecdotally, the exact incidence is not reported. The cause is thought to be multifactorial: a combination of dehydration, low intake of fiber, behavioral avoidance of defecation due to the cold, the inconvenience of removing layers of protective clothing, and lack of suitable private sanitary facilities above timberline. Constipation is a well-known problem during military deployments in general and may be exacerbated during deployment to high mountains. Diagnosis and treatment are the same as at low altitude. While not usually not life-threatening, the condition can become severe enough to affect morale and performance. Preventive measures include increase in fiber in the diet, proper hydration, and provision of warm and protected sanitary facilities.

SUMMARY

In addition to the classic altitude illnesses (ie, AMS, HACE, and HAPE), the constellation of medical problems associated with deployment to mountain regions of the world includes a number of other conditions, some of which are related to hypoxia and others that are not but all of which medical support personnel will have to manage. Although many seem relatively benign, all can contribute to the disease and nonbattle injury decrement in unit fighting strength and degrade military performance. Environmental factors other than hypoxia that contribute to injury and illness in mountainous areas include rugged terrain, thermal stress, low humidity, and often violently inclement weather. Medical problems in which hypoxia plays a significant role include peripheral edema, high-altitude eye problems, sleep disturbances, thromboembolic disorders, suppression of cell-mediated immunity, and high-altitude pharyngitis/bronchitis with coughing severe enough to cause rib fractures. Chronic medical conditions that are present prior to deployment can be exacerbated by the hypoxia at high altitude, or they can increase the degree of hypoxia and worsen altitude illness. All hypoxia-related conditions can be improved by descent or supplemental oxygen. Medical problems that are not directly related to hypoxia but are common in mountain terrain include trauma, cold injury, sunburn and snowblindness, lightning strikes, carbon monoxide poisoning, some infectious diseases, poor hydration and nutrition, and constipation. Because hypoxia is not the major cause of these conditions, they are generally managed at high altitude in the same manner as at low altitude.

REFERENCES

1. Steele P. Medicine on Mount Everest, 1971. *Lancet*. 1971;ii:32–39.

2. Ward MP, Milledge JS, West JB. *High Altitude Medicine and Physiology*. 2nd ed. London, England: Chapman & Hall Medical; 1995.

3. Waterlow JC, Bunjé HW. Observations on mountain sickness in the Colombian Andes. *Lancet*. 1966;ii:655–661.

4. Singh I, Khanna PK, Srivastava MC, Lal M, Roy SB, Subramanyam CSV. Acute mountain sickness. *N Engl J Med*. 1969;280:175–184.

5. Sheridan JW, Sheridan R. Tropical high-altitude peripheral oedema. *Lancet*. 1970;ii:242.

6. Hultgren HN. High altitude medical problems. *West J Med*. 1979;131:8–23.

7. Hackett PH, Rennie D, Grover RF, Reeves JT. Acute mountain sickness and the edemas of high altitude: A common pathogenesis? *Resp Physiol*. 1981;46:383–390.

8. Hackett PH, Rennie D, Hofmeister SE, Grover RF, Grover EB, Reeves JT. Fluid retention and relative hypoventilation in acute mountain sickness. *Respiration*. 1982;43:321–329.

9. Hackett PH, Rennie D. Rales, peripheral edema, retinal hemorrhage and acute mountain sickness. *Am J Med*. 1979;67:214–218.

10. Bärtsch P, Shaw S, Franciolli M, Gnädinger MP, Weidmann P. Atrial natriuretic peptide in acute mountain sickness. *J Appl Physiol*. 1988;65:1929–1937.

11. Bärtsch P, Maggiorini M, Schobersberger W, et al. Enhanced exercise-induced rise of aldosterone and vasopressin preceding mountain sickness. *J Appl Physiol*. 1991;71:136–143.

12. Hackett P, Rennie D. Acute mountain sickness. *Lancet*. 1977;i:491–492.

13. Richalet J-P, Hornych A, Rathat C, Aumont J, Larmignat P, Rémy P. Plasma prostaglandins, leukotrienes and thromboxane in acute high altitude hypoxia. *Resp Physiol*. 1991;85:205–215.

14. Roach JM, Muza SR, Rock PB, et al. Urinary leukotriene E_4 levels increase upon exposure to hypobaric hypoxia. *Chest*. 1996;110:946–951.

15. Krasney JA. A neurogenic basis for acute altitude illness. *Med Sci Sports Exerc*. 1994;26:195–208.

16. Swenson ER, Duncan TB, Goldberg SV, Ramirez G, Ahmad S, Schoene RB. Diuretic effect of acute hypoxia in humans: Relationship to hypoxic ventilatory responsiveness and renal hormones. *J Appl Physiol*. 1995;78:377–383.

17. Anand IS, Chandrashenkhar Y, Rao SK, et al. Body fluid compartments, renal blood flow, and hormones at 6,000 m in normal subjects. *J Appl Physiol*. 1993;74:1234–1239.

18. Milledge J, Bryson E, Catley D, et al. Sodium balance, fluid homeostasis, and the renin aldosterone system during the prolonged exercise of hill walking. *Clin Sci.* 1982;62:595–604.

19. Anand IS, Malhotra RM, Chandrashekhar Y, et al. Adult subacute mountain sickness—A syndrome of congestive heart failure in man at very high altitude. *Lancet.* 1990;335:561–565.

20. Hultgren HN. *High Altitude Medicine.* San Francisco, Calif: Hultgren Publications; 1997.

21. Sedan J. Hermorrhagies retiniennes survenues chez ds hypertendus au cours de vol en avion [in French]. *Ann d'ocul.* 1938;175:307.

22. Frayser R, Houston CS, Bryan AC, Rennie ID, Gray G. Retinal hemorrhages at high altitude. *N Engl J Med.* 1970;282:1183–1184.

23. McFadden DM, Houston CS, Sutton JR, Powles ACP, Gray GW, Roberts RS. High-altitude retinopathy. *JAMA.* 1981;245:581–586.

24. Wiedman M. High altitude retinal hemorrhage. *Arch Ophthalmol.* 1975;93:401–403.

25. Wiedman M, Tabin G. High-altitude retinal hemorrhage as a prognostic indicator in altitude illness. *Int Ophthalmol Clin.* 1986;26:175–186.

26. Rennie D, Morrissey J. Retinal changes in Himalayan climbers. *Arch Ophthalmol.* 1975;93:395–400.

27. Vogt C, Greite JH, Hess J. Netzhautblutungen bei Teilnehmern an Hochgebirgs-Expeditionen [High-altitude retinal hemorrhages in mountain climbers]. *Klin Monatsbl Augenheilk.* 1978;172(5):770–775.

28. Schumacher GA, Petajan JH. High altitude stress and retinal hemorrhage. *Arch Environ Health.* 1975;30:217–221.

29. Butler FK, Harris DJ Jr, Reynolds RD. Altitude retinopathy on Mount Everest, 1989. *Ophthalmology.* 1992;99:739–746.

30. Clarke C, Duff J. Mountain sickness, retinal hemorrhages, and acclimatization on Mount Everest in 1975. *Br Med J.* 1976;2:495–497.

31. Shults WT, Swan KC. High altitude retinopathy in mountain climbers. *Arch Ophthalmol.* 1975;93:404–408.

32. Rock PB, Meehan RT, Malconian MK, et al. Operation Everest II: Incidence of retinal pathology during simulated ascent of Mt Everest [abstract]. *Fed Proc.* 1986;45:1030.

33. Cusick PL, Benson OO Jr, Boothby WM. Effect of anoxia and of high concentrations of oxygen on the retinal vessels: A preliminary report. *Proceedings of the Staff Meetings of the Mayo Clinic.* 1940;15:500–502.

34. Meehan RT, Taylor GR, Rock P, Mader TH, Hunter N, Cymerman A. An automated method of quantifying retinal vascular responses during exposure to novel environmental conditions. *Ophthalmology.* 1990;97(7):875–881.

35. Kobrick JL, Appleton B. Effects of extended hypoxia on visual performance and retinal vascular state. *J Appl Physiol.* 1971;31:357–362.

36. Brinchmann-Hansen O, Myhre K. Blood pressure, intraocular pressure, and retinal vessels after high altitude mountain exposure. *Aviat Space Environ Med.* 1989;60:970–976.

37. Mader TH, Friedl KE, Mohr LC, et al. Conjunctival oxygen tension at high altitude. *Aviat Space Environ Med.* 1987;58:76–79.

38. Wiedman M, Tabin GC. High-altitude retinopathy and altitude illness. *Ophthalmology.* 1999;106:1924–1927.

39. Duane TD. Valsalva hemorrhagic retinopathy. *Trans Am Ophthalmol Soc.* 1972;70:298–313.

40. Fanin LA, Thrasher JB, Mader TH. Valsalva retinopathy associated with trans-rectal prostate biopsy. *Br J Urol.* 1994;74:391–392.

41. Hunter DJ, Smart JR, Whitton L. Increased capillary fragility at high altitude. *Br Med J.* 1986;292(6513):298.

42. Lubin JR, Rennie D, Hackett PH. High altitude retinal hemorrhage: A clinical and pathological case report. *Ann Ophthalmol.* 1982;14:1071–1076.

43. Wise GN, Dolery CT, Henkind P. *The Retinal Circulation.* New York, NY: Harper & Row; 1971: Chap 2.

44. Henkind P. The radial peripapillary capillaries of the retina, I: Anatomy: Human and comparative. *Br J Ophthalmol.* 1967;51:115.

45. Henkind P. New observations on the radial peripapillary capillaries. *Invest Ophthalmol.* 1967;6:103.

46. Henkind P. Microcirculation of the peripapillary retina. *Trans Am Acad Ophthalmol Otolaryngol.* 1969;73:890.

47. Sharma RC. Ocular manifestations of high altitude. *Indian J Ophthalmol.* 1981;29:261–262.

48. Mader TH, Blanton CL, Gilbert BN, et al. Refractive changes during 72-hour exposure to high altitude after refractive surgery. *Ophthalmology.* 1996;103:1188–1195.

49. Lang GE, Kuba GB. High-altitude retinopathy. *Am J Ophthalmol.* 1997;123:418–420.

50. Hayreh SS, Hayreh MS. Optic disc edema in raised intracranial pressure, II: Early detection with fluorescein fundus angiography and stereoscopic color photography. *Arch Ophthalmol.* 1997;95:1245–1254.

51. McLeod D, Marshall J, Kohner EM, et al. The role of oxoplasmic transport in the pathogenesis of retinal cotton-wool spots. *Br J Ophthalmol.* 1977;61:177–191.

52. Gray GW, McFadden DM, Houston CS, et al. Effect of altitude exposure on platelets. *J Appl Physiol.* 1975;39:648–652.

53. White LJ, Mader TH. Refractive changes with increasing altitude after radial keratotomy. *Am J Ophthalmol.* 1993;115:821–823.

54. Mader TH, White LJ. Refractive changes at extreme altitude after radial keratotomy. *Am J Ophthalmol.* 1995;119:733–777.

55. Winkle RK, Mader TH, Parmley VC, et al. The etiology of refractive changes at high altitude following radial keratotomy: Hypoxia versus hypobaria. *Ophthalmology.* 1998;105(2):282–286.

56. Ng JD, White LJ, Parmley VC, Hubickey W, Carter J, Mader TH. Effects of simulated high altitude on patients who have had radial keratotomy. *Ophthalmology.* 1996;103(3):452–457.

57. Snyder RP, Klein P, Solomon J. The possible effect of barometric pressure on the corneas of an RK patient: A case report. *International Contact Lens Clinics.* 1988;15:130–132.

58. White LJ, Mader TH. Effects of hypoxia and high altitude following refractive surgery. *Ophthalmic Practice.* 1997;15:174–178.

59. Mader TH, White LJ. High-altitude mountain climbing after radial keratotomy. *Wilderness Environ Med.* 1996;1:77–78.

60. Davidorf JM. LASIK at 16,000 feet [letter]. *Ophthalmology.* 1997;104:565–566.

61. Nelson ML, Brady S, Mader TH, White LJ, Parmley VC, Winkle RK. Refractive changes caused by hypoxia after Laser In Situ Keratomileusis surgery. *Ophthalmology.* 2001;108:542–544.

62. Mader TH, Blanton CL, Gilbert BN, et al. Refractive changes during 72-hour exposure to high altitude after refractive surgery. *Ophthalmology*. 1996;103:1188–1195.

63. Mertens HW, Collins WE. The effects of age, sleep deprivation, and altitude on complex performance. *Hum Factors*. 1986;28:541–551.

64. Ravenhill TH. Some experience of mountain sickness in the Andes. *J Trop Med Hyg*. 1913;16:313–320.

65. Weil JV, Kryger MH, Scoggin CH. Sleep and breathing at high altitude. In: Guilleminault C, Dement WC, eds. *Sleep Apnea Syndromes*. New York, NY: Alan R Liss; 1978: Chap 7.

66. Powles ACP, Sutton JR. Sleep at altitude. *Seminars in Respiratory Medicine*. 1983;5:175–180.

67. Reed DJ, Kellogg RH. Effect of sleep on hypoxic stimulation of breathing at sea level and altitude. *J Appl Physiol*. 1960;15:1130–1134.

68. Sutton JR, Houston CS, Mansell AL, et al. Effect of acetazolamide on hypoxemia during sleep at high altitude. *N Engl J Med*. 1979;301:1329–1331.

69. Dill DB. Physiological adjustments to altitude changes. *JAMA*. 1968;205:123–129.

70. Bärtsch P, Maggiorini M, Ritter M, Noti C, Vock P, Oelz O. Prevention of high altitude pulmonary edema by nifedipine. *N Engl J Med*. 1991;325:1284–1289.

71. West JB, Peters RM Jr, Aksnes G, Maret KH, Milledge JS, Schoene RB. Nocturnal periodic breathing at altitudes of 6,300 and 8,050 m. *J Appl Physiol*. 1986;61:280–287.

72. Eichenberger U, Weiss E, Riemann D, Oelz O, Bärtsch P. Nocturnal periodic breathing and the development of acute high altitude illness. *Am J Respir Crit Care Med*. 1996;154:1748–1754.

73. Matsuzawa Y, Kobayashi T, Fujimoto K, et al. Nocturnal periodic breathing and arterial oxygen desaturation in acute mountain sickness. *Wilderness Environ Med*. 1994;5:269–281.

74. Reite M, Jackson D, Cahoon RL, Weil JV. Sleep physiology at high altitude. *Electroencephalogr Clin Neurophysiol*. 1975;38:463–471.

75. Waggener TB, Brusil PJ, Kronauer RE, Gabel RA, Inbar GF. Strength and cycle time of high-altitude ventilatory patterns in unacclimatized humans. *J Appl Physiol: Respirat Enviro Exercise Physiol*. 1984;56:576–581.

76. Kryger M, Glas R, Jackson D, et al. Impaired oxygenation during sleep in excessive polycythemia of high altitude: Improvement with respiratory stimulation. *Sleep*. 1978;1:3–17.

77. Masuyama S, Kohchiyama S, Shinozake T, et al. Periodic breathing at high altitude and ventilatory responses to O_2 and CO_2. *Japanese Journal of Physiology*. 1989;39:523–535.

78. Anholm JD, Powles ACP, Downey R III, et al. Operation Everest II: Arterial oxygen saturation and sleep at extreme simulated altitude. *Am Rev Respir Dis*. 1992;145:817–826.

79. White DP, Gleeson K, Pickett CK, Rannels AM, Cymerman A, Weil JV. Altitude acclimatization: Influence on periodic breathing and chemoresponsiveness during sleep. *J Appl Physiol*. 1987;63:401–412.

80. Berssenbrugge A, Dempsey J, Iber C, Skatrud J, Wilson P. Mechanisms of hypoxia-induced periodic breathing during sleep in humans. *J Physiol*. 1983;343:507–524.

81. Lahiri S, Maret K, Sherpa MG. Dependence of high altitude sleep apnea on ventilatory sensitivity to hypoxia. *Respir Physiol*. 1983;52:281–301.

82. Goldenberg F, Richalet JP, Onnen I, Antezana AM. Sleep apneas and high altitude newcomers. *Int J Sports Med*. 1992;13(suppl 1):S34–S36.

83. Hackett PH, Roach RC, Harrison GL, Schoene RB, Mills WJ Jr. Respiratory stimulants and sleep periodic breathing at high altitude. *Am Rev Respir Dis*. 1987;135:896–898.

84. Fujimoto K, Matsuzawa Y, Hirai K, et al. Irregular nocturnal breathing patterns at high altitude in subjects susceptible to high-altitude pulmonary edema (HAPE): A preliminary study. *Aviat Space Environ Med*. 1989;60:786–791.

85. Nicholson AN, Smith PA, Stone BM, Bradwell AR, Coote JH. Altitude insomnia: Studies during an expedition to the Himalayas. *Sleep*. 1988;11:354–361.

86. Normand H, Barragan M, Benoit O, Bailliart O, Raynaud J. Periodic breathing and O_2 saturation in relation to sleep stages at high altitude. *Aviat Space Environ Med*. 1990;61:229–235.

87. Williams ES. Sleep and wakefulness at high altitudes. *Br Med J*. 1959;i:197–198.

88. Weil JV. Sleep at high altitude. *Clin Chest Med*. 1985;6:615–621.

89. Miller JC, Horvath SM. Sleep at altitude. *Aviat Space Environ Med*. 1977;48:615–620.

90. Pugh LGCE, Gill MB, Lahiri S, et al. Exercise at great altitude. *J Appl Physiol*. 1964;19:431– 440.

91. Powles ACP, Anholm JD, Houston CS, Sutton JR. Sleep and breathing at simulated extreme altitude. In: Sutton JR, Houston CS, Coates G, eds. *Hypoxia: The Tolerable Limits*. Indianapolis, Ind: Benchmark Press; 1988: Chap 13.

92. Phillipson EA. Control of breathing during sleep. *Am Rev Respir Dis*. 1978;118:909–939.

93. Strohl KP, Fouke JM. Periodic breathing at altitude. *Seminars in Respiratory Medicine*. 1983;5:169–174.

94. Sutton JR, Gray GW, Houston CS, Powles ACP. Effects of duration at altitude and acetazolamide on ventilation and oxygenation during sleep. *Sleep*. 1980;3:455–464.

95. Horii M, Takasaki I, Ohtsuka K, et al. Changes of heart rate and QT interval at high altitude in alpinists: Analysis by Holter ambulatory electrocardiogram. *Clin Cardiol*. 1987;10:238–242.

96. Cummings P, Lysgaard M. Cardiac arrhythmia at high altitude. *West J Med*. 1981;135:66–68.

97. Malconian M, Hultgren H, Nitta M, Anholm J, Houston H, Fails H. The sleep electrocardiogram at extreme altitudes (Operation Everest II). *Am J Cardiol*. 1990;64:1014–1020.

98. Karliner JS, Sarnquist FN, Graber DJ, Peters RM Jr, West JB. The electrocardiogram at extreme altitude: Experience on Mt Everest. *Am Heart J*. 1985;109:505–513.

99. Berssenbrugge A, Dempsey J, Skatrud J. Hypoxic versus hypocapnic effects on periodic breathing during sleep. In: West JB, Lahiri S, eds. *High Altitude and Man*. Baltimore, Md: American Physiological Society; 1984: Chap 10.

100. Bisgard GE, Forster HV. Ventilatory responses to acute and chronic hypoxia. In: Fregly MJ, Blatteis CM, eds. *Handbook of Physiology*. Section 4. *Environmental Physiology*. Vol 2. New York, NY: Oxford University Press; 1996: Chap 52.

101. Georgopoulos D, Bshouty Z, Younes M, Anthosnisen NR. Hypoxic exposure and activation of the afterdischarge mechanism in conscious humans. *J Appl Physiol: Respir Environ Exerc Physiol*. 1990;69:1159–1164.

102. Lahiri S, Maret KH, Sherpa M, Peters RM Jr. Sleep and periodic breathing at high altitude: Sherpa natives vs sojourners. In: West JB, Lahiri S, eds. *High Altitude and Man*. Baltimore, Md: American Physiological Society; 1984: Chap 7.

103. Young T, Palta M, Dempsey JA, Skatrud J, Weber S, Badr MS. The occurrence of sleep disordered breathing among middle-aged adults. *N Engl J Med*. 1993;328:1230–1235.

104. Dempsey JA, Morgan BJ. Sleep apnea leads to chronic hypertension via intermittent hypoxia. In: Houston CS, Coates G, eds. *Women at Altitude. Proceedings of the 10th International Hypoxia Symposium*. Burlington, Vt: Queen City Printers; 1997: Chap 28.

105. Pugh LGCE, Ward MP. Some effects of high altitude on man. *Lancet*. 1956;ii:1115–1121.

106. Swenson EK, Leatham KL, Roach RC, Schoene RB, Mills WJ Jr, Hackett PH. Renal carbonic anhydrase inhibition reduces high altitude sleep periodic breathing. *Respir Physiol*. 1991;86:333–343.

107. Hackett PH, Roach RC. High-altitude medicine. In: Auerbach PS, ed. *Wilderness Medicine: Management of Wilderness and Environmental Emergencies*. 3rd ed. St Louis, Mo: Mosby; 1995: Chap 1.

108. Meehan RT, Zavala DC. The pathophysiology of acute high-altitude illness. *Am J Med*. 1982;73:395–403.

109. Houston CS, Sutton JR, Cymerman A, Reeves JT. Operation Everest II: Man at extreme altitude. *J Appl Physiol*. 1987;63:877–882.

110. Sutton JR, Gray GW, Houston CS, Powles ACP. Effects of acclimatization on sleep hypoxemia at altitude. In: West JB, Lahiri S, eds. *High Altitude and Man*. Baltimore, Md: American Physiological Society; 1984: Chap 12.

111. Andrew M, O'Brodovich H, Sutton J. Operation Everest II: Coagulation system during prolonged decompression to 282 Torr. *J Appl Physiol*. 1987;63:1262–1267.

112. Houston C, Bates R. *K2: The Savage Mountain*. Seattle, Wash: Mountaineers; 1979.

113. Dickinson J, Heath D, Gosney J, Williams D. Altitude-related deaths in seven trekkers in the Himalayas. *Thorax*. 1983;38:646–656.

114. Houston CS, Dickinson J. Cerebral form of high-altitude illness. *Lancet*. 1975;ii:758–761.

115. Ward M. *Mountain Medicine: A Clinical Study of Cold and High Altitude*. London, England: Crosby Lockwood Staples; 1975.

116. Wilson R. Acute high-altitude illness in mountaineers and problems of rescue. *Ann Int Med*. 1973;78:421–428.

117. Wohns RNW. Transient ischemic attacks at high altitude. *Crit Care Med*. 1986;14:517–518.

118. Song S-Y, Asaji T, Tanizaki Y, Fujimaki T, Matsutani M, Okeda R. Cerebral thrombosis at altitude: Its pathogenesis and the problems of prevention and treatment. *Aviat Space Environ Med*. 1986; 57(1):71–76.

119. Aoki T, Tsuda T, Onizuka T, et al. A case of high-altitude illness with pulmonary and cerebral infarction [in Japanese]. *Japanese Journal of Thoracic Diseases*. 1983;21(8):770–774.

120. Nayak NC, Roy S, Narayanan TK. Pathologic features of altitude sickness. *Am J Pathol*. 1964;45:381–391.

121. Hultgren, H, Spikard W, Lopez C. Further studies of high altitude pulmonary edema. *Br Heart J*. 1962;24:95–102.

122. Staub NC. Pulmonary edema—Hypoxia and overperfusion. *N Engl J Med*. 1980;13:725–732.

123. Rennie D. Splinter hemorrhages at high altitude [letter]. *JAMA*. 1974;228(8):974.

124. Heath D, Harris P, Williams D, Krüger H. Nail haemorrhages in native highlanders of the Peruvian Andes. *Thorax*. 1981;36:764–766.

125. Shuping L, Weiss EL. High altitude hemorrhage syndromes. *Wilderness Environ Med*. 1993;4:115–117.

126. Litch JA, Basnyat B, Zimmerman M. Subarachnoid hemorrhage at high altitude. *West J Med.* 1997;167:180–181.

127. Breddin HK. Thrombosis and Virchow's triad: What is established? *Thromb Haemost.* 1989;3:237–239.

128. Chohan IS, Singh I, Balakrihsnan K. Fibrinolytic activity at high altitude and sodium acetate buffer. *Thromb Diath Haemorrh.* 1974;32:65–70.

129. Singh I, Chohan IS. Adverse changes in fibrinolysis, blood coagulation and platelet function in high-altitude pulmonary oedema and their role in its pathogenesis. *Int J Biometeorol.* 1974;18:33–45.

130. Sharma SC. Platelet count and adhesiveness on induction to high altitude by air and road. *Int J Biometeorol.* 1982;26:219–224.

131. Sharma SC, Vijayan GP, Suri ML, Seth HN. Platelet adhesiveness in young patients with ischaemic stroke. *J Clin Path.* 1977;30:649–652.

132. Cucinell SA, Pitts CM. Thrombosis at mountain altitudes. *Aviat Space Environ Med.* 1987;58:1109–1111.

133. Bärtsch P, Waber U, Haeberli A, et al. Enhanced fibrin formation in high-altitude pulmonary edema. *J Appl Physiol.* 1987;63:752–757.

134. Bärtsch P, Haeberli A, Hauser K, Gubser A, Straub PW. Fibrinogenolysis in the absence of fibrin formation in severe hypobaric hypoxia. *Aviat Space Environ Med.* 1988;59:428–432.

135. Bärtsch P, Haeberli A, Franciolli M, Kruithof EKO, Straub PW. Coagulation and fibrinolysis in acute mountain sickness and beginning pulmonary edema. *J Appl Physiol.* 1989;66:2136–2144.

136. Dahlback B. Factor V gene mutation causing inherited resistance to activated protein C as a basis for venous thromboembolism. *J Intern Med.* 1995;237:139–151.

137. Emonson DL. Activated protein C resistance as a "new" cause of deep venous thrombosis in aviators. *Aviat Space Environ Med.* 1997;68:606–608.

138. Meehan RT. Immune suppression at high altitude. *Ann Emerg Med.* 1987;16:974–979.

139. Singh I, Chohan IS, Lal M, et al. Effects of high altitude stay on the incidence of common diseases in man. *Int J Biometeorol.* 1977;21:93–122.

140. Sarnquist FH. Physicians on Mount Everest: A clinical account of the 1981 American Medical Research Expedition to Everest. *West J Med.* 1983;139:480–485.

141. Meehan RT, Duncan U, Neale L, et al. Operation Everest II: Alterations in the immune system at high altitudes. *J Clin Immunol.* 1988;8:397–406.

142. Chohan IS, Singh I, Balakrihsnan K, Talwar GP. Immune responses in human subjects at high altitude. *Int J Biometeorol.* 1977;21:93–122.

143. Biselli R, Le Moli S, Matricardi PM, et al. The effects of hypobaric hypoxia on specific B cell responses following immunization in mice and humans. *Aviat Space Environ Med.* 1991;62:870–874.

144. Knighton DR, Halliday B, Hunt TK. Oxygen as an antibiotic: The effect of inspired oxygen on infection. *Arch Surg.* 1984;119:199–204.

145. Gong H Jr, Tashkin DP, Lee EY, Simmons MS. Hypoxia-altitude simulation test: Evaluation of patients with chronic airway obstruction. *Am Rev Respir Dis.* 1964;130:980–986.

146. Pitts GC, Pace N. The effect of blood carboxyhemoglobin on hypoxic tolerance. *Am J Physiol.* 1947;148:139–151.

147. Malhotra MS, Selvamurthy W, Purkayastha SS, Murkerjee AK, Mathew L, Dua GL. Responses of the autonomic nervous system during acclimatization to high altitude in man. *Aviat Space Environ Med.* 1976;47:1076–1079.

148. Lane PA, Githens JH. Splenic syndrome at mountain altitudes in sickle cell trait: Its occurrence in nonblack persons. *JAMA.* 1985;253:2251–2254.

149. Hultgren, HN. Coronary disease and trekking. *Wilderness Environ Med.* 1990;1:154–161.

150. Jenzer G, Bärtsch P. Migraine with aura at high altitude. *Wilderness Environ Med.* 1993;4:412–415.

151. Moore LG. Altitude aggravated illness: Examples from pregnancy and prenatal life. *Ann Emerg Med.* 1987;16:965–973.

152. Niermeyer S. The pregnant altitude visitor. *Adv Exp Med Biol.* 1999;474:65–77.

153. Pandolf K, Burr RE, Wenger CB, Pozos RS, eds. *Medical Aspects of Harsh Environments, Volume 1.* In: Zajtchuk R, Bellamy RF, eds. *Textbook of Military Medicine.* Washington, DC: Department of the Army, Office of The Surgeon General, and Borden Institute; 2001. Also available at www.armymedicine.army.mil/history/borden/default.htm.

154. Schussman LC, Lutz LJ, Shaw RR, Bohnn CR. The epidemiology of mountaineering and rock climbing accidents. *Wilderness Environ Med.* 1990;1:235–248.

155. Baird RE, McAninch GW. High altitude penetrating chest trauma: A case report. *Mil Med.* 1989;154:337–340.

156. Rosario PG, Fernandes S. Trekker's shoulder. *N Engl J Med.* 1990;322(22):1611.

157. Holtzhausen LM, Noakes TD. Elbows, forearm, wrist, and hand injuries among sport rock climbers. *Clin J Sport Med.* 1996;6:196–203.

158. Roeggla M, Wagner A, Moser B, Roeggla G. Hiking sticks in mountaineering [letter]. *Wilderness Environ Med.* 1996;7:258.

159. Rao KS, Natesan R, Singh KPB. The morbidity pattern in a high altitude hospital. In: Manchanda SK, Selvamurthy W, eds. *Advances in Physiological Sciences. Proceedings of the Second Congress of the Asian and Oceanic Physiological Societies, November 12–15, 1990.* New Delhi, India. Delhi, India: MacMillan India Limited; 1992: Chap 45.

160. Deeter DP, Gaydos JC, eds. *Occupational Health: The Soldier and the Industrial Base.* In: Zajtchuk R, Bellamy RF, eds. *Textbook of Military Medicine.* Washington, DC: Department of the Army, Office of The Surgeon General, and Borden Institute; 1993.

161. James WJ, ed. *Military Dermatology.* In: Zajtchuk R, Bellamy RF, eds. *Textbook of Military Medicine.* Washington, DC: Department of the Army, Office of The Surgeon General, and Borden Institute; 1994. Also available at www.armymedicine.army.mil/history/borden/default.htm.

162. Lomax P, Thinney R, Mondino BJ. Solar radiation. In: Dubas F, Vallotton J, eds. *Color Atlas of Mountain Medicine.* Boston, Mass: Mosby–Year Book; 1991: 67–71.

163. Brandt F, Malla OK. Eye problems at high altitudes. In: Brendel W, Zink RA, eds. *High Altitude Physiology and Medicine.* New York, NY: Springer Verlag; 1982: Chap 32.

164. Duclos PJ, Sanderson LM. An epidemiological description of lightning-related deaths in the United States. *Int J Epidemiol.* 1990;19:673–679.

165. Dusek ER, Hansen JE. Biomedical study of military performance at high terrestrial elevation. *Mil Med.* 1969;134:1497–1507.

166. Cherington M. Lightning injuries. *Ann Emerg Med.* 1995;25:516–519.

167. Leikin JB, Aks SE, Andrews S, Auerbach PS, Cooper MA. Lightning injuries. *Dis Mon.* 1997;43:871–892.

168. Cwinn AA, Cantrill S. Lightning injuries. *J Emerg Med.* 1985;2:379–388.

169. Cherington M, Yarnell PR, London SF. Neurologic complications of lightning injuries. *West J Med.* 1995;162:413–417.

170. Cooper MA. Emergent care of lightning and electrical injuries. *Semin Neurol.* 1995;15:268–278.

171. Kelley PW, ed. *Military Preventive Medicine: Mobilization and Deployment.* In: Zajtchuk R, Bellamy RF, eds. *Textbook of Military Medicine.* Washington, DC: Department of the Army, Office of The Surgeon General, and Borden Institute; 2001. In press. Also available at www.armymedicine.army.mil/history/borden/default.htm.

172. US Department of the Army. *Medical Problems of Man at High Terrestrial Elevations.* Washington, DC: DA; 1975. Technical Bulletin MED 288.

173. Bruce-Chwatt LJ. Malaria at high altitudes in Africa. *Br Med J.* 1985;291:280.

174. Hershey DW, McGregor JA. Low prevalence of Toxoplasma infection in a Rocky Mountain prenatal population. *Obstet Gynecol.* 1987;70:900–902

175. Basnyat B, Litch JA. Medical problems of porters and trekkers in the Nepal Himalaya. *Wilderness Environ Med.* 1997;8:78–81.

176. Schwartz E, Innis BL, Shlim DR, Snitbhan R. Viral hepatitis in foreign residents and travelers in Nepal. *Wilderness Environ Med.* 1991;2:88–93.

177. Tomkins LS. *Bartonella* infections including cat-scratch disease. In: Fauci AS, Braunwald E, Isselbacher KJ, et al, eds. *Harrison's Principles of Internal Medicine.* 14th ed. New York, NY: McGraw-Hill; 1998: Chap 165.

178. Marriot BM, Carlson SJ, eds. *Nutritional Needs in Cold and in High-Altitude Environments.* Washington, DC: National Academy Press; 1996.

179. Pandolf KS, Burr RE, eds. *Medical Aspects of Harsh Environments, Volume 3.* In: Zajtchuk R, Bellamy RF. *Textbook of Military Medicine.* Washington, DC: Department of the Army, Office of The Surgeon General, and Borden Institute; 2003. In press.

180. Butterfield GE, Gates J, Fleming S, Brooks GA, Sutton JR, Reeves JT. Increased energy intake minimizes weight loss in men at high altitude. *J Appl Physiol.* 1992;72:1741–1748.

181. Mawson JT, Braun B, Rock PB, Moore LG, Mazzeo RS, Butterfield GE. Women at altitude: Energy requirement at 4,300 m. *J Appl Physiol.* 2000;88:272–281.

182. Rose MS, Houston CS, Fulco CS, Coates G, Sutton JR, Cymerman A. Operation Everest II: Nutrition and body composition. *J Appl Physiol.* 1988;65:2545–2551.

183. Foutch RG, Henrichs W. Carbon monoxide poisoning at high altitudes. *Am J Emerg Med.* 1988;6:596–598.

184. Turner WA, Cohen MA, Moore S, Spengler JD, Hackett PH. Carbon monoxide exposure in mountaineers on Denali. *Alaska Med.* 1988;30:85–90.

185. Keyes LE, Hamilton RS, Rose JS. Carbon monoxide exposure from cooking in snow caves at high altitude. *Wilderness Environ Med.* 2001;12:208–212.

186. Roughton FJW, Darling RC. The effect of carbon monoxide on the oxyhemoglobin dissociation curve. *Am J Physiol.* 1944;141:17–41.

187. Thomas MF, Penny DG. Hematologic responses to carbon monoxide and altitude: A comparative study. *J Appl Physiol.* 1977;43:365–369.

188. Pandolf KB. Air quality and human performance. In: Pandolf KB, Sawka MN, Gonzalez RR, eds. *Human Performance Physiology and Environmental Medicine at Terrestrial Extremes.* Indianapolis, Ind: Benchmark Press (now Traverse City, Mich: Cooper Publishing Group). 1988: Chap 16.

189. Kelley JS, Sophocleus GJ. Retinal hemorrhages in subacute carbon monoxide poisoning. *JAMA.* 1978;239:1515–1517.

Chapter 27

MILITARY MEDICAL OPERATIONS IN MOUNTAIN ENVIRONMENTS

PAUL B. ROCK, DO, PhD[*]; AND EUGENE J. IWANYK, MD[†]

INTRODUCTION

ESTIMATING DISEASE AND NONBATTLE INJURY AND PERFORMANCE
DECREMENTS
Disease and Nonbattle Injury
Performance Decrements

HEALTH MAINTENANCE
Prevention of Environmental Injury and Illness
Treatment of Environmental Injury and Illness

DEPLOYMENT OF MEDICAL SUPPORT ASSETS
Environmental Effects on Medical Support
General Principles for Deployment of Medical Assets

SUMMARY

[*]Colonel, Medical Corps, US Army (Ret); Associate Professor of Medicine, Center for Aerospace and Hyperbaric Medicine, Oklahoma State University Center for the Health Sciences, Tulsa, Oklahoma 74132; formerly, US Army Research Institute of Environmental Medicine, Natick, Massachusetts 01760
[†]Lieutenant Colonel, Medical Corps, US Army (Ret); Ellis Eye and Laser Medical Center, El Cerrito, California 94530

INTRODUCTION

One of the fundamental challenges faced by medical personnel supporting military units deployed in mountain regions is to deal with the effects of the environment on the health service support mission. Mountain environments have an impact on virtually all aspects of the mission. On one hand, mountains add to the spectrum of disease and injury that normally occurs during military operations. Indeed, in the absence of combat, environmental injuries are the biggest source of casualties that reduce unit fighting strength. On the other hand, they affect the health service support system itself, constraining the options for prevention or treatment of casualties. Factors in the mountain environment degrade the performance of medical personnel and equipment and limit the ways in which medical assets can be deployed. If the effects of mountain environments are not anticipated and successfully avoided or abated, the health support mission, and with it possibly the tactical mission, will be jeopardized.

The purpose of this chapter is to provide information that will help medical personnel successfully manage the impact of mountain environments on the health service support mission. In its simplest form, that mission is to conserve the fighting strength of the tactical unit by

- advising the unit commander about the potential impact of the environment on unit personnel and operations, and recommending means, countermeasures, or both to lessen that impact;

- providing a health maintenance program to (*a*) prevent environmental medical problems and (*b*) treat them effectively when they occur; and
- managing the field medical support assets to allow efficient treatment and return to duty or evacuation of casualties.

In this general formulation, the mission is applicable to most organizational levels of medical support to most tactical units.

The information presented here is organized around the simple formulation of the health service support mission stated above. The first section of this chapter reviews the potential impact of mountain environments on military units and countermeasures that can be recommended to lessen environmental effects. The next section discusses health maintenance in units deployed to high altitude. The final section deals with the effect of the mountain environment on the medical support system itself. The considerations underlying the concepts presented are based on providing support to "traditional" ground combat units such as infantry, light infantry, armor, and cavalry units. Although many of the general concepts are relevant to other types of military units, including special operations units, the unique aspects of medical support of special operations are discussed in Chapter 37, Medical Support of Special Operations, and Chapter 38, Organizational, Psychological, and Training Aspects of Special Operations Forces of this textbook.

ESTIMATING DISEASE AND NONBATTLE INJURY AND PERFORMANCE DECREMENTS

Military leaders need good estimates to plan effectively for their unit's mission. Combat leaders need estimates of the unit's fighting strength (manpower) and performance capabilities in the environment in which the unit will operate. In the mountains, they need estimates of the extent to which the mountain environment itself will degrade unit strength (ie, disease and nonbattle injury [DNBI]) and performance over time. Medical support personnel need estimates of the number of casualties so that they can plan for the care of those casualties. In the mountains, they need estimates of the effects of the mountain environment on manpower and performance to accurately brief the combat commander, guide health maintenance activities, and allocate the medical support resources.

Useful estimates of the effects of mountain envi-

ronments on unit strength and performance ideally would be based on experience, in the same way as the most useful estimates of battle casualty rates are derived from "experience tables" based on data from previous battles. Unfortunately, there are few useful data about medical problems available from the mountain warfare experience. For instance, although Houston's excellent review of the effects of the environment on past military campaigns in the mountain regions of Europe and Asia (Chapter 20, Selected Military Operations in Mountain Environments: Some Medical Aspects) graphically illustrates the deleterious impact that mountains can have (eg, what commander today would want to suffer the nearly 50% reduction in force that Hannibal experienced while crossing the Alps), much of that historical information is not particularly applicable to current military operations, owing to differences in equipment, transportation, and medical technology. Similarly, the information on combat injuries from previous battles with swords and shields is not especially applicable to the present-day battlefield, with its high-velocity ballistic weapons. Of the conflicts that took place in the mountains during the 20th century and, therefore, might be more applicable, the only readily available data on environmental casualties are from the Sino–Indian border conflict (1962–1963).[1] Additionally, some data are also available from studies of military training activities in the mountains,[2–5] but the information is based on limited numbers of individuals.

Even in the absence of extensive experience-based data, medical personnel can make reasonable estimates of the effects of mountain environments on unit strength and performance by combining some general concepts with extrapolations of the limited data available. Estimates are, after all, *estimates*. Considerations for making reasonable estimates of DNBI and performance decrements for mountain terrain are presented below.

Disease and Nonbattle Injury

The major components of DNBI in high mountain terrain are listed in Exhibit 27-1 and extensively discussed in Chapters 24, 25, and 26, which deal with acute mountain sickness (AMS), high-altitude cerebral edema (HACE), high-altitude pulmonary edema (HAPE), and other edematous and nonedematous illnesses. They include conditions that are caused by the hypobaric hypoxia that is characteristic of high-altitude and conditions related to other environmental factors. That both hypoxia and other environmental factors play a role during military operations in the mountains was strikingly demonstrated during a training exercise at 3,600 to 4,000 m altitude in the Colorado mountains.[3] The number of soldiers evacuated during 5 days of mountain operations was more than 10-fold that for the same unit doing the same maneuvers for the same amount of time in North Carolina. The casualties at altitude were caused by AMS and HAPE, both related to hypobaric hypoxia; traumatic and overuse injuries, related to the rugged topography; and one fatality and five injuries from a lightning strike.

A reasonable method to estimate DNBI for military operations in mountains is to start with estimates for a nonmountainous region, add hypoxia-related conditions, and then make appropriate adjustments for other factors that change in the mountains but

are not necessarily related to hypoxia (eg, increased chance of lightning injury, decreased chance of mosquito-borne diseases). Experience tables for DNBI are available for the United States[6] and most other military forces. Estimates of DNBI for temperate climate operations are a reasonable starting point for altitudes from 1,500 to 4,000 m because the climate conditions at those elevations are fairly similar. Estimates for arctic regions may be a better baseline for mountain regions above 4,000 m elevation, where increasingly cold ambient temperatures prevail.

Considerations for estimating the additional effect of altitude on incidence of hypoxia-related and other environmental injuries are drawn from the military and civilian experience in the mountains. Reports from civilian experience are mostly related to recreational activity, however. Because tactical considerations dictate the timing, duration, and location of environmental exposure during military operations, civilian recreational exposure is not

---

EXHIBIT 27-1

HEALTH THREATS TO MILITARY PERSONNEL FROM MOUNTAIN ENVIRONMENTS

Hypoxia Related

    Acute mountain sickness (AMS)

    High-altitude cerebral edema (HACE)

    High-altitude pulmonary edema (HAPE)

    High-altitude peripheral edema

    High-altitude eye problems

    Sleep problems with sleep deprivation

    Thromboembolism

    Exacerbation of preexisting disease

    High-altitude pharyngitis/bronchitis

    Performance decrements

Not Related to Hypoxia

    Trauma

    Thermal injury (especially cold injury)

    Ultraviolet (UV-A, UV-B) radiation energy

    Lightning strikes

    Carbon monoxide poisoning

    Infections

    Hypohydration

    Inadequate nutrition

entirely equivalent.[7] Estimates can be made from this data, however, by considering activities that might be roughly equivalent to military activities. For example, trekking and backpacking in the mountains (ie, long journeys on foot carrying camping equipment; see Exhibit 19-1 in Chapter 19, Mountains and Military Medicine: An Overview) are roughly equivalent to an approach march, although, owing to tactical contingencies, soldiers often carry more equipment and set a faster pace.

Altitude illness, which includes AMS, HACE, and HAPE, is the only component of DNBI that is unique to the mountains. As detailed in Chapter 24, Acute Mountain Sickness and High-Altitude Cerebral Edema, and Chapter 25, High-Altitude Pulmonary Edema, the incidence of altitude illness is increased with increasing severity of altitude exposure, as determined by the elevation achieved and the speed of ascent. In general, the altitude at which personnel sleep is the most important one in determining the incidence of altitude illness. Additionally, altitude illness decreases over time as individuals acclimatize. Information presented in Chapters 24 and 25 suggests that for ascent rates of 1 to 2 days, the incidence of individuals with AMS symptoms can be as high as 20% at 2,000 m and 67% at 3,000 m; the incidence of HACE may be 0.1% at 2,000 m and as high as 1.8% at 5,500 m; and the incidence of HAPE, 0.1% at 2,500 m and 15% at 5,500 m. Many of those with AMS will not be casualties but will be "medically noneffective" for as long as several days. Dusek and Hansen[3] found that 6% of soldiers in a Special Forces unit were incapacitated with AMS at 3,600 to 4,000 m, while Pigman and Karakla[2] reported that 1.4% of Marines were incapacitated at 2,000 to 2,600 m. For purposes of estimating unit strength decrement, all casualties with HACE and HAPE should be considered as needing evacuation for treatment.

Cases of altitude illness will be clustered in space and time. The units that ascend the highest in the least amount of time will have the most altitude illness, and the prevalence of illness will be greatest during the first several days to a week or more after ascent. An extremely important point is that because exposure to hypobaric hypoxia is ubiquitous at high altitude, all unit members are equally susceptible to altitude illness, including command staff and medical and other support personnel.

Most components of DNBI that are not related to hypoxia also vary with altitude. Cold, ultraviolet (UV) -radiation injury, and trauma are common in many environments other than mountains (interested readers should consult Section II: Cold Environments [Chapters 10–18 and Appendix 1] of *Medical Aspects of Harsh Environments, Volume 1*[8]), and the incidence, prevalence, or both in those situations could provide a baseline reference point for estimating altitude rates. UV radiation exposure is increased with increasing elevation, and consequently the estimated rate of injury should be increased. The potential for cold injury increases with elevation because ambient temperatures drop, and the rugged ("nonlinear") mountain topography will increase the accidental trauma and overuse injury. The magnitude of increase for these factors is not well established but it is substantial. Additionally, environmental causality rates will be higher, because of the interaction of factors. Thus, increasing hypobaric hypoxia may contribute to an increased incidence of cold injury by decreasing plasma volume and impairing cognitive performance and judgment.

Unlike most components of DNBI, the incidence of infectious disease in the mountains is more or less inversely related to altitude (ie, the greater the altitude, the less risk of infectious disease; see Chapter 26, Additional Medical Problems in Mountain Environments). This is largely due to the decrease in arthropod disease vectors and decreased survival of bacteria in the open environment at altitudes above approximately 4,500 m. Diseases that are spread by person-to-person transmission, including fecal–oral transmission of diarrheal diseases, that age-old scourge of military field operations, can occur at virtually any altitude, however. Consequently, rate calculations for the infectious disease component of DNBI can ignore arthropod vector–related diseases at very high altitudes but should retain rate estimates for diseases transmitted person-to-person.

Performance Decrements

Degradation of individual and group military performance during high-altitude exposure has been documented in controlled studies.[3,4,9,10] Most military activity involves behaviors with varying degrees of physical exertion and psychological functioning, combined or in rapid serial sequence. The hypobaric hypoxia of high altitude impairs both physical and psychological performance (see Chapter 22, Physical Performance at Varying Terrestrial Altitudes, and Chapter 23, Cognitive Performance, Mood, and Neurological Status at High Terrestrial Elevation). It is the major cause of decrements in soldier and unit function, although other factors such as cold exposure and hypohydration also contribute.

Because the decrease in oxygen content of ambient air is ubiquitous at high altitude, the effects are universal and they affect all members of a unit deployed to the mountains, including command staff and medical support personnel. Although performance decrements increase with increasing elevation because the degree of hypoxia increases, the effects of hypoxia improve over time as the body acclimatizes to altitude. Medical officers must apprise unit commanders of both the threat from altitude-related performance decrements, which threatens a unit's ability to accomplish its mission, and the means to lessen the impact of those decrements on operations.

Physical Performance

The main effect on physical performance of hypobaric hypoxia at high altitude is decreased maximal aerobic exercise capability and endurance (see Chapter 22, Physical Performance at Varying Terrestrial Altitudes). Muscular strength and anaerobic activity are not much affected. Because the energy required to do a specified amount of work (ie, the metabolic cost) does not change with altitude but the maximum amount of energy that can be expended goes down, individuals have to work at a higher percentage of their maximal aerobic capability to accomplish any physical task. This means that those tasks will either require relatively more effort, take longer to complete, or both, compared with the same tasks done at lower altitudes. The amount of decrement in any specific task is a function of the mix of aerobic and anaerobic activity required to do the job. Tasks that have a greater anaerobic component are less affected.

The threshold for onset of altitude effects on physical performance is low, but meaningful effects do not begin until altitudes higher than 2,400 m are reached. The rate of decline in maximal exercise capacity is dramatic above 6,000 m. Importantly, physically fit individuals suffer a greater decrement in their maximal exercise capacity at high altitude than less fit individuals. They may still be able to do more work than less-fit individuals, however, owing to their higher starting sea-level work capacity.

The effect of physical performance decrements on mission is an interaction of the type of performance entailed by the task and the contribution of the task to the mission. For example, military tasks that require only a small aerobic energy output at sea level will require an increasing percentage of the diminished maximal energy capacity at higher altitudes, but they can still be accomplished. On the

other hand, tasks that require a large energy output may not be possible to perform. If the mission depends on tasks that do not require a large energy output, the altitude-induced performance decrement will not create a problem. If it depends on energy-intensive tasks that cannot be done at high altitude, then the mission will be in jeopardy.

Exhibit 22-2 in Chapter 22, Physical Performance at Varying Terrestrial Altitudes, provides specific examples. For a task that entails prolonged standing on a circulation (traffic) control point (see number 1 in Exhibit 22-2, which pertains to Task #3, MOS 95B [Military Police]), the percentage of maximal oxygen uptake increases only from 9% to 13% between sea level and 5,000 m. Consequently it is unlikely that the physical aspects of that task will be significantly degraded by altitude exposure. However, the energy required to carry tube-launched, optically tracked, wire-guided (TOW) missile system equipment up a 20% grade at a rate of 0.89 m/s exceeds the maximal oxygen uptake at 5,000 m and is greater than 95% of the maximal uptake at 4,000 m (see number 32 in Exhibit 22-2; Task #1, MOS 11H [Heavy anti-armor weapons, Infantry]). In theory, the task cannot be accomplished at 5,000 m. If the mission success depends on standing on a traffic control-point at 5,000 m, there will be little problem. But if mission success depends on carrying equipment up a slope at 5,000 m, then the mission is in jeopardy and alternative means to do the task will have to be found.

Once acclimatization has been achieved, maximal exercise capacity improves somewhat with altitude acclimatization and with physical training at high altitude, but it *never* regains sea-level values. It is important that commanders know that maximal performance decrement will *always* occur at high altitude, so they can plan for it. Submaximal physical performance decrements can be negated by expending more effort, but the cost of doing so is increased fatigue. Chapter 21, Human Adaptation to High Terrestrial Altitude, suggests that submaximal physical performance decrements are best approached by (1) increasing the amount of time allowed to complete the task, (2) decreasing the intensity of the work, and/or (3) taking more-frequent rest breaks.

Psychological Performance

High-altitude exposure alters a number of psychological parameters, including cognitive and psychomotor function, visual parameters, and mood and personality adjustments, in ways that can have a negative impact on military performance (see Chapter 23, Cognitive Performance, Mood, and Neurological Status Effects at High Terrestrial Altitude). As with physical performance decrements, the psychological effects are primarily due to hypobaric hypoxia and tend to increase with increasing altitude and improve with acclimatization. Additionally, there is a large individual variability in these effects.

Cognitive function and psychomotor skills are progressively diminished above 3,000 m and are very noticeably affected over 5,500 m. In general, cognitive processes are more affected than psychomotor function. As a result, complex tasks are more affected than simple ones, and tasks requiring decisions or strategy are more affected than more "automatic" ones. There is some improvement in function with acclimatization, but there is always an element of intellectual "dulling" at very high altitudes. This results in an increased number of errors, an increase in the time needed to complete a task, or both.

A common functional strategy for countering the effects of altitude on task performance is to increase the time taken to do the job to decrease the number of errors. Many individuals adopt this strategy on their own volition. As a consequence, more time to complete most tasks should be anticipated at high altitude. Increasing proficiency by training before deployment and maintaining proficiency while deployed at high altitude by frequent practice also help improve performance. Important or critical

tasks always should be carefully checked for errors.

The most important sensory decrement from the standpoint of military performance is a persistent decrease in night vision that begins as low as 2,500 m and does not improve with acclimatization. This diminished night vision will increase the possibility for accidents during night travel and may make it more difficult to detect enemy movements at night. Because the decrement is persistent, methods will need to be instituted to lessen its impact (eg, provisions for guidance during night travel, increased reliance on nonvisual means for detecting enemy activity at night).

Mood changes and personality-trait adjustments that occur at high altitude can affect the interpersonal relationships among unit members and disrupt unit cohesion. The euphoric response that many individuals experience during the first few hours after ascent can predispose them to accidents. Once the euphoria subsides, a depressed mood, irritability, or apathy can appear. A number of factors in addition to hypoxia, including the person's underlying psychological makeup, weather, and social bonds will influence mood and personality adjustments in high mountain environments. Symptoms of altitude illness can also influence mood, motivation, and performance. Building high morale and esprit de corps prior to deployment will help lessen the impact of negative mood and personality-trait changes. Prophylaxis to prevent symptoms of altitude illness will also help.

HEALTH MAINTENANCE

Medical support activity to sustain the health and performance of personnel in military units deployed to high mountain areas is directed toward (1) prevention of illness and injury and (2) effective detection and treatment of those illnesses and injuries that occur despite preventive efforts. Effective treatment facilitates rapid return to duty or evacuation of the sick or injured unit member (see Exhibit 27-1 for an array of potential illnesses and injuries found in mountain environments). Specific information on how to prevent, diagnose, and treat those conditions is presented in the previous chapters of the Mountain Environments section of this textbook and in *Medical Aspects of Harsh Environments, Volume 1*,[8] and *Volume 3*.[11] General considerations about ways in which that information can be used to maintain the health of members of a unit deployed in mountain terrain are presented here.

Prevention of Environmental Injury and Illness

Prevention of medical problems caused by the mountain environment can be accomplished by limiting exposure to the mountain environment, by providing ways to counter its adverse effects, or both. High altitude is the major factor conferring risk in the mountains. Increasing altitude not only increases the level of hypoxia and altitude illness but also increases risk of cold injury, UV radiation exposure, lightning, trauma, and most other environment-related conditions. Limiting altitude exposure means controlling the elevation, the rate of ascent, or both. This may not always be possible for military units deploying into mountainous regions because the mission or the tactical situation may be an overriding priority that dictates unit movement. In that instance, increased reliance will have to be placed on protective measures.

Activities by medical personnel to facilitate prevention in a unit deploying to the mountains include (*a*) recommending countermeasures to the unit commander, (*b*) providing medical screening, (*c*) providing training to unit members, and (*d*) facilitating the provision of necessary equipment and supplies to unit personnel.

Recommending Countermeasures

General countermeasures for hypoxia-related illness and performance decrements function either to promote acclimatization or to protect unacclimatized individuals against effects of hypoxia. Different countermeasures have advantages and disadvantages in specific tactical situations. The unit commander must choose the best option based on the mission and tactical constraints.

Options for using altitude acclimatization as a countermeasure are (1) to promote acclimatization through appropriate ascent rates (ie, profiles) or (2) to maintain previously acquired acclimatization until the next ascent (see Chapter 24, Acute Mountain Sickness and High-Altitude Cerebral Edema). Two ascent profiles promote acclimatization and prevent altitude illness: (1) slow or gradual ascent and (2) a staged ascent. The recommended profile for a slow ascent is to sleep 2 or 3 nights at 3,000 m and then spend 2 nights for every 500- to 1,000-m increase in sleeping altitude thereafter. The recommendation for staged ascent is to stop for 3 or more days to acclimatize at one or more intermediate elevations before ascending to the final destination altitude. As previously noted, the altitude at which unit members sleep is the most important factor (ie, the lower the sleeping altitude, the better). The disadvantage of both of these ascent profiles is that they take time, which may not be available to a unit in a rapidly evolving tactical situation.

Maintaining previously acquired altitude acclimatization would allow rapid deployment of a unit without risking altitude illness. The best way to achieve this from a physiological standpoint would be to station soldiers at high altitude so that they would always be in an acclimatized state. This strategy might be appropriate for a unit with a significant ongoing altitude mission. The other way to maintain altitude acclimatization would be to expose unit members to altitude at regular intervals. The schedule for doing that is not known, but could require at least weekly exposures.[12] Like stationing units at high altitude, this strategy might require a significant ongoing mission to justify the effort and expense involved.

When means to acquire or maintain altitude acclimatization are not available, successful rapid deployment to high mountains depends on pharmacological prophylaxis or supplemental oxygen to prevent altitude illness and increase performance. The logistical problems entailed in providing supplemental oxygen to units much larger than a squad probably prohibit this alternative as a realistic option for military deployment. Pharmacological prophylaxis, on the other hand, is a practical means for allowing rapid insertion of unacclimatized military personnel into high mountain environments.

At present, the most suitable pharmacological prophylaxis for military personnel deploying to high mountains is acetazolamide (see Chapter 24, Acute Mountain Sickness and High-Altitude Cerebral Edema). The recommended regimen is 125 to 250 mg twice a day or 500 mg slow-release formulation once a day, beginning 24 hours before ascent and continuing for several days after reaching altitude until soldiers acclimatize. Acetazolamide is both safe and effective in this prophylactic role. It is sanctioned by the US Food and Drug Administration (ie, it is FDA-approved) for prophylaxis against AMS. It also prevents altitude-induced, sleep-disordered breathing, which can cause daytime performance decrements (see Chapter 26, Additional Medical Problems in Mountain Environments). In most individuals, acetazolamide has only minor, easily tolerable side effects. Prophylaxis with acetazolamide should be used in individuals with a history of previous altitude illness. Given its effectiveness and relative safety, it should be strongly considered for all military unit members deploying to altitudes where the incidence of AMS can exceed 25% (ie, > 3,000 m) except for those individuals in whom the drug is explicitly contraindicated. There are currently no other recommended means of pharmacological prophylaxis in a military setting.

Medical Screening

Medical screening identifies individuals at increased risk for medical problems in mountain environments. If the risk to these individuals is high, they can be precluded from deploying. Those with lesser degrees of risk can be deployed with special precautions, surveillance to prevent problems, or both; or they can be identified and treated early before becoming casualties. Screening can identify two general types of problems: (*a*) the potential for environmental injury and (*b*) medical conditions that could be exacerbated by hypobaric hypoxia.

Environmental Injury. Altitude illness and cold injury are the main environmental disorders to which individuals deploying to the mountains might have increased susceptibility. Although several methods to predict susceptibility to altitude illness have been investigated (see Chapter 25, High-Altitude Pulmonary Edema, and Chapter 26, Additional Medical Problems in Mountain Environments), they involve measurements of a person's ventilatory response to hypoxia, and are neither very sensitive nor practical for use on large numbers of people. In the setting of a military deployment, a positive history of a previous episode of altitude illness may be the most practical predictor of susceptibility. Unfortunately, many individuals have not had sufficient prior exposure to high altitude to determine if they are susceptible. For small units with a committed high-altitude mission, measurement of the cardiac and respiratory response to normobaric hypoxia (11.5% inspired oxygen) at rest and during 50% of maximum exercise may allow detection of individuals at high risk of altitude illness.[13]

Exacerbation of Preexisting Medical Conditions. Preexisting medical conditions that can be exacerbated by altitude exposure are primarily those that affect respiration and oxygen transport. These conditions are not common in most military populations because they are not compatible with active service and are either screened out prior to entering the military or at the time the problem develops. Conditions that might be found in military personnel and that should be screened for prior to deployment to high altitude are listed in Table 27-1.

Sickle cell trait may be relatively common in military populations and is thought to confer a risk of splenic infarct during exposure to altitudes over 2,500 m.[14,15] There has been some debate about the risk conferred by sickle trait during altitude exposure, owing, in some reported cases,[16] to possible inaccurate identification of the precise hemoglobinopathy. Because splenic infarct or incapacitation due to sickling at altitude would be a significant problem for the afflicted individual, the unit, and medical resources, screening for the presence of sickle cell trait by history or laboratory testing should be done if deployment to high altitude is a possibility. Those identified as having sickle cell trait can then be further evaluated on an individual basis to determine their specific risk. If they have a mixed he-

moglobinopathy, a high percentage of sickling under hypoxic conditions, or both, then the medical officer should give strong consideration to giving those individuals a formal medical profile that limits their exposure to altitudes higher than 2,500 m.

Two general options are possible for individuals who are determined by screening to be at high risk for medical problems during altitude deployment. If the condition for which they are at risk can be prevented by appropriate prophylactic measures, then consideration should be given to allowing that individual to deploy *with prophylaxis*. Examples include use of nifedipine for HAPE or acetazolamide for severe AMS symptoms. Conditions that do not respond to prophylaxis should be evaluated for a medical profile to limit altitude exposure.

Individuals with history of life-threatening HAPE or HACE should be evaluated for a medical profile to limit their altitude exposure. Likewise, those with a history of thromboembolic event at high altitude should also be considered for a medical profile. Individuals with mixed hemoglobinopathies or a high percentage of sickling when their blood is exposed to hypoxic conditions should be considered for a profile to limit their exposure. Pregnant women should receive a temporary medical profile to limit their altitude exposure to lower than 2,500 m while they are pregnant.

TABLE 27-1

MEDICAL SCREENING FOR DEPLOYMENT TO ALTITUDE

Condition or System	Example
History of Environmental Injury	Altitude illness Cold injury
Cardiovascular Disease	Essential hypertension Coronary artery disease
Pulmonary Disease	Chronic obstructive pulmonary disease Asthma Pulmonary hypertension
Neurological Disease	Seizures Migraine headache
Hematological Disease	Anemia Sickle cell trait
Musculoskeletal System	Overuse injury
Pregnancy	—
Medications	Any that cause respiratory depression

In units with an altitude mission, initial medical screening can be done when an individual joins the unit. Prior to any altitude deployment, medical records for all deploying unit members should be screened to identify new conditions that may have developed and that could confer risk. All medical waivers that allow an individual to stay on active duty with an otherwise disqualifying medical condition should be examined to determine whether that condition confers a risk at altitude.

Training

Adequate training is an essential ingredient of an effective health maintenance program for military personnel deployed to a high mountain environment. Three types of training are needed during the predeployment period. First, all unit personnel should be familiarized with the health threats of the mountain environment and the countermeasures for those threats. Second, the military tasks and skills that might be used during deployment should be trained and practiced to the highest degree of proficiency, to lessen the impact of altitude-induced physical and cognitive performance decrements. Specific strategies to decrease errors and increase performance should be briefed (see Chapter 23, Cognitive Performance, Mood, and Neurological Status at High Terrestrial Elevation, and Chapter 24, Acute Mountain Sickness and High-Altitude Cerebral Edema). Third, physical training should be ongoing to maintain a high level of fitness. With regard to physical training, however, it is important that unit leaders understand that fitness will *not* prevent altitude illness, and that the altitude-induced decrement in maximum physical performance will be relatively greater in physically well-conditioned individuals (see Chapter 22, Physical Performance at Varying Terrestrial Altitudes). Training on environmental health threats is the responsibility of medical support personnel. The military task and physical training will be provided through the unit command structure, but it is the responsibility of medical personnel to ensure that the importance of that training to the unit capabilities is understood.

Adequate training on health threats in mountain environments includes recognition of major environmental factors and the injury or illness and performance decrements they cause, the preventive measures that can be taken, and first aid (self care and buddy aid). Environmental factors and the health problems they cause are listed in Exhibit 27-1; they are discussed in detail along with the specific countermeasures in the previous chapters of the Mountain Environments section of this textbook.

In addition to presenting specific environmental health threats and countermeasures, some key concepts should be emphasized. Soldiers should understand that mountains are a complex and inherently dangerous environment. They must realize that hypoxia is ubiquitous, that no one is entirely immune to its effects, and that the physical and cognitive performance decrements it causes can exacerbate risks from other environmental factors. Knowing the usual time course of acclimatization helps people tolerate symptoms of AMS more easily. If pharmacological prophylaxis with acetazolamide is required, then soldiers should understand its purpose, safety, and side effects so that they are comfortable taking the drug.

Factors common to all deployments should also be reviewed in training, not only the factors specific to mountain environments. These include personal hygiene, skin care, and maintenance of hydration and nutrition. Most of this training should take place prior to deployment. Consideration should be given to refresher training during deployment, when specific problems noted by medical surveillance can be emphasized.

Provisions for Protective Equipment and Supplies

Medical support personnel need to facilitate the supply and distribution of items necessary for health maintenance of unit members during deployment to mountain environments. Clothing and shelter suitable for the cold weather conditions are obvious requirements. A consideration with clothing supply is the issue of scarves or balaclavas through which individuals can breathe at very high altitudes to help prevent high-altitude pharyngitis and bronchitis due to drying of the upper respiratory passages. Adequate sun block for the skin and lips is necessary, as are UV-blocking sunglasses with side shields to prevent eye damage from light reflected off snowfields and rocks. Sunglasses, gloves, and other items that can be easily misplaced should have cords to attach them to the person so that they are less easily lost when the individual is hypoxic. Hiking sticks or staffs will help prevent trauma from falls in rugged mountain terrain (Figure 27-1). If prophylaxis with acetazolamide is to be used, then adequate supplies will have to be obtained and issued.

Provisions for adequate water, nutrition, and field sanitation are critical elements of health maintenance in any military deployment—and no less in deployment to mountain regions; medical personnel should be intimately involved in planning

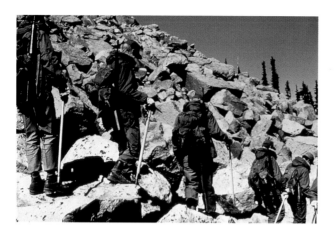

Fig. 27-1. Special equipment may help decrease environmental injuries in mountain environments. Hiking staffs (sticks) can help prevent falls when military personnel move through rugged mountain terrain. Medical personnel should recommend procurement and issue of items that could prevent injury, even if these items are not available in the normal military supply chain. Much useful mountaineering equipment for recreational mountaineering is available in the civilian marketplace. Photograph: Reproduced from *Medical Problems of Military Operations in Mountainous Terrain.* US Army Training Film TF8-4915; 197–.

for them. As discussed in the chapter by Montain in *Medical Aspects of Harsh Environments, Volume 3,*[11] although the fluid requirement at high altitude is increased, assuring an adequate supply is fraught with potential difficulties. Likewise, the caloric requirement is increased in high mountains, but, due to a variety of factors, the tendency is for decreased food consumption. Increasing the carbohydrate content of the diet (to ~70%) will make the rations more palatable and help prevent symptoms of altitude illness.

Poor sanitation, the leading source of noncombat disease and manpower losses for military units from the beginnings of organized warfare through the most recent conflicts, is as least as great a problem—if not a greater one—at high altitude as in any other harsh environment. The combined effects of cold air temperatures, limited water, and hypoxia-related decrements in cognition and mood constrain both the opportunity and the motivation for maintaining good personal hygiene. Rugged terrain and limited water can force personnel to rely on ice and snow within small, confined areas for both their water supply and disposal of waste, creating a high potential for contamination. In addition, reduced ambient air pressure at high altitudes lowers the boiling point of water, making heat sterilization of water progressively inefficient at higher altitudes.

Treatment of Environmental Injury and Illness

When preventive measures are unable to preclude the occurrence of DNBI, the key to maintaining unit fighting strength is either effective treatment with return to duty or timely evacuation. Methods for treating of the constellation of DNBI likely to occur during deployment in mountains (see Exhibit 27-1) are discussed in Chapters 24, 25, and 26. The medical support elements needed to provide adequate treatment include (*a*) a surveillance system to detect illness and injury as early as possible, (*b*) trained medical personnel to provide the treatment, (*c*) appropriate equipment and supplies, and (*d*) treatment and evacuation facilities. Surveillance, training, and equipment and supply needs are discussed here; treatment and evacuation facilities are discussed below in the Deployment of Medical Support Assets section of this chapter.

Medical Surveillance

Medical surveillance is an important tool for medical personnel to use at all echelons of the field medical support system. It serves a dual purpose in that it facilitates early detection of illness and injury and also helps identify developing health threats so that preventive action can be taken. Effective surveillance can be accomplished by (*a*) actively monitoring parameters of health in unit members and (*b*) recording the incidence of injury and illness to facilitate identification of developing problems so that preventive measures can be taken.

To actively monitor a unit deployed in the mountains, medical personnel must see the unit members frequently enough to have some basis for judging their state of health. The signs and symptoms of environmental illness are indicators to which medical personnel obviously should be highly attuned. For instance, the absence of an altitude-induced diuresis in the first day or so following ascent should alert the medical officer to the possible development of serious altitude illness. Likewise, truncal ataxia is a sensitive sign of developing altitude illness. One of the simplest indications of overall health status of individuals at high altitudes is body weight. Weight gain or failure to lose a small amount of weight in the first few days of deployment may signal onset of altitude illness, for it is an indicator that the altitude-induced diuresis necessary for successful acclimatization has not occurred. Over a longer period of time, body weight reflects nutrition and hydration status. Obtaining accurate body weights in the field may not be practical or necessary, however. Most individuals are capable of detecting meaningful weight change in themselves, so that it may be sufficient for medical personnel to merely inquire about weight change rather than actually measure it. Severe weight loss at very high altitudes (climber's cachexia; see Figure 26-7 in Chapter 26, Additional Medical Problems in Mountain Environments) will be apparent from physical appearance. Hydration status can also be monitored fairly simply by noting the color of the urine (as described in Section I: Hot Environments, and Section II: Cold Environments, in *Medical Aspects of Harsh Environments, Volume 1.*[8])

Awareness of the incidence of environmental injury and illness is best achieved by keeping written records and reviewing them regularly to look for increasing incidence, clusters of events, or specific types of illness or injury that indicate a developing threat (ie, sentinel events). This activity is appropriate at all echelons of medical support in mountain environments.

Training

Because the unique constellation of medical problems and the rugged topography associated with mountain terrain present special challenges to providing medical support for military units deployed in the mountains, medical personnel require extra training to function successfully. The training should (*a*) furnish the information necessary to diagnose and treat the injuries and illness associated with high mountain environments and (*b*) teach the specific techniques and skills needed to operate specialized equipment and perform rescue and evacuation from rugged terrain features.

The specific injuries and illnesses that medical personnel are likely to have to treat during deployment to mountain regions are listed earlier in this chapter (see Exhibit 27-1). The techniques for diagnosis and treatment of these are presented in Chapters 24, 25, and 26 of this textbook and are also found in other sources.[7,17–19] In addition to the information on diagnosis and treatment, the key concept, that *hypobaric hypoxia has a pervasive influence in all activity at high altitude,* must be stressed. Medical personnel should know that the first step in treating any altitude-related illness is to either evacuate the victim to a lower elevation or provide supplemental oxygen. Additionally, medical officers should consider the potential for a harmful interaction of hypoxia with any medications they administer. And finally, they need to realize the extent to which hypobaric hypoxia can degrade their own physical and mental performance and take appropriate steps to limit the consequences of those effects.

Techniques for evacuation of casualties during military operations in mountain terrain are found in US Army publications[20,21] and in myriad civilian sources. Some of the subjects that should be covered are techniques for manual carries and litter carries on steep slopes and cliffs (Figure 27-2). Triage and evacuation for a mass casualty situation should be reviewed in the specific context of avalanche and rock slides. In addition to specific tech-

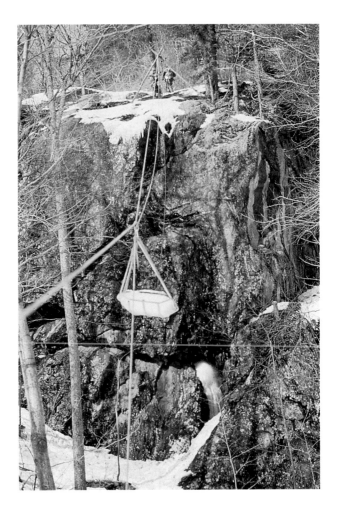

Fig. 27-2. Evacuating casualties and moving medical supplies in mountain terrain can involve techniques that require special training to perform with competence and safety. Training should be accomplished prior to deployment. Refresher training and practice during deployment will help make the skills more automatic and less vulnerable to hypoxia-induced decrements in physical and cognitive performance. Photograph: Courtesy of Murray Hamlet, DVM, Chief, Research Support Division, US Army Research Institute of Environmental Medicine, Natick, Mass.

niques, the trainer should emphasize several important concepts about mountain evacuation. Personnel must realistically assess their own capabilities in the context of hypoxia-induced performance decrements and plan accordingly. Because weather, terrain, and operational conditions can vary greatly in the mountains, personnel involved in evacuations should always have alternative plans and be skilled in the use of field expedients. Finally, to prevent shock or further trauma, they should make the utmost effort to protect the casualty from the harsh environmental conditions.

Ideally, training of medical personnel should take place prior to deployment. The mountains, however, are the best place to train for mountain operations. Consequently, refresher training or practice sessions should be given during deployment whenever feasible. Personnel with an ongoing mission to support units that deploy should train in mountain environments as frequently as possible.

Provision for Equipment and Supplies

The mountain environment affects medical logistical requirements for treatment and evacuation of patients in two ways. First, the characteristic types of medical problems found in the mountains determine the equipment and supplies that will be needed. Second, environmental parameters can alter drug action and the normal operation of some medical equipment. Additionally, environmental factors such as cold temperature and decreased atmospheric pressure can have direct detrimental effects on some supplies and equipment (eg, freezing of liquid medications, volume expansion of air in intravenous bags or bottles of medication). Planning for medical support operations in mountain terrain will have to take these effects into consideration.

The major medical problems caused by the mountain environment are listed previously (see Exhibit 27-1); deployment planning should provide for sufficient medical supplies to treat the projected incidence of these problems. Special consideration should be given to the means for treating altitude illness because those conditions are not found in deployment to other environments. Supplemental oxygen supplies should be made available whenever possible and by whatever means, as oxygen can be used in treating all altitude illnesses and it may be helpful as an adjunctive treatment for other medical conditions at altitude. "Bottled" oxygen (in metal tanks) has the disadvantages of being heavy, cumbersome, and possibly explosive if struck by gunfire or shell fragments. In relatively fixed facilities with adequate power supplies to run the devices, oxygen molecular concentrators are a good alternative to oxygen tanks.[22] In the most forward echelons, the amount of oxygen a patient breathes can be increased through use of lightweight, portable, cloth hyperbaric chambers (PHC; eg, the Gamow bag), and these devices should be made available. Drugs that should be available for treating altitude illness include acetazolamide for treating AMS and altitude-related sleep disorders, dexamethasone for treating severe AMS and HACE, and nifedipine for treating HAPE.

Altitude effects on drug action are primarily a function of hypoxia-induced changes in body physiology. Altitude effects on medical equipment function are largely due to hypobaria. Both effects play a role in general anesthesia for surgery.[23,24] The practical limits for useful general anesthesia are not known precisely, but surgical services should probably not be located higher than 4,000 m, and much lower would be preferable.[25] Ketamine is a reasonable choice for intravenous anesthesia because it has minimal effects on the airway and the respiratory drive.[25]

DEPLOYMENT OF MEDICAL SUPPORT ASSETS

Effective deployment of medical assets is essential to successful support of military units operating in high mountain environments. The assets that are available are a function of organization level, but general principles apply to most levels. The major factors that affect how medical resources are used in the mountains are the tactical mission and the environment. In a sense, the tactical mission determines the support requirements, while the environment sets constraints on how those requirements can be met.

Medical assets must be deployed to conform to the tactical plan within the often significant constraints imposed by the mountain environment.

Environmental Effects on Medical Support

Conformity to the tactical plan is a fundamental principle of medical support. The rugged, nonlinear topography of mountain regions shapes tactical plans in a general way, for it severely limits the ability of large units to maneuver. As a result, combat commanders place increased reliance on smaller, separate maneuver units that act more independently within the overall tactical plan. Medical assets must be configured and deployed to support these units.

The mountain environment imposes constraints on virtually all aspects of medical support activities from the ability to establish medical treatment facilities with appropriate proximity to the supported units, to establishing and maintaining effective evacuation and resupply. Environmental factors that have the major impact are (*a*) the rugged terrain, (*b*) the decrease in ambient oxygen, and (*c*) the cold temperature and frequent harsh weather.

Rugged terrain severely limits mobility and lines of communication. The amount of time required for overland transportation or evacuation of casualties can be greatly increased. The routes for movement forward, evacuation, and resupply are often limited by terrain features. Routes that are determined by features of the terrain are susceptible to disruption by enemy action, or by natural events such as rock slides and avalanches. Vertical terrain also limits space for medical facilities.

Low oxygen content in ambient air causes performance decrements in medical personnel and also in any equipment powered by fuel combustion. Personnel suffer decrements in both physical work and cognitive function. Casualties may need supplemental oxygen at high altitude for conditions that would not require it at lower altitude. Internal combustion engines on vehicles, generators, and cooking equipment are progressively less efficient at higher altitudes. In addition to low oxygen content, low ambient air pressure may also degrade performance of equipment. Helicopters and propeller-driven aircraft have progressive difficulty operating at higher altitudes. The problems are especially significant for takeoffs and landings, where both types of aircraft may lack lift, and sufficient runway space may not be available. Low ambient air pressure may alter the operating characteristics of medical equipment. Anesthesia and respiratory support equipment, for example, are progressively inefficient at higher altitudes.

Like low oxygen content, the cold ambient air temperatures at high altitude can effect personnel, equipment, and many medical supplies. Harsh climate conditions affect transportation and may limit options for evacuation and resupply. This means that casualties at forward echelons will be held there longer, and that larger supply stores are needed there also.

General Principles for Deployment of Medical Assets

The major constraints to medical support in the mountains are (*a*) the need to support smaller and disconnected tactical units, (*b*) the facts that transportation may be difficult and mobility limited, and (*c*) significant performance decrements of personnel and equipment. The primary means to counter these constraints are to "fix forward" to maintain proximity to the supported units, to maintain as much flexibility as possible in transportation options, and to augment personnel and equipment.

To provide support to smaller and more isolated maneuver units, the echelons of the medical support within the combat zone may have to be reconfigured and moved far forward. If the maneuver units are widely separated, then forward echelons of medical support may need to be augmented to provide adequate proximity to supported units. Increased reliance may need to be placed on buddy aid training and other multipliers of medical capabilities in small, isolated units. These individuals will need to be trained to care for environmental injuries prior to deployment. Location of assembly points, aid stations, clearing stations, and other elements of support at confluences of natural lines of patient drift and evacuation routes along creeks, streams, and small rivers may allow coverage of units that are dispersed in a wider area, but locating routes at these points also increases the opportunity for disruption by enemy action or by catastrophic environmental events such as flooding or avalanches.

The fundamental principle of flexibility is the key to dealing with transportation problems in mountain terrain. Both alternative routes and alternative methods of transportation must be planned for and maintained. As previously noted, the rugged topography of mountains limits the number of natural transportation routes for evacuation and resupply and makes those routes susceptible to disruption by enemy action or natural catastrophes. To assure continued operations, medical personnel should identify and carefully plan for use of all possible land routes within their area of responsibility.

In addition, all alternative methods of transport should also be considered and planned for. Air transportation circumvents many of the problems inherent in overland travel, but it is severely limited by the landing zone requirements for fixed-wing aircraft and by altitude-ceiling limitations for many military rotary-wing aircraft (ie, helicopters).

Frequent bad weather conditions in the mountains also limit the use of aircraft.

Rugged terrain and the lack of adequate roads may severely limit the use of vehicles in many mountain regions. Many areas will not be accessible by motor vehicles or air transportation. In those areas transportation of patients and supplies will have to be by humans or pack animals (Figure 27-3). Most medical units have contingencies for casualty and supply transport by litter bearers in the forward battle area, but in mountain regions this contingency may have to be used to support areas further to the rear. Many modern military units have not used pack animals, but their use is an option that could be considered in difficult mountain terrain.

In addition to flexibility in routes and in means of transportation in the mountains, flexibility must also be maintained to deal with times when no transportation is possible, owing to weather conditions, blocked routes, or both. Medical support planners must make provisions for the possible extension of normal maximum hold times for casualties at all forward echelons of medical support.

Medical support to military operations will require augmentation of personnel and provisions for specialized equipment and training (Figure 27-4). Augmentation of personnel in forward elements of medical support will be required because of the necessity to support smaller, dispersed combat maneuver units, and because of the decreased reliance on vehicle transport and the hypoxia-induced decreased physical performance. Decrease in physical performance capacity means an increase to 6-man litter teams (from the standard 4-man teams) and shorter distance carries. Litter relay points may be needed. Special training for mountain litter-carrying techniques will be necessary to function in rugged terrain.

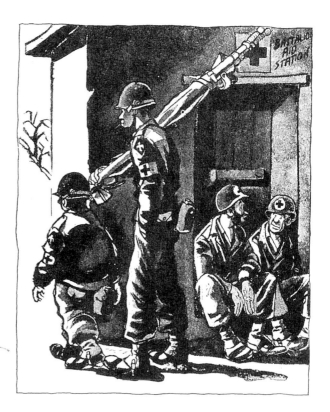

Fig. 27-3. *"I calls her Florence Nightingale."* As this Bill Mauldin cartoon from World War II points out, pack animals are an alternative method of transportation of casualties and supplies in rugged mountain terrain. Copyright 1944. By Bill Mauldin. Reprinted with permission by Bill Mauldin.

Fig. 27-4. *"That's our mountain team."* Bill Mauldin's cartoon from World War II uses humor to emphasize the need for augmentation of personnel in medical units supporting military units operating in mountain terrain. For example, this tall–short team of stretcher bearers could carry a casualty up or down a slope and always keep the stretcher level. A more cynical interpretation could be that Mauldin is ridiculing the Army's seeming predeliction to view soldiers as interchangeable parts. Copyright 1944. By Bill Mauldin. Reprinted with permission by Bill Mauldin.

SUMMARY

Medical support in mountain environments requires familiarity with the threat and adequate planning to accomplish the mission. Mountain environments cause a specific constellation of medical problems and performance decrements, in which hypobaric hypoxia plays a significant role. To apprise the tactical commander of possible loss of unit strength and to plan adequate medical support, medical personnel should estimate the DNBI and environmentally induced performance decrements prior to deployment. Health maintenance of military units deployed to high mountain terrain requires preventive measures and effective treatment of injury and illness, with return to duty or evacuation of the casualty being the two best outcomes. Medical screening can identify those at high risk for environmental injury in the mountains. Appropriate ascent profiles or pharmacological prophylaxis for altitude illness will help maintain unit fighting strength. Unit personnel should be trained to recognize environmental threats and be provided with appropriate countermeasures to protect themselves. Medical personnel should be trained to treat the constellation of environmental medical problems in the mountains and provisioned with appropriate equipment and supplies to do so. The mountain environment can severely hamper the function of medical support. To conform to the tactical mission and to operate efficiently under the restrictions imposed by the mountain topography and climate, medical support units will need to be augmented and to maintain flexibility in their configuration and deployment.

REFERENCES

1. Singh I, Khanna PK, Srivastava MC, Lal M, Roy SB, Subramanyam CSV. Acute mountain sickness. *N Engl J Med*. 1969;280:175–184.

2. Pigman EC, Karakla DW. Acute mountain sickness at intermediate altitude: Military mountainous training. *Am J Emerg Med*. 1990;8:7–10.

3. Dusek ER, Hansen JE. Biomedical study of military performance at high terrestrial elevation. *Mil Med*. 1969;134:1497–1507.

4. House JL, Joy RJT. Performance of simulated military tasks at high altitude. *Percept Mot Skills*. 1968;27:471–481.

5. Hackney AC, Kelleher DL, Coyne JT, Hodgdon JA. Military operations at moderate altitude: Effects on physical performance. *Mil Med*. 1992;157:625–629.

6. US Department of the Army. *Staff Officers' Field Manual—Organizational, Technical, and Logistic Data*. Washington, DC: DA; 1987. Field Manual 101-10-1.

7. Cymerman A, Rock PB. *Medical Problems in High Mountain Environments: A Handbook for Medical Officers*. Natick, Mass: US Army Research Institute of Environmental Medicine; 1994. T94-2.

8. Pandolf K, Burr RE, Wenger CB, Pozos RS, eds. *Medical Aspects of Harsh Environments, Volume 1*. In: Zajtchuk R, Bellamy RF, eds. *Textbook of Military Medicine*. Washington, DC: Department of the Army, Office of The Surgeon General, and Borden Institute; 2001. Also available at www.armymedicine.army.mil/history/borden/default.htm.

9. Tharion WJ, Hoyt RW, Marlowe BE, Cymerman A. Effects of high altitude and exercise on marksmanship. *Aviat Space Environ Med*. 1992;63:114–117.

10. Muza SR, Jackson R, Rock PB, Roach J, Lyons T, Cymerman A. *Effects of High Terrestrial Altitude on Physical Work Performance in an NBC Protective Uniform*. Natick, Mass: US Army Research Institute of Environmental Medicine; 1997. T97-7.

11. Pandolf KS, Burr RE, eds. *Medical Aspects of Harsh Environments, Volume 3*. In: Zajtchuk R, Bellamy RF. *Textbook of Military Medicine*. Washington, DC: Department of the Army, Office of The Surgeon General, and Borden Institute; 2003. Forthcoming.

12. Lyons TP, Muza SR, Rock PB, Cymerman A. The effect of altitude preacclimatization on acute mountain sickness during reexposure. *Aviat Space Environ Med*. 1995;66:957–962.

13. Rathat C, Richalet J-P, Herry J-P, Larmignat P. Detection of high-risk subjects for high altitude diseases. *Int J Sports Med*. 1992;13(suppl 1):S76–S78.

14. Lane PA, Githens JH. Splenic syndrome at mountain altitudes in sickle cell trait: Its occurrence in nonblack persons. *JAMA*. 1985;253:2251–2254.

15. Goldberg NM, Dorman JP, Riley CA, Armbruster EJ. Altitude-related splenic infarction in sickle cell trait. *West J Med*. 1985;143:670–672.

16. Caldwell CW. The sickle cell trait: A rebuttal. *Mil Med*. 1984;149:125–129.

17. Hackett PH, Roach RC. High-altitude medicine. In: Auerbach PS, ed. *Wilderness Medicine: Management of Wilderness and Environmental Emergencies*. 3rd ed. St Louis, Mo: Mosby; 1995: Chap 1.

18. Hultgren HN. *High Altitude Medicine*. Stanford, Calif: Hultgren Press; 1997.

19. Ward MP, Milledge JS, West JB. *High Altitude Medicine and Physiology*. 2nd ed. London, England: Chapman & Hall Medical; 1995.

20. US Department of the Army. *Mountain Operations*. Washington, DC: DA; 1980. Field Manual 90-6.

21. US Department of the Army. *Military Mountaineering*. Washington, DC: DA; 1989. Training Circular 90-6-1.

22. Litch JA, Bishop RA. Oxygen concentrators for the delivery of supplemental oxygen in remote high-altitude areas. *Wilderness Environ Med*. 2000;11:189–191.

23. James MFM, White JF. Anesthetic considerations at moderate altitude. *Anesth Analg*. 1984;63:1097–1105.

24. Safar P, Tenicela R. High altitude physiology in relation to anesthesia and inhalation therapy. *Anesthesiology*. 1964;63:515–531.

25. Nunn JF. Anaesthesia at altitude. In: Ward MP, Milledge JS, West JB. *High Altitude Medicine and Physiology*. 2nd ed. London, England: Chapman & Hall Medical; 1995: 523–526.

MEDICAL ASPECTS of HARSH ENVIRONMENTS
VOLUME 2
SECTION IV: SPECIAL ENVIRONMENTS

Section Editor:

SARAH A. NUNNELEY, MD
Senior Scientist, Wyle Laboratories
Brooks Air Force Base
San Antonio, Texas

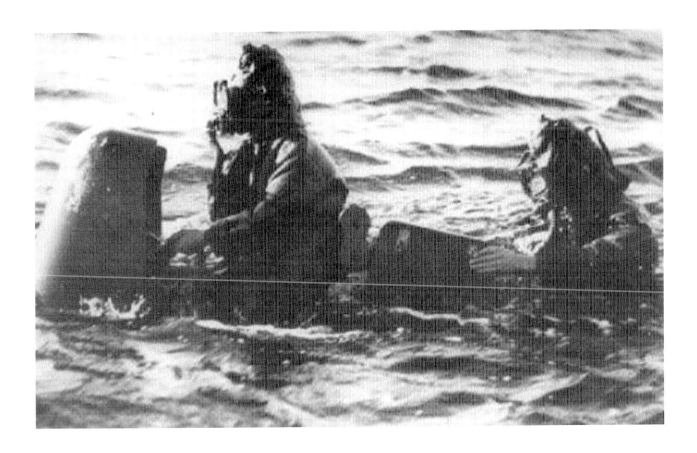

Surely the "human topedoes" of World War II must rank among the archetypal Special Operations warriors of military history. This photograph is of a British Mark I Human Torpedo, better known as the Royal Navy's *chariot*, two of which made an unsuccessful attack on the German battleship *Tirpitz* in October 1942. Far more successful were the submersible frogman delivery vehicles of the Italian Navy, the *maiali* (pig or swine), three of which sank two British battleships (HMS *Valiant* and the flagship of the Mediterranean Fleet, HMS *Queen Elizabeth*; the latter was disabled for 17 mo) in the harbor at Alexandria, Egypt, in December 1941. Amazingly, no one, including the six Italian human torpedoes and the crews of the Royal Navy battleships, was killed in this most spectacular special operations action. Photograph: Royal Navy; available at http://www.geocities.com/waratsea/midgets.htm.

Chapter 28

INTRODUCTION TO SPECIAL ENVIRONMENTS

SARAH A. NUNNELEY, MD[*]

[*]Senior Scientist, Wyle Laboratories, 2504 Gillingham Road, Brooks Air Force Base, Texas 78235; formerly, Research Medical Officer, Biodynamics and Protection Division, Air Force Research Laboratory, 2504 Gillingham Road, Brooks Air Force Base, Texas 78235

BACKGROUND

The mammalian body evolved to withstand the constant pull of gravity, motion due to walking or running, a variety of climates, and changes in altitude achieved on foot. Thus it is that humans possess considerable ability to adapt to a range of activities in varied climates and at high terrestrial elevations, natural environments which were discussed in earlier sections of this book. In contrast, the special environments involve artificial production, amplification or prolongation of environmental stress, and are based on the ability of the human mind to drive the body beyond the envelope for which it evolved. This can be viewed as a form of self-imposed stress, voluntarily undertaken for a variety of motives which may include altruism, ambition, curiosity and greed.

Historically, many types of exposure to special environments first appeared with the Industrial Revolution (Table 28-1). New challenges to physiology and medicine arose at each step as humans learned to sail on the sea or dive beneath it, speed over the ground, fly in the air, and launch themselves into space. In fact, many of the problems addressed in this Special Environments Section of *Medical Aspects of Harsh Environments, Volume 2*, result from the development of mechanized transportation. Rapid movement over long distances involves upsetting motion, changes in circadian timing, and abrupt exposure to thermal conditions and altitudes that are poorly tolerated because there is no time for adaptation. Paradoxically, problems also arise through artificially induced reduction in accustomed stress, as when sailors suffer *mal de debarkment* (sickness of disembarkation) or astronauts lose bone mass in orbit.

The natural limits of human adaptability sometimes curtail the use of technology, as when a pilot must ease off on an aerobatic maneuver to avoid blacking out. Such biological limits on system performance may be reduced by enhancing innate defense mechanisms or avoided by adding still more technology in the form of protective clothing and life-support systems. To return to the example, fighter pilots now increase their acceleration tolerance through a combination of systematic strength-training and pneumatic anti-G trousers.

ACADEMIC CONSIDERATIONS

Of the small numbers of physicians who concentrate their efforts on the special environments, many are trained and make their careers in the military services. Some possess additional qualifications as engineers or pilots, but the majority train in the fields of Aerospace Medicine, Hyperbaric Medicine, or Occupational Medicine—all of which fall under the purview of the American Board of Preventive Medicine (Table 28-2). These specialists focus on the prevention of environmental injury to healthy persons and the identification and protection of persons made more vulnerable by preexisting medical conditions. They must thoroughly understand normal responses to stress, adaptation processes, tolerance limits, and the mechanisms of decompensation and injury. These physicians often function as members of multidisciplinary teams, which may also include physiologists, engineers, human factors experts, and others with special knowledge related to technology and the interactions between humans and machines. The difficulty in communication among disciplines led to the development of compendia such as the *Bioastronautics Data Book*.[1]

Many physicians and physiologists have themselves served as pioneers in pushing the envelope for human exposure to hostile or potentially lethal environments. A French physician, Pilâtre de Rozier, piloted the first free ascent in a hot-air balloon in 1783, only to die 2 years later in the explosion of a hydrogen balloon. The French physician and physiologist Paul Bert demonstrated on himself a century later the usefulness of oxygen-enriched air at simulated altitude, then went on to provide supplementary oxygen for balloon ascents to very high altitudes; this extraordinary scientist also described oxygen toxicity and recognized that the new phenomenon, termed "compressed-air illness," was a consequence of bubble formation in body fluids during decompression.[2] Dr John Paul Stapp rode a rocket sled in repeated experiments to delineate the upper limits of human tolerance for sudden deceleration, and Dr Joseph W. Kittenger tested life-support equipment and parachutes at altitudes exceeding 100,000 ft.[3] More recently, a physician was launched into space with a central venous line in place to study the immediate effects of entry into zero gravity.[4]

Because of its multidisciplinary nature, the literature concerning work in special environments (sometimes termed "environmental ergonomics") is scattered through a large number of journals sponsored by a variety of learned societies in the

TABLE 28-1

NOTABLE EVENTS IN SPECIAL ENVIRONMENTS

Year	Special Environment				Event
	Float	Dive	Fly	Other	
1690		x			Diving bell with air resupply
1783			x		Balloon ascent
1800		x			Air pump for continuous supply to divers
1823				G	Passenger railroad train*
1830		x			Hard-hat diving suit to 100-ft depth
1841		x			Caisson for compressed air work
1854		x			Account of "compressed air illness"
1870s		x			Hyperbaric and hypobaric chambers developed and used to treat various ailments
		x			Submarine developed
	x				Steamship crossing of the Atlantic Ocean
	x				Armored ships
1874			x		Supplemental oxygen via pipe stem for balloonists
1893				G	Automobile*
1900		x			Submarine diver lockout system
1903			x		Flight of heavier-than-air craft
1906		x			Staged decompression schedules
1919			x		Oxygen mask for aviators
1927			x		Solo flight across the Atlantic Ocean
1929			x		Instrument flight
1930			x		Pressure suit for high-altitude flight
			x		Round-the-world flight
1934			x		High-G flight maneuvers (dive bombing)
			x		Human centrifuge
			x		Anti-G suit
1939		x			Helium used for deep diving
1942			x		Jet airplane
1943		x			Fully automatic scuba
	x				Aircraft carrier
1946	x				Hypothermia risk in sinkings recognized
			x		Pressurized aircraft
1954	x	x			Nuclear submarine
1960			x		Hyperbaric oxygen used to treat altitude decompression sickness
1961				O	Orbital flight
		x			Saturation diving
1968				O	Moon landing

*Not usually thought of as a special environment but notable for the motion sickness and rapid change in altitude its passengers experienced
G: ground; O: orbit

TABLE 28-2

PERTINENT ACADEMIC SOCIETIES IN SPECIAL ENVIRONMENTS

Organization	Headquarters	Web Site
Aerospace Medical Association	Alexandria, Virginia	www.asem.org
Undersea and Hyperbaric Medical Society	Kensington, Maryland	www.uhms.org
American College of Sports Medicine	Indianapolis, Indiana	www.acsm.org
American College of Occupational and Environmental Medicine	Arlington Heights, Illinois	www.acoem.org
American Board of Preventive Medicine	Washington, DC	www.abpm.org

US and overseas. Relevant American societies include the Aerospace Medical Association (founded in 1929 as the Aviation Medical Association), the Undersea and Hyperbaric Medical Society, and the American Academy of Occupational Medicine. Related research in basic science appears in the journals of the American Physiological Society and the American College of Sports Medicine, as well as publications by various engineering and ergonomics organizations (see Table 28-2).

ORIGINS AND LIMITATIONS OF RESEARCH

Special environments are often linked to military operations. Many of the technologies which create the special environments were originally developed to meet military requirements, only later finding their way into civilian industry, recreation, and exploration. Aerospace and undersea medicine received major infusions of effort in association with the two world wars (see Table 28-1). Indeed, much of our current knowledge regarding human stress physiology and protective technologies comes from research performed in military laboratories or supported through Department of Defense funding to universities and industry. Because this military orientation reinforced cultural bias, past research on special environments focused almost exclusively on the responses of healthy young men, using as subjects either military members or college students. This began to change in the late 1970s with gradually increasing interest in the stress tolerance of women and older individuals.

Women have always pioneered in special environments, although often in unofficial or unrecognized capacities and sometimes even disguised as men. Women flew in balloons beginning in 1784 and piloted early monoplanes[5]; they took up scuba and saturation diving and passed the qualification tests for the first astronauts (although only men were then allowed to apply to the program). With increasing numbers of women entering the ranks of serious athletes, explorers, military recruits, astronauts, and combat pilots, many of the old assumptions regarding women's supposed vulnerability to stress have been reexamined. This has been accomplished through replication of classic studies or design of new experiments for direct comparison of men and women who are reasonably well matched with respect to physical characteristics and conditioning. Other chapters in *Medical Aspects of Harsh Environments* provide references to such studies for physical work, heat, and cold (*Volume 1*) and high terrestrial altitude (*Volume 2*); landmark works in special environments include diving[6] and altitude decompression sickness.[7] Elements of the debate on inclusion of women in combat crews aboard ships and aircraft and their continued exclusion from Special Operations appear in the report of the Presidential Commission on Women in Combat.[8] Much of the recent research in this area was supported through congressionally mandated funding under the direction of the Defense Women's Health Research Panel.

COMMON THEMES AND SELECTED TOPICS

Although sea, air, and space are widely different environments, they are alike in their hostility to human life and thus share many aspects of physical and psychological stress. For instance, the submariner and the astronaut each dwell in a sealed capsule made habitable by sophisticated systems that closely control atmospheric pressure and gas composition as well as ambient temperature; pressurized aircraft differ from submarines and spacecraft only in that aircraft can use outside air to ventilate the cabin and scavenge oxygen. Divers, flyers, and astronauts all are subject to decompression sickness and may be required to wear impermeable protective clothing that not only impedes movement but also can cause body heat storage with attendant discomfort and hyperthermia.

Crews who dwell in special environments face high levels of physical risk, cramped quarters, and forced interpersonal closeness, all of which are combined with isolation from their families and society at large; these stressful conditions are found in ships, submarines, and saturation diving habitats, at Antarctic stations, aboard aircraft on globe-girdling flights, and in spacecraft. The development of these environments has gradually led to the need to select individuals who are resistant to stress or at least not unusually susceptible to stress-induced disability. Thus, submariners, pilots, and astronauts undergo initial screening examinations with inclusion and exclusion criteria designed to select individuals who are physically healthy and psychologically stable (see Santy P, *Choosing the Right Stuff*, in the Recommended Reading List at the end of this chapter). For such individuals, relatively minor variations from optimal health may have serious implications for their careers and livelihoods, and selection is usually followed by rigorous periodic examinations and aggressive programs of education in health and wellness to minimize the effects of self-induced stress such as tobacco, drugs and alcohol, obesity, and physical inactivity. Fortunately, research that focuses on seemingly exotic occupations such as space flight often provides major advances in general clinical medicine, including improved health risk appraisal, lifestyle modification, and the understanding of normal aging. Another outgrowth of work in special environments is improved understanding of human factors and accident investigation.

The Special Environments Section in this textbook is limited to selected areas that relate to military deployment and topics with which any military physician should have some acquaintance. It does not include areas that are covered in other volumes of the Textbook of Military Medicine series or are discussed extensively in textbooks on occupational medicine. Thus, we did not include noise, vibration, impact, radiation, or the problems of handling toxic fuels. However, we hope that the reader will be sufficiently intrigued to explore these and related topics in standard texts.

Afloat

The oldest of the special environments is the ship designed for long voyages. In the early days of sail, vessels traveled within sight of land and put in to shore at night, but commerce and curiosity—together with growing navigational skills—eventually took sailors across oceans and around the world, a progression described in detail by Boorstin.[9] Provisioning expeditionary vessels was the first human experience with the requirement to anticipate every need of a crew isolated for weeks or months in hazardous surroundings. Whether the craft were Chinese, European, or Polynesian, voyagers had to deal with confinement, water supply, food, and sanitation, as well as occupational risks and psychological stress.

The wooden ships of 18th-century Europe represented a combination of floating domicile and complex machine. The problems of provisioning and crewing the ships of the Royal Navy during the Napoleonic wars are well described in Rodger's *Wooden World*,[10] while an extraordinary feel for life on board as well as the problems encountered by the ship's surgeon (rarely a physician) can be obtained from the "Aubrey–Maturin" novels by Patrick O'Brian. Although we no longer "press" crews or provide grog (strong alcohol) as part of

the ration at sea, a careful reading of Chapter 29, Shipboard Medicine, reveals that many of the old medical problems persist in some form aboard modern warships.

Under Water

Diving inspired the earliest development of an artificial life-support system for work in an inherently lethal environment (see Table 28-1). Humans had used breath-hold diving to harvest the sea floor since prehistoric times, and it is said that Alexander the Great had himself lowered into the Bosphorus in a glass barrel. The desire to reach beyond breath-hold limits prompted the development of diving bells: air-filled containers with open bottoms that were lowered to working depth to provide the diver with access to a limited volume of air, which was naturally compressed to ambient pressure. While work with bells was at first limited to the initial trapped air, divers soon learned to use barrels for resupply and later added air that was hand-pumped through a hose from the surface. This was followed in the 1800s by development of "hard-hat" diving suits tethered to an umbilical, which supplied a flow of compressed air to the helmet.

The advent of mechanized compressors permitted deeper, longer dives and the use of caissons filled with compressed air for construction of underwater bridge footings and tunnels. Medical problems arose when caisson workers and divers began to develop a crippling and sometimes fatal condition known as "caisson disease" or "bends." In 1874, Bert recognized that this illness (now termed decompression sickness, or DCS) was a consequence of decompression to 1 atm.[2] However, decades passed before prevention of DCS was made possible by the development in 1906 of the first schedules for staged decompression.

With increasing depth, decompression times came to exceed bottom time, and this inefficiency eventually became a limiting factor, which motivated the development during the 1960s of saturation diving, in which divers used pressurized living quarters as a base for a series of work bouts without the need for intervening decompression. Further complexities were added by the use of artificial gas mixtures (nitrox, heliox) to avoid nitrogen narcosis and the more dramatic high-pressure nervous syndrome. Recently, research on very deep saturation diving has dwindled with the development of practical unmanned systems for observation and work at great depth. Interested readers can find more detail on deep diving in the Recommended Reading list at the end of this chapter, particularly Bennett and Elliott's *Physiology and Medicine of Diving*, and Bove's *Bove and Davis' Diving Medicine*.

The material on diving in this section appears in two linked chapters, the first (Chapter 30, Physics, Physiology, and Medicine of Diving) presenting the special challenges of diving and hyperbaric environments, and the second (Chapter 31, Military Diving Operations and Medical Support) focusing on medical aspects of diving and submarine operations. Readers may wish to seek more detail in one of the several major textbooks on diving and hyperbaric medicine. These texts also provide information on the growing use of hyperbaric oxygen to treat medical and surgical conditions of particular interest to the military, including DCS, gas gangrene and necrotizing infection, crush injury, and nonhealing wounds.[11] A recent addition to the literature is a brief pictorial history of hyperbaric chambers.[12]

In Flight

As mentioned above, human flight began with balloon ascents in 1783. The first escape system was not far behind; in 1797 an aeronaut deliberately parachuted 2,000 ft from his balloon to a safe landing. Although balloons were generally regarded as showpieces for public spectacle, the armed forces adopted them as observation platforms in the American Civil War (1861–1865) and the Franco–Prussian War (1870–1871). In addition, balloons were used by scientist-aeronauts to explore the characteristics of the atmosphere at high altitudes, beginning with ascents above 20,000 ft in the 1860s and continuing to the edge of space in the 1970s.[3]

Powered flight was pioneered in the United States by the Wright brothers and was also quickly adopted for military purposes. Airplanes were employed for aerial observation early in World War I, but they soon began carrying machine guns and even hand-dropped bombs. Increased aircraft power and maneuverability soon brought a new set of medical problems (see Gibson and Harrison's "Into Thin Air: A History of Aviation Medicine in the RAF" in the Recommended Reading Section in this textbook). While birds are naturally adapted to aerial maneuvers and the rigors of high altitude, humans are not, and military commanders in World War I soon realized that more pilots were being lost to accidents than to enemy action. Aviation medicine was born as a specialty as physicians sought to reduce noncombat casualties by improving tech-

niques for pilot selection and training as well as designing better personal equipment. Today, aerospace medicine encompasses all aspects of military and civil aviation as well as space flight (see DeHart's *Fundamentals of Aerospace Medicine* and Ernsting and colleagues' *Aviation Medicine* in the Recommended Reading Section at the end of this chapter).

First balloons and later powered aircraft achieved altitudes where hypoxia impaired mental function and then induced unconsciousness and death. Provision of oxygen in flight is a good example of the multidisciplinary problems of providing life support in a hostile environment. It began with Paul Bert's simple bladder of oxygen to be sucked through a pipe stem; unfortunately, laboratory tests with this system failed to allow for the increased oxygen requirement associated with physical activity and cold during actual flights, and fatalities ensued when balloonists received insufficient oxygen or exhausted their supply. Interest in high-altitude air operations in World War II led to major studies of respiratory physiology and the development of highly engineered oxygen systems: The pipe stem was replaced by the oronasal mask supplied by a demand regulator, followed by positive-pressure systems, partial pressure suits, and ultimately full pressure suits, as pioneered by Wiley Post.

Three chapters in this section present selected topics from aerospace medicine. Hypoxia and hypobaria (Chapter 32, Pressure Changes and Hypoxia in Aviation) are critical, intertwined challenges to flight at very high altitude. The piece on acceleration (Chapter 33, Acceleration Effects on Fighter Pilots) illustrates the combined use of autonomic mechanisms, crew training, and mechanical devices to enhance human tolerance to artificially induced stress. The chapter on space flight (Chapter 34, Military Spaceflight) summarizes the challenges to the US Air Force's emerging role as "the space and air force." Although US military use of space is currently limited to observation satellites, future developments may well parallel the progression of balloons and aircraft from passive to active roles.

The Trouble With Motion

Motion sickness poses a vexing problem associated with all forms of mechanized transportation (Chapter 35, Motion Sickness). The oculovestibular axis, which evolved to keep land animals oriented and their vision stabilized, becomes counterproductive in the face of artificially amplified or conflicting sensory inputs such as the "cross-coupling" produced by certain aerobatic maneuvers. A related syndrome, known as "simulator sickness," often limits the ability of personnel to train or work with realistic visual displays that lack corresponding motion inputs. While the evolutionary origin of motion sickness remains a matter for speculation, it is clear that the mechanisms are so embedded in the neurological system that there is little possibility for technological intervention to reduce or ameliorate these responses. Pharmacological agents offer some relief, but their use is limited by side effects including drowsiness or visual changes.

Studies of motion effects and related therapies are difficult for several reasons. Few subjects will volunteer for repeated-measures protocols that induce severe nausea or vomiting. Furthermore, data are noisy because the incidence and severity of symptoms vary widely between individuals and from day to day in the same person, and also show a strong relationship to expectation and emotional state. These psychophysiological linkages foster the public's acceptance of unproven therapies such as wrist bands and magnets.

Vulnerability to motion-induced symptoms can be minimized among pilots and other specialists by selecting resistant individuals and training them through repetitive, escalating exposure to the offending stimulus. Space flight presents special challenges in this regard, since astronauts often feel ill in the first hours or days after arrival in orbit; there is no way to simulate sustained zero gravity conditions on the ground, nor is the incidence of symptoms in orbit reduced among experienced test pilots (Chapter 34, Military Spaceflight).

Motion sickness is a far worse problem among nonspecialists. Consider the problems faced by operators of passenger ferries and cruise ships in rough weather, especially in these litigious times. Carnival rides and theme-park simulators cater to individuals who enjoy the thrill of vertiginous experiences but do not expect to have their day ruined. More relevant to this textbook, motion-induced discomfort and even incapacitation can have enormous impact on military deployments (eg, among troops brought to combat by ship or special operations forces transported aboard low-flying aircraft).

Clothing as Protective Burden

Personal protection and life-support systems play a variety of roles ranging from limited emergency back-up for cabin systems to primary defense against lethal environments, as in salvage diving, work in contaminated atmospheres, or extravehicular activity in space. All systems of personal protection share certain undesirable characteristics, including the hobbling effect of the clothing, limitations on environmental heat exchange, and restricted breathing, as well as adverse effects on visual fields, manual dexterity, and interpersonal communication. Thus, equipment intended only for emergencies must be evaluated for cost-to-benefit ratio. A classic example is the antiexposure (immersion) suit worn by military pilots flying over cold water: how does one balance the discomfort of wearing a hot, bulky suit for hundreds of hours of normal flight against the remote possibility that it may save a life in case of ditching? Analogous considerations apply to clothing worn by troops working in environments potentially contaminated by nuclear, biological, or chemical agents, where heat stress and other clothing-related problems may severely reduce operational capability (Chapter 36, Protective Uniforms for Nuclear, Biological, and Chemical Warfare: Metabolic, Thermal, Respiratory, and Psychological Issues). Personnel who are forced to wear protective clothing too often take unsanctioned measures to make themselves more comfortable, by loosening seals or removing a layer, even though such actions often render the item ineffective in a real emergency.

Special Operations

All four military services train units of highly selected personnel for Special Operations, ranging from aggressive military action to humanitarian missions. As described in the last two chapters of this textbook (Chapter 37, Medical Support of Special Operations, and Chapter 38, Organizational, Psychological, and Training Aspects of Special Operations Forces), Special Operations constitute a microcosm combining all the problems involved in deployment to harsh environments. In the course of training for and carrying out Special Operations, personnel may require the support of flight surgeons, diving medical officers, specialists in occupational medicine, and experts in sports medicine and rehabilitation.

A common thread for combat operations is the use of uncomfortable or risky modes of transportation so that troops arrive at the site of operations already stressed by some combination of anxiety, motion, dehydration, nutritional deficit, sleep deprivation, and circadian dysrhythmia. They may then be expected to carry out a mission that would represent a maximum effort for unstressed troops. Medical care of casualties can pose particularly difficult challenges owing to the minimal level of support available during a remote and sometimes secret operation.

CONCLUSION

For physicians and physiologists, the special environments pose unique challenges to their understanding of the effects of many kinds of stress. Military operations often present problems that deal with human limitations at the interface between biology and engineered systems.

REFERENCES

1. Webb P, ed. *Bioastronautics Data Book.* Vol SP 3006. Washington, DC: National Aeronautics and Space Administration; 1964: 400.

2. Bert P. *Barometric Pressure.* Hitchcock MS, Hitchcock FA, trans. Bethesda, Md: Undersea Medical Society; 1978: 1053. Originally published in 1878.

3. Engle E, Lott A. *Man in Flight.* Annapolis, Md: Leeward Publications; 1979: 396.

4. Buckey JC, Gaffney DA, Lane LD, et al. Central venous pressure in space. *J Appl Physiol.* 1996;81(1):19–35.

5. Dille JR. Women in civil and military aviation: The first 125 years (1804–1929). *Aviat Space Environ Med.* 2000;71(9):957–961.

6. Fife W, ed. *Women in Diving: Proceedings of the 35th UHMS Workshop.* Kensington, Md: The Undersea and Hyperbaric Medical Society; 1987: 162.

7. Webb JT, Pilmanis AA, Krause KK, Kannan N. Gender and altitude-induced decompression sickness susceptibility. *Aviat Space Environ Med.* 1999;70(4):364.

8. Herres RT, ed. *Women in Combat: Report to the President.* McLean, Va: Brassey's (US); 1993: 120.

9. Boorstin DJ. *The Discoverers.* New York, NY: Random House; 1983: 745.

10. Rodger NAM. *Wooden World: An Anatomy of the Georgian Navy.* London, England: WW Norton and Company; 1986: 343.

11. Kindwall EP, Whelan HT, eds. *Hyperbaric Medicine Practice.* 2nd ed. Flagstaff, Ariz: Best; 1999: 950.

12. Haux GFK. *History of Hyperbaric Chambers.* Flagstaff, Ariz: Best; 2000: 153.

RECOMMENDED READING

Bennett P, Elliott D, eds. *Physiology and Medicine of Diving.* Durham, NC: Duke University; 1993.

Boorstin DJ. *The Discoverers.* New York, NY: Random House; 1983.

Bove A, ed. *Bove and Davis' Diving Medicine.* Philadelphia, Pa: Saunders; 1997.

DeHart RL, ed. *Fundamentals of Aerospace Medicine.* 2nd ed. Baltimore, Md: Williams & Wilkins; 1996.

Ernsting J, Nicholson A, Rainford D, eds. *Aviation Medicine.* London, England: King's College; 1999.

Fife W, ed. *Women in Diving: Proceedings of the 35th UHMS Workshop.* Kensington, Md: The Undersea and Hyperbaric Medical Society; 1987.

Gibson T, Harrison M. *Into Thin Air: A History of Aviation Medicine in the RAF*. London, England: Robert Hale; 1984.

Haux GFK. *History of Hyperbaric Chambers*. Flagstaff, Ariz: Best; 2000.

Herres RT, ed. *Women in Combat: Report to the President*. McLean, Va: Brassey's (US); 1993.

Kindwall EP, Whelan HT, eds. *Hyperbaric Medicine Practice*. 2nd ed. Flagstaff, Ariz: Best; 1999.

Rodger NAM. *Wooden World: An Anatomy of the Georgian Navy*. London, England: WW Norton and Company; 1986.

Santy PA. *Choosing the Right Stuff: The Psychological Selection of Astronauts and Cosmonauts (Human Evolution, Behavior, and Intelligence)*. Westport, Conn: Praeger; 1994.

Chapter 29

SHIPBOARD MEDICINE

TERRENCE RILEY, MD[*]

*Captain, Medical Corps, US Navy (Ret); Professor of Neurology, Department of Neurology, Baylor College of Medicine, One Baylor Plaza, Houston, Texas 77030

INTRODUCTION

The demands of the environment exert extraordinary influence on the practice of medicine at sea. Even at sea, medicine is still medicine: history and examination are necessary for diagnosis, use of diagnostic adjuncts must be weighed against resources, and treatment is based on universal principles of surgery and medication. And yet, being at sea is different. The stress of close living quarters, isolation, and a hazardous environment are unequaled short of space travel. The prolonged absence from home, community, and normal environment creates profound emotional stress. It also precludes normal exposure to minor infections, rendering an entire crew not only immunologically isolated but also immunologically naïve, compared with shore populations. The cramped living and working spaces create complicated and unnatural challenges for hygiene, nutrition, and the control of contagion. It is also a unique industrial environment, which carries yet further medical concerns.

Although there are no diseases unique to ships, several factors make shipboard medicine unique:

- Medical personnel are fully integrated with their patients (ie, the crew) and the life of the ship.
- The Medical Officer (MO) must not only plan for every medical eventuality but also interact fully with all other departments for everything the ship or battle group may do.
- Medical operations vary widely with the different phases of the ship's cycle.
- Roles that customarily belong to public health departments, industrial hygienists, and hospitals belong to the ship's Medical Department.

The demands of the environment exert extraordinary influence on the practice of medicine on a ship at sea. Although there are few books on shipboard medicine,[1,2] the US Navy's Virtual Naval Hospital (VNH) constitutes a comprehensive digital library of medical information tailored to the Sea Service. Its home page (http://www.vnh.org) lists the following topical headings: Common Medical Problems; Dentistry; Pharmacy; Health Promotion; Occupational and Environmental Health; Medical Intelligence and Medical Plannng; Procedures; First Aid; Textbooks; Administrative Manuals; MEDLINE and Medical Journals; Continuing Education; Professional Health Organizations; Palm Handheld Computer Medical Resources; and Navy and DOD Resources. Specific sources of information available through VHN will be cited below, together with relevant journal publications.

This chapter focuses on military surface ships; medical problems aboard submarines are substantially similar[3] and will not be addressed here. Medical professionals on cruise ships find that the care of large numbers of passengers mimics the caseload of civilian emergency medicine.[4]

Organization Aboard Ship

The ship as an organization has many of the same departments and key positions seen in other large military units. However, the traditions of the Sea Service and unique features of seafaring have evolved special roles and titles, so that terminology sometimes differs from other services. For example, in the US Army a quartermaster is a storekeeper; on a ship, he or she is a navigational expert. "First Lieutenant" is the title but not the rank of the officer who runs the Deck Department, which takes care of all the lines (ropes), deck appliances, boats, and the architectural concerns of the ship. And the Captain of a small ship may hold a lower rank, such as commander.

The ship has a special document, the *Watch Quarter and Station Bill,* which assigns every crewmember to watch-standing rotations and to specific positions and duties for military action or emergencies at sea. The *Bill* for each department is posted where everyone can check it, and crewmembers are expected to memorize their own assignments and those of their buddies. Watch standing has special meaning at sea. Survival of the ship and its crew depends on the vigilance of the sailor on the watch in certain positions. Watch standers may be alone for long periods and fatigued from their ordinary work; staying awake on watch can be difficult, and staying alert may be even more so. Therefore, the culture and responsibility of watch standing are immeasurably important in the Sea Service. They are important issues for the Medical Department as well, both for the safety and health of the crew and because medical watch standers are the first line of treatment in an emergency.

Ships and Missions

While ultimate responsibility for everything on a ship rests with the Captain, it is the responsibility of the MO to thoroughly assess the medical needs of a ship. A coastal freighter with a crew of 15 has less need, fewer resources, and an entirely different class of medical threats than an aircraft carrier with a hundred jet aircraft and several thousand crewmembers. Only through a thorough understanding of the ship, the ship's cycle, and its specific mission can the MO give the Captain necessary advice and optimize care of the crew.

There are as many types of ships as there are reasons for sailing on the oceans. Several classes of ship from the US Navy are described in Table 29-1; they have parallels in the navies of other nations. Ships of war are unique for their complex surveillance programs, training requirements, and dangerous environment. In many cases, the medical responsibility is not limited to the ship's company: an am-

TABLE 29-1

SOME CLASSES OF SHIPS AND THEIR MEDICAL DEPARTMENTS

Ship	Function	Total Personnel	Medical Department Personnel
Destroyers, DD class; Frigates, FF class; 4,500–8,000 tons	Surface patrol and combat, ASW	200–300	2–3 corpsmen, at least one an IDC. Small sick bay with 1 operating table and ≤3 infirmary beds. 2–3 BDSs.
Nuclear powered cruiser, CGN class; 8,000–10,000 tons	Anti–air warfare, surface patrol and combat, missle warfare	450–600	1 GMO, 3 corpsmen (1 IDC), 4 ward beds. Sick bay slightly larger than on DD or FF. 3 BDSs. No full OR or ICU
Auxiliary (service) ships, AD, AGF, AOE, AOR, AR, AS classes; 10,000–20,000 tons	Logistics, supply: general replenishment, ordnance, fuels	300–500	1 GMO, 1 PA or nurse practitioner; often a dental officer (DO). 5–10 corpsmen. Larger sick bay with 1 operating table and 1–2 examining tables, 1 dental operatory. Usually 5–13 infirmary beds. 2–3 BDSs.
Aircraft carrier, CV and CVN (nuclear power) classes; 75,000–92,000 tons	Tactical aircraft, ASW helicopters, power projection and joint operations	> 5,300	6 MOs (1 a general surgeon); 3 flight surgeons from embarked airwing. 1 RN, 1 CRNA or anesthesiologist, 1 PA, 4 dentists (1 an oral surgeon), 30 corpsmen, 13–14 dental technicians. 1 OR; audiology booth; endoscopy, pharmacy, and X-ray facilities; and laboratory. 4–6 BDS.
Command Control ship, LCC class; 19,000 tons	Command and Control of fleet, theater, and Amphibious Task Force Operations	720–900	1 MO and 1 dentist (plus a senior MO on the embarked flag staff for staff planning), 12 corpsmen (at least 1 IDC), and often a PA, 3 dental techs. 20 ward beds, and 4 "quiet beds" that can be more intensive.
Tank Landing ships, LST class; 8,450 tons	Transport and land amphibious vehicles, tanks, and combat vehicles and equipment	> 700	5 corpsmen, 1 IDC. Embarked Marines may bring 12–20 corpsmen. Occasionally, embarked Marines may also have 1 GMO. Med Dept has lab and X-ray capability. 9 ward beds.
Amphibious Assault ships, LHA and LHD classes; 40,000 tons	Primary landing ships, and sea control, large troop carrying helicopters and VSTOL jets (Harriers)	> 3,000 (ship's company and troops)	Ship's company has 1 MO, 1 dentist, 15–17 corpsmen. Embarked troops have 1–2 flight surgeons, 2 GMOs, and 12–20 corpsmen. Embarked surgical team to operate the large operating and ward suites: 3 MOs, including at least 1 surgeon, 1 anesthesia provider, 2 RNs (1 a perioperative specialist), 1 medical regulator, 10–12 corpsmen. Medical suite 4–6 ORs, 17 ICU beds, 40–50 ward beds, and 300–500 overflow beds.
Hospital ships, T-AH class; 69,400 tons	Mobile, flexible, surgical and intensive full hospital for combat and other operations	1,300 + patient census	12 ORs, 80 ICU beds, 20 recovery beds, 280 intermediate beds, 120 light care, 500 limited care. Lab, X ray, pharmacy, and blood bank facilities. 55 MOs, 6 dentists, 172 nurses, 20 MSCs, 674 corpsmen, 16 dental techs.

ASW: antisubmarine warfare; BDS: battle dressing station; CRNA: certified registered nurse anesthetist; GMO: general medical officer; ICU: intensive care unit; IDC: independent duty corpsman; MO: medical officer; MSC: Medical Service Corps; OR: operating room; PA: physician assistant; RN: registered nurse; VSTOL: vertical/short take-off and landing

phibious attack vessel may start with a crew of about 1,000, but when it embarks 2,000 Marines with 70 helicopters and jet aircraft, a larger Medical Department is required simply to take care of all the people aboard. Furthermore, when the ship enters amphibious operations, it becomes a hospital for ground troops, many of whom arrived on other ships.

Life on Board

From the time a ship is commissioned until it is decommissioned, it is never "turned off" or left unmanned. Personnel assigned to ships are surrounded by hazards at all times as they work, eat, and sleep. Hazards on deck include helicopters, cables, fuel lines, and other items (Figure 29-1). Excessive heat and noise pervade the engineering spaces, boiler rooms, and machinery compartments. Steam pipes present the threat of asbestosis from insulation and danger from the steam itself if the pipes break. All kinds of equipment constitute electrical hazards. Toxic fumes and materials are ubiquitous from welding, paints, batteries, and even the

mercury used by the Dental Department for fillings.

In addition to those hazards, shipboard life presents challenges simply because of the confined space. Although habitability has improved on military ships in the last 50 years, life on board is still more arduous than is living ashore or in barracks. Even with the very largest ships, space is always critical. Enlisted crew racks (ie, beds) typically have only 20 to 36 inches of vertical clearance between them, and usually are stacked three to five high. On amphibious ships, the embarked troops may have racks with even less clearance stacked up to six high.

The sailor's only private place is his or her rack; most ships have curtains that can close off each rack for further privacy and darkness. Racks are usually arranged in rows that form small, roomlike enclaves to permit a sense of community and some privacy. Berthing assignments customarily place people with members of their own department in similar pay grades. The inclusion of women in crews requires more ingenuity to maintain departmental and rank-based berthing that separates men and women. Since the ship operates around the

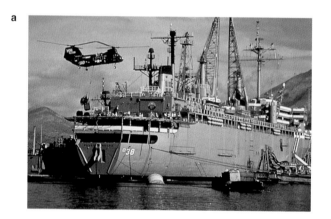

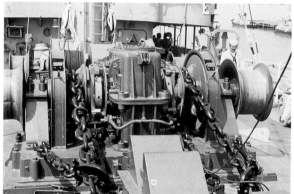

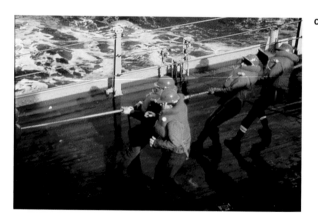

Fig. 29-1. Sailors encounter numerous hazards on the deck of a ship. (**a**) When a ship is being resupplied by helicopter, hazards include hovering aircraft, pallets being carried underneath helicopter, and the designated area in which pallets can be delivered. (**b**) Machinery for lifting anchor. Hazards include the sheer weight of an anchor and the mass of chains to attach it to the ship. Anyone who gets entangled with the chain will be crushed. (**c**) Sailors hauling fueling lines onboard a ship. Hazards include slippery decks and the wet, windy environment, both of which increase the risk for falling overboard. The tension on the lines that hold the two ships together during the fueling maneuver can be extremely hazardous for nearby sailors, particularly if the lines break or snap back: sailors could easily sustain severe injuries, such as amputation or decapitation from the lines. Photographs: Navy Imaging Command, Anacostia Naval Air Station, Washington, DC. Figure legend: Courtesy of Louis Kroot, MD, Department of Emergency Medicine, University of Kentucky Chandler Medical Center, Lexington, Ky.

clock, invariably some crewmember is beginning a watch or regular work duties in the middle of an adjacent shipmate's sleeping period. This traffic adds to the already difficult challenge of sleep hygiene and accommodation to schedules.

Ventilation is critical in the confined berthing compartments, so many vents are located in the overhead (ie, the ceiling). Many other projections dangle from the overhead and intrude into the space above the top rack. The berthing areas are crowded with racks, lockers, projecting ship fittings, and other sailors. Simple daily events such as dressing are made difficult when the 6 to 12 people in a cubicle try to accomplish it at the same time in a deck space that may be only 3 or 4 ft by 8 or 10 ft.

Showers, sinks, and commodes are called "heads" on a ship and are usually distributed among berthing departments. With several dozen sailors per shower and commode, heavy utilization can overwhelm the ventilation in those compartments. If showers do not dry between uses, fungi, soapy residue, and bad odors accumulate; sailors then avoid the bad shower and begin using one in a different area, driving up the use there so that it, too, will be overwhelmed.

Tight living conditions have obvious health implications. Many jobs on the ship cause sweating during exposure to petroleum products and dirt. Prevention of eczema and contact dermatitis requires clean, dry garments, yet clothing and boots do not dry well in crowded spaces. Lice and other parasites are a constant threat. So clean garments become a more important issue at sea than under other circumstances, and the crew must have frequent and ready access to laundry service.

Primary prevention is critical for diseases spread by respiratory routes or personal contact, which can infect dozens of sailors within a few hours. An outbreak of influenza could be rapidly devastating, so vaccination of the entire crew must be done yearly. Secondary prevention is no less important once index cases of respiratory illness are detected. Whenever possible, a sailor with even mild respiratory disease should be admitted to the medical ward. Barriers to droplet transmission, such as surgical masks, may sometimes be required for sailors with respiratory symptoms.

Sea sickness is a major problem for new crewmembers and in high seas, and is aggravated in berthing or working spaces where sailors lose sight of the horizon. In the cramped living spaces, whether a ship pitches or rolls, some of the racks will unavoidably be oriented in the axis of motion most conducive to sea sickness (for further infor-

mation, see Chapter 35, Motion Sickness).

The loss of privacy aboard ship is terribly stressful to many people. The feeling of being only one of a multitude can threaten a young person's self-esteem and cause a paradoxical sense of loneliness. The psychological consequences of this kind of living are all the more threatening to immature sailors and those with personality or anxiety disorders.

The Ship's Cycle

A ship has a recurring cycle much like a living organism. The components of the cycle include the following:

* Workups. The term "workups" denotes the formal process of testing and training that occurs in the months before a ship departs on extended deployment. Workups consist of a series of underway periods that make increasingly complex demands on ship and crew. The first short outings teach the crew to work the ship's power and navigational systems. Longer cruises follow to test maneuver, weapons, communications, and tactics. Finally, periods are spent at sea coordinating with other ships in the task force, embarked amphibious forces, or other branches of the armed forces. At each step, evaluations and inspections are held to certify the ship's readiness to move on to the next phase.
* Deployment. The ship's mission or patrol, deployment involves many months away from home port.
* Maintenance. On the ship's return from deployment, maintenance and minor upgrades are performed in the yard. This work may require only a few weeks for a small ship or 6 months for a large, complex ship such as an aircraft carrier.
* Major overhaul. After two to five complete cycles, the ship needs a major overhaul to implement technological advances and repair accumulated wear and tear. Large ships may require more than a year in the yard.

The crew also has a cycle. Because military crewmembers are assigned to a ship for periods of only 2 to 4 years, at least one third of the crew turns over every year. Extensive training is necessary for new crewmembers and for incumbents after a long deployment and a time in the yard; new technology and tactics for a planned deployment may require new skills for the entire crew.

Like a moth and a caterpillar, the ship is an entirely different organism in each phase of its cycle. The medical problems of each phase differ too. In the yard, the ship becomes an intense, crowded, dangerous industrial plant. Ordinary ventilation, plumbing, and electrical systems are compromised. Passageways are crowded and cramped with people and equipment. Sandblasting, other respiratory hazards, paint, and solvents are everywhere. Welding being done all over the ship causes risks of fire and hazards to vision. Grinding equipment creates hearing and ocular hazards. Workers are vulnerable to falling tools and metal objects; common injuries include head trauma, burns, crushed extremities, and lacerations. Workers unfamiliar with the ship can wander into unventilated spaces and die of asphyxia.

When the ship goes to sea for workups, the safety of all systems must be checked, certified, and treated with great respect. New crewmembers are likely to trip over unfamiliar projections on decks and are vulnerable to falls down ladder wells and holds. Burns and lacerations are common; puncture wounds and fractures of wrists and ankles occur, too. And new crewmembers encounter the problems of life at sea: sea sickness, loneliness, cramped spaces, unprecedented stress, and long working hours. Depression, acting out, and suicidal gestures emerge as important clinical problems. In addition, the Medical Department must implement a major teaching program to train all crewmembers in ship hygiene, first aid, cardiopulmonary resuscitation, the locations of first aid boxes, and their mass casualty roles.

During the cruise, the ship is almost always deployed outside its home waters, away from families and domestic ports for several months. Although the pace of activity during a cruise is often less harried than it was on workups, the atmosphere is more serious because action is imminent. The Medical Department must manage all of the ship's routine medical care, pursue required preventive medicine programs, maintain its own working and berthing spaces, and be prepared to care for mass casualties even if major portions of the ship—possibly including the main Medical Department—are destroyed in battle. The Medical Department must also manage the details of any necessary medical evacuations. Depending on the type of ship and its mission, port calls are often made to foreign nations, where the crew carries the home nation's culture and image to other peoples and is in turn exposed to the local culture—and its endemic diseases. Morale and readiness are usually at their highest at the early part of the cruise and before port calls.

THE MEDICAL DEPARTMENT ABOARD SHIP

The term "Medical Department" may apply to one person and his or her equipment on a small ship or as many as 70 people staffing a virtual hospital on a large amphibious ship. Regardless of size, the department is obliged to look after its own spaces, the personal needs of its members, and its budget. Every department also has to take a role in shipwide business, which includes berthing arrangements, watch standing, cleaning passageways and common areas, scheduling of meetings, and interacting with all other departments (eg, supply, deck, weapons, and navigation). In some ships, departments also share housekeeping chores such as preparing food, loading supplies, and painting.

The Medical Officer's Line and Staff Roles

As in any military organization, the ship has both line and staff functions. Department heads are line officers and usually report to the Executive Officer (XO), who is second in command and responsible for the daily activities of the ship. Staff officers such as the lawyer and chaplain report directly to the Captain to provide expert advice in matters that affect the crew broadly across department boundaries. The aggregate volume of directives and policies from higher authority is staggering, and the topics are frequently so technical that the Captain, who is ultimately responsible for compliance with all of them, must rely on the department heads and staff officers to carry them out and to advise him of any shortcomings.

The head of the Medical Department is unique in fulfilling both line and staff functions. In this chapter we will refer to this person as the Medical Officer, although that role may be filled on small ships by an Independent Duty Medical Corpsman, a Physician's Assistant, or a Nurse Practitioner. Although the MO's daily job is the line function of running the Medical Department, the staff role is often paramount, because planning and preventive medicine are more important to the overall health of the command than is medical treatment after the fact. The MO must serve as Captain's eyes and conscience for medical matters and must have the trust of the Captain to deviate from medical directives when necessary, but should always notify the Captain when that happens. Doing this effectively requires that the MO develop a solid relationship of confidence and trust with both the Captain and the XO.

Everything the ship does has medical ramifications, which can be fully understood by the MO only in the context of (1) the physical threats and stresses involved in naval operations and (2) a thorough knowledge of the ship. The MO must be prepared to recognize and point out to the heads of other departments when proposed operations might affect crew health, require extra medical attention, or threaten to exceed the ship's medical capabilities. A representative of the Medical Department must be included in all interdepartmental conferences and planning sessions. Although many operational topics are classified or confidential, the MO always has a "need to know."

To build relationships of mutual confidence, members of the medical staff must mingle with their counterparts in other departments for meals, casual conversation, and off-duty activities. MOs and chief petty officers (CPOs) should visit the bridge and all working spaces on the ship as often as possible, and study how others do their jobs. The word "shipmate" denotes an abiding relationship unlike any other. Trust, esteem, reliance, compatibility—ingredients for the deepest kind of teamwork—are necessary to build a place for the Medical Department among all others on the ship. This process may be especially challenging on a small ship where the head of the Medical Department is a corpsman and all the other department heads are officers. In such cases, the corpsman must develop strong relationships with the Captain and the XO to gain acceptance by other department heads.

Medical Staffing

The size and composition of the medical staff depend on the number of the crew and the mission of the ship. As a rule of thumb, there should be one independent provider per 800 to 1,000 crewmembers but at least one on every ship. On small ships, the sole provider is usually an Independent Duty Corpsmen, a senior petty officer with a minimum of 6 years of experience as a corpsman followed by a year of intensive medical training. On larger ships with several providers, three fourths should be physicians. A ship with women embarked needs at least one provider with special skills in gynecological diagnosis.

Every medical provider on a ship needs to be proficient and certified in both Advanced Trauma Life Support (ATLS)[5] and Advanced Cardiac Life Support (ACLS).[6] Falls, burns, and lacerations are frequent aboard ship and can require endotracheal intubation, emergency crichothyrotomy, insertion of chest tubes, diagnostic peritoneal lavage, and venous cutdowns. The presence on a small ship of intensive treatment spaces that resemble operating rooms does not imply true operating capability. On the other hand, an aircraft carrier is fitted with a full operating room staffed by a general surgeon, an oral surgeon, and an anesthesiologist or a nurse anesthetist, as well as a qualified operating room nurse and at least two fully trained surgical technicians.

Ships with continuous air operations and embarked aviation groups of squadron size or larger need a flight surgeon and at least one aeromedical technician. On aircraft carriers and amphibious attack ships, embarked aviation units bring their own flight surgeons. On an aircraft carrier, the Senior MO is also an experienced flight surgeon. Destroyers, frigates, cruisers, and auxiliary ships with a one- or two-helicopter detachment rarely have a flight surgeon on board, and aviation personnel must obtain aeromedical services from other elements of the battle group.

An example of the complex organizational relationships aboard ship is the surgical team that usually embarks with a Marine Amphibious Ready Group. Although the surgical team reports operationally to the Commander of the Amphibious Task Force, it is assigned administratively to the ship's Medical Department. The team's credentials and privileges are managed by higher military medical authority, but they must also be reviewed and certified for the Captain by the ship's MO.

The MO on any large ship serves as the chief of the medical staff, which requires medical training beyond residency as well as several years of practice including bona fide hospital experience. The ability to interface with senior officers and other ships requires several years in the Navy and at least one prior tour at sea. These are responsibilities of being the department head, in which role the MO reports to the XO. It bears repeating that the role of staff officer and adviser to the Captain, although requiring fewer hours, is often more important to the command and also requires years of naval experience. When medical resources fall short of supporting the required standard of care, the MO has the demanding task of convincing the Captain or higher military authority that corrective measures must be taken.

Standards of Care

It was once accepted that arduous, isolated environments such as military deployments or ships at sea could function at lower standards of medical care than those in the home community. Throughout the 1980s, deployable medical systems in the US military were held to a standard called "austere but adequate," which meant sufficient to preserve life and limb without frills. Not much insight is needed to recognize that this really implied "not quite as good as in civilian settings but *good enough.*" Today, the only standard acceptable to military patients, the department of defense, and the US Congress is the state of the art. The expectation is that injured or diseased personnel who survive to reach medical attention will be healed, and that medical or surgical outcomes at sea will match the standards of civilian facilities. However widely held, experienced professional military medical officers know that this outlook is naïve and utopian. Therefore, it is incumbent on the military medical services that they help educate members of congress, journalists, and the public regarding the limitations imposed by the combat environment. We must ensure that the populace and its leaders understand that the austere military surgical and medical capabilities on a battlefield—on land and at sea—are far different from those at a civilian Level 1 trauma center.

The ship's Medical Department must be able to handle all contingencies that could foreseeably occur in the mission, either providing definitive care on board or managing expeditious transport of patients to more capable facilities. The Medical Department must assure that the training of all medical personnel as well as sanitation and equipment in the Medical Department meet the standards of any medical facility of similar size in the home community. The department must be able to treat—at contemporary standards—any illnesses or injuries—or be able to expeditiously and safely transport the patient to a capable medical facility within a timely interval. If the foregoing conditions cannot be met, the MO must either take steps to remedy the situation or notify the Captain of the deficiency. Although the Captain has the authority to decide that military necessity overrides concerns for medical care, the MO must be sure that the Captain understands all the potential medical consequences.

Credentials, Inspections, and Higher Military Medical Authority

The procedures for establishing credentials and delineating privileges for independent providers are the same as on shore and are usually managed by the medical staff of the Fleet Commander.[7] Although shipboard medical departments do not require accreditation by civilian agencies such as the Joint Commission for Accreditation of Healthcare Organizations, naval inspections at every phase of the ship's cycle resemble their civilian equivalents and are in many regards more stringent.

During shipyard periods, the Naval Occupational Safety and Health Agency makes frequent surveys of the conditions and surveillance programs on the ship. Before beginning workups, the Squadron Medical Officer and the Type Commander's medical staff perform Medical Readiness Assessments, which include checking the ship's medical equipment, storerooms, pharmacy, and condition of the medical spaces, as well as inspecting the health records of the crew and the Medical Department's logs and training records. Providers on naval vessels must document their active state licensure as well as currency in continuing medical education and life support. During workups, the Fleet Training Group conducts a specific battery of evaluations and inspections called Refresher Training. For the Medical Department, this focuses particularly on how well the crew at large performs in first aid and mass casualty drills, the department's response to medical emergencies, and how well individual members of the Medical Department know the functions of all of the ship's other departments. At the end of workups, after preparation of the entire Battle Group, the Fleet or Type Commander's medical staff conducts a thorough evaluation of each ship's individual Medical Department together with coordination throughout the Battle Group, including medical communication, patient transport and evacuation, and emergency preparedness.

Many layers of oversight affect the Medical Department. Each administrative and operational command has its own medical staff, which periodically sends direction, guidance, and inquiries to its ship. Of course, such higher authority is expected to route communications through the ship's command channels. However, telephone lines in port and satellite transmission at sea allow direct contact between the MO and medical authorities outside the ship; while such communications surely improve medical care, the MO must inform both the XO and the Captain of contact with higher medical authority. On those rare occasions when there is incompatibility or disagreement between the ship's command and guidance from higher military medical authority, the MO faces a difficult dilemma: professionally, he or she may be inclined to side with superior medical officers; nonetheless, if the MO cannot persuade the Captain to adopt the medical viewpoint, the Captain's decision prevails.

Education and Training for the Crew

In the many inspections and evaluations by higher authority, the Medical Department is graded on how the entire crew performs in first aid and in mass casualty and medical evacuation drills. All crewmembers must be trained in CPR and the resuscitation of an unconscious victim of electrocution. In addition, all must master the treatment of the "Five Basic Wounds," which were chosen because they are severe injuries that are likely to occur in a major explosion or fire[8] and because victims can be saved by fast action. In addition, the skills involved can be used for all other traumatic injuries. The five wounds are

1. sucking chest wound (chest puncture with pneumothorax),
2. traumatic amputation of the hand,
3. maxillofacial trauma with compound fracture of the mandible,
4. abdominal wound with penetration of viscera, and
5. compound fracture of the leg or ankle.

Most ships have a closed-circuit television (CCTV) system, an invaluable way to spread medical and safety information. Many entertaining and understandable video tapes on medical topics are available. In addition, the MO should frequently have "call in" sessions to discuss current health topics such as the annual influenza vaccinations, outbreaks of illness, or health issues in upcoming port calls. Notwithstanding the frenetic work schedule in all ship departments, medical staff should schedule frequent classes with small groups on subjects such as diet, hearing protection, responsible sex practices, prevention of unwanted pregnancy and sexually transmitted diseases (STDs), smoking cessation, substance abuse, and the importance of water intake at sea. The medical staff also provides health training for special occupational groups on the ship such as barbers, food handlers, and laundry workers.

PREDEPLOYMENT PLANNING

Predeployment planning is the critical test of the MO and the Medical Department. When the ship leaves the pier, it must have on board everything the medical staff could possibly need throughout the deployment. Training, information gathering, and planning must be accomplished in advance, because once the ship is under way, the entire crew works 12- to 16-hour days, with full attention required by daily workload and rapidly unfolding events.

General guidance on planning a medical inventory can be found in the *International Medical Guide for Ships*[1] and the *Handbook of Nautical Medicine*.[2] In the US Navy, medical supplies required for each type of ship are listed in a document called the *Authorized Medical Allowance List*. The required stocks of medical equipment, medicines, and other consumable supplies are staggering; even for small ships, the lists run to dozens of pages and thousands of line items. Predeployment planning includes advance knowledge of locations where medical resupply can be obtained if the need arises. Nevertheless, the Medical Department must be fully stocked before deployment because even if the ship will be in a part of the world where needed items should be available, replenishment can be prevented by operational necessity or weather.

Nearly every action of the ship carries health and medical consequences, yet line officers who are discussing tactics, weapons systems, or sailing plans may not realize the medical implications of those activities. For instance, certain operations may require exposing the crew to physiological hazards such as hypothermia and exhaustion, or the ship's routing may reduce the possibilities for medical evacuation. The MO needs to recognize such problems and insist that this information be considered by the other department heads in all military and operational planning. The MO must also be able to tell the Captain where proposed operations may exceed the Medical Department's capabilities and the foreseeable consequences for the crew. The Captain may then either adapt operational plans to reduce medical risks or decide that they are acceptable when balanced against other considerations, but such difficult decisions can only be made correctly with full counsel from the MO.

Many deployments involve a number of ships traveling in company. Destroyers or other ships with limited medical departments may be part of a task force that includes larger ships with extensive facilities. Under these conditions, potential interaction among the ships in the group must be carefully planned. During the yard and workup phases of the cycle, the MOs of the different ships in a battle group should get to know one another by name and training, and should exchange visits to acquire first-hand familiarity with the facilities and equipment on the other ships in the group. If visits cannot be arranged, then it is imperative to engage in the fullest possible exchange of letters and direct telephone communication. Systems for medical consultation and communication should be exercised, as well as methods of patient transfer between ships. Because emergencies during deployment invariably entail cooperation among the ships traveling in a task force, medical aspects of mass casualty and damage control drills must be inserted into group training plans during workups.

Medical Intelligence

Medical intelligence can be used for both medical and military planning.[7] The MO should anticipate being called on to interpret information on immunization campaigns or disease outbreaks to help the Operations and Intelligence departments understand the condition of a nation and its preparedness for war. For purposes of medical planning, the MO gathers data about ports or countries that the ship will visit. This must be done well enough in advance to allow for the procurement and administration of immunizations, and plans for such prophylactic measures as antimalarial medications and gamma globulin for protection from hepatitis. Intuitively, it seems that ships should encounter infectious diseases only during port calls when crewmembers go ashore. However, the risk of disease has increased with the frequent use of aircraft for logistics and mail flights as well as transport of replacement crewmembers and visitors. All new arrivals will have traveled through intermediate countries and are potential carriers of infection. In addition, crates and bags of vegetables brought on board may carry rodents and insects. To take the necessary precautions, the MO must be familiar with endemic conditions in all areas of planned operation.

The main sources of medical intelligence for the US Navy are

1. the Armed Forces Medical Intelligence Center in Frederick, Maryland, which is oriented toward biological and medical sources of intelligence, and
2. the Naval Environmental and Preventive Medicine Units (NEPMUs), which focus on medical threats and health concerns for naval ships in a specific region.

The two sources provide slightly different information; the Medical Department must keep the latest compact disk issued by each. Early in the planning cycle and again immediately before departure, the MO must communicate directly with the NEPMU nearest the ship's planned area of operations and ask the theater or fleet medical staffs for information about recent disease outbreaks and epidemiology. Finally, information should be sought from medical representatives at embassies and consulates in nations where the ship expects port calls and near passage, although information from State Department sources is often less authoritative than from military sources.

Planning for Medical Evacuation

Everything about medical evacuation must be planned and written into operating procedures before the cruise begins.[7] To begin with, the ship's medical staff must articulate the exact capabilities and limitations of their skills and equipment and decide what kinds of diseases and injuries, levels of severity, and numbers of patients would exceed their capacity and thereby trigger medical evacuation. The MO should obtain the medical evacuation plans prepared by theater or fleet staffs and should notify them of the ship's medical resources and when to expect it in their area. All of these issues must then be explained to the Captain, who needs to understand clearly the requirements of modern medical care and the limitations of his Medical Department.

If the ship's planned movements will take it beyond the reach of air transportation or to areas where shore hospitals offer limited care, the Captain must be given a clear understanding of the potential cost of inability to evacuate certain classes of patients for definitive treatment. He may then want to reconsider the plans for deployment.

Crew Preparation and Screening

Medical screening of assigned personnel is the first step in preparing the crew for deployment. Ships are hazardous and some people do not belong on board: in an emergency at sea, one person's limitations or illness can put many crewmates at risk. In the US Navy, the *Manual of the Medical Department*[9] establishes physical and medical standards for sea duty. Vision and hearing are critical to perception of hazards; although hearing aids and eyeglasses may be acceptable, everyone on the ship must be able to see well enough under poor lighting conditions to avoid injury while moving about and must be able to hear alarms even while asleep. Crewmembers must be agile enough to use the narrow passageways and steep ladders that typify military ships. A person with a chronic medical condition can be accepted for a cruise only if the Medical Department and its staff can deal with the condition and the consequences of its deterioration over time.

Some classes of ships such as aircraft carriers and amphibious assault ships carry large numbers of embarked troops (see Table 29-1). Although they require the same immunizations and preparation as the ship's company, such troops are seldom available in advance to the ship's Medical Department. The MO must therefore arrange details early by communicating with the medical staffs of all commands that will embark troops. It is imperative that the XO or Captain participate in this discussion, because the ship could be at risk later if the command fails to insist on medical clearance before deployment.

Most military ships today embark numbers of nonmilitary personnel, including dignitaries and journalists on familiarization visits, technical representatives from industry, law enforcement agents, and educators under contract to teach college or vocational courses to crewmembers. These people, usually civilians, are easily overlooked by the Medical Department. Although they may not have the same physical requirements as sailors, they should be evaluated for limitations on mobility and screened for chronic medical conditions that could lead to emergencies; coronary artery disease is the most frequent and most frightening example.

The Medical Department must make the command and the entire crew aware of the need to acquire certain types of personal items well before going to sea on workups. Most important are eyeglasses, contact lenses, medications not in the ship's formulary, and special clothing items such as shoe inserts or orthotics; these and other items that may be taken for granted at home may be difficult or impossible to obtain once deployed.

Contact lenses can be problematic in the dust and fumes encountered below decks, and crewmembers with long duty hours often forget to change contacts as advised, especially the long-wear and soft varieties. Crewmembers who use contact lenses must bring several pairs of them and sufficient supplies of cleaning and lubricant solutions for the duration of the cruise. Moreover, all crewmembers who require refraction, even if they use contact lenses, must bring with them at least two pairs of shatterproof, current-prescription eyeglasses. Personnel who are required to wear safety glasses on the job must also bring two pairs of those.

During both the yard and workup phases, sailors can seek medical attention ashore. It is critical that the Medical Department be aware of all diagnoses and treatments from either civilian or military sources. Sailors have a knack for seeking out forms of treatment unacceptable to the Navy or obtaining inappropriate medical counsel from providers (sometimes even in the military) who have no knowledge of shipboard conditions.

Personality disorders are a serious cause of problems at sea.[10–12] Sailors with personalities of the antisocial, narcissistic, and borderline types who have acted out or required disciplinary action should be detached from the ship before deployment, because the incidence of suicidal gestures and disruptive behavior is so high among people with significant personality disorders. Unfortunately, these personality disorders often cannot be recognized until the combination of sleep deprivation, demanding work, and congested living cause enough stress to precipitate calamitous behavior. Whenever such problems are revealed, the MO must persuade the command that although a personality disorder is not a medical illness, it is evidence of unsuitability for sea duty and that the sailor must be reassigned as soon as possible. A sailor with any prior suicide attempt—ever—should not go to sea except with the strongest supportive endorsement by a qualified military psychiatrist, preferably one familiar with the stresses and limitations of duty at sea.

SHIPBOARD ENVIRONMENT IN THE YARDS, UNDERWAY, AND DURING PORT CALLS

The environment aboard changes in significant ways in the different phases of the ship's cycle. Although the close spaces, noise, and high risk for trauma remain constant, the work tempo, industrial activities, and food services differ. The psychological environment changes too, producing different manifestations among the crew.

The traditional concerns of occupational and pre-ventive medicine are intertwined on a ship, both because the crew lives in the workspace and because the same medical personnel are responsible for both preventive and occupational programs.[13] The Medical Department shares responsibility for most prevention and surveillance programs with at least one other department. For example, if a ship is large enough to carry an industrial hygienist, he or she is assigned to the Safety Officer but works closely with medical and engineering personnel. Responsibility for food service is shared by the Supply and the Medical departments; heat protection, ventilation, and hearing conservation are overseen by the Engineering Department, while the medical staff provides monitoring, related equipment, and record keeping.

Heat and Noise

Protection from both heat stress and excessive noise are primarily the responsibility of engineers, with help from the Medical Department for monitoring and treatment; both heat illness and hearing loss can be prevented far more easily than they can be treated. The differences are that acoustical injury can be both cumulative and permanent—and heat stroke can be fatal.

Thermal stress is a special problem on ships.[12] Weather decks and flight decks may be exposed to severe conditions of heat and cold as the ship moves through different climatic zones. However, the most common concern is excessive heat and humidity below decks. Although modern ships have complex ventilation and air conditioning systems that reach most spaces, it is not possible to completely control the climate in engine rooms, galleys, sculleries, and laundries. Galleys are areas of insidious heat stress, with their hot appliances and surprisingly high work loads, and sailors work long hours in sculleries with high humidity and heat from basins of hot water and dishwashers. Laundries also require special attention; large amounts of heat are generated by dryers and pressing machines, and ventilation may be inadequate, especially when equipment has been upgraded or the laundries occupy spaces originally designed for other uses. The operation of certain large items of ship's equipment can create high heat loads in adjacent spaces where the work would not otherwise be stressful. For example, the steam catapults on aircraft carriers can raise the temperature and humidity in the layer of spaces immediately below the flight deck, which are occupied by offices, living spaces, and ready rooms.

Appropriate engineering design and insulation of heat-generating equipment are the first steps in prevention, but they can only be accomplished during ship construction or a major overhaul. Ventilation is more tractable and depends not only on fans and ducts but also on open doors, hatches, and scuttles. Under conditions of threat when watertight integrity is required, many of these must be secured, and the resulting decline in air flow can raise thermal stress to dangerous levels. The Medical Department can help prevent heat illness by visiting all spaces on the ship and seeing that sailors keep themselves well hydrated and avoid physical exhaustion. In the engine spaces and flight decks, water loss can exceed 6 to 8 quarts per day, so water intake has to be encouraged and its importance constantly reinforced to the crew. The final means of protection against heat stress is to restrict exposure; the Wet Bulb Globe Temperature Index is routinely used aboard ship. (Heat-related problems in military operations is the subject of the Hot Environments section of *Medical Aspects of Harsh Environments, Volume 1*.[14])

Naval crewmembers can incur cumulative acoustical trauma over many years. Individual hearing protection must take into account any existing hearing loss (1) so that extra protection can be prescribed as needed and (2) to document the hearing status of each member when assigned to the ship and again when they leave it. Audiograms should be recorded at the time of first reporting to the ship and at predetermined intervals during the period of assignment. If the ship does not carry audiology equipment and technicians, the Medical Department must diligently schedule audiograms elsewhere.

Standards for required hearing protection are outlined in the many directives available to medical and engineering departments. Engine spaces, flight decks, hangar decks, and machine shops always require hearing protection; in the very loudest environments, double protection with both internal and external devices may be necessary.

Isolation and Confinement

The environment on a ship at sea is, paradoxically, both crowded and isolated. The crew is packed close together without much privacy in their living quarters and they see the same faces day after day during meals and at work, never able to get away. At the same time, people feel isolated because there are few opportunities to communicate with family or friends back home. Time at sea means being away from land, vegetation, and most ordinary diversions. This is especially stressful for the young people on naval vessels, many of whom have left their families and homes for the first time. Common reactions include shortness of breath, insomnia, anxiety reactions, depression, panic attacks, and prolonged sea sickness. Bedwetting is less common and headaches usually have other causes. Materials on psychiatric symptoms and emergencies are useful at sea.[11,12]

The ship's command must take measures to minimize psychological problems and to ensure that crewmembers will recognize symptoms of stress in themselves and others. Otherwise, a young sailor who reports to sick call with symptoms and is told that the cause is stress may interpret that as dismissive or disrespectful. The Captain should address the psychological effects of confinement and isolation at Captain's Calls and in talks to the crew early in each cruise. Division officers and CPOs should bring up the topic early and often at daily muster in quarters.

The command's other tools are recreation and distraction. The command must make special efforts to promote vigorous exercise and recreational programs that focus on getting the sailors out of their berthing and working spaces. Most ships other than submarines or mine sweepers have decks or flight decks that permit jogging, basketball, and calisthenics. Group sports are valuable to provide vigorous interaction with crewmembers other than bunk mates or workers from the same shop, although injuries from such activities also cause a significant proportion of lost duty time.[15] Diverse interactions reduce the sensation of being trapped with only a small circle of friends. Movies and television provide views of land, communities, and automobiles, as well as diversion, but they are passive and can keep a sailor in the berthing area when it would be better to get away.

Historically, sailors looked forward to a daily tot of rum or grog, and some navies still allow small amounts of alcohol at mealtime. The US Navy strictly prohibits alcohol, and sneaking it is now quite rare on naval vessels. However, drinking on liberty (shore leave) can be a problem, and alcohol withdrawal can become a medical concern from the second day underway. Alcohol withdrawal must be suspected in sailors with new tremors, autonomic symptoms, insomnia, or seizures in the first few weeks at sea. The ship will have an alcohol abuse counselor who has special training in recognizing and helping with substance abuse problems, but he or she must call for medical evaluation of potential clients so that the MO can rule out neurological diseases, endocrine or metabolic disturbances, and psychiatric problems.

Epidemiology and Epidemics

Information on epidemiology and methods of tracking of disease outbreaks may be found in the *Manual of Naval Preventive Medicine*.[13] *Health Information for International Travel*[16] is also a useful re-source. (*Military Preventive Medicine: Mobilization and Deployment*,[17] another volume in the Textbook of Military Medicine series, also contains information on these matters.) The commonest outbreaks on ships are food-borne illnesses, respiratory diseases, and skin conditions. Outbreaks of water-borne illness are less common and are more likely to be caused by chemicals than by infectious agents. Any outbreak of infectious disease must be reported immediately to the Fleet Commander and the NEPMU. Tracking of outbreaks begins with a clear diagnosis or at least a detailed description of the symptoms and time course of the index case or cases. It is imperative to confirm that the problem represents physical illness, since in close environments, outbreaks of hysterical somatic complaints can spread rapidly and be just as devastating as physical illness.

Most food-borne outbreaks can be traced to food storage problems and the mixing of foods that should be kept apart.[13] The main defenses are good personal hygiene among food workers, cleanliness of work spaces and equipment, and proper practices in the storage and serving of foodstuffs. The commonest symptoms are acute gastroenteritis with cramps and diarrhea. Taking a careful dietary history from each crewmember should enable medical personnel to identify the food items, meal shift, and galley common to affected members. Patients must be adequately hydrated; oral rehydration salts are preferable to intravenous fluids. Antispasmodic medications may be helpful for severe cases. It is usually impractical to identify specific bacterial or viral agents aboard ship; if bacterial culturing is available, it may be useful to identify the genera *Shigella*, *Salmonella*, or *Vibrio*, which can require antibiotics for effective treatment. Widespread use of antibiotics among the crew is seldom warranted.

The closely confined quarters and compromised ventilation aboard ship foster the rapid spread of respiratory illnesses, and respiratory symptoms are among the commonest reasons for visits to sick call. Zones of harsh contrast between cool–dry and hot–humid spaces cause cough and local mucosal irritability, which can be so widespread as to both mimic infectious outbreaks and make the crew more vulnerable to them. Although respiratory infections are usually mild and self-limited, influenza and tuberculosis are much feared at sea. Primary prevention of tuberculosis consists of proper screening of the crew and an active program of skin testing.[12] Vigorous enforcement of annual influenza vaccinations is critical despite the youth of ship's crews, because epidemic influenza could put the ship itself at risk. Secondary prevention of respiratory diseases is relatively ineffective because they are usually infectious before symptoms develop. There is often a clamor for cough suppressants and decongestants or antihistamines, none of which reliably hasten recovery and all of which may have side effects that can be dangerous on a ship. The most important measures are to provide bed rest for as many of the affected crew as possible, encourage high fluid intake, control air conditioning, and prevent cigarette smoking. The temptation to prescribe antibiotics for everyone with a cough must be resisted unless there is good evidence for a susceptible pathogen; fostering the emergence of an antibiotic-resistant organism in a crew who will work together for the next several months can be more hazardous than the effects of a judicious delay for diagnosis before starting an appropriate antibiotic.

Pests and Vectors

External parasites, insects, and rodents are recurrent problems aboard ships, and their control is addressed in the *US Navy Shipboard Pest Control Manual*.[18] Scabies, lice, and other external parasites are best prevented by crew education and hygiene. Bathing and laundry standards are most important. Skilled preventive medicine technicians should frequently inspect berthing areas, with special attention to bed linens. There must be a high level of suspicion during sick call; any sailor who complains of itching or other skin symptoms must be disrobed and examined with particular attention to hairy areas and spaces between digits. Whenever a case is detected, the affected individual must be treated immediately and berthed in an isolated area such as the medical ward, if possible. All linen in his or her berthing compartment must be laundered immediately, and mattresses may need to be discarded.

Cockroaches thrive in the warm, damp areas of a ship and where nutrients are available; eating in the berthing compartments must be prohibited and the rule enforced. Traps should be maintained in most heads and in all food preparation areas, but it must be emphasized that the traps are intended for detection rather than eradication. Control of cockroaches is achieved by the elimination of standing water and moisture by means of vigorous cleaning and ventilation of heads, galleys, and sculleries. Insecticide sprays add a margin of control but are still only secondary to cleanliness and prevention.

Rodents are a serious problem for ships. Rats usually get aboard in port areas with their abundant hiding spaces and litter. Vigilance at brow walkways and installation of rat cones on lines are the main preventive measures. Since rats can swim, preventive medicine technicians need to work with the Deck Department and local authorities to inspect the hull at the water line at least daily and preferably several times per day. Mice usually enter the ship in crates of stores, especially grain and flour products. All new stores should be inspected for breaks in containers and the presence of mouse droppings. As with roaches, the main control of rodents on board is to deprive them of food by careful food storage and by confining food and eating to mess decks. Rats and mice both live in storerooms, especially where food is kept; stores should be stacked and arranged so that inspectors can see all areas where rodents might enter or hide. Rodents and other vermin can usually be eliminated by traps and careful use of poisons. If the infestation is so severe or resistant that fumigation is required, that can only be performed by certified technicians.

Hypoxic Spaces

A ship that has many sealed or unventilated spaces that can become hypoxic or can accumulate toxic or explosive gases. For example, stored vegetables consume oxygen, so that whenever a worker goes into a food storeroom, someone must be on watch outside with oxygen breathing apparatus nearby. Crewmembers are trained to be aware of such hypoxic hazards, but civilian workers in the yards may open doors or bolted covers in the course of their work or simply to sneak off for a nap—with fatal consequences.

An additional hazard arises during the yard phase of the ship's cycle because welding consumes oxygen at a high rate, and compartments where welding is being done are often closed to forestall interruptions. Because welding requires a watcher in adjacent compartments in case a fire is started by heat conducted through a metal bulkhead, the "firewatcher" should also be trained to monitor the welder for signs of hypoxia.

Flying Operations at Sea

Although aircraft carriers and large amphibious ships are well known for their flight operations, many other ships also have flight decks and carry one or two helicopters at sea. All the hazards inherent in military flight operations pertain at sea, including windblast, collisions, fires, and explosions. However, the naval environment exaggerates some of these risks and adds some unique problems.[19] For the flight crew, a failed landing—which runs an aircraft into the grass on land—produces a rapidly sinking metal coffin at sea, since jet canopies are difficult to open and helicopters that land in water invert and sink immediately, owing to the weight of their overhead engines. Jet blast can blow a sailor over the side, and the fall from the flight deck—30 to 40 feet—can be incapacitating. Pneumothorax from impact, abdominal injuries, and hypothermia have to be anticipated from any accident that puts a person into the water. Therefore, everyone who works on the flight deck of a ship must wear a survival vest or jacket with a self-inflating mechanism, as well as locator beacons, sea dye markers, and shark repellant.

Medical crews need to be on the deck during flight operations to assist in rescue, and the main Medical Department assumes a high level of alert. On aircraft carriers and large amphibious assault ships, CCTV allows the main Medical Department to monitor flight operations for immediate medical response to mishaps.

Workers on the flight deck are exposed to extremes of wind and weather. Since any ship conducting flight operations turns into the wind to add lift for the aircraft, wind chill is a serious problem in cold climates. However, heat, sun, and the black-painted metal deck more often cause problems, which are amplified by the fact that all crewmembers on deck are required to wear protective head gear, long-sleeved jerseys, and flotation vests. The combination of intense work, high temperature, and protective garments causes overheating and dehydration. In addition, the pace of work is so high that crewmembers must be reminded to drink; supervisors and corpsmen must mingle frequently with workers on the flight deck to encourage fluid intake and watch for fatigue and signs of overheating.

Although major mishaps with mass trauma and severe burns are a constant concern during flight operations, less dramatic injuries are more common and still dangerous. They include musculoskeletal injuries and fractures, eye trauma, contusions, lacerations, crush injuries, and severe sunburn. Ubiquitous fatigue and sleep deprivation can lead to fatal inattention. The machinery on the flight deck is particularly dangerous. On aircraft carriers, arresting cables stretch across the deck to catch the tailhook from landing jets. A sailor whose foot is in the way of the cable when it catches an airplane or retracts suffers severe fractures of the ankle or leg; if those high-tension cables snap from a rough landing, the whipping action can slice off a limb or head. Tractors for towing aircraft, in the crowded on-deck environment, pose a significant hazard for colliding with deck workers. Steam catapults with their rapidly shuttling transoms are further sources of injury.

MEDICAL CARE AT SEA

The spaces assigned to the Medical Department on virtually all ships are confined and constrained (Figure 29-2). Even on large ships, pipes, valves, and over-

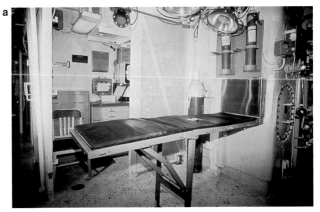

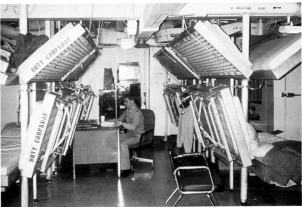

Fig. 29-2. (**a**) A battle dressing station is equivalent to an examination room in a hospital emergency department. The two small green canisters above and one large green canister to the right of the examination table contain oxygen. An emergency water tank to be used if power fails aboard the ship is located above the ceiling lamps. The yellow lights in the ceiling are also emergency lights that will be used in case of loss of power. Against the far wall is a portable suction machine and a wall-mounted autoclave (partially obscured). Below these are drawers where intravenous equipment, bandages, medicines, and surgical supplies are kept. Unless the ship is rigged for battle (ie, General Quarters), when not in use the examination table is folded flat against the wall, and the wire mesh partitions around the autoclave and drawers are closed and locked to prevent damage and pilferage. (**b**) Space is limited aboard a ship, and a physician's examining area may be an unused part of an inpatient ward. Unoccupied berths (beds) are folded toward the overhead (ceiling) to provide additional floor space. Photographs and figure legend: Courtesy of Louis Kroot, MD, Department of Emergency Medicine, University of Kentucky Chandler Medical Center, Lexington, Ky.

EXHIBIT 29-1

MOST COMMON MEDICAL PROBLEMS AT SEA

Abdominal pain

Asthma

Concussion/head trauma

Cutaneous abscess

Dermatitis

Fracture diagnoses and treatment

Gastroenteritis/vomiting and diarrhea

Hand injuries

Headache

Minor wounds and lacerations

Muscle strains/sprains/jams

Myocardial infarction

Pelvic pain

Personality disorder

Pharyngitis

Routine immunizations

Sexually transmitted diseases

Shoulder dislocation

Tooth abscess

Toothache

Upper respiratory infection

Adapted with permission from D'Alessandro DM, D'Alessandro MP, Hendrix MJC, Bakalar RS. Information needs of naval primary care providers and patients at sea. *Mil Med.* 1999;164(2):128.

---

suggest taking over medical space for nonmedical purposes. The change may indeed be necessary for the good of the ship, but the MO must protect the medical capability of the ship and be sure that the Captain and XO clearly understand the possible adverse effects of any such change.

Sick Call

Sick call is the period each day when the clinic is open for routine visits and treatment. Sick call is far more important on a ship than in other military settings, because minor problems must be treated early to keep them from worsening beyond the ship's treatment capacity. In addition, sick call must provide over-the-counter medications, band aids, and the like, which the sailor would find in a drugstore at home.

Rates of particular complaints and injuries vary with the type and mission of the ship, the climate, the phase of the ship's cycle, and the time of year (Exhibit 29-1). Sick call provides the most fundamental means for monitoring the health of the crew. The number of sailors treated and their diagnoses are reported daily to the XO and Captain in the "Sick List" or "Binnacle List," so named because historically the names of all sick sailors were posted on the ship's compass (binnacle) on the bridge. One of the commonest "prescriptions" from sick call is a note or chit recommending light duty or rest; although the sailor's division officer or CPO nearly always honors such a chit, it is important for both the medical personnel and their patients to realize these chits are not orders but only *recommendations* to the command.

head structures intrude into the working space in every battle dressing station (BDS), creating nooks and corners that are used to brace and store medical equipment. The medical team must become thoroughly familiar with the layout and the location of supplies and equipment to allow their rapid, efficient use when required. Ship overhaul may provide an opportunity to improve medical spaces, but it also may be the occasion for another department or a naval architect to

Fig. 29-3. *Sick, Lame, and Lazy: Sick Bay Line Aboard USS Oriskany (CVA-34) During the Gulf of Tonkin, Aug 71.* Painting by Charles Waterhouse. With no chairs and no magazines to read, a long line of men waits for sick call; privacy is scarce to nonexistent. The title seems to reflect the artist's perception that malingerers may be among those who attend sick call. Painting: Courtesy of US Naval Historical Center, Washington, DC.

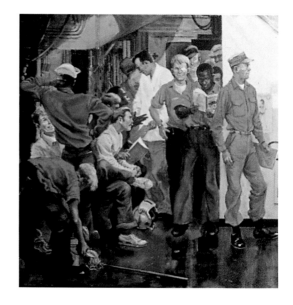

On most ships, sick call is open two or three times each day to accommodate crew working and sleeping schedules. Patients are usually seen first by junior corpsmen; a standing operating procedure details treatment for specific problems and lists those complaints that require the attention of a physician or a senior corpsman. On large ships, many sailors gather at the clinic door for sick call and form a long line that extends down the passageway (Figure 29-3). Such lines are wasteful of the ship's manpower and demoralizing to the crew; standing in line conveys an image of inefficiency and lack of respect that undermines the crew's confidence in the Medical Department. One way to reduce waiting is to have an appointment system that allows sailors to sign up for a sick call visit the same day. An alternative is to triage the people who are waiting; those who feel acutely ill or have new injuries are brought to the front of the line, others with less-urgent problems are asked to return about 30 minutes later, and members who are there for follow-up visits are asked to return after the second group.

Privacy is hard to provide on a ship but is essential in sick call. It is necessary to have a sign-in method that allows sailors to state their medical complaint where others cannot hear it, and the sign-in log must not be visible to other patients. Because most sailors are reluctant to discuss medical history or emotional topics if they can be overheard by shipmates, there must be a consultation room with a door that can be closed. Sick call is a haven for sailors who need sympathy or respite; they should feel that they can trust "the docs"—a term used for corpsmen as well as physicians—to provide a sympathetic ear as well as prompt treatment. Knowing that even minor aches and pains will be taken seriously and treated in a private, dignified manner is terribly important to young people who have few distractions aboard ship and can be prone to worry and ponder about physical problems.

Some sailors come to sick call so often that they win a reputation as slackers or "sick bay commandos" and it is important for the medical staff to avoid becoming cynical or hardened to these sailors. When a large number of hypochondriacal complaints appear, it may well be the sign of a morale problem that is as important to the command as an outbreak of physical illness. Also, of course, physical illness may cause subtle symptoms for some time before it becomes evident on physical examination or laboratory tests. A patient who is dismissed or becomes discouraged at the first visit to sick call may not return until the illness grows much worse. Most important, however, the crew must fully trust the Medical Department if they are to be open and honest in giving medical histories and feel confident at times of emergency or personal crisis. While the Medical Department needs to help people return to work and discourage hypochondriasis, it is far better to tolerate "sick bay commandos" than to build a reputation for skepticism or insensitivity.

During times of busiest operational tempo, sailors are less likely to come to sick call for minor problems. At these times, members of the medical staff must walk through all work spaces to assess levels of fatigue and find people who need treatment. It is at these times that special efforts to push fluids are also necessary.

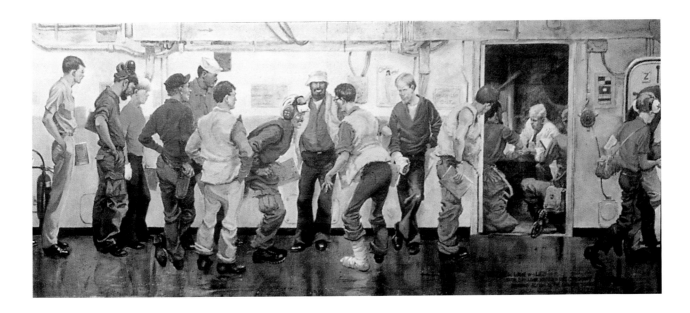

Disposition of the Sick Sailor

The MO at sea must consider proper treatment of the patient in the context of both occupational and military requirements. To determine whether a sick or injured sailor can return to duty requires understanding of his or her job and familiarity with the workspace. Often the MO needs to visit the patient's work area before deciding. Allowance must be made for the fact that work is harder and duty hours longer at sea than on shore, and that sleep deprivation and fatigue impair recovery from almost every ailment. Bed rest is the oldest and still the most reliable treatment for many ills at sea. The value of rest and repeat examination cannot be overemphasized for cases of nonspecific illness. Crewmembers with fever or general weakness, or who require intravenous fluid for any reason, should be berthed in the medical ward when possible. On some ships, the Sick Bay does not have ward beds or the number of patients may exceed the berths in the Medical Department. Any sailor who must be confined to his or her own rack should have an attendant from the same department and berthing area. Medical personnel should visit the patient several times a day to record vital signs.

The maximum period that a sick sailor can be kept on the ship will have been established by the theater evacuation policy and the ship's own predeployment plan. Even the most sophisticated Medical Department on a ship lacks the diagnostic capability of a hospital ashore, and a smoldering illness that eludes diagnosis or a sailor who cannot return to duty can be demoralizing to the crew, deprives the ship of a useful member, and consumes important resources. Medical staff must not allow indecision to tempt them into keeping a sick sailor beyond the predetermined time limit.

Telemedicine

Experience shows that corpsmen and young physicians do not seek consultation as often as they should, and they should be taught that consultation not only improves treatment but can also prevent unnecessary patient transfers and evacuations.[20,21] Voice communication among Medical Departments in a battle group is the first level of consultation. Even when a ship is steaming independently, satellite communication often allows consultation with physicians or specialists on distant ships or at major shore facilities. Procedures for medical communication may be specified in predeployment plans or arranged at need.

Satellite television transmission for medical use is available on an increasing number of ships. While the consultant cannot touch or palpate patients, the ability to interview them and see facial expressions adds great value. These medical systems can transmit electrocardiograms and include appliances for auscultation as well as otoscopic and ophthalmoscopic examinations. The image allows very good dermatological diagnosis and visualization of endoscopy. All of this can be done in real time to assist the isolated medical provider, even in emergencies.

Medical Evacuation

The best way to transfer a patient is from a pier. Because all forms of transportation at sea incur risk, and most are rough compared with transportation on land, patients should be evacuated at sea only when predetermined medical criteria are met, opportunities for consultation and telemedicine have been fully exploited, and the risks of transport are outweighed by the patient's needs.

In years past, transfer at sea was by Stokes litter or boatswain's chair on high-tension cable strung between ships. Today, patient transport at sea is usually by helicopter (Figure 29-4). Most military ships have landing areas; if not, the helicopter can hover over the deck and winch the patient aboard in a litter cage. However, the latter process is terrifying for most patients and can be a rough ride, so it should be used only when no other transport is available. When the patient can wait long enough for evacuation to be arranged by higher military medical authority, the Medical Department contacts the fleet's Medical Regulating Officer, who arranges for the best treatment facility, transportation, and itinerary. The possibility of a long stay, further transport, or even reassignment cannot be predicted, so all medical and personnel records must accompany the patient at the time of transfer.

Preparation is critical in cases of urgent evacuation: the patient must be stable and it must be confirmed that the receiving ship or facility is prepared to receive the patient and capable of delivering the required treatment. The definition of "stable" is elusive, but in general it means that the patient will not deteriorate hemodynamically during transport and is either breathing spontaneously or ventilated by a method that can be reliably sustained throughout the transfer. At sea as anywhere else, medical care must "first do no harm," and this includes transport. The only reason to evacuate an unstable patient is that he or she will certainly die without it.

Safety is the first consideration in preparing a

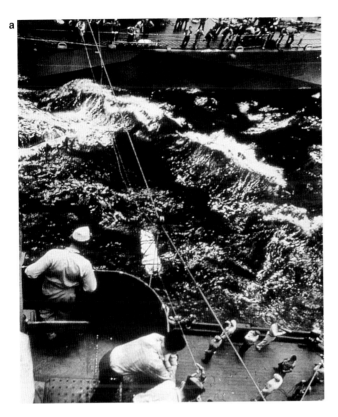

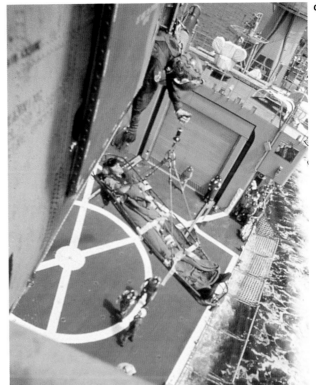

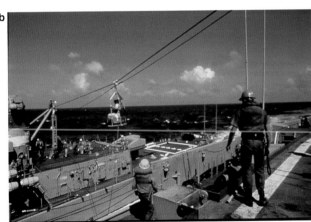

Fig. 29-4. Casualty transport at sea is a dangerous, arduous undertaking. (**a**) A casualty on a Stokes litter is being transferred from ship to ship during World War II. (**b**) A peacetime ship-to-ship transfer of a casualty using a boatswain's chair. (**c**) This peacetime casualty is being transferred from ship to helicopter on a Stokes litter because the flight deck is too small for the helicopter to land. (**d**) In this World War II mass casualty situation, a large number of casualties is being transferred back to ships by a landing craft. Photographs a and d: Official Historian, Bureau of Medicine and Surgery, Department of the Navy, Washington, DC. Photographs b and c: Navy Imaging Command, Anacostia Naval Air Station, Washington, DC. Figure legend: Courtesy of Louis Kroot, MD, Department of Emergency Medicine, University of Kentucky Chandler Medical Center, Lexington, Ky.

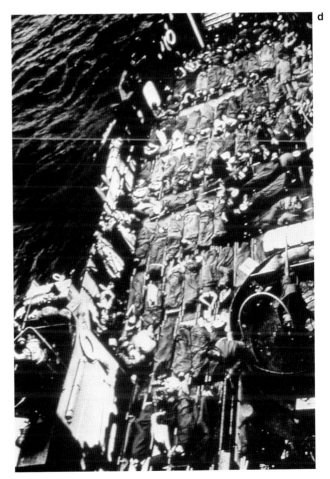

patient for transport. A medical escort must accompany the patient to provide care in flight. The patient must wear a survival vest, preferably one that does not require inflation. An ambulatory patient should walk aboard the aircraft and strap in like any other passenger. Litter patients must be secured with straps that permit quick release in an emergency. Tubes for fluids or oxygen must not dangle where they can become entangled with anything else on the aircraft, and intravenous fluids and blood must be contained in plastic bags without air pockets. If the patient could not survive ditching at sea, the necessity for transfer should be reconsidered.

Most patients sick enough to warrant evacuation should have supplemental oxygen, since even low-attitude helicopter flight can drop the partial pressure of oxygen too low for a patient with blood loss or compromised pulmonary function. The medical escort should watch the patient with an oxygen mask for vomiting and aspiration. A pneumothorax must be vented through a chest tube attached to a flutter valve or other mechanism to prevent backflow. Neither inflatable casts nor military antishock trousers can be used because they will expand in flight.

Port Calls

The MO should have reviewed local disease surveillance reports long before the ship approaches any port of call.[7] An advance party usually visits the port to take care of diplomatic issues and arrange for docking and replenishment. It should include a medical representative, but if that is not possible, the MO must consult with the members of the advance party to assure that they gather the necessary information. General epidemiological information must be updated with particular attention to the following:

- current outbreaks of disease;
- incidence of tuberculosis, arthropod-borne diseases, malaria, hepatitis, and STDs;
- occurrence of any disease with antibiotic-resistant organisms;
- the capabilities and standards of local hospitals;
- local water purification standards;
- food and restaurant sanitation standards; and
- incidence of recreational drug use in the area.

Before allowing sailors to go ashore, the CPOs or division officers of every department briefs their members. These briefings must include persuasive remarks about malaria prophylaxis, warnings about food- and water-borne illnesses, and safe sex practices. Unless the MO is satisfied regarding food safety and potable water supplies, the crew should be advised to avoid eating or drinking in the local economy and to take on liberty bottled water from the ship.

In areas with significant malaria risk, the MO should try to persuade the Captain either to select an alternate port for rest and recreation or to keep the crew onboard the ship. Crewmembers who are required to go ashore for operational reasons must follow strict measures to prevent malaria, including the use of insect repellant, long-sleeved garments treated with permethrin, mosquito nets when it is necessary to sleep ashore, and rigorous adherence to malaria chemoprophylaxis.[22] Because chloroquine-resistant malarial strains are spreading over the world, it is essential that the MO review current information.

On arrival in port, the MO must visit the nearest hospital to which crewmembers will be referred if hospitalization is necessary. In this visit, the MO can assess the standards and capabilities of local medical practice and establish the method of payment for medical treatment on shore. The MO must also explain to local providers the requirements and limitations of the ship so they will not overestimate the onboard medical facilities and return to the ship sailors who should have been treated at the hospital.

Most STDs are contracted on shore. Sexual relations among crewmembers is forbidden with mixed-gender crews but carries less social opprobrium than homosexual relations. However, experience suggests that sexual activity between shipmates occurs predominantly on shore. Educational programs that encourage abstinence, monogamous relations, and barrier (condom) protective measures are still the best ways to prevent STDs.

It is frequently suggested that the ship distribute condoms at the brow or quarterdeck as crewmembers depart on liberty, but this is not as good an idea as it first seems. All crewmembers should be provided with an appropriate and thorough educational program long before any port call. It is not the quick availability of condoms that determines whether sailors will use them but a decision in advance to practice safe sex. Modern sailors may be enlightened about sex, but many would be embarrassed to have condoms thrust upon them in public, and others are offended that someone expects them to have sex with a stranger (even though some will). Finally, both families in the United States and people in the port communities may fail to appreciate the preventive medicine perspective and interpret condom distribution as encouraging casual sex. The most effective way to help sailors avoid STDs is to provide education in advance and make condoms easily available in private.

Special Medical Concerns Aboard Ship

Conditions aboard ship place many medical issues in a special context. The inclusion of increasing numbers of women in US Navy crew means that medical departments must be able to provide advice and care in areas of gynecology and obstetrics never before of concern aboard ship. The availability of highly capable, fully staffed operating rooms aboard large warships not only improves the level of care available but also obligates staffs to provide colposcopy and other services for women and also raises the question of the propriety of performing elective surgery on board instead of transferring patients to hospitals on shore. Other unusual concerns include the implementation of a "walking blood bank" to support emergency transfusions at sea and the proper disposal of medical waste in an era of concern over protecting ocean ecology.

Medical Care of Women

Women have served on auxiliary US Navy ships as integrated members of the crew since 1978 and began serving aboard combat ships in 1994. The ability of a ship to provide obstetrical and gynecological care must be consistent with the general level of medical and surgical care on board. If the sole provider is a corpsman, he or she should be knowledgeable regarding differential diagnosis, the effects of hormonal cycles, hazards of pregnancy, diagnosis of pelvic pain and pelvic infections, and when consultation and transport are necessary. Larger ships with at least one physician—especially if more than 200 women are on the ship—should also have a provider such as a nurse practitioner who has specialized training in the care of women. Ships with personnel capable of performing abdominal operations must have at least one provider aboard who is trained in colposcopy, and in the very near future pelvic and vaginal ultrasound will also be required.

From the medical planner's standpoint, the primary issues about healthcare for women are as follows:

- availability of personal hygiene items (a Supply Department issue with health implications);

- privacy for medical history taking, screening programs, and examinations;
- staff competence and proficiency in reproductive and routine gynecological care;
- equipment for appropriate gynecological examinations and procedures; and
- contraception and pregnancy.

Contraception should always have been a concern for male crewmembers, but the personal significance and medical consequences of contraception are much greater for women.

There is some evidence that women utilize medical services more often than men on land and at sea, although (with the exception of gynecological issues) the medical complaints are generally similar.[23] These results imply that as increasing numbers of women are included in naval crews, medical staffs may need to be increased and sick call lengthened to accommodate women's legitimate need for medical care. It remains to be seen whether naval women in traditionally male occupations will follow their civilian sisters in adopting high-risk lifestyles.[24]

Present US Navy policy permits women to remain assigned to sea duty for the first 20 weeks of pregnancy, *as long as the patient remains within 6 hours of definitive gynecological, surgical, and obstetrical care.* This limitation reflects the risks of spontaneous abortion and hemorrhage from ectopic pregnancy during the first 20 weeks.[25] This rule permits pregnant women to remain aboard on deployments in the Mediterranean and Caribbean, within several hundred miles of most coasts, and worldwide when assigned to a hospital ship. During those first 20 weeks, a pregnant woman should be able to perform her ordinary job, although those whose work includes considerable bending and heavy lifting may need some duty limitations and may have an increased rate of musculoskeletal strain. Discovery of a pregnancy more advanced than 20 weeks requires the earliest possible gentle transfer to shore.

Babies should not be delivered on naval ships. However, women have been able to conceal pregnancy for many months, and some have gone into labor at sea. Therefore, on any ship that has women aboard, at least one member of the Medical Department should be competent to perform a vaginal delivery, including a low-forceps delivery, if necessary. Ships with an operating room should have a physician able to perform a caesarian section. Neonates cannot be properly managed on a military ship, so if a baby is delivered, the ship must return to port as soon as possible to disembark the mother and child at the pier. Evacuation by helicopter is a distant second choice, owing to difficulties with keeping an infant warm, performing resuscitation en route, and ensuring survival at sea in case of an aircraft mishap.

Elective Surgery

Many surgical operations are well within the capabilities of a large ship, which carries a competent operating room, a qualified surgical staff, and modern anesthesia. Emergency operations that can be performed include appendectomy, repair of an acute or strangulated inguinal hernia, resection of perforated bowel, and a number of other urgent procedures. However, the propriety of performing truly elective surgery is controversial, as is any procedure while the ship is within reach of a hospital.[26] The argument against elective surgery is that even the best medical department at sea lacks the ability of a real hospital to cope with unusual complications. On the other hand, performing selected procedures maintains the skills of the surgeons, trains and exercises the surgical team, and keeps sailors on the ship where they can quickly return to duty.

The debate over elective surgery continues because both sides have strong arguments; however, a fatality during elective surgery aboard ship is intolerable. So, despite the great challenge of maintaining surgical skills aboard ship, I recommend that elective procedures be delayed until the procedure can be scheduled in a hospital on shore.

"Competence for Duty" Examinations

Sometimes a supervisor observes unusual clumsiness or poor work performance by a sailor and suspects that he or she is physically impaired because of some form of misconduct or dereliction such as consuming alcohol or drugs or staying out too late the previous night. The supervisor may then bring the sailor to the Medical Department for a formal examination to determine competence for duty. This is not a question of medical diagnosis and treatment but rather a legal requirement for disciplinary or personnel action; such an examination should be performed only on written order of the Captain or a duly designated officer in the sailor's chain of command. The MO is expected to perform a clinical examination and state whether the crewmember is physically able to perform his or her duties and whether the crewmember is under the influence of alcohol, drugs, or other incapacitating substances, or is sleep-deprived. The MO should order only those laboratory tests that are necessary to formulate a *clinical* conclusion. For example,

if the sailor appears to be drunk and smells of alcohol without evidence of neurological disease, then a clinical diagnosis of intoxication can be made without a blood alcohol measurement. The MO may ethically provide a professional opinion as legal evidence, but the Medical Department does not perform legally binding blood alcohol or drug screens and medical staff must not be placed in the role of investigators or enforcement agents.

Mass Casualty Situations

A mass casualty event is one in which the number and severity of injuries exceeds the capacity of the Medical Department to care for them, so that response requires coordination throughout the ship and rationing of care for the injured.[7] Although civilian triage is performed to preserve as many lives and limbs as possible, on a military ship the overarching goal must be to save the mission or perhaps the ship itself (Exhibit 29-2). Therefore, the highest priority is to return the greatest possible number of injured to their duties in order to keep the ship afloat and in action. All crewmembers assigned to moving or treating patients must thoroughly understand this rationale.

A mass casualty situation requires immediate removal of the injured from the scene to a clear area where they can be laid out for quick evaluation and triage. At the triage station, casualties receive initial first aid measures such as intravenous lines, pain medication, and dressings. Some of the injured who receive adequate first aid may be released directly from triage for return to duty.

Coordination is critical in any mass casualty situation. A senior member of the Medical Department must move immediately to Damage Control (DC) Central to determine the best locations for triage, a staging area if required, and the main medical treatment site or BDS. These decisions must be coordinated from DC Central because it has the best information about the state of the ship; areas that have been damaged; and routes for moving patients when many doors, passageways, and hatches are secured for General Quarters. Members of the Medical Department must know how to use sound-powered telephones, which use wire strung during the emergency to bypass damaged communications and power systems. In addition, runners must be designated in advance from among the litter bearers; in case of complete communications failure, they carry messages, questions, and information among the triage, staging, and treatment sites and to DC Central.

EXHIBIT 29-2

THE *FORRESTAL* FIRE

On 29 August 1967 the USS *Forrestal*, CV 59, was off the coast of Vietnam, preparing to launch attack aircraft. A Zuni rocket malfunctioned and set an A-4 Skyhawk afire on the flight deck. Within minutes several other armed aircraft caught fire, and the subsequent explosions and fuel fires set the entire flight deck ablaze (Exhibit Figure 1). Dozens of flight crew and workers on the flight deck were killed within minutes; many others were severely burned. The fires and explosions extended down many deck levels on the after half of the ship, trapping and wounding sailors in the after mess decks and in several berthing compartments.

Over the several days of the ordeal, 134 *Forrestal* sailors died and several hundred others suffered severe burns, inhalation injury, and fractures. The two after auxiliary battle dressing stations were destroyed. At the same time that firefighting was begun, a staging and triage area was set up in the forward hangar bay and forward mess decks. All flight operations were impossible, so evacuation was delayed for several days. The first casualties arrived in the main medical area within 10 minutes, and the operating room was in constant use for several days. Major treatment areas had to be set up in the forward battle dressing stations on the O-3 deck just below the flight deck and in the forward mess decks. The 53 beds in the medical ward were quickly filled, so patients were treated in makeshift holding beds in mess decks—and some commandeered berthing compartments.

As tragic as the loss of life was in this fire, the rapid action of the Medical Department was responsible for saving the lives of dozens of patients. By returning most of the casualties to duty to fight the fires and control damage, the Medical Department also indirectly helped save the lives of others on the ship.

a

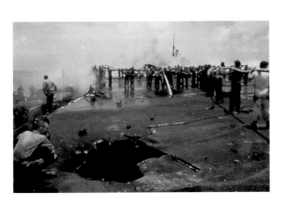

b

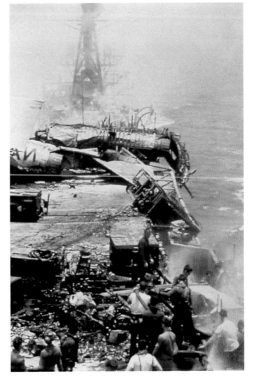

c

Exhibit Figure 1. (a) On 29 August 1967, armed US Navy aircraft exploded and burned as they sat on the flight deck of the USS *Forrestal*; crews attempted to extinguish the fires while the aircraft burned, but the explosions and ensuing conflagration claimed the lives of 134 sailors. **(b)** The exploding bombs detonated by the fires blew holes through the flight deck of the *Forrestal*. In an attempt to cool parts of the wreckage below in the hangar deck, crews cut holes through the flight deck and hosed water down to the wreckage below. **(c)** Cleanup proceeded in the aftermath of the fire. The ghostlike structure at the top of the photograph is the mast of another ship astern of the USS *Forrestal*. Photographs: Navy Imaging Command, Anacostia Naval Air Station, Washington, DC. Figure legend: Courtesy of Louis Kroot, MD, Department of Emergency Medicine, University of Kentucky Chandler Medical Center, Lexington, Ky.

Corpses

The unpleasant but necessary topic of disposition of human remains aboard ship is frequently misunderstood and can cause confusion and discord at very difficult times. The XO and all department heads must understand before the ship leaves the pier that the Medical Department does not take care of corpses. The fact that death certificates, medical records, and autopsies are handled by medical specialists can be misleading. In operational and doctrinal terms, however, a human body ceases to be a person at the time of death and can no longer be a patient. *Management and transport of corpses is NOT the job of the Medical Department.* Procurement and storage of materiel such as coffins, transport boxes, or body bags are the responsibility of the Supply Department.

Death at sea is difficult for a crew regardless of the circumstances. Soon after a death occurs is not a good time to discuss with the XO or Captain the best way to handle human remains, so they must understand the issue beforehand. When the XO asks the MO about topics such as the inventory of coffins or refrigerators for corpses, the MO must quickly and persuasively redirect the questions to the Supply Officer.

The Walking Blood Bank

A modern blood bank is simply not available at sea except on hospital ships and sometimes on large amphibious attack ships. Even carrying supplies of Type O, Rh negative blood is impractical for technical and logistical reasons. Dried frozen blood and synthetic oxygen-carrying fluids may soon provide blood replacement at sea, but as of this writing, severe blood loss at sea can only be treated by using blood from shipmates. The term "walking blood bank" refers to a group of prescreened, registered volunteers with known blood types who are prepared to donate blood for emergency transfusions at sea. Such blood does not meet the standards of the safe blood supply found in modern medical centers. For example, there is always a risk that a donor has acquired a pathogen such as the human immunodeficiency virus (HIV) between the last set of tests and donation; such a risk is unacceptable in ordinary medical circumstances. Critics of the walking blood bank argue that planning for the use of blood in this manner constitutes an endorsement of substandard practice. On the other hand, the walking blood bank is a source of vital oxygen-carrying fluid when blood replacement is absolutely necessary to preserve life and limb.

The roster of the potential donors should begin with volunteers, but it is understood that all crewmembers

expected to participate if necessary. All members of the crew must have a known, confirmed record of blood type and receive annual screening tests for syphilis and HIV as well as tuberculosis skin tests. Additional screening of volunteers for the blood bank is time-consuming; it must be done before going to sea and repeated at least annually. Medical history should exclude members who have ever had malaria, leishmaniasis, or any other blood-borne disease. Laboratory procedures should include examination of a blood smear, a hepatitis panel, and tests to screen out blood dyscrasias and hemoglobin variants such as sickle cell trait, thalassemia minor, or glucose-6-phosphate dehydrogenase deficiency. Use of the walking blood bank must be rehearsed during workups and periodically during the cruise to ensure that all donors and their supervisors are familiar with the procedures.

Disposal of Medical Waste

In the past, ships disposed of all trash and refuse at sea, but times have changed. Now, only that which is biologically degradable and harmless to ocean ecology and the sea floor is thrown over the side. No plastic is disposed of at sea and great efforts are made to limit the amount of plastic that is even allowed aboard. Ships are now very concerned with how to limit the amount of, and how to handle, the seven classes of waste:

1. human elimination products, which pass through commodes and sinks into the ocean at sea or into holding tanks in port;
2. garbage and food waste, which are thrown into the sea to be eagerly and safely devoured;
3. degradable trash, such as some paper, which is incinerated or dissipated safely into the ocean;
4. metal and other recyclable material, which must be stored and brought to shore for proper disposition;
5. hazardous materials, such as paint, chemicals, batteries, some plastics, and expired medications, which are stored and disposed of ashore by authorities or certified agents;
6. medical waste that contains specific medical and biological material, certain medicines, spent needles and scalpels, and all tissues, which are held in designated medical spaces until released to capable disposal agencies; and
7. infectious waste or material, which requires special handling by the Medical Department.

SUMMARY

Few undertakings in the medical profession are as challenging or as rewarding as running a Medical Department at sea. Anyone who has done so remembers it as the high point of a career. Nowhere do the patients and the entire community depend more on the skills and compassion of the healers. The demands of life at sea, the very environment of the ship, define medical care just as much as do the basic principles of medicine. Only by thoroughly integrating the Medical Department with the crew, by careful and continuous planning, and by adapting to the ship's cycle can the MO give the crew and the ship the best possible medical care.

The organization of the ship, its physical structure, and its specific mission form the working environment for the crew and the Medical Department. Life on board is constrained by limited space for work and tight living quarters with very little privacy. The kind of work and the tempo vary markedly with the ship's cycle, consisting of workups and training; deployment; maintenance periods in the yards; and major overhauls, which take the ship out of service for many months.

The Medical Department aboard ship is configured and staffed to meet the needs of the specific ship and its mission, and it ranges from a single corpsman on a small ship to a staff of about 70, including staff for the operating room aboard an aircraft carrier or large amphibious landing ship. The MO is unique in serving both line and staff roles. The line function consists of running the Medical Department on a daily basis; the staff role requires that the MO provide sage advice to the Captain and the XO concerning medical aspects of military planning and the overall health and morale of the crew, an important aspect of the ship's readiness for action.

Medical care aboard ship is expected to meet the standards of a community hospital of comparable size on shore, reflecting the widespread public misperceptions about medical capabilities during combat; provider credentials and privileges are closely monitored, and the adequacy of the Medical Department and its preparation for emergencies are frequently inspected by higher medical authority within the Navy. The medical staff is also responsible for training the crew with respect to first aid, mass casualty response, and personal health issues.

Predeployment planning is the bedrock of medical preparedness for a cruise. Everything the ship will need for the entire deployment must be on board when the ship leaves the pier. Planning includes obtaining up-to-date medical intelligence regarding health risks in the area of the cruise and especially in ports of call. The MOs of ships that will travel in company should get to know each other and are required to define the medical capabilities of each ship and its staff, to allow planning for consultation and appropriate transfer of patients whose clinical condition is beyond the capabilities of the ship. Detailed plans for medical evacuation must be coordinated with fleet operations. And the crew must be screened for acute and chronic medical conditions, some of which may be disqualifying, and receive necessary immunizations before departure.

The shipboard environment changes in many ways with the ship's cycle. A ship in the yard has on board not only its crew but also numerous civilian workers. Activities of heavy industry prevail, with heat, noise, grinding, and welding throughout the ship. The Medical Department shares with the Engineering and Safety officers the responsibility for preventing injuries. When the ship is at sea, the pressure of work and long hours prevail; confinement in crowded spaces together with a paradoxical loneliness often precipitate psychological crises, especially among young crewmembers leaving home for the first time. Outbreaks of food-borne illness, respiratory disease, and skin conditions are common problems that require immediate action by the medical staff. Constant vigilance and careful hygiene in heads and galleys are required to control cockroaches and rodents. Closed spaces aboard ship readily become hypoxic and pose a serious risk to the unwary, especially during periods in the yard. The Medical Department must always be on alert during flight operations because of multiple hazards, including the risk of aircraft crashing into the sea and jet blast blowing a deckhand overboard.

Medical care at sea is based on daily sick call, which provides routine care for physical ills and a haven for stressed sailors. It is also a tool for monitoring the overall health and well-being of the crew. Sick sailors may be recommended for light duty or bed rest, or they may be admitted to sick bay. Anyone who remains ill beyond a predetermined time limit must be transferred to a more-capable medical facility. Telemedicine should be readily used for consultation to improve medical care and to prevent unnecessary medical evacuation. Only stable patients can be transferred except in life-threatening situations, and the receiving facility must always be warned in advance of the incoming patient. The smoothest transfer of a patient is made at the pier; most transport at sea is by helicopter and requires special preparation of the patient for flight. Port calls require medical planning to provide appropriate health advice to crewmembers and coordinate medical care with authorities ashore.

Shipboard medicine includes a number of special concerns. Inclusion of women in crews requires provision of basic gynecological care and the capability to deliver a baby if required. Large ships have true operating rooms and carry surgical staffs; performance of elective procedures on board is sometimes advocated as a means of maintaining staff competence, but this is inadvisable because the limited facilities on a ship cannot deal with rare but potentially fatal complications. The medical staff may be asked to perform "Competence for Duty" examinations and needs to understand the legal ramifications of this task. The Medical Department is a key element in planning and drills for mass casualty situations, including triage, patient transportation, and emergency communication in a heavily damaged ship. Other issues include the disposition of corpses (not a medical responsibility), the organization of a walking blood bank, and the disposal of medical waste.

ACKNOWLEDGMENT

The author thanks Louis Kroot, MD, Department of Emergency Medicine, University of Kentucky Chandler Medical Center, Lexington, Kentucky, for assembling the figures and providing the figure legends in this chapter.

REFERENCES

1. World Health Organization. *International Medical Guide for Ships, Including the Ship's Medicine Chest.* 2nd ed. Geneva, Switzerland: WHO; 1988.

2. Goethe WHG, Watson EN, Jones DT, eds. *Handbook of Nautical Medicine.* New York, NY: Springer-Verlag; 1984.

3. Thomas TL, Parker AL, Horn WG, et al. Accidents and injuries among US Navy crewmembers during extended submarine patrols, 1997 to 1999. *Mil Med.* 2001;166(6):534-540.

4. DiGiovanna T, Rosen T, Forsett R, Sivertson K, Kelen GD. Shipboard medicine: A new niche for emergency medicine. *Ann Emerg Med.* 1992;21(12):1476–1479.

5. Committee on Trauma, American College of Surgeons. *Advanced Trauma Life Support Program for Physicians: Instructor Manual.* 5th ed. Chicago, Ill: American College of Surgeons; 1993.

6. Cummins RO. *Advanced Cardiac Life Support: ACLS Provider Manual.* Dallas, Tex: American Heart Association; 2001.

7. Surface Warfare Medicine Institute. *Fleet Medicine Pocket Reference.* Washington, DC: Bureau of Medicine and Surgery, Department of the Navy; 1999: 14. Available at http://www.vnh.org.

8. Department of the Navy. *Standard First Aid Course.* Washington, DC: DN; n.d. NAVEDTRA 13119. Available at http://www.vnh.org.

9. Department of the Navy. *Manual of the Medical Department.* Washington, DC: Bureau of Medicine and Surgery, DN; 2000. NAVMED P-117. Available at http://www.vnh.org.

10. Hourani L, Warrack G, Coben G. *Demographic Analysis of Suicide Among US Navy Personnel.* San Diego, Calif: Naval Health Research Center; 1997. NHRC-97-30.

11. Clancy G; adapted and revised by Bakalar NL. *Emergency Psychiatry Service Handbook.* Washington, DC: Department of the Navy; 1998. Available at http://www.vnh.org.

12. Department of the Navy. *General Medical Officer Manual.* Washington, DC: Bureau of Medicine and Surgery, DN; 2000. NAVMED P-5134. Available at http://www.vnh.org.

13. Department of the Navy. *Manual of Naval Preventive Medicine.* Washington, DC: Bureau of Medicine and Surgery, DN; 1999. NAVMED P-5010. Available at http://www.vnh.org.

14. Pandolf K, Burr RE, Wenger BC, Pozos RS, eds. *Medical Aspects of Harsh Environments, Volume 1.* In: Zajtchuk R, Bellamy RF, eds. *Textbook of Military Medicine.* Washington, DC: Department of the Army, Office of The Surgeon General, Borden Institute; 2001. Available at www.armymedicine.army.mil/history/.

15. Krentz MJ, Li G, Baker SP. At work and play in a hazardous environment: Injuries aboard a deployed US Navy aircraft carrier. *Aviat Space Environ Med.* 1997;68(1):51–55.

16. Centers for Disease Control and Prevention. *Health Information for International Travel 1999–2000 (The Yellow Book).* Atlanta, Ga: Centers for Disease Control and Prevention, US Department of Health and Human Services, Public Health Service; 1999.

17. Kelley PW, ed. *Military Preventive Medicine: Mobilization and Deployment.* In: Zajtchuk R, Bellamy RF, eds. *Textbook of Military Medicine.* Washington, DC: Department of the Army, Office of The Surgeon General, Borden Institute; 2002. In press. Available at www.armymedicine.army.mil/history/.

18. Navy Disease Vector Ecology and Control Center. *US Navy Shipboard Pest Control Manual.* Washington, DC: Bureau of Medicine and Surgery, Department of the Navy; 2000. Available at http://www.vnh.org.

19. Society of US Naval Flight Surgeons. *US Naval Flight Surgeon's Handbook.* 2nd ed. Pensacola, Fla: Society of US Naval Flight Surgeons; 1998. Available at http://www.vnh.org.

20. Nice DS. US Navy medical communications and evacuations at sea. *Mil Med.* 1987;152(9):446–451.

21. Stoloff PH, Garcia FE, Thomason JE, Shia DS. Cost effectiveness analysis of shipboard telemedicine. *Telemed J.* 1998;4(4):293–204.

22. Naval Environmental Health Center. *Navy Medical Department Pocket Guide to Malaria Prevention and Control.* Norfolk, Va: NEHC, Bureau of Medicine and Surgery, Department of the Navy; 1998. Technical Manual NEHC-TM6250.98-2. Available at http://www.vnh.org.

23. Means-Markwell M, Hawkins R, Reichow K, et al. A survey of women's health care needs on US Navy ships. *Mil Med.* 1998;163(7):439–443.

24. Hansen HL, Jensen J. Female seafarers adopt the high risk lifestyle of male seafarers. *Occup Environ Med.* 1998;55(1):49–51.

25. Garland FC, Garland CF, Gorham ED. A model of the expected occurrence of adverse pregnancy outcomes aboard US Navy ships. *Mil Med.* 2000;165(9):691–697.

26. Fontana M, Lucha P, Snyder M, Liston W. Surgery aboard ship: Is it safe? *Mil Med.* 1999;164(9):613–615.

Chapter 29: ATTACHMENT

SHIPBOARD MEDICINE DURING WAR

Prepared for this textbook by Louis Kroot, MD, Commander, Medical Corps, US Navy (Ret), Surface Warfare Medical Department Officer; currently, Department of Emergency Medicine, University of Kentucky Chandler Medical School, Lexington, Kentucky 40536-0298.

Unlike ground combat, there are no echelons of medical care during naval warfare within a given ship. Medical care in ground combat begins with immediate basic care given at squad level. Should the injured require more definitive care, they are transported to next level of care. In naval warfare, medical care is limited initially to what is aboard the ship. Unlike an army division, a ship cannot detach a portion of its medical assets while the remainder of the division continues on with its primary mission. If the decision is made that one ship has to assist another, its entire primary mission must be subordinated to transporting its medical assets to assist another vessel that is already unable to meet its mission requirements. Assisting a disabled vessel during wartime *effectively doubles* the number of vessels unavailable to the operational commander.

Battle Damage to Surface Ships

As Captain Richard R. Cooper wrote in his article, "Medical Support to the Fleet"[1]:

Medical support during battle at sea cannot be implemented effectively unless the scenario includes the following:

- Casualties are injured or wounded rather than killed.
- A ship that has been hit stays afloat long enough for the casualties to be medically managed.
- Medical personnel and equipment in the damaged ship remain functional.
- Treatment is focused upon supporting those who are able to fight the ship.
- Transfer to another unit is feasible despite the isolation of the ship, bad weather or an ongoing battle.
- The receiving unit has its own medical capabilities, a place to hold the wounded and the ability either to treat the patient or to transfer him out of the battle force.

The delivery of medical care during battle is completely different from that of peacetime naval medical practice because *saving the ship has first priority*. The two main threats to a ship's survival during combat are fire and flooding. More ships have been lost to fire and flooding than have been sunk by the immediate effects of the weapons causing the damage. During General Quarters (the condition when a ship is ready to go into battle), ships compartments and air shafts are sealed to control fire and flooding. All movement is coordinated and cleared through Damage Control Central to ensure that air and watertight integrity are maintained, thus minimizing and controlling damage from enemy missiles, torpedoes, shells, and mines. When the ship is damaged by enemy action or accidents, repair parties (which are preassigned and trained) for specific areas of the ship will respond to control the threat. The threat of fire and flooding are so great that if casualties are in a space that is damaged, the repair party will only move them out of their way in order to control the damage. *Only when the threat is contained will the injured be removed for medical assistance.*

Other important factors differentiate shipboard battle casualties from ground casualties, namely, the circumstances of wounding (how they occur) and the nature of the wounds. Unlike ground combat, in which the occurrence of casualties is usually continuous, shipboard casualties are generated suddenly and in large numbers. Naval history abounds in examples of what happens to the crew when a warship sustains sudden catastrophic damage. For example, after a magazine explosion broke HMS *Hood* into two parts that sank within 3 minutes, only 3 survived of a crew of 1,400.[2]

More-manageable examples of battle damage and the associated casualties are found in the following examples. In March 1945, the flight deck of the USS *Franklin* was struck by two bombs, which exploded in the ship's hanger and detonated the *Franklin's* aircraft ordinance and fuel. The resultant secondary explosions and fires destroyed the aft portion of the ship down to but not including the ship's machinery, killing 724 and wounding 264 of the ship's crew (Attachment Figure 1). The main battle dressing station

(BDS) was destroyed and all the ship's doctors but one were trapped below deck for hours.[3] The experience of the one doctor who was able to care for the wounded aboard the *Franklin*—Samuel Robert Sherman, Medical Corps, US Naval Reserve—is well worth reading for its graphic description of the realities of shipboard medicine during war.[3]

During the Okinawa campaign in World War II, the USS *Princeton* took a kamikaze hit that caused 292 casualties: 9 killed in action (KIA), 191 wounded in action (WIA), and 92 missing. The USS *Birmingham* came to assist the *Princeton*. When the *Princeton* exploded, she caused 50% of the *Birmingham*'s crew to be killed or wounded. The *Birmingham*'s Medical Department, which consisted of 1 medical officer and 14 corpsmen, provided care for 420 wounded men from both ships. Only 8 of the wounded died (DOW). Five had to be operated on and of those, two died.[4]

The USS *New Mexico* also took a kamikaze hit, resulting in 30 KIA and 129 WIA. The tactical situation prevented the evacuation for nearly 2 weeks. The severely injured were forced to wait until night for definitive treatment. These extreme circumstances caused great anxiety among the injured as well as adversely affecting the morale of the crew; according to the Senior Medical Officer aboard the USS *New Mexico*,

Too much emphasis cannot be placed upon the importance of early evacuation of the wounded from a damaged ship.[4]

A listing of more-recent combatlike incidents aboard US Navy vessels and the associated casualties is found in Attachment Table 1.

US Navy data on casualty generation have been extensively studied; interested readers can consult C. G. Blood's seminal work on the subject, *Analysis of Battle Casualties by Weapon Type Aboard US Navy Warships*.[5] Although Blood's analysis is based on World War II data (that is to say, damage to ships of World War II design by World War II–era weapons), the results—with qualifications such as the disappearance of heavily armored and protected ships and the replacement of large-caliber guns by guided missiles—remain applicable to the present. The most common weapons that struck American warships in World War II were as follows[5]:

1. kamikaze-piloted planes, 37%
2. gunfire, 23%
3. bombs, 16%
4. torpedoes, 14%
5. multiple kinds of weapons, 6%, and
6. mines, 4%.

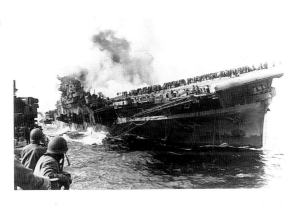

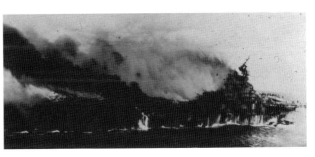

Attachment Fig. 1. (**a**) This famous photograph was taken from aboard the USS *Santa Fe* as that cruiser came alongside the damaged USS *Franklin* several hours after the successful Japanese bombing attack. The entire aft portion of the ship above the machinery space is engulfed by fire. The list to starboard resulted not from damage to the hull but from the accumulated weight of water used to fight the fires. (**b**) Billowing smoke nearly obscures the *Franklin* in this photograph, which was taken about the same time from a low-flying airplane. Some of the *Franklin*'s surviving crew, seen in both views, await rescue by the *Santa Fe*. The damage incurred by the *Franklin* was of the same magnitude as that sustained by the four Japanese aircraft carriers that were sunk in the Battle of Midway. Photographs: Courtesy of US Navy.

ATTACHMENT TABLE 1

SELECTED SHIP DISASTERS AND CASUALTIES AT SEA

Ship	Date	Type of Disaster and Casualty Information
USS *Franklin*[1]	1945	1,000 casualties: 800 died, 210 from burns, 133 from asphyxiation
USS *Oriskany*[2]	1966	Fire and explosion on the hangar deck; 44 dead, 24 from smoke inhalation
IDF destroyer *Eliat*[3]	1967	Hit and sunk by a cruise missile. A second missile exploded in the water. Of the casualties, 32 sailors who were in the water at the time were rescued and transferred to a hospital in Cyprus within 5–6 h; 24 developed signs of abdominal injury; 23 had tears in the viscera or bleeding intestines; 4 died postoperatively; and 19 had significant lung injury.
USS *Forrestal*[2,4]	1968	Fire and explosion on the flight deck; 134 dead, 168 injured
USS *Enterprise*[5]	1969	Fire on the flight deck; 27 dead, 85 injured
USS *Belknap*/USS *Kennedy*[6]	1975	Collision; on the *Belknap*, 8 dead, 45 injured; on the *Kennedy*, 1 dead, 2 injured
Sir Galahad Auxiliary[4]	1982	Sunk during Falkland War; 179 casualties, 83 with burns
HMS *Sheffield*[4]	1982	Heat from an *unexploded* Exocet cruise missile caused fire in 15–20 sec; 20 dead, 24 with burns and smoke inhalation
USS *Stark*[1,6]	1984	Hit by two Exocet cruise missiles; total dead = 37, total injured = 15. Two of the injured had 23% and 42% TBSA burns. Of the 37 fatalities, 17 had blast injuries, 13 had burn injuries, 3 had blast/burn injuries, 2 had smoke inhalation, 1 had asphyxia, and 1 body was never recovered.
USS *Bonefish*[7]	1988	Fire; 22 injured from burns and smoke, 3 died of smoke inhalation

IDF: Israeli Defence Forces; TBSA: total body surface area

Sources for casualty data: (1) Pinkstaff CA, Sturtz DL, Bellamy RF. USS *Franklin* and the USS *Stark*: Recurrent problems in the prevention and treatment of naval battle casualties. *Mil Med*. 1989;154(5):229–233. (2) Foster WF. Fire on the hangar deck: *Oriskany*'s tragedy, October 1966. *The Hook*. 1988;Winter:38–53. (3) Smith AM. Getting them out alive. *Naval Proceedings*. 1989;Feb:41–46. (4) Smith AM. Any navy can go to war alone, but staying there is another thing. *Navy Medicine*. 1990;Nov-Dec;9–15. (5) Bellamy RF. Colonel, Medical Corps, US Army (Ret). Personal experience, January 1969. (6) Smith AM. Lecture at Uniformed Services University of the Health Sciences on the USS *Belknap*/USS *Kennedy* collision and USS *Bonefish* casualties. Bethesda, Md; 1991. (7) Hooper RR. Medical support for the fleet. *Naval War College Review*. 1990; Summer:43–54.

During World War II, the KIA to WIA ratio aboard a ship was 1:1, except when the weapon was torpedoes or torpedoes with multiple weapons, when the ratio was 2:1 (in ground forces, the KIA:WIA ratio is 1:4).[6] Cruisers had the largest absolute number of casualties, followed by carriers and then by escort carriers. The average number of casualties on any ship hit was 38 KIA and 34 WIA. Casualties surviving to be treated included 39% with penetrating wounds; 21% burns; 11% with both burns and penetrating wounds. No other significant grouping of types of wounds was seen, although crewmen of torpedoed or mined ships may sustain extremity fractures that are caused by rapid translation motion of the deck due to blast. Kamikaze attacks generated 37% penetrating wounds, 30% burns, 9% multiple wounds.[5] Medical officers need to understand that kamikaze attacks have considerable relevance to modern naval warfare because of their similarity to today's guided antiship missiles (kamikaze attacks can be thought of as roughly equivalent to modern Cruise missiles [ie, the organic guidance systems—the human pilots—were replaced by silicon guidance systems—computers]). Thus, blast and burn with associated inhalation injuries can be expected to be more common than in the past.

In order not to lose all medical assets in a single hit, the Medical Department mans BDSs throughout the ship, in addition to the main medical spaces (see Figure 29-2 in Chapter 29, Shipboard Medicine). It has also been recognized that trying to move medical supplies and litters to the injured from the sickbay and assuming that power will not be interrupted during combat are unrealistic. Therefore, scattered throughout the ship are first aid boxes; portable medical lockers (PMLs; also called a BDS in a box); decontamination boxes; and litters, their numbers being prescribed by Navy regulations (Attachment Exhibit 1). Each BDS is equipped with a 50-gal gravity-fed water tank; multiple battery-powered lanterns, which are being recharged while there is power; and is on the emergency backup power system and has emergency communication lines. *All communications and evacuations are cleared through Damage Control Central first; the safety of the ship must take priority over individual medical care or everyone may perish.* Maintaining watertight integrity and fire boundaries may require four litter bearers 20 to 30 minutes to move a single casualty 500 ft and the same amount of time to return. One key factor that optimizes shipboard medicine during war that is directly dependent on the ship's medical officers is crew training (Attachment Exhibit 2).

Sinking, Immersion, and Survival

Despite the horrific nature of immediate, direct damage inflicted on ships in naval warfare, the experience of both the Royal Navy[7] and the US Navy[8] has been that 66% of deaths occurred *after* the crew had successfully abandoned a sinking ship. Unless a sinking occurs in tropical waters, the main threat to a sailor's survival is the environment. The most critical items for survival after sinking are extra clothing and blankets. The critical need for water and food occurs in days for water (the record is 11 days without water) and weeks for food. The hazards associated with immersion are listed in Attachment Exhibit 3. Water conducts heat 25-fold faster than air; the problem with sudden exposure to cold is induced sympathetic reflex, which causes tachycardia, hypertension, tetany, and hyperventilation. In choppy water, this can lead to drowning. Death occurs from drowning before death from hypothermia because the hypothermic, lethargic sailor loses the ability to protect his airway and turn his back to a choppy sea. A sailor's survival after abandoning a ship is dependent on the water temperature, sea state, swimming ability, physical conditioning, and acclimatization to the cold. According to Royal Navy data, many deaths from hypothermia occurred within the first 24 hours after immersion, even in the English Channel. But if a sailor survived the first 24 hours of immersion, his chances for survival improved dramatically.[7]

The next greatest time of risk for the survivors after a ship sinks occurs shortly after they are rescued from the water. During World War II and continuing to the present, the syndrome of sudden collapse and death after the rescue has been observed, usually within the first 15 minutes of rescue but occasionally up to several hours later. When the Argentinean cruiser *General BelGrano* was torpedoed and sunk during the Falkland War (1982), 71 life raft survivors were rescued; of these, 69 had hypothermia and 18 died of exposure; about 600 men had already been killed when the ship sank. After the British *Atlantic Conveyer* sank, 12 of her crew, most of whom were in the water, died; 2 sailors drowned after the HMS *Coventry* was sunk.[9] Both the Royal Navy and the US Navy have made recommendations for maximizing the survival of sailors who have suffered from immersion (Attachment Exhibit 4).

After the environment, the next greatest threat to survival at sea is lack of potable water. The Royal Navy has found that 150 mL of water per day was associated with a 22% mortality for a 6-day period. However, when water consumption was between 150 and 450 mL/day, the mortality was 0.6% for the same period.[7] Their recommendation is that no water be drunk the first day except by the injured, and that the water be given three times a day in a measured beaker. In the tropics the Royal Navy recommends that work be done *only* during the cool of the day. Soaking clothing in sea water can decrease sweating by 83%,[7] but the clothing must be allowed to dry before sunset to avoid heat loss at night.

The concentration of body fluids is approximately 1% saline. The maximum concentration of salts in urine is 2%, half of which is sodium chloride and half urea. Drinking seawater increases the concentration of salt in the body fluid, further aggravating dehydration. The only way to get rid of the excess salt is by sacrificing internal water. Additionally, mixing salt water with freshwater does not help because of the obligatory shift from intracellular to extracellular water. Both of these scenarios hasten death.[7] *An absolute prohibition is needed against drinking seawater or mixing it with freshwater.* The mortality of survivors of a sinking who did and did not drink seawater is given in Attachment Table 2.

ATTACHMENT EXHIBIT 1

SHIPBOARD REQUIREMENTS FOR SPECIFIC MEDICAL EQUIPMENT

Medical Equipment per 100 Personnel	No. of Personnel
1. First Aid Boxes	
4	< 500
5/100	500
8/100	1,500–3,000
10/100	> 3,000
2. Stokes Litters	
1.5/100	< 1,500
3/100	1,500–3,000
4.5/100	> 3,000

3. Neil Robertson Litters: 1 located adjacent to each vertical trunk, machine room, and shop space

4. Portable Medical Lockers (PMLs): located adjacent to each repair party station; 1 PML per 250 personnel

5. Battle Dressing Stations: number determined by class of ship; minimum: 2 (frigates) to 6 (aircraft carriers); (see Figure 29-2 in Chapter 29, Shipboard Medicine)

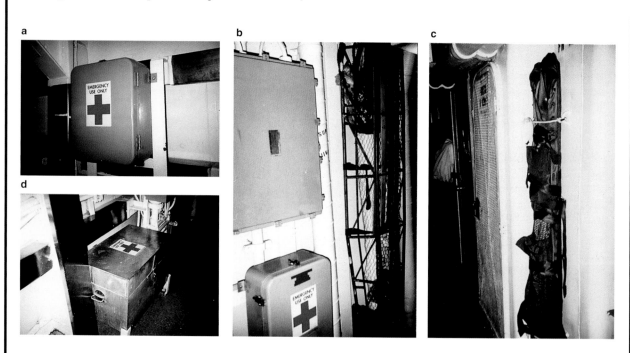

Exhibit Fig. 1. (**a**) A first aid box; these are located throughout the ship. (**b**) The Stokes litter and (**c**) the Neil Robertson litter are especially useful onboard ships, because once a casualty is securely fastened on the litter and the wire cage is in place (Stokes litter), he can be transported in any direction (eg, from ship to ship or up and down vertical ladders to the battle stations). (**d**) A portable medical locker, which is sometimes called a "battle dressing station in a box." Exhibit text adapted from US Navy. *Shipboard Medical Procedure Manual.* Washington, DC: US Navy. COMNAVSURFLANT/PAC Instruction 6000.1. Photographs: Naval Imaging Command, Anacostia Naval Air Station, Washington, DC.

ATTACHMENT EXHIBIT 2

CREW TRAINING IN PREPARATION FOR BATTLE

Crewmembers to be trained:

- Corpsmen
- Litter bearers

Training tools and techniques:

- Closed-circuit television (CCTV) lectures
- Navy training films
- First aid (self and buddy aid)
- American Heart Association's Basic Life Support course

Training content in preparation for battle:

- Battle bill
- Battle dressing stations
- Repair parties
- Portable medical lockers
- Decontamination lockers
- First aid boxes
- "Gun" bags

Amphibious Operations

Amphibious operations against a defended beachhead are the most arduous and dangerous type of military campaign. On the first day of amphibious assault at Tarawa, Saipan, Peleliu, and Iwo Jima, the WIA rate per 1,000 men was, respectively, 55, 75, 63, and 60.[8] The reason there are so many medical assets and spaces aboard amphibious ships is that, in reality, two separate crews are assigned, Navy and Marine. The problem of caring for casualties aboard ships was summed up best in the *History of The Medical Department of The United States Navy in World War II*:

> It was part of a pattern of thought which permeated the forces afloat and influenced the establishment of hospital facilities ashore. It was the "bed for a casualty" type of thinking; in other words as long as the wounded man was in a bunk and out of sight of the troops, part of the medical mission was accomplished. It must be recognized that war wounds are surgical problems, best handled by a trained surgeon during the golden hours of early surgery. When one considers the facilities and personnel required to care for 150 seriously wounded patients, as well as for 325 patients with minor wounds, it becomes apparent that *three medical officers with limited equipment, regardless of their talent or heroic efforts, will not suffice.*[4]

Naval and Marine leaders are well aware of the difficulties in amphibious operations. There are accepted manuals and protocols for effective command, communication, control, and logistical support for formal amphibious operations. With time for adequate planning, practice, and support, medical resources can be integrated effectively into amphibious operations and mistakes of the past avoided.[4]

From the invasion of Tarawa, where all the casualties on litters were placed aboard a single amphibious tractor that was sunk before it reached the beach, we learned not to concentrate medical resources in one location. In the invasion of Saipan, without medical advice, casualties were evacuated in aircraft by line officers. The aircraft arrived at its destination with casualties who had died of their wounds or were in poor condition. In the subsequent invasion of Iwo Jima, before an airhead had been established, casualties were placed on a landing craft for transport to a ship.

ATTACHMENT EXHIBIT 3

HAZARDS OF BEING SUNK AT SEA

Hypothermia

Drowning

Entanglement in or traumatic contact with a sinking ship

Inhalation of and contamination with fuel oil

Trauma from surfacing objects

Underwater explosions

Source: *Handbook for Royal Naval Officers*. London, England: Ministry of Defense, Medical Directorate General (Naval); July 1981. BR 2193.

ATTACHMENT EXHIBIT 4

CARE OF SURVIVORS OF VESSELS SUNK AT SEA

Assist survivors out of the water into the rescuing vessel[†]
* Conscious:

    Never leave unsupervised for first 72 h

    Prevent postural hypotension

    Avoid alcohol consumption

    Minimize ambulating to rewarming area

    Rewarm survivors by seating them, clothed, under a hot shower, and gradually remove clothing[*]

* Unconscious:

    Maintain the airway

    Place under warm blankets after wet garments have been removed

Notes on near-drowning:

    60% vomit during resuscitation

    Pulmonary edema may occur between 15 min to 72 h after rescue from water

---

[*]There is currently no other accepted therapy for treating hypothermia.
[†]During World War II, many sailors were lost when they attempted to climb the net up the side of the rescuing vessel. The effort was too great; they fell back into the sea and were lost. During the latter stages of the Battle of the Atlantic, lifeboats were lowered and sailors pulled into them; they were then hoisted aboard ships. Also, special ships at the end of convoys were outfitted with large booms with netting; these were swung out to sea for sailors to grab onto. The booms were swung back in and the sailors lifted to safety.
Adapted from *Handbook for Royal Naval Officers*. London, England: Ministry of Defence, Medical Directorate General (Naval); July 1981. BR 2193.

Some casualties were aboard the landing craft for up to 8 hours without medical attendants or supplies. Later, after airfields had been established, 2,500 casualties received medical clearance before being evacuated by air from Iwo Jima. The medical clearance process decided which casualties were stable enough for transport; this resulted in no deaths during this air evacuation.[4] As these examples demonstrate, casualties are not static problems, like broken equipment; the physical conditions of casualties will generally deteriorate over time if no medical intervention occurs.

Today's Navy does not have the quantity of dedicated medical resources to support amphibious operations that were available at the end of World War II and the Korean War. Additionally, with the improvement in satellite communication and surveillance, the time to recognize and respond to a threat has decreased dramatically, and the distance at which the US military can successfully intervene has correspondingly

ATTACHMENT TABLE 2

MORTALITY ASSOCIATED WITH DRINKING SEAWATER

Seawater	No. of Life Craft Voyages	No. of Men	No. of Deaths	Died (%)
Drank	29	997	387	38.8
Did Not Drink	134	3,994	133	3.3

Adapted from *Handbook for Royal Naval Officers*. London, England: Ministry of Defence, Medical Directorate General (Naval); July 1981. BR 2193.

increased. The need for operational security, the tension between the operational plan and the logistical support, and the priority to deploy combat power quickly have resulted in amphibious operations suddenly commencing with only peacetime medical resources available to support the operational commitments. For example, during Operation Urgent Fury (the 1983 invasion of Grenada), the USS *Guam* received 37 casualties. There had been no prior triage before the casualties were sent to the ship. Twenty-three cases of lactated Ringer's solution were used in 1 day, and the inventory had to be replaced three times from other ships. The 50 units of blood in the blood bank were inadequate and had to be resupplied—initially from the walking blood bank of the *Guam*'s crew. The blood bank was later supplemented from the USS *Independence*'s walking blood bank. According to the Medical Officer of the USS *Guam*,

at one point I got so desperate [from the volume and rate of casualty arrival that] I merely matched blood type from the patient's dog tag and drew from one [the crewmember of the USS Guam] and transfused to another [the casualty].[9]

The capability of launching amphibious operations from "over the horizon," which involve both landing craft and aircraft, brings new vulnerabilities. The accelerated pace and depth of which today's military is capable have created increased demands on medical support to sustain military operations and to care for casualties from both military and civilian victims of a conflict.

SUMMARY

Shipboard medicine during war differs from combat casualty care on land because of the following characteristics: the occurrence of sudden and potentially catastrophic damage to the ship; the grave risk that the ship will sink; a mass casualty situation dominated by thermal, blast, and inhalation injuries; and, frequently, the destruction of the medical treatment facilities. And when ships sink, the risk to the surviving crew is not over. Death from drowning, hypothermia, and dehydration are common occurrences. It is no exaggeration to say that shipboard medicine during war provides the greatest challenge likely to be faced by the military physician.

REFERENCES

1. Cooper RR. Medical support for the fleet. *Naval War College Review*. 1990;43(3):43–54.

2. Smith AM. Any navy can go to war alone, but staying there is another thing. Navy Medicine. 1990;Nov–Dec:9–15.

3. Sherman SR; Herman JK, interviewer. Flight surgeon on the spot: Aboard USS *Franklin* 19 March 1945. *Navy Medicine*. 1993;84(4)4–10.

4. *The History of The Medical Department of The United States Navy in World War II*. Vol 1. Washington, DC: Government Printing Office; 1953. NAVMED P-5031.

5. Blood CG. *Analysis of Battle Casualties by Weapon Type Aboard US Navy Warships*. Washington, DC: Naval Medical Research and Development Command, DN; 1991. Report 91-1.

6. Beebe GW, De Bakey ME. *Battle Casualties: Incidence, Mortality, and Logistic Considerations*. Springfield, Ill: Charles C Thomas; 1952: 20–22.

7. *Handbook for Royal Naval Officers*. London, England: Ministry of Defence, Medical Directorate General (Naval); July 1981. BR 2193.

8. Blood CG. *Shipboard and Ground Troop Casualty Rates Among Navy and Marine Corps Personnel During World War II Operations*. Washington, DC: Naval Medical Research and Development Command, DN; 1990. Report 9016.

9. Llewellyn CH, Smith AM. Tactical and logistical compromise in the management of combat casualties: There is no free lunch! *Naval War College Review*. 1990;43(1):53–66.

Chapter 30

PHYSICS, PHYSIOLOGY, AND MEDICINE OF DIVING

JAMES VOROSMARTI, Jr, MD[*] AND RICHARD D. VANN, PhD[†]

*Captain, Medical Corps, US Navy (Ret); Consultant in Occupational, Environmental, and Undersea Medicine, 16 Orchard Way South, Rockville, Maryland 20854
†Captain, US Navy Reserve (Ret); FG Hall Hypo/Hyperbaric Center, Box 3823, Duke University Medical Center, Durham, North Carolina 27710

INTRODUCTION

Diving as a military activity is sufficiently common that any military physician has a probability—and those in Special Operations Forces have a high probability—of involvement in diving operations or in treating or examining divers during his or her career and certainly should have some familiarity with diving medicine. In addition, military physicians may be called on to treat civilian recreational divers with diving-related problems when no appropriate facilities exist in the civilian community.

Diving is not new to military operations. The first recorded use of breath-hold divers for military purposes dates from the 5th century BC, when Scyllus[1] and his daughter Cyane saved the fleet of Xerxes by freeing the ships' anchors and allowing them to get underway rapidly when threatened by a sudden storm. The Syracusans[2] are said to have trained divers to swim under water and damage enemy ships. Divers of Tyre[3] were employed to cut the anchor ropes of Alexander the Great's ships during the siege of Tyre

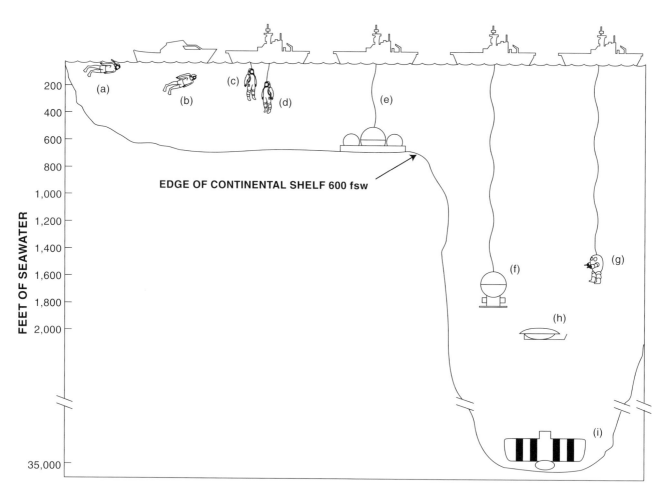

Fig. 30-1. Various forms of diving and other submarine activities in relation to ocean depth. (**a**) Breath-hold diving is usually not deeper than 45 fsw, although some divers can go deeper. (**b**) Self-contained underwater breathing apparatus (scuba) diving on air is usually limited to 130 fsw. (**c**) Surface-supported air diving is usually limited to 180 fsw, US Navy, or for commercial diving in the United States, 220 fsw. (**d**) Surface-supported helium–oxygen diving without a bell is usually to a depth of about 300 fsw, because of the problems of long decompressions; (**e**) the deepest habitat operation, 520 fsw; (**f**) the deepest saturation diving at sea operation, 1,510 fsw; (**g**) the deepest dive in an armored 1-atm suit, 1,440 fsw. (**h**) Research submersibles can operate to depths of about 2,000 fsw; (**i**) the bathyscaphe *Trieste* has been to the deepest-known depth of the ocean, 35,800 fsw, in the Marianas trench. Note that the ordinate, marking depth, has been shortened. If this graphic were drawn to scale, a page at least 1.26 m long would be required to display ocean depth to the bottom of the Marianas trench.

in 332 BC. However, not until the 19th century, after many technological advances, did diving became a military as well as an industrial specialty. Military diving operations today include Special Operations; explosive ordnance disposal and mine clearance; salvage of ships; location and retrieval of aircraft or other equipment lost in the water; clearance of wrecks and debris from harbors and waterways; ship-hull maintenance and repairs (ship's husbandry); repair of piers, locks, dams, and other associated structures; and reconnaissance. The military services employ military and civilian divers to fulfill these varied missions worldwide.

Figure 30-1 shows the relationship of the depth of the oceans to the attempts that man has made to enter them. Water is an unforgiving and difficult environment in which to work. Most diving operations are done in cold water with a minimum of visibility. The diver's ability to work is also degraded by the equipment required, increased breathing resistance, and other effects of pressure such as nitrogen narcosis. The diver is prone to diseases due to pressure changes, which are much greater underwater than those experienced by the aviator.

PHYSICAL PRINCIPLES

Certain fundamental physical principles need to be understood before the deleterious effects specific to diving can be appreciated. Foremost among these physical principles are the descriptions of the behaviors of gases under pressure. Buoyancy is also a consideration.

Barometric pressure is the force per unit surface area exerted by the atmosphere. Under natural conditions, this pressure is the result of gravity acting on the column of air that stands several miles above the surface of Earth; its value was initially measured against a column of mercury and was given a value of 760 mm Hg at sea level under standard conditions.

The primary unit of pressure in the International System of Units (SI units, Système International d'Unités) is the pascal (Pa, a unit derived from newtons per square meter), where 1 atmosphere (atm) equals 101.3 kPa. In addition, other units are sometimes used (Exhibit 30-1).

Many pressure gauges read zero at ambient (surface) pressure, thereby measuring only differential pressure (eg, a blood pressure gauge). However, physiological calculations require the use of absolute pressure, where zero corresponds to a complete vacuum. Therefore, every expression of pressure must be designated as gauge (g) or absolute (a). Conversion between the two requires knowledge of ambient barometric pressure at the time the measurement was made.

Actual pressure underwater differs between fresh and salt water and varies slightly from one area of the ocean to another, depending on local salinity and temperature. One atmosphere is equivalent to 10.13 meters of depth in sea water (msw) or 33.08 feet of depth in sea water (fsw). In fresh water, however, 1 atm = 10.38 msw, or 33.83 fsw.

The following formula may be used when convert-

EXHIBIT 30-1

PRESSURE UNITS AND EQUIVALENTS

1 atm	=	1.013250 bar
1 atm	=	101.3250 kPa
1 atm	=	760.0 torr[*]
1 atm	=	14.6959 psi
1 atm	=	33.08 fsw
1 atm	=	10.13 msw
1 bar	=	100.00 kPa[*]
1 bar	=	32.646 fsw[†,§]
1 bar	=	10.00 msw
1 msw	=	10.000 kPa[‡,§]

[*]Signifies a primary definition from which other equalities were derived.

[†]Primary definition for feet of seawater (fsw); assumes a density for seawater of 1.02480 at 4°C, which is the value often used for calibration of a depth gauge.

[‡]Primary definition for meters of seawater (msw); assumes a density for seawater of 1.01972 at 4°C.

[§]These primary definitions for fsw and msw are arbitrary because the pressure below a column of seawater depends on the density of the water, which varies from point to point in the ocean. These two definitions are consistent with each other if the appropriate density correction is applied.

Adapted with permission from the pressure conversion table published on the last page of each issue of *Undersea & Hyperbaric Medicine,* the journal of the Undersea and Hyperbaric Medical Society, 10531 Metropolitan Avenue, Kensington, Md.

ing from diving depth to atmospheres (Equation 1):

(1)   absolute pressure = (D + De) / De

where D represents the depth in units of length and De represents the number of those units equivalent to 1 ata. NOTE: this equation assumes a pressure of 1 atm at the surface of the water and requires correction for high-altitude diving.

Gas Laws

Changes in barometric pressure and the composition of inspired gas affect the human body in ways that reflect the physical behavior of gases in gaseous mixtures and liquid solutions. A good grasp of the gas laws and related physical principles is therefore prerequisite to understanding the physiological effects of the acute pressure changes imposed by flying and diving.

Pressure Effect (Boyle's Law)

The volume of a given mass of gas varies inversely with absolute pressure when temperature is held constant. In mathematical terms (Equations 2a and 2b),

(2a) $P_1 / P_2 = V_2 / V_1$

or the formula can be rewritten:

(2b) $P_1 \bullet V_1 = P_2 \bullet V_2$

where P represents pressure, V represents volume, and the subscripts 1 and 2 refer to the condition before and after a pressure change. For example, if a flexible container is filled with 1 L of gas at 1 ata and then subjected to increasing pressure, at 2 ata the volume will be halved (0.5 L) and at 3 ata it will be one third of its original volume (0.33 L). Ascent to an altitude of 18,000 ft (0.5 ata) would cause the volume to double (2 L).

Because gas in body cavities is saturated with water vapor at body temperature, Boyle's law is often applied in the following form (Equation 3):

(3) $(P_1 - P_{H_2O}) / (P_2 - P_{H_2O}) = V_2 / V_1$

where P_{H_2O} represents water vapor pressure at body temperature (47 mm Hg). The addition of the term P_{H_2O} is important when doing respiratory studies and in high-altitude work but is insignificant when calculating pressure volume relationships in diving.

Temperature Effect (Charles's Law)

The volume of a given mass of gas is directly proportional to its absolute temperature when pressure is held constant. According to Charles's law, this relationship can be expressed mathematically (Equations 4a and 4b):

(4a) $P_1 / P_2 = T_1 / T_2$

or the formula can be rewritten:

(4b) $P_1 \bullet T_2 = P_2 \bullet T_1$

where T_1 and T_2 represent initial and final temperature, respectively. For this purpose the temperatures must be expressed in absolute units, which can be calculated as T°K (Kelvin) = T°C (Celsius) + 273.

Universal Gas Equation

Boyle's and Charles's laws are often expressed in a single equation for calculating the effects of concurrent changes in pressure and temperature, as follows (Equation 5):

(5) $(P_1 \bullet V_1) / T_1 = (P_2 \bullet V_2) / T_2$

Partial Pressure in Gaseous Mixtures (Dalton's Law)

The total pressure exerted by a mixture of gases is equal to the sum of the pressures that each gas would exert if it alone occupied the container. According to Dalton's law, this can be expressed mathematically (Equation 6):

(6) $P_t = P_1 + P_2 + P_3 + P_n$

where P_t represents the total pressure of the mixture, and $P_1 + P_2 + P_3 + P_n$ represent the component partial pressures. The partial pressure of a single gas in a mixture may be calculated from the following relationship (Equation 7):

(7) $P_x = F_x \bullet P_t$

where P_x represents the partial pressure of gas x, and F_x represents the fractional concentration of that gas in the mixture. At 1 ata, oxygen and nitrogen exert partial pressures of 0.21 and 0.79 atm, respectively. On raising barometric pressure to 3 ata, these partial pressures triple, to 0.63 and 2.37 atm.

Related Physical Principles

Gas-Filled Compartments. The gas laws are discussed above in terms of a flexible container that fully accommodates alterations in volume due to changes in pressure and temperature. For gas in a rigid container, however, increasing ambient pressure will eventually cause structural collapse of the container, while decreasing pressure will force the walls to burst. For this reason, the inability to ventilate semirigid, gas-filled body compartments such as the lungs and middle ear during severe pressure changes can cause incapacitating or fatal injury in the form of a diving "squeeze" or overinflation.

Transmission of Pressure in a Liquid (Pascal's Law). Pressure exerted at any point on a confined liquid is transmitted uniformly in all directions. Because solid organs are mostly liquid, pressure exerted on them is distributed equally throughout the body and does not change tissue volume.

Gases in Solution (Henry's Law). The quantity of a gas that dissolves in a liquid is directly proportional to its partial pressure in the gas phase, assuming that temperature remains constant and that no chemical reaction takes place. When the partial pressure of the gas is reduced, a proportional amount of that gas will emerge from solution and may form bubbles in the liquid phase.

Buoyancy

Buoyancy is important to a diver, as it affects the amount of work needed to change or maintain depth. A positively buoyant diver rises, and a negatively buoyant diver sinks. If the buoyancy is not appropriate, a catastrophic accident may occur. As stated in Archimedes' principle, any object immersed in liquid will be buoyed up by a force equal to the weight of the water displaced. For example, an object that weighs 100 lb in air and displaces 90 lb of water will—being 10 lb heavier than the water displaced—therefore, sink. If the amount of water displaced is equal in weight to the object, its depth remains constant, as it is neutrally buoyant.

The desired state of buoyancy depends on operational requirements. For example, a combat diver swimming into an enemy harbor at 20 fsw will try to achieve neutral buoyancy—both to make the best speed and to conserve breathing gas. If negatively buoyant, he might swim too deep and develop oxygen toxicity; if positively buoyant, he might break the surface and be detected. On the other hand, a diver doing salvage work on a hull of a ship may want to be strongly negatively buoyant so that he can handle the equipment and tools required without being unsteady or easily movable in the water.

Control of buoyancy is achieved by various methods. The most common is by adding or removing gas from the diving dress (a garment that provides thermal and mechanical protection) or the buoyancy compensator (an inflatable vest for adjusting buoyancy). Weights or weighted equipment are also used to provide initial negative buoyancy for entering the water. When a diver wishes to return to the surface, he may establish positive buoyancy by dropping weights or inflating the buoyancy compensator. Certain types of protective clothing, such as the closed-cell neoprene suit, are positively buoyant at shallow depths but become less so at greater depths as the material collapses. Buoyancy increases as the gas in diver-worn tanks is used.

UNDERWATER PERTURBATIONS OF THE SPECIAL SENSES

Vision

Vision underwater is affected by the mask a diver wears; absorption of light by the water; intensity of light; and turbidity of the water, which depends on the amount of material suspended in it.

Looking through a diving mask or helmet magnifies objects underwater by 25% to 35% and therefore makes them look closer (Figure 30-2). This displacement of the image is a result of refraction of light as it passes from water through the faceplate material to gas, and it can be confusing to novice divers. A mask or helmet also restricts the peripheral vision of the diver by as much as 50%. Masks or helmets with larger viewing areas increase the field of view but introduce annoying visual distortion. Stereoacuity or depth perception, the ability to determine the relative distance between objects, is also adversely affected. This is especially noticeable in clear, well-illuminated water and worsens with decreasing illumination and increasing turbidity. Decreased contrast underwater, even in clear water, is thought to contribute to this phenomenon.

Absorption of light affects underwater vision by decreasing available illumination. In clear (nonturbid) water, only about 20% of incident light penetrates to 33 ft (10 m). Available light also decreases with a decreasing angle of incidence of sunlight to the water surface (as the sun approaches the horizon), and more light is reflected instead of penetrating the surface. However, in clear water with a high sun angle, useful illumination may be found as deep as

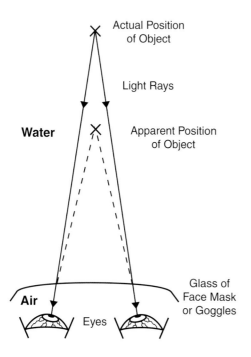

Fig. 30-2. When seen underwater, images are displaced toward the diver. The closer apparent position is caused by the refraction of light rays as they pass through the water, the material of the face mask, and the gas inside the mask.

198 to 297 ft (60–90 m). As the turbidity increases, the penetration of light decreases. In many rivers, lakes, and harbors, there may be no usable light, even within a few feet of the surface.

Changes in color perception occur because water selectively absorbs the very short and very long wavelengths of light. At fairly shallow depths, the red–orange spectrum is lost and most objects will appear blue–green. For example, at a depth of about 10 ft (3 m) blood will appear greenish rather than red. If an underwater light source is used, however, the colors appear normal.

Vision in dry, hyperbaric environments is not significantly changed. The only vision-related problems that may arise in repetitive or prolonged saturation dives (see Chapter 31, Military Diving Operations and Medical Support) are a slight loss in visual acuity and a tendency to esophoria.

Hearing

In a dry, hyperbaric environment the only effect on hearing appears to be an increase in the hearing threshold with increasing depth. This is not due to changes in bone conduction, which remains normal at depth, but to changes in conductivity in the middle ear as a result of increasing gas density. It reverses with decreasing pressure. This is true of both nitrogen–oxygen and helium–oxygen environments.

Hearing underwater is a completely different situation. Because the densities of tissue and water are similar, a submerged head is "transparent" to sound energy. In addition, water in the external ear canal damps the vibrations induced in the tympanic membrane. Therefore, hearing underwater occurs through bone conduction rather than through the middle ear, with a 50% to 75% decrease in the hearing threshold.

Sound is difficult to localize underwater. It travels much faster in water than in air, reducing the difference in time at which sound arrives at each ear. Without this difference, localization can often be impossible.

Speech intelligibility is a problem in diving. In water, it is almost impossible for divers to converse without a communications device, because too much power is required for through-water sound transmission by voice alone. Divers wearing rigid helmets can converse by touching helmets, so that sound is transmitted directly from helmet to helmet. While speech intelligibility decreases somewhat as the density of a nitrogen–oxygen mixture increases, speech is almost impossible when a helium–oxygen mixture is used, because helium shifts the resonance of vocalizing structures and gas-filled cavities and thus drastically changes the timbre of the vowels. This results in a high pitched, nasal quality referred to as "Donald Duck" speech. Most saturation divers find that their understanding of such speech improves after several days under pressure, but it is still poor.

Permanent hearing loss was a common problem among divers in the past because of high noise levels in helmets and chambers. Although divers who wear the "hard hat" (the classic rigid diving helmet) may still have this problem, the newer diving equipment is quieter and hearing loss is not common. If a decompression chamber does not have muffling for the compression and exhaust systems, divers inside the chamber and operators outside should use individual hearing protection to prevent temporary or permanent hearing loss.

A submarine's sonar (*so*und *n*avigation *a*nd *r*anging) uses sound signals propagated into water for certain aspects of operation (eg, active sonar). Standards for diving operations near active sonar sources are defined in NAVSEA Instruction Series 3150.2. Exposure to sonar can produce both auditory and nonauditory effects. Exposure to high sound pressure in water is similar to exposure to loud noise in air, causing either a temporary threshold shift or sensorineural deafness. Whether the decreased hearing is temporary or permanent depends on the sound pressure level and the frequency of the sonar signal. Unless a sonar signal is unexpectedly energized at close range there is little danger, because a diver who is swimming in the area of a sonar source can hear or feel the signal and can stay clear of the danger zone.

Divers exposed to sonar have reported feeling vibrations (in parts of or the entire body), vertigo, nausea, general discomfort, disorientation, decreased ability to concentrate, fatigue, and transient joint pain. The vibration is a mechanical phenomenon, whereas the vertigo, nausea, and discomfort indicate effects on the vestibular system. Similarly, nausea, vomiting, and vertigo are occasionally described in patients with vestibular signs or symptoms induced by loud noise (the Tullio phenomenon). The combination of disorientation, decreased concentration, and fatigue are similar to those symptoms seen in motion sickness and probably result from sound stimulation of the vestibular system. The cause of joint pain is uncertain. Adherence to the published exposure standards should prevent these symptoms.

PATHOPHYSIOLOGICAL EFFECTS OF PRESSURE: BAROTRAUMA

Barotrauma refers to injury caused by changes in pressure. Barotrauma can occur on descent or ascent when a gas-filled cavity fails to equilibrate with changing ambient pressure. Almost any gas-filled cavity in the body can be affected by barotrauma. For example, gastrointestinal barotrauma can occur if gas is swallowed. The gas will expand during ascent causing abdominal distress, cramping, flatus, or eructation. No therapy is usually required as the gas will be expelled over a short time, but several cases of gastric rupture after decompression have required emergency attention.[4]

Less-obvious body cavities are restored dental caries and gingivitis, which can also be gas-filled. Often referred to as aerodontalgia, dental barotrauma—as the result of poor or eroded fillings or gum infection—can occur on both ascent and descent. On descent, an air space can be filled with gum tissue or blood, and pain may occur. Descent also may cause the thinned filling or cementum over a carious tooth to collapse. If gas has become trapped under a filling during a dive, the pressure change during ascent may cause the cavity walls to explode.

Barotrauma that occurs when pressure increases is commonly referred to as a "squeeze." For example, suit squeeze occurs in a poorly fitted wetsuit or in a drysuit with an insufficient gas supply to keep it slightly expanded. There may be no symptoms at all, or the diver may notice some pinching of the skin. Upon removal of the suit, irregular linear wheals or ecchymoses may be seen where the skin was pinched in folds of the suit material. No therapy is required. Mask squeeze can occur if a diver fails to equalize the pressure in the mask during descent. The space inside the mask is subjected to a relative vacuum and the skin under the mask becomes puffy, edematous, and may show small hemorrhages. Mask squeeze is more common around the eyes and in the conjunctivae. A severe squeeze will bruise the entire area under the mask.

Middle Ear Barotrauma (Descent)

The most common form of barotrauma is middle ear squeeze. Anyone who has flown in an airplane or ridden in an elevator in a tall building has felt fullness in the ears during descent to ground level. This usually resolves by swallowing or yawning, which opens the eustachian tube and allows pressure equalization of the air on both sides of the tympanic membrane: ambient air and the air within the middle ear. The consequences of nonequilibration are much worse in diving, where pressure changes far exceed the 1 atm maximum change in descent from altitude. The initial symptom of fullness in the ear progresses to pain if descent continues without equalization. The tympanic membrane retracts and small hemorrhages occur (Figure 30-3). If the process continues, the relative vacuum in the middle ear causes serum and blood to fill the space, and eventually the tympanic membrane ruptures. Should cold water then enter the middle ear, sudden severe vertigo may occur, producing disorientation, nausea, vomiting, and panic.

Predisposing factors to eustachian tube dysfunction and middle ear squeeze are conditions that prevent easy opening and closing of the eustachian tube, such as upper respiratory tract infections, allergies, mucosal polyps, mucosal irritation from smoking, otitis media, or anatomical variations.

The diver should begin equilibration as soon as descent begins and continue every few feet. If the pressure differential is allowed to become too large, the eustachian tube will collapse to a point where it is "locked" and cannot be opened by any method. Methods of opening the eustachian tubes, or "clearing" the ears, include sliding the jaw around, opening the mouth, yawning, swallowing, and performing the Valsalva and Frenzel maneuvers. The Valsalva maneuver consists of closing the mouth, blocking the nostrils, and exhaling gently to in-

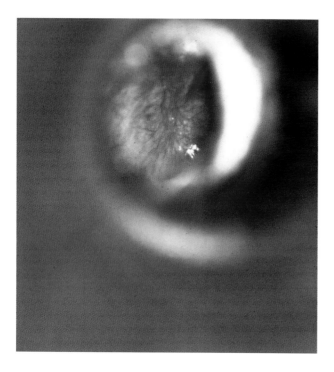

Fig. 30-3. Photograph showing moderate barotrauma of the middle ear. Note the hemorrhaging around the handle of the malleus and surrounding tympanic membrane, and the slight retraction and dullness of the tympanic membrane.

crease internal gas pressure. A forceful Valsalva maneuver may produce pressure high enough to cause rupture of the round window with cochlear and vestibular damage (see Inner Ear Barotrauma, below). The Frenzel maneuver consists of closing the mouth, glottis, and nose, and contracting the muscles of the mouth and pharynx or swallowing. If these maneuvers do not work, the diver should ascend a few feet and try again. If repeated attempts do not allow equilibration, the dive should be aborted. For unknown reasons, clearing the ears in a head-up position is easier than in a head-down position.

Prevention of middle ear barotrauma includes not diving when any condition exists that prevents proper eustachian tube function. Some divers often have, and most sometimes have, "sticky ears," a condition in which eustachian tube function is present but equilibration is difficult to achieve. Oral, nonsedative decongestants can be helpful but may not be effective in certain cases. Topical decongestants should be used with care, as overuse can make matters worse.

There is no specific therapy for middle ear barotrauma except the prohibition of significant pressure change or the use of autoinflation techniques until the problem resolves. In the case of tympanic membrane rupture, close observation is needed to detect infection when it first occurs. For severe barotrauma, serial audiograms are recommended to exclude hearing loss that may require further investigation and therapy. Generally, a diver who has had an ear squeeze without perforation can return to diving within 2 weeks. The basis for return is complete resolution of signs and symptoms as well as demonstration of the ability to equilibrate pressure in the middle ear. If rupture has occurred, a month or longer may be needed before return to diving can be allowed. Recurrence is common if exposure to pressure is allowed too soon after rupture.

Middle Ear Barotrauma (Ascent)

Middle ear barotrauma of ascent is infrequent, as the middle ear can normally vent passively through the eustachian tube when its pressure reaches about 50 cm H_2O over ambient. When it does occur, middle ear barotrauma of ascent is usually a consequence of middle ear barotrauma of descent. If blockage is severe, ascent without trauma may be impossible. Symptoms are pressure or pain, tinnitus, vertigo, or hearing loss. Vertigo, which is due to a pressure differential between the left and right middle ears (alternobaric vertigo), is a particular danger, as it can lead to disorientation and the inability to locate the surface. Pressure equalization during ascent, if necessary, uses the same maneuvers—Valsalva and Frenzel—as during descent. Descending a few feet before attempting equalization may be helpful. There is usually little to observe clinically, but hyperemia or hemorrhage in the tympanic membrane may occur. No specific therapy is required unless the vertigo persists after pressure equalization. Continued vertigo requires immediate investigation, especially if there is hearing loss.

Inner Ear Barotrauma

Any diver who has had difficulty equalizing the ears or has had barotrauma of the middle ear may also develop inner ear barotrauma, probably due to a rupture of either the round window or the vestibular membrane. Tinnitus is the most common manifestation, but hearing loss may occur at the time of barotrauma or within a few days. Some divers may experience vertigo, nausea, and vomiting. Hearing loss is usually sensorineural and is probably due to cochlear membrane rupture or hemorrhage. If deafness is instantaneous and present in all frequencies, it is probably due to severe round-window rupture. If it is mild and develops over several days, a round-window fistula may be present. If air leaks into the perilymph, the deafness may change with head position. If the deafness is limited to high frequencies (4,000 Hz) and does not change over several days, it is probably due to hemorrhage or trauma in the cochlea. Immediate referral to an otolaryngologist is recommended to prevent permanent hearing loss. Bed rest with the head elevated is required. The diver should be cautioned not to do anything that will raise the pressure of the cerebrospinal fluid, such as nose blowing, performing a Valsalva maneuver, straining at the stool, or coughing.

If there is no improvement within 24 to 48 hours or if the casualty's condition deteriorates, then surgical therapy should be considered. If improvement is steady, bed rest is continued until 1 week after improvement plateaus. Air evacuation, if required, should occur in an aircraft that can be pressurized to sea level. If helicopter transfer is the only method available, the pilot should be instructed not to ascend above 200 ft (61 m). If deafness, vertigo, or tinnitus persist despite all therapy, the casualty should be advised against any future diving. Inner ear barotrauma and inner ear decompression sickness (DCS; discussed below) can have similar symptoms, and their differentiation is important because DCS is treated by recompression, which is contraindicated in barotrauma.

Sinus Barotrauma

Sinus barotrauma during descent is probably the next most common problem after ear squeeze and involves the same predisposing factors. Symptoms include a feeling of pressure or tightness and pain over the face during descent. If the maxillary sinuses are affected, pain may be referred to the teeth. Often the diver may not realize that a mild squeeze has occurred until ascent, when the ostia may open, expelling blood and fluid. Sometimes the fluid, blood, or gas can be felt escaping from the sinuses. Divers who are unfamiliar with the problem can become panicky and extremely worried should this occur. Although pain is usually relieved on ascent, it may persist for several hours. Persistent pain indicates that equilibration has probably not occurred and there is a risk of acute sinusitis. Valsalva maneuvers will usually allow equilibration of the sinuses. Nasal decongestants may also be used.

Sinus barotrauma rarely occurs during ascent. However, if the pressure in the sinuses is high enough, there may be a painful rupture of the ostia or mucosa into the nasal cavities. Fracture of the sinus walls, allowing gas or fluid to enter the soft tissues, is a rare event. Treatment is the application of nasal decongestants.

Palsies of the fifth and seventh cranial nerves can result from as a result of sinus barotrauma (cranial nerve V) or middle ear barotrauma (cranial nerve VII).

Pulmonary Barotrauma of Descent

Pulmonary barotrauma of descent occurs under two circumstances:

1. when a hard-hat diver accidentally descends faster than the gas can be supplied to the helmet or suit; and
2. in breath-hold diving at depths so great that gas in the lungs is compressed to less than the residual volume.

The second circumstance is a very rare event in conscious divers, as chest pain alerts the diver of excessive depth. For most people the maximum breath-hold depth is about 100 fsw (30 msw), although a few individuals have exceeded 300 fsw (90 msw). One factor believed responsible for these deeper dives in certain individuals is their bodies' unusual ability to pool blood in the veins of the thoracic cavity (up to 1 L), which compensates for the inability to further decrease the volume of gas below residual volume. (Also see Chapter 31, Military Diving Operations and Medical Support.)

Pulmonary Barotrauma of Ascent

Pulmonary barotrauma of ascent is potentially the most severe of all types of barotrauma and can occur in all types of diving and in submarine escape (as well as in rapid decompression to high altitudes; see Chapter 32, Pressure Changes and Hypoxia in Aviation). Pulmonary barotrauma of ascent is caused by overinflation of the lung as the gas expands during ascent, either by breath-holding or by some local pathology that prevents gas from escaping from a portion of the lung. Pulmonary barotrauma is believed to be the second most common cause of mortality in divers (drowning is the most common). It has been reported[5] in ascent from a depth as shallow as 6 ft (1.8 m) of water. During naval submarine escape training, the incidence of pulmonary barotrauma is about 1 in 2,300, with death occurring in about 1 in 53,000 ascents.[6] These ascents are done under close supervision after medical screening, with emergency medical care immediately available. Predisposing conditions for pulmonary barotrauma are breath-holding during ascent, previous spontaneous pneumothorax, asthma, cysts, tumors, pleural adhesions, infections, pulmonary fibrosis, or any other disease that weakens the lung tissue or interferes with the free passage of gas.

Pulmonary barotrauma may result in local or wide damage to lung tissue, characterized by disruption of the alveolar–capillary membrane and consequent passage of alveolar gas (*a*) into the mediastinum, causing mediastinal emphysema; (*b*) into the pleural space, causing pneumothorax; and (*c*) into the capillaries, with probable resultant cerebral arterial gas embolism (CAGE). These traumata can occur alone or in combination. Patients with pulmonary barotrauma but no signs or symptoms of CAGE should be kept under observation for at least 24 hours, even if no therapy is required, to ensure that medical attention is available if the patient worsens, or if a new condition, such as DCS, should emerge.

Pulmonary Tissue Damage

There may be no symptoms with local pulmonary tissue damage, but if the damage is widespread, the diver may surface with cough, hemoptysis, and dyspnea. Respiratory failure may result if enough alveoli have been ruptured. Severe symptoms of pulmonary damage require immediate respiratory support with 100% oxygen, as in the treatment of near-drowning or acute respiratory distress syndrome. If pulmonary barotrauma is suspected, positive-pressure breathing is not recommended unless it is absolutely necessary for survival, to avoid the possibility of further lung damage or producing other complications of pulmonary barotrauma. Recompression is not needed unless symptoms or signs of CAGE or DCS are present.

Mediastinal Emphysema

Mediastinal emphysema occurs when gas enters the mediastinum along perivascular sheaths or tissue around the airways. The gas may extend to the subcutaneous tissue of the neck (subcutaneous emphysema), the pericardium (pneumopericardium), or the retroperitoneal space (pneumoperitoneum). There may be no symptoms in mild cases, or symptoms may appear immediately or over hours, depending on the severity of the condition. Symptoms include a fullness in the throat, retrosternal discomfort, voice changes, dyspnea, dysphagia, syncope, shock, and unconsciousness. Signs include crepitus under the skin, faint heart sounds, paralysis of the recurrent laryngeal nerve, tachycardia,

hypotension, cyanosis, and coma. Crepitus that is heard over the precordium and is related to heart sounds is called Hamman's sign. Gas that has dissected into the pericardial sac or between the pleura and pericardium may cause cardiac tamponade. A chest roentgenogram will confirm the diagnosis, or it may be the only evidence of mediastinal emphysema. In our experience, mediastinal emphysema and the variants listed above are not very common. This is a diving problem that is generally not life-threatening and usually requires no treatment. Breathing 100% oxygen will accelerate absorption of the gas in mild cases and is required in severe cases for life support. Severe cases may benefit from recompression to reduce the volume of gas in the tissues. An oxygen treatment table for shallow depths, such as US Navy Treatment Table 5,[7] (see Figure 31-23 in Chapter 31, Military Diving Operations and Medical Support) should suffice.

Pneumothorax

Pneumothorax occurs when increased pressure in the lung ruptures the pleura with results similar to a spontaneous pneumothorax. A hemopneumothorax may occur if blood vessels are torn. Symptoms, should they occur, include sudden onset of chest pain (possibly pleuritic) and dyspnea. Bilateral pneumothoraces may be present after a fast ascent, as in submarine escape training or in an emergency ascent from a dive. Signs include increased respiratory rate, decreased breath sounds, and increased resonance. If a tension pneumothorax is present, the classic tracheal shift to the unaffected side may occur, with shock and severe respiratory distress. If the pneumothorax is small, no therapy is necessary, although breathing 100% oxygen at the surface should accelerate pleural gas absorption.

If the patient is under pressure and decompression continues, a tension pneumothorax will result. If in a chamber, treatment includes recompression to reduce symptoms, 100% oxygen breathing (or a gas mix with increased partial pressure of oxygen), and the insertion of a chest tube or valve to allow decompression while avoiding expansion of the pneumothorax. If the diver is in the water when the pneumothorax occurs, however, none of the above treatments are possible.

If the patient is on the surface and severe symptoms are present, recompression should not be initiated unless required for treatment of CAGE or DCS. Treatment at sea level does not differ from that of a pneumothorax resulting from other causes. If recompression is required for therapy of CAGE or

DCS, a chest tube should be inserted before recompression. For emergency recompression, a needle with a nonreturn valve should be inserted and later converted to the usual chest tube with suction or underwater drainage. If recompression is needed and a chest tube with drainage is in place, care is required to prevent sucking water and gas into the chest during compression. If the system allows gas or fluid into the chest, the chest tube should be clamped close to the chest wall until treatment depth is reached. Because of the possibility of infection, we recommend that chest tubes not be used in a recompression chamber unless absolutely necessary.

Cerebral Arterial Gas Embolism

CAGE can be life-threatening or result in permanent injury, and requires immediate recompression. CAGE is a complication of pulmonary barotrauma caused by the entry of gas through tissue tears into the pulmonary venous system, with further distribution through the left side of the heart to the arterial system. The gas bubbles generally come to rest in the cerebral circulation, or, uncommonly, in the coronary circulation. The bubbles block small blood vessels, with concomitant serious results. In the coronary system, immediate death can result through cardiac failure. In the cerebral circulation, the typical signs are of sudden arterial block, as in a cardiovascular accident. The onset of signs and symptoms is sudden and dramatic, appearing during the ascent or always within a few minutes of surfacing. The most common signs are semiconsciousness, unconsciousness, disorientation, and paresis. Paresis can occur in any distribution but is most often unilateral. Other symptoms, depending on the anatomical location of the blockage, include vertigo, visual disturbances, dysphasia, sensory abnormalities, and convulsions. If the coronary system is involved, cardiac chest pain and dysrhythmias may be present.

Arterial gas emboli, whether in the brain or elsewhere, cause ischemia in the surrounding tissue and induce coagulopathies, hemorrhages, and endothelial damage. Protein and cells are deposited on the bubble surface. If treatment—recompression—is long delayed, reperfusion injury may occur once the circulation has been reestablished.

Studies may show abnormal electrocardiographic, electroencephalographic, and brain scan findings, but if CAGE is suspected, there is no reason to delay treatment while these tests are obtained. Immediate recompression is the key to adequate treatment of this syndrome. If treatment is delayed, the chances for a good outcome decrease and therapy becomes more difficult. Surveys show that delay of recompression for more than a few hours results in a 50% decrease in the cure rate.[8(p107)] In severe cases, even immediate and aggressive therapy may not produce a good result, and death may follow. In mild cases, the symptoms may resolve without any therapy. In some cases, a patient may improve after initial symptom onset but relapse despite treatment. There is no way to predict which case will resolve and which will fail. Therefore, all cases of suspected CAGE should be recompressed as soon as possible.

Iatrogenic CAGE has occurred during open heart surgery, brain surgery, and kidney dialysis. Treatment in these cases is no different from that in cases resulting from ambient pressure changes.

The treatment for CAGE is immediate recompression. There is some controversy about whether recompression should be to low pressure, 60 fsw (18 msw, or 2.8 ata) (in accordance with US Navy Treatment Table 6),[7] or to high pressure, 165 fsw (50 msw, or 6 ata) (in accordance with US Navy Treatment Table 6A).[7] (See Figures 31-24 and 31-25 in Chapter 31, Military Diving Operations and Medical Support.) At the present time the *US Navy Diving Manual*[7] recommends initial recompression to 60 fsw on 100% oxygen. If the symptoms resolve, treatment may be completed in accordance with US Navy Treatment Table 6. If the patient does not respond satisfactorily, further compression to 165 fsw (50 msw) is an option in an effort to make remaining bubbles smaller. If immediate recompression is not available, 100% oxygen breathing by mask and intravenous fluid administration should be initiated. The patient should be positioned on his back or side on a horizontal plane. In the past, it was advised that the patient be placed in the Trendelenburg position to prevent more gas from entering the cerebral circulation. This is no longer recommended, as it has been determined[9] that the head-down position increases central venous and cerebral venous pressure and cerebral edema. Increased venous pressure may also make it more difficult for bubbles to pass into the venous circulation.

If convulsions are present, Valium (diazepam; manufactured by Roche Products Inc, Manati, Puerto Rico) may be useful. Lidocaine hydrochloride has been shown[10] to increase cerebral vasodilation and decrease the rise in intracranial arterial pressure. It is also a useful drug in the treatment of cardiac dysrhythmias. The use of parenteral steroids, once thought to reduce cerebral edema, is controversial. Their utility has not been verified as of this writing, and some claim[8(p109)] that they actually are detrimental. In any case, CAGE causes immediate damage and steroids take hours before an effect is evident.

Transportation to a recompression facility should be done as gently and quickly as possible to prevent further distribution of bubbles to the brain or else-where. Air evacuation, if required, should occur at an altitude no higher than 800 ft (242 m), and preferably in an aircraft that can be pressurized to sea level. Other supportive therapy should be used as required.

In certain cases, there may be difficulty in determining whether the diver has CAGE or cerebral DCS (see the Decompression Sickness section, below).

PATHOPHYSIOLOGICAL EFFECTS OF COMMON DIVING GASES

Gases used in diving should be free of contaminants. A small fraction of contaminants cause increased toxicity at high barometric pressure because the partial pressures increase with depth, as described by Dalton's law (see above). The current US Navy standards for the purity of air, oxygen, nitrogen, and helium are found in the *US Navy Diving Manual*.[11] Breathing gases that do not meet these standards are not to be used for diving. This section deals with the pathological condition associated with commonly used breathing gases and some common contaminants (CO_2, CO).

Oxygen Toxicity

The pathophysiology of all metabolically active gases (O_2, CO_2, CO) depend on the partial pressure, not on the percentage of that gas in the breathing mixture. For example, at 1 atm, a mixture containing 5% oxygen is not compatible with life but at 5 atm is perfectly adequate. Breathing high partial pressures of oxygen can cause two types of toxicity: pulmonary and cerebral.

Pulmonary Oxygen Toxicity

Pulmonary oxygen toxicity was first described by Lorrain-Smith[12] in 1899 as the result of breathing pure oxygen at sea level for a prolonged time (usually 2–3 d). We now know that this can occur at inspired partial pressures of oxygen (P_{IO_2}) as low as 0.5 to 0.6 atm, either at 1 atm or at higher pressures. Clinically, patients first report the symptoms of tracheobronchitis, such as tracheal burning and cough following deep inspiration. If oxygen administration continues, actual breathlessness will occur. A measurable sign of pulmonary oxygen toxicity is a decrease in vital capacity, with increasing loss of inspiratory capacity and increasing residual volume. Atelectasis occurs and increases as the pathology worsens. The pathophysiology includes endothelial thickening, proliferation of cells, loss of surfactant, exudate, hemorrhage, and consolidation. Even though the patient may be breathing pure oxygen, the cause of death is asphyxia.

Although pulmonary oxygen toxicity is an uncommon problem, gas content must be carefully planned in saturation diving, where divers are exposed to a P_{IO_2} in the range of 0.4 to 0.5 atm for days with intermittent exposures to higher levels for diving excursions (see Chapter 31, Military Diving Operations and Medical Support, for a discussion of saturation diving). Pulmonary oxygen toxicity can also occur in prolonged recompression therapy for DCS or CAGE. When this occurs, the P_{IO_2} must be reduced to at least 0.5 atm to allow recovery.

The effect of oxygen exposure on the vital capacity can be estimated by the unit pulmonary toxicity dose (UPTD),[13] which is based on the experimental measurement of changes in vital capacity in human subjects. This concept assumes no decrement in lung function when breathing oxygen at a partial pressure of 0.5 atm or less. The results of such calculations should be considered to be no more than a rough guide to pulmonary effects, as there are large individual differences, but it is useful as a guide to limiting prolonged oxygen breathing at partial pressures higher than 0.5 atm.

Cerebral Oxygen Toxicity

Cerebral oxygen toxicity was discovered by Paul Bert[14] in 1878 and is referred to as acute oxygen poisoning because of its rapid onset. Acute toxicity occurs only while breathing oxygen under pressure at P_{IO_2} greater than 1.3 atm. The lowest documented P_{IO_2} at which convulsions have occurred during diving with 100% oxygen is 1.74 atm, as opposed to 1.6 atm during mixed-gas diving. The first sign of trouble is often a grand mal convulsion. Other symptoms of central nervous system (CNS) oxygen toxicity include muscular twitching around the mouth or of the abdominal wall, nausea, dizziness, tunnel vision, and anxiety, but these are rare and cannot be relied on to precede seizures. The treatments for CNS oxygen toxicity are to remove the patient from the high-level oxygen source and to prevent self-injury. Rarely, a convulsion may occur within minutes after stopping oxygen breathing.

This is known as the "off effect" and has no accepted explanation, but it may represent the culmination of a process that began during oxygen breathing.

Because oxygen toxicity is dose-related, oxygen can safely be used so long as time and depth are limited. This allows the use of oxygen at greater than 1 atm partial pressure to reduce inert gas absorption at depth, both to accelerate inert gas elimination during decompression and for recompression therapy. The latent period prior to the onset of symptoms can be extended by periodically breathing a gas with a reduced oxygen partial pressure. Therefore, treatment tables at 60 fsw (18 msw) utilize oxygen breathing periods of 20 to 25 minutes, separated by 5-minute air breaks (see Chapter 31, Military Diving Operations and Medical Support, for a discussion of treatment tables).

A number of factors affect sensitivity to oxygen toxicity. These include the extreme variation among individuals and within the same individual from day to day. There is no guarantee that someone who did not have an oxygen convulsion today will not have one tomorrow. Immersion and exercise decrease the latent period, and this increases the risk of a working diver compared with that of a diver at rest in a dry hyperbaric chamber. Increased inspired or arterial carbon dioxide decreases the latency, and individuals prone to retain carbon dioxide may be at greater risk. Modern underwater breathing apparatuses (UBAs) have less breathing resistance and dead space than earlier UBAs, but heavy work at great depth appears to cause carbon dioxide retention and to potentiate oxygen toxicity. Increased gas density also decreases ventilation and can lead to retention of carbon dioxide.

The mechanism by which oxygen causes these pulmonary and cerebral derangements is still not understood. The most accepted explanation is that reactive oxygen species, such as superoxide, hydroxyl radicals, and hydrogen peroxide, are generated and may interfere with cellular metabolism and electrical activity. Oxygen can inactivate many enzymes and metabolic pathways, with enzymes containing a sulfhydryl group being especially sensitive. It is puzzling that the time required to effect these changes in vitro is much longer than the time required to produce convulsions in intact animals, although the partial pressure of oxygen in the in vivo tissue is much lower than the P_{IO_2}. Another possibility is lipid peroxidation and depression of the prostaglandin I_2 system, leaving the thromboxane A_2 system intact. Lipid peroxidation can affect cell membrane function causing decreased glutamate uptake, increased potassium retention, decreased active sodium transport, and inactivation of the sodium–potassium adenosine triphosphatase pump. In lung tissue, decreases occur in serotonin and norepinephrine uptake; pulmonary capillary endothelium function; and prostaglandin E_2, bradykinin, and angiotensin metabolism. Other nonbiochemical effects of oxygen include vasoconstriction-induced reduction in peripheral blood flow, decreased carbon dioxide carrying capacity by hemoglobin, and increased red blood cell fragility, but these subtle changes do not generally cause concern.

The probability of clinical oxygen toxicity is reasonably low if the time–depth limits in the *US Navy Diving Manual*[11] are observed (Table 30-1). In routine air diving the oxygen exposures are not high enough to produce either CNS or pulmonary toxicity, but the recent use of nitrogen–oxygen mixes with more than 21% oxygen (nitrox, enriched air) by recreational divers has led to a number of CNS oxygen-toxicity episodes and some fatalities.[15]

The *US Navy Diving Manual*[11] also allows making one excursion as deep as 50 fsw (15.1 msw) during dives on 100% oxygen, but only for 5 minutes and only under the following conditions:

- The maximum dive time cannot exceed 240 minutes.
- Only one excursion is allowed.
- The diver must return to 20 fsw (6.1 msw) or less by the end of the excursion.
- The excursion must not exceed 15 minutes at 21 to 40 fsw (6.4–12.1 msw) or 5 minutes at 41 to 50 fsw (12.4–15.1 msw).

TABLE 30-1

SINGLE-DEPTH OXYGEN EXPOSURE LIMITS

Depth (fsw)	Maximum Oxygen Time (min)
20	240
30	80
35	25
40	15
50	10

Reproduced from US Department of the Navy. *US Navy Diving Manual.* Vol 2. Washington, DC: DN; 1991. NAVSEA 0994-LP-001-9020. Rev 3.

The US Navy closed-circuit mixed gas UBA (the Mk 16 UBA) is designed to control the oxygen partial pressure to 0.7 atm. CNS oxygen toxicity is not a problem at this level (various other types of UBAs are discussed in Chapter 31, Military Diving Operations and Medical Support). During saturation diving, the US Navy maintains the oxygen partial pressure in the chamber at 0.40 and 0.45 atm; for diving excursions, the allowable partial pressure is 0.40 to 1.2 atm.

NOTE: The partial pressure and depth–time limits given here are subject to change. Readers should refer to the latest appropriate standards for the diving operation at hand. In addition, if the diving is conducted under other than US Navy authority (ie, another government agency or a foreign government), different limits may be used. American divers may be prohibited from diving under procedures other than those specified by the US Navy.

Carbon Dioxide Toxicity

The effects of increased carbon dioxide include hyperventilation, dyspnea, tachycardia, headache, lightheadedness, and dizziness progressing to mental confusion and unconsciousness (Table 30-2). As with other gases, the effects are dependent on the partial pressure of the gas, not the percentage.

Increased carbon dioxide levels and toxicity can be caused by the following conditions:

- increased carbon dioxide in the breathing gas due to compression of contaminated gas

TABLE 30-2

ACUTE EFFECTS OF INCREASED INSPIRED CARBON DIOXIDE

Carbon Dioxide (%,SLE)	Effects
0–3	No adverse effects
~ 5	Mild hyperventilation
5–10	Shortness of breath, panting, confusion, drowsiness
10–20	Extreme respiratory distress, unconsciousness, muscle twitching and spasms, convulsions, death

*SLE: sea-level equivalent; increasing pressure causes increasing partial pressure and therefore the physiological effect of gas, although the percentage remains constant

in open-circuit breathing apparatus or failure of the carbon dioxide absorbent in a closed-circuit apparatus;

- increased respiratory dead space owing to poor equipment design, or inadequate ventilation of chamber or helmet;
- voluntary hypoventilation (divers hold their breath after inhalation or "skip-breathe" to increase the duration of the open-circuit gas supply);
- increased partial pressure of oxygen, which decreases the ventilatory response to carbon dioxide; and
- increased breathing resistance, either intrinsic (diver's lungs) or extrinsic (breathing equipment); the latter is more common than the former. Added breathing resistance decreases ventilatory response to elevated carbon dioxide.

Carbon Monoxide Toxicity

The acute toxic effects of carbon monoxide at depth depend on its partial pressure and are the same at depth as at sea level. Absolute pressure has no effect on the binding of carbon monoxide to hemoglobin or on symptoms, but the increased partial pressure of oxygen at depth decreases carbon monoxide's binding to hemoglobin, somewhat lessening its effects.

Carbon monoxide contamination of compressed air is rare but dangerous when it occurs. The commonest source of contamination is an air compressor whose intake is near the exhaust of an internal combustion engine, perhaps the compressor's motor. Compressors lubricated with oil are also a potential source of carbon monoxide. A small amount of carbon monoxide is produced during the metabolism of hemoglobin, and smokers exhale even larger quantities for the first 24 hours that they are confined in a chamber. These amounts of carbon monoxide can accumulate in a saturation diving complex. Contamination of breathing air with carbon monoxide from any source prevents normal saturation of hemoglobin with oxygen. Table 30-3 lists the ranges of carboxyhemoglobin levels commonly associated with symptoms.

As carbon monoxide binds to myoglobin as well as to hemoglobin, carboxyhemoglobin concentrations do not always correlate with symptomatology. The length of exposure, inspired carbon monoxide partial pressure, and physical activity are also important. A short exposure of a resting person to a high level of

TABLE 30-3

ACUTE EFFECTS OF INCREASED INSPIRED CARBON MONOXIDE

COHb*(%)	Effects
< 10	None obvious; heavy smokers often reach this level. Subtle changes in vision and cognition have been detected by sophisticated testing.
10–20	Mild headache may be present. Skin flushing sometimes occurs.
20–30	Definite, often throbbing, headache.
30–40	Weakness, nausea, vomiting, drowsiness, dizziness, sweating, blurred vision.
> 40	Unconsciousness, Cheyne-Stokes respiration, convulsions, coma, death.

*COHb: hemoglobin in the form of carboxyhemoglobin in the arterial blood

carbon monoxide may produce a lower blood level than a long exposure of a working person to a relatively low inspired carbon monoxide concentration.

Because carbon monoxide and oxygen compete for binding sites on hemoglobin, oxygen breathing, particularly at increased pressure, is an effective treatment for carbon monoxide poisoning. The half-life of carbon monoxide is 4 to 5 hours breathing room air at rest, but this is reduced to 40 to 80 minutes breathing 100% oxygen at sea level, and to 20 minutes breathing 100% oxygen at 3 ata. The rates at which carbon monoxide is eliminated from myoglobin and cellular compartments are unknown.

Nitrogen Narcosis

Nitrogen narcosis (rapture of the deep) is the progressive intoxication that develops as a diver descends and the partial pressure of nitrogen increases. Depending on individual sensitivity, each 1 to 2 atm increase in air pressure is said to be equivalent to one gin martini, the so-called "martini law." While perhaps not absolutely correct, this analogy does reflect the subtle changes that begin at 50 to 100 fsw and include increased reaction time, decreased manual dexterity, and mild impairment in reasoning. At 100 to 150 fsw (30–45 msw), most divers will become light-headed and euphoric with loss of fine discrimination. Deeper than 150 fsw (45 msw), the symptoms progress to joviality, garru-

lousness, and dizziness with uncontrolled laughter, loss of concentration, and mistakes in simple, practical, and mental tasks. Additional symptoms and signs include peripheral numbness and tingling and poor attention to personal safety, which is particularly hazardous to divers in the water. Responses to signals and other stimuli are slow. At 300 fsw (90 msw), mental depression, loss of clear thinking, and impaired neuromuscular coordination occur. At 350 fsw (105 msw), many divers lose consciousness. Severe narcosis may result in amnesia lasting for several hours. Sleepiness after the dive is common.

Factors that exacerbate nitrogen narcosis are inexperience, anxiety, alcohol, fatigue, and increased inspired carbon dioxide. Ameliorating factors are experience, strong will, and fixation on a task. The evidence for adaptation to narcosis with frequent exposure is limited and controversial. If it does occur, the effect appears small.

As narcosis is a threat to diver safety, most agencies limit air diving with self-contained underwater breathing apparatus (scuba) to around 130 fsw (40 msw) and with hard-hat tethered air diving to around 165 to 180 fsw (50–55 msw).

The mechanism of nitrogen narcosis, which is similar to anesthesia, is still under study. Anesthetic potency shows some relationship to the ratio of the gas solubilities in oil and water and also to their effects on surface tension. These were formerly thought to cause cell membranes to swell, thereby influencing ion transport. This is consistent with the lack of narcosis from helium with its low solubility and low surface tension. More-recent studies, on the other hand, have focused on neurotransmitter release at presynaptic or postsynaptic sites as the active sites for anesthetic action.

Helium and Other Inert Gases

Although the noble gases (group zero in the periodic table of chemical elements) are chemically inert, they are physiologically active. Substitution of helium for nitrogen in breathing gas has four major effects. The first, described previously, is the effect on the voice. The second is the absence of narcosis. The third is decreased work of breathing, owing to the lower density of helium. This, and the lack of narcosis, make helium particularly useful at depths greater than 150 fsw (45 msw). The fourth effect is the loss of heat through the skin and the lungs, owing to helium's high heat capacity and conductivity. Both the skin and the breathing gas must be heated during prolonged helium–oxygen diving to prevent hypothermia. Hot water is usually used for this purpose. Hypothermia can also occur in a dry, helium–oxygen filled chamber if the temperature is not raised above the normal comfort level for air. The required temperature increases with increasing gas density. A full discussion of these effects can be found in the section on saturation diving in Chapter 31, Military Diving Operations and Medical Support.

Of the other noble gases, neon has been used in deep diving experiments but is not used for diving operations, as it is expensive and has a higher density than helium (or than hydrogen), which causes greater respiratory work. Argon, xenon, and krypton are narcotic at 1 ata and therefore not appropriate for diving. Because of its high insulating properties, argon is sometimes used to inflate dry diving suits.

Hydrogen

Interest in hydrogen diving has been renewed because engineering advances in handling hydrogen–oxygen mixtures have reduced the danger of explosion. These techniques take advantage of the fact that hydrogen cannot ignite if mixed with less than 5.5% oxygen. Hydrogen is inexpensive, readily available, and less narcotic and of lower density than nitrogen. The decompression properties of hydrogen appear to be between those of helium and nitrogen.

Physiological Effects of Pressure: High-Pressure Nervous Syndrome

Because helium does not cause narcosis, it is the gas of choice for dives deeper than 150 to 180 fsw (45–54 msw). However, an effect called the high-pressure nervous syndrome (HPNS) begins at depths greater than 600 fsw (180 msw). HPNS is characterized by hyperexcitability, including tremors, poor sleep, loss of appetite, and psychosis at depths greater than 2,000 fsw (600 msw). Initially, HPNS was believed to be caused by helium per se ("helium tremors"), but subsequent experiments with liquid-breathing animals indicated that pressure is the responsible agent. Indeed, the excitatory effects of pressure and the narcotic effects of nitrogen are partially counteractive, and 5% nitrogen in a helium–oxygen breathing gas is sometimes used to ameliorate HPNS effects, which can be debilitating deeper than 1,000 fsw (300 msw).

The use of nitrogen in breathing gases for very deep diving is disadvantageous because its high density imposes ventilatory resistance and therefore reduces exercise capacity. Up to 20 bars of hydrogen have been used[16] to reduce both HPNS and breathing resistance at a record depth of 2,343 fsw (710 msw), but hydrogen narcosis, perhaps exacerbated by HPNS, appears to be a limiting factor. HPNS and low exercise capacity, particularly with UBAs, limit the maximum practical working depth to somewhere in the range of 1,500 to 2,000 fsw (450–600 msw).

DECOMPRESSION SICKNESS

Decompression sickness (DCS) refers to the overt illness that follows a reduction in environmental pressure with the development of endogenous gas bubbles. This condition is distinguished from cerebral arterial gas embolism (CAGE), in which bubbles originate from the lungs or external sources and enter the vasculature through disruptions in the pulmonary membranes. DCS occurs in diving, caisson work, rapid ascent to high altitude, and following hyperbaric chamber work. DCS can occur at any time following the start of decompression and can be subtle or catastrophic. The initiating cause is the formation of bubbles of the inert gases dissolved in the tissues. Diagnosis can be difficult, as the signs and symptoms of DCS resemble not only nondiving diseases but also CAGE. Symptoms and signs may disappear spontaneously but return unpredictably hours later. DCS should be the topmost diagnosis in the physician's mind when a patient presents with complaints following any dive.

DCS is traditionally classified into two types:

- Type I, which is minor, includes only limb or joint pain, itch, skin rash, or localized swelling; and
- Type II, which is serious, includes presentations with neurological and pulmonary symptoms or signs.

The term *decompression illness* has been suggested to be used for any diving accident involving pressure reduction, including Type I DCS, Type II DCS, and CAGE, and does not differentiate among these entities. There is a good deal of controversy over whether this terminology is advantageous.

In certain cases, it may be impossible to distinguish between CAGE and DCS with signs of cerebral dysfunction, or a combination of both, as Exhibit 30-2 illustrates. Table 30-4 provides some guidance, but differentiation is often not possible. Clinically, this is not a significant issue, as the current *US Navy Diving Manual*[7] specifies the same symptom-based therapy, including saturation therapy, for both CAGE and severe neurological DCS: recompression with oxygen to 60 ft (18 m), or to deeper depths with air or a breathing gas with an increased oxygen content (eg, 50% oxygen–50% nitrogen). The depth and duration of therapy are determined by the clinical progression. Another term, Type III DCS, has also been suggested[17] as an appropriate designation to describe these very serious cases: when CAGE is suspected and both cerebral and spinal signs and symptoms of DCS are present.

For treatment purposes, the most important point is how these symptoms respond to therapy, not the initial classification. In fact, as therapy progresses, the diagnosis may change. For example, a diver with severe pain may not notice local weakness or sensory loss until recompression relieves the pain. The pain may also mask the signs to an examiner. Immediate recompression of patients with serious

signs and symptoms should take precedence over a detailed physical examination that may reveal less-obvious signs.

Inert Gas Exchange

When an inert gas is breathed at elevated pressure, its partial pressure in the lungs initially exceeds that in the tissues. As the time at pressure lengthens, the inert gas is progressively absorbed by the tissues until its partial pressure there equals that in the lungs. The principal factors governing the rate of gas absorption by tissue are perfusion and solubility. Lipid tissues, such as fat, with high inert gas solubility and poor perfusion, absorb (and eliminate) inert gas much more slowly than low-solubility aqueous tissues, such as muscles, that are well perfused. Diffusion is not as important as per-

---

EXHIBIT 30-2

DECOMPRESSION SICKNESS, ARTERIAL GAS EMBOLISM, OR BOTH?

An adult male diver was decompressing at 10 to 15 fsw after a 25-minute dive to 110 ft. A swell running had made it difficult to hold his depth, and near the end of the decompression stop (length of time unknown), he noted numbness and weakness of his right arm. After surfacing, the weakness increased, his right leg became weak, and both hands became numb. He was also dysphasic and had intermittent loss of consciousness. He was immediately given 100% oxygen and taken ashore, where he became disoriented with twitching of the muscles of the arms and left leg. On arrival at the nearest emergency room the disorientation had cleared but the other symptoms and signs remained. He was transported to a hospital with a recompression chamber. This took about 4 hours, during which oxygen and intravenous fluids were administered. On reaching the chamber, he was oriented, had mild weakness in his right arm and marked weakness in his right thigh, and now noted mild weakness in his left leg. He was initially treated in accordance with an extended US Navy Treatment Table 6[1] (see Figure 31-29 in Chapter 31, Military Diving Operations and Medical Support), near the end of which he developed bilateral loss of sensation from T-2–T-3 down, weakness of the left upper extremity, and weakness of both lower extremities. He was unable to urinate and required a Foley catheter. Over the next 2 weeks, he improved in all areas during subsequent recompression therapies, but still had mild weakness of all four limbs and required a Foley catheter for bladder drainage. Sensation at this time was normal. He was transferred for physical rehabilitation as there was no further improvement from hyperbaric oxygen treatments. The final outcome of all therapy is unknown.

The early onset of cerebral symptoms in this case is compatible with a cerebral arterial gas embolism (CAGE), which possibly occurred because of pulmonary barotrauma due to a sudden decrease in pressure from the heavy swell. The improvement with time and oxygen administration without recompression is not unusual in cases of mild CAGE. The bilateral numbness in the hands probably signaled the onset of spinal cord decompression sickness (Type II DCS), which developed into bilateral loss of sensation, quadriplegia, and loss of bladder function near the end of the first recompression. A number of factors may have contributed to the clinical presentation: the lack of adequate decompression time; the long delay to recompression, which led to further tissue damage; inadequate initial recompression therapy; and bubbles in the spinal circulation as a result of venous or arterial gas emboli from the pulmonary barotrauma or bubbles arising from elsewhere in the body, causing overwhelming DCS. The mechanisms are uncertain but appear to have involved both DCS and CAGE

---

(1) US Department of the Navy. *US Navy Diving Manual*. Vol 1. Washington, DC: DN; 1993. NAVSEA 0994-LP-001-9110. Rev 3.

TABLE 30-4

COMPARISON OF DECOMPRESSION SICKNESS AND CEREBRAL ARTERIAL GAS EMBOLISM

Factor	Decompression Sickness (DCS)	Cerebral Arterial Gas Embolism (CAGE)
Occurrence	A dive of sufficient depth and duration to cause absorption of significant inert gas	Any dive
Onset	Immediate or delayed	Immediate
Cause	Inert gas bubbles in tissue, veins, or arteries	Bubbles in arteries only as a result of pulmonary barotrauma
Bubbles	From dissolved gas	From alveolar gas
Usual First Symptom	Localized pain or numbness	Unconsciousness or paralysis
Neurological Signs	Usually bilateral	Usually unilateral
Prognosis	Mild to serious	Serious

fusion, but it can influence gas exchange any time that areas of tissue have different inert gas tensions. For example, diffusion shunts can occur between adjacent arterial and venous vessels, resulting in slower inert gas exchange in a tissue than would be expected on the basis of perfusion alone. Diffusion between adjacent sections of tissue may lead to apparently anomalous results, as when the absorption of a tracer gas continues in one region of tissue as a result of diffusion from another region, when the tracer gas is no longer present in the inspired gas. Such effects and variations in perfusion rate make inert gas exchange a complex and unpredictable phenomenon.

Bubble formation that follows decompression isolates inert gas from the circulation and reduces the effectiveness of perfusion in eliminating the inert gas in the vicinity of the bubble. An effective method for accelerating the elimination of an inert gas from tissues or bubbles is to increase the partial pressure of oxygen in the inspired gas, which increases the difference between inert gas in the lungs and in the tissue.

Bubble Formation

In experiments with animals performed during the 1870s, Paul Bert[14] of France demonstrated that the most severe forms of DCS are caused by bubbles in the blood and tissues. Bubbles are less obvious in the milder forms of DCS and this has led to the suggestion of other etiologies, but none of these theories has been sustained. The presence of bubbles, after even very mild dives, can be detected using ultrasonic detectors.

In both living and nonliving systems, a primary factor that determines whether a bubble will appear is the level of supersaturation, or the sum of the partial pressures of all vapors and dissolved gases, minus the local absolute pressure. The level of supersaturation that leads to bubble formation is a clue to how bubbles form. Supersaturations of gases on the order of 100 to 1,000 atm in nonliving systems is evidence for de novo nucleation (ie, the formation of bubbles where no gas phase previously existed). During physiological decompression, however, supersaturation rarely exceeds several atmospheres, and the lowest supersaturation at which DCS occurs is about 0.5 atm. Under these conditions, bubbles probably expand from preexisting gaseous micronuclei, or gas nuclei, which exist in all aqueous fluids. It is difficult to understand the origin of gas nuclei in closed living systems, but some are probably mechanically generated by de novo nucleation that results from both viscous adhesion in tissue and shear forces during the relative motion of articular surfaces. Such motion causes the local pressure to transiently decrease to hundreds of negative atmospheres and creates vaporous bubbles that make audible sounds as they collapse ("cracking" joints). Stable gas bubbles also form as result of this process. The population of some

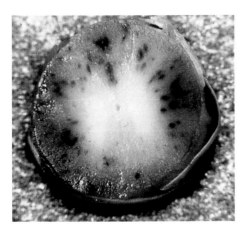

Fig. 30-4. This gross cross-section of a spinal cord shows the hemorrhages in the white matter that are typical of decompression sickness.

gas nuclei in the body appears to be normally in a state of dynamic equilibrium, wherein their creation by mechanically induced nucleation is balanced by their elimination due to surface tension.

Pathophysiology of Decompression Sickness

DCS results from a reduction in ambient pressure with the subsequent formation of stable bubbles. Despite the common occurrence of bubbles in the circulatory system, bubbles probably do not originate in blood but form extravascularly and seed the microcirculation as they expand. These bubbles grow by the inward diffusion of nitrogen as they are carried in the venous blood to the heart and lungs. The lungs filter small quantities of bubbles, but if the volume of gas becomes overwhelming, as can occur in accidental ascent from great depth, blood can be displaced from the heart, leading to death by asphyxia.

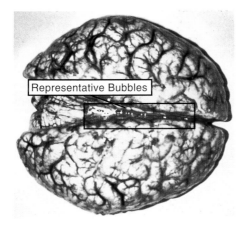

Fig. 30-5. Brain from a patient who died of severe decompression sickness, showing bubbles in the surface vasculature.

Venous bubbles have the potential for reaching the arterial circulation by passing through the pulmonary circulation or by-passing the lungs altogether through arteriovenous shunts or a patent foramen ovale. Venous bubbles can also pass to the arterial circulation if the number or volume of bubbles exceeds the filtering capacity of the lungs.

Large numbers of emboli in the arterial circulation can arise, of course, owing to pulmonary barotrauma, should a diver hold his breath during ascent. While this gas can have serious consequences if carried to the brain, the situation is worse if the barotrauma should occur at the *end* of a dive when the tissues contain excess inert gas. Bubbles that enter the arterial circulation can expand if they reach supersaturated tissue. This may explain a devastating form of DCS (Type III DCS), which involves both the brain and spinal cord after relatively mild dives that end with pulmonary barotrauma (Figures 30-4 and 30-5).

Bubbles have both mechanical and biochemical effects, which may be extravascular or intravascular (arterial and venous). Extravascular bubbles can compress or stretch tissue and nerves. Intravascularly, they can cause embolic obstruction, stasis, ischemia, hypoxia, edema, hemorrhage, and tissue death (Figure 30-6). En-

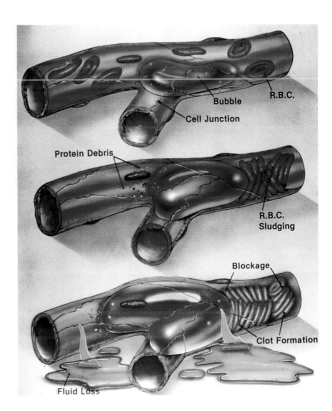

Fig. 30-6. Bubble formation in a blood vessel. (**a**) The lodging of a bubble at a vascular junction, with (**b**) sludging of the red blood cells (RBCs) and formation of protein debris, and (**c**) blood clot and extravascular fluid loss. Bubbles in blood vessels are typically not spherical.

943

dothelial cell membranes are stripped by the passage of bubbles. Bubbles may block lymph channels, causing tissue edema. The most serious of these events are rare, except in cases of severe DCS or CAGE, and mild cases are the rule when modern dive procedures are used. The human body appears to tolerate a certain volume of bubbles with no symptoms or only mild symptoms.

The biochemical effects of bubbles relate to their surface active properties, which cause enzyme activation and protein denaturation leading to thrombosis and complement activation. Together, the mechanical and biochemical effects of bubbles can increase blood viscosity, postcapillary resistance, transcapillary fluid loss, and hematocrit. These interactions can produce reperfusion injury, which occurs when toxic oxygen species such as superoxide, hydrogen peroxide, and hydroxyl radicals are generated after circulation has been re-established. Reperfusion injury may explain a poor response to hyperbaric therapy or relapse after initially successful treatment of DCS or CAGE. Relapse may occur due to the aggregation of leukocytes on damaged endothelium.

Clinical Presentation

Whether provoked by diving or by rapid ascent to altitude, DCS is a protean disease that can present with subtle symptoms and no signs. These may or may not worsen over minutes to hours. DCS may also present as a sudden catastrophic event with multiple symptoms and signs and multiple organ involvement. Table 30-5 lists the signs and symptoms reported in a series of naval and civilian cases of DCS.[18] The five most frequent signs or symptoms reported by Rivera[18] were pain (91.8%), numbness/paresthesia (21.2%), weakness (20.6%), rash (14.9%), and dizziness or vertigo (8.5%). A more recent study by Vann and colleagues[19] of 3,150 cases of DCS in recreational divers reported to the Divers Alert Network revealed the following five most frequent signs and symptoms: numbness (56.3%), limb pain (47.0%), weakness (24.9%), dizziness (22.9%), and fatigue (21.3%). Comparison of the two studies indicates that the number of DCS cases involving pain was less in the Vann series,[19] and that the number of cases with neurological symptoms (numbness/paresthesia, dizziness, and fatigue) was greater. The reasons for these differences are not clear. In Rivera's series,[18] most of the divers were military and probably reported their symptoms and were treated earlier, thereby preventing more serious symptoms. Military divers are also under more strict control regarding adherence to decompression schedules and may be more conservative than recreational divers

in selecting decompression schedules. Recreational divers also tend to make more repetitive dives, which could predispose them to more serious problems. Half of the divers in the Vann series[19] reported past medical diagnoses and 25% reported current medical disease. Whether these contributed to causing more serious DCS has not been established. Military divers are usually in excellent physical condition and are routinely screened for medical problems.

A minor symptom, itching skin (pruritus), known as "skin bends," is most common in dry chamber dives. Itching may be accompanied by an urticarial rash and is usually localized in well-perfused, exposed skin such as the ears, although it can occur anywhere on the body. Skin bends does not require treatment, but the diver should be observed for at least an hour for the onset of more-serious symptoms. A severe form of rash called "marbling" or "mottling" (cutis marmorata) appears as a pale area with cyanotic mottling. The area may enlarge, become hyperemic, and show swelling. Marbling does not require therapy but may be a harbinger of more-severe symptoms or signs that do require treatment.

Lymphatic obstruction appears as painless local edema, usually on the trunk. If it is severe the skin may have a "pigskin" appearance. Unilateral breast swelling and swelling of specific muscles may occur. In these cases, recompression may or may not help. Obstruction of the lymphatics usually disappears in a few days with or without treatment.

Joint pain and numbness are the most common DCS symptoms. The onset of pain may be gradual or abrupt, and its nature mild, severe, paroxysmal, aching, or boring. Severe cases may be associated with a cold sweat. Pain commonly increases with motion. Occasionally, the pain can be reduced by the application of local pressure with a sphygmomanometer cuff. A painful joint will sometimes have an associated area of numbness or altered sensation that may reflect a peripheral nerve lesion, but this is difficult to diagnose.

Divers with neurological symptoms should be recompressed as soon as possible to achieve the most complete relief and to forestall the onset of more-severe problems. Abdominal pain occurring in a circumferential pattern (girdle pain) signals the onset of spinal cord DCS. The pain may disappear after a short time but be followed within an hour or so by severe symptoms, usually paralysis of the lower extremities (see Exhibit 30-2).

In diving, DCS occurs in the upper extremities two to three times more often than in the lower extremities. The opposite is true for caisson workers, saturation divers, and ground-based altitude exposures simulating astronaut extravehicular activity. The reason for this difference may be due to the weight-bearing stresses of gravity in the latter cases. In divers, these stresses are relieved by immersion in water, which could reduce the formation and expansion of bubbles in the legs. CNS symptoms vary with the site of the tissue insult and are similar to those found in CNS disease from other causes. There is a wide range of symptoms (see Table 30-5). Any CNS symptom following diving is serious, and the patient should be recompressed as soon as possible for best results.

Only about 10% of symptoms begin during decompression, and usually only after longer, deeper dives. About 45% of symptoms occur within the first hour after surfacing, with an additional 12% (approximately) in the second hour. About 85% of symptoms appear within the first 6 hours. Occasionally the onset time is longer, but few symptoms appear after more than 24 hours Even though a symptom does not occur until 24 hours or longer after diving, the patient should be presumed to have DCS until this cause is ruled out. Symptoms with very long onset times sometimes respond to recompression and should not be dismissed as not dive-related, although this probability becomes small for symptoms that appear several days after surfacing.

Sequela: Aseptic Bone Necrosis

Aseptic bone necrosis is a delayed consequence of DCS that may not be evident until years after exposure (Figure 30-7). The condition is related to the occurrence of DCS and to the length of the diving career. Bone necrosis is found in 1% to 4%[8(p199)] of divers who observe standard diving practice. In divers who do not, the incidence can be as high as 50%.[20] Most of the lesions are in the midshaft of the humerus and femur, never cause symptoms, and are only identified by radiography. No treatment is required for lesions that do not cause symptoms. The most serious lesions are juxtaarticular. If these areas become necrotic and collapse, it may be necessary to replace the joint with a prosthesis.

Diving at Altitude and Altitude Exposure After Diving

There is increased danger of DCS whenever the barometric pressure is reduced soon after, or in association with, diving. Circumstances can include diving at altitude, mountain travel after diving, and flying after diving.

Diving at altitude requires reduced time on the bottom (bottom times) for no-stop decompression dives, and more decompression time for dives requiring decompression stops. The US Navy tables are not

TABLE 30-5

FREQUENCY OF SIGNS AND SYMPTOMS OF DECOMPRESSION SICKNESS

Sign or Sympton	Percentage of Patients With a Given Sign or Symptom (n=933)
Pain	91.8
Numbness/paresthesia	21.2
Weakness	20.6
Rash	14.9
Dizziness or vertigo	8.5
Nausea or vomiting	7.9
Visual distrubances	6.8
Paralysis	6.1
Headache	3.9
Unconsciousness	2.7
Urinary disturbance	2.5
Dyspnea or "chokes"	2.0
Personality change	1.6
Agitation, restlessness	1.3
Fatigue	1.2
Muscular twitching	1.2
Convulsions	1.1
Incoordination	0.9
Disturbance of equilibrium	0.7
Local edema	0.5
Intestinal disturbance	0.4
Auditory disturbance	0.3
Cranial nerve disturbance	0.2
Aphasia	0.2
Hemoptysis	0.2
Subcutaneous emphysema	0.1

Adapted with permission from Rivera JC. Decompression sickness among divers: An analysis of 935 cases. *Military Medicine: International Journal of AMSUS.* 1964;129(4):320.

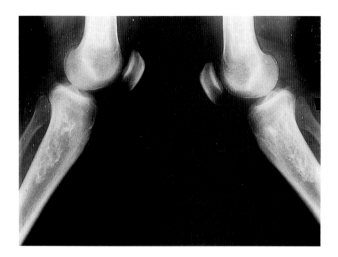

Fig. 30-7. A composite roentgenogram shows an abnormal pattern of calcification—shaft lesions—in both proximal tibias as a result of aseptic bone necrosis, a sequela of decompression sickness.

approved for use at altitudes higher than 2,300 ft (700 m). Because some depth gauges do not compensate for altitude, the depth of the dive should always be physically measured and the appropriate conversion made for fresh water (1 atm = 34 fsw). Decompression tables developed by Boni and colleagues[21] for use at altitude have received limited testing. No other tested tables exist. Ad hoc guidelines for adjusting sea level schedules for altitude have also been published in the recreational diving literature, but the adjustments simply increase the actual depth by a fraction to arrive at a corrected depth for table selection. There is no documentation of the efficacy of this method. Diving should be delayed for at least 12 hours after arriving at a high dive site to allow the nitrogen absorbed in the body to equilibrate to the reduced pressure. Without equilibration, the situation is similar to making a repetitive dive after decompression from a saturation dive at 1 ata.

Flying is common after recreational diving trips that may have lasted several days and involved many dives. During the subsequent flight home in a commercial aircraft, a diver may be exposed to a cabin altitude of as much as 8,000 ft (2,438 m), the maximum altitude permitted by the Federal Aviation Administration. To avoid DCS as a result of flying after diving, a diver must wait at sea level a sufficient time to allow excess nitrogen from diving to leave his body. A number of recommended preflight surface intervals have been published for single dives with no underwater stops for decompression; for example, 2 hours, US Navy; 12 hours, Divers Alert Network; and 24 hours, US Air Force.[22] The wide range of these guidelines indicates how few experimental data are available on which to base them. Recent experiments,[22] however, suggest that 2 hours is too short, while 12 hours may be satisfactory for some single dives and 24 hours conservative. Following multiple dives, on the other hand, a surface interval of at least 17 hours may be needed.

If air evacuation of a diving casualty is required, an aircraft capable of pressurization to 1 atm should be used. If such an aircraft is unavailable, and particularly for helicopter evacuation, the cabin altitude should not exceed 800 ft (242 m), and the diver should receive 100% oxygen during the flight. The administration of 100% oxygen is recommended during all types of transport of all casualties as a standard practice. The administration of 100% oxygen (not less) is particularly important as first aid for diving accidents.

Factors Affecting Individual Susceptibility

Several factors are known or suspected to affect susceptibility to DCS, among them inadequate decompression; exercise and body temperature as they affect perfusion; and individual characteristics such as age, obesity, and dehydration. The most common cause of DCS is inadequate decompression, which can result from ignorance or misapplication of the decompression schedules, panic, equipment failure, and other causes. Omitted decompression does not necessarily result in DCS, and DCS may occur even if the prescribed decompression is followed exactly. DCS has also occurred after dives that ordinarily do not require decompression stops. The severity of DCS does not correlate well with the amount of omitted decompression. Neurological DCS is more common after deeper dives than shallow dives. Repetitive diving (more than one dive in 12–24 h) may increase the risk of DCS.

Any physiological or environmental factor that changes local perfusion (eg, exercise, body temperature) also changes regional inert gas exchange. A change in perfusion may have a different effect on DCS risk depending on the phase of the dive in which it occurs (ie, at pressure, during decompression, or after decompression). For example, a factor that increases perfusion while a diver is at depth will increase inert gas uptake, but this same factor will increase its elimination if present during decompression. Factors that increase peripheral perfusion include exercise, immersion, and heat, while cold and dehydration decrease perfusion. Immersion and exercise at pressure have been demonstrated[23] to increase gas uptake and DCS risk. When multiple factors exist that change during a dive, the results may be difficult to anticipate. Mild exercise during decompression appears beneficial but may be confounded by exercise at pressure. The most disadvantageous situation probably occurs during a decompression dive, wherein the diver works at pressure and rests during decompression. In this instance, work at pressure increases the perfusion and warms the diver, while rest during decompression decreases perfusion and causes vasoconstriction from cooling.

Temperature and exercise also have effects unrelated to perfusion. Inert gas solubility decreases as the temperature rises. As a diver warms on the surface after a dive, the inert gas solubility falls and the dissolved gas tension and supersaturation rise. This fact may explain the anecdotal observations that hot showers precipitate DCS.

Exercise may mechanically aggravate the formation and expansion of bubbles by reducing the local absolute pressure in tissue and thus increasing the local supersaturation, which expands existing bubbles or micronuclei and may cause new nuclei to form. Human experimental evidence[23] indicates that exercise after decompression from diving or to altitude increases the DCS incidence. Note the distinction between exercise during and after decompression (or while breathing oxygen before altitude decompression). Exercise during decompression increases the elimination of inert gas by raising perfusion, while exercise after decompression, when bubbles are already present, can initiate or accelerate bubble expansion.

There is no demonstrated relationship between physical fitness and DCS risk. A high level of physical fitness, however, is essential for the diver to be able to manage the rigors of the underwater environment and deal with occasional emergencies.

Increasing age increases the risk of DCS. This has been variously reported[23] to be 2- to 9-fold higher in older (> 45 y) individuals; the lower figure appears to us to be more reasonable. The age effect may be related to decreased inert gas exchange efficacy and increased formation of gas nuclei.

Early observations of humans and animals indicated that obesity increases the risk of DCS, presumably because inert gas is more soluble in fatty than in aqueous tissue. These observations have not held up in recent studies,[23] however, perhaps because modern diving exposures are less severe than earlier exposures.

Dehydration reduces perfusion and inert gas elimination. Divers with DCS are often found to have elevated hematocrit values, perhaps from dehydration but perhaps also from increased capillary permeability resulting from DCS. Typical causes of dehydration in diving are alcohol consumption, low fluid intake, sweating in hot climates or diving suits, sea sickness, and cold or immersion-induced diuresis.

Experience with caisson workers[24] shows that the incidence of DCS is greatest during the first few days of repeated exposure to increased pressure. This may result from a depletion of the gas nuclei that appear to be the origin of bubbles. No acclimatization effect has been found in air diving, but it may be present in helium–oxygen diving.[25]

Several studies[26] suggest that women have a somewhat higher risk for DCS than men, both in aviation and during hyperbaric exposure. One study[27] showed that, at least in exposures to high altitudes, there was no difference between genders for DCS suseptibility. Whether the perceived differences are of clinical or operational significance is unknown at present, as are the causes of these differences, if they are real.

Other factors that have been proposed but not proven to increase the risk of DCS are previous injury (trauma or previous DCS), body position during decompression, increased carbon dioxide in the breathing gas, and fatigue.

Predicting and Preventing Decompression Sickness

Decompression Tables

The most important factors in reducing the risk of DCS are (*a*) limiting the time at depth to reduce inert gas uptake and (*b*) allowing for slow ascent so that inert gas may be harmlessly eliminated through the lungs. Death or permanent disability were common among divers and caisson workers in the 19th century, before this was understood. By the end of the century it was recognized that some type of slow decompression had to be used to prevent injury. Not until after the turn of the 20th century in England, when J. S. Haldane[28] began studying the problem systematically, were decompression schedules as we know them today constructed. Haldane realized that the manner of decompression used at the time, steady decompression at rates between 1.5 and 5 fsw/min, was too slow at deeper depths and too rapid at shallow. This allowed more inert gas to be absorbed at depth and not enough time for inert gas to be eliminated in shallow water. He devised the now-familiar staged decompression schedules, which use progressively longer stops near the surface. Modifications of the Haldane calculation methods are still the basis of many modern decompression schedules.

A decompression table contains multiple decompression schedules for a particular dive depth and bottom time. Each schedule defines the depths and duration of the decompression stops, and tables are available for diving with different inert gases and oxygen concentrations. Most were derived from empirical data with little testing in water, and testing has usually been done with only physically fit young men as subjects. Some schedules or parts of schedules have been tested and the rest calculated mathematically to fill in the gaps. Different environmental conditions and individual physiology were not considered. Nevertheless, current procedures make DCS a rare event and diving a relatively safe activity. Estimates of DCS incidence during actual diving are uncertain because record keeping is difficult. The DCS incidence when using the US Navy diving tables,[7,11] which all US military diving operations are required to use, is about 0.1%. We have reviewed various reports and, depending on the types of diving, commercial diving companies have had a rate of 0.1% to 3% in the past. The current rate of DCS in commercial diving in the United States is about 0.1% or less.[29]

Dive Computers

A dive computer measures the water pressure and automatically computes the diver's decompression requirement. Early pneumatic and analog dive computers were unreliable and were not widely accepted. Improvements in pressure transducer and digital technology coupled with the increasing popularity of recreational diving in the 1980s have made reliable mass-produced dive computers possible at reasonable cost. (Dive computers and computer models are also discussed and illustrated in Chapter 31, Military Diving Operations and Medical Support; see Figures 31-19 and 31–24.

The first commercially successful digital dive computer was tested without incident in 1983 dur-

ing 110 chamber dives. Many mass-produced dive computers are now available, their programs all using variants of the Haldane decompression algorithm, but no further decompression trials of dive computers have been conducted. The decompression "safety" of computer model and table diving is debated vigorously, but accident reports do not offer compelling evidence for a higher DCS incidence with computers. Accident data[30] compiled by the Divers Alert Network indicate that DCS occurs after deeper dives and after more multilevel and decompression dives with computers, but such data are insufficient for quantifying DCS risk.

Dive computers minimize errors in table selection by accurately tracking actual depth–time profiles. Also, because table selection no longer depends on using the deepest depth of the dive for the entire dive time as when using the standard tables, time underwater can usually be increased without a significant increase in decompression time. Therefore, dive computer models often provide very different diving guidelines than the US Navy tables.

Probability of Decompression Sickness and Acceptable Risk

Any dive profile might be called "safe" if an individual diver completes it without DCS. But is a dive safe if DCS occurs in 1 of 10 divers, or in 1 of 100? The answer depends on the definition of safety. Many human activities would be impossible if absolute safety—the complete absence of risk—were required. Safety is based on the level of risk a person is willing to accept. Thus, *safety* is defined as the *acceptable risk.*

Establishing acceptable risk is a two-part process. The first part determines the probability and severity of an injury and is a scientific problem that diving researchers are only beginning to understand. The second part decides what level of risk is acceptable and is a political activity. An individual might choose an acceptable risk for himself or might rely on the judgment of an organization such as the US Navy or the National Oceanic and Atmospheric Agency.

ADDITIONAL THREATS TO DIVERS

Thermal Stress

Divers are exposed to both heat and cold, although cold is a far more common environmental stress, and

diving is one of only a few situations in which healthy, active individuals may suffer serious hypothermia. This section discusses thermal stress only in divers. Immersion hypothermia in the wider population is discussed in detail in Chapter 18, Cold Water Immersion, in *Medical Aspects of Harsh Environments, Volume 1*.[31]

For a nude human at rest, the thermal comfort zone during immersion lies between 30°C and 35°C, depending on the individual's amount of subcutaneous fat. Therefore, diving in even tropical water (20°C–25°C) allows the body to lose heat faster than it can be generated. This is because the thermal conductivity and specific heat of water are, respectively, 25- and 1,000-fold greater than those of air. For the unprotected diver, it is cold rather than decompression that usually limits the dive time. Divers will be comfortable and require minimal protective clothing during several hours of moderate work at water temperatures of 23°C to 30°C. Thermal protection is required in water colder than 23°C.

The first indication of impending hypothermia is the feeling of being uncomfortably chilly. As hypothermia progresses, the hands become insensitive and manual dexterity decreases. With continuing exposure, the core temperature drops, the body increases heat production by shivering, the respiration rate rises, and gas consumption increases. Subsequently, coordination degenerates, thinking becomes difficult, and unconsciousness follows.

The most common thermal protection is passive, as with a wetsuit that traps a stagnant layer of warm water to prevent cold water from washing over the diver's skin. Wetsuits are made of closed air-filled cells that have the disadvantage of collapsing and providing less insulation as the water pressure increases. The drysuit is another passive system that allows no water to contact the diver's skin; it is commonly worn over underwear, which provides additional insulation. Wetsuits and drysuits are used by free-swimming divers. Tethered divers can have the advantage of active heating provided from the surface, and the hot-water wetsuit is common in military and commercial diving. A hot-water wetsuit fits the diver loosely, allowing hot (105°C) water to flow over the body. The hot water is exhausted through the wrist and ankle seals into the gloves and boots to keep the hands and feet warm. Close control of the water temperature is important to prevent skin burns.

Divers breathing helium–oxygen deeper than 300 fsw (91 msw) also lose heat through respiration even if the skin is comfortably warm. The breathing gas must be heated to avoid this problem.

Although the condition is much less common than hypothermia, divers can become hyperthermic while working in water warmer than 35°C, such as in the outflow of a power plant or the Red Sea.

Under these conditions, the temperature difference between the water and the diver's body is insufficient to eliminate metabolic heat by conduction or convection. Hyperthermia can also occur in a suited diver or a recompression chamber in a hot environment. Two saturation divers died of hyperthermia in the late 1970s or early 1980s when their chamber overheated (—JV, Jr, personal information). Shading the chamber or spraying cool water on it can reduce this problem.

The treatment for hypothermia or hyperthermia following diving is no different than that used to treat these conditions arising from other circumstances.

Underwater Blast Injury

Even in peacetime, divers work with explosives and may inadvertently be exposed to underwater blast. Blast is more dangerous in water than in air because the greater density and incompressibility of water allow the shock waves to travel further and lose less energy. A shock wave is reflected by tissue in air but is transmitted underwater. If the transmitted wave reaches a gas-filled cavity in the human body, the wave's energy is dissipated at the interface and great injury can occur. Multiple factors affect the severity of injury, including the size and type of explosive, thermal profile of the water, bottom composition, underwater banks or shoals, a nearby ship or structure, reflection from the sea bottom and the surface, and location of the explosive in the water column relative to the position of diver (Figure 30-8).

The out-rushing gas from an underwater detonation produces a shock wave called the initial pulse, which is characterized by a sudden pressure rise with exponential collapse. The initial pulse is followed by second and third expansions called the subsidiary and the bubble pulses. These cause less injury than the initial pulse unless they are reinforced by reflection from the bottom, the surface, or nearby structures. They may also cancel each other out.

Calculation of peak shock wave pressures is controversial and requires knowledge of empirical constants for each explosive. There is general agreement that injury is unlikely for peak shock wave pressures lower than 50 psi (< 345 kPa). Injury is likely for peak pressures between 50 and 500 psi (345–3,447 kPa), whereas serious injury occurs at 500 to 2,000 psi (3,447–13,790 kPa), and death is certain at pressures higher than 2,000 psi (> 13,790 kPa).

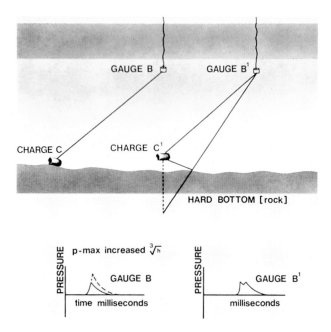

Fig. 30-8. The difference produced in a pressure wave-form by moving an explosion from the hard, rock bottom of a waterway (charge C) to slightly above the bottom (charge C¹). Because of the reflection of the original pressure wave from the hard, rock bottom (waveform, bottom right), a diver located in the position of pressure gauge B¹ (top) would experience two pressure peaks from an explosion at charge C¹. Compare this waveform with the one that a diver at gauge B would receive from an explosion at charge C (waveform, bottom left). Adapted with permission from Wakeley CPG. Effect of underwater explosives on the human body. *Lancet.* 1945;June 9:715.

Injury occurs by tissue shear in air-filled organs and by motion in solid organs. A shock wave travels through water and tissue at the same speed but compresses on reaching a tissue–gas interface (eg, in the middle ear, lungs, intestines) and tears (or "spalls") the tissue. The sudden motion of tissue by abdominal compression may damage solid organs, but only rarely.

Blast injury to the lung results from transmission of the shock waves through the chest rather than through the airways, with alveolar disruption, lacerations, and pinpoint-to-massive hemorrhage. A blast casualty may exhibit dyspnea, chest pain, and slowed breathing. Complications of lung damage include pulmonary edema and pneumonia. Lung damage can affect the heart, circulation, and nervous system. Vagal reflex may cause a transient bradycardia or asystole. Myocardial damage may occur due to gas embolism of the coronary arteries.

There may be hemothorax or pneumothorax, mediastinal emphysema, and contraction of the pulmonary capillary bed with an increase in pulmonary capillary pressure. Hemorrhages in the mucosa of the trachea and bronchial tree are common. Severe lung damage may lead to circulatory collapse. The CNS may be affected by transmission of the pressure to the cerebrospinal fluid, causing rupture of blood vessels in the brain. Other CNS damage may occur from gas embolism or hypoxia, owing to circulatory dysfunction. Transient paralysis, headaches and disorientation, delirium, amnesia and other symptoms of CNS damage can occur.

The gastrointestinal tract is thought to be more sensitive to blast injury than the lungs. The abdomen may be distended and silent. Intestinal vessels rupture, causing microhemorrhages in the gut wall and large bands of hemorrhage in the wall or massive hemorrhage into the lumen. Paralytic ileus can be present. The gastrointestinal tract can rupture and peritonitis ensue. Liver contusion probably occurs only in the most severe cases. Rectal bleeding may be the first sign of gastrointestinal problems.

Injury to the upper airway and the sinuses is not common, but there are records of tympanic membrane rupture and ossicle derangement, so the ear should not be overlooked as a site for damage.

A victim of underwater blast with no apparent injury should remain under observation, as late complications may occur. Treatment is the same as for acute total body trauma. All standard measures should be undertaken to combat shock and maintain respiration. Oxygen should be administered. Abdominal surgery must be considered if the clinical signs point to severe abdominal distress. Appropriate laboratory studies should be done as soon as possible. If cerebral or coronary gas embolism is suspected, recompression therapy must be considered, but this will require air evacuation to a medical center that can provide critical care in a recompression chamber.

Drowning and Near-Drowning

Drowning is defined as death from suffocation caused by immersion in a liquid, usually water. Near-drowning is defined as survival, at least temporarily, after suffocation by immersion. Three immersion suffocation syndromes are recognized: wet, dry, and salt-water aspiration. About 85% of drowning or near-drowning victims have aspirated water into their lungs (ie, the lungs are "wet"). The remaining 15% are "dry." In dry suffocation, the casualty becomes hypoxic because of laryngospasm or breath-holding. Death from the respiratory distress syndrome after a near-drowning is known as *secondary* drowning and is the cause of death in 10% to 25% of cases. In the third syndrome, called the salt-water aspiration syndrome, the severity of the effects of immersion is not sufficient to classify the case as one of near-drowning. These three syndromes are part of a common process with gradations in severity that depend on the extent of the pathophysiological changes.

The early stages of drowning and near-drowning are the same. During initial submersion or loss of respirable gas, breath-holding continues until the increasing concentration of arterial carbon dioxide forces inspiration or causes unconsciousness. If aspiration with laryngospasm occurs, the lungs will remain dry. Water is often swallowed at this point and may induce vomiting with aspiration of water or vomitus. As hypoxemia progresses, unconsciousness, arrhythmia, and circulatory arrest follow. However, most casualties involuntarily inspire water and will die if not immediately removed from the water. Survival is possible with adequate treatment. Factors associated with a poor prognosis after rescue are the following:

- age less than 3 years,
- submersion longer than 5 minutes,
- resuscitation delayed for longer than 15 minutes after rescue,
- seizures with posturing and fixed or dilated pupils,
- cardiopulmonary resuscitation required on admission to the emergency department,
- arterial pH lower than 7.10, and
- persistent coma.

The pathophysiology of drowning and near-drowning can be complex. Bradycardia and peripheral vasoconstriction may occur due to the mammalian diving reflex. Recovery is usually rapid if no fluid is aspirated. If more than 22 mL of water per kilogram of body weight have been aspirated, electrolyte changes may occur. Near-drowning victims will usually have aspirated less than 4 mL/kg, so electrolytes are usually within the normal range. Aspirated fresh water is absorbed rapidly through the alveolar membranes and can cause transient hypervolemia. Fresh water decreases pulmonary surfactant, leading to poorly ventilated or unventilated alveoli. Salt-water aspiration causes increased osmolality, with rapid fluid movement into the alveoli and loss of surfactant. The result in either case is hypoxemia. With

aspiration of as little as 1 to 3 mL of fluid per kilogram of body weight, the arterial oxygen tension can fall to 50% or less.

The clinical picture is largely a result of hypoxia or anoxia. The CNS may be undamaged, or the patient may show a decorticate or decerebrate response. Symptoms and signs of pulmonary pathology include dyspnea, retrosternal chest pain, frothy sputum (may be blood-tinged), tachypnea, cyanosis, crepitations, rales, and rhonchi. Chest roentgenograms may be normal or show patchy infiltrates or evidence of pulmonary edema. Adult respiratory distress syndrome, pneumonitis, bronchopneumonia, pulmonary abscess, and empyema may be secondary or late complications. Common cardiac problems are supraventricular rhythms or other dysrhythmias, hypotension, and shock. Cardiac output may be low, and failure of the right side of the heart may occur, owing to increased pulmonary vascular resistance. Other complications include decreased urinary output, renal failure, hemolysis with hemoglobinuria, and disseminated intravascular coagulation.

The single most important factor influencing long-term survival is immediate life support. Cardiopulmonary resuscitation, using 100% oxygen with positive pressure, should start as soon the casualty is removed from the water. If the patient is unconscious and appears to have cardiac arrest, intubation is recommended with administration of intravenous fluids. If hypothermia is present, further loss of body heat should be prevented until active rewarming can be done, if required by the degree of hypothermia. Drowning victims should be transferred to a medical treatment facility as soon as possible and placed on 100% oxygen even if they are in no apparent difficulty. Serious complications often arise up to 24 hours after near-drowning. As there are "miraculous" recoveries after 40 minutes of submersion, cardiopulmonary and other resuscitative measures should be continued until normal body temperature has been restored and death is without question. Factors that improve the chances of recovery from prolonged immersion include hypothermia, laryngospasm with gas in the lungs, and continuing pulmonary gas exchange despite fluid in the lungs. Hypothermia has a well-known protective effect against hypoxia, and when present, death cannot be assumed until the casualty has been rewarmed to normal body temperature.

Salt-water aspiration syndrome refers to events beginning with aspiration of small amounts of salt water, as may occur during buddy-breathing, breathing through a defective regulator, air-breathing on the surface, or snorkeling. The initial symptom is coughing with or without sputum. A latent period of 1 to 15 hours (most commonly 1–2 h) follows, after which the cough returns with dyspnea, retrosternal pain on inspiration, a feverish feeling, malaise, headache, anorexia, tachycardia, and shivering. The shivering may sometimes be severe and may be alleviated by a hot shower. Generalized aches and pains may be present. Signs include a mildly increased temperature, elevated heart rate, and generalized or localized rhonchi in the chest. The chest roentgenogram may show patchy consolidation or increased pulmonary markings. During the first 6 hours, the forced expiratory volume in 1 second and vital capacity may be decreased. Blood gases may show a decreased arterial oxygen partial pressure with normal or low arterial carbon dioxide partial pressure while breathing air. These signs and symptoms rarely continue for more than 24 hours. Treatment consists of oxygen administration to alleviate the pulmonary signs and symptoms, rest, and warmth. The major difficulty with the salt-water aspiration syndrome is differentiating it from other causes, including a lung or other infection, DCS, pulmonary barotrauma, or the effects of immersion in cold water. The diagnosis can be made on the basis of the confirmation of aspiration by the diver, a latent period between initial coughing and later symptoms, a rapid response to oxygen administration without recompression, and delayed symptom onset that is not compatible with the rapid onset of pulmonary barotrauma or gas embolism.

Pulmonary edema without aspiration of water has been reported[32] and termed *cold-induced pulmonary edema,* because all of the original cases appeared to be associated with diving in water temperatures of less than 12°C. However, the same authors reported a case that occurred in 27°C water, and reported several cases in divers who were in cold water but fully protected with drysuits. These same authors also reported multiple episodes in some divers. The cause for this is unknown. In the divers studied, no cardiac disease was found and there was no history of severe exertion. Clinically, severe dyspnea occurs at depth and is associated with cough, weakness, chest discomfort, wheezing, hemoptysis, expectoration of froth, and other usual symptoms of pulmonary edema. Signs include rales and roentgenographic evidence of pulmonary edema. The episodes last from 24 to 48 hours and may require standard therapy for pulmonary edema, although cases have resolved without treatment.

SUMMARY

Since the earliest days of breath-hold diving, the underwater environment has posed unique risks due to large pressure changes, hypoxia, and drowning. Immersion also distorts human vision and hearing. The introduction of compressed air and artificial gas mixtures extend diving range and duration but also create problems related to inert-gas effects and rapid ascent to the surface. A series of gas laws represented by simple equations describe the physical effects of pressure and temperature on gas volume and constituent partial pressures. Pressure change creates the potential for barotrauma in closed or functionally trapped gas pockets including the face mask, middle ear, inner ear, sinuses, and lungs, all of which are subject to problems on descent (compression or "squeeze") and ascent (expansion and possible rupture). Inhalation of compressed air or artificial gas mixtures at increased pressure readily leads to problems with oxygen toxicity, excess carbon dioxide, carbon monoxide poisoning, and narcosis due to nitrogen and other inert gases. At extreme depth, pressure itself produces effects collectively described as high-pressure nervous syndrome.

Early work with compressed air produced syndromes (called "caisson disease" or "bends") that were eventually recognized as the result of relatively rapid decompression. Ascent to the surface reduces ambient partial pressure of nitrogen or other inert gases, and the now-supersaturated tissues and blood tend to form bubbles, which underlie clinical problems ranging from cutaneous mottling to joint pain and a range of neurological problems. In addition, leakage of expanding gas from the pulmonary system into the circulation (arterial gas embolism) can lead to circulatory collapse and/or severe cerebral damage and death. Fortunately, these problems can be avoided by correct use of diving equipment and implementation of staged decompression to allow gradual desaturation of tissues without bubble formation. Treatment of decompression problems requires return to pressure in a hyperbaric chamber to shrink existing bubbles, followed by gradual decompression combined with inhalation of 100% oxygen to wash out inert gases. All military physicians, and not just those practicing Special Operations medicine, should be aware of the pathophysiology, prevention, and, if necessary, treatment of the unique hazards found in the underwater environment.

REFERENCES

1. Herodotus. *Urania.* Vol 3, Book 8. Beloe W, trans. New York, NY: Harper Bros; 1844. Cited by: Larson HE. *A History of Self-Contained Diving and Underwater Swimming.* Washington, DC: National Academy of Sciences, National Research Council: 1959: 5.

2. Beebe W. *Half Mile Down.* New York, NY: Duell, Sloane, and Pierce; 1934. Cited by: Larson HE. *A History of Self-Contained Diving and Underwater Swimming.* Washington, DC: National Academy of Sciences, National Research Council: 1959: 5.

3. Bachrach AJ. A short history of man in the sea. In: Bennett PB, Elliott DH, eds. *The Physiology of Diving and Compressed Air Work.* 2nd ed. Baltimore, Md: Williams & Wilkins; 1975: Chap 2.

4. Molenat FA, Boussages AH. Rupture of the stomach complicating diving accidents. *Undersea Hyperb Med.* 1995;22:87–96.

5. Waite CL. *Case Histories of Diving and Hyperbaric Accidents.* Bethesda, Md: The Undersea and Hyperbaric Medical Society; 1988: 52.

6. Greene KM. *Causes of Death in Submarine Escape Training Casualties: Analysis of Cases and Review of Literature.* Alverstoke, Gosport, England: Admiralty Marine Technology Establishment; 1978. AMTE(E) Report R78-402.

7. US Department of the Navy. *US Navy Diving Manual.* Vol 1. Washington, DC: DN; 1993. NAVSEA 0994-LP-001-9110. Rev 3.

8. Edmonds C, Lowry C, Pennefeather J. *Diving and Subaquatic Medicine.* 3rd ed. Oxford, England: Butterworth-Heinnemann; 1992.

9. Dutka AJ, Polychronides JE, Mink RB, Hallenbeck JM. *The Trendelenburg Position After Cerebral Air Embolism: Effects on the Somatosensory Evoked Response, Intracranial Pressure and Blood Brain Barrier.* Bethesda, Md: Naval Medical Research Institute; 1990. Report 90-16.

10. Evans DE, Catron PW, McDermott JJ, et al. Effect of lidocaine after experimental cerebral ischemia induced by air embolism. *J Neurosurg.* 1989;70:97–102.

11. US Department of the Navy. *US Navy Diving Manual.* Vol 2. Washington, DC: DN; 1991. NAVSEA 0994-LP-001-9020. Rev 3.

12. Smith JL. The pathological effects due to increase of oxygen tension in the air breathed. *Journal of Physiology, London.* 1899;24:19–35.

13. Wright WB. *Use of the University of Pennsylvania Institute for Environmental Medicine Procedures for Calculation of Pulmonary Oxygen Toxicity.* Panama City, Fla: US Navy Experimental Diving Unit; 1972. NEDU Report 2-72.

14. Bert P. *Barometric Pressure.* Hitchcock MA, Hitchcock FA, trans. Columbus, Ohio: College Book Co; 1943: 709–754, 859–890. Originally published in 1878.

15. Vann RD. Nitrox diving data review. In: Lang M, ed. *Diver's Alert Network Nitrox Workshop Proceedings.* Durham, NC: DAN; 2000: 19–29.

16. Lafay V, Barthelemy P, Comet B, Frances Y, Jammes Y. EDB changes during the experimental human dive HYDRA 10 (71 atm/7200 kPa). *Undersea Hyperb Med.* 1995;22:51–60.

17. Neuman TS, Bove AA. Combined arterial gas embolism and decompression sickness following no-stop diving. *Undersea Biomed Res.* 1990;17:429–436.

18. Rivera JC. Decompression sickness among divers: An analysis of 935 cases. *Mil Med.* 1964;129(4):314-334.

19. Vann RD, Bute BP, Uguccioni DM, Smith LR. Prognostic indicators in DCI in recreational divers. In: Moon R, Sheffield P, eds. *Treatment of Decompression Illness: 45th Undersea & Hyperbaric Medical Society Workshop.* Kensington, Md: The Undersea and Hyperbaric Medical Society; 1996: 352–363.

20. Oiwa H, Itoh A, Ikeda T, Sakurai S. Osteonecrosis of the long bones in diving fishermen. In: *Proceedings of the 9th International Symposium on Underwater and Hyperbaric Physiology.* Bethesda, Md: The Undersea and Hyperbaric Medical Society; 1987: 893–902.

21. Boni MM, Schmidt R, Nussberger P, Buhlmann AA. Diving at diminished atmospheric pressure: Air decompression tables for different altitudes. *Undersea Biomed Res.* 1976;3:189–204.

22. Vann RD, Gerth WA, Denoble PJ, Sitzes CR, Smith LR. A comparison of recent flying after diving experiments with published flying after guidelines. Proceedings of the Annual Scientific Meeting, The Undersea and Hyperbaric Medical Society, May 1996; Bethesda, Md. *Undersea Hyperb Med.* 1996;23(suppl):36.

23. Vann RD, Thalmann ED. Decompression physiology and practice. In: Bennett PB, Elliott DH, eds. *The Physiology and Medicine of Diving.* 4th ed. Philadelphia, Pa: WB Saunders; 1993; Chap 14.

24. Hempleman V. History of decompression procedures. In: Bennett PB, Elliott DH, eds. *The Physiology and Medicine of Diving.* 4th ed. Philadelphia, Pa: WB Saunders; 1993: Chap 13.

25. Eckenhoff RG, Hugher JS. Acclimatization to decompression stress. In: Bachrach AJ, Matzen MM, eds. *Proceedings of the 8th Symposium on Underwater Physiology.* Bethesda, Md: Undersea Medical Society; 1984: 93–100.

26. Taylor MB. Women and diving. In: Bove AA, Davis J, eds. *Diving Medicine.* 2nd ed. Philadelphia, Pa: WB Saunders; 1990: Chap 13: 157.

27. Webb JT, Pilmanis AA, Kraus KM, Kannen N. Gender and altitude-induced decompression sickness susceptibility. *Aviat Space Environ Med.* 1999;70:364.

28. Boycott AE, Damant GDD, Haldane JS. The prevention of compressed air illness. *J Hyg (Cambridge).* 1908;8:342–443.

29. Reedy J. Past President, Association of Diving Contractors, Labadieville, La. Personal communication, March 2001.

30. Diver's Alert Network. *Report on Decompression Illness and Diving Fatalities.* Durham, NC: DAN; 1997.

31. Pandolf KS, Burr RE, Wenger CB, Pozos RS, eds. *Medical Aspects of Harsh Environments, Volume 1.* In: Zajtchuk R, Bellamy RF, eds. *Textbook of Military Medicine.* Washington, DC: Department of the Army, Office of The Surgeon General, and Borden Institute; 2001. In press.

32. Hampson NB, Dunford RG. Pulmonary edema of scuba divers. *Undersea Hyperb Med.* 1997;24:29–33.

RECOMMENDED READING

Shilling CW, Carlston CB, Mathias RA. *The Physician's Guide to Diving Medicine.* New York, NY: Plenum Press; 1984.

Chapter 31

MILITARY DIVING OPERATIONS AND MEDICAL SUPPORT

RICHARD D. VANN, PhD[*]; AND JAMES VOROSMARTI, JR, MD[†]

[*]Captain, US Navy Reserve (Ret); Divers Alert Network, Center for Hyperbaric Medicine and Environmental Physiology, Box 3823, Duke University Medical Center, Durham, North Carolina 27710
[†]Captain, Medical Corps, US Navy (Ret); Consultant in Occupational, Environmental, and Undersea Medicine, 16 Orchard Way South, Rockville, Maryland 20854

INTRODUCTION

Divers breathe gases and experience pressure changes that can cause different injuries from those encountered by most combatant or noncombatant military personnel. This chapter places diving hazards and the therapy of diving casualties in historical and operational context. There are no formal data from which accurate estimates of diving populations can be estimated, but recreational dive training statistics suggest there are currently some 2 to 4 million active divers in the world, most participating in sport or recreation. Those of concern in this chapter are the 4,000 to 5,000 divers of the US military, a number that appears to be in decline since the end of the Cold War. An informal survey suggests there are some 5,000 to 10,000 military divers in other nations of the world.

The US Navy has responsibility for all diving by US forces, and most US military divers are in the Navy. All diving operations by US forces must be conducted in accordance with the *US Navy Diving Manual*[1] and related directives. As of this writing, approximately 3,000 Navy divers typically conduct some 100,000 dives annually. About 1,500 divers are in diving and salvage and 1,500 are in Naval Special Warfare (NSW). Diving and salvage forces include four ARS-50 *Safeguard*-class salvage ships, Explosive Ordnance Disposal (EOD) units, two Mobile Diving and Salvage Units (MDSUs), two Underwater Construction Teams (UCTs), a Consolidated Diving Unit, and teams assigned to submarine tenders and shore-based ship repair facilities. The diving and salvage forces conduct salvage, search and recovery, underwater mine clearance, underwater construction, security inspections, and ships husbandry tasks such as hull cleaning and maintenance.

Salvage divers receive basic training at the Navy Diving and Salvage Training Center (NDSTC), Panama City, Florida, and some qualify in the Mark (Mk) 21 Mod 1 mixed-gas diving helmet (Figure 31-1) to a depth of 90 meters of seawater (msw; equivalent to 300 feet of seawater [fsw]). EOD divers receive basic training at the Explosive Ordnance Disposal School, Indian Head, Maryland, and later qualify in the Mk 16 Underwater Breathing Apparatus (UBA), which is used for mine clearance. About 100 US Navy divers specialize in saturation diving using Personnel Transfer Capsules (PTCs) and Deck Decompression Chambers (DDCs).

Of the 1,500 combat swimmer and divers in Naval Special Warfare, most are in six SEAL (*sea*, *air*, *land*) teams and two SEAL delivery vehicle (SDV) teams. SEALs are trained for reconnaissance and direct action missions at rivers, harbors, shipping, and coastal facilities in restricted or denied waters. SEAL divers operate from surface craft, submerged submarines, and miniature wet submersibles (which are SDVs). Insertion by fixed or rotary wing aircraft is also possible. All SEALs qualify in open-circuit and closed-circuit oxygen scuba (self-contained underwater breathing apparatus), and those assigned to SDV teams receive additional training in the Mk 16. SEALs are part of the Special Operations Forces that include about 1,000 US Army, Air

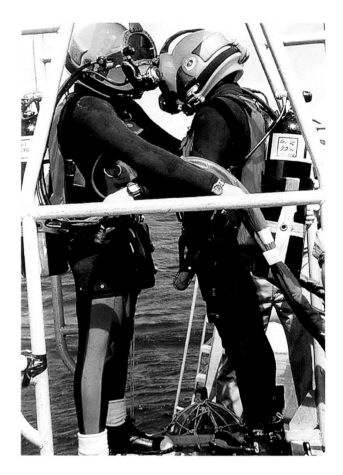

Fig. 31-1. Both divers are wearing the US Navy Mark (Mk) 21 Mod 1 Underwater Breathing Apparatus for helium–oxygen diving to 90 msw (300 fsw). Reprinted from US Department of the Navy. *US Navy Diving Manual.* SS521-Ag-PRO-010. Washington, DC: Naval Sea Systems Command. Rev 4 (20 Jan 1999); Change A (1 Mar 2001): p13-12. NAVSEA 0994-LP-100-3199.

Force, and Marine Corps divers, who have narrower training and missions and dive less frequently. SEALs train at the Naval Special Warfare Center (NSWC), Coronado, California, while divers from other services train at NDSTC, Panama City, or at the US Army Underwater Swim School, Key West, Florida.

Other military divers include about 100 from the US Air Force for rescue, about 100 from the US Army for port facility maintenance, and fewer than 50 from the US Coast Guard for rescue and pollution response. The military also employs civil service divers and contracts with commercial diving companies for specific projects. Military personnel and dependents with military or civilian diving training are an unofficial military diving population who participate in recreational diving and can develop diving-related illnesses not in the line of duty.

Training in diving medicine for military physicians is conducted by the US Navy for all US forces and occasionally for foreign militaries. Instruction includes 6 weeks of practical diving training and 3 weeks of diving medicine in Panama City. Navy Undersea Medical Officers (UMOs) receive 12 weeks of additional training in submarine-specific issues at the Naval Undersea Medicine Institute (NUMI), New London, Connecticut. Training is followed by an operational tour with a submarine squadron, fleet diving unit, or NSW command. Operational tours are typically succeeded by assignment to administrative positions, graduate education, research at the Navy Experimental Diving Unit

(NEDU), Panama City, or medical specialty residency training. There are fewer than 100 UMOs on active duty but others are in the reserves. Diving medicine training for noncommissioned officers is conducted by the Navy in Coronado and Panama City and by the Army in Key West.

The unique medical support requirements for diving are a result of the physiological, engineering, and environmental challenges present underwater. These challenges are nicely illustrated by examples from diving history. Breath-hold is the simplest form of diving and although uncommon in current military operations except for submarine escape training, its physics and physiology are a good basis for understanding many of the respiratory and circulatory adjustments to UBAs. A UBA extends the time at elevated pressure leading to the potential for hypothermia, nitrogen narcosis, oxygen toxicity, carbon dioxide poisoning, arterial gas embolism (AGE), and decompression sickness (DCS). Military diving physicians require broad training for the wide range of missions they may support, but military physicians may also consult concerning civilian diving casualties, as many military personnel or their dependents are recreational divers. In addition to these hazards, divers must cope with threats posed by various forms of marine life. Medical officers need to be mindful of all the problems, not the respiratory ones exclusively, that military divers and swimmers may encounter in the marine environment.

BREATH-HOLD DIVING

Breath-hold diving, or free diving, requires little equipment and provides examples of many physical and physiological constraints of the underwater environment. Free diving was an essential operational technique in the Pacific Theater of Operations during World War II (Exhibit 31-1) and remains a fundamental skill for present-day combat swimmers.

Figure 31-2 shows pressures to which a diver must adapt during descent. The pressure at sea level is 1 atmosphere absolute (1 ata; 14.7 pounds per square inch [psi] absolute [psia]). With each 10 msw (33 fsw) of descent, a diver is exposed to an additional atmosphere of pressure. The forward escape trunk of a submarine during lock-out and lock-in operations of combat swimmers (ie, entering and leaving a submarine via an escape trunk that can be flooded or drained and the pressure increased or decreased; discussed below in Submarine Res-

cue and Escape) is at about 9 msw (30 fsw; 1.9 ata [which refers to the absolute, or total, pressure; atm, on the other hand, refers to the partial pressure of gases]). The standard depth for treating DCS (see Chapter 30, Physics, Physiology, and Medicine of Diving) is 18 msw (60 fsw; 2.8 ata). For diving with scuba in the US Navy and in civilian recreational diving, the usual depth limit is 39 msw (130 fsw; 4.9 ata).

The breath-hold diver must anticipate and compensate for the compression of gas-containing spaces in the body that occurs during descent according to Boyle's law: the volume of a given mass of gas varies inversely with absolute pressure when temperature is held constant (the gas laws are described in Chapter 30, Physics, Physiology, and Medicine of Diving). The middle ear requires active inflation to avoid otic or aural barotrauma (ear squeeze), which is the most common medical prob-

---

EXHIBIT 31-1

AMPHIBIOUS WARFARE IN THE PACIFIC

When the landing craft bottomed-out and the bow ramps dropped on the island of Tarawa on November 20, 1943, US Marines waded off a barrier reef and into a deep lagoon. Many drowned and more were killed or wounded during the long walk to the beach. This disaster gave rise to the Underwater Demolition Teams (UDT), whose mission was to chart off-shore waters and destroy natural or man-made obstacles that could impede an invasion force.[1]

Under cover of heavy naval gunfire on the morning before an invasion, UDT swimmers wearing facemasks and swim fins were dropped about half a mile off-shore and swam to and from the beach recording the water depths shallower than 3.5 fathoms (6.4 msw; 21 fsw) with lead-lines and slates while examining the bottom for obstacles. On returning seaward, they formed a pick-up line and were snared by a passing boat, one by one, with a rubber loop thrown over an outstretched arm. The rare swimmer who missed his pick-up swam to sea hoping for a passing destroyer.[1]

Information obtained from the hydrographic reconnaissance was converted into a beach chart for planning the amphibious landing. The swimmers returned the following morning and fixed demolition charges to preassigned obstacles during breath-hold dives. When all obstacles were connected by detonating cord, the swimmers retired to seaward while a pair of fuse-pullers attached and ignited firing assemblies with 10 to 15 minute delays. The fuse-pullers—usually the fastest swimmers—freestyled seaward. This was the only time that underwater recovery strokes were not required.[1]

In 1983, the Underwater Demolition Teams were converted to SEAL teams or SDV teams. Today's students at Basic Underwater Demolition/SEAL (BUD/S) training are still taught breath-hold diving, hydrographic reconnaissance, and combat demolition, but these techniques see only occasional use such as the 1983 combat hydrographic reconnaissance conducted in Grenada (*Operation Urgent Fury*) or the decoy combat demolition during the 1991 invasion of Kuwait in the Gulf War (*Operation Desert Storm*).

Source: (1) Fane FD. *The Naked Warriors*. Annapolis, Md: Naval Institute; 1995.

---

lem in diving, but the lungs are also affected, sometimes fatally, in breath-hold diving (Case Study 1).

Case Study 1: Fatal Lung Squeeze. A 28-year-old US Navy Underwater Demolition Team diver was free-diving in 24 msw (80 fsw) in Subic Bay, Philippines, in 1968. After a series of uneventful dives, he was found unconscious and face-up at 12 msw (40 fsw) while sinking slowly. On rescue, he was apneic and bleeding frothy, bright, red blood from the mouth. He became coherent 45 minutes later but developed progressive dyspnea and cyanosis and died 3 hours later. At autopsy, his lungs were congested and edematous with interstitial and intraalveolar hemorrhage.[2]

Figure 31-3 represents a breath-hold diver with a total lung capacity of 6 L and a residual lung volume of 1.5 L. If this diver performed a maximal inhalation on the surface (1 ata) and descended for a free dive, Boyle's law predicts that the lung volume would decrease to 3 L at 10 msw (33 fsw; 2 ata) and 2 L at 20 msw (66 fsw; 3 ata). On reaching 30 msw (99 fsw; 4 ata), the lung volume equals the 1.5-L residual volume.

With greater descent, the elasticity of the chest wall resists further reduction in volume and the alveolar pressure becomes less than the absolute pressure, which is transmitted equally throughout all solid and liquid tissues in accordance with Pascal's law: pressure exerted at any point on a confined liquid is transmitted uniformly in all directions. This phenomenon causes a relative vacuum between alveolar gas and alveolar capillary blood and leads to engorgement of the alveolar capillaries as blood shifts from peripheral tissues into the thorax. Further descent is possible because these fluid shifts reduce the residual volume.

The fluid-shift effect is illustrated by record free dives to depths in excess of 100 msw (330 fsw). Suppose, for example, a diver with a 7.22-L total lung capacity and a 1.88-L residual volume achieved a depth of 105 msw (346 fsw).[3] By Boyle's law, the ratio of these volumes specifies 28 msw (93 fsw) as the depth at which the lungs are compressed to residual volume. To reach 105 msw, the residual volume would have to be reduced to 0.63 L, representing a 1.25-L shift of blood from peripheral vessels

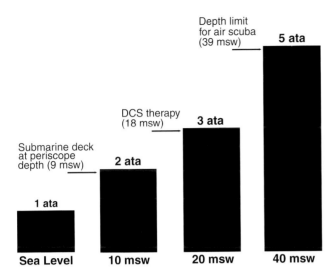

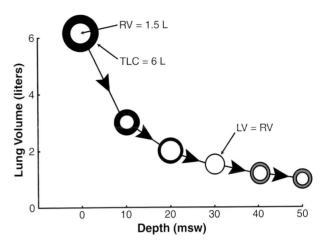

Fig. 31-2. Benchmark seawater pressures. The standard pressure at sea level is defined as 1 atmosphere absolute (1 ata, or 760 mm Hg). Each 10 meters of seawater (msw) (equivalent to 33 ft of seawater [fsw]) of descent adds an additional atmosphere of pressure. The deck of a submarine at periscope depth during lock-out and lock-in of combat swimmers is at about 9 msw (30 fsw). (Divers "lock-out" from and "lock-in" to a submarine when they enter and leave through an escape trunk that can be flooded or drained while the pressure is increased or decreased to allow transition from lower submarine pressure to higher sea pressure.) Decompression sickness (DCS) is usually treated at a pressure of 2.8 ata (18 msw; 60 fsw). The depth limit for open-circuit compressed air scuba is 39 msw (130 fsw).

Fig. 31-3. Compression of the lungs during descent on a breath-hold dive. The diver with a residual lung volume (RV) of 1.5 L (white center of circles) begins on the surface with a 4.5 L vital capacity inhalation (black circles) to a total lung capacity (TLC) of 6 L. During descent, the lung volume (LV) decreases in inverse proportion to the absolute pressure, as described by Boyle's law. At 4 ata (30 msw; 99 fsw), the lung volume equals the residual volume. With additional descent, the elasticity of the thorax impedes further compression, leading to a relative vacuum in the lungs. Blood from the peripheral circulation shifts into the pulmonary capillaries (gray circles), which then reduces the residual lung volume (white centers) and allows descent to 40 and 50 msw (132 and 165 fsw).

to pulmonary capillaries. There is indirect evidence that such blood shifts do occur, but reductions in residual volume may also result from elastic compression of the chest wall and upward shift of the abdominal contents.

Descent to too great a depth causes compression of the thorax to beyond its elastic limit, and the resulting chest pain signals the diver to ascend, as in Case Study 2, below. Failure or inability to heed this warning pain could cause lung squeeze, thoracic squeeze, or chest squeeze, in which chest wall compression, intraalveolar vacuum, or both, damage the thorax and lungs. Thoracic squeeze is rare because of chest pain, but the diver in Case Study 1, above, appears to have lost consciousness, exhaled passively, and descended due to negative buoyancy according to Archimedes' principle: any object immersed in liquid will be buoyed up by a force equal to the weight of the water displaced. In such a circumstance, the warning chest pain would have gone unnoticed.

Case Study 2: Unconsciousness on Ascent. A 29-year-old Underwater Demolition Team diver making a breath-hold dive in the US Navy Submarine Escape Tower in Hawaii in 1971 noted chest pain at 27 msw (90 fsw) during descent, and he began his ascent. On reaching 12 msw (40 fsw), he experienced severe dyspnea followed by euphoria at 6 msw (20 fsw). Just before surfacing, he became unconsciousness and convulsed after being pulled from the water. Recovery was uneventful.

The symptoms reported in Case Study 2 are clues to the mechanisms responsible for the not-uncommon "breath-hold blackout" that occurs in breath-hold swimming and diving. (Breath-hold blackout is sometimes called "shallow-water blackout." The term "shallow-water blackout" originated during World War II and is discussed below in Closed-Circuit Oxygen Scuba.) There is an inherent risk of unconsciousness during diving or breath-hold swimming in shallow water if time underwater is prolonged inadvertently, by hyperventilation, or by will power. This has been a causative factor in many cases of unconsciousness or drowning.[3]

Hypercapnia and hypoxia are the principal causes of the ventilatory drive that is responsible for dyspnea. In severe hypoxia, euphoria often precedes unconsciousness, and hypoxic seizures are not uncommon (as in Case Study 2.) In the early 1960s, Edward H. Lanphier, MD, and Hermann Rahn, PhD, conducted experiments in a hyperbaric chamber to demonstrate the changes that occur to gases in the lungs during breath-hold and breath-hold diving. Figure 31-4a illustrates the progressive rise in end-tidal carbon dioxide partial pressure and the fall in oxygen partial pressure during a breath-hold experiment at sea level.[4] Gases were sampled from a bag into which the subject exhaled (and reinhaled) every 10 seconds. Hypoxic and hyper-

capnic ventilatory drive caused a break in breath-hold at 60 seconds at well above the 20 to 30 mm Hg (0.04 atm) alveolar oxygen partial pressure at which there is a risk of unconsciousness.

In another experiment (Figure 31-4b),[5] a subject made a breath-hold dive to 10 msw (33 fsw). The end-tidal oxygen and carbon dioxide partial pressures increased during descent, as described by Dalton's law of partial pressures: the total pressure exerted by a mixture of gases is equal to the sum of the pressures that each gas would exert if it alone occupied the container. While at depth, the oxygen partial pressure decreased owing to the subject's

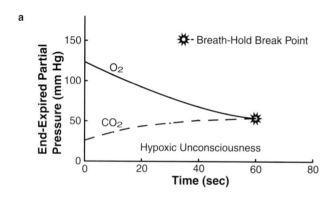

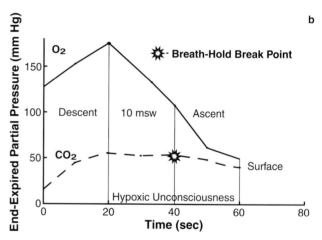

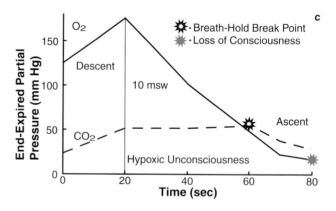

Fig. 31-4. (a) Effects of breath-hold at sea level on end-tidal oxygen and carbon dioxide. End-exhalation oxygen and carbon dioxide partial pressures were measured at 10-second intervals when the subject exhaled into a bag and then reinhaled. There was a progressive decrease in the oxygen partial pressure and an increase in the carbon dioxide partial pressure. Breath-hold breakpoint occurred when the sum of the hypoxic and hypercapnic ventilatory drives became too great to withstand. **(b)** Effects of breath-hold on end-tidal oxygen and carbon dioxide during a 10 msw (33 fsw) dive. The oxygen and carbon dioxide partial pressures increased on descent to 10 msw (33 fsw) according to Dalton's law of partial pressures: the total pressure exerted by a mixture of gases is equal to the sum of the pressures that each gas would exert if it alone occupied the container. While at depth, oxygen was continually removed from the lungs by the circulation to replenish metabolic consumption. Carbon dioxide remained relatively constant, as its alveolar partial pressure was greater than that in the arterial blood. Breath-hold breakpoint occurred entirely as a result of hypercapnic ventilatory drive, since the oxygen was well above the onset point of hypoxic drive. The oxygen and carbon dioxide partial pressures decreased on ascent, again according to Dalton's law. **(c)** Effects of breath-hold on end-tidal oxygen and carbon dioxide during a 10 msw (33 fsw) dive after hyperventilation. Hyperventilation eliminates carbon dioxide and delays the onset of hypercapnic ventilatory drive, which is responsible for the breath-hold breakpoint. Additional oxygen is consumed during the extended breath-hold, and on ascent, the oxygen partial pressure falls below the level needed to sustain consciousness. Graph a: Adapted with permission from Lanphier EH, Rahn H. Alveolar gas exchange during breath-hold diving. *J Appl Physiol*. 1963;18:471–477. Graphs b and c: Adapted with permission from Lanphier EH, Rahn H. Alveolar gas exchange during breath holding with air. *J Appl Physiol*. 1963;18:478–482.

metabolism, but it remained above the 50 to 60 mm Hg level at which the hypoxic ventilatory drive begins. Carbon dioxide actually diffused from the lungs into the blood because of its higher alveolar partial pressure. Hypercapnic ventilatory drive forced the subject to ascend after 40 seconds at 10 msw (33 fsw), and the oxygen and carbon dioxide partial pressures decreased, again due to Dalton's law.

In yet another experiment,[5] the subject dived to 10 msw (33 fsw) after hyperventilating to eliminate carbon dioxide and delay the onset of the hypercapnic ventilatory drive (Figure 31-4c). This extended his dive time by 20 seconds, during which oxygen metabolism continued but without inducing hypoxic ventilatory drive. When hypercapnia finally caused the diver to ascend, his oxygen partial pressure fell to below 40 mm Hg, and he exhibited cyanosis, confusion, and loss of control.

Lanphier and Rahn's experiments took place under close supervision in a dry, hyperbaric chamber. Underwater, the outcome might have been different. The diver in Case Study 2 could have drowned, for example, or met a fate similar to that described in Case Study 1, had he not been rescued.

CENTRAL NERVOUS SYSTEM OXYGEN TOXICITY IN COMBAT DIVERS

During World War II, Italian and British divers used oxygen diving effectively for hydrographic reconnaissance, ship attack, and with submersible craft, but fatalities were common due to loss of consciousness and subsequent drowning in both training and combat. Cerebral oxygen toxicity (gas toxicities are discussed in Chapter 30, Physics, Physiology, and Medicine of Diving) was one cause of these difficulties, and recommended maximum exposures of 120 minutes at 15 msw (50 fsw) or 30 minutes at 27 msw (90 fsw) provided inadequate protection. To better define safe limits for oxygen diving, the Royal Navy established a program that exposed human volunteers to various oxygen pressures and durations. The experience of one volunteer, quoted below, is instructive Case Study 3:

Case Study 3: Oxygen Convulsions During 30 Minutes at 50 fsw. I suddenly felt a violent twitching of my lips. ... [M]y mouth was blown out like a balloon. ... The twitching ... increased, and I felt a terrific tingling sensation at the side of my mouth as if someone were touching it with a live wire. This ... became a definite pain ... . [M]y lips became so distorted ... as if my mouth were stretched to my right ear. ... Although my lips formed words, no sound came. ... [B]lackness closed in on me—I was out.[6(pp60–61)]

A seizure is the most spectacular and objective sign of central nervous system (CNS) oxygen toxicity, but there is no evidence that it leads to permanent damage if the oxygen exposure is promptly discontinued (assuming, of course, that drowning and physical injury are avoided). Experimental oxygen exposures are often terminated by the subject when symptoms, including abnormal breathing, nausea, twitching, dizziness, incoordination, and visual or auditory disturbances, are noted. These symptoms also occur during operational exposures but do not necessarily precede convulsions.

Factors that elevate cerebral blood flow also augment oxygen delivery to the brain, which appears to increase susceptibility to oxygen toxicity. These factors include immersion, exercise, and carbon dioxide. Carbon dioxide may be present in the inspired gas or may be retained in the body, owing to inadequate ventilation caused by high gas density or external breathing resistance. Some people appear to have a lower than normal response to hypercarbia and are known as "carbon dioxide retainers." The primary treatment for all forms of oxygen toxicity is to reduce the partial pressure of inspired oxygen to a nontoxic level.

Oxygen exposure limits have been established to reduce the risk of convulsions for divers breathing pure oxygen or the oxygen in nitrogen–oxygen gas mixes; Figure 31-5 shows the exposure limits for pure oxygen[1] and for oxygen in mixed gas.[7] Oxygen exposure limits are based on very few data, and these data can be highly variable (compare Figures 31-5 and 31-18). Chamber trials and experience in open water indicate that convulsions occasionally occur near or within the accepted oxygen exposure limits. The incidents of convulsions or symptoms of CNS oxygen toxicity that have occurred in US Navy experiments are shown in Figure 31-5. Incidents with nitrogen–oxygen gas mixes were observed at lower oxygen partial pressures than incidents with pure oxygen. This is the reason that the oxygen exposure limits are more conservative for nitrogen–oxygen mixes than for pure oxygen. Nitrogen–oxygen mixes have higher gas densities than oxygen, as they are used at greater depths. The higher gas densities are believed to cause greater carbon dioxide retention within the body, which increases susceptibility to oxygen toxicity.

Fig. 31-5. Central nervous system (CNS) oxygen toxicity exposure limits for 100% oxygen and nitrogen–oxygen mixes. The dashed line describes the US Navy limits for single dives with 100% oxygen.[1] The solid line describes the National Oceanographic and Atmospheric Administration's (NOAA's) limits for exposure to oxygen in mixed gas.[2] The triangles represent CNS oxygen toxicity symptoms or convulsions during experiments with 100% oxygen that were conducted by the US Navy, and the squares represent symptoms or convulsions with nitrogen–oxygen mixes.[3–8] The mixed-gas limits are more conservative than the 100% limits because symptoms and convulsions occurred at lower oxygen partial pressures when nitrogen–oxygen mixes were breathed.

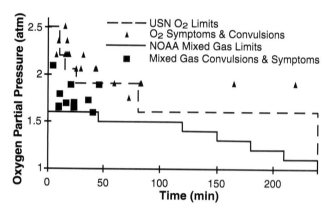

Data sources: (1) US Department of the Navy. *US Navy Diving Manual*. SS521-Ag-PRO-010. Washington, DC: Naval Sea Systems Command. Rev 4 (20 Jan 1999); Change A (1 Mar 2001): p18-14. NAVSEA 0994-LP-100-3199. (2) National Oceanographic and Atmospheric Administration. *NOAA Diving Manual*. 4th ed. Washington, DC: US Department of Commerce; 2001: 16-9. (3) Lanphier EH. *Nitrogen-Oxygen Mixture Physiology: Phases 1 and 2*. Panama City, Fla: Navy Experimental Diving Unit; 1955. NEDU Report 7-55. (4) Butler FK Jr, Thalmann ED. CNS oxygen toxicity in closed-circuit scuba divers. In: Bachrach AJ, Matzen MM, eds. *Underwater Physiology, Vol 8*. Bethesda, Md: Undersea Medical Society, Inc; 1984. (5) Butler FK Jr, Thalmann ED. CNS oxygen toxicity in closed-circuit scuba divers: II. *Undersea Biomed Res*. 1986;13(2):193–223. (6) Butler FK. *Central Nervous System Oxygen Toxicity in Closed-Circuit Scuba Divers: III*. Panama City, Fla: Navy Experimental Diving Unit; 1986. NEDU Report 5-86. (7) Piantadosi CA, Clinton RL, Thalmann ED. Prolonged oxygen exposures in immersed exercising divers at 25 fsw (1.76 ata). *Undersea Biomed Res*. 1979;6:347–356. (8) Schwartz HJC. *Manned Testing of Two Closed-Circuit Underwater Breathing Apparatus: US Navy Emerson Rig and Fenzy PO.68*. Panama City, Fla: Navy Experimental Diving Unit; 1984. NEDU Report 13-84.

UNDERWATER BREATHING APPARATUSES

A UBA provides the diver with a continuous and reliable supply of physiologically safe breathing gas. The use of such devices by the military became prominent in World War II, when they were used by the "human torpedoes" (see the Section IV frontispiece in this textbook) and by the divers who cleared the Normandy beaches of German countermeasures before the D day invasion (Exhibit 31-2). There are two broad categories of UBAs, surface supplied (or tethered) and self-contained, and each of these has a number of subcategories with advantages and disadvantages that lend to a particular operational utility.

Open-Circuit Self-Contained Underwater Breathing Apparatus: The Aqualung

The most familiar and common UBA in use today is the open-circuit, compressed-air self-contained underwater breathing apparatus (scuba), also known as the aqualung. This concept was first conceived and implemented in the 19th century[8] but did not become practical until Cousteau and Gagnan applied 1940s technology (Exhibit 31-3).[9] Improvements have been continuous since then, and compressed-air scuba is presently used by millions of divers throughout the world.

Open-circuit scuba consists of one or more tanks

of gas compressed to a pressure of 137 to 341 ata (2,000–5,000 psi gauge [psig]). A first-stage pressure regulator attached to the tanks reduces their high pressure to an intermediate pressure of about 7 atm (100 psig) over the ambient water pressure. During inhalation, a second-stage regulator, held in the diver's mouth, reduces the intermediate pressure to ambient. The system is described as "demand" and "open-circuit" because the diver inhales on demand and exhales directly into the water.

The partial pressures of oxygen and nitrogen change with depth for divers breathing air or 100% oxygen (Figure 31-6). With pure oxygen, there is a significant risk of CNS oxygen toxicity at 10 msw (33 fsw), while with compressed air, which is only 21% oxygen, there is no oxygen CNS toxicity risk until depths of about 57 to 66 msw (187–218 fsw) are reached.

Surface-Supplied Diving

UBAs became possible with the invention of the air compressor in the 18th century during the industrial revolution, but the first practical equipment did not appear until about 1828, when the Deane brothers in England developed an open helmet that rested on the diver's shoulders.[10] Hand-driven pumps on the surface supplied the helmet with air through a hose, and excess air escaped around the shoulders, but the helmet would flood if the diver leaned over too far. When the men operating the hand-pumps on the surface became tired or when the diver was deeper than about 45 msw (150 fsw), work became impossible, as the air supply was insufficient to remove carbon dioxide.

Further developments by the Siebe-Gorman Div-

EXHIBIT 31-2

AMPHIBIOUS WARFARE IN NORMANDY: OPERATION OVERLORD

Hydrographic reconnaissance and obstacle clearance in the English Channel before the invasion of Europe on June 6, 1944, in Operation Overlord, were quite different than they were in the Pacific. The tidal zone off the Normandy beaches was 300 yd broad, with a tidal range of 25 ft and a speed of rise of 8 min/ft. Row after row of steel, concrete, rock, and wooden obstacles had been emplaced by German forces, in anticipation of an invasion.[1]

Hydrographic reconnaissance was conducted at night by divers (using oxygen rebreathers) who were launched from Royal Navy X-craft (dry midget submarines). The divers, who were from several nations, departed the surfaced submarines at about 1,500 yd off-shore, taking soundings and bottom samples as they approached the beach. On reaching the obstacles, they made detailed drawings of their location, arrangement, and associated mines.[2]

During clearance operations on D day, US Naval Combat Demolition Units (NCDU) at Omaha and Utah beaches loaded demolitions on their obstacles while wading in the rising tide. On Omaha Beach, direct exposure to hostile fire caused more than 50% casualties in NCDU personnel. On Sword and Gold beaches, the British used divers and had fewer than 5% casualties.[3]

The US landing force did not have an oxygen diving capability at the time of Operation Overlord. This technique was declined by the Navy in 1940 when offered it by Christian Lambertsen, who was a medical student at the time. Dr Lambertsen subsequently developed military oxygen diving teams for the Office of Strategic Services (OSS) and trained Navy Underwater Demolition Teams and Army engineers in oxygen diving after the war[4] (Exhibit Figure 1).

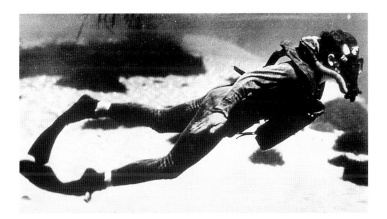

Exhibit Fig 1. An Office of Strategic Services (OSS) swimmer is pictured underwater using the Lambertsen Amphibious Respiratory Unit (LARU) Mark 10, also called the Lambertsen rebreather, on a training exercise in 1943. Photograph: Courtesy of C. J. Lambertsen, Philadelphia, Pa.

1. Fane FD. *The Naked Warriors*. Annapolis, Md: Naval Institute; 1995.
2. Brou W-C. *Combat Beneath the Sea*. New York, NY: Thomas Y. Crowell; 1957.
3. Kelly O. *Brave Men—Dark Waters*. Novato, Calif: Presidio; 1992.
4. Larsen HE. *A History of Self-Contained Diving and Underwater Swimming*. Washington, DC: National Academy of Sciences—National Research Council; 1959. Publication 469.

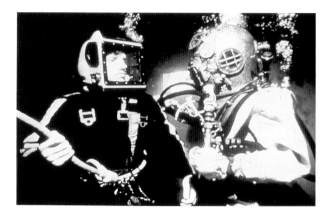

Fig. 31-7. US Navy Mark (Mk) 12 (left) and Mk V (right) diving helmets. The Mk V was used until 1980, when it was replaced by the Mk 12. The Mk 21 replaced the Mk 12 in 1993. Reprinted from US Department of the Navy. *US Navy Diving Manual.* SS521-Ag-PRO-010. Washington, DC: Naval Sea Systems Command. Rev 4 (20 Jan 1999); Change A (1 Mar 2001): p1-9. NAVSEA 0994-LP-100-3199.

ing Company of England in the mid 19th century added a closed suit to the helmet, which prevented flooding and improved thermal protection. This became the traditional "hard-hat" deep-sea diving dress, which remained the primary equipment for military and commercial diving until the 1970s. The US Navy diving helmet, the Mk V (Figure 31-7), was introduced 1905 with improvements in 1916 and 1927 and was the system of choice until 1980, when it was replaced by the Mk 12. The Mk 12 was used until replaced by the Mk 21 in 1993 (see Figure 31-1). The Mk 21 incorporates a demand regulator from open-circuit scuba but instead of a mouthpiece, uses an oronasal mask that allows spoken communications. The oronasal mask in the Mk 21 has much less respiratory dead space than the Mk V and Mk 12 and permits lower gas-supply flow rates without carbon dioxide retention. This was an important improvement.

The Mk 21 Mod 1 helmet has a depth limit of 57 msw (190 fsw) when used for air diving. Its principal applications are search, salvage, inspection, ship's husbandry, and enclosed-space diving. The Mk 21 Mod 1 may also be used to a depth of 90 msw (300 fsw) with helium–oxygen mixtures (see Figure 31-1). Another tethered diving system in the US Navy inventory is the lightweight Mk 20 Mod 0 (Figure 31-8), which is used to a maximum depth of 18 msw (60 fsw) for diving in mud tanks or enclosed spaces. For saturation diving, the Navy uses

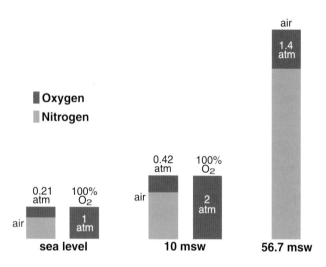

Fig. 31-6. Nitrogen and oxygen partial pressures for air and 100% oxygen. When diving with 100% oxygen, the threshold depth for central nervous system oxygen toxicity is quite shallow, about 6 to 7.6 msw (20–25 fsw; 1.6–1.76 atm). With air, the threshold is on the order of 56.7–66.2 msw (187–218 fsw), where the oxygen partial pressure is 1.4 to 1.6 atm. The "thresholds" are poorly defined owing to lack of data, and the threshold concept may not be entirely valid because of various factors that influence susceptibility, such as exercise, immersion, and inspired carbon dioxide.

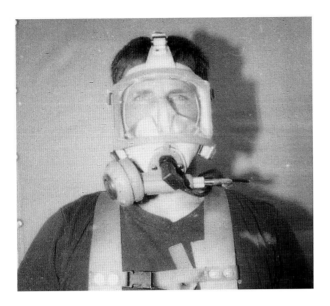

Fig. 31-8. The US Navy Mark 20 Mod 0 surface-supplied, open-circuit, lightweight system with full facemask is limited to a depth of 60 fsw for applications such as diving in mud tanks and enclosed spaces. Reprinted from US Department of the Navy. *US Navy Diving Manual.* SS521-Ag-PRO-010. Washington, DC: Naval Sea Systems Command. Rev 4 (20 Jan 1999); Change A (1 Mar 2001): p6-55. NAVSEA 0994-LP-100-3199.

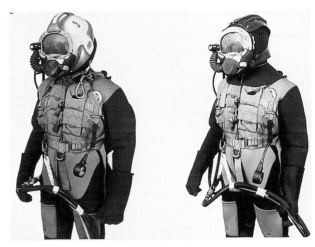

Fig. 31-9. The US Navy Mark (Mk) 21 Mod 0 helmet with hot water suit (left) and Mk 22 Mod 0 band mask with hot water suit and shroud (right) for heating breathing gases. These are the primary underwater breathing apparatuses for saturation diving. Reprinted from US Department of the Navy. *US Navy Diving Manual.* SS521-Ag-PRO-010. Washington, DC: Naval Sea Systems Command. Rev 4 (20 Jan 1999); Change A (1 Mar 2001): p15-6. NAVSEA 0994-LP-100-3199.

the Mk 21 Mod 0 helmet and Mk 22 Mod 0 band mask (Figure 31-9) with hot water suit and hot water shroud for breathing-gas heating.

Closed-Circuit Oxygen Scuba

Closed-circuit oxygen scuba was invented by Henry Fleuss in 1878, when chemical agents that absorbed carbon dioxide were discovered.[11] This device allowed a diver to rebreathe expired gas after carbon dioxide had been removed and oxygen added. There were further developments by the Siebe-Gorman Diving Company in England, but the only apparent use of oxygen rebreathers before World War II was for clearing a flooded tunnel under the Severn River in 1882.[11] Closed-circuit oxygen diving became firmly established as an operational technique as a result of activity during World War II (Exhibit 31-4).

Closed-circuit oxygen scuba is relatively simple and produces no bubbles in the water to disclose the diver's location when used correctly, but its hazards have relegated it largely to military operations. During World War II, unconsciousness from mysterious causes was common during closed-circuit oxygen div-

ing and was known as "shallow-water blackout."[12] Factors contributing to this problem included

- dilution hypoxia from failure to initially purge nitrogen from the lungs and the breathing loop;
- CNS oxygen toxicity at depths deeper than about 7.5 msw (25 fsw);
- carbon dioxide poisoning caused by the design, malfunction, or exhaustion of the CO_2 absorbent; and
- flooding of the breathing loop, leading to both loss of buoyancy and chemical burns from wet absorbent ("caustic cocktail").

The safety of closed-circuit oxygen diving equipment is determined, to large degree, by its design. Early units were pendulum rebreathers in which the diver inhaled and exhaled through a single hose into a CO_2 scrubber and "counterlung" (breathing bag). Figure 31-10 shows the pendulum unit used by X-craft divers to attack the *Tirpitz* and *Takeo*[6] (see Exhibit 31-4). Oxygen from a high-pressure cylinder was added to the breathing bag to make up for metabolic consumption. In this configuration, the mouthpiece and hose were a dead space in which carbon dioxide accumulated. The dead space volume increased as the

---

EXHIBIT 31-4

CLOSED-CIRCUIT OXYGEN DIVING IN COMBAT

The first extensive use of closed-circuit oxygen diving was by the Italian navy in the Mediterranean Sea during World War II. Attack swimmers from Italian "Gamma" units sank or disabled about 20 British merchantmen in Algiers, Algeria; Alexandretta, Turkey; and the Bay of Gibraltar, while piloted torpedolike submersibles known as "Maiali" (literally, "Sea Swine," in the Italian) disabled or sank about 15 ships in Alexandria, Egypt, including the British battleships HMS *Valiant* and HMS *Queen Elizabeth*.[1,2]

The British retaliated with their divers, known as Chariots or Human Torpedoes, who sank two Italian cruisers and several merchantmen moored near Palermo, Sicily. British divers also operated from midget submarines, known as X-craft, conducting successful operations in Norway, the Normandy region of France, and the Pacific Ocean. A dry-dock, a transport, and the German battleship *Tirpitz* were sunk or disabled in Norway. Divers also conducted hydrographic reconnaissance of the Normandy landing beaches prior to the invasion of Europe. They also disabled the Japanese cruiser *Takeo* in the Singapore harbor, and cut undersea telegraph cables to Hong Kong and Singapore.[1,2]

Since that time, public knowledge of closed-circuit oxygen diving in combat has been rare. A recent example was the sinking of a patrol craft by US Navy SEALs in the Panama Canal Zone. The US Navy also has applied the concept of Maiale and Chariots in developing the SEAL Delivery Vehicle (SDV) (see the Frontispiece of the Special Environments section of this textbook). An SDV is a wet submersible designed to carry combat swimmers on missions that include underwater mapping, recovery of lost objects, reconnaissance, and destruction of enemy harbor facilities or the naval order of battle. SDV divers use compressed air, closed-circuit oxygen, or closed-circuit mixed gas scuba. SDVs often operate off nuclear submarines that are equipped with Dry Deck Shelters (DDSs). A DDS has three pressure chambers and mates to an escape trunk or missile tube on the submarine. One chamber can be flooded to allow the submerged launch of an SDV, a second is a recompression chamber, and a third provides access to the submarine.[3]

---

1. Brou W-C. *Combat Beneath the Sea*. New York, NY: Thomas Y. Crowell; 1957: 132–146.
2. Halberstadt H. *US Navy SEALs*. Osceola, Wis: Motorbooks; 1993.
3. Wood MP. Silent but deadly: The *USS Kamehameha* Dry Deck Shelter. *Full Mission Profile*. 1994;Spring:48-51.

CO_2 absorbent nearest the diver became depleted. Accumulating carbon dioxide gas led to carbon dioxide poisoning or potentiated CNS oxygen toxicity, both of which were causes of shallow-water blackout.[13]

The carbon dioxide retention problem due to dead space in the pendulum unit was corrected by the recirculating (ie, closed-circuit) rebreather, in which exhaled gas passes through the oxygen absorbent (O_2 scrubber) and into the breathing bag prior to reinhalation (Figure 31-11). This is the design of the Mark 25 UBA Draeger Lar V closed-circuit oxygen rebreather that is currently used by North Atlantic Treaty Organization (NATO) combat swimmers. About 10,000 Mark 25s have been produced. Another configuration placed the CO_2 scrubber between inhalation and exhalation breathing bags, which decreased the work of breathing by reducing the gas flow rate through the absorbent bed (Figure 31-12). This allowed more physical exertion with less carbon dioxide retention and was the design of the US Navy Emerson-Lambertsen

oxygen rebreather that was used for about 20 years, from the 1960s through the 1980s.

The location of the breathing bag or bags relative to the lungs can cause carbon dioxide retention and reduce the diver's exercise capacity (Figure 31-13). A back-mounted bag is at a lower pressure than the lungs with the diver in a prone swimming position. This imposes a negative static lung load (as in breathing through a snorkel) and requires extra work during inspiration but less work during expiration. A chest-mounted bag imposes a positive static lung load, which assists inhalation but imposes extra work during exhalation. Of the two types of lung load, a small positive load causes less carbon dioxide retention and is preferable to a negative load.

Semiclosed Mixed-Gas Scuba

After the Normandy landings in World War II, European ports were found to be heavily mined and had to be cleared to allow war materiel to move for-

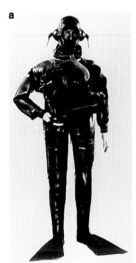

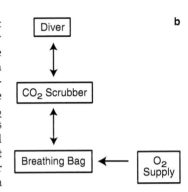

Fig. 31-10. (a) A diver wearing the pendulum closed-circuit oxygen rebreather used during World War II by Royal Navy X-craft divers. This rebreather was an adaptation of the Davis Submarine Escape Device (DSEA) manufactured in England by the Siebe-Gorman Diving Company. **(b)** Schematic diagram of a pendulum oxygen rebreather. The mouthpiece and hose, which connect the diver to the CO_2 scrubber, are a dead space in which carbon dioxide builds up during bidirectional ventilation. The diver exhales and inhales through a single hose connected to a CO_2 absorbent scrubber. The scrubber is built into a breathing bag (or counterlung) into which the diver exhales and from which he inhales. Fresh oxygen from the compressed gas supply below the breathing bag is added to compensate for metabolic consumption. The distal end of the scrubber is unused, while the proximal end adds to the dead space as absorbent is consumed. The rising concentration of carbon dioxide increases cerebral blood flow, thereby augmenting oxygen delivery to the brain and potentiating oxygen toxicity.

Fig. 31-11. (a) Schematic diagram of a closed-circuit oxygen rebreather. Equipment dead space is reduced by one-way valves, which ensure that gas flows in only one direction through the breathing hoses and the CO_2 absorbent (ie, the CO_2 scrubber). This eliminates all but a small dead space in the mouthpiece and results in more even use of the CO_2 scrubber. **(b)** The Mark (Mk) 25 UBA (Underwater Breathing Apparatus—Draeger Lar V) closed-circuit oxygen rebreather. This equipment has been the standard unit used by the North Atlantic Treaty Organization since the 1980s, and about 10,000 have been manufactured since 1981. Photograph b: US Navy.

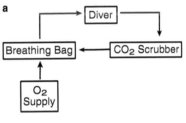

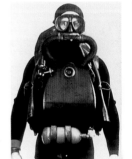

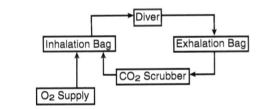

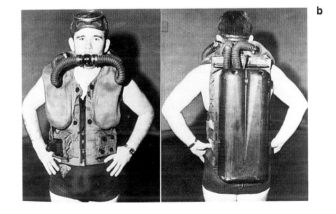

Fig. 31-12. (a) Schematic diagram of a split-bag closed-circuit oxygen rebreather. The split bag (ie, the inhalation bag is worn on the front; the exhalation, on the back) decreases peak gas flows through the CO_2 absorbent canister (the CO_2 scrubber). Separating the inhalation and exhalation bags reduces breathing resistance and prolongs gas residence time, which improves canister efficiency. **(b)** US Navy Emerson-Lambertsen closed-circuit oxygen rebreather. This is a split-bag, recirculating unit based on a design by Dr Christian Lambertsen that evolved from the Lambertsen Amphibious Respiratory Unit (LARU) Mark 10 (see Exhibit 31-2). The US Navy used the Emerson-Lambertsen unit from the 1960s through the 1980s. Photograph b: US Department of the Navy. *US Diving Manual.* Washington, DC: Navy Dept. March 1970: p573. NAVSHIPS 0994-001-9010.

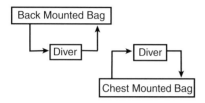

Fig. 31-13. Chest- and back-mounted breathing bags relative to a diver swimming in the prone position. The position of the breathing bag determines the static lung load, which significantly affects respiratory performance, particularly during exercise. A back-mounted bag imposes negative-pressure breathing, which is more deleterious to ventilatory function than the positive-pressure breathing imposed by a chest-mounted bag. The absolute magnitude of the static lung load is greater with the back-mounted bag, which floats off the diver's back instead of being pressed to the chest, as with the chest mount.

ward in support of the Allied advance. Closed-circuit oxygen scuba was unsatisfactory for this purpose, as oxygen toxicity limited its use to about 10 msw (33 fsw). To overcome the problem, the Royal Navy developed a breathing apparatus in which a mixture of nitrogen and oxygen (typically 40%–65% oxygen) rather than pure oxygen was added to the counterlung.[13] The apparatus was known as *semiclosed*, because some gas had to be exhausted to the sea as the diver did not metabolize the nitro-

gen. Thus, semiclosed scuba is not as bubble-free as oxygen scuba.

The same respiratory design constraints apply to semiclosed scuba as to closed-circuit oxygen scuba, and single or split breathing bags may be used with chest or back mounting. The chest-mounted, two-bag, semiclosed-circuit Mk VI unit that was employed by the US Navy from the 1960s through the 1980s and a schematic diagram of the Mk VI are shown in Figure 31-14. The inspired oxygen partial pressure of semiclosed scuba is a function of depth, the percentage of oxygen in the supplied gas, the gas injection rate, and diver's oxygen consumption. There is an optimal oxygen percentage for each depth to achieve a maximum gas-supply duration, and the diver must adhere to specific depth limits for each gas mixture to avoid CNS oxygen toxicity. If a diver works too hard, more oxygen may be consumed than is added, and the "dilution hypoxia" that results can cause unconsciousness. Dilution hypoxia may also occur if the supply gas is exhausted without the diver's knowledge.

Closed-Circuit, Mixed-Gas Scuba

Many of the difficulties of semiclosed-circuit scuba—oxygen toxicity, tell-tale bubbles, and gas-supply duration—are corrected by closed-circuit, mixed-gas scuba, which maintains a nearly constant oxygen partial pressure in the inspired gas. Figure

a

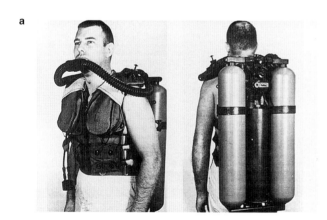

b

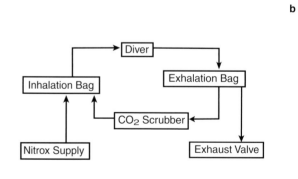

Fig. 31-14. (**a**) A Mark (Mk) 6 semiclosed-circuit, mixed-gas rebreather. This is a split-bag, recirculating unit, based on a Lambertsen design, which was used by the US Navy from the 1960s through the 1980s. (**b**) A schematic of the Mk 6 underwater breathing apparatus. Note the similarity of the Mk 6 shown here to the Emerson-Lambertsen closed-circuit oxygen rebreather (see Figure 31-12). The principal difference between the two designs is that the Mk 6 has a relief valve for venting excess gas because nitrogen from the supply gas is not metabolized and collects in the breathing circuit. Photograph a: US Department of the Navy. *US Diving Manual.* Washington, DC: DN. March 1970: 594. NAVSHIPS 0994-001-9010.

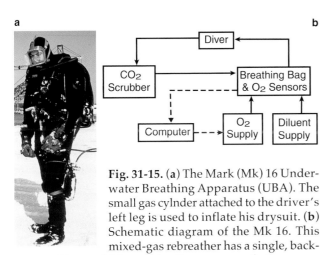

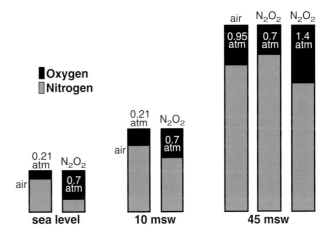

Fig. 31-15. (**a**) The Mark (Mk) 16 Under-water Breathing Apparatus (UBA). The small gas cylnder attached to the driver's left leg is used to inflate his drysuit. (**b**) Schematic diagram of the Mk 16. This mixed-gas rebreather has a single, back-mounted bag, which contains three sensors that measure the oxygen partial pressure. The dotted lines represent electrical signals to and from the computer. If the mean partial pressure falls below the set point (0.7 ata for the Mk 16), the computer adds oxygen to the breathing loop. The diluent supply is air or 16% oxygen in helium and serves to inflate the breathing bag during descent. Photograph a: US Navy.

31-15 shows the US Navy Mk 16 UBA, which has a back-mounted breathing bag, and a schematic of the Mk 16. Closed-circuit, mixed-gas rebreathers have one or more oxygen sensors (the Mk 16 has three) that measure the inspired oxygen partial pressure. This partial pressure is compared to the desired oxygen set point (0.7 atm for the Mk 16) by an ana-log or digital computer, which adds oxygen to the breathing bag when the partial pressure falls be-low the set point.

Figure 31-16 shows how the oxygen and nitro-gen (or other inert gas) partial pressures change with depth for an Mk 16 with an oxygen set point of 0.7 atm (compare Figure 31-6 with Figure 31-16.) Shallower than 77 fsw, a diver breathes a nitrogen–oxygen mixture that contains less nitrogen than air and, consequently, provides a decompression ad-vantage (see below). Deeper than 77 fsw, the reverse is true, and the diver absorbs more nitrogen with the Mk 16. This disadvantage can be remedied by raising the set point to 1.3 or 1.4 atm.

Perhaps the greatest advantage of a closed-circuit mixed-gas rebreather is gas conservation. At a fixed depth, the gas consumption of a closed-circuit rebreather equals the diver's metabolic rate (between 0.5 L/min for rest and 3.0 L/min for work), which a small oxygen supply can support for hours. The purpose of the diluent supply (see Figure 31-15) is to fill the counterlung during descent, but the

Fig. 31-16. Oxygen and nitrogen partial pressures when using a Mark (Mk) 16 mixed-gas rebreather. With an oxy-gen set point of 0.7 atm, the diver breathes 70% oxygen at sea level instead of 21% in air. The fraction of oxygen decreases with increasing depth for the Mk 16 and is 35% at 10 msw (33 fsw). At 23.3 msw (77 fsw), the gas in the Mk 16 is 21% oxygen. Deeper than 23.3 msw (77 fsw), the Mk 16 oxygen fraction becomes less than 21% (eg, 12.7% at 45 msw [150 fsw]). The Mk 16 is at a decom-pression disadvantage for dives deeper than 23.3 msw (77 fsw) and at an advantage shallower than 23.3 msw (77 fsw) or during shallow decompression stops. The disadvantage for deeper dives can be removed by rais-ing the oxygen set point to 1.4 atm.

diluent can be quickly exhausted by multiple ver-tical excursions. The diluent is usually air for depths shallower than about 45 msw (150 fsw), and 12% oxygen in helium to prevent nitrogen narcosis to a depth of 90 msw (300 fsw). Both air and 12% oxygen (but not less) can be breathed in an open-circuit mode at the surface in the event of equip-ment malfunction. The use of rebreathers in the open-circuit mode is one of a number of emergency procedures that must be mastered during diver training.

Closed-circuit mixed-gas rebreathers are signifi-cantly more complex than open-circuit oxygen scuba, and malfunctions are more frequent. Among the disadvantages are a generally greater breath-ing resistance, additional training requirements for divers and maintenance personnel, and costs of ini-tial purchase and subsequent maintenance. Closed-circuit mixed-gas scuba is still evolving and will al-ways be a specialty that is most appropriate for divers who are highly trained, well funded, and willing to assume risks beyond those encountered with open-circuit scuba.

THE ROLE OF RESPIRATION IN DIVING INJURIES

Divers who make emergency ascents to the surface are at risk for arterial gas embolism (AGE) or decompression sickness (DCS), and those who lose consciousness underwater are at risk of drowning. Loss of consciousness when breathing air or nitrogen–oxygen has been called "deep-water blackout," as opposed to shallow-water blackout, which occurs with oxygen rebreathers. The causes of these events can be difficult to determine, but nonfatal occurrences and unplanned laboratory incidents indicate that respiration plays an important role, as Edward H. Lanphier, MD, describes in Case Study 4, quoted below. Knowledge of the underlying mechanisms is incomplete, as experimental investigations are understandably rare.

Case Study 4: Carbon Dioxide Retention and Dyspnea. We were testing a new bicycle ergometer at 7.8 ata (67 msw; 224 fsw) in the dry chamber. Nitrogen narcosis is very evident on air at that pressure, but we were doing OK until we started breathing on the measuring circuit that gave us only about half the air we needed. Herb stopped pedaling after about three minutes, out cold with his eyes rolled back. I took the bike. I knew I wasn't getting nearly enough air, but I was too narc'd to think straight and was determined to finish the test. I pedaled myself right into oblivion and coming around slowly afterwards with a horrible feeling of suffocation was the worst experience of my entire life. Both of us surely would have drowned if such a thing had happened when we were underwater.[14(pp67–69)]

Carbon Dioxide Retention and Dyspnea

Respiration is designed to maintain physiologically acceptable levels of oxygen and carbon dioxide in the blood and tissues, and healthy people breathing free air at sea level adjust their ventilation unconsciously to match their exertion. This is not always so during diving, where the effects of nonphysiological levels of oxygen, nitrogen, and carbon dioxide can interact and are exacerbated with increasing depth by work, breathing resistance, and gas density.[12]

Exercise capacity at sea level is limited by the cardiovascular system, whereas the respiratory system is usually the limiting factor during diving. Immersion shifts blood from the legs to the thorax, which reduces vital capacity and maximum ventilatory capacity. A regulator decreases the ventilatory capacity still further by increasing the work of breathing. Work of breathing is caused, in part, by resistance to gas flow in the airways and breathing apparatus. This resistance increases with depth as the gas density increases. Carbon dioxide is retained when ventilation is inadequate.

Carbon dioxide is the primary ventilatory stimulus in diving. The hypoxic ventilatory drive is generally absent, as most diving gases are hyperoxic. Blood is designed to carry oxygen and carbon dioxide at normoxic pressures, not at elevated oxygen partial pressures. At sea level pressure, where the venous oxygen is low, carbon dioxide is tightly bound to hemoglobin. At high oxygen partial pressures during diving, carbon dioxide is more loosely bound to hemoglobin, causing its tension in the blood and tissues to rise. This is known as the Haldane effect.

Dyspnea generally results if increased ventilation does not reduce the elevated carbon dioxide tension, but carbon dioxide can accumulate in the body without the increased ventilation that occurs at sea level. An interesting environment, frightening experience, or nitrogen narcosis (see Case Study 4) may inhibit ventilation, and divers sometimes consciously override the hypercapnic ventilatory stimulus and hypoventilate ("skip-breathe") to conserve air. Skip-breathing also can be responsible for headaches after diving.

The importance of adequate respiration is not usually stressed during diver training, and a diver who expects the same respiratory performance at depth as on land may be surprised by the breathlessness that can occur should sudden exertion be required in an emergency. As Case Study 4 indicates, dyspnea is a frightening experience, and panic is a common response. Newly trained divers are particularly susceptible to making emergency ascents when dyspnea occurs. A diver overcome by an overwhelming desire to surface and breathe free air may ascend too rapidly and risk AGE, DCS, or both.

An episode of respiratory insufficiency underwater can be a learning experience, but it is not an ideal lesson (Case Study 5). Since the normal unconscious regulation of respiration at sea level may be compromised during diving, divers should beware of incipient dyspnea, ventilate adequately, and minimize exertion. Sufficient ventilatory reserve should be maintained so that sudden, unexpected activity does not cause breathlessness and panic. If breathlessness occurs, the best way to avoid becoming in extremis is to stop all activity and let the ventilation return to normal.

Case Study 5: Deep-Water Blackout. During a dive to 54 msw (180 fsw) in a water-filled pressure chamber, a

Fig. 31-17. Deep air diving is dangerous because interactions of depth, work, oxygen, nitrogen, and carbon dioxide affect respiration and consciousness. Carbon dioxide is the primary factor controlling respiration during diving when the hypoxic ventilatory drive is absent in the presence of hyperoxia (P_{O_2}). Various factors contribute to increased P_{CO_2} in blood (center of diagram). Hyperoxia shifts the carbon dioxide dissociation curve to the right (the Haldane effect), which increases the P_{CO_2}. Gas density increases as depth increases, which raises the work of breathing and decreases ventilation. Nitrogen narcosis increases with depth and may depress ventilation, as do other anesthetics. (Because this effect is hypothetical, it is shown as a dashed line.) Some divers reduce ventilation voluntarily to save gas, whereas others have poor ventilatory response to elevated carbon dioxide. Elevated carbon dioxide potentiates both nitrogen narcosis and central nervous system oxygen toxicity, and carbon dioxide itself is narcotic. In the presence of hyperoxia, dyspnea caused by carbon dioxide is less effective as a warning of altered consciousness. The risks of unconsciousness from oxygen and carbon dioxide toxicity and nitrogen narcosis (all of which increase with depth) are exacerbated by physiological interactions among oxygen, nitrogen, and carbon dioxide.

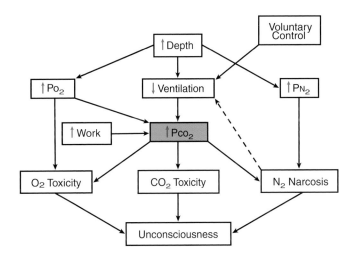

diver performed moderate exercise while swimming against a trapeze at an oxygen consumption of 2 L/min. He was using an Mk 15 UBA (similar to the Mk 16 [see Figure 31-15]) with an oxygen partial pressure of 1.4 ata in nitrogen. Despite orders from the Diving Supervisor to slow down, he increased his workload until he became unconscious. He revived immediately on removal from the water.

Interactions Between Gases and Impaired Consciousness

Carbon dioxide retention is exacerbated as depth increases by greater work of breathing. Inspired carbon dioxide partial pressures of 10% to 15% surface equivalent are narcotic and can affect a diver's consciousness.[1] When the oxygen partial pressure is elevated, hypercapnia loses its effectiveness as a warning signal of respiratory embarrassment or of impending unconsciousness. Excess carbon dioxide potentiates nitrogen narcosis, and narcosis can cause the hypercapnic ventilatory drive to be overlooked (see Case Study 4). Elevated carbon dioxide increases cerebral blood flow and raises oxygen delivery to the brain, increasing the risk of CNS oxygen toxicity.

Thus, diving can impair consciousness through the combined effects of nitrogen narcosis, carbon dioxide intoxication, and oxygen toxicity. These effects are exacerbated by exercise and gas density, which further increase carbon dioxide retention. Figure 31-17 illustrates the interactions among gases, exercise, and depth that increase the risk of unconsciousness.

Individual Susceptibility to Impaired Consciousness

Susceptibility to carbon dioxide retention, oxygen toxicity, and nitrogen narcosis vary widely from one individual to another. Some divers—the carbon dioxide retainers—have poor ventilatory response to inspired carbon dioxide[11]; they are believed to be at el-

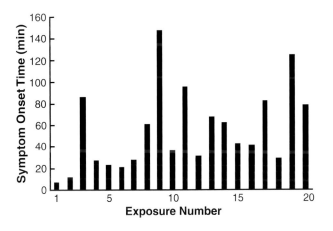

Fig. 31-18. Variation in individual susceptibility to symptoms of CNS oxygen toxicity. The time to symptom onset is illustrated for a single individual who was exposed to 100% oxygen at 21 msw (70 fsw) on 20 days over 3 months. The average onset time was 44 minutes, with a range of 7 to 148 minutes. Data source: Donald K. *Oxygen and the Diver.* Welshpool, Wales: The SPA Ltd; 1993: 45, 46.

evated risk of CNS oxygen toxicity due to increased cerebral oxygen delivery. Studies also have shown wide variability of the latent period before CNS toxicity for the same individual. Experiments[13] by the British during World War II found that the time to symptom onset varied randomly from 7 to 145 minutes for a single diver who made 20 exposures at 21 msw (70 fsw) while breathing 100% oxygen (Figure 31-18).

A few individuals have made compressed air

(21% O_2) dives to depths of 90 to 150 msw (300–500 fsw) and have returned safely, despite nitrogen and oxygen stresses that would incapacitate most people. Other divers have developed severe DCS or have not returned, probably owing to loss of consciousness. There are individual differences in susceptibility among divers but no way to predict who is susceptible or resistant or how individual susceptibility varies from day to day.

DECOMPRESSION PROCEDURES

From the point of view of DCS, diving today is a relatively safe activity, especially when compared with the situation at the turn of the 20th century, when permanent paralysis and death were common (Case Study 6):

Case Study 6. Fatal Decompression Sickness in 1900. A Royal Navy diver descended to 45 msw (150 fsw) in 40 minutes, spent 40 minutes at depth searching for a torpedo, and ascended to the surface in 20 minutes with no apparent difficulty. Ten minutes later, he complained of abdominal pain and fainted. His breathing was labored, he was cyanotic, and he died after 7 minutes. An autopsy the next day revealed healthy organs but gas in the liver, spleen, heart, cardiac veins, venous system, subcutaneous fat, and cerebral veins and ventricles.[15]

By the present US Navy Standard Air Decompression Tables, this diver should have had 174

minutes of decompression time.[1] Decompression risk is relatively low for divers who follow standard decompression tables, such as those published in the *US Navy Diving Manual*,[1] but even divers who adhere to accepted tables may develop the less-serious forms of the disease and, occasionally, severe problems. Decompression tables specify rules for the time at maximum depth, decompression stops, and surface intervals between dives. More recently, diver-worn digital computers have automated the process of decompression calculations, making them simpler and less prone to the kinds of errors that divers make when working with tables. Neither dive tables nor dive computers guarantee freedom from risk of DCS, however, and both are the subjects of controversy, particularly as their specified safety limits disagree widely.

In 1993, the rate of ascent to the first decompres-

TABLE 31-1

NO-STOP DIVE TIMES AT FIVE DEPTHS

Dive Table or Computer	Longest (No-Stop) Bottom Time Allowed at the Indicated Depth Without Required Decompression Stops				
	15 (msw)	18 (msw)	24 (msw)	30 (msw)	39 (msw)
	Time (min)				
56 USN Tables	100	60	40	25	10
RN Tables	85	60	30	20	11
DSAT Tables	80	55	30	20	10
DCIEM Tables	75	50	20	10	5
BSAC Tables	74	51	30	20	13
EDGE	73	52	31	20	10
DataMaster	70	51	29	19	10
Datascan2	65	49	30	19	5
Aladin	62	45	23	15	7
Monitor	61	45	23	15	9

BSAC: British Sub Aqua Club; DCIEM: Defense Civil Institute of Environmental Medicine [United States]; DSAT: Diving Science and Technology [Canada]; EDGE: Electronic Dive Guide Experience; RN: Royal Navy; USN: US Navy
Data source: Lewis JE, Shreeves KW. *The Recreational Diver's Guide to Decompression Theory, Dive Tables, and Dive Computers.* Santa Ana, Calif: Professional Association of Diving Instructors; 1990.

sion stop was changed in the *US Navy Diving Manual* from 18 msw/min (60 fsw/min) to 9 msw/min (30 fsw/min).[1] The safety stop, a development in recreational diving during the 1990s, interrupts ascents from no-stop dives with a 3- to 5-minute stage at 3 to 6 msw (10–20 fsw).[16] Slower ascent rates and a safety stop can reduce the incidence of venous gas emboli, but their effect on the risk of DCS is uncertain. Studies with animals indicate that the effects of ascent rate can be complex.

No-Stop (No-Decompression) Dives

No-stop (ie, no-decompression) dives are the simplest, safest, and most common form of exposure. No-stop dives are short enough that the diver can return directly to the surface with an acceptably low risk of DCS. Unfortunately, there is considerable variability in the no-stop exposure limits given both by tables and dive computers. Table 31-1, for example, lists the no-stop limits at five depths for five decompression tables and five dive computer models.[17] The longest no-stop limits for any given depth are 1.4 to 3.6 times greater than the shortest limits.

In-Water Decompression Stops

If the bottom time at a given depth exceeds the stated no-stop limit for a decompression table or dive computer, the diver must remain at a shallower depth (a decompression stage or stop) long enough to allow inert gas to be eliminated harmlessly through the lungs. If the decompression stops are too short, excessive formation and growth of bubbles in the blood and tissues may result in DCS. In-water decompression stops are traditionally at 3 msw (10 fsw) intervals, with the most shallow stop being at 3 or 6 msw (10 or 20 fsw). With dive computers, however, decompression may be conducted during continuous ascent.

Experiments and observations (see a review by Vann and Thalmann[18]) have found that decompression time can be reduced by 30% to 50% with about the same or a lower risk of DCS if oxygen is used instead of air during in-water decompression stops, but this benefit comes with the risk of CNS oxygen toxicity. In-water oxygen decompression is not recommended deeper than 6 msw (20 fsw) and then only with careful attention to depth control. A back-up decompression plan should be available for times when in-water oxygen cannot be used. Air should be available as a back-up breathing gas in the event of oxygen-toxicity symptoms, and an emergency plan should be available to manage convul-

sions. British[19] and Canadian[20] tables have in-water oxygen decompression options but those developed and used by the US Navy do not.

Surface Decompression

During salvage of silver and gold in World War I, the weather or the military situation sometimes forced British divers to surface before completing their required in-water decompression stops (reviewed by Vann and Thalman[18]). Experience showed that this was possible if the divers were rapidly recompressed in a shipboard pressure chamber within 5 to 10 minutes of reaching the surface. Surface decompression was initially conducted with air, but subsequent studies by the US Navy (reviewed by Vann and Thalman[18]) found that decompression with oxygen was more effective. Surface decompression with oxygen (Sur-D O_2) is typically conducted with recompression on 100% oxygen to a depth of 12 msw (40 fsw). Oxygen breathing has been found acceptable at 12 msw (40 fsw) in a dry chamber, rather than 6 msw (20 fsw) for divers in the water, because dry divers are at a lower risk of oxygen toxicity (reviewed by Vann and Thalman[18]). The US Navy has surface decompression tables for both air and oxygen, but the air table is used only in emergencies.[1]

Repetitive and Multilevel Diving

If two dives are made in close succession, inert gas remaining in the body from the first dive requires that the second dive have a reduced bottom time or longer decompression time to avoid increased DCS risk. The second exposure is known as a *repetitive dive*, and the time between the two dives is called a *surface interval*. Complete elimination of inert gas from the body can take as long as 12 to 24 hours, depending on the diver's recent dives. The US Navy Air Decompression Tables treat all dives with surface intervals of less than 12 hours as repetitive dives, but this time is as short as 6 hours for some recreational dive tables, and as long as 18 hours for the Canadian tables.[20] Repetitive diving is common among recreational divers, and four or more no-stop dives per day are not unusual over several days. Repetitive diving is thought to increase the risk of DCS, but this appears to depend on the dive table or computer that is used. Definitive data to resolve the issue are unavailable.

Multilevel diving is a variant of repetitive diving in which the diver does not return directly to the surface but ascends in stages that take advantage of the longer no-decompression times at shallow depths (see Table 31-1) while avoiding mandatory decompression stops. Commercial, recreational, and military diving (with submersibles, in Special Operations) are frequently multilevel. There are a number of multilevel dive tables, but multilevel dives are most efficiently conducted when dive computers are part of divers' equipment.

Dive Computers

The common term for a digital computer that a diver carries underwater for decompression guidance is a *dive computer*. The computer is worn on the wrist where it can be easily viewed. (An alternative term sometimes used by the US Navy is Underwater Decompression Monitor [UDM]). The first commercially successful, mass-produced digital dive computer appeared in 1983, and many others are now available. All dive computers are programmed with models, or algorithms, that are derived from the same or similar mathematical calculations as decompression tables.

A decompression model is a mathematical representation of the kinetics of inert gas exchange in body tissues with rules to preclude ascents that might result in unsafe bubble formation or growth. Because the physiology of decompression is not completely understood and because of differences between individuals, decompression models are not totally effective in avoiding DCS, although the incidence appears to be less than 1%.[21]

Figure 31-19 shows a dive computer developed for use with SEAL Delivery Vehicles (SDVs) and a schematic diagram of a typical dive computer. Its principal components include a pressure transducer that reads the diver's depth; a temperature transducer for compensating the pressure transducer for temperature change; a timer for measuring dive time; memory to store a mathematical model (ie, an algorithm) of the decompression process; a microprocessor to sample depth and temperature and to compute the diver's decompression status; and a display for presenting the current depth and decompression status to the diver. Optional components measure the diver's gas-supply pressures and allow the dive's depth–time profile to be recorded for later recall on a personal computer.

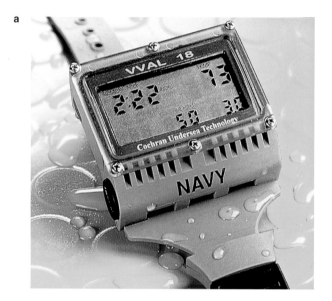

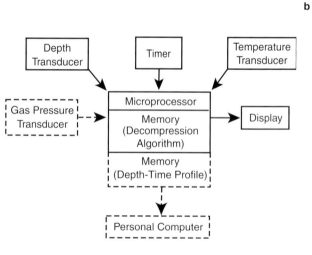

Fig. 31-19. (a) A dive computer for use with SEAL Delivery Vehicles (SDVs). Dive computers help a diver track his decompression status and guide his ascent to the surface. This is particularly useful for multilevel diving, wherein the diver does not return directly to the surface but varies his depth during the dive. Dive computers are easier to use than dive tables, but neither totally eliminates the risk of decompression illness. (b) Schematic diagram of a dive computer. Solid lines indicate mandatory components, which include depth and temperature transducers to measure and temperature-compensate the diver's depth; a timer, microprocessor, and decompression algorithm to compute decompression status; and a display to report the diver's decompression requirements. Dashed lines indicate optional components, which include a transducer to measure gas supply pressure and memory to store the depth–time profile for later recall by a personal computer. Photograph: Reprinted with permission from Cochran UnderSea Technology, Richardson, Tex.

Dive computers accurately track depth–time profiles and minimize the human errors that can occur in table selection. Dive computers are reasonably reliable, but hardware failures occasionally occur and backup computers or tables are recommended. The decompression "safety" of dive computers and tables is vigorously debated, but there are presently no data that offer compelling evidence of a higher incidence of DCS for either. Reports to the Divers Alert Network (DAN) suggest that among recreational divers with decompression injuries, AGE is less common among those who rely on their dive computers rather than conventional tables,[22] but dive computer safety has been questioned for multiple repetitive dives with short surface intervals.[23] To resolve the issue of safety will require knowledge of how the risk of decompression injury is affected by depth–time exposure. Dive computers with the capability for recording depth and time may ultimately provide data on which this knowledge can be based.

Nitrogen–Oxygen Diving

Many breathing devices can be used with gases other than air. The most common mixtures are of nitrogen and oxygen (often called *nitrox*) in which the oxygen percentage is greater than the 21% in air. Such mixes are also known as enriched air nitrox (EAN). Semiclosed- or closed-circuit rebreathers (see Figures 31-14 and 31-15) use nitrox, but the oxygen fraction varies with the depth. Nitrox mixes that contain less nitrogen than air reduce the risk of DCS if used with standard decompression procedures; however, the bottom time is often extended instead, which negates the reduction in decompression risk.

The advantages of fixed-percentage nitrox are as follows:

- reduced nitrogen absorption at depth, and
- accelerated nitrogen elimination during decompression.

And the disadvantages are

- the need for oxygen-clean equipment to limit fire hazard,
- the complexity of gas mixing,
- the requirement for accurate gas analysis, and
- the importance of depth control to stay within the mixed-gas oxygen-exposure limits for CNS oxygen toxicity (see Figure 31-5).

Figure 31-20 illustrates the oxygen and nitrogen partial pressures at various depths with air and with 36% nitrox. The 36% nitrox has a clear decompression advantage over air, owing to its lower nitrogen partial pressure, but the depth limitation due to increased risk of oxygen toxicity is also obvious. Ignoring depth limits in nitrox diving has led to fatal convulsions. Nitrox diving can be conducted with reasonable safety, but additional training in physics, physiology, and gas mixing and analysis is advisable.

The most widespread application of fixed-percentage nitrox diving is the National Oceanic and Atmospheric Administration's (NOAA's) adaptation of the US Navy Standard Air Tables[1] for 32% oxygen.[7] The no-stop exposure limit at 15 msw (50 fsw) is 200 minutes with 32% nitrox, for example, while the limit is only 100 minutes with air. Nitrox is not suitable for deep diving because of the increased risk of CNS oxygen toxicity. NOAA's upper limit for oxygen partial pressure exposure is 1.6 atm, which makes 39 msw (130 fsw) the greatest allowable depth with 32% oxygen. If the oxygen partial pressure is limited to 1.4 atm, the maximum depth is reduced to 33.8 msw (111 fsw).

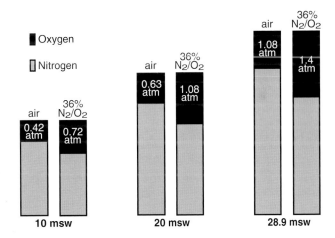

Fig. 31-20. Oxygen partial pressures in air and 36% nitrogen–oxygen mixture (nitrox). The 36% nitrox provides a decompression advantage over air by reducing the nitrogen partial pressure to which a diver is exposed. Thus, 36% nitrox at 10 msw (33 fsw) has the same nitrogen partial pressure and is the decompression equivalent of breathing air at 6.2 msw (20.5 fsw). This is known as the equivalent air depth (EAD). The EAD at 20 msw (66 fsw) is 14.3 msw (47 fsw), and the EAD at 28.9 msw (95 fsw) is 21.5 msw (71 fsw). NOTE: the deepest recommended depth for 36% nitrox is 28.9 msw (95 fsw), because at this depth the oxygen partial pressure rises to 1.4 atm; the risk of central nervous system oxygen toxicity may be excessive above this pressure.

Helium–Oxygen and Trimix Diving

For diving deeper than about 45 msw (150 fsw), *heliox* (a mixture of helium and oxygen) or *trimix* (a mixture of helium, nitrogen, and oxygen) are used to eliminate or reduce nitrogen narcosis. The oxygen fraction in these mixtures is often less than 21% and is chosen to avoid oxygen partial pressures above 1.3 to 1.4 atm, which are potentially toxic to the CNS at the planned maximum depth. The US Navy developed helium–oxygen tables for bottom times of up to several hours' duration (known as *bounce* dives), but these tables are not frequently used. The commercial diving industry developed its own helium tables in the 1960s and 1970s for off-shore oil work, but commercial tables are unpublished and not readily available. Helium–oxygen bounce diving became uncommon in commercial operations of the 1980s and 1990s and has been replaced by saturation diving (see below), which is more efficient.

Omitted Decompression

A diver who surfaces before completing a decompression stop is subject to increased risk of DCS. Decompression may be omitted as a result of hypothermia, wave action, tidal flow, equipment failure, dangerous marine life (Exhibit 31-5), or running out of air. Out-of-air situations are more common with scuba than with surface-supplied equipment. The US Navy requires an on-site recompression chamber (within a travel time of 30 min) for decompression diving because of possible omitted decompression and because the risks of decompression dives are greater than those of no-stop dives.[1] No-stop dives are safer than decompression dives because decompression *cannot* be omitted.

Flying After Diving and Diving at Altitude

DCS can occur independently of diving during altitude exposures above about 5,490 m (18,000 ft; a barometric pressure of 0.5 ata). Nitrogen dissolved in the tissues at sea level has a tension of about 0.79 atm and leaves solution to form bubbles at altitude. Flying after diving increases the risk of DCS if additional nitrogen remains in the tissues after a dive. To reduce the DCS risk from flying too soon after diving, divers are advised to wait long enough at sea level until nitrogen dissolved in their tissues is eliminated harmlessly through the lungs. The *US Navy Diving Manual*[1] provides a table of preflight surface intervals before flying is considered safe. These surface intervals range from 0 to 24 hours depending on the flight altitude and the severity of the previous diving exposures. The US Air Force re-

---

EXHIBIT 31-5

HAZARDOUS MARINE LIFE

Hazards to humans in the marine environment in order of frequency of injury are (*a*) dermal irritations or infections, (*b*) stings or envenomations, (*c*) poisonings from ingestion, and (*d*) trauma or attack. The first category includes coral or barnacle cuts, seaweed dermatitis, sea cucumber or sponge irritation, sea louse or annelid worm bite, bristleworm sting, bathers' itch, fish handlers' disease, marine granuloma, and parasites. Envenomations result from stingray, scorpionfish, toadfish, catfish, weeverfish, starfish, sea urchins, jellyfish, fire coral, cone shells, octopus, sea snake, crown of thorns, and various worms. Poisonings include or can occur from scromboid (pseudoallergic), tetrodotoxin/fugu (pufferfish), ciguatera, paralytic shellfish, hallucinatory fish, and fish blood, roe, or liver. Attacks or trauma can occur from sharks, barracuda, moray eels, sea lions, triggerfish, surgeonfish, crocodiles, electric eels, swordfish, and giant clams.

The sources listed below should be consulted for specific recommendations, but the usual ABCs of first aid—ensure that the casualty's *a*irway is patent, is *b*reathing without assistance, and *c*irculation is intact—are the rescuer's primary concern, followed by evacuating the casualty to a competent medical facility. Wound cleansing and antibiotics can be particularly important to remove debris and bacteria and to control infection. Allergic reactions are usually minor but can be life-threatening. The Divers Alert Network can be called at (919) 684-8111 or (800) 684-4DAN for advice or referral to local authorities.

Sources: (1) Edmonds C. *Dangerous Marine Creatures*. Flagstaff, Ariz: Best Publishing Co; 1995. (2) Auerbach PS. *Hazardous Marine Life*. Flagstaff, Ariz: Best Publishing Co; 1997.

quires a 24-hour wait after any diving before flight.[24]

Diving at altitude also increases the risk of DCS. Two factors are relevant:

1. Because the bodies of sea-level residents are in equilibrium with the 0.79 atm of nitrogen in atmospheric air, rapid ascent to an altitude of, say, 5,486 m (18,000 ft), where the atmospheric nitrogen is only 0.4 atm, would cause a supersaturation of some 0.39 atm. The supersaturated nitrogen dissipates over about 24 hours, but while it is present, no-stop dive times (see Table 31-1) must be reduced or additional decompression time must be given.

2. After equilibration is complete, the no-stop times are still shorter than those given in Table 31-1 because bubbles grow larger at reduced barometric pressure than at sea level. There are empirical modifications to existing decompression tables and dive computer models for altitude diving. The *US Navy Diving Manual*[1] contains altitude diving procedures relevant to military diving.

The decompression problem can be avoided entirely by diving with pure oxygen if the depth is limited to about 10 msw (33 fsw). As oxygen scuba weighs less than compressed-air scuba, this is an important consideration for altitude expeditions, whose members must carry their own equipment.

The Safety of Decompression Practice

Advances in our knowledge of decompression physiology since 1950 have been of little help in developing the decompression algorithms used by dive tables and dive computers. These algorithms are largely empirical, and their uncertainty is reflected by the dissimilarity of the computed dives (see Table 31-1). Dives are still classified as "safe" or "unsafe" according to whether some calculated measure of the excess inert gas supersaturation exceeds a threshold, but this approach has started to change with the introduction of probabilistic decompression modeling by the US Navy.[25] Although the absolute accuracy of probabilities estimated by these methods is uncertain, they allow dissimilar dives to be compared and are helpful for understanding the ambiguity of existing tables and dive computers.

Figure 31-21 shows a series of two no-stop dives to a depth of 16.5 msw (55 fsw), separated by a surface interval of 57 minutes.[17] The bottom times of both dives were chosen to give the longest allowed

no-stop exposures. Residual nitrogen remaining from the first dive makes the second dive shorter. Table 31-2 gives the bottom times of the two dives for the 11 dive tables and dive computers listed in Table 31-1. The first dive times range from 50 to 77 minutes, while the times for the second dive range from 0 to 45 minutes. The wide range of the second dive times underscores the uncertainty of our knowledge of decompression safety and the underlying mechanisms of DCS. We know which time is safest (0 min), but we must make a subjective judgment as to which times are safe *enough* (ie, of acceptable DCS risk; see Chapter 30, Physics, Physiology, and Medicine of Diving).

The probabilities that DCS will develop are also given in Table 31-2, estimated at the end of the second dive by the US Navy decompression algorithm.[25] Second-dive times of 0 to 45 minutes correspond to DCS probabilities of 1.9% to 3.2%. Thus, DCS probability appears to vary gradually over a wide range of dives, and dissimilar dive profiles can have similar DCS probabilities. At present, insufficient experimental or observational data are available to confirm the estimated probabilities, although the estimates are suspected to exceed the true values. As such data and more powerful microprocessors become available, probabilistic algorithms are expected to replace the algorithms currently used by dive tables and dive computers.

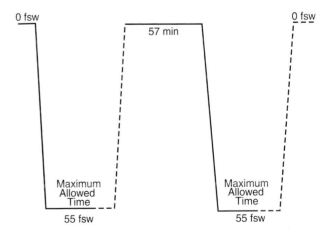

Fig. 31-21. A two-dive profile for comparing the repetitive dive exposure limits of the dive tables and dive computers listed in Table 31-1. Two no-stop exposures to 16.5 msw (55 fsw) are separated by a surface interval of 57 minutes. The maximum allowable exposure times (indicated by dashed lines) are chosen for each dive according to the requirements of the particular dive table or dive computer.

TABLE 31-2

NO-STOP BOTTOM TIMES FOR TWO DIVE PROFILES IN FIGURE 31-21*

Dive Table or Computer Model	1st Dive[†] (min)	2nd Dive[‡] (min)	PDCS[§] (%)
EDGE	62	45	3.2
Aladin	51	41	3.2
DataMaster	61	39	3.2
Monitor	51	35	2.9
DSAT Tables	54	26	2.7
DCIEM Tables	50	23	2.5
93 USN Tables	75	17	3.2
56 USN Tables	60	8	2.3
Datascan II	57	5	2.1
RN Tables	60	0	1.9
BSAC Tables	51	0	1.9

*times as specified by 6 dive tables and 5 dive computers (see Table 31-1).
[†]depth: 16.5 msw (55 fsw); surface interval between dives: 57 min
[‡]depth: 16.5 msw (55 fsw)
[§]Probabilities of decompression sickness (PDCS) estimated from USN 93 algorithm in Weathersby PK, Survanshi SS, Homer LD, Parker E, Thalmann ED. Predicting the time of occurrence of decompression sickness. *J Appl Physiol.* 1992;72(4):1541–1548
BSAC: British Sub Aqua Club; DCIEM: Defense Civil Institute of Environmental Medicine [Canada]; DSAT: Diving Science and Technology (United States); EDGE: Electronic Dive Guide Experience; RN: Royal Navy; USN: US Navy
Data source: Lewis JE, Shreeves KW. *The Recreational Diver's Guide to Decompression Theory, Dive Tables, and Dive Computers.* Santa Ana, Calif: Professional Association of Diving Instructors; 1990.

SATURATION DIVING

After about 24 hours at any depth, the inert gas tension in the body reaches equilibrium with the inert gas partial pressure in the ambient atmosphere, and the decompression time achieves its maximum length, independent of dive duration. While saturation dives are logistically complex, they avoid the stresses of multiple bounce dive decompressions in circumstances where long working times are desirable. Saturation diving is used most often in commercial diving, occasionally in scientific diving, and by the Navy for submarine rescue.

Saturation divers usually live in a surface chamber known as a Deck Decompression Chamber (DDC) at a "storage" pressure that is shallower than the dive site at which they work. If the chamber is on a surface ship, the divers transfer to a Personnel Transfer Capsule (PTC) through a mating hatch in the DDC, and the PTC is lowered to above or below the dive site. Figure 31-22 shows a saturation diving system with one PTC and two DDCs. Saturation diving may also be conducted from sea-floor habitats, but few of these are now in use as they are expensive and difficult to maintain.

If a diver is stored at a given depth and the worksite is deeper than the storage depth, he makes a descending, or downward, excursion to the worksite. Ascending, or upward, excursions from storage depth are usually made from underwater habitats. The *US Navy Diving Manual*[1] provides tables for excursions from various saturation depths, following which divers may return to the storage pressure without decompression stops. Downward excursions are most common, with the DDC storage depth chosen as shallow as the operation of the excursion tables allow. This minimizes the pressure at which the divers must live and the length of the final decompression to the surface. Oxygen partial pressures during excursions range from 0.4 to 1.2 atm, depending on the breathing apparatus used and the type of operation. Because helium is expensive and not readily available and because open-circuit equipment (scuba or surface-supplied) uses large gas volumes as the depth increases, exhaled gases are sometimes returned to the PTC or the surface, where they are reconditioned for reuse by removing carbon dioxide and adding oxygen.

Atmospheric Control

A saturation chamber is a closed environment whose atmosphere must be carefully controlled to maintain diver health. As the saturation depth increases, the oxygen percentage decreases so that the oxygen partial pressure does not exceed 0.5 atm, which is the approximate threshold for pulmonary oxygen toxicity (see Chapter 30, Physics, Physiology, and Medicine of Diving, for a discussion of breathing gas toxicities). At a depth of 300 msw (1,000 fsw), for example, the oxygen percentage must not exceed 1.6%.

The balance of the pressure is made up by inert gas, which is nitrogen for dives to depths of about 36 msw (120 fsw) and helium at greater depths. Most saturation diving occurs deeper than 61 msw (200 fsw), with helium as the inert gas. At depths of 300 msw (1,000 fsw) and deeper, a trimix of helium–nitrogen–oxygen or a mix of hydrogen–helium–oxygen is sometimes used to reduce the high-pressure nervous syndrome (HPNS), but it is uncertain if the nitrogen ameliorates the HPNS or only relieves some of its symptoms. The Navy currently has procedures only for helium–oxygen.[1]

Accurate gas analysis is essential to maintain safe levels of oxygen and carbon dioxide. The carbon dioxide level is typically controlled to less than 0.5% surface equivalent (SEV) by absorbent material in a closed-loop life-support system. Chamber ventilation must be adequate to keep the atmosphere mixed. In a helium atmosphere, heavier gases such as carbon dioxide and oxygen tend to pool in low or poorly ventilated areas, and toxic levels of carbon dioxide have occurred in bunks that are isolated by curtains.

Toxic atmospheric contaminants such as carbon monoxide or hydrocarbons can be eliminated only by flushing the chamber and piping systems with fresh gas, but this is costly and may be impossible on a ship with limited gas supplies. Contaminants must be prevented from entering the chamber. Carbon monoxide is produced at a rate of 8 to 10 mL per person per day by the metabolism of hemoglobin and must be monitored, but unsafe levels from this source are unusual.

Hydrocarbons can be introduced from petroleum lubricants, leaks in life-support refrigeration units, or improperly cleaned piping. Petroleum lubricants are a fire hazard as well as source of pollution. Divers produce methane at a rate of 300 to 500 mL per person per day. Some chamber systems lock out human waste immediately; others hold it in a sanitary tank. Human waste allowed to sit in a sanitary tank produces ammonia, indole, skatole, sulfur dioxide, hydrogen sulfide, chlorine, and carbon dioxide; therefore, sanitary tanks should be vented externally to prevent contaminating the chamber atmosphere. Many naturally occurring contaminants can be removed by filters in the life-support loop. Mercury is prohibited, and instruments or components such as mercury thermometers and electrical mercury switches must be avoided. The basic rule for preventing contamination is "if in doubt, keep it out."

Infection

Hygiene is important in a closed environment. High humidity leads to external otitis and skin infection. The current recommendation for preventing external otitis is to instill a solution of aluminum acetate with 2% acetic acid into each ear every morning and evening, and before and after diving. The external ear canals are filled with this solution for 5 minutes while the diver lies on one side and then the other. Bed linen should be changed every 48 hours and daily showers taken whether diving or not. Chamber surfaces require daily cleaning with a nonionic detergent solution, and the bilges should be rinsed and drained at the same time. Food

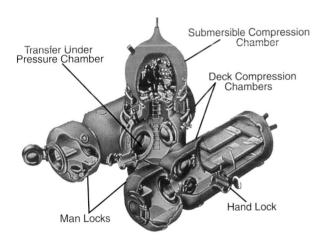

Fig. 31-22. A saturation diving system (diameter ~ 2 m) with two deck compression chambers (DDCs), two man locks, two medical (hand) locks, and a personnel transfer capsule (PTC, called a submersible compression chamber in this figure). The transfer under pressure chamber allows working divers to be moved between the worksite and living chambers (called deck compression chambers in this figure) without disturbing the off-duty divers. The man and medical locks are for transferring personnel, food, medicine, reading material, laundry, and the like to and from sea level.

spills and the like should be cleaned immediately. Divers should wear their own thermal protection suits to prevent the spread of skin infections. Suits should be rinsed with nonionic detergent and water and be hung to dry.

Hyperbaric Arthralgia

Hyperbaric arthralgia is joint discomfort or pain that occurs during compression and decreases in intensity during 24 hours or more at constant depth. Symptoms include joint cracking, a sensation of "dry and grainy" joints (sometimes described as "no joint juice"), and a feeling similar to sprain. In order of severity, affected joints are the shoulders, knees, wrists, hips, and back. Least affected joints are the ankles, fingers, and elbows. Hyperbaric arthralgia can occur during short bounce dives but is more common during deep saturation dives. Its frequency, severity, and duration increase with depth and compression rate, but task performance is usually not affected. The condition is less common with the slow compression rates used to alleviate HPNS. The origin of hyperbaric arthralgia is unknown but suggested causes are (1) changes in the nature of bubble formation with increasing pressure and (2) changes in joint fluid osmolarity leading to dehydrated articular cartilage. There is no evidence that hyperbaric arthralgia leads to joint degeneration or aseptic bone necrosis.

Depth Limits

HPNS begins at about 180 msw (600 fsw) and is manifested by tremor, decreased motor and intellectual performance, dizziness, nausea, vomiting, and, occasionally, psychosis. Focal reflex changes sometimes occur and balance may be affected. Deeper than 300 msw (1,000 fsw), electroencephalograms may have slow theta waves, and alpha activity may be depressed. Divers easily fall into microsleep if not continually aroused. HPNS symptoms can be reduced but not eliminated by slowing or interrupting compression as depth increases.

Although there is considerable individual variability, HPNS imposes a limit of not much more than 600 msw (2,000 fsw) as the maximum depth that humans can tolerate under dry conditions. The maximum depth at which practical work in the water is possible is less than 600 msw owing to excess work of breathing in the UBA, particularly during exhalation.

Decompression

Saturation decompression must occur very slowly to avoid DCS. For helium–oxygen, the US Navy uses a continuous reduction of pressure according to the following schedule:

- 1.8 msw/h from 480 to 60 msw (6 fsw/h from 1,600–200 fsw);
- 1.5 msw/h from 60 to 30 msw (5 fsw/h from 200–100 fsw);
- 1.2 msw/h from 30 to 15 msw (4 fsw/h from 100–50 fsw); and
- 0.9 msw/h from 15 to 0 msw (3 fsw/h from 50–0 fsw).[1]

To minimize decompression during sleep, the US Navy schedule stops decompression from midnight to 0600 and from 1400 to 1600. The oxygen partial pressure is maintained at 0.4 to 0.45 atm until 10 msw (33 fsw) and at 20% to 30% to the surface. The Royal Navy decreases the pressure in stages with periodic drops of 5 msw (16.5 fsw) over 5 minutes. Divers are required to remain near a recompression chamber for at least 2 hours after decompression and within 30 minutes' travel time to a chamber for 48 hours. Flying is prohibited for 72 hours.

THERMAL PROTECTION AND BUOYANCY

Most of Earth's waters are well below body temperature, and except for short exposures, the unprotected diver is at risk of hypothermia; *hyper*thermia, on the other hand, is an unusual hazard for divers (Exhibit 31-6). The *US Navy Diving Manual*[1] gives allowable exposure durations as a function of temperature and the means of thermal protection. Buoyancy control is closely linked to thermal protection, as almost all thermal protection methods use gas for insulation.

Historically, the hard-hat diver wore heavy woolen underwear beneath a canvas outer suit. The suit was supposed to remain dry but frequently leaked. Because the suit was filled with air, the diver wore heavy boots and weights to achieve the negative buoyancy needed to walk on the bottom. To maintain proper buoyancy the suit had to be inflated during descent and deflated during ascent. Hard-hat divers could suffer severe injury from suit squeeze (ie, barotrauma that occurs when a poorly

---

EXHIBIT 31-6

DIVING IN WARM WATER AND IN CONTAMINATED WATER

Hyperthermia is rare but can occur in special circumstances. At remote diving sites in hot climates, recompression chambers that treat diving casualties and deck decompression chambers (DDCs) that support saturation diving may be outdoors and exposed to the sun. This resulted in two fatalities during a saturation diving operation in the 1980s. Hyperthermia is less likely during open water diving, but US Navy divers in the Persian Gulf during the Persian Gulf War in 1991 were exposed to water temperatures in excess of 32°C (90°F) and wore ice vests to prevent overheating. Divers in confined waters (eg, in or around power plants) may also be exposed to temperatures that can cause hyperthermia. This is a particular problem in hazardous environments such as nuclear reactors, where special suits and breathing apparatuses are worn to prevent inward leaks of water contaminated by radioactive material. These suits may incorporate closed-circuit cooling water to prevent the divers' overheating. In addition to being leak proof, suits used in water or other liquids that are contaminated with biological agents or toxic chemicals must be made of materials that will not degrade during exposure. Before the diver undresses, the suits are thoroughly washed down to prevent harmful exposure of the diver himself or of support personnel.

---

fitting suit is insufficiently expanded; see Chapter 30, Physics, Physiology, and Medicine of Diving) if the air supply was inadequate to maintain suit volume during descent. During ascent, gas was vented from the suit to avoid uncontrolled positive buoyancy (ie, blow-up) in which the diver was propelled to the surface and risked air embolism, DCS, or mechanical injury from collision.

The wetsuit is the most common form of thermal protection used today. Made of air-filled, closed-cell neoprene foam, wetsuits are satisfactory for several hours at temperatures of 10°C to 15.5°C (50°F–60°F) but provide less protection with increasing depth as the air-filled cells compress. Minor suit squeeze sometimes occurs with tight-fitting wetsuits. As a diver descends, wetsuit compression reduces buoyancy by several pounds. A buoyancy compensator (BC) to which gas can be added or removed is typically used to make adjustments from slightly positive to slightly negative buoyancy, according to whether ascent or descent is desired. With open-circuit scuba, buoyancy increases by several pounds as compressed gas is consumed from the tanks. Swimming with fins is the common mode of propulsion with scuba and helps a diver remain warm for several hours.

The next level of thermal protection, the drysuit, is a waterproof outer garment over insulating underwear that is sufficiently warm for brief periods of ice diving. Drysuit diving requires training in buoyancy control to avoid suit squeeze or blow-up. For an untethered scuba diver in deep water, moreover, an uncontrolled descent in a drysuit could be

fatal. For an untethered scuba diver in deep water wearing a drysuit, a suit squeeze could make the diver negatively buoyant, resulting in a fatal, uncontrolled descent. A blow-up from overinflation of the suit with uncontrolled ascent, on the other hand, could result in serious or fatal AGE or DCS. A diaper or other urine-collection device is essential if the drysuit is to remain dry during a dive of several hours' duration. Drysuits provide inadequate thermal protection during 6- to 8-hour exposures in –1.1°C to 4.4°C (30°F–40°F) water for resting divers, such as the operators or passengers of SDVs. Because of its greater bulk, a drysuit is more difficult to swim in than a wetsuit.

Drysuits can be inflated from the diver's breathing gas or from a separate gas supply. Argon is sometimes used for this purpose because of its good insulating properties. Helium, on the other hand, offers particular thermal challenges in diving. Helium is a poor insulator because its thermal conductivity is 4.8 times greater and its heat capacity 2.3 times greater than that of air. These characteristics cause heat loss to increase with depth. Most heat loss occurs by convection through the skin and lungs; as a result, for normal body temperature to be maintained, the ambient temperature in a saturation chamber must be 29.4°C to 32.2°C (85°F–90°F). The range of thermal comfort narrows with increasing depth. Water vapor diffuses slowly at high pressure, and evaporation provides little cooling, which makes the skin feel wet without evidence of sensible water. The comfort range for relative humidity is 50% to 70%.

Wetsuits and drysuits provide passive insulation, which delays but does not prevent body cooling. Active heating is the most effective thermal protection. The most common active heat source is hot water (not to exceed 43°C) supplied from the surface or PTC to a loose-fitting wetsuit through which hot water flows before it exits at the hands and feet (see Figure 31-9). An even distribution of flow and careful temperature control are critical for adequate heating without causing hot spots or thermal burns. During deep helium–oxygen diving, the breathing gas must be heated to prevent convective heat loss through the lungs, as this can cause a progressive hypothermia that may go unnoticed. Electric suits are under development as an alternative active heat source (particularly for SDVs) but are complex and expensive.

TREATMENT OF DECOMPRESSION SICKNESS AND ARTERIAL GAS EMBOLISM

AGE is the result of pulmonary barotrauma, while DCS is caused by the formation of bubbles in the blood and tissues. As such, the immediate goal of therapy is to reduce the volume of the offending bubbles. This may be possible for patients who are treated shortly after symptom onset, but long delays are common, and gas bubbles may have caused physical or biochemical damage that persists after the bubbles themselves have resolved. In such situations, therapy can still be beneficial by oxygenating poorly perfused tissue or by reducing edema.

The definitive treatment for DCS and AGE is increased atmospheric pressure and 100% oxygen. The additional pressure serves to reduce the size of the bubbles, and oxygen accelerates their resolution by causing nitrogen to diffuse from bubble to blood. On reaching the lungs, excess nitrogen from the blood is exhaled. Pressure (or recompression) was first used in 1909 to treat DCS (what was then called caisson disease), but oxygen was not routinely used during recompression until the 1960s.[26]

The best first aid for AGE or DCS is 100% oxygen delivered by mask. Inspired oxygen percentages near 100% are essential for the greatest effect. As injured divers are often dehydrated, owing either to the illness or to lack of sufficient fluids, rehydration is also important—orally if possible and intravenously if necessary. There are no proven adjuvant therapies, although aspirin is sometimes recommended to inhibit platelet aggregation, and steroids, to reduce edema. Lidocaine has been proposed for DCS with spinal cord involvement.

As there is no definitive test for DCS or AGE, a differential diagnosis is important to rule out other conditions that can have similar signs and symptoms (eg, stroke, myocardial infarction, or musculoskeletal injury). One of the first questions the medical officer should ask is whether the patient has a recent history of diving or altitude exposure. Signs or symptoms with onsets of later than 48 hours after diving or altitude exposure are probably unrelated to decompression.

Therapy According to US Navy Treatment Tables

The standard US Navy therapy for DCS or AGE is recompression to 18 msw (60 fsw; 2.8 ata) while the patient is breathing 100% oxygen. Typically, the course of treatment is determined by the response of the signs and symptoms. US Navy Treatment Table 5 (Figure 31-23) may be used if

- the only symptoms are joint or limb pain, itching, rash, or local swelling;
- the absence of neurological findings is verified by physical examination; and
- the symptoms are completely relieved within 10 minutes of oxygen breathing at 18 msw (60 fsw).

Treatment Table 5 requires 135 minutes to administer, with two oxygen periods at 18 msw (60 fsw) and one oxygen period at 9 msw (30 fsw).[1] The oxygen periods at 18 msw are 20 minutes long followed by 5 minutes of air breathing to reduce the risk of CNS oxygen toxicity. Ascent from 18 to 9 msw (60–30 fsw) and 9 to 0 msw (30–0 fsw) occurs at 0.33 msw/min (1 fsw/min).

US Navy Treatment Table 6 (Figure 31-24) is used if

- a neurological exam has not been conducted;
- Treatment Table 5 fails to provide complete resolution of symptoms within 10 minutes; and
- any neurological or cardiopulmonary signs or symptoms are present.

Treatment Table 6 requires 285 minutes to administer and has three 25-minute cycles at 18 msw (60 fsw) and two 75-minute cycles (60 min O_2, 15 min air) at 9 msw (30 fsw). Treatment Table 6 can be extended by up to two cycles at 18 msw (60 fsw) and two cycles at 9 msw (30 fsw).[1]

For patients with serious or life-threatening conditions, particularly those suggesting AGE, the option

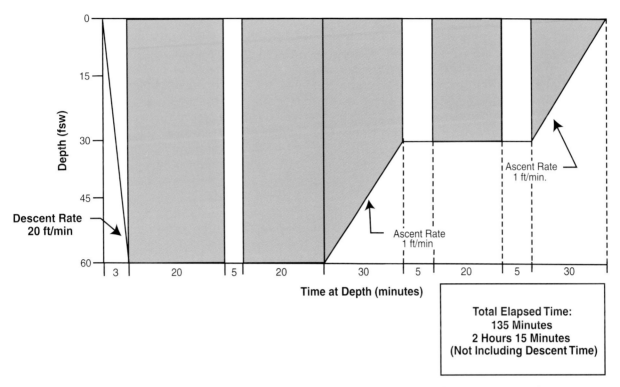

Fig. 31-23. The US Navy Treatment Table 5 Depth/Time Profile can be used only if the diving casualty has no neurological symptoms and if all symptoms are relieved within 10 minutes at 18 msw (60 fsw). Consult the *US Navy Diving Manual* before using this or other treatment tables. Reprinted from US Department of the Navy. *US Navy Diving Manual.* SS521-Ag-PRO-010. Washington, DC: Naval Sea Systems Command. Rev 4 (20 Jan 1999); Change A (1 Mar 2001): p21-40. NAVSEA 0994-LP-100-3199.

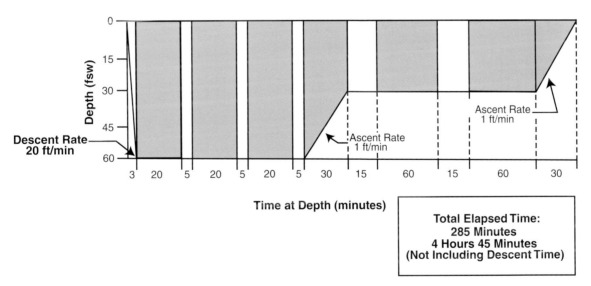

Fig. 31-24. In the US Navy Treatment Table 6 Depth/Time Profile, three 25-minute oxygen cycles at 18 msw (60 fsw) are standard, but two additional cycles may be added. Two additional 75-minute oxygen cycles may also be added at 9 msw (30 fsw). The decompression requirements of inside attendants must also be considered so that they do not themselves develop decompression sickness. Consult the *US Navy Diving Manual* before using this or other treatment tables. Reprinted from US Department of the Navy. *US Navy Diving Manual.* SS521-Ag-PRO-010. Washington, DC: Naval Sea Systems Command. Rev 4 (20 Jan 1999); Change A (1 Mar 2001): p21-41. NAVSEA 0994-LP-100-3199.

is available for further compression from 18 to 50 msw (60–165 fsw) if the patient does not stabilize during the first oxygen period at 18 msw (60 fsw). A recompression to 50 msw (165 fsw) is known as Treatment Table 6A (Figure 31-25 and Exhibit 31-7).[1] Compression to 50 msw (165 fsw) can be accomplished with air or 40% to 50% oxygen in nitrogen. The high-oxygen mix is beneficial for reducing nitrogen narcosis and additional nitrogen uptake at 50 msw (165 fsw). If relief is complete at 50 msw (165 fsw) within 30 minutes, the patient can be decompressed at 0.91 msw/min (3 fsw/min) to 18 msw (60 fsw) (NOTE: procedures for Treatment Table 6 are now followed).

Should relief at 50 msw (165 fsw) be unsatisfactory after 30 minutes, the time at depth can be extended to 120 minutes, after which decompression to 18 msw (60 fsw) is accomplished using US Navy Treatment Table 4 (Figure 31-26).[1] When the patient arrives at 18 msw (60 fsw), decompression may continue according to Treatment Table 4 if either the patient's condition is satisfactory or the recompression chamber can be held at 18 msw (60 fsw) for at least 12 hours, followed by decompression according to US Navy Treatment Table 7 (Figure 31-27). Patients with residual symptoms at the end of an

extended treatment on Treatment Table 6 or Treatment Table 6A, or patients who cannot tolerate further oxygen due to pulmonary toxicity, may be given repetitive treatments on subsequent days. (Mild pulmonary toxicity is reversible within hours to a day.) Typically, one to six additional treatments are given, which may be according to Treatment Tables 5 or 6, or sometimes at 9 msw (30 fsw) for 60 to 90 minutes. The rule of thumb is that repetitive treatments end when no clinical improvement can be demonstrated during two successive recompressions.

For a seriously ill patient, saturation therapy is an alternative to multiple repetitive recompressions. During saturation treatment, the patient is maintained at 18 msw (60 fsw) until he or she stabilizes. This avoids the nontherapeutic decompression to sea level, which may cause symptoms to return. After at least 12 hours at 18 msw (60 fsw) during which the patient may breathe oxygen and air in 25-minute cycles (pulmonary toxicity allowing), decompression is conducted according to Treatment Table 7 over 56 hours.[1] Saturation therapy should not be attempted without adequate facilities and personnel. A scrubber for removing carbon dioxide is required, as is staffing to support 24-hour opera-

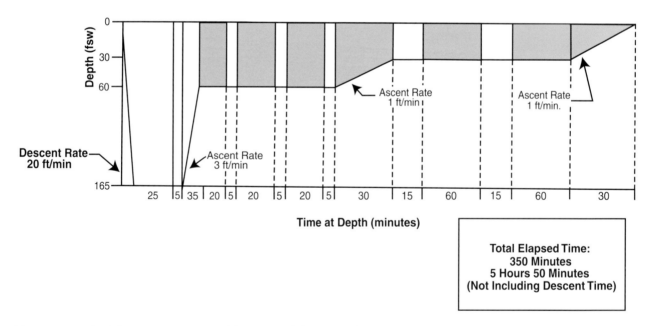

Fig. 31-25. In the US Navy Treatment Table 6A Depth/Time Profile, as long as 20 minutes may be spent at 18 msw (60 fsw) before making the decision to compress to 50 msw (165 fsw). The advantage of compression to 50 msw (165 fsw) over 18 msw (60 fsw) is greater reduction in bubble volume. A spherical bubble is compressed to 35% of its original volume at 18 msw (60 fsw) and to 17% at 50 msw (165 fsw). At 50 msw (165 fsw), high-oxygen treatment gas may be breathed to reduce nitrogen uptake. Consult the *US Navy Diving Manual* before using this or other treatment tables. Reprinted from US Department of the Navy. *US Navy Diving Manual.* SS521-Ag-PRO-010. Washington, DC: Naval Sea Systems Command. Rev 4 (20 Jan 1999); Change A (1 Mar 2001): p21-42. NAVSEA 0994-LP-100-3199.

EXHIBIT 31-7

IS RECOMPRESSION TO 50 MSW NECESSARY, OR IS RECOMPRESSION TO 18 MSW ADEQUATE?

When Treatment Tables 5, 6, and 6A were introduced in the 1960s, Table 6A was specifically prescribed for treating arterial gas embolism (AGE). Subsequently, AGE was recognized to be difficult to diagnose, and treatment at 18 msw (60 fsw) was found in experiments with animals to be as good as treatment at 50 msw (165 fsw). Some people recommended that treatment at 50 msw (165 fsw) be abandoned in favor of treatment at 18 msw (60 fsw), but others argued that success was not always achieved at 18 msw (60 fsw) and further recompression to 50 msw (165 fsw) was sometimes required. This unresolved controversy was reviewed by Thalman in 1996.[1] The *US Navy Diving Manual*[2] adopted a compromise in which treatment for all forms of decompression illness could begin at 18 msw (60 fsw) with the option for further descent to 50 msw (165 fsw) if indicated by inadequate resolution at 18 msw (60 fsw).

The drawbacks of recompression to 50 msw (165 fsw) must be recognized. The patient and attendants are subject to nitrogen narcosis, fatigue can be significant for those inside and outside the chamber, and there is additional risk of decompression sickness. The use of helium–oxygen has been proposed as an alternative gas to air for recompression deeper than 18 msw (60 fsw) and is undergoing study.

1.Thalmann ED. Principles of US Navy recompression treatments for decompression sickness. In: Moon RE, Sheffield PJ, eds. *Treatment of Decompression Illness*. Kensington, Md: 45th Undersea and Hyperbaric Medical Society Workshop, June 1996: 75–95.
2.US Department of the Navy. *US Navy Diving Manual*. SS521-Ag-PRO-010. Washington, DC: Naval Sea Systems Command. Rev 4 (20 Jan 1999); Change A (1 Mar 2001). NAVSEA 0994-LP-100-3199.

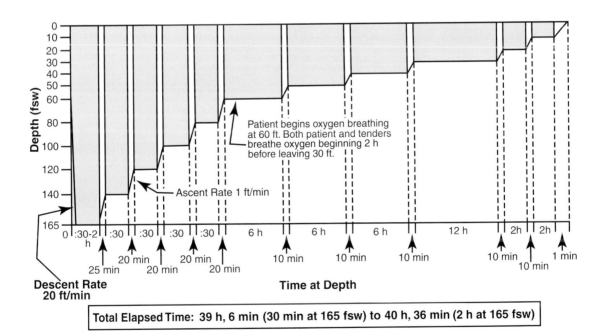

Fig. 31-26. In the US Navy Treatment Table 4 Depth/Time Profile, time at 50 msw (165 fsw) is from 30 minutes to 2 hours. At 50 msw (165 fsw), high-oxygen treatment gas may be breathed to reduce oxygen uptake. Oxygen breathing at 18 msw (60 fsw) is in cycles of 25 minutes interrupted by 5 minutes of air breathing. Consult the *US Navy Diving Manual* before using this or other treatment tables. Reprinted from US Department of the Navy. *US Navy Diving Manual*. SS521-Ag-PRO-010. Washington, DC: Naval Sea Systems Command. Rev 4 (20 Jan 1999); Change A (1 Mar 2001): p21-43. NAVSEA 0994-LP-100-3199.

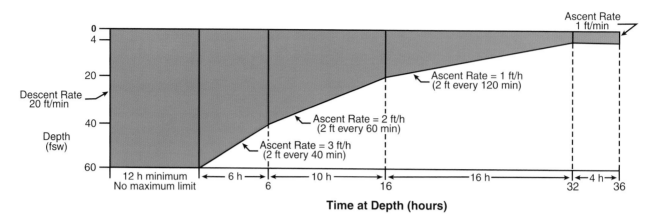

Fig. 31-27. The US Navy Treatment Table 7 Depth/Time Profile is an extension at a depth of 60 fsw of Treatment Tables 6, 6A, and 4 (Figures 31-24 through 31-26). At 50 msw (165 fsw), high-oxygen treatment gas may be breathed to reduce nitrogen uptake. Oxygen breathing at 18 msw (60 fsw) is in cycles of 25 minutes interrupted by 5 minutes of air breathing. Consult the *US Navy Diving Manual* before using this or other treatment tables. Reprinted from US Department of the Navy. *US Navy Diving Manual.* SS521-Ag-PRO-010. Washington, DC: Naval Sea Systems Command. Rev 4 (20 Jan 1999); Change A (1 Mar 2001): p21-43. NAVSEA 0994-LP-100-3199.

tions. During complex or extended treatments, careful planning is required to ensure that the decompression status of the inside attendants remains satisfactory, as they generally do not breathe as much oxygen as the patient.

The best type of chamber for treating a patient with DCS is large enough to accommodate a medical attendant as well as the patient. The closest available chamber, however, may be used for hyperbaric oxygen therapy and can accommodate only a single person. Such "monoplace" chambers and hyperbaric oxygen therapy are described in Exhibit 31-8.

Decompression Sickness in Saturation Diving

DCS that occurs during or after the slow decompression from saturation dives usually manifests as mild knee or leg pain. Neurological symptoms are very rare. The onset of DCS is subtle and may begin with aching or a feeling in the anterior thighs similar to that after hard exercise. This is treated by recompression and administration of high oxygen partial pressures. For occurrences under pressure, oxygen partial pressures of 1.5 to 2.5 atm in helium–oxygen are administered as in Treatment Table 6, with a cycle of 20 minutes of high–partial pressure oxygen (1.5–2.5 atm and 5 min of low–partial pressure oxygen [0.3–0.5 atm]).

Recompression can occur in 3-msw (10-fsw) stages until attaining the depth of relief at which the diver is held for 2 to 6 hours, depending on response. The standard saturation decompression schedule is resumed on relief of symptoms. Relief usually occurs within 10 msw (33 fsw) of the onset depth, but further recompression is not recommended if symptoms are not relieved within 20 msw (66 fsw), as the pain may not be caused by DCS, and other causes should be investigated. For DCS that occurs after reaching the surface and breathing air, a diver may be treated according to Treatment Table 6.

DCS that occurs 60 minutes or more after an ascending excursion can be treated as described above, but DCS that occurs within 60 minutes of ascent from an excursion dive deeper than the saturation depth should be considered serious, even if pain is the only symptom. Neurological symptoms, particularly those related to the inner ear, are not uncommon after rapid ascent from excursions. Recompression to at least the excursion depth should be immediate, and further recompression is warranted if symptoms do not improve significantly within 10 minutes. High oxygen partial pressures should be administered for at least 2 hours as described above, after which the patient should be held at depth for 12 hours before resuming standard saturation decompression.

MEDICAL STANDARDS FOR DIVING

Diving medical officers (DMOs) examine candidates for initial diving training, provide advice to diving officers concerning the medical aspects of diving operations, examine divers before or after dives, offer routine medical care, and treat divers for diving injuries. Some conditions (eg, epilepsy)

EXHIBIT 31-8

RECOMPRESSION CHAMBERS AND HYPERBARIC OXYGEN THERAPY

There are two principal types of hyperbaric chambers: multiplace and monoplace. Multiplace chambers are steel or aluminum, can accommodate two or more people, and are usually compressed with air. Their depth capability is often greater than 18 msw (60 fsw). Multiplace chambers generally have two or more compartments that allow personnel to be transferred in or out while at pressure. Depending on size, a compartment may accommodate as many as 12 patients who receive 100% oxygen by mask or "head-tent." The compartment is periodically ventilated with air to keep the carbon dioxide level below 1.5% surface equivalent and to maintain the oxygen level below 23% to limit the fire hazard. Critical care nursing can be provided should mechanical ventilation or intravenous drug infusion be required.

A monoplace chamber is generally an acrylic cylinder that is compressed with 100% oxygen and accommodates a single patient in the supine position. Its depth capability is often 13.5 to 18 msw (45–60 fsw). Monoplace chambers do not allow for direct patient access although air breaks during oxygen breathing often can be given by mask for conscious patients. Monoplace chambers have been used effectively for decompression illness therapy, but depending on depth capability, they may not be able to provide therapy in accordance with the standard treatment tables. Because of their lower cost, there are many more monoplace chambers than multiplace chambers. Lightweight, inflatable monoplace chambers that can be compressed with air are under development. These will provide the capability for on-site treatment in remote locations or for transport under pressure to larger recompression facilities.

Decompression illness is a relatively rare phenomenon, and most recompression facilities are used more frequently to provide hyperbaric oxygen therapy for other indications. Hyperbaric oxygen therapy is recommended for conditions caused by gas bubbles, inadequate perfusion, and metabolic poisons, including

- decompression sickness, arterial gas embolism, or iatrogenic gas embolism;
- crush injury, compartment syndrome, or acute traumatic ischemia;
- blood-loss anemia;
- necrotizing soft-tissue infections such as gas gangrene or nonclostridial fasciitis;
- refractory osteomyelitis;
- osteoradionecrosis;
- compromised skin grafts or flaps;
- thermal burns;
- intracranial abscess;
- selected problem wounds; and
- carbon monoxide, cyanide, or smoke inhalation.

Recompression facilities can be located by calling The Undersea and Hyperbaric Medical Society, Bethesda, Md, at (301) 942-2980, or the Divers Alert Network, Durham, NC, at (919) 684-2948 or (919) 684-4DAN.

The rationale and methods for using hyperbaric oxygen in these conditions are described in Hampson NB. *Hyperbaric Oxygen Therapy: 1999 Committee Report*. Bethesda, Md: The Undersea and Hyperbaric Medical Society; 1999.

---

are absolute contraindications for diving, while others (eg, upper respiratory infection) are temporarily disqualifying or disqualifying until corrected. Table 31-3 summarizes the recommended relative and absolute contraindications. Conditions that might be allowed for recreational divers may be disqualifying for military divers; the US Navy regulations guide the practice of military diving for all services.

The *US Navy Diving Manual*[1] provides general guidelines for return to diving after DCS or AGE, but each case requires review by a DMO. For example, a diver who had complete relief of Type I DCS during Treatment Table 5 may return to diving 48 hours after therapy is complete, and a diver who required therapy with Treatment Table 6 for complete relief of Type I (minor) symptoms may resume diving after 7 days. If there is any question about the presence of Type II (serious) symptoms,

TABLE 31-3

RECOMMENDED* ABSOLUTE AND RELATIVE CONDRAINDICATIONS TO DIVING

System	Absolute Contraindications	Relative Contraindications
Ears and Upper Respiratory	Open tympanic perforation Inability to equalize the middle ear Tube myringotomy Inner ear surgery (eg, stapedectomy, ossicular chain) Permanent obstruction of the external canal Meniere's disease or other inner ear disease Chronic mastoiditis or mastoid fistula History of vestibular barotrauma Inability to retain mouthpiece Deafness in one ear	Middle ear barotrauma Recurrent or chronic sinus, external canal or middle ear infections Allergies of the nose and upper respiratory tract
Pulmonary	History of spontaneous pneumothorax Reactive airways disease (asthma) of any origin Chronic obstructive pulmonary disease Restrictive lung disease History or radiographic evidence of pulmonary blebs, bullae, or cysts	Childhood asthma without residual hyperactivity or air trapping Pneumothorax due to barotrauma, penetrating injury, or surgery without air trapping _____
Cardiovascular	Aortic or mitral stenosis History of myocardial infarction Angina or coronary artery disease Cardiac septal defects Complete or fixed second-degree heart block Wolf-Parkinson-White syndrome with paroxysmal atrial tachycardia or syncope Exercise induced tachyarrhythmias Fixed-rate pacemaker Hypertension with evidence of end-organ damage Drugs that inhibit normal exercise Peripheral vascular disease that limits exercise	
Neurological	Seizure disorder Brain or spinal cord tumor Cerebrovascular accident or transient ischemic attack Demyelinating disease Spinal cord trauma with neurological deficit Head injury with sequelae Intracranial surgery Central nervous system aneurysm or vascular malformation Migraine headaches Episodic loss of consciousness	History of head trauma with loss of consciousness but no sequelae Chronic headaches History of neurological decompression sickness with residual
Hematological	Unexplained anemia Polycythemia or leukemia Sickle cell disease	Acute anemia
Endocrine	Insulin-dependent diabetes mellitus Diabetes mellitus treated by diet or oral agents with history of hypoglycemia	Non–life-threatening hormonal excess or deficiency Renal insufficiency Obesity
Reproductive	Pregnancy in any stage	_____

(*Table 31-3* **Continues**)

Table 31-3 **Continued**

Psychiatric	Inappropriate motivation
	Claustrophobia or agoraphobia
	Active psychosis or psychosis while receiving
	  psychotropic drugs
	Panic disorder
	Alcohol or drug abuse
	Suicidal ideation with or without severe
	  depression
	Significant anxiety state
	Manic state
		____

Ophthalmological	Radial keratotomy
	Uncorrected visual acuity inadequate to find
	  diving buddy or boat if corrective lenses
	Corrected visual acuity inadequate to read
	  instruments
		____

Gastrointestinal	Uncorrected abdominal wall hernia Paraesophageal or hiatal hernia Chronic or recurrent obstruction Severe gastroesophageal reflux	Peptic ulcer disease Malabsorption Functional bowel disorders Inflammatory bowel disease
Musculoskeletal	Low back pain with neurological symptoms Disability that would hamper work in the water or with diving equipment Juxtaarticular aseptic bone necrosis	Acute sprain or strain Acute trauma

*Sources for the rationales for these recommendations: (1) Bove AA, Davis JC. *Diving Medicine.* 2nd ed. Philadelphia, Pa: WB Saunders; 1990. (2) Davis JC, Bove AA. *Medical Examination of Sports SCUBA Divers.* Flagstaff, Ariz: Best; 1986. (3) Linaweaver PG, Vorosmarti J. *Fitness to Dive: 34th UHMS Workshop Report.* Kensington, Md: The Undersea and Hyperbaric Medical Society; 1987.

the diver should be examined by a DMO.

For Type II symptoms that were completely relieved after the second oxygen-breathing period at 18 msw (60 fsw) during Treatment Table 6, the diver may resume diving after 14 days with a DMO's concurrence, if the symptoms involved only patchy peripheral paresthesias (numbness, tingling, or decreased sensation). However, if there were symptoms suggesting AGE, cardiorespiratory involvement, or neurological involvement other than patchy peripheral paresthesias, diving should not be allowed for 4 weeks—and then only after further examination. If the symptoms required treatment according to Treatment Tables 4 or 7, diving should not be allowed for 3 months. Up-to-date regulations should be consulted, as these proscriptions can change and may differ among the services.

SUBMARINE RESCUE AND ESCAPE

If a submarine is disabled and cannot surface, the crew may be rescued by a submersible chamber or small submarine, or may be required to leave the submarine through an "escape trunk" that allows passage from low submarine pressure to higher water pressure, from which they ascend through the water to the surface. While not specifically a diving activity, submarine rescue and escape expose sailors to pressure changes that cause illnesses associated with diving. Submarine rescue has not been needed by the US Navy since 1939 (Exhibits 31-9 and 31-10).

The US Navy has two methods for rescuing the crew of a disabled submarine. One method uses the Submarine Rescue Chamber (SRC), which is lowered from a surface vessel and mated to a hatch on the downed submarine. The SRC, which was developed in 1931, saved 33 men from the *USS Squalus* in 1939.

The second method, which is the primary rescue method, uses the Deep Submergence Rescue Vehicle (DSRV), a submersible that mates with the disabled submarine and transfers surviving crewmembers to the surface or another submarine (Figure 31-28). The DSRV can be pressurized internally if the submarine itself is under pressure, but as there are currently no surface chambers that allow transfer under pressure, rescued personnel must be decompressed to sea level and recompressed in a surface-based chamber for subsequent saturation decompression. The initial decom-

EXHIBIT 31-9

THE RATIONALE FOR SUBMARINE
ESCAPE AND RESCUE

Given the paucity of recent US Navy submarine disasters ... one might conclude it is not prudent to devote too much of the Navy's resources ... to submarine rescue or escape. Submarine sailors, as well as airline passengers, wisely do not spend much time pondering the possibility that they may be embarking on a one way trip. Statistically speaking, submarine and commercial airline travel is very safe.

. . . .

It is frequently argued that since US submarines spend 95 percent of their time operating in waters [in which the ocean bottom is] deeper than the hull crush depth, discussions of escape or rescue are for the comfort of wives and mothers back home. Nevertheless, the chance of a mishap is much greater while the submarine is over the continental shelf because of the increased risks associated with sea trials, diving and surfacing, and transiting with open hatches and other hull penetrations in areas with greater sea traffic density, such as near major seaports.

Reproduced from: Molé DM. *Submarine Escape and Rescue: An Overview* [thesis]. Washington, DC: Department of the Navy, Submarine Development Group One; 1990: 1.

EXHIBIT 31-10

SUBMARINE ESCAPE AND LOCK-OUT
TRAINING IN THE US NAVY

There has been no need for submarine rescue in the US Navy since the sinking of the USS *Squalus* in 1939. The USS *Thresher*, which sank in 2,520 msw (8,400 fsw) in 1963, and the USS *Scorpion*, which sank in 3,000 msw (10,000 fsw) in 1968, were too deep for rescue. The Navy conducted submarine escape training until the 1980s in two 100-ft-tall fresh-water towers in Groton, Connecticut, and Pearl Harbor, Hawaii, but these have been decommissioned due to concern over the incidence of arterial gas embolism (about 1 in every 22,000 exposures). Other navies continue submarine escape training in land-based towers. The US Navy presently has three 50-ft towers that are used primarily for submarine lock-out (leaving the submarine through an escape hatch) training for Special Operations personnel.

Source: Molé DM. *Submarine Escape and Rescue: An Overview* [thesis]. Washington, DC: Department of the Navy, Submarine Development Group One; 1990: 1.

pression to sea level may result in a high incidence of DCS. The DSRV is expensive to maintain, requires dedicated aircraft for transportation, takes at least 24 hours to arrive at a nearby port, and must be carried by ship or submarine to the disabled submarine.

To escape from a disabled submarine, several sailors enter an escape trunk, which is then isolated from the submarine by closing an inner hatch. The escapees don an appliance known as the Steinke hood, which is a life jacket with an attached hood that allows continuous breathing. The hood is plugged into an air-charging system, and the escape trunk is flooded with sea water and compressed to ambient sea pressure. The outer hatch of the trunk is opened, and the escapee leaves the trunk and is carried to the surface by the positive buoyancy of the hood. Air expanding in the hood vents to the sea during ascent. The risk of air embolism is small if the escapee breathes normally. This system has several drawbacks, however:

- if compression of the escape trunk is slow and the depth is great, the risk of DCS is significant;
- the escapees operate the trunk themselves, which may be difficult if they are frightened or compromised by contaminated air, carbon dioxide, hypoxia, pulmonary oxygen toxicity, or nitrogen narcosis;
- if an escapee is caught in the trunk, it becomes unusable by others; and
- unless rescue is immediate when the escapee reaches the surface, the chance of survival is small because no thermal protection is provided.

Medical officers who supervise training exercises or actual escapes must be prepared to manage casualties from cerebral air embolism, DCS, trauma, burns, and exposure.

The Royal Navy has a different escape system: a one-man lock that can be flooded and pressurized very quickly. This system offers some advantages. The escapee is completely enclosed by a hood that is attached to a survival suit. On entering the lock, the escapee plugs into an air supply, and the lock is automatically flooded and pressurized to eliminate the possibility of operator error. During compression, the pressure doubles every 4 seconds, which

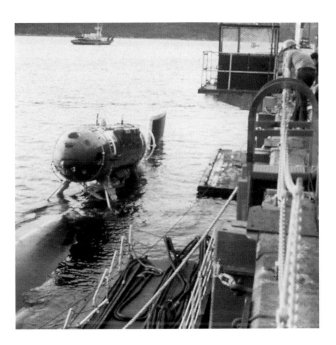

Fig. 31-28. One of the US Navy's Deep Submergence Rescue Vehicles (DSRVs; center, in 1985) is locked-on to (ie, mated with) the after escape trunk of a surfaced submarine. Photograph: US Navy.

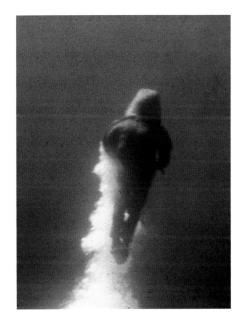

Fig. 31-29. An escapee, enclosed in a survival suit and hood, ascends from a submerged submarine using the Royal Navy method. The US Navy is in the process of adopting this escape method. Photograph: Royal Navy, London, England.

reduces nitrogen uptake and the risk of DCS. (The middle ear space seems to equilibrate passively during this rapid compression, or rupture of the tympanic membrane is not noticeable.) The outer hatch opens when the lock reaches ambient pressure, and the escapee is buoyed rapidly to the surface without risk of entanglement in the trunk (Figure 31-29). The survival suit is designed for at least 24 hours in cold seas and bad weather. This system has been tested at sea from a depth of 180 msw (600 fsw). The US Navy plans to retrofit its submarines with the British escape system.

SUMMARY

Military diving operations have special medical requirements because of the physiological stresses imposed by barometric pressure, breathing gas composition, and immersion. Personnel at risk include some 4,000 to 5,000 divers in the US military (Navy, Marine Corps, Army, Air Force, Coast Guard) and 5,000 to 10,000 military divers from other nations. For US forces, the *US Navy Diving Manual*[1] provides guidance on the conduct of diving operations and associated medical assistance. In addition to diving, UMOs in the US Navy support the escape and rescue of crewmembers who may be trapped in disabled submarines.

Diving history provides a useful context in which the interactions of mission and environment can be appreciated from a medical perspective, and examples drawn from combat swimming and diving operations during World War II serve to illustrate the problems of breath-hold and oxygen diving. UBAs, which provide a reliable source of breathing gas and extends the dive time, introduce additional problems that can occur with increasing depth, including the need for thermal protection and alterations of consciousness from interactions of oxygen, carbon dioxide, and nitrogen.

Ascent from depth must become progressively slower as the surface is approached to avoid DCS from bubbles that form in the diver's body. Decompression schedules and diver-worn computers provide guidance concerning how to ascend with acceptable DCS risk. After 12 to 24 hours, divers become saturated with inert gas and may remain at depth indefinitely without accruing additional decompression time. Saturation dives require special pressure chambers in which the divers live while not actively working underwater.

Failure to follow the decompression prescriptions of dive schedules or computers (and sometimes even if these prescriptions are followed) can lead to DCS or AGE. These conditions usually can be successfully treated by recompression while the patient breathes 100% oxygen, which causes bubbles to resolve. The pulmonary, cardiovascular, and neurological systems require particularly close evaluation during medical examinations to determine fitness to dive for initial training or for the return to diving after DCS or AGE.

REFERENCES

1. US Department of the Navy. *US Navy Diving Manual.* SS521-Ag-PRO-010. Washington, DC: Naval Sea Systems Command. Rev 4 (20 Jan 1999); Change A (1 Mar 2001). NAVSEA 0994-LP-100-3199.

2. Strauss MB, Wright PW. Thoracic squeeze diving casualty. *Aerospace Med.* 1971; 42(6):673-675.

3. Lin Y-C, Hong SK. Hyperbaria: Breath-hold diving. In: Fregley MJ, Batteis CM, eds. *Handbook of Physiology.* Section 4, Vol 3. *Environmental Physiology.* New York, NY: Oxford University Press; The American Physiology Society; 1996: 979–995.

4. Lanphier EH, Rahn H. Alveolar gas exchange during breath-hold diving. *J Appl Physiol.* 1963;18:471–477.

5. Lanphier EH, Rahn H. Alveolar gas exchange during breath holding with air. *J Appl Physiol.* 1963;18:478–482.

6. Woollcott S. Quoted by: Waldron TJ, Gleeson J. *The Frogmen.* London, England: Evans Brothers Ltd; 1950: 60–61.

7. National Oceanographic and Atmospheric Administration. *NOAA Diving Manual.* 4th ed. Washington, DC: US Department of Commerce; 2001.

8. Larsen HE. *A History of Self-Contained Diving and Underwater Swimming.* Washington, DC: National Academy of Sciences—National Research Council; 1959. Publication 469.

9. Cousteau JY, Dumas F. *The Silent World.* New York, NY: Harper Brothers; 1953.

10. Bevan J. *The Infernal Diver.* London, England: Submex; 1996.

11. Davis RH. *Deep Diving and Submarine Operations: A Manual for Deep Sea Divers and Compressed Air Workers.* 7th ed. London, England: Saint Catherine Press; 1962.

12. Lanphier EH, ed. *The Unconscious Diver: Respiratory Control and Other Contributing Factors.* Bethesda, Md: Undersea Medical Society; 1982. Publication 52WS (RC) 1-25-82.

13. Donald K. *Oxygen and the Diver.* Welshpool, Wales: The SPA Ltd; 1993.

14. Lanphier E. The story of CO_2 build-up. *aquaCorps.* 1992;3(1):67–69.

15. Admiralty Report. *Deep-Water Diving.* London, England: His Majesty's Stationery Office; 1907.

16. Hamilton RW, Rogers RE, Powell MP, Vann RD. *The DSAT Recreational Dive Planner: Development and Validation of No-Stop Decompression Procedures for Recreational Diving.* Tarrytown, NY: Diving Science and Technology, Inc, and Hamilton Research, Ltd; 1994.

17. Lewis JE, Shreeves KW. *The Recreational Diver's Guide to Decompression Theory, Dive Tables, and Dive Computers.* Santa Ana, Calif: Professional Association of Diving Instructors; 1990.

18. Vann RD, Thalmann ED. Decompression physiology and practice. In: Bennett PT, Elliott DH, eds. *The Physiology of Diving and Compressed Air Work.* 4th ed. Philadelphia, Pa: WB Saunders; 1992: 376–432.

19. Ministry of Defence. *Royal Navy Diving Manual*. London, England: Her Majesty's Stationery Office; 1972. MOD BR 2806.

20. Universal Dive Techtronics. Defense Civil Institute of Environmental Medicine *Diving Manual*. Richmond, Ontario, Canada: Universal Dive Techtronics; 1992. DCIEM 86-R-35.

21. Dear G de L, Uguccioni DM, Dovenbarger JA, Thalmann ED, Cudahy E, Hanson E. Estimated DCI incidence in a select group of recreational divers. *Undersea Hyperb Med*. 1999;26(suppl):19. Abstract 34.

22. Divers Alert Network. *Report on Decompression Illness and Diving Fatalities*. Durham, NC: DAN; 1998.

23. Hamilton RW, ed. *Effectiveness of Dive Computers in Repetitive Diving*. Bethesda, Md: The Undersea and Hyperbaric Medical Society; 1995. 81(DC)6-1-94.

24. Sheffield PJ. Flying after diving guidelines: A review. *Aviat Space Environ Med*. 1990;61:1130–1138.

25. Weathersby PK, Survanshi SS, Homer LD, Parker E, Thalmann ED. Predicting the time of occurrence of decompression sickness. *J Appl Physiol*. 1992;72(4):1541–1548.

26. Bennett PB, Elliott DH, eds. *The Physiology of Diving*. 4th ed. London, England: WB Saunders; 1993.

Chapter 32

PRESSURE CHANGES AND HYPOXIA IN AVIATION

R. M. HARDING, BSc, MB BS, PhD[*]

[*]Principal Consultant, Biodynamic Research Corporation, 9901 IH-10 West, Suite 1000, San Antonio, Texas 78230; formerly, Royal Air Force Consultant in Aviation Medicine and Head of Aircrew Systems Division, Department of Aeromedicine and Neuroscience of the UK Centre for Human Science, Farnborough, Hampshire, United Kingdom

INTRODUCTION

The physiological consequences of rapid ascent to high altitude are a core problem in the field of aerospace medicine. Those who live and work in mountain terrain experience a limited range of altitudes and have time to adapt to the hypoxia experienced at high terrestrial elevations. In contrast, flyers may be exposed to abrupt changes in barometric pressure and to acute, life-threatening hypoxia (see also Chapter 28, Introduction to Special Environments).

In 1875, a landmark balloon flight to 28,820 ft ended in tragedy when the three young French aeronauts on board failed to use their supplemental oxygen effectively; Tissandier survived, but his colleagues, Sivel and Crocé-Spineli, became the first known fatalities due to in-flight hypoxia. In early aviation, too, the lack of oxygen took a regular toll of both lives and aircraft; many military crewmembers were killed by hypoxia, and the performance of many more was significantly impaired in flight. Historic ascents over many years demonstrated that even with inhalation of 100% oxygen, unpressurized flight above 42,000 ft was impractical because of the effects of hypoxia and extreme cold. It was found that humans cannot adapt to hypoxia in flight but must instead be provided with life-support systems that (*a*) maintain physiological normoxia under routine operating conditions and (*b*) protect from significant hypoxia in emergencies.

Pioneering research by physicians, physiologists, and life-support engineers has established reliable techniques for safe flight at high altitudes, as demonstrated by current atmospheric flight in all its forms, military and civilian, from balloon flights to sail planes to supersonic aircraft and spacecraft. Although reliable cabin pressurization and oxygen delivery systems have greatly reduced incidents and accidents due to hypoxia in flight, constant vigilance is required for their prevention.

The aims of this chapter are, therefore, to present a distillation of our current comprehension of the physics and physiology of rapid ascent to high altitude and to describe the technology required to support human existence in that most hostile of environments. To this end, the chapter briefly characterizes the atmosphere within which flight takes place, then describes normal physiological responses to acute hypobaria and hypoxia, and finally describes the life-support systems that enable flyers to operate safely at high altitudes.

Military requirements drove much of the early research in aviation physiology as well as the development of robust life-support systems. Prominent centers for aviation altitude research included the US Air Force School of Aerospace Medicine, San Antonio, Texas; the now-defunct Royal Air Force Institute of Aviation Medicine, Farnborough, Hampshire, England; and various universities whose hypobaric chambers were supported with military research funds.

THE ATMOSPHERE

Earth's atmosphere is vital to our existence: it provides a moderate temperature environment at the surface, a protective barrier against the effects of radiation, and the oxygen needed for the release of biological energy. Flyers depart from the safety of this surface cocoon at their peril.

The physical characteristics of the atmosphere are a complex product of solar heating, ionizing radiation, and ozone formation (Figure 32-1). The upper atmosphere reflects some solar radiation and absorbs the rest, re-radiating infrared energy into the lower atmosphere and thence to Earth's surface. This "greenhouse" effect ensures that Earth's surface is warmer than it would be if it received only direct solar heating.

High-energy particulate material (cosmic radiation) continuously bombards the atmosphere. This primary ionizing radiation collides with atoms in the upper atmosphere at high velocity to create secondary radiation. Fortunately, the atmosphere further reduces the level of this radiation so that it has little effect on life at the surface, but high-altitude flight can produce significant cumulative radiation exposure for flyers.

Structure

The outer limit of the atmosphere is determined by two opposing factors: solar heating tends to expand gases from the outer atmosphere into the surrounding vacuum of space, while gravity tends to pull the gases toward Earth's surface. The structure of the atmosphere is conventionally described in terms of several concentric shells with differing thermal profiles and other characteristics:

- The *troposphere* (0–40,000 ft) is characterized by a steady decrease in temperature with altitude, the presence of varying amounts of water vapor, and the occurrence of large-scale turbulence (weather). This is the realm of most conventional aviation, including

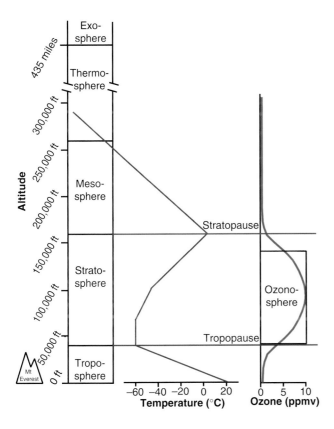

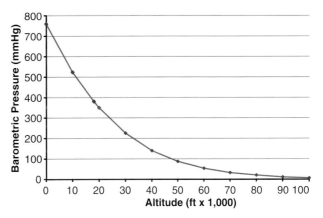

Fig. 32-2. The exponential relation of barometric pressure to altitude. Note that at 18,000 ft (380 mm Hg), barometric pressure is half that at sea level.

Fig. 32-1. The structure of the atmosphere and the relation of altitude to temperature and ozone concentration. Note that at the top of Mount Everest, the highest point on Earth (29,028 ft), the temperature is about –40°C and ozone concentration is about 1 ppmv. For the next 125,000 ft the temperature becomes more moderate while ozone becomes more, then again less, concentrated. The temperature at the top of Mount Everest, –40°C, is not reached again until about 100,000 ft. Adapted with permission from Harding RM. The Earth's atmosphere. In: Ernsting J, King P. *Aviation Medicine.* 2nd ed. London, England: Butterworths; 1988: 5.

balloon flights.

- The *stratosphere* (40,000–160,000 ft) includes a lower *isothermal* layer, above which temperature increases with altitude. Ozone is formed in the stratosphere, and flight in this region is generally limited to military aircraft.
- The *mesosphere* (160,000–260,000 ft) exhibits a rapid decline in temperature with altitude.
- The *thermosphere*, also called the *ionosphere* (260,000 ft to ~ 435 mi [700 km, the outer limit of the atmosphere]), exhibits extreme temperatures, which vary with solar activity.
- The *exosphere* (≥ 435 mi), where the tempera-

ture approaches absolute zero, extends beyond the atmosphere to the vacuum of space.

The pressure exerted by the atmosphere, termed *barometric pressure* (PB), falls exponentially with altitude (Figure 32-2), producing a proportional decrease in the partial pressures of oxygen and other constituent gases. The International Civil Aviation Organization's (ICAO's) Standard Atmosphere is an agreed description of the relation among PB, temperature, and altitude at a latitude of 45° north (Table 32-1).[1] This description forms the basis for calibration of pressure-measuring flight instruments and allows precise comparisons between the performances of different aircraft and aircraft systems. The measurement of physiological variables such as volume and mass of gas, gas flow, and metabolic rate, as well as the related specifications for life-support systems, are profoundly affected by changes in body temperature, PB, and saturation of water vapor in the lungs. The conditions of measuring physiological variables at altitude are summarized in Exhibit 32-1. (Related information on the larger changes in PB associated with diving is found in Chapter 30, Physics, Physiology, and Medicine of Diving.)

Composition

The atmosphere is made up of a remarkably constant mixture of nitrogen and oxygen, with traces of other gases (Table 32-2). In addition, the lower troposphere may contain significant amounts of carbon dioxide and toxic gases, reflecting human activity and natural phenomena such as volcanic eruptions. It may also contain increased quantities of water vapor, de-

TABLE 32–1

INTERNATIONAL CIVIL AVIATION ORGANIZATION STANDARD ATMOSPHERE

Altitude (ft)	Altitude (m)	Pressure (mm Hg)	Temperature (°C)	Altitude (ft)	Altitude (m)	Pressure (mm Hg)	Temperature (°C)
0	0	760	+15.0	25,000	7,620	282	–34.5
1,000	305	733	+13.0	30,000	9,144	226	–44.4
2,000	610	706	+11.0	35,000	10,668	179	–54.2
3,000	914	681	+9.1	40,000	12,192	141	–56.5
4,000	1,219	656	+7.1	45,000	13,716	111	–56.5
5,000	1,525	632	+5.1	50,000	15,240	87.3	–56.5
6,000	1,829	609	+3.1	55,000	16,764	68.8	–56.5
7,000	2,134	586	+1.1	60,000	18,288	54.1	–56.5
8,000	2,438	565	–0.9	65,000	19,812	42.3	–56.5
9,000	2,743	543	–2.8	70,000	21,336	33.3	–55.2
10,000	3,048	523	–4.8	80,000	24,384	20.7	–52.1
15,000	4,572	429	–14.7	90,000	27,432	13.0	–49.1
20,000	6,096	349	–24.6	100,000	30,480	8.2	–46.0

Adapted with permission from International Civil Aviation Organization. *Manual of the ICAO Standard Atmosphere.* 2nd ed. Montreal, Quebec, Canada: ICAO; 1964.

pending on the temperature of the air mass and whether it has recently passed over water.

Ozone is the highly reactive, triatomic form of oxygen that may adversely affect the respiratory tract[2]; its formation and destruction in the atmosphere are therefore of great physical and biological importance. Ozone forms in the stratosphere when molecular oxygen absorbs ultraviolet radiation, a process that greatly reduces harmful ultraviolet radiation at lower altitudes. Ozone concentration reaches approximately 10.0 parts per million by volume (ppmv) at 100,000 ft but falls to less than 1.0 ppmv at altitudes below 40,000 ft and to about 0.03 ppmv at sea level (see Figure 32-1).

THE PHYSIOLOGICAL CONSEQUENCES OF RAPID ASCENT TO ALTITUDE

The physiological consequences associated with the physical changes in the atmosphere seen on rapid ascent to altitude include hypoxia and hyperventilation, as a result of reduction in the partial pressure of oxygen (Po_2); barotrauma and the decompression illnesses, as a result of reduction in total pressure; and thermal injury, as a result of decreased temperature (Figure 32-3). Cold (thermal) injury is discussed in *Medical Consequences of Harsh Environments, Volume 1*[3]; the remaining potential problems are addressed below. To a large extent, our understanding of these problems has only been made possible with the help of experimental hypobaric chambers in military and university laboratories worldwide.

Hypoxia

Oxygen is one of the most important requirements for the maintenance of normal function by living systems, as energy for biological processes is generated by the oxidation of complex chemical foodstuffs into simpler compounds, usually with the eventual formation of carbon dioxide, water, and other waste products. Human beings are extremely vulnerable and sensitive to the effects of oxygen lack, and severe deprivation leads to a rapid deterioration of most bodily functions. If the situation persists, death is inevitable. Not without reason is hypoxia generally held to be the most serious single physiological hazard encoun-

---

EXHIBIT 32-1

VOLUME, TEMPERATURE, PRESSURE, AND WATER VAPOR IN RESPIRATORY MEASUREMENT

BTPS. Gas in the lungs is said to be at *body temperature and pressure, saturated* (BTPS). Body temperature is usually regarded as constant at 37°C; water vapor at that temperature reaches a pressure of 47 mm Hg at saturation.

ATPS. Ambient air is usually cooler and dryer than gas in the lungs and is designated as *ambient temperature and pressure* (ATP). If respiratory volumes are measured using a water spirometer, calculations are made from ambient temperature and pressure, saturated (ATPS), where water vapor pressure is calculated as the saturation value at the temperature of the spirometer.

Conversion from ATPS to BTPS can be expressed mathematically:

$$V_{BTPS} = V_{ATPS} \bullet \frac{273 + 37}{273 + T_{db}} \bullet \frac{P_B - P_{H_2O}}{P_B - 47}$$

where *V* represents volume; *273* = melting point of ice, expressed in °K; *37* = body temperature, expressed in °C; T_{db} represents ambient dry bulb temperature, expressed in °C; P_B represents barometric pressure, expressed in mm Hg; P_{H_2O} represents saturated water vapor pressure at T_{db}; and *47* = P_{H_2O} at body temperature.

STPD. Metabolic calculations require knowledge of the number of molecules (ie, the mass) of oxygen used and carbon dioxide produced. For this purpose, the gas volumes are expressed as standard temperature and pressure, dry (STPD), where the standard temperature is 273°K (O°C) and the standard pressure is 760 mm Hg (1 atm). Under these conditions, gases comply with Avogadro's law (ie, 1 g-mol of a gas has a volume of 22.4 L_{STPD}), so that the number of molecules contained within the STPD volume can readily be calculated.

Likewise, conversion from ATPS to STPD can be expressed mathematically:

$$V_{STDP} = V_{ATPS} \bullet \frac{273}{273 + T_{db}} \bullet \frac{P_B - P_{H_2O}}{760}$$

Other Conditions. Specifications for life-support systems may quote gas volumes as atmospheric temperature and pressure, dry (ATPD); and gas consumption figures may be quoted as normal temperature and pressure (NTP). The need to express gas quantities under NTP conditions arises because gases expand on exposure to low barometric pressure, thereby altering the relationship between volume flow and mass flow of a gas. For example, at an altitude of 18,000 ft (0.5 atm), a mass flow of 5.0 L_{NTP}/min will provide a volume flow of about 10.0 L_{ATPD}/min. Because respiration is a volume-flow phenomenon, mass flow versus volume flow has particular relevance for respiratory physiology at altitude.

---

tered during flight at altitude.

The absence of an adequate supply of oxygen to the tissues, whether in mass or in molecular concentration, is termed *hypoxia* and may be defined in several ways. In aerospace medicine, the concern is with *hypoxic* hypoxia, which is the result of a reduction in oxygen tension in the arterial blood (PaO_2), and of which acute *hypobaric* hypoxia is one cause.

In military aviation, the principal causes of hypoxia in flight are the following[4(p46)]:

- ascent to altitude without supplementary oxygen (about 10% of casualties);
- failure of personal breathing equipment to deliver oxygen at an adequate concentra-

tion or pressure (about 68%); and

- decompression of the pressure cabin at high altitude (about 20%).

The physiological consequences of hypoxia in flight are dominated by the changes seen in three main areas: the respiratory and cardiovascular responses to hypoxia, and the neurological effects of both hypoxia itself and the cardiorespiratory responses to it.[4] The clinical consequences reflect changes seen in all three systems. It is worth remembering that in healthy individuals at sea level, alveolar ventilation is the prime determinant of tissue carbon dioxide level, and local blood flow is the prime determinant of tissue oxygen tension.

TABLE 32-2

ATMOSPHERIC COMPOSITION OF DRY AIR

Gas	Percentage by Volume in Dry Air[*]
Nitrogen	78.09
Oxygen	20.95
Argon	0.93
Carbon Dioxide	0.03
Neon	$1.82 \bullet 10^{-3}$
Helium	$5.24 \bullet 10^{-4}$
Krypton	$1.14 \bullet 10^{-4}$
Hydrogen	$5.00 \bullet 10^{-5}$
Xenon	$8.70 \bullet 10^{-6}$

[*]For most practical purposes, however, dry air may be regarded as a mixture consisting of 21% oxygen and 79% nitrogen.
Reproduced with permission from Harding RM. The Earth's atmosphere. In: Ernsting J, King P. *Aviation Medicine*. 2nd ed. London, England: Butterworths; 1988: 5.

Respiratory Responses to Hypoxia

The respiratory responses to hypoxia clearly depend on the manner in which the insult is delivered. Thus, the changes that accompany a slow ascent to altitude when breathing air are different from those seen if the ascent is undertaken when breathing oxygen, and different again if hypoxia is

the result of a rapid loss of cabin pressure.

Alveolar Gases When Breathing Air. As described above, ascent to altitude is associated with an exponential fall in P_B (with parallel reductions in both air density and temperature) and also, therefore, in the partial pressures of the component gases of the atmosphere. The fall in the partial pressure of oxygen in the inspired gas (P_{IO_2}) produces a corresponding reduction in the partial pressure of oxygen in the alveoli (P_{AO_2}). But the main determinant of the difference between P_{IO_2} and P_{AO_2} is the partial pressure of carbon dioxide in the alveoli (P_{ACO_2}), as shown in Equation 1:

$$(1) \qquad P_{IO_2} - P_{AO_2} = P_{ACO_2}\left(F_{IO_2} + \frac{1 - F_{IO_2}}{R}\right)$$

where F_{IO_2} represents the fraction of inspired oxygen, and R represents the respiratory exchange ratio.

P_{ACO_2} is itself determined by the ratio of carbon dioxide production to alveolar ventilation, a ratio that is independent of environmental pressure. Provided that this ratio is undisturbed, P_{ACO_2} will remain constant on ascent to altitude. This is indeed what happens during ascent from sea level to about 10,000 ft: P_{ACO_2} remains constant and P_{AO_2} falls linearly with the reduction in environmental pressure.

Above 10,000 ft, however, the partial pressure of oxygen in arterial blood (P_{aO_2}) falls to a level that stimulates respiration via the arterial chemoreceptors, and so P_{ACO_2} decreases as alveolar ventilation increases. Because there is little if any change in metabolic production of carbon dioxide under these circumstances, the ventilatory response to hypoxia is *hyperventilation* (discussed below). As a consequence of the reduction in P_{ACO_2}, the difference between P_{IO_2} and P_{aO_2} is less than it would have been had no stimulation of ventilation occurred. So the

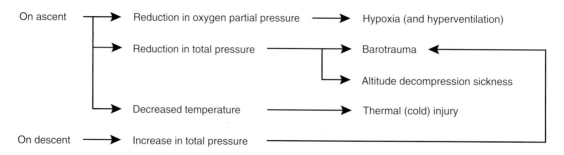

Fig. 32-3. The environmental changes associated with ascent to altitude are dominated by the development of hypoxia as a result of reduced oxygen partial pressure. Those asociated with descent are dominated by the possible development of otic and sinus barotrauma as a result of increased total pressure. Adapted from Harding RM, Mills FJ. Problems of altitude. In: Harding RM, Mills FJ, eds. *Aviation Medicine*. 3rd ed. London, England: British Medical Association; 1993: 71.

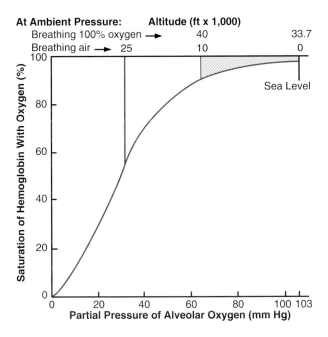

At Ambient Pressure: **Altitude (ft x 1,000)**

Breathing 100% oxygen →   40   33.7

Breathing air →   25   10   0

Fig. 32-4. The relation between oxygen saturation of hemoglobin and oxygen partial pressure, as reflected in the sigmoid shape of the dissociation curve, minimizes the physiological effects of a fall in partial pressure. The plateau represents an in-built reserve, or buffer zone, which provides protection for healthy individuals up to an altitude of 10,000 ft, and is exploited by aircraft designers, who maintain commercial aircraft cabins at an altitude below this. Above 10,000 ft, and especially above 25,000 ft, percentage saturation of hemoglobin falls and hypoxia results (unless enriched oxygen is provided). Note that, in this regard, sea level and 33,700 ft, and 10,000 ft and 40,000, can be described as physiologically equivalent altitudes. Adapted from Harding RM, Mills FJ. Problems of altitude. In: Harding RM, Mills FJ, eds. *Aviation Medicine*. 3rd ed. London, England: British Medical Association; 1993: 61.

increase in ventilation is "protective" against hypoxia insofar as it reduces the fall in P_{AO_2} that would otherwise be seen on ascent; however, the magnitude of the effect is itself a compromise between the demand for an adequate oxygen supply (ventilation stimulated via chemoreceptors) and the need to maintain a normal acid–base balance (ventilation inhibited by hypocapnia).

Reaching an altitude of 10,000 ft is consequently a crucial stage in the development of the physiological changes associated with an ascent. A consideration of the oxyhemoglobin dissociation curve helps to show why this should be (Figure 32-4). The relation between the partial pressure of oxygen (P_{AO_2}) and the percentage saturation of hemoglobin with oxygen describes a sigmoid curve. The plateau at the top of the curve represents a physiological reserve, whereby a fall in P_{O_2} (however produced) from the normal 100 mm Hg to about 60 to 70 mm Hg produces very little desaturation. In healthy individuals, a fall in P_{O_2} of this magnitude is seen during an ascent from sea level to 10,000 ft. Above this altitude, the steep part of the dissociation curve takes effect: hemoglobin rapidly desaturates and significant hypoxia develops.

Alveolar Gases When Breathing Oxygen. If ascent is undertaken when breathing 100% oxygen, and provided that P_{ACO_2} remains constant, then P_{AO_2} will fall linearly with environmental pressure until such time as hypoxia stimulates respiration. Thus, when 100% oxygen is breathed, not until an altitude of 33,700 ft does P_{AO_2} fall to 103 mm Hg (ie, to its sea level value [equivalent] when breathing air). And not until an altitude of about 39,000 to 40,000 does P_{AO_2} fall to 60 to 65 mm Hg (ie, to the value seen at 10,000 ft when breathing air). Above 40,000 ft, P_{AO_2}, and therefore P_{aO_2} too, fall to levels that stimulate respiration even though 100% oxygen is being inspired. Once again, the resulting fall in P_{ACO_2} (ie, hyperventilation) is "protective" against hypoxia, and P_{AO_2} will rise by 1 mm Hg for every 1 mm Hg reduction in P_{ACO_2}. The concept of physiologically equivalent altitudes when breathing air or 100% oxygen is of considerable value in the design of life-support systems (see the discussion below in the Personal Oxygen Equipment section).

If hypoxia is induced by a change from breathing gas with a high oxygen content to air, then P_{AO_2} falls progressively as the nitrogen concentration in the inspired and alveolar gas rises to about 80%. There is frequently a phase during this process when P_{AO_2} is lower than P_{aO_2}, and so oxygen passes out of the pulmonary circulation into the alveolar gas, thus briefly counteracting the original fall.

Alveolar Gases During Rapid Decompression. The sudden fall in P_B that accompanies a rapid decompression (RD) of an aircraft cabin (that is, a decompression over a period of seconds or less) produces equally severe falls in the partial pressures of alveolar gases. The magnitude of this effect will depend not only on the ratio of the environmental pressure before decompression to that after the event, but also on the composition of the gas being breathed at the moment of decompression.[5]

For example, a decompression from 8,000 ft to 40,000 ft in 1.6 seconds while air is breathed produces a fall in P_{AO_2} from 65 mm Hg to 15 mm Hg, and a fall in P_{ACO_2} to only 10 mm Hg. Although the latter quickly recovers to about 25 to 30 mm Hg, P_{AO_2} remains at about 18 mm Hg for as long as air is breathed (because at 40,000 ft, P_{IO_2} is only 20 mm Hg).

But a fall in P_{AO_2} to below 30 mm Hg will inevitably be accompanied by profound neurological hypoxia, and such a fall is an equally inevitable consequence of breathing air during an RD to a final altitude greater than 30,000 ft. This is the case even if delivery of 100% oxygen commences at the moment of decompression. Although subsequently, breathing 100% oxygen will cause a rapid rise in P_{AO_2}, the greater the final altitude and the longer the delay in delivering 100% oxygen, the more profound will be the degree of hypoxia. Thus, it is clear that breathing an oxygen-rich mixture before an RD will reduce the severity of hypoxia after it. Indeed, for example, P_{AO_2} will at no time fall below about 60 mm Hg if 100% oxygen is breathed before, during, and after an RD from 8,000 ft to 40,000 ft. These rapid physiological changes have important implications for the design of personal oxygen equipment because an oxygen-rich inspirate must be provided before the event. Furthermore, delivery of 100% oxygen must be initiated within 2 seconds of the start of an RD if significant hypoxia is to be avoided.

Cardiovascular Responses to Hypoxia

Cardiovascular responses to hypoxia involve general and regional changes. In the resting subject, heart rate starts to rise when breathing air at altitudes above 6,000 to 8,000 ft, and is approximately doubled at 25,000 ft. Cardiac output also rises, but stroke volume and mean arterial blood pressure are unchanged. Systolic blood pressure and pulse pressure are usually elevated but peripheral resistance is reduced, overall, with a redistribution of flow by local and vasomotor mechanisms.

Hypoxia causes vasodilation in most vascular beds, but there are some important features in the responses of certain regional circulations. Thus, the redistribution of cardiac output results in an increase in blood flow to the heart and brain at the expense of other, less vital, organs such as the bowel, the skin, and the kidneys. Flow to skeletal muscle is unchanged. Flow in the coronary circulation increases in parallel with cardiac output, but there is a reduction in cardiac reserve such that a profound fall in P_{AO_2} can cause myocardial depression and, in some cases, a severe compensatory vasoconstriction with cardiac arrest. Electrocardiographic changes are a feature only during profound hypoxia.

Predictably, the cerebral circulation is acutely sensitive to changes in both P_{AO_2} and P_{ACO_2}. When P_{AO_2} is greater than 45 to 50 mm Hg, cerebral blood flow is exclusively determined by P_{ACO_2}, to which it bears a directly linear relation over the physiologically tolerable range (20–80 mm Hg). A fall in P_{AO_2} below 45 mm Hg induces a hypoxic vasodilation, so that a P_{AO_2} of 35 mm Hg will cause a 50% to 100% increase in cerebral blood flow. A conflict therefore exists between the *vasodilating* effect of hypoxia and the *vasoconstricting* influence of hypocapnia, itself caused by the ventilatory response to hypoxia.

Hypoxic desaturation of the blood by just 20% is sufficient to produce a generalized and rapid vasoconstriction in the pulmonary circulation, which, in the presence of an increased cardiac output, produces a rise in pulmonary artery pressure.

Neurological Effects of Hypoxia

Although the neurological consequences of a gross fall in P_{AO_2} are usually the cause of loss of consciousness in hypoxia, a simple vasovagal syncope occurs in about 20% of cases. In these individuals, loss of peripheral resistance in the systemic circulation is accompanied by a profound bradycardia, a fall in arterial blood pressure, and a failure of cerebral blood flow.

The ability of tissues to function normally will depend critically on tissue oxygen tensions. Once again, the implications of the oxyhemoglobin dissociation curve are highly relevant (see Figure 32-4). In this case, the steep part of the curve reflects the enhanced and protective ability of hemoglobin to unload oxygen at low levels of P_{O_2}. Thus, for example, when breathing air at sea level (where P_{AO_2} = 100 mm Hg), the delivery of 5 mL of oxygen from every 100 mL of blood results in an arteriovenous difference of 60 mm Hg. The extraction of the same quantity of oxygen when breathing air at 18,000 ft (where P_{AO_2} = 32 mm Hg) results in an arteriovenous difference of only 10 mm Hg.

The neurological effects of hypoxia are obviously of great practical significance in aviation. Exhibit 32-2 summarizes the covert features of early cerebral hypoxia, when air is breathed; medical officers should keep in mind, though, the wide variability in individual behavior, which is primarily a consequence of differences in the respiratory responses to hypoxia.

In more-severe hypoxia, provided that vasovagal syncope does not preempt the issue, loss of consciousness occurs when jugular venous oxygen tension falls to 17 to 19 mm Hg, reflecting significant cerebral hypoxia. The cerebral arterial oxygen tension at which this point is reached depends on cerebral blood flow, and so will vary according to the degree of accompanying hypocapnia: it may lie anywhere between 20 and 35 mm Hg.

EXHIBIT 32-2

COVERT FEATURES OF ACUTE HYPOBARIC HYPOXIA

Psychomotor Function
- Choice reaction time is impaired significantly by 12,000 ft.
- Eye-hand coordination is impaired by 10,000 ft, even for well-learned tasks.
- Muscular incoordination increases > 15,000 ft.
- Simple reaction time is affected only > 18,000 ft.

Cognitive Function
- Performance at novel tasks may be impaired at 8,000 ft.
- Memory is increasingly impaired > 10,000 ft.

Visual Function
- Light intensity is perceived as reduced.
- Visual acuity is diminished in poor illumination.
- Light perception threshold is increased.
- Peripheral vision is narrowed (ie, tunneling).

Adapted with permission from Ernsting J, Sharp GR. Harding RM, rev-eds. Hypoxia and hyperventilation. In: Ernsting J, King PF, eds. *Aviation Medicine*. 2nd ed. London, England: Butterworths, 1988: 57.

Again, consciousness will inevitably be lost if P_{AO_2} falls below 30 mm Hg (eg, following an RD to an altitude above 30,000 ft). Even in these instances, however, circulation and brain equilibration times are such that consciousness persists for 12 to 14 seconds after the event.

Clinical Features of Acute Hypobaric Hypoxia

The clinical features of acute hypobaric hypoxia are a combination of the respiratory and cardiovascular responses and the neurological effects described above; consequently, the symptoms and signs are extremely variable. The speed and order of the appearance of signs and of the severity of symptoms produced by a lowering of the P_{IO_2} depend on (1) the rate at which, and the level to which, the oxygen tension falls and (2) the duration of the reduction. Even when these factors are kept constant, however, there is considerable variation among individuals; although for the same individual the pattern of effects does tend to remain similar—a phenomenon that increases the value of routine exposure of aircrew

to hypoxia in a training environment. Exhibit 32-3 summarizes the clinically obvious features of hypobaric hypoxia (and of hyperventilation). Several additional factors may influence an individual's susceptibility to hypoxia and so modify the pattern of symptoms and signs produced. These factors include

- physical activity (exercise exacerbates the features of hypoxia),
- ambient temperature (a cold environment reduces tolerance to hypoxia),
- intercurrent illness (the additional metabolic load imposed by ill health increases susceptibility to hypoxia), and
- drugs (many pharmacologically active substances have effects similar to those of hypoxic hypoxia and so mimic or exacerbate the condition; proprietary preparations containing antihistamine constituents are particularly likely to cause problems, as is alcohol).

Although the greater the altitude the more marked will be the features seen, rapid ascent can allow high altitudes to be reached before severe symptoms and signs occur. In such circumstances, however, sudden unconsciousness may precede the classic features. Accordingly, it is useful to consider the clinical picture seen during slower ascents to various altitudes (Table 32-3).

The *Time of Useful Consciousness* (TUC) denotes the interval between the onset of reduced P_{IO_2} and the point at which there is a specified impairment of performance. The latter is most usefully defined as the point beyond which the hypoxic individual can no longer act to correct the situation. The TUC for a resting subject who changes from breathing oxygen to breathing air at 25,000 ft is about 3 to 6 minutes but is reduced to about 1 to 2 minutes if the subject is exercising. The corresponding times at 40,000 ft are 30 seconds (resting) and 15 to 18 seconds (exercising). Quick corrective action is critical during the TUC, and the importance of a rapid, accurate self-diagnosis followed by emergency action cannot be overemphasized. The nature of hypoxia must be taught and demonstrated regularly to aircrew so that they may learn to recognize their individual symptomatology and take appropriate action. For example, a pilot who instantly identifies an RD can switch to 100% oxygen before the inevitable loss of consciousness, thus increasing the likelihood of recovery in time to regain control of the aircraft before it crashes.

Acute hypobaric hypoxia is rapidly and completely reversed if oxygen is administered or if P_{AO_2} is elevated as a consequence of sufficiently in-

EXHIBIT 32-3

SIGNS AND SYMPTOMS OF ACUTE HYPOXIA (AND OF HYPERVENTILATION)

Hypoxia

- Personality change
- Lack of insight[*]
- Loss of judgment[*]
- Feelings of unreality
- Loss of self-criticism[*]
- Euphoria
- Loss of memory
- Mental incoordination
- Muscular incoordination
- Sensory loss
- Cyanosis

- Hyperventilation[*]

- Semiconsciousness
- Unconsciousness
- Death

(Signs and Symptoms of Hyperventilation)[†]
- °Dizziness
- °Lightheadedness
- °Feelings of apprehension
- °Neuromuscular irritability
- °Paresthesias of the face and extremities
- °Carpopedal spasm

[*]Because of their sinister covertness, these items have special significance in the early phase of hypobaric hypoxia.
[†]Although a sign of hypoxia, hyperventilation also has its own signs and symptoms, which are separate from those of hypoxia.
Adapted with permission from Ernsting J, Sharp GR. Harding RM, rev-ed. Hypoxia and hyperventilation. In: Ernsting J, King PF, eds. *Aviation Medicine.* 2nd ed. London, England: Butterworths, 1988: 57.

creased environmental pressure. There are no sequelae other than a persistent generalized headache if the exposure was prolonged. Occasionally, a temporary (15–60 s) worsening of the clinical features may occur as P_{AO_2} is restored, a phenomenon known as the "oxygen paradox," which is probably caused by a combination of arterial hypotension and persistent hypocapnia, and may manifest as clonic spasms and even loss of consciousness. It is, however, usually mild with some decrement in psychomotor performance accompanying a flushing of the face and hands. In the event of a paradox, it is essential that delivery of oxygen is maintained despite the decline in clinical state.

Hyperventilation

Hyperventilation is a condition in which pulmonary ventilation is greater than that required to eliminate the carbon dioxide produced by body tis-

sues. There is a consequent excessive fall in carbon dioxide levels within alveolar gas, the blood (hypocapnia), and the tissues. A reduction in P_{ACO_2} will also lead to a fall in hydrogen ion concentration (that is, to a rise in pH) so that hyperventilation causes a respiratory alkalosis.

The causes of hyperventilation may be summarized thus:

- Hypoxia (hyperventilation is a normal response to a fall in P_{AO_2} below 55–60 mm Hg).
- Emotional stress—particularly anxiety, apprehension, or fear—is the commonest cause of hyperventilation. Anyone can be affected; hyperventilation occurs in student aircrew during training, in experienced air crew (eg, on change of role), and in passengers.
- Pain, motion sickness, environmental stress

TABLE 32-3

SIGNS AND SYMPTOMS OF HYPOXIA RELATED TO ALTITUDE

Breathing Air	Breathing 100% Oxygen	Signs and Symptoms
≤ 10,000 ft	≤ 39,000 ft	No symptoms, but impaired performance of novel tasks.
10,000–15,000 ft	39,000–42,500 ft	Few or no signs and symptoms are present when resting. Any impairment of performance at skilled tasks is unappreciated. Physical work capacity is severely reduced.
15,000–20,000 ft	42,500–45,000 ft	All the overt signs and symptoms in Exhibit 32-3 may appear, and those due to hyperventilation may dominate. Signs and symptoms are severely exacerbated by physical activity.
> 20,000 ft	> 45,000 ft	Marked signs and symptoms are seen, with rapid decline in performance and sudden loss of consciousness. Hypoxic convulsions are likely.

(eg, high ambient temperatures), and whole-body vibration (as produced by clear air turbulence) at 4–8 Hz when flying at low level, can all produce hyperventilation.
• Positive-pressure breathing (see below).

The physiological consequences of hyperventilation comprise cardiovascular responses and neurological effects.[4] Hypocapnia has no effect on either cardiac output or arterial blood pressure, although the former is redistributed. Thus, blood flow through skeletal muscle is increased, while that through the skin and cerebral circulation is reduced. The intense cerebral vasoconstriction acts to reduce local Pa_{O_2}, and the neurological features of profound hyperventilation are probably due to a combination of cerebral hypoxia and alkalosis. A reduction in Pa_{CO_2} to below 25 to 30 mm Hg produces significant decrements in the performance of both psychomotor and complex mental tasks, while the ability to perform manual tasks is compromised by the neuromuscular disturbance associated with a fall in Pa_{CO_2} below 20 mm Hg. There is gross clouding of consciousness and then unconsciousness if Pa_{CO_2} falls below 10 to 15 mm Hg. The increased sensitivity and spontaneous activity in the peripheral nervous system are consequences of the local rise in pH and produce sensory (eg, paraesthesias) and motor (eg, spasms) disturbances.

The clinical features of hyperventilation relate to the extent of the reduction in Pa_{CO_2} and are summarized in Exhibit 32-4. In those rare cases where extreme anxiety-induced hyperventilation leads to unconsciousness, recovery naturally occurs as autonomic respiratory control reasserts itself and carbon dioxide levels return to normal. Unfortunately, the hyperventilation associated with hypoxic hypoxia in flight is not subject to such self-correction. Because most of the early symptoms of hypoxia are similar to those of hypocapnia (and indeed the features of hypocapnia frequently dominate the early stages of hypoxia), hypoxia must always be suspected when symptoms or signs of hypocapnia occur at altitudes above about 10,000 ft. Therefore, aircrew have to appreciate that corrective procedures must be based on the assumption that the condition is caused by hypoxia until proven otherwise. In combat aircraft, the appropriate corrective action in cases of suspected hypoxia is the emergency oxygen drill (which selects an alternative supply of gas) as laid down in the aircraft flight procedures. Although a common course of action, it is not appropriate or acceptable to select 100% oxygen from the main aircraft system as a "trial" treatment.

Barotrauma: The Direct Effects of Pressure Change

The human body may be considered to be at a constant temperature, and any gas within closed or semiclosed body cavities will obey Boyle's law on ascent to altitude. So, for example, any such gas will double in volume if it is free to do so on ascent from

EXHIBIT 32-4

SYMPTOMS AND SIGNS OF HYPERVENTILATION

Partial Pressure of Alveolar Carbon Dioxide (mm Hg)	Symptoms and Signs of Hyperventilation
P_{ACO_2} 20–25:	Lightheadedness, dizziness, anxiety (which may produce a vicious circle), and paraesthesias of the extremities and around the lips
P_{ACO_2} 15–20:	Muscle spasms of the limbs (carpopedal) and face (risus sardonicus)
	Augmentation of the tendon reflexes (positive Chvostek's sign)
	General deterioration in mental and physical performance
P_{ACO_2} < 15:	General tonic contractions of skeletal muscle (tetany)
P_{ACO_2} < 10–15:	Semiconsciousness, then unconsciousness

sea level to 18,000 ft. The lungs, the teeth, and the bowel may be affected by gas expansion during ascent (although aerodontalgia is now rare), while the middle ear cavities and sinuses are particularly affected by compression during descent.[6] A more-complete discussion of barotrauma can be found in Chapter 30, Physics, Physiology, and Medicine of Diving. The problems in lungs, teeth, and bowel are more severe in diving than flight because the pressure changes are greater.

Pulmonary Barotrauma

Expansion of gas within the lungs does not usually present a hazard on ascent because increasing volume can easily vent through the trachea. However, RD with a closed glottis can potentially produce catastrophic aeroembolism. (This topic is also discussed in Chapter 30, Physics, Physiology, and Medicine of Diving).

Gastrointestinal Distension

Expansion of gas within the small intestine can cause pain of sufficient severity to produce vasovagal syncope. Although this is unlikely to occur at normal rates of ascent in both transport and combat aircraft, it is a possibility after rapid loss of cabin pressurization at high altitude in the latter. In military aircrew, gut pain of this nature can also occur during RD undertaken for training purposes; indeed, this is the commonest cause of failure in such training. Gaseous expansion in the small bowel is aggravated by gas-producing foods (eg, beans, curries, brassicas, carbonated beverages, and alcohol). Gas in the

stomach and large intestine does not usually cause problems because it can easily be released.

Otic Barotrauma

Expanding gas in the middle ear cavity easily vents through the eustachian tube on ascent and only rarely causes any discomfort. The symptoms of otic barotrauma develop during descent because air cannot pass back up the tube so readily.[7] Pain, which begins as a feeling of increased pressure on the tympanic membrane, quickly becomes increasingly severe unless the eustachian tube is able to open, an event colloquially known as "clearing" the ears. Many experienced aircrew can achieve such opening merely by swallowing, yawning, or moving the lower jaw from side to side. Others perform a deliberate technique to open the tube by raising the pressure within the pharynx. Some people have great difficulty in learning these procedures, and some may be unable to do so even after much coaching and practice.

The most useful of these techniques is the Frenzel maneuver, which is performed with the mouth, nostrils, and epiglottis closed. Air in the nasopharynx is then compressed by the action of the muscles of the mouth and tongue. The Frenzel maneuver not only generates higher nasopharyngeal pressures than the Valsalva maneuver, discussed below, but also achieves opening of the eustachian tube at lower pressures.[7]

In the Toynbee maneuver, pharyngeal pressure is raised by swallowing while the mouth is closed and the nostrils occluded. This is the best technique to use when evaluating eustachian function under physiological conditions: under direct vision, the observer sees a slight inward movement of the tympanic membrane, followed by a more marked outward movement.

The Valsalva maneuver consists of a forced expiration through an open glottis while the mouth is shut and the nostrils occluded. The increase in intrathoracic pressure is transmitted to the nasopharynx and hence to the eustachian tubes. The rise in intrathoracic pressure is a disadvantage, however, because it impedes venous return to the heart and may even induce syncope.

The acute angle of entry of the eustachian tube into the pharynx predisposes to closure of the tube by increasing P_B during descent. By causing inflammation and edema of the lining of the eustachian tube, upper respiratory tract infections increase the likelihood of developing otic barotrauma and of its ultimate result: rupture of the tympanic membrane. Aircrew are made fully aware of this condition during training and are instructed not to fly if they are unable to clear the ears during an upper respiratory tract infection. In doubtful cases, a nonmoving tympanic membrane can be detected by direct vision. Treatment of otic barotrauma, particularly if blood or fluid is present in the middle ear cavity, should include analgesia, a nasal decongestant, and a broad-spectrum antibiotic.

Sinus Barotrauma

The etiology of sinus barotrauma is the same as that of its otic counterpart. On ascent, expanding air vents easily from the sinuses through their ostia. On descent, however, the ostia are readily occluded, especially if the victim has an upper respiratory tract infection. Characteristically, a sudden, severe, knifelike pain occurs in the affected sinus. The pain continues if descent is not halted and epistaxis may result from submucosal hemorrhage. The development of sinus barotrauma is related to the rate of descent, and its prevention is part of the rationale behind the slow rate of descent employed in transport and civilian aircraft. The possibility of a sinus problem cannot be predicted prior to flight, but flying with a cold will clearly increase the risk. As with otic barotrauma, treatment of sinus barotrauma should include analgesia, nasal decongestants, and a suitable antibiotic.

Altitude Decompression Sickness

Altitude decompression sickness (DCS) is that syndrome produced by exposure to altitude that is not due to low P_{IO_2}, to expansion of trapped or enclosed gas, or to intercurrent illness. Altitude DCS is therefore a diagnosis of exclusion; although it is conventionally regarded as a syndrome similar to the classic diving affliction, there are some fundamental and vitally important differences (Table 32-4).

The etiology of altitude DCS is not fully understood but certainly involves supersaturation of body tissues with nitrogen.[8] Ascent to altitude is associated with a fall in the partial pressure of inspired nitrogen and a corresponding fall in the partial pressure of alveolar nitrogen. Nitrogen consequently starts to leave body stores but, since it is poorly soluble in blood, the partial pressure of nitrogen in tissue falls at a slower rate than does the partial pressure of inspired nitrogen in blood. The tissues and blood may therefore become supersaturated with nitrogen, and bubbles begin to form around pre-existing microscopic nuclei, such as vessel wall irregularities. The bubbles grow as blood gases diffuse into them and can be carried to other parts of the body where they may or may not manifest clinically. Bubble formation is more likely if the partial pressure of nitrogen in tissue is high (notably in fat, which has high nitrogen solubility and low blood flow) or if P_B is low. Bubbles apparently need to reach a critical size before clinical features develop.

Many factors can influence the *occurrence* of clinical DCS; these are summarized in Exhibit 32–5. The clinical *features* of DCS may include any or all of the following[9]:

- Joint and limb pains (the "bends"). Bends pain is the commonest manifestation of altitude DCS and is seen in about 74% of cases. The pain is deep and poorly localized, made worse on movement, and frequently likened to having glass in the joint. Although single, large joints are most frequently affected, more than one joint can be involved and at any site. The pain usually resolves during descent to ground level.
- Respiratory disturbances (the "chokes"). Respiratory involvement is seen in about 5% of cases and has serious implications. Feelings of constriction around the lower chest, with an inspiratory snatch, paroxysmal cough on deep inspiration, and substernal soreness, is followed by malaise and collapse unless descent is initiated.
- Skin manifestations (the "creeps"). Dermal manifestations in the form of an itchy, blotchy rash (perhaps with formication) are seen in

TABLE 32-4

IMPORTANT FACTORS IN COMPARING AVIATORS' AND DIVERS' DECOMPRESSION SICKNESS

Factor	Flying	Diving
Preventive Denitrogenation	Denitrogenation can be used before the mission to reduce the risk of decompression sickness (DCS)	Not applicable to diving
Preexisting Degree of Saturation	Decompression starts from a saturated state	Saturation remains constant during the diving and intervening periods
Inspired Gas	Inspired gas usually contains high oxygen concentration	Diving mixtures must limit oxygen concentration to prevent toxicity
Composition of Gas Bubbles	Bubbles contain nitrogen, oxygen, carbon dioxide, and water	Nitrogen and the noble gases predominate
Pressure in Bubbles (Compared With Sea Level)	Pressure can be very low	Pressure can be very high
Duration of Dysbaria	Time of exposure to altitude is limited	Duration depends on the dive profile
Onset of DCS	DCS occurs during the mission	Risk of DCS on return to surface
Symptoms	Symptoms are usually mild and limited to joint pain	Severe pain and neurological symptoms are frequent
Repeat Exposure	Recompression to ground level is therapeutic	Return to depth is limited and hazardous
Individual Susceptibility	Individual susceptibility varies widely	Individual susceptibility is less varied
Sequelae	There are no documented cumulative effects	Chronic bone necrosis and neurological changes found in divers

about 7% of cases but are of little significance except in association with respiratory symptoms, when urticaria and mottling of the skin of the thorax may be present.
- Visual disturbances. Visual symptomatology is seen in about 2% of cases. Blurring of vision, scotomata, and fortification spectra (zigzag bands of light resembling, at the edges of scintillating scotomata, the walls of a fortified medieval castle, which are most usually seen in migraine attacks) may be reported. There is usually no disturbance

of the other special senses (hearing, smell, taste, and touch).
- Neurological disturbances (the "staggers"). Neurological involvement is rare, being seen in only about 1% of cases. Regional paralysis, paraesthesias, anaesthesia, and seizures may all be features.
- Cardiovascular collapse. Occasionally, a profound cardiovascular collapse may occur either without warning (primary) or subsequent to any of the other manifestations of altitude DCS (secondary). The features of

---

EXHIBIT 32-5

FACTORS INFLUENCING THE OCCURRENCE OF DECOMPRESSION SICKNESS

Altitude. In healthy individuals who start near sea level, clinical decompression sickness (DCS) is not usually seen at altitudes below 18,000 ft. It is rare between 18,000 and 25,000 ft but becomes increasingly common at altitudes above 25,000 ft.

Duration of Exposure. DCS usually develops after at least five minutes at altitude, with the maximum incidence at 20–60 min after exposure.

Rate of Ascent. The rates of ascent employed in routine military aviation have little if any significant effect on the occurrence of DCS.

Underwater Diving. The increases in pressure sustained during diving (particularly to depths > 15 ft) lead to compression of additional nitrogen in the tissues. Although some of this will evolve into gas during ascent (decompression) to the water's surface, more nitrogen than usual will be present to form more gas bubbles if a further ascent to altitude is undertaken shortly afterwards (also see Exhibit 32-6).[1,2,3]

Reexposure. Repeated exposure over a short time to altitudes at which DCS may occur (eg, paratroop training) will predispose to DCS.

Temperature. The risk of developing DCS increases if environmental temperatures are low.

Exercise. The altitude at which clinical DCS may develop is reduced by exercise.

Hypoxia. The presence of coexisting hypoxia increases both the incidence and the severity of DCS.

Age. The risk of developing DCS increases with age, approximately doubling every decade.

Body Build. Those with much adipose tissue appear to have an increased susceptibility to DCS.

Previous Injury. Physical damage to tissues may predispose to DCS by encouraging formation of nuclei around which bubbles may form.

General Health. Drugs, alcohol, smoking, and intercurrent illness will all increase susceptibility to DCS.

Individual Susceptibility. There appears to be a true individual variation in susceptibility to DCS.

Sources: (1) Furry DE, Reeves E, Beckman E. Relationships of SCUBA diving to the development of aviator's decompression sickness. *Aerospace Med.* 1967;38:825-828. (2) Blumkin D. Flying and diving—A unique health concern. *Flight Safety Foundation's Human Factors and Aviation Medicine.* 1991;Sep/Oct:21-28. (3) Sheffield PJ. Flying after diving guidelines: A review. *Aviat Space Environ Med.* 1990;61:1130-1138.

---

such a collapse include malaise; anxiety; diminution of consciousness; and pale, clammy, sweaty skin. A bradycardia leads to loss of consciousness. Recovery is usually accompanied by vomiting and a frontal headache.

Although the natural history of altitude DCS is that symptoms and signs resolve on descent—approximately 95%[9] of volunteer subjects affected in hypobaric chamber studies have recovered on reaching ground level—there may very rarely be a persistence or even a worsening of features several hours after return. Such a delayed collapse is usually only seen if severe symptoms and signs of DCS (such as chokes or bends) were present at altitude.

In addition to the features of collapse described above, there may be general and focal neurological signs and mottling of the skin. The hematocrit rises, as does the white blood cell count and temperature. Should unconsciousness develop, the outcome is almost invariably fatal.

Arterial Gas Embolism

In addition to the constellation of features colloquially described above as the "staggers," a second neurological syndrome—cerebral arterial gas embolism (CAGE)—may very rarely be associated with RD to high altitude (although it is more common in the hyperbaric environment). In this condition, overinflation of pulmonary tissue results in rupture of alveoli and escape of gas directly into the arterial circulation. Subsequent embolization to the brain can produce a clinical picture very similar to cerebral decompression sickness, or CNS DCS.[10] (Because of this similarity, the global term decompression *illness* [DCI] has been recommended as a replacement for the more-familiar DCS[10]; this textbook, however, uses the terms DCS and CAGE.)

Diagnosis and Treatment of Decompression Sickness

The differential diagnosis of DCS must include flight stresses such as hypoxia, hyperventilation, abdominal distension, alternobaric vertigo (ie, sudden, powerful vertigo caused by pressure change within the middle ear; the condition usually occurs at low altitude during ascent and may be a potent cause of spatial disorientation), motion sickness, and acceleration atelectasis (ie, the rapid collapse of oxygen-filled basal alveoli due to the ventilation–perfusion abnormalities associated with high +Gz acceleration [ie, positive acceleration along the body's z, or head-to-toe, axis; see Figure 33-1 in Chapter 33, Acceleration Effects on Fighter Pilots]); and intercurrent illness such as ischemic heart disease, spontaneous pneumothorax, and cramp of or injury to the limbs. Although it is usually easy to exclude these conditions, it may be necessary to monitor the hematocrit, white blood cell count, and temperature.

Recovery from altitude DCS is usually complete, but the management of the established condition occurs in several stages. In-flight management involves descent to as low an altitude as circumstances permit (and at least to below an aircraft altitude of 18,000 ft), administering 100% oxygen, keeping still and warm if practicable, and landing as soon as possible where medical aid is available and has been alerted.

The casualty must be seen by a medical officer immediately after landing and be kept under observation for at least 4 hours, even if symptoms improved markedly during descent or have completely disappeared. Failure of symptoms or signs to improve, or any deterioration in condition, or the appearance of new symptoms and signs during the observation period all suggest the possibility of impending collapse,

and active treatment should be initiated immediately. Important symptoms suggesting deterioration include headache, nausea, visual disturbances, anxiety, and sweating; signs of significance include hemoconcentration, pyrexia, and peripheral vascular failure (pallor, cyanosis, and weak distal pulses in the presence of near-normal blood pressure). Although the form of active treatment depends on both geographical location and the availability of recompression resources, the order of preference is as follows:

1. Immediate hyperbaric compression with or without intermittent oxygen breathing.
2. Institution of treatment for established or incipient circulatory collapse, followed by early transfer to a hyperbaric facility if possible within reasonable time (< 6 h) or distance. Transport should be by road or low-level flight (< 1,000 ft if possible but not > 3,000 ft).
3. Full supportive treatment for collapse (essential if there is no chance of prompt transfer to a hyperbaric facility). Such treatment should include expansion of plasma volume, administration of 100% oxygen and intravenous steroids, correction of blood electrolytes, and drainage of pleural effusions.

The ideal way in which to prevent altitude DCS is to limit the pressure environment to less than 18,000 ft. This may not always be possible, however, in which case time above 22,000 ft should be kept to a minimum, and the influence of predisposing factors should be minimized. For experimental and training purposes in decompression chambers, DCS can be prevented by denitrogenation (ie, reducing body nitrogen content by breathing 100% oxygen before or during ascent to high altitude, a process also termed "prebreathing"), although such prebreathing is often impracticable for operational purposes. And the possibility of developing DCS as a consequence of operating fixed-wing aircraft out of and into airfields at high terrestrial locations, and of rotary wing operations in mountainous regions, must always be kept in mind (Exhibit 32-6).

LIFE-SUPPORT SYSTEMS FOR FLIGHT AT HIGH ALTITUDE

The means by which protection against the hazards of altitude are provided for the occupants of aircraft include (*a*) the cabin pressurization systems of large transport and civilian aircraft, and of small

military combat aircraft, and (*b*) the requirements and design of personal oxygen equipment. The ways in which the requirements for protection in each class of aircraft are achieved and interrelate

EXHIBIT 32-6

FLYING AFTER DIVING

There is a bewildering number of published guidelines from which divers can seek advice about flying after diving: at least 30 published sets of recommendations exist for those who wish to fly after diving within standard air tables; 5 more for saturation divers; and a further 12 to guide those concerned with the in-flight management of decompression sickness or with flying after hyperbaric therapy. It is wise to select a single reference and, in the United Kingdom, the *Royal Navy Diving Manual*, although aimed primarily at service divers, is well-known and authoritative. Article 5122 of the Manual provides simple advice on the minimum intervals between diving and flying, for dives without or with stops (see table). And Article 5121 gives advice for those who intend to fly after diving at altitude (eg, in mountain lakes). In the United States, similar guidelines are recommended by the Federal Aviation Administration (FAA) and the Undersea and Hyperbaric Medicine Society (UHMS). More stringent regulations apply to aircrew who may have participated in sports diving.

Type of Dive	Time Interval Between Diving and Flying (h)	Maximum Altitude[*]
Without Decompression Stops	≥1	~ 1,000 ft (300 m)[†]
	1–2	~ 5,000 ft (1,500 m)
	> 2	Unlimited flying in commercial aircraft (usually no more than an effective 8,000 ft [2,400 m])
With Decompression Stops	≤ 4	~ 1,000 ft (300 m)[†]
	4–8	~ 5,000 ft (1,500 m)
	8–24	~ 16,500 ft (5,000 m)
	> 24	Unlimited

[*](or effective altitude in pressurized aircraft)
[†]eg, flying in helicopters
Adapted from Harding RM, Mills FJ. Problems of altitude. In: Harding RM, Mills FJ, eds. *Aviation Medicine*. 3rd ed. London, England: British Medical Association; 1993: 69.

TABLE 32-5

PROTECTIVE SYSTEMS FOR TRANSPORT AND COMBAT AIRCRAFT

Aircraft	Protection	
	Primary	Secondary
Transport	Cabin pressurization system (high differential)[*]	Personal oxygen system for flight deck crew and passengers
Combat	Personal oxygen system	Emergency oxygen supply *plus* Cabin pressurization system (low differential)[†]

[*]Large pressure difference between cabin and outside
[†]Small pressure difference between cabin and outside: cabin pressurized to approximately 22,000 ft because of considerable risk of rapid decompression

are summarized in Table 32-5.

Cabin Pressurization Systems

Cabin pressurization maintains the inside of an aircraft at a higher pressure (and hence lower effective altitude) than that outside the aircraft. The physiological ideal would be to pressurize the cabin to sea level at all times, but this is not cost-effective, so the minimum acceptable level of pressurization is determined by the need to prevent hypoxia, gastrointestinal distension, and altitude DCS, as well as to minimize the possible consequences of sudden loss of pressurization. In addition, the maximum rates of cabin ascent and descent are determined by effects on the middle ear cavities and sinuses.[11] Each of these factors imposes altitude limits (Table 32-6).

The difference between the absolute (or total) pressure within the aircraft and that of the atmosphere outside is termed the *cabin differential pressure*, the magnitude of which depends on the type of aircraft. In large passenger aircraft, where comfort and mobility are important and the risk of RD is small, the cabin is pressurized to about 6,000 ft. Such aircraft are said to have high-differential-pressure cabins because, when the aircraft is flying at high altitudes, a large difference exists between pressure within the cabin and the pressure outside. In combat aircraft, however, where only minimal weight can be devoted to life-support equipment and where there may be a considerable risk of RD, cockpits are pressurized to about 22,000 ft and are called low-differential-pressure cabins.

The relation between the effective cabin altitude and the actual, changing aircraft altitude is termed the *pressurization schedule* (Figure 32-5). For example, US combat aircraft use an isobaric schedule in which cabin altitude is held constant as the aircraft ascends until the maximum differential pressure is reached, after which cabin altitude rises linearly with aircraft altitude. In passenger aircraft, on the other hand, cabin differential pressure initially increases gradually with aircraft altitude until maximum differential pressure is attained. Thereafter, cabin altitude again rises linearly with aircraft altitude.

The cabin pressurization system controls not only the pressure of air within the cabin but also its humidity, mass flow, volume flow (ie, ventilation), and temperature (Figure 32-6). In fact, most of the demand for compressed air provides for cabin ventilation rather than pressurization. Passenger aircraft carry redundant systems and controls, while combat aircraft have a single pressure controller.

Loss of Cabin Pressurization

Loss of cabin pressurization (decompression) is usually the result of a system malfunction that either reduces inflow (as in a compressor failure) or increases outflow (as in leaks through open valves). Such losses are usually slow and are soon recognized and corrected by the crew. RDs are rare events and result from structural faults (eg, a failure of canopy seals, or loss of transparencies, doors, or windows) or enemy or terrorist action. An added complication is the possible Venturi effect of air

TABLE 32-6

CABIN ALTITUDE LIMITS AND PERFORMANCE IMPOSED BY PHYSIOLOGICAL FACTORS

Physiological Factors*	Cabin Altitude Limits and Performance (ft)		
	Transport Aircraft	Both	Combat Aircraft
Hypoxia	8,000		20,000–22,000
Decompression Sickness		< 22,000	
Gastrointestinal Distension	< 6,000		< 25,000
Middle Ears and Sinuses: Ascent Descent		5,000–20,000 ft/min < 500 ft/min	

*The predicted consequences of rapid decompression on the lungs must also be taken into account

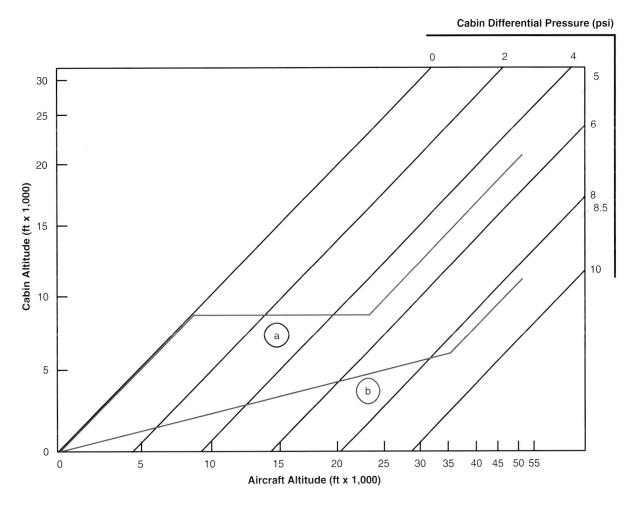

Cabin Differential Pressure (psi)

Fig. 32-5. The relation between cabin altitude and aircraft altitude, and the change in differential pressure for two general types of aircraft. Curve (**a**) is an isobaric schedule, of the type used in US combat aircraft. After a period of parallel rise in aircraft and cabin altitude, near Earth's surface, cabin altitude is thereafter kept constant (in this example, at 8,000 ft) until the maximum differential pressure is reached (here, at 5 psi), and cabin altitude again increases with aircraft altitude. Curve (**b**) is an example of the pressurization schedule used for commercial aircraft, in which passenger comfort is an important issue. In this form, cabin altitude is allowed to rise only slowly from ground level with aircraft altitude. Because a high differential pressure can be accommodated, cabin altitude can be maintained at a physiologically acceptable level throughout the aircraft's normal flight profile. Should the aircraft reach its maximum differential pressure altitude (here, 8.5 psi at 36,000 ft), cabin altitude change thereafter is obliged to parallel the change in aircraft altitude. Adapted from Harding RM, Mills FJ. Problems of altitude. In: Harding RM, Mills FJ, eds. *Aviation Medicine.* 3rd ed. London, England: British Medical Association; 1993: 61.

rushing over the defect in the pressure cabin: this "aerodynamic suck" can further reduce cabin pressure and thus increase effective altitude by as much as 10,000 ft.

The biological effects of RD include gas expansion, hypoxia, cold, and decompression sickness. Lung damage can occur if the occupants hold their breaths during the event or if the decompression is so severe that it produces a transthoracic pressure differential of 80 to 100 mm Hg. The profile of the

decompression depends on both the differential pressure at the moment of pressure loss and the ratio of cabin volume to the size of the defect. The high-differential systems used in passenger aircraft dictate the need for small windows and fail-safe doors: following the loss of a typical passenger window at 40,000 ft, cabin pressure falls gradually to ambient in about 50 seconds, during which the pilot can accomplish emergency descent. In combat aircraft, on the other hand, decompression to am-

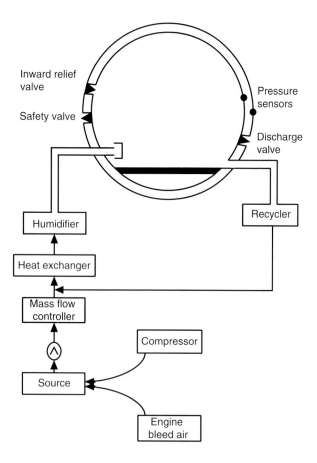

Inward relief valve

Safety valve

Pressure sensors

Discharge valve

Recycler

Humidifier

Heat exchanger

Mass flow controller

Compressor

Source

Engine bleed air

Fig. 32-6. A cabin pressurization system controls not only air pressure within the cabin but also its relative humidity, mass flow, volume flow (ventilation), and temperature. Most of the demands on such a system are based on the requirements for cabin conditioning rather than pressurization. In combat aircraft, the system is simplified by the omission of the humidifier and the recycler.

bient may be almost instantaneous, and the low differential pressure systems of combat aircraft are used in part to mitigate the effect of a large defect in a small cabin volume. In any RD, wind and flying debris within the cabin and through the defect promote confusion and difficulty with hearing and vision.

Personal Oxygen Equipment

The primary purpose of personal oxygen equipment for use in aircraft is to prevent the hypoxia associated with ascent to altitude by maintaining P_{AO_2} at its sea-level value of about 103 mm Hg. In achieving this aim, however, a number of other factors of both a physiological[12,13] and a general[14] nature must be considered. The physiological requirements of oxygen systems, discussed below, include

adequate oxygen, nitrogen, and ventilation and flow, all at adequate pressure; positive-pressure breathing; minimum added external resistance; and a means to disperse the expirate. The general requirements of oxygen systems are summarized in Exhibit 32-7.

Physiological Requirements of Oxygen Systems

Adequate Oxygen at Adequate Pressure. Sea-level P_{AO_2} can be maintained during ascent by progressively increasing the percentage of oxygen in the inspired gas (termed *airmix*) until 100% oxygen is provided at 33,700 ft. At this altitude, P_B is 190 mm Hg, P_{AO_2} is 103 mm Hg, the partial pressure of water vapor in alveoli (P_{AH_2O}) is 47 mm Hg, and P_{ACO_2} is 40 mm Hg. Thus, P_{AO_2} at 33,700 ft when breathing 100% oxygen will be the same as P_{AO_2} at sea level when breathing air; this is an example of the concept of equivalent altitudes. Continued ascent will reduce P_{AO_2} even when 100% oxygen is breathed, but healthy individuals will not experience severe hypoxia until 40,000 ft is reached, where P_B is 141 mm Hg and P_{AO_2} is 54 mm Hg (note that the values of P_{AH_2O}, 47 mm Hg, and P_{ACO_2}, 40 mm Hg, are unchanged from 33,700 ft and in fact are unchanged from sea level). This altitude is the upper limit for safe ascent while breathing air at ambient pressure. It would simplify matters if 100% oxygen could be provided at all altitudes, but this would be wasteful as well as producing potential problems with acceleration atelectasis and ear blocks (ie, oxygen ear).

Positive-Pressure Breathing. Above 40,000 ft, hypoxia can be prevented only by providing 100% oxygen under pressure that exceeds P_B by enough to maintain alveolar pressure at 141 mm Hg (called positive-pressure breathing, or PPB). PPB may be applied to the airway using a tightly fastened oronasal mask, but this is uncomfortable and causes distension of the upper respiratory tract, difficulty with speech and swallowing, and spasm of the eyelids due to pressurization of the lachrymal ducts. Whether pressure is applied by mask or by other means (see below), PPB distends the lungs and expands the chest. Overdistension can be prevented by training in the technique of PPB, but even so there is a tendency for inspiratory reserve volume to fall and expiratory reserve volume to rise: pulmonary ventilation may increase by 50% when breathing at a positive pressure of 30 mm Hg. The associated fall in P_{ACO_2} means that hyperventilation is a feature of PPB, although this too can be mini-

---

EXHIBIT 32-7

GENERAL REQUIREMENTS OF OXYGEN SYSTEMS

Safety Pressure. A slight but continuous overpressure in the system ensures that any leaks will be outboard and prevents the inspiration of hypoxic air.

Optional 100% Oxygen. The ability to select 100% oxygen and positive pressure manually at any altitude provides emergency protection from smoke and fumes. The selection of 100% oxygen is also the first line of treatment should decompression sickness occur.

Simplicity. Insofar as possible, the system should be convenient to use and automatic in operation.

Confirmation of Integrity. The system should allow the user to test its integrity before take-off, confirm normal gas supply in flight, and provide clear warning of any degradation in performance.

Back-up Systems. Military aircraft generally provide a secondary breathing regulator, for use should the primary device fail, as well as a small bottle of reserve oxygen for use if the primary supply fails or is contaminated.

Protection During High-Altitude Escape. A reserve oxygen supply is mounted on the ejection seat of combat aircraft to provide 100% oxygen for use after aircraft abandonment during descent to below 10,000 ft. This reserve, which is usually physically the same as the back-up system described above, is termed the emergency oxygen supply (known colloquially as the EO or Green Apple).

Ruggedness. All items of personal oxygen equipment must function satisfactorily in the extreme environmental conditions of flight (ie, pressure, temperature [especially cold], acceleration, vibration, and windblast). The plight of aircrew whose craft have entered water must also be considered, and antidrowning valves, to prevent water inhalation, are frequently incorporated in components that may be immersed in such circumstances. Antisuffocation valves in the facemask ensure that air breathing remains possible.

---

mized by training. The cardiovascular effects of PPB include peripheral pooling, impaired venous return, and reduced central blood volume; if there is a loss of peripheral arteriolar tone, then tachycardia and a gradual fall in blood pressure will lead to a collapse resembling a simple vasovagal syncope.[15]

Counterpressure garments provide external support to the chest, abdomen, and limbs to minimize the adverse effects of PPB. An oronasal mask alone can be used only to a pressure of 30 mm Hg, but the addition of an inflated pressure vest and anti-G suit (also called G trousers) raise the level of tolerable PPB to 70 mm Hg. Breathing pressures progressively above this require the use of a pressurized enclosed helmet and then a full-pressure suit. The overall result is that PPB has such severe disadvan-

---

EXHIBIT 32-8

GET-ME-DOWN AND KEEP-ME-UP

Get-me-down: an emergency life-support system designed to maintain pilot function only long enough for controlled descent of the aircraft to an altitude where ambient barometric pressure and partial pressure of oxygen are sufficient to make cabin pressurization unnecessary. An example is a positive-pressure breathing system for use at very high altitudes, where the required mask pressure can be tolerated for only a limited time.

Keep-me-up: a backup life-support system that allows the pilot to continue flying at normal altitude and perhaps complete the mission before returning to base.

---

tages that flyers use it for altitude protection only as an emergency "get-me-down" procedure (Exhibit 32-8). The physiology of PPB for enhancement of tolerance to sustained +Gz accelerations (PPB for G [acceleration]: PBG) will clearly be much the same as for altitude protection (PPB for altitude: PBA). But the routine use of the technique for PBG places additional constraints on systems designed for PBA, both in terms of the level of positive pressure delivered and on the design of the counterpressure garments used (see also Chapter 33, Acceleration Effects on Fighter Pilots). The physiological requirements for oxygen during acute ascent to altitude are summarized in Table 32-7.

Adequate Nitrogen. To avoid acceleration atelectasis, the inspired gas should contain at least 40% nitrogen, provided that the requirements to protect against hypoxia are not compromised. Figure 32-7 depicts the physiological requirements for the composition of inspired gas (airmix) in relation to cabin and aircraft altitude.[16] The aircraft and cabin altitude areas are directly related to each other

TABLE 32-7

PHYSIOLOGICAL REQUIREMENTS FOR OXYGEN DURING ASCENT

Altitude (ft)	Source of Oxygen Required to Maintain Physiological Normality During Ascent
0–8,000	Air
8,000–33,700	Air enriched with O_2
33,700–40,000	100% O_2
> 40,000	100% O_2 under pressure

(and so create a representative or typical cabin differential profile). They are, therefore, also both related to both of the curves in the figure.

Adequate Ventilation and Flow. The requirements for aircrew breathing systems may surprise

Fig. 32-7. This figure is based on the physiological requirements for inspired gas composition that are summarized in Table 32-7, and relates cabin altitude to the needed oxygen concentration. A representative cabin pressurization profile is generated by the inclusion of aircraft altitude as the upper horizontal axis. It is on this approach that design requirements for oxygen systems are based. The lower curve in the graph represents the *minimum* concentration of oxygen required to prevent hypoxia; the upper curve represents the *maximum* oxygen concentration acceptable if acceleration atelectasis is to be avoided. The kink in the "hypoxia" (lower) curve, the precise position of which will vary with the cabin pressurization profile of the aircraft, reflects the additional oxygen concentration in the inspired gas required to prevent hypoxia should a rapid decompression (RD) occur from within that band of cabin altitude. Similarly, the increase in the "atelectasis" (upper) curve from 60% oxygen at a cabin altitude of about 15,000 ft (in this example) to 80% and then 100% by 20,000 ft reflects the need to breathe 100% oxygen during or immediately after an RD. The slope-to-vertical element is present because of the need to accommodate design and engineering shortfalls in breathing system performance, which would otherwise have to cope with a choke point in this physiologically critical area. Sources: (1) Ernsting J. Prevention of hypoxia—Acceptable compromises. *Aviat Space Environ Med.* 1978;49:495–502. Harry G. Armstrong Lecture. (2) Ernsting J. The ideal relationship between inspired oxygen concentration and cabin altitude. *Aerospace Med.* 1963;34:991–997.

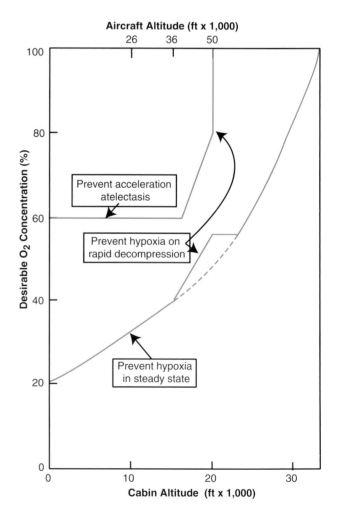

medical officers. Current international requirements,[17] based on in-flight studies, state that an oxygen system for use by military aircrew should be able to deliver a respiratory minute volume of at least 60 L and accommodate peak instantaneous flows of 200 L/min at a maximum rate of change of 20 L/s^2 (all volumes are at ambient temperature and pressure, dry [ATPD]). The greatest demand placed on a breathing system is on the ground prior to take-off, especially if the pilot ran to the aircraft. Unfortunately, breathing system performance is optimized for function at altitude and so is usually at its worst in this situation.

Minimum Added External Resistance. Added external resistance, whether it affects the inspiratory or the expiratory phase of the respiratory cycle, produces unwanted physiological effects including reduction in minute volume, increase in the work of breathing, and feelings of suffocation. It is therefore most important that the external resistance imposed by a breathing system be kept as low as possible by using (wherever feasible) low-resistance valves and wide-bore hoses and connectors.

Dispersal of Expirate. The breathing system must disperse expired carbon dioxide to ambient (ie, to the cabin), and dead space must be kept as low as possible to avoid significant rebreathing of carbon dioxide.

Personal Oxygen Systems

Personal oxygen systems in military aviation are almost exclusively of the simple, open-circuit type (ie, expired gas is dispersed to the environment). Closed-circuit systems are inherently unsuitable for the robust world of military flying, in that they are complex, their components tend to freeze readily, and nitrogen and carbon dioxide may accumulate.

There are two main types of open-circuit system: continuous-flow systems, which provide gas at a fixed flow throughout the respiratory cycle, and demand-flow systems, which provide gas flow to the user only when an inspiratory demand is made. Demand-flow systems are found in most high-performance military aircraft and as the emergency supply on the flight decks of transport aircraft.

Oxygen is provided either from an onboard store of gaseous or liquid oxygen, which is replenished when the aircraft is on the ground, or from an onboard system (eg, a molecular sieve, discussed below), which produces oxygen in flight.[14] Solid, inert, chemical forms of oxygen storage are used for some emergency systems for passenger use. Whatever the source, however, the oxygen delivered must be of a very high standard; for systems other than molecular sieves, the gas must be at least 99.5% pure with a water content, at standard temperature and pressure, lower than 0.005 mg/L and with defined (low) levels of toxic contaminants.

Gaseous Oxygen Storage. Oxygen gas is stored in steel cylinders of various capacities (400–2,250 L), usually at a pressure of 1,800 psi. The size and number of cylinders depend on the type of aircraft and its role. Oxygen gas storage has the advantages of being simple in construction, easily replenished worldwide, available for use immediately after charging, and secure from loss when not in use. But it also has the great disadvantages of being heavy and bulky. Such storage is therefore used when weight and bulk are of less importance: in some military training aircraft; in transport aircraft, where the supply is intended for use by crew and passengers should cabin pressurization fail, or as the supply for small, portable, and therapeutic oxygen sets; and in combat aircraft as the (small) emergency oxygen supply.

Liquid Oxygen Storage. Liquid oxygen (LOX) is stored in double-walled, insulated, steel containers (rather like vacuum flasks)—called LOX converters—at a pressure of 70 to 115 psi and at a temperature lower than –183°C. Above that temperature, 1 L of LOX vaporizes to produce 840 L of oxygen gas. This expansion ratio makes LOX an attractive source of breathing gas for small combat aircraft, where weight and bulk are at a high premium. The capacity of the LOX converter will depend on the size of the aircraft and its role, but is usually 3.5, 5.0, 10.0, or 25.0 L.

Operation of a LOX system is complex and involves three distinct phases:

1. *filling*, during which liquid oxygen is delivered from an external supply until evaporation and consequent cooling reduces the temperature of the system to –183°C, at which point the converter fills with the liquid;
2. *buildup*, during which LOX is allowed into an uninsulated part of the circuit to evaporate before passing in gaseous form back into the converter, and in so doing raising the operating pressure of the system to the required level; and
3. *delivery*, during which oxygen gas is withdrawn from the system by the user.

LOX storage systems have considerable disadvantages, including

- dangers of handling,
- wastage of oxygen (because much LOX is lost before ever reaching a converter),
- continuous loss after charging because insulation is (necessarily) imperfect ($\leq 10\%$ can be lost in 24 h),
- a finite time requirement to reach operating pressure (which means that the storage system is not usable immediately after charging), and
- a potential for the buildup of toxic contaminants with boiling points higher than that of oxygen.

LOX systems are also prone to temperature stratification, a phenomenon whereby layering of LOX at different temperatures occurs within the converter. Subsequent agitation during taxi or flight causes disturbance of these layers, such that colder LOX comes into contact with the gaseous phase, with resulting condensation of the latter and a fall in system pressure. This problem is overcome in some combat aircraft by disturbing the stratification (ie, bubbling a small supply of oxygen gas back through the liquid from which it evolved, so agitating the fluid and eliminating any strata within it) so that the temperature is slightly elevated and uniform throughout the LOX: the system is then said to be stabilized. Despite all of these drawbacks, LOX remained the storage medium of choice for small combat aircraft until recent years, when molecular sieve technology provided a realistic alternative.

Solid Chemical Storage. When ignited with finely divided iron, sodium chlorate burns to produce copious amounts of pure oxygen (Equation 2):

$$(2) \qquad NaClO_3 + Fe \longrightarrow FeO + NaCl + O_2$$

This exothermic reaction is the basis of the solid chemical storage of oxygen used in some passenger-carrying aircraft as a source of emergency supply. Additional advantages include the simplicity, convenience, and long shelf-life of such devices (known as *candles*), although the nature of the reaction makes it unsuitable for use as a supply for a primary oxygen system. (Combustion of oxygen candles in the cargo hold is presumed to be the basis of the loss in the Florida Everglades of the ValuJet DC-9 aircraft in May 1996.)

Onboard Oxygen Production. The onboard production of oxygen overcomes all the logistical and operational penalties of conventional storage systems. Although many physicochemical techniques have been investigated in the search for an effective means of producing oxygen onboard an aircraft, the adsorption of nitrogen by molecular sieve material has proven to be the most successful and has led to the development of molecular sieve oxygen concentrating (MSOC) systems.[14]

Molecular sieves are alkali metal aluminosilicates of the crystalline zeolite family with an extremely regular structure of cages, the size of which determines the size of the molecules that can be held in the sieve. The sieving process is exothermic and depends crucially on pressure, an increase in which enhances adsorption. Pressurization of the sieve (by compressed air from the aircraft engines) causes adsorption of nitrogen molecules and allows oxygen and argon to pass through as the product gas (to a maximum concentration, at present, of 94% oxygen). However, once all the cages are occupied by nitrogen molecules, then nitrogen, too, will appear in the product gas. Depressurization of the sieve allows adsorbed nitrogen to be released from its cages, so that the technique is reversible. An MSOC therefore consists of two or more beds of sieve material used alternately to concentrate oxygen and clear out nitrogen. Because a two-bed MSOC capable of providing the needs of two crewmembers has the same weight and volume as a 10-L LOX converter, requires no coolant, and consumes just 50 W of 28-V direct electrical current, it is an overwhelmingly attractive alternative to conventional storage devices.

The use of an MSOC system does, however, raise some difficulties, including failure of the sieve to produce oxygen if engine power is lost (there is no reserve oxygen in the sieve), or if the aircrew eject from the aircraft at high altitude. Both cases require instantaneous switching to a small gaseous oxygen bottle. Similarly, if the aircraft cabin decompresses at high altitude, a supply of oxygen gas is required during the time needed for the MSOC to respond to the new pressure–altitude condition. In addition, during routine flight, 94% oxygen is too rich to breathe, and a means to dilute it is necessary. This can be accomplished either by prolonging the pressurization cycle time of the MSOC beds, thereby allowing nitrogen to appear in the product gas, or by increasing the flow of gas through the MSOC beds, which has the same effect.

These relatively minor difficulties are outweighed by the clear operational and logistical benefits of MSOC, compared with those of conventional systems. Such benefits include

- the elimination of ground recharging of the oxygen store, and therefore promotion of speedier and safer turnaround of aircraft;
- the elimination of ground manufacture, storage, and transport of oxygen;
- the elimination of the risk of contamination of breathing gas, which exists with LOX; and
- an increase in the overall reliability of the oxygen system, with a consequent reduction in the frequency of routine maintenance.

Oxygen Delivery. The simplest way in which breathing gas from any source can be delivered to the user is by a *continuous-flow* system. Although wasteful, such systems are used to provide oxygen for bail-out and emergency use, and some have been adapted for use by high-altitude parachutists. The interposition of a reservoir between the oxygen supply and the user decreases consumption by 50% to 70%, and although such systems are used for passengers in commercial aircraft, they are not suitable for more-complex applications. Some of these systems, also, have been adapted for use by high-altitude parachutists.

The *demand-flow* system, on the other hand, is more complex. In this system, the flow of gas varies in direct response to inspiration by the user, and it is possible to provide controlled airmix, PPB, safety pressure, and an indication of supply and flow. The key component in the provision of these requirements is the regulator, which is termed a *pressure-demand oxygen regulator* if it is capable of delivering gas under increased pressure.[14] Originally, demand regulators needed to be relatively large to accommodate the size of the control diaphragm and mechanical linkages required to maintain inspiratory resistance at a tolerable level, and so were panel-mounted (ie, they were located in a convenient place on a console). This continues to be the site of choice in most US combat aircraft, as well as in transport and commercial aircraft, where space is less critical. In other countries, the evolution of pneumatic engineering and the ability to miniaturize control surfaces, driven by the increasing demand placed on console space by avionics, led first to man-mounted and then to seat-mounted regulators. Man-mounted regulators are very expensive and complex, prone to damage, and one is required for each crewmember. Seat-mounted regulators overcome these drawbacks and the fault-correction drills are less complicated for the aircrew to

follow: the ejection seat is now the site of choice for this component in many non-US combat aircraft.

All demand regulators, wherever located within the cockpit, are designed similarly to enable them to provide various specific automatic and manual functions (Exhibit 32-9). The precise routing of breathing gas to the user from the regulator will depend on the location of the latter and whether an ejection seat is used.

Oxygen Delivery Mask. The final component of a personal oxygen system is the oxygen mask.[14] Masks designed for continuous use by aircrew must satisfy several design requirements, including stability and comfort over long periods, small size to avoid restriction of visual fields, and minimum dead space to avoid rebreathing exhaled carbon dioxide. The mask must be available in an appropriate range of dimensions to fit and seal against all shapes and sizes of face, and the material from which it is made should neither sensitize skin nor itself be adversely affected by human secretions.

All masks designed for use with pressure-demand regulators are of a similar basic design, which includes a flexible molded facepiece (sometimes with a reflected edge) that seals against the face when the mask cavity is pressurized. The facepiece contains openings (ports), in which are mounted the valves appropriate to its role, and the mask microphone; the whole is supported by webbing straps or a rigid exoskeleton, which also provides the means by which the mask is suspended from the protective helmet or headset.

It is clear that the mask used in all open-circuit oxygen systems will require at least a simple expiratory valve so that cabin air cannot be inspired. If, however, the system is capable of delivering safety pressure or PPB, then the expiratory valve must be compensated to prevent its opening under conditions of raised mask cavity pressure. The associated inspiratory valve should be placed high in the mask to minimize the risk of obstruction by debris and to reduce the chance of contact with moist expirate, which can freeze.

Specialized Systems: Pressure Clothing

Extreme altitudes may require additional personal protection by means of pressure clothing.[14,18] In aviation, such clothing is usually worn uninflated and is pressurized only if the cabin altitude exceeds a certain level or if it is necessary to abandon the aircraft at high altitude (> 40,000 ft). Pressure clothing ranges from a full-pressure suit, which applies pressure to the whole person, to partial-pressure

EXHIBIT 32-9

AUTOMATIC AND MANUAL FUNCTIONS OF DEMAND REGULATORS

- Demand regulators provide breathing gas as needed and are essentially boxes divided into two compartments by a flexible control diaphragm: one compartment is open to the environmental pressure of the cockpit, while the other (the demand chamber) communicates at one end with the delivery hose to the user, and at the other with the oxygen supply line. A demand valve in the regulator governs the latter communication. The inspiratory demand of the user creates a negative pressure within the demand chamber, draws the diaphragm inward, and, by a pivot mechanism, opens the demand valve. Gas flows into the regulator and thence to the user until inspiration ceases. Pressure within the demand chamber then rises until the control diaphragm returns to its original position, thereby closing the demand valve.

- Air dilution (airmix) is required to avoid unnecessary wastage of stored gas and to overcome the undesirable effects of breathing 100% oxygen when it is not needed. In systems based on gaseous or liquid storage of oxygen, dilution is achieved by mixing stored gas with cabin air inside the regulator. Oxygen enters the demand chamber through an air inlet port and injector nozzle, which entrains cabin air by a Venturi effect. With altitude, the degree of entrainment must decline so that the valve that allows entry of cabin air is progressively closed by the expansion of an aneroid capsule. The injector dilution mechanism delivers 40% to 50% oxygen during quiet breathing at low altitudes. If toxic fumes are present in the cockpit or if decompression sickness is suspected, then 100% oxygen can be selected manually at any altitude. Many modern oxygen regulators also incorporate a pressure-loaded valve at the air inlet so that air cannot be drawn in unless oxygen pressure is present. This facility removes the risk of unwittingly breathing hypoxic air through the air inlet port should the oxygen supply fail.
In systems based on molecular sieves, air dilution is accomplished by manipulating oxygen concentration upstream of the regulator. Regulators in such systems therefore have no airmix facility.

- Safety pressure is the slight overpressure (usually ~ 1–2 mm Hg) generated within the mask cavity, which ensures that any leak of breathing gas as a result of an ill-fitting mask will be outboard, thus preventing the risk of hypoxia by inadvertent dilution of breathing gas with cabin air. Safety pressure is achieved by applying an appropriate spring load to the regulator control diaphragm so that the demand valve opens slightly, gas flows downstream, and the required pressure builds up. Once pressure is attained, the diaphragm returns to its resting position and the demand valve shuts. Because the presence of safety pressure within the mask will slightly increase the resistance to expiration, it is usually only initiated (by means of an aneroid control) at cabin altitudes higher than 10,000 ft.

- Pressure breathing is also achieved by spring loading the regulator control diaphragm. The load is once again determined by the expansion of an aneroid, but in this case it progressively increases with altitude so that the magnitude of pressure breathing likewise increases. As a safety margin, pressure breathing usually commences at about 38,000 ft instead of at the theoretical level of 40,000 ft. In regulators that are also capable of providing pressure breathing for G (the unit of acceleration) protection, loading of the pressure breathing module for that purpose is accomplished by a signal from the G valve.
The presence of a raised pressure within the mask, whether it be safety pressure or pressure breathing, requires that the nonreturn expiratory valve be suitably modified to prevent the continuous loss of pressurized gas from the mask. This is achieved by delivering gas to the back of the expiratory valve at the same (inspiratory) pressure as that passing into the mask, a technique known as compensation. The presence of a connection between the inspiratory pathway and the expiratory valve in turn mandates the need for an inspiratory nonreturn valve if the pressure of expiration is not to be transmitted to the back of the expiratory valve and so hold it shut.

- Function of the demand valve can be confirmed visually by the operation of a flow indicator, which usually takes the form of an electromagnetic circuit completed by the deflection of a small diaphragm in response to flow of gas into the regulator. The presence of flow completes the circuit and causes the magnetic indicator to show white. When flow ceases, the circuit breaks and the indicator shows black. The device therefore operates in time with respiration, and correct function should be confirmed at regular intervals throughout flight. The magnetic indicator is usually an integral part of a panel-mounted regulator but, for obvious reasons, is placed on a visible console in man-mounted or seat-mounted systems.

(**Exhibit 32-9** *continues*)

garments, which pressurize the respiratory tract simultaneously with a greater or lesser part of the external surface of the body.

In most circumstances, in the event of a failure of cabin pressurization, an immediate descent will be initiated. But operational constraints may require that a military aircraft remain at high altitude until its mission is completed. Thus, pressure clothing may be used either to provide the short-term protection needed until descent can be made to a safe altitude, or to provide long-term protection so that the aircraft and its crew can remain safely at high altitude. The latter can only be attained by using a garment that maintains a pressure equal to or greater than 280 mm Hg around the body, both to prevent hypoxia and altitude DCS and to provide heat to maintain a satisfactory thermal environment. The only form of garment that can fulfil these requirements is a full-pressure suit (for further discussion, please see Chapter 34, Military Space Flight). If the aircraft is able to descend rapidly, however, physiological protection is needed only against hypoxia. Again, a full-pressure suit is the ideal solution because

- it applies the required pressure in an even manner to the respiratory tract and to the entire external surface of the body, and
- pressure gradients between different body parts do not occur; therefore,
- no serious physiological disturbances arise in the cardiovascular system or in the respiratory system.

A full-pressure suit is bulky and all-enveloping, however, and hinders routine flying even when uninflated; for this reason, partial-pressure garments are often a rational alternative. From the physiological standpoint, counterpressure should be applied to as much of the body as possible, but the advantages of the "partial" principle, however (low thermal load, less restriction when unpressurized, and greater mobility when pressurized), make it desirable that counterpressure should be applied to the minimum area of the body. Thus, the proportion of the body

covered by partial-pressure garments is a compromise between physiological ideal and operational expediency. Furthermore, because partial-pressure assemblies for high-altitude protection are only used for very short exposures, certain compromises with regard to moderate hypoxia are also acceptable: different considerations apply to the use of such assemblies when used in support of PPB as a means of enhancing tolerance to high, sustained +Gz accelerations.

Using a mask alone, the maximum breathing pressure that can be tolerated is about 30 mm Hg. For a P_{AO_2} of 60 mm Hg to be maintained (ie, an absolute lung pressure [which equals breathing pressure plus environmental pressure] of 141 mm Hg), respiratory protection to an altitude of 45,000 ft is possible. A P_{AO_2} of 45 to 50 mm Hg is acceptable, however, and will provide protection for 1 minute against the effects of loss of cabin pressurization up to 50,000 ft, provided that descent is undertaken to below 40,000 ft within 1 minute. The combination of a PPB mask and a suitable oxygen regulator is widely used to provide this level of get-me-down protection (see Exhibit 32-8).

Trunk counterpressure may be applied by a partial-pressure vest, which comprises a rubber bladder restrained by an outer inextensible cover. The bladder usually extends over the whole of the thorax and abdomen as well as the upper thighs (to avoid the risk of inguinal herniation at high breathing pressures). The bladder is inflated to the same pressure as that delivered to the respiratory tract, but PPB at 70 mm Hg with counterpressure to the trunk alone may induce syncope as a consequence of the large displacement of blood to all four limbs. This circulatory disturbance can be reduced by applying counterpressure to the lower limbs via G trousers. Both the vest and the G trousers may be inflated to the same pressure, or the latter may be inflated to a greater pressure than that being delivered to the vest and mask. If the absolute pressure within the lungs is maintained at 141 mm Hg, the combination of mask, vest, and G trousers will provide protection to a maximum altitude of 54,000 ft. Again, however, a certain degree of hypoxia is acceptable, and a breathing pressure of 68 to 72 mm Hg can be employed at 60,000 ft, where it will provide an absolute pressure in the lungs of 122 to

126 mm Hg, and a P_{AO_2} of 55 to 60 mm Hg. The combination of the discomfort of a high breathing pressure in the mask and a certain degree of hypoxia limits the duration of protection afforded by this ensemble to about 1 minute at 60,000 ft, followed immediately by descent at a rate of at least 10,000 ft/min to 40,000 ft for a total of 3 minutes.

When the required level of PPB exceeds the physiological limits associated with the use of an oronasal mask, use is made of oxygen delivery via a partial-pressure helmet, while a vest provides counterpressure to the trunk, and G trousers to the lower limbs. Partial-pressure helmets give support to the cheeks, the floor of the mouth, the eyes, and most of the head, thereby eliminating the uncomfortable pressure differentials that develop between the air passages and the skin of the head and neck when an oronasal mask is employed. Even when a partial-pressure helmet is used, however, severe neck discomfort may occur during PPB at pressures greater than 110 mm Hg. Finally, it would be physiologically beneficial to include the upper limbs in the areas to which counterpressure is applied (the vest being sleeveless), and a wide variety of garments have been employed to provide this extensive coverage in combination with a pressure helmet.

SUMMARY

The substrate for all aviation is Earth's atmosphere. Although its gas composition is essentially constant, ascent from ground level to the edge of space is accompanied by an exponential decrease in P_B and large, predictable changes in temperature and radiation. As balloons and then airplanes carried humans high above Earth, problems were encountered that were caused by hypoxia, hyperventilation, and altitude DCS; the advent of pressurized aircraft, with their potential for RD, added barotrauma to this list.

Although altitude DCS involves the same mechanisms as diving DCS, there are differences in symptom patterns and treatment: descent to ground level while breathing 100% oxygen constitutes the first and often sufficient line of therapy for victims of altitude DCS, whereas divers must be returned to a hyperbaric environment for treatment. The physiological problems of atmospheric flight are prevented by means of pressurized aircraft cabins, inhalation of oxygen-enriched gas through a mask or pressurized garments, or both. Oxygen supplies may be carried on board as a compressed gas or in liquid form, generated by chemical reactions or scavenged from outside air by onboard molecular sieves.

REFERENCES

1. International Civil Aviation Organization. *Manual of the ICAO Standard Atmosphere*. 2nd ed. Montreal, Quebec, Canada: ICAO; 1964.

2. Young WA, Shaw DB, Bates DV. Effect of low concentrations of ozone on pulmonary function in man. *J Appl Physiol*. 1964; 19: 765–768.

3. Pandolf K, Burr RE, Wenger CB, Pozos RS, eds. *Medical Aspects of Harsh Environments, Volume 1*. In: Zajtchuk R, Bellamy RF, eds. *Textbook of Military Medicine*. Washington, DC: Washington, DC: Department of the Army, Office of The Surgeon General, and Borden Institute; 2001: In press. Available at www.armymedicine.army.mil/history.

4. Ernsting J, Sharp GR. Harding RM, rev-ed. Hypoxia and hyperventilation. In: Ernsting J, King PF, eds. *Aviation Medicine*. 2nd ed. London, England: Butterworths; 1988: 46–59.

5. Ernsting J. The effect of brief profound hypoxia upon the arterial and venous oxygen tensions in man. *J Physiol*. 1963;169:292–311.

6. Harding RM, Mills FJ. Problems of altitude. In: Harding RM, Mills FJ, eds. *Aviation Medicine*. 3rd ed. London, England: British Medical Association; 1993: 58–72.

7. King PF. The eustachian tube and its significance in flight. *J Laryngol Otol*. 1979;93:659–678.

8. Ernsting J. Decompression sickness in aviation. In: Busby DE, ed. *Recent Advances in Aviation Medicine*. Dordrecht, The Netherlands: D Reidel Publishing; 1970: 177–187.

9. Fryer DI. Subatmospheric decompression sickness in man. Slough, England: Technivision Services; 1969.

10. Francis JR. The classification of decompression illness. In: Pilmanis AA, ed. *Proceedings of the 1990 Hypobaric Decompression Sickness Workshop*. San Antonio, Tex: Air Force Systems Command Armstrong Laboratory; 1992: 489–493. AL-SR-1992-0005.

11. Macmillan AJF. The pressure cabin. In: Ernsting J, King PF, eds. *Aviation Medicine*. 2nd ed. London: Butterworths; 1988: 112–126.

12. Ernsting J, Sharp GR. Macmillan AJF, rev-ed. Prevention of hypoxia. In: Ernsting J, King PF, eds. *Aviation Medicine*. 2nd ed. London, England: Butterworths; 1988: 60–71.

13. Ernsting J. Prevention of hypoxia—Acceptable compromises. *Aviat Space Environ Med.* 1978;49:495–502.

14. Harding RM. Oxygen equipment and pressure clothing. In: Ernsting J, King PF, eds. *Aviation Medicine*. 2nd ed. London, England: Butterworths; 1988: 72–111.

15. Ernsting J. Some effects of raised intrapulmonary pressure. *AGARDograph No 106*. Maidenhead, England: Technivision Ltd; 1966.

16. Ernsting J. The ideal relationship between inspired oxygen concentration and cabin altitude. *Aerospace Med.* 1963;34:991–997.

17. Air Standardization Coordinating Committee. *The Minimum Physiological Design Requirements for Aircrew Breathing Systems.* Washington DC: Air Standardization Coordinating Committee; 1982. Air Standard 61/22.

18. Sheffield PJ, Stork RL. Protection in the pressure environment: Cabin pressurization and oxygen equipment. In: DeHart RL, ed. *Fundamentals of Aerospace Medicine*. 2nd ed. Baltimore, Md: Williams & Wilkins; 1996: 126129.

RECOMMENDED READING

DeHart RL, ed. *Fundamentals of Aerospace Medicine*. 2nd ed. Baltimore, Md: Williams & Wilkins; 1996.

Edholm OG, Weiner JS, eds. *The Principles and Practice of Human Physiology*. London, England: Academic Press; 1981.

Ernsting J, King PF, eds. *Aviation Medicine*. 2nd ed. London, England: Butterworths; 1988.

Gillies JA, ed. *A Textbook of Aviation Physiology*. Oxford, England: Pergamon Press; 1965.

Harding RM, Mills FJ. *Aviation Medicine*. 3rd ed. London, England: British Medical Association; 1993.

Chapter 33

ACCELERATION EFFECTS ON FIGHTER PILOTS

ULF I. BALLDIN, MD, PhD, Dr hc*

*Senior Scientist, Wyle Laboratories, Air Force Research Laboratory, 2504 Gillingham Drive, Suite 25, Brooks Air Force Base, Texas 78235-5104

INTRODUCTION

Acceleration (G) is one of the major physical stresses associated with combat flying. More than 10% of pilots of fighter aircraft reported experiencing unexpected loss of consciousness (LOC) while flying aerobatic maneuvers[1]; the real incidence is probably higher because such events often induce amnesia. While such loss of consciousness resembles ordinary syncope, the consequences can be fatal, and the US Air Force cited sudden unconsciousness as the cause of 18 fatal accidents during the years 1982 through 1990.[2]

LOC during steep turns was first reported in 1918 as "fainting in the air" and became a problem during early air races.[3] Significant acceleration peaks became common experience for pilots flying improved aircraft between World War I and World War II, although the combination of high aerodynamic drag and low engine thrust in aircraft of that period made such acceleration a transient phenomenon. Nevertheless, concerns related to pilot blackout and loss of consciousness led to operational restrictions on the turn rates of some aircraft during the 1920s.

Aggressive dive-bombing techniques that were developed during the 1930s produced severe acceleration during the pull-up at the end of the bombing run.[4] Sporadic reports began to appear of blackout during these maneuvers as well as concern about acceleration-induced loss of consciousness (G-LOC). These problems were correctly attributed to "cerebral anemia produced by centrifugal action," and the Royal Air Force determined that 4 G (acceleration 4-fold greater than the force of gravity) was the limit of human acceleration tolerance.[5] In 1934 the US Navy developed a pneumatic "acceleration belt" consisting of an abdominal bladder, which the pilot inflated prior to the dive-bombing run, but this device probably had only marginal effect on acceleration tolerance.

Laboratory research on responses to acceleration was made possible by the development of human centrifuges, machines that produce acceleration by rotating an arm 20 to 30 ft long, at the end of which is mounted a capsule in which the subject sits or reclines. Although centrifuges had existed in earlier times, the first machines designed for aviation-related research were built in Germany and the United States during the 1930s, followed later by centrifuges at institutes of aviation medicine in Japan, the Soviet Union, Australia, and several European countries. Extensive research at the Mayo Clinic, Rochester, Minnesota, during the 1940s led to the development of both the five-bladder pneu-

matic anti-G suit (also called "G trousers") and the straining maneuvers (Exhibit 33-1) that significantly increased human ability to withstand acceleration. These techniques were adopted by military pilots worldwide over the next 3 decades, a period during which fighter aircraft remained capable of only limited periods of acceleration at peak levels of about 7 G.

The current challenge to pilot acceleration tolerance began in the 1980s with the introduction of fighter aircraft with greatly increased engine thrust and wingload capacity that allowed sustained accelerations of 9 G or more. LOC again became a problem and was identified as the cause of a number of fatal crashes. For the first time since the 1920s, the pilot's limitations began to restrict aircraft maneuverability, a serious problem in aerial combat situations where ability to turn hard and climb fast may be the key to survival. Furthermore, sudden onset of high acceleration can reduce the pilot to unconsciousness without warning. In response to these problems, during the 1990s research centrifuges have been upgraded to achieve the rapid onsets (6 G/s) and high accelerations (12 G) found in new aircraft. Recent developments include extended-coverage anti-G suits and systems for balanced pressure breathing to better counteract the circulatory effects of high acceleration. In addition, several nations now use centrifuge training to ensure that each fighter pilot makes optimal use of straining maneuvers. With these improvements, most pilots can now maintain vision and consciousness for extended periods at acceleration levels of 9 G.

Readers need to understand certain conventions and terminology that are used in discussing acceleration and its physiological effects (see Exhibit 33-1). Acceleration vectors are described in relation to three body axes (Figure 33-1), and the orientation is designated positive (+) or negative (–): Gz (head-to-foot), Gx (front-to-back), and Gy (side-to-side). The dominant acceleration for a seated pilot is +Gz, which occurs in ordinary turns and pull-ups and forces blood to pool in the legs and feet. Its reverse, –Gz, accompanies outside loops and forces blood toward the head.

Astronauts experience +Gx during launch, as do pilots in semireclining seats. Lateral (Gy) forces have been of little concern until now but may become a problem with the introduction of a new type of agile fighter aircraft, which will be able to slew its nose toward a target while continuing on its original flight path.

EXHIBIT 33-1

TERMS USED IN HIGH-ACCELERATION AVIATION

g:	Acceleration equal to gravity at the surface of Earth, 9.80665 m/s^2.
G:	A unit of convenience calculated as the observed acceleration divided by *g*; thus, acceleration of 29.4 m/s^2 is expressed as 3 G. "G" is also used as shorthand for the word "acceleration." For positive and negative directional designations and x, y, and z body axes used with the abbreviation G, see Figure 33-1.
Grayout:	Dimming of vision due to reduced retinal perfusion. It is usually accompanied by narrowing of visual fields (tunneling).
Blackout:	Loss of vision during acceleration due to insufficient retinal perfusion; it precedes loss of consciousness because eye perfusion is opposed by normal intraocular pressure.
Redout:	Reddish fogging of vision due to venous pooling and increased perfusion pressure in the eye during exposure to –Gz.
Acceleration-induced loss of consciousness (G-LOC):	Loss of consciousness during sustained acceleration due to inadequate cerebral perfusion.
Anti-G suit:	Trousers fitted with pneumatic or hydrostatic bladders over the abdomen and legs; an inelastic outer layer assures that increased bladder pressure during +Gz is transmitted to the adjacent tissues to minimize venous pooling.
Pressure breathing (PBG):	Continuous positive pressure applied to the airway during +Gz to increase intrathoracic pressure and thereby raise arterial blood pressure.
Balanced pressure breathing:	Use of a bladder contained in a vest to reduce the work of pressure breathing. The bladder is inflated to airway pressure and prevents over-expansion of the chest as well as making it easier to exhale against pressure. Also called "assisted" pressure breathing.
Straining maneuvers:	(1) Voluntary isometric contraction of major muscle groups (especially in the abdomen and legs) to prevent venous pooling and preserve cerebral perfusion during acceleration. (2) Valsalva maneuvers used to increase intrathoracic pressure and arterial pressure to preserve cerebral perfusion during acceleration.

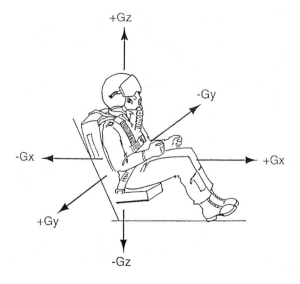

Fig. 33-1. The drawing shows the three standard axes (x, y, z) used to describe inflight acceleration (G) and their positive (+) and negative (–) directional designations. In each instance, the motion of the aircraft produces an opposite reaction in the human body. For example, for a seated pilot, the commonest acceleration is "head-to-foot," or +Gz, in which the aircraft turns sharply with the pilot's head aimed toward the inside of the turn: the headward pull of the aircraft causes soft tissue to sag downward and blood to pool in the legs. Negative Gz occurs less often when the pilot's head is pointed toward the outside of the turn. Positive Gx is commonly experienced when a powerful vehicle accelerates forward, while –Gx occurs with braking. Historically, lateral acceleration (+/–Gy) has not been a problem. Drawing: Courtesy of Mark Regna, Technical Sergeant, US Air Force.

PHYSICAL EFFECTS OF ACCELERATION

Acceleration (+Gz) has mechanical effects on soft tissues and compresses the spine. It also affects the cardiovascular and pulmonary systems, creating increased risks for visual symptoms, G-LOC, and pulmonary atelectasis. The less-common "negative" acceleration (–Gz) causes visual and cardiovascular disturbances and can also cause G-LOC.

Mechanical Effects

Acceleration causes soft tissues to sag; one obvious result is that the face appears to age remarkably—fortunately, a reversible change (Figure 33-2). Acceleration in any axis makes movement diffi-

cult. Above +2.5 G it is difficult to rise from a seat and at +3 G the limbs can hardly be raised, so that emergency escape from an aircraft requires an ejection seat. At +8 G any gross movement is impossible, but a pilot whose arms are supported can operate a properly designed control stick and buttons to +12 G and beyond.

Helmets and helmet-mounted equipment (Figure 33-3) create special mechanical problems because they alter the center of gravity of the head and their acceleration-magnified weight may overstress the cervical muscles. At +8 Gz a helmeted pilot can keep the head erect, but should it tip forward, the chin drops onto the chest and cannot be raised until acceleration is released.[6] Transient compression of the spinal column by up to 5 mm has been demonstrated after flights involving +7 Gz.[7]

Hydrostatic Effects and Cardiovascular Compensation

Acceleration increases the weight of the blood and so raises the pressure gradient in the hydrostatic column along the axis of acceleration. For example, the acceleration due to ordinary turns is

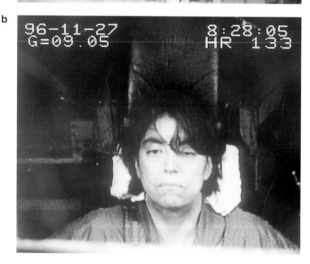

Fig. 33-2. The face of a subject exposed to (**a**) +1 G and (**b**) +9 G. Notice the aged appearance of the subject as she executes a straining maneuver at the higher level of acceleration.

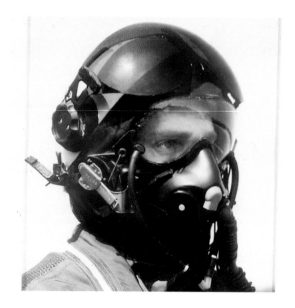

Fig. 33-3. A pilot wearing a Swedish-developed helmet and breathing mask system (mfg by FFV Aerotech AB, Sweden) with chemical–biological protection equipment for use in combination with assisted pressure breathing during acceleration (G). Photograph: FFV Aerotech AB, Sweden.

oriented in the +Gz direction for a sitting pilot, and so increases the pressure gradient from head to foot. Even moderate acceleration has relatively great effects on the venous circulation, greatly increasing venous pressure and therefore pooling below the heart, where "below" varies with the acceleration vector. These effects on the low-pressure side of the circulation in turn compromise venous return and therefore reduce cardiac output to regions above the heart. Heart–head distance has a significant negative correlation with acceleration tolerance, as demonstrated by studies involving a variety of seat-back angles.[3] Tall individuals have a slight disadvantage when sitting upright.

Hydrostatic effects on the arterial side of the circulation become important only at high accelerations.[8] For instance, at +9 Gz, arterial pressure in the feet of a sitting pilot might theoretically reach 630 mm Hg. Although peripheral vasoconstriction and precapillary sphincter constriction prevent some of this rise in pressure, edema and petechiae (also called "G-measles") are commonly found in dependent areas. Prolonged exposure to very high acceleration may induce hematoma in the feet, scrotum, or other dependent body regions.

Exposure to +Gz decreases arterial pressure in the head; in the absence of compensating mechanisms, perfusion to the brain would approach zero

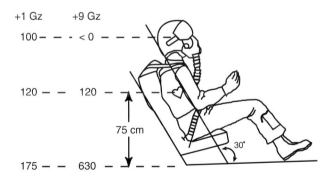

Fig. 33-4. Acceleration alters arterial blood pressure (BP, shown in mm Hg) by increasing the weight of blood and thus the hydrostatic pressure gradient along the axis of acceleration. The model shown here calculates the resulting pressures without considering physiological compensatory mechanisms. In a seated subject at +1 Gz (see Figure 33-1), if BP is 120 mm Hg at the heart, hydrostatic effects reduce the pressure to approximately 100 mm Hg at the head and raises it to 175 mm Hg at the feet. Exposure to +9 Gz increases the hydrostatic gradient: although the body maintains a BP of 120 mm Hg at the heart, pressure at the head decreases to approximately zero, while that at the feet increases to 630 mm Hg.

at +5 Gz (Figure 33-4). The rigidity of the skull and negative venous pressure above the heart are thought to create a siphon effect, which helps to maintain cerebral circulation, but the eyes have no such protection and are further disadvantaged by the intraocular pressure of 20 mm Hg. It is for this reason that gradual onset of acceleration typically produces visual symptoms before LOC.

During exposure to high +Gz (also called high *G-loads*), when blood is forced in the head-to-foot direction, baroreflexes in the carotid and aortic regions above the heart compensate for declining blood pressure with an increased heart rate and a moderate rise in peripheral resistance. This compensation requires 5 to 10 seconds to take effect and may be too slow to affect tolerance for rapid-onset acceleration.[9] It is therefore during the first few seconds of increasing acceleration that a pilot is most vulnerable to LOC. Recent research shows that tolerance for +Gz decreases markedly in a "push–pull" maneuver, when a brief period of mild –Gz precedes the +Gz stress.[10]

Pulmonary Effects

Acceleration (+Gz) makes breathing difficult by pulling down the diaphragm and exaggerates the ventilation–perfusion mismatch in the lungs. Basal congestion tends to close off lower airways, a tendency that is increased by compression from the abdominal bladder of an anti-G suit. Should the pilot also be breathing a high percentage of oxygen for protection from hypoxia, the rapid absorption of this gas from poorly ventilated basal alveoli may lead to symptomatic pulmonary atelectasis (Figure 33-5).[11]

Negative Acceleration

A pilot is exposed to negative acceleration (–Gz) during an outside loop (ie, when the pilot's head points to the outside of the turn) or the transition from a steep climb into a dive. Increased venous pressure and pooling of the blood in the head and face cause a sensation of fullness and sometimes headache. With longer exposures, facial edema develops, along with lacrimation, blurred vision, and a red-colored visual fog. A high level of –Gz is extremely uncomfortable and the eyes may feel as if they will pop out. Various cardiac arrhythmias may occur, including bradycardia followed by asystole and unconsciousness. While a stress of –2 Gz may be tolerated for up to 5 minutes, –3 Gz can be borne for only 30 seconds, and –4 Gz for only a few seconds.

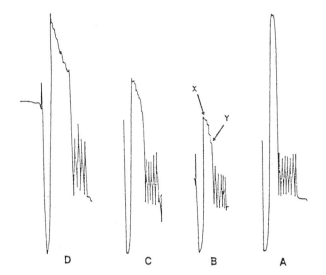

D · · · C · · · B · · · A

Fig. 33-5. Changes in vital capacity for a human subject (**a**) before and (**b, c, d**) after a 4-minute exposure to varied levels of acceleration while breathing 100% oxygen. Note that spirometry tracings are recorded from right to left. A sharp atelectasis-induced reduction in vital capacity occurred immediately (**b**) after the ride and (**c**) 1 minute later. The tracings reveal two components: stable atelectasis (x) and labile atelectasis (y). (**d**) The final tracing shows return to normal vital capacity after the subject took several deep breaths to clear the atelectasis. Reproduced with permission from Tacker WA, Balldin UI, Burton RR, Glaister DH, Gillingham KK, Mercer JR. Induction and prevention of acceleration atelectasis. *Aviat Space Environ Med.* 1987;58:71.

TOLERANCE TO ACCELERATION

Tolerance for high acceleration has been extensively studied in volunteers who are riding human centrifuges. Exceeding an individual's tolerance limits leads to G-LOC. Because a variety of factors help determine acceleration response, tolerance varies widely between individuals and fluctuates for the same person from day to day.

Tolerance Limits

Tolerance limits for +Gz acceleration are usually signaled by visual symptoms including tunneling, dimming, grayout, and blackout (Figure 33-6). During slow onset of acceleration, a relaxed subject not wearing an anti-G suit typically experiences initial visual symptoms at +4 Gz (range: +2 to +7 Gz) followed by blackout with a further +1 Gz; with faster onset, visual symptoms occur at lower acceleration levels. A subject can remain conscious through rapid onset to a transient high-G peak with immediate deceleration, but if the high acceleration persists, he will lose consciousness without any warning visual symptoms.

G-LOC (discussed in greater detail below) is often seen on the centrifuge, when the experimental subject fails to stop the run at onset of visual symptoms. The subject's head drops to the chest and seizure-like flailing motions may occur. Consciousness returns immediately as the centrifuge slows; the subject begins to raise the head, looks briefly confused, and then can respond to questions.[12] Subjects frequently do not remember the incident and may deny losing consciousness. Repeated episodes of G-LOC in healthy individuals appear to have no acute

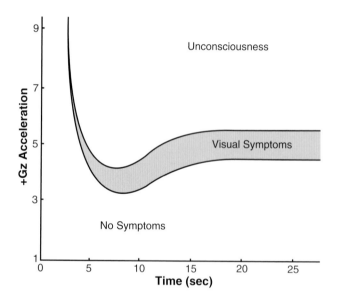

Fig. 33-6. Generalized human time–tolerance curve for +Gz acceleration (see Figure 33-1). The curves were developed from a large number of centrifuge experiments using relaxed human volunteers. The left side of the curve indicates relatively high tolerance levels for exposures that are so short that there is not enough time for development of venous pooling or cerebral hypoxia. The right side of the curve shows that tolerance is around 5 G for exposures of 15 to 30 seconds, which allow full activation of cardiovascular defense mechanisms; visual symptoms (first grayout, then blackout) precede loss of consciousness. The dip in tolerance for exposures of 5 to 15 seconds reflects the interval when venous pooling and cerebral hypoxia develop before cardiovascular defense mechanisms are fully activated. Reproduced with permission from Stoll AM. Human tolerance to positive G as determined by the physiological end-points. *J Aviat Med.* 1956;27:356-367.

or chronic aftereffects.[13]

During flight, an episode of G-LOC means that the pilot (1) unexpectedly ceases to control the aircraft for a critical period of time and (2) may not realize what has happened. G-LOC is a cause of accidents in high-performance aircraft[2]; however, because G-LOC is a transient functional state, its role in a fatal accident is always difficult to ascertain, as no evidence will be available at autopsy. G-LOC accidents are characterized by the crash of a mechanically intact aircraft that is both performing a high-G maneuver and lacks appropriate pilot response for recovery from the situation. The abrupt cessation of voluntary straining maneuvers can be detected in cockpit sound recordings and provides evidence of G-LOC.

Factors That Lower Tolerance

General fatigue, sleep deprivation, and any form of hangover or illness may significantly reduce acceleration tolerance. Pilots should therefore avoid flying high-G missions when they are ill or recovering from illness. Pilots should also be aware that their tolerance for high acceleration diminishes during any substantial layoff period during which they are not flying high-G maneuvers.

Heat stress and dehydration measurably decrease acceleration tolerance, owing to the combined effects of increased peripheral vasodilation and reduced plasma volume. A 3% level of dehydration significantly reduces tolerance for high acceleration even with the use of an anti-G suit and straining.[14] Extensive sunburn, with its peripheral cutaneous vasodilation, would likely decrease tolerance to acceleration in a similar way.

Hyperventilation due to anxiety, mental stress, hypoxia, and pressure breathing (see Exhibit 33-1) may decrease acceleration tolerance through cerebral vasoconstriction and peripheral vasodilation.

Countermeasures for Acceleration Effects

The adverse effects of high acceleration may be reduced by use of semireclining seats to the extent that they are compatible with aircraft design. Other countermeasures include voluntary straining maneuvers, anti-G suits, and pressure breathing.

Seat Configuration

The standard, chairlike seat in most cockpits has many advantages, such as easy adaptation to ejec-

tion requirements, but the upright back maximizes the length of the hydrostatic column subjected to +Gz acceleration. The change to a 30° seat-back angle in the US Air Force F-16 and French Rafale fighter planes reduces heart–brain distance and leads to a small but measurable increase in the threshold for visual symptoms.[3] Greater effects might be produced by further reclining the seat to 70° and elevating the feet; it would be even better to place the pilot in the prone position. However these more horizontal positions create difficulties in aircraft design and combat flying. Most fighter pilots crouch forward in combat, thus slightly reducing the heart-to-head distance.

Straining Maneuvers

Acceleration tolerance can be increased by 3 to 4 G through skilled use of straining maneuvers, which include (1) muscular contractions of the abdomen and legs, and (2) specialized respiratory techniques. The large-muscle component consists of strong, sustained isometric contractions of the muscles of the abdomen and limbs, producing a reflex increase in blood pressure and a mechanical decrease in peripheral pooling. The respiratory component involves use of Valsalva and related respiratory maneuvers to raise intrathoracic pressure and hence the arterial pressure at the heart.

These maneuvers must be taught to pilots, who learn to tense all major muscle groups while adopting a breathing pattern that involves straining against a closed glottis for 3 to 4 seconds, taking a quick breath and returning to straining. Regular practice is required to maximize both skill and stamina for these maneuvers, and strength training of major muscle groups has been found to significantly increase tolerance for sustained high-G profiles. Straining was formerly taught on an ad hoc basis during flight instruction, but much more consistent results are now obtained by training pilots on a human centrifuge (Figure 33-7).[15]

Physical Training

Various strength training programs have been developed in attempts to increase acceleration tolerance and stamina.[16] It appears that effective training can be accomplished without inducing muscle hypertrophy. Possible mechanisms include improved neuromuscular efficiency, which is seen during the initial phases of any strength training program. Despite the important role of abdominal

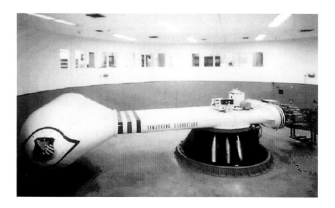

Fig. 33-7. The human centrifuge at Brooks Air Force Base, San Antonio, Texas. The closed gondola seen at the left carries one subject strapped into an aircraft seat, as well as a variety of measurement devices. The centrifuge operators, medical monitor, and investigators sit behind the windows seen above the centrifuge; they communicate with the subject by intercom and observe him or her through closed-circuit television. The machine is driven by hydraulic motors connected to an enormous "bull gear" under the center of rotation. The gondola swings on its fore-to-aft axis so that the resultant acceleration is always oriented from floor to ceiling; at rest the capsule floor is horizontal like the floor of the room, but during centrifugation it rotates out to parallel the wall. Study of different acceleration axes is accomplished by repositioning the chair within the gondola. Subjects experience significant, nauseogenic Coriolis effects during changes in centrifuge speed.

tensing in anti-G straining maneuvers, training limited to these muscles is not effective; training programs must include all of the major muscles of the legs, arms, and abdomen. Muscle biopsies of subjects trained on a centrifuge show no correlation of tolerance with the proportion of slow- or rapid-twitch muscle fibers.

A moderate level of aerobic fitness is thought to enhance acceleration tolerance and reduce overall fatigue. However, some authorities believe that excessive aerobic conditioning can reduce acceleration tolerance, perhaps because the athletic heart, with its very low resting rate, takes longer to respond to sudden acceleration stress. As a result, pilots of high-performance aircraft are now expected to follow a regular exercise program that combines moderate aerobic exercise with strength training, adding special exercises to maximize the strength of neck muscles.

Drugs

Pharmacological modalities have been examined

for their potential to improve tolerance to acceleration but without much success. They usually have only marginal, transient effects and many have undesirable side effects. Ephedrine and amphetamine sulfate may reduce the fatigue caused by repeated fighter sorties, but their adverse effects outweigh any benefit and make their use inappropriate during ordinary high-performance aircraft operations.

Anti-G Suits and Positive-Pressure Breathing

As stated above, anti-G suits were initially developed during World War II and changed little over the ensuing 40 years. These suits consist of trousers made of two layers of nonstretch material, with rubber bladders inserted at the calf, thigh, and abdomen (Figure 33-8). The bladders are interconnected, and the abdominal bladder is fitted with an umbilical hose that is connected to a special regulator (the G-valve), which provides gas pressure to the anti-G suit in proportion to the +Gz level. The suit pressurizes automatically when the G-valve senses acceleration; this inflation tightens the trousers around the limbs and abdomen and thus reduces dependent pooling. In addition, the abdominal bladder enhances the return of blood from the

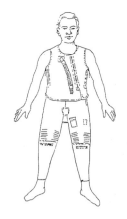
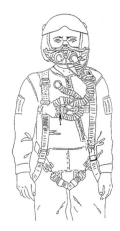

Fig. 33-8. An example of a modern US Air Force anti-G system. A pneumatic valve automatically inflates the bladders covering the legs to reduce venous pooling and delivers positive pressure to the mask to elevate intrathoracic pressure and hence blood pressure. The use of a counterpressure vest reduces the work of exhalation associated with positive pressure breathing. The valve delivers pressure that is proportional to the G load; pressure in the vest and mask is always slightly lower than that delivered to the leg bladders.

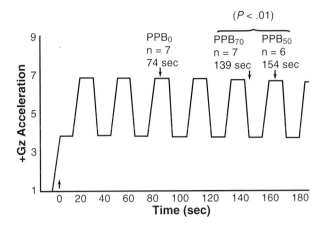

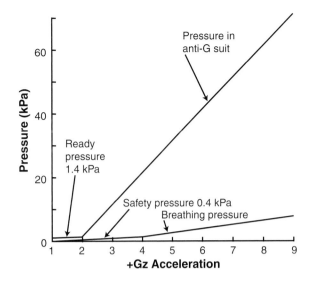

Fig. 33-9. Acceleration profile for a simulated air-combat maneuver on the centrifuge at Brooks Air Force Base, San Antonio, Tex. Alternating 5- and 9-G intervals of 10 seconds represent the acceleration experienced by a pilot engaged in a dynamic dogfight with another aircraft. Volunteer subjects were highly trained to become accustomed to the centrifuge; they wore anti-G suits and performed straining maneuvers to maintain consciousness while riding the repetitive profile to the point of exhaustion or impending blackout. Marks indicate mean endurance time without pressure breathing (PPB_0) and with pressure breathing levels of 50 and 70 mm Hg (PPB_{50} and PPB_{70}). Note that PPB significantly lengthens endurance by reducing the need for voluntary straining. There is a significant advantage for the higher level of PPB. The arrows represent times and do not coincide with plateaus. Reproduced with permission from Burns J, Balldin UI. Assisted positive-pressure breathing for augmentation of acceleration tolerance time. *Aviat Space Environ Med.* 1988;59:229.

Fig. 33-10. A schedule for automatic delivery of pressure to an anti-G suit and positive-pressure breathing system. A slight residual pressure is maintained in both mask and leg bladders in normal flight (1–2 Gz) to allow instantaneous delivery of increased pressure on sudden onset of high acceleration (G). The profiles shown are for the life support system of the Swedish Air Force Gripen (Griffin) fighter aircraft; US Air Force equipment and pressure schedules are similar. Reproduced with permission from Balldin UI, Dahlback G, Larsson L-E. *Full Coverage Anti-G Suit and Balanced Pressure Breathing.* Stockholm, Sweden: FOA Report C50065-5.1; 1989. ISSN 0347-7665.

abdomen to the thorax and reduces the downward movement of the diaphragm and heart at high acceleration.

As explained above, the development of advanced fighter aircraft during the 1980s created a demand for improved anti-G protection. Anti-G valves were modified to provide faster inflation profiles. Experimental suits were made to produce sequential pressurization of bladders, and other variations were explored. However, the major improvement came with the development of full-coverage anti-G suits, in which the bladders entirely surround the legs.

Recent experimental work on human centrifuges[17] showed that balanced positive-pressure breathing during acceleration (PBG), can be substituted for respiratory straining maneuvers (Figure 33-9). The advantages of PBG include substantially diminished fatigue as well as restoration of ability to talk at high acceleration. Because inspiratory

pressures during PBG usually exceed 30 mm Hg and can reach 60 mm Hg, a counterpressure bladder over the chest is used to ease the work of expiration. The resulting combination of positive-pressure breathing and chest counterpressure is sometimes termed "assisted PBG." New anti-G valves were required to control the differing but related pressures needed in the anti-G suit and the mask–vest system (see Chapter 32, Pressure Changes and Hypoxia in Aviation). A typical pressure schedule used for PBG appears in Figure 33-10.

The combination of full-coverage suits and assisted PBG increases the maximum level of acceleration that can be tolerated.[18] A major effect of this combination lies in reducing fatigue. Centrifuge subjects can ride relaxed at up to +8 to +9 Gz, and their endurance time for continuous sequences of high-G maneuvers increases 4-fold or more. Experienced fighter pilots have endured more than 12 minutes on a centrifuge-simulated aerial combat profile consisting of alternating 10-second periods at +5 and +9 Gz.

ACCELERATION-RELATED PHYSIOLOGICAL PERTURBATIONS

Acceleration effects on pilots may include motion sickness, cardiovascular and pulmonary effects, and neck and back pain. Protective equipment such as anti-G suits and pressure-breathing systems may produce unwanted side effects. Although men and women have similar tolerance levels, anatomical differences can produce gender-specific problems. Medication of various types can reduce G tolerance.

Motion Sickness

Rapid changes in acceleration stimulate the semicircular canals and may be accompanied by spatial disorientation, vertigo, and motion sickness, especially if the subject makes simultaneous movements of the head. This topic is discussed more completely in Chapter 35, Motion Sickness.

Cardiac Dysrhythmias

There is no scientific evidence that acute or chronic acceleration exposure damages the heart.

Mild acceleration, like exercise, often eliminates the occasional premature ventricular contractions seen in healthy individuals. On the other hand, high acceleration on the centrifuge often stimulates more-serious dysrhythmias, including frequent premature atrial contractions and premature ventricular contractions, and, more rarely, ventricular tachycardia.[19,20] An electrocardiograph used with a centrifuge may also record relative bradycardias that proceed to asystole. Any of these arrhythmias may lead to LOC; fortunately, they routinely revert to normal as the centrifuge is brought to a halt (Figure 33-11).

These arrhythmias are not a result of pathology but reflect functional problems caused by displacement of the heart and diminished blood supply to the cardiac muscle and nodes. Medical observers are trained to immediately halt any centrifuge run in which a subject exhibits relative bradycardia, prolonged ventricular bigeminy or trigeminy, multiple paired or multifocal PVCs, or more than three beats of ventricular tachycardia. Pilots should be discour-

G-LOC

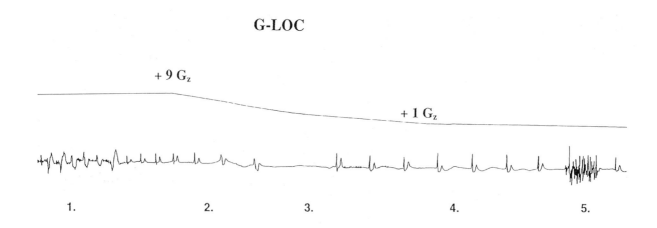

Fig. 33-11. The electrocardiogram for a human subject during and after a centrifuge run that peaked with several seconds at +9 Gz (see Figure 33-1) and was terminated when the subject suddenly lost consciousness (G-LOC). The upper line shows the decreasing acceleration (G) level as the centrifuge was slowed and stopped. Note (**1**) the onset of ventricular tachycardia at +9 Gz followed by (**2**) bradycardia of 45 beats per minute, (**3**) asystole lasting 7 seconds and (**4**) a further period of bradycardia at 35 beats per minute as the level of acceleration fell. (**5**) The subject regained consciousness and a normal cardiac rhythm on return to +1 Gz and had no sequelae. Although occasional premature ventricular contractions are a common occurrence at high acceleration, the response shown here is rare. Acceleration-induced arrhythmias correct themselves when the stress is discontinued but could still prove fatal to the pilot of a single-seat aircraft.

aged from using caffeine because of its tendency to produce arrhythmias.

Pulmonary Shunts and Atelectasis

The redistribution of blood in the lungs during acceleration amplifies ventilation–perfusion mismatching and reduces oxygen saturation.[21] During typical +Gz acceleration, blood pools at the base of the lungs, causing edema and constriction of the distal airways, reducing local ventilation. The acceleration also displaces lung tissue, stretching and expanding the apical alveoli. This displacement can occasionally be sufficient to cause pneumothorax and mediastinal emphysema. Pilots who breath an oxygen-rich mixture (> 70% O_2) during high-G maneuvers may experience bronchial irritation, substernal pain, cough, and shortness of breath. Laboratory studies have demonstrated a decrease in vital capacity under such conditions, and it has been shown[11] that the underlying problem is pulmonary atelectasis due to the rapid absorption of oxygen from closed-off, highly perfused alveoli near the base of the lung. Usually these symptoms diminish and disappear following several deep breaths. The problem can be prevented by keeping at least 30% nitrogen in the inspired gas unless altitude exposure dictates otherwise.

Pain, Petechiae, and Edema

Fit problems with helmets, anti-G suits, and vests, which seem minor on the ground, may lead to painful pinching, friction, and bruising at high acceleration. The increased intravascular pressures in the body during high G-loads, straining, and pressure breathing may cause petechiae, edema, and even hematoma formation in unprotected areas below the heart, including the arms, hands, crotch, and feet. Prolonged exposure to high G-loads can cause severe arm pain, especially when PBG is used in aircraft with a control stick placed well below the heart. Proteinuria may be seen following severe acceleration exposures.

Disorders of the Back and Neck

Fighter pilots often complain of acute neck pain, especially following aerobatic maneuvers accompanied by rapid head movements.[6] Chronic problems may also develop, especially in crew members who wear helmets loaded with electronic devices. The lower cervical spine seems to be most vulnerable to injury, especially in navigators or weapons officers who are subject to unexpected acceleration. Regular strength training of the neck muscles seems to diminish the number of complaints; nevertheless, serious injuries can occur; documented acceleration-induced injuries include torn ligaments as well as fractures of the cervical vertebral bodies and spinous processes.

A slight possibility for cervical disc problems exists when a fighter pilot moves his head during lower but more sustained acceleration. A fully loaded helmet (ie, a helmet mounted with displays, sights, laser eye protection, night vision goggles, etc) adds to the weight and increases the probability for neck injuries. Neck pain is reported in more than one third of the pilots who fly high-performance fighter aircraft.[6,7] Magnetic resonance imaging occasionally shows bulging cervical discs among symptomatic fighter pilots, and there are indications of an increased risk of degenerative changes with chronic exposure.

Back pain has also been reported[8,16] among fighter pilots, but this condition is so common in the nonflying population that it is difficult to relate it to acceleration exposure. A study[22] using magnetic resonance imaging (MRI) investigated two groups: 22 asymptomatic males who had previously been subjects in Gz centrifuge experiments and 19 age-matched, asymptomatic, nonaccelerated controls. Individuals of both groups were seen on MRI to have disc bulges, herniated nucleus pulposus, disc degeneration or desiccation, and Schmorl's nodule. Most of the abnormalities occurred from the mid-thoracic through the lumbar spine (one subject from each group had a bulge or a herniated nucleus pulposus in the cervical spine), but no significant differences were found between the two groups. Thus, exposure to acceleration per se does not appear to result in spinal column abnormalities. In extreme cases, spinal column trauma has been seen after exposures to high acceleration in aircraft as well as in centrifuges. The severe +Gz acceleration on the spine during ejection with gun-type seats exceeds +25 G for 0.12 to 0.15 seconds and is known to cause compression fractures of the vertebral bodies and herniated intervertebral discs. With rocket-assisted ejection seats, the acceleration peak is reduced to +15 G or less during 0.2 to 0.5 seconds, thus reducing the risk for spinal injuries. In addition, windblast during high-velocity ejections may cause injuries when the arms and legs are flailing.

Continuing improvements in aircraft performance have produced a need to look at acceleration up to +12 Gz. To minimize the risk to human subjects, several laboratories sought improved methods for documenting the integrity the vertebral column. However, neither conventional methods nor magnetic resonance imaging shows a good correlation between disc pathology and subjective symptoms.[22]

Side Effects of Using Acceleration-Protective Equipment

While new anti-G equipment increases acceleration tolerance to match current flight profiles, it will also likely lead to expectations for further increases in aircrew tolerance for long-duration, high-G exposure. These more-severe exposures to acceleration will likely lead to the reappearance of known problems as well as create new ones. For instance, prolonged centrifuge experiments reveal the need for anti-G suits that include pressure socks to control pain, petechiae, and edema in the feet. Other problems include arm, neck, and back pain; motion sickness; and generalized fatigue. Many of these symptoms persist long after flight and will become troublesome challenges for commanders and flight surgeons as they accumulate during prolonged flights or surge operations.

Gender-Specific Medical Risks

The risks for women exposed to high G-loads are not particularly well studied but are generally similar to the risks for men.[23] However, the need for correct fitting of protective equipment is an important issue; anti-G suits must be tailored to fit women to prevent the abdominal bladder from compressing the lower ribs, causing pain and restricting breathing.[24] Men, on the other hand, may have a slight risk of high-G-related discomfort to their genitalia, such as scrotal pain and hemorrhage.

Women may experience increased menstrual flow or bleeding (spotting) between menses during acceleration stress.[25] The effects of acceleration on a fetus are also mostly unknown, and the potential for fetal injury, malformation, spontaneous abortion, or fetal death cannot be excluded. Rarely, oral contraceptives may cause formation of thrombosis, which might become dislodged and advance to the lungs with possible fatal results. If there is an augmented risk of dislodging thromboses during increased G-load, it is currently unknown; however, the lower hormone content of modern oral contraceptives may have substantially minimized this risk.

ACCELERATION-INDUCED LOSS OF CONSCIOUSNESS

G-LOC develops gradually during slow onset of acceleration. The subject usually experiences dimming or tunneling of vision followed by blackout before actual unconsciousness occurs (see Figure 33-6). However, with sudden onset of acceleration and high G levels, G-LOC may occur without warning. In centrifuge experiments in which the machine is immediately slowed to a halt, unconsciousness typically lasts 10 to 15 seconds and is followed by an equal or longer period of mental confusion that is often accompanied by convulsive movements.

Subjects may report having vivid dreams during this period.[13] Amnesia is also a frequent occurrence, so that subjects deny that they lost consciousness and are dumbfounded when shown video tapes of the episode.

MEDICATIONS FOR PILOTS OF HIGH-PERFORMANCE AIRCRAFT

Few systemic medications are acceptable for pilots of high-performance aircraft, as drugs might interfere with the flying and mission capabilities. Exceptions include single doses of aspirin, antacids for mild epigastric distress, hemorrhoidal suppositories, and bismuth subsalicylate for mild afebrile diarrhea. Decongestant nasal sprays may be used to treat ear block for get-me-down purposes (see Exhibit 32-8 in Chapter 32, Pressure Changes and Hypoxia in Aviation). Oral antibiotics and topical acyclovir (Zovirax, mfg by Burroughs Wellcome, Research Triangle Park, NC) may also be allowed, if prescribed by a flight surgeon.

Other drugs may be approved after a waiver has been received from the appropriate command level when the potential for idiosyncratic reactions is excluded and with certain restrictions:

- malaria prophylaxis,
- scopolamine and ephedrine for airsickness in flying trainees,
- doxycycline for mild diarrhea (after 72 h ground testing),
- completion of oral antibiotics for asymptomatic streptococcal pharyngitis and other specified infections,
- vaginal creams or suppositories, and
- some medications for treatment of acute urinary tract infection or prostatitis (after symptoms have abated).

Waivers may also be obtained for use of other, less commonly indicated medications such as chlorothiazide or hydrochlorothiazide for controlling hypertension, and triamterene, probenecid, and allopurinol for gout.

SUMMARY

Crews of fighter aircraft encounter severe physical stress due to the acceleration produced by aerobatic maneuvers. G-LOC was first recognized early in the development of military aviation and has re-emerged as a problem with the recent introduction of increasingly powerful, agile aircraft. Acceleration effects include increased weight of head and extremities, sagging of soft tissue, spinal compression, and amplified hydrostatic gradients in the cardiovascular system. With slow onset of acceleration, cardiovascular reflexes provide some protection, and visual changes precede loss of consciousness. For rapid onset and higher acceleration levels, voluntary straining maneuvers and protective clothing are used to increase tolerance. Relaxed tolerance for head-to-foot acceleration (normally about 4 +Gz) can be substantially increased by tensing the limbs and abdominal muscles combined with respiratory maneuvers to increase intrathoracic pressure. Introduction of PBC, combined with extended-coverage anti-G suits, has improved acceleration tolerance by reducing the fatiguing effort required.

Crews who fly fighter aircraft are expected to engage in regular physical training to increase neck strength and improve the efficacy of limb contractions; regular acceleration exposure in flight or on a centrifuge are required to optimize the combination of limb tensing, abdominal contractions, and respiratory maneuvers. Many factors can reduce acceleration tolerance, including fatigue, loss of training effects, illness, and medication or hangover.

Medical problems associated with exposure to acceleration include skin manifestations (petechiae or bruising), dependent edema, back and neck pain, and muscle strains. In addition, cardiac arrhythmias may occur during exposure, although these normally disappear when acceleration abates.

REFERENCES

1. Johansen DC, Pheeny HT. A new look at the loss of consciousness experience within the US naval forces. *Aviat Space Environ Med*. 1988;59:6–8.

2. Lyons TJ, Harding R, Freeman J, Oakley C. G-induced loss of consciousness accidents: USAF experience, 1982–1990. *Aviat Space Environ Med*. 1992;63;60–66.

3. Burton RR, Whinnery JE. Operational G-induced loss of consciousness: Something old, something new. *Aviat Space Environ Med*. 1985; 56:812–817.

4. Harsch V. German acceleration research from the very beginning. *Aviat Space Environ Med*. 2000;71:854–856.

5. Gibson TM, Harrison MH. "... too much acceleration." In: *Into Thin Air: A History of Aviation Medicine in the RAF*. London, England: Robert Hale; 1984: chap 9.

6. Hämäläinen O, Vanharanta H, Bloigu R. +Gz-related neck pain: A follow-up study. *Aviat Space Environ Med*. 1994;65(1);16-18.

7. Hämäläinen O, Vanharanta H, Hulpi M, Karhu M, Kuronen P, Kinnunen H. Spinal shrinkage due to +GZ forces. *Aviat Space Environ Med*. 1996;67:659–661.

8. Balldin UI. Factors influencing G-tolerance. *Clin Physiol*. 1986;6:209–219. Editorial review.

9. Stoll AM. Human tolerance to positive G as determined by the physiological end-points. *J Aviat Med*. 1956;27:356–367.

10. Banks RD, Grissett JD, Turnipseed GT, Saunders PL, Rupert AH. The "push–pull" effect. *Aviat Space Environ Med*. 1994;65:699–704.

11. Tacker WA, Balldin UI, Burton RR, Glaister DH, Gillingham KK, Mercer JR. Induction and prevention of acceleration atelectasis. *Aviat Space Environ Med*. 1987;58:69–75.

12. Whinnery JE. *Acceleration Induced Loss of Consciousness: A Review of 500 Episodes.* Warminster, Pa: Naval Air Development Center, Air Vehicle and Crew Systems Technology Department (code 602C); 1988. Report NADC-88100-60.

13. Jones DR. A review of central nervous system effects of G-induced loss of consciousness on volunteer subjects. *Aviat Space Environ Med.* 1991;62(7):624–627.

14. Nunneley SA, Stribley RF. Heat and acute dehydration effects on acceleration response in man. *J Appl Physiol.* 1979;47:197–200.

15. Gillingham KK, Fosdick JP. High-G training for fighter aircrew. *Aviat Space Environ Med.* 1988;59:12–19.

16. Balldin UI. Physical training and G-tolerance. *Aviat Space Environ Med.* 1984;55:991–992. Guest editorial.

17. Burns J, Balldin UI. Assisted positive pressure breathing for augmentation of acceleration tolerance time. *Aviat Space Environ Med.* 1988;59:225–233.

18. Harding RM, Bomar JB Jr. Positive pressure breathing for acceleration protection and its role in prevention of inflight G-induced loss of consciousness. *Aviat Space Environ Med.* 1990;61:845–849.

19. Balldin UI, Tong A, Marshall JA, Regna M. Premature ventricular contractions during +Gz with and without pressure breathing and extended coverage anti-G suit. *Aviat Space Environ Med.* 1999;70;209–212.

20. Whinnery JE. The electrocardiographic response to high +Gz centrifuge training. *Aviat Space Environ Med.* 1990; 61:716–721.

21. Glaister DH. *Effects of Gravity and Acceleration on the Lung.* London, England: Technivision Services. North Atlantic Treaty Organization Advisory Group on Aerospace Research and Development; 1970. AGARDograph 133.

22. Burns JW, Loecker TH, Fischer JR Jr, Bauer DH. Prevalence and significance of spinal disc abnormalities in an asymptomatic acceleration subject panel. *Aviat Space Environ Med.* 1996;67:849–853.

23. Gillingham K, Schade C, Jackson W, Gilstrap L. Women's G tolerance. *Aviat Space Environ Med.* 1986;57:745–753.

24. Dooley JW, Hearon CM, Shaffstall RM, Fischer MD. Accommodation of females in the high-G environment: The USAF Female Acceleration Tolerance Enhancement (FATE) project. *Aviat Space Environ Med.* 2001;72(8):739–746.

25. Heaps CL, Fischer MD, Hill RC. Female acceleration tolerance: Effects of menstrual state and physical condition. *Aviat Space Environ Med.* 1997;68:525–530.

RECOMMENDED READING

Burton RR, ed. Panel on deliberate G-induced loss of consciousness. *Aviat Space Environ Med.* 1991:62;609–637.

Burton RR, Whinnery JE. Sustained acceleration. In: DeHart RL, ed. *Fundamentals of Aerospace Medicine.* 2nd ed. Baltimore, Md: Williams & Wilkins; 1986; 201–260.

Wood EH. *Evolution of Anti-G Suits and Their Limitations.* 2 vols. Rochester, Minn: Mayo Foundation; 1990.

Chapter 34

MILITARY SPACEFLIGHT

F. ANDREW GAFFNEY, MD*; AND JAMES P. BAGIAN, MD†

*Colonel, US Air Force Reserve, Medical Corps; Senior Flight Surgeon and Astronaut; Division of Cardiology, Vanderbilt University School of Medicine, Nashville, Tennessee
†Colonel, US Air Force Reserve, Medical Corps; Senior Flight Surgeon and Astronaut; Director, Department of Veterans Affairs, National Center for Patient Safety, Ann Arbor, Michigan 48106

INTRODUCTION

Support of life in space is surely the most demanding technical challenge undertaken by humankind, and requires close collaboration among physicians, physiologists, engineers, and professionals with a variety of other skills. This chapter is designed to help the reader develop a basic understanding not only of the challenges of life support in the space environment but also of the medical issues related to health maintenance in physiological readaptation on return to the planetary surface. The topics should be of interest to all military physicians as well as to those specializing in aerospace and occupational medicine.

Long before human spaceflight was technically possible, aeromedical physicians were considering its possibilities and discussing the problems that humans would face when leaving Earth. Probably the best early discussion of aeromedical problems of space travel occurred at a symposium sponsored by the US Air Force and the National Research Council of the National Academy of Sciences in the late 1940s.[1] The authors of the report of that symposium, who included General Harry Armstrong, Dr Heinz Haber, and Dr Hubertus Strughold, noted that human physiological responses "will play a more decisive role in the initial stages of space travel than it did during the early stages of aviation."[1] These prescient scientists identified potential problems with acceleration, radiation, rapid decompression from collisions with orbital debris, temperature extremes, sensorimotor and neurological changes, psychological stresses, and the dangers of fire with hyperoxic environments. They actually divided these problems into two phases: (1) adaptation to microgravity and (2) readaptation on return to Earth or another celestial body's gravity field. Their discussion concluded with the telling observation that "We can only guess the facts here: experiments must be the final answer."[1]

More than 1 decade later (12 Apr 1961 and 20 Feb 1962, respectively), the brief orbital flights of Yuri Gagarin (1 h, 48 min) and John Glenn (4 h, 55 min) showed that human orbital flight was indeed possible. The close confinement and short duration of early flights limited the development of medical data; several more decades were required to acquire precise data regarding specific physiological changes associated with acute and chronic exposure to microgravity.

The early astronauts and cosmonauts were recruited from military flying programs. Military physicians provided a substantial component of the medical expertise for developing and supporting human spaceflight, and much of the medical and physiological testing of early astronaut candidates took place at the US Air Force School of Aerospace Medicine, Brooks Air Force Base, San Antonio, Texas. Military facilities have continued to provide research and testing support to the US space program, and resources from all of the uniformed services have been used to support launch, recovery, and contingency planning for piloted orbital flight. Although the US Air Force Space Command does not now have a defined role for humans in orbit, this is almost certain to change with the continuing evolution of sophisticated orbital reconnaissance capabilities and single-stage–to–orbit spacecraft.

ORBITAL MECHANICS AND FREE FALL

How do spacecraft remain in orbit and why do astronauts find themselves "weightless"?[2] It is a popular misconception that microgravity is caused by the spacecraft's distance from Earth. In fact, if a spacecraft were simply lifted into space, it would fall back to Earth as a ball dropped from the hand would, owing to the pull of gravity. Orbital flight occurs when the pull due to gravity ($A_{gravity}$) equals the centripetal acceleration that is related to the object's tangential velocity ($V_{tangent}$) as described in Equation 1, where the radius of the orbit (r_{orbit}) is measured from the center of Earth (Equation 1):

1. $$A_{gravity} = (V^2_{tangent}) / r_{orbit}$$

A typical low-Earth orbit of 170 miles' altitude requires a speed of approximately 17,400 mph

(25,520 fps) and yields an orbit with approximately a 90-minute period. As in any orbital condition, the spacecraft is in "free fall" on a curved path that continuously misses Earth. Although this condition is often called "zero G" ($0g$) because astronauts do not feel the pull of gravity, the subtleties of orbital mechanics actually impose *microgravity* on the order of a few millionths of a *g* (the Systéme International d'Unités symbol representing units of gravity and acceleration).

Because orbital flight involves a balance of forces, returning from orbit is a matter of decelerating the spacecraft to destroy this equilibrium and allowing gravity to alter the orbital altitude. A small decrease in tangential velocity causes a reduction in the craft's orbital altitude; drag from the upper atmosphere further decelerates the craft, which con-

Fig. 34-1. A diagram of the orbital path of the Skylab space station. Note that the craft crosses the Equator at approximately 50°; this results in a groundtrack extending from 50°N to 50°S in latitude. Higher orbital inclinations provide overflight of a larger portion of Earth's surface but substantially increase the energy required to reach orbit. Photograph: Courtesy of National Aeronautics and Space Administration, Washington, DC.

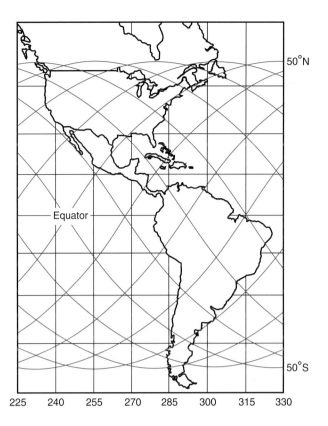

tinues to reduce its speed (and therefore its altitude) until it eventually lands on Earth's surface.

All known human spaceflight missions have utilized equatorial low-Earth orbits. These launches point toward the east to take advantage of the tangential velocity provided by Earth's spin, reducing the energy, and more importantly, the fuel and mass needed to achieve orbit. The closer the launch site is to the equator, the greater this effect. The precise direction of launch sets the orbital inclination, which is the angle at which the orbital plane crosses the equator (Figure 34-1). A large angle is desirable for Earth observation flights because it increases the maximal northern and southern latitudes of the track over the ground and allows direct observation of a large percentage of Earth's land mass. However, available inclinations have been limited by considerations of safety of people and objects on the ground under the launch track. Shuttle launches from the Kennedy Space Center in Cape Canaveral, Florida, are generally restricted to a band between 28.5°N and 62°N. Russian crewed flights launched from Kazakhstan are 51.6°N. Shuttle launches from Vandenberg Air Force Base in southern California would have permitted polar orbits overflying 100% of the planetary surface, but the required launch facilities were never completed.

LIVING IN SPACE

Living and working in space poses a number of medical and physiological challenges. These stem from conditions created by the microgravity environment as well as other factors that are created by the technical details of the methods used to deal with the hostile physical environment. The following section provides a brief overview of the unique medical-support requirements associated with spaceflight operations and identifies some directions for aerospace medicine in the 21st century.

Life Support

Space is a near-vacuum with temperatures ranging from −156°C (−250°F) in shade to +120°C (+250°F) in direct sunlight. Humans must be protected from this hostile environment by means of sophisticated spacecraft or suits for extravehicular activity (EVA) (Figure 34-2). Both use insulation and reflective materials to minimize direct heat gain and loss and have thermal control systems to properly compensate for the radiative heat gain and loss, as well as heat generated by the people and/or the equipment onboard the spacecraft.

Early US spacecraft utilized a cabin atmosphere of 100% oxygen at 5.0 psi. This low-pressure, high-oxygen system permitted lighter weight spacecraft that were within the lift capabilities of existing US ballistic missiles.[3] However, the elevated partial pressure of oxygen (Po_2) presented significant risk due to flammability and contributed to the Apollo 1 fire, which took the lives of three astronauts. The atmosphere was subsequently changed to a sea-level composition for launch, then depressurized to 5.0 psi, and gradually increased to 100% oxygen once in space. Skylab was the first US spacecraft to use a two-gas, hyperoxic, hypobaric system. A molecular sieve was utilized for removal of carbon dioxide, replacing the CO_2 absorption canisters that had been used in previous spacecraft.

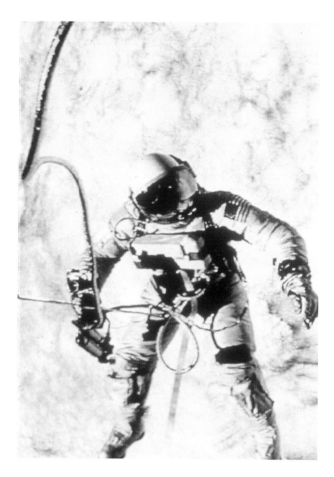

Fig. 34-2. Astronaut Edward White II performing the United States's first extravehicular activity during the Gemini IV mission, 3–7 June 1965. Photograph: Courtesy of National Aeronautics and Space Administration, Washington, DC. Photograph S65-30427.

The US Shuttle and current Russian spacecraft use an atmosphere similar to air at sea level. A simple sensing system controls inflow of nitrogen and oxygen, the former to maintain barometric pressure and the latter, the vessel's Po_2. Carbon dioxide is removed from the Shuttle with lithium hydroxide canisters, while the Russians utilize both absorption compounds and a molecular sieve system.

Initial EVA suits were air-cooled but this proved inadequate, and water-cooled suits were quickly developed to provide adequate heat transport. Current US and Russian EVA suits are constructed with multiple layers of fabric, which provide pressure retention, thermal insulation, and some degree of protection from penetration by sharp edges and micrometeoroids. A water-cooled undergarment is used to reject excess body heat to the exterior through the backpack. Suit pressure is reduced below that in the spacecraft because a higher level of inflation would make movement difficult or impossible, but pressure reduction is limited by the requirement to maintain an adequate inspired pressure of oxygen and the need to prevent decompression sickness. The current US suit, the Extravehicular Maneuvering Unit (EMU), utilizes 100% oxygen at 4.3 psi, while the Russian suit (Orlan-DMA) operates at 4.0 to 5.88 psi; the lower pressure is intended for use during periods when enhanced manual dexterity is required. The reduced pressure option is not being incorporated in the design of the next version of Russian suit (Orlan-M).[4]

EVA imposes increased physical demands on astronauts, especially of their upper extremities and hands, because the inflated suit resists movement and requires the use of awkward gloves. Heart rates were measured during the United States's first EVA mission, in 1965 on Gemini IV (see Figure 34-2). This and subsequent Skylab data showed pulse rates averaged 110 to 155, with peak rates up to 180 beats per minute.[5,6] No oxygen utilization data were obtained from those flights. Apollo lunar surface EVAs (1969–1972) were associated with an average energy consumption of 185 W (159 kcal/h). Energy levels during orbital EVAs ranged from 175 to 585 W (151–504 kcal/h) in the Apollo flights, while those of the 3 Skylab missions averaged 267 W (230 kcal/h).

Development of New Space Suits

One of the principal challenges of constructing the space station will be the necessity for routine, prolonged EVAs. The current space suits are extremely complex and require extensive maintenance on the ground between uses. In addition, the combination of reduced pressure and hard exercise during EVA dictates that astronauts spend hours "prebreathing" 100% oxygen to minimize the risk of decompression sickness (see Chapter 32, Pressure Changes and Hypoxia in Aviation). Engineers and scientists are working to develop suits that do not require prebreathing, can be repaired and refurbished aboard the spacecraft, and require only occasional major maintenance on Earth.

Spacecraft Contamination

Contamination of the spacecraft environment (by normal activity and by accident) is another problem that deserves attention. Spacecraft contamination may come from a broad range of sources, including metabolic waste products from the astronauts, off-gassing of materials, products of air and water reclamation systems, and chemicals used in onboard experiments. Unrecognized effects of contamination on astronaut performance or behavior could have catastrophic consequences, with loss of life and equipment costing billions of dollars. Because astronauts live continuously in their working environment, threshold limit values for inhaled or contacted substances aboard the spacecraft are generally far more conservative than Earth-based occupational safety limits, which assume exposures of a few hours per day. The effects of common environmental contaminants in such chronic settings are not known, and in most cases there are insufficient data on which to base recommendations. A method for determining spacecraft environmental guidelines has been developed by the National Research Council's Committee on Toxicology[7]; this monograph also contains an extensive discussion of terms, relevant compounds, and an excellent bibliography.

Physiological Adaptation to Microgravity

Concerns about the possible rigors of space travel produced an extensive (and in retrospect, perhaps excessive) screening program for early astronauts. Although the US and Soviet space programs had accomplished experimental flights with both dogs and monkeys, the absence of human data dictated extreme caution in planning the initial orbital flights. Substantial emphasis was placed on tolerance to the hypergravitational, thermal, vestibular, and psychological stresses thought to characterize spaceflight.[8] As Patricia A. Santy notes in her comprehensive description of early astronaut selection, it was difficult to develop specific astronaut screening criteria because there had been no experience with humans in space.[8] This concern for crew health and safety and its resultant batteries of medical testing did little to improve the relationship between flight medicine physicians and astronauts, but it did lead to the development of space-age telemetry. Electrocardiographic telemetry and extensive postflight medical examinations and debriefings documented only minimal physiological effects of short orbital flights and reassured program managers that longer orbital and lunar flights were medically feasible. The lack of physiological "showstoppers" contributed to the operational focus that characterized the Mercury, Gemini, and Apollo programs (1961–1972).[9–11]

Skylab, the world's first space station, followed the lunar Apollo program and provided a magnificent microgravity laboratory, with an extensive array of medical experiments examining the physiological effects of long-duration flights lasting up to 84 days in duration.[12,13] Blood, urine, and stool specimens were collected in flight, and onboard medical equipment included a multilead electrocardiograph system, an automated sphygmomanometer, an exercise bicycle, a lower-body negative pressure (LBNP) device for studying cardiovascular deconditioning, a rotating chair for vestibular experiments, an electroencephalography system, and a mass spectrometer for respiratory gas analysis. Findings from the Skylab II, III, and IV missions, which lasted 28, 59, and 84 days, respectively, became the basis for long-duration missions conducted over the next decade. Those results and data from a series of Spacelab missions, especially Spacelab Life Sciences (SLS) 1 and 2 and NeuroLab, conducted almost 2 decades later, have provided a detailed characterization of microgravity-induced physiological changes and their underlying mechanisms.

Physiological adaptation to microgravity can be characterized by three principal physical effects: a redistribution of fluids toward the head (cephalad), an unloading of the musculoskeletal system, and a dramatic alteration of somatosensory and vestibular inputs. Several major reviews have been published,[14–16] so only a brief summary will be provided here. The actual adaptive processes are complex, and the affected organ systems appear to change over different time courses. Vestibular symptoms[17] and cardiopulmonary changes appear within minutes after reaching orbit, but may stabilize after a few days or within 1 to 2 weeks, respectively, whereas changes in the musculoskeletal system may take days to weeks to become manifest and continue for months to years, if not the entire time the astronaut remains in orbit.[18]

Fluid Redistribution

On a typical US Space Shuttle flight in low-Earth orbit, the time from lift-off to orbit is approximately 8 minutes, with maximal acceleration of 3g. This acceleration is almost all +Gx in direction, although a small component of –Gz is present. (The positive and negative acceleration vectors are Gx, front to back; Gy, left side to right side; and Gz, head to foot; see Figure 33-1 in Chapter 33, Acceleration Effects on Fighter Pilots.) The change from 3g to microgravity at main-engine cutoff (MECO) is virtually instantaneous, with facial edema and engorged neck veins observable within minutes of reaching orbit. These fluid shifts last the entire flight, regardless of its duration. Leg volume, measured as early as 2 to 3 hours in space, is significantly decreased and has a downward trend. Initially, losses in leg volume are due to fluid loss from interstitial tissues, but this stabilizes after a few days. Subsequent decrease in leg volume is caused by muscle atrophy.[19–21] Surprisingly, central venous pressure (CVP) does not appear to be elevated despite the obvious clinical signs documenting major cephalad fluid shifts and increased jugular venous distention.[22–24] Cardiac chamber dimensions and ventricular function have been assessed by several investigators[22–24]:

- M-mode echocardiographic measurements made by Atkov[25] on 15 cosmonauts during 7- to 237-day flights on a series of Salyut missions demonstrated an absence of change in myocardial contractility. No consistent alterations of resting ventricular volume were noted.

- Two-dimensionally guided M-mode measurements from Shuttle astronauts, reported by Bungo and colleagues,[26] showed a decrease in ventricular volumes and a slight increase in heart rates, compared with supine, 1*g* control values. Cardiac dimensions, estimated from two-dimensional echocardiographic measurements on the SLS-1 and SLS-2 flights, showed significant increases in left atrial and left ventricular diastolic dimensions and stroke volumes when measured early in flight. This combination—of a low, near-zero CVP and increased cardiac dimensions and stroke volume—was surprising, given that these normally change in parallel. This finding, confirmed on three separate Spacelab Shuttle flights (SLS-1, SLS-2, and D-2) in four astronauts, suggests that intrapleural pressure decreased, or cardiac compliance increased, or both. Although it is theoretically possible that intrapleural pressure falls in space, there are no data to suggest that it is does. It is more likely that (1) redistribution of pulmonary blood volume away from the lungs' bases and the heart and (2) the absence of myocardial muscle and blood weight in microgravity are the basis for the paradoxically low CVP with increased left ventricular volume.

Carotid baroreflex function, assessed by measuring heart rate changes caused by mechanically altered carotid sinus transmural pressures, is depressed by spaceflight (as it also is during periods of prolonged bedrest).[27,28] The onset of change in space seems to be more rapid than is seen during the bedrest studies. It is not known how or why microgravity produces baroreflex dysfunction or the extent to which the dysfunction contributes to cardiovascular deconditioning following spaceflight.

The cephalad fluid shift that occurs with microgravity does not seem to decrease total body water, although a major redistribution of fluids within the body's various compartments does occur.[29] Plasma volume decreases approximately 17% within the first 24 hours of flight and remains approximately 10% below preflight values for at least 1 to 2 weeks on orbit (Figure 34-3). Plasma volumes measured after landing following flights of short or long duration show similar reductions, suggesting that this probably represents a stable, adapted volume state. Transient increases in plasma proteins

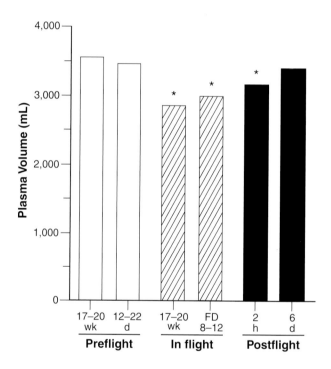

Fig. 34-3. Plasma volume was measured in six Spacelab Life Sciences 1 (SLS-1) and SLS-2 astronauts with injection of iodine 125–labeled serum albumin. Values before, during, and after flight are shown. Plasma volume is significantly reduced during flight. The decrease in plasma (and blood) volume contributes to the postflight orthostatic hypotension seen after essentially all orbital flights. Reproduced with permission from Alfrey CP, Udden MM, Leach-Huntoon CS, Driscoll T, Pickett MH. Control of red blood cell mass in space flight. *J Appl Physiol.* 1996;81:99.

*Significantly less than both preflight and 6-d postflight mean values

FD: Flight day

early in the flight probably reflect hemoconcentration, while subsequent decreases suggest increased vascular permeability with migration of plasma proteins out of the vascular compartment. The extravasated fluids seem to move into the extravascular and intracellular compartment. No diuresis occurs early in flight.

Much of the initial intravascular volume loss is probably caused by decreases due to immediate prelaunch intake restriction, along with associated nausea, vomiting, and space motion sickness. Renal function has been studied with intravenous injections of inulin and *para*-aminohippuric acid (PAH).[29] Glomerular filtration increases early in flight, while effective renal plasma flow appears to be unchanged throughout the flight. Urinary antidiuretic hormone increases early in flight but quickly normalizes. Aldosterone and plasma renin activity both decrease early in flight but normalize as the flight continues.

Spaceflight anemia was identified as a problem in the earliest days of the space program. In-flight studies published in 1975[30] and 1996[31] utilizing chromium 51–tagged red blood cells (RBCs) and iron 59 injections have provided a clear understanding of RBC production and destruction in space and have shown the anemia to be a physiological response to cephalad fluid shifts.[30,31] RBC mass in space decreases approximately 10%. The cephalad fluid shift and hemoconcentration early in flight cause an increase in central blood volume and effective increase in RBC mass sensed by the body. This increase, in turn, produces an almost immediate decrease of erythropoietin to levels associated clinically with little or no RBC production (Figure 34-4). Thus, there is a significant depression in RBC production and an inhibited maturation of newly formed RBCs prior to their release from the bone marrow. RBC production appears to normalize once a new equilibrium is established with a "normal" hematocrit associated with a significantly reduced plasma volume. The reduced RBC mass, appropriate for microgravity, persists until the astronaut returns to Earth. Subsequent gravitationally driven redistribution of blood and fluids within the various body compartments and increased fluid retention lead to hemodilution and anemia. This anemia then contributes to the orthostatic hypotension seen in astronauts after spaceflight. Erythropoietin is again stimulated and the anemia is resolved without medical intervention.

Pulmonary function on Earth is influenced, to a major extent, by gravity-dependent inequalities of ratio between ventilation and perfusion ($\dot{V}/\dot{Q}$). These $\dot{V}/\dot{Q}$ variations account for commonly observed clinical findings such as tuberculosis affecting the oxygen-rich apices of the lungs and atelectasis occurring in the relatively less-well-ventilated basal regions. Thus, microgravity would be expected to produce substantial changes in pulmonary gas exchange and spirometry. Vital capacity decreased approximately 10% in Skylab astronauts, but there was concern that Skylab's hyperoxic, hypobaric atmosphere could have caused this change.[32] More extensive studies subsequently confirmed these early observations and extended the range of tests performed.[33] Expiratory flow rates also decrease approximately 10% in the first week of flight but seem to normalize after that. Diffusing capacity, as estimated by uptake of carbon monoxide, increases approximately 28% (Figure 34-5).[34] Although the in-

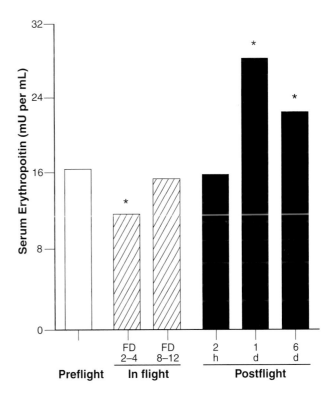

Fig. 34-4. Serum erythropoietin levels were measured in six Spacelab Life Sciences 1 (SLS-1) and SLS-2 astronauts. The initial decrease in plasma volume is associated with a transient hemoconcentration, which leads to depressed serum erythropoietin levels. Values rebound briskly as intravascular volume is restored after the flight to preflight levels. Reproduced with permission from Alfrey CP, Udden MM, Leach-Huntoon CS, Driscoll T, Pickett MH. Control of red blood cell mass in space flight. *J Appl Physiol.* 1996;81:101.
*Significantly different from preflight mean
FD: Flight day

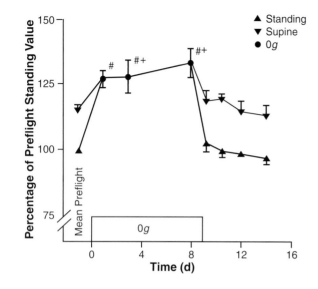

Fig. 34-5. The diffusing capacity of lung for carbon monoxide (D$_{LCO}$), a simple test of alveolar–capillary lung function, was measured before, during, and after spaceflight. The in-flight values were significantly higher than those measured either standing or supine in 1*g*. Changes in pulmonary capillary blood volume were not sufficient to explain such a large increase in D$_{LCO}$. The investigators postulated that a substantial increase in alveolar–capillary surface area occurs in space. Reproduced with permission from Prisk GK, Guy HJB, Elliott AR, Deutschman RA III, West JB. Pulmonary diffusing capacity, capillary blood volume and cardiac output during sustained microgravity. *J Appl Physiol.* 1993;75:19.
#:Significant difference (*P* < .05) between preflight standing average and average data from individual days in-flight and standing postflight
+:Significant difference (*P* < .05) between preflight supine average and average data from individual days in-flight and supine postflight.

crease in diffusion capacity correlates significantly with an increase in pulmonary capillary blood volume, the change is not sufficient to explain the improved gas exchange as measured by the diffusing capacity of lung for carbon monoxide (D$_{LCO}$). It appears that a substantially larger effective capillary surface area is available in microgravity because more capillaries are perfused in the absence of gravity gradients in the pulmonary arterial circulation (Figure 34-6). It was expected that microgravity would eliminate all $\dot{V}/\dot{Q}$ inequalities, but tracings of expired carbon dioxide concentrations continue to demonstrate evidence of inhomogeneities within lung, even in the absence of gravity.[35] Studies comparing the pulmonary distribution of inhaled helium and sulfur hexafluoride also documented the persistence of what were previously thought to be

gravity-dependent inhomogeneities in pulmonary ventilation.[36] These pulmonary function data from space demonstrate that a component of the $\dot{V}/\dot{Q}$ mismatch always seen on Earth is anatomically determined and+ not solely due to gravity. Airway closing volumes were not altered by microgravity, although residual volume decreased almost 18%.[37] Table 34-1 provides a summary of microgravity-induced changes in lung function.

Vestibular Inputs and the Space Adaptation Syndrome

Because of extensive linkages between gravity and otolith stimulation, significant alterations in vestibular function during and after spaceflight could be expected (see Chapter 35, Motion Sickness). Neurovestibular symptoms are most notable in the first few days of flight. These symptoms are called the space adaptation syndrome (SAS) and are clinically similar but not identical to ordinary motion sickness. Extensive in-flight testing was first conducted on the Skylab missions.[38] These investigators utilized a rotating chair and programmed head movements during rotation to test the Skylab astronauts' susceptibility to motion sickness following their adaptation to microgravity. A remarkable decrease in sensitivity was documented both inflight and immediately after the flight. The investigators also noted that the greater freedom of movement possible in the spacious workshop of the Skylab was more likely to produce vestibular symptoms than had been seen in earlier flights in more confined spacecraft, and they suggested that prevention of symptoms would require both drugs and adaptive training.

Further testing in cosmonauts and astronauts from Salyut, Mir, and Shuttle missions has documented major changes in otolith function and oculovestibular responses.[39–43] It appears that astronauts in space initially increase their dependence on visual and tactile stimuli. As the flight continues, however, they appear to "internalize" the reference system for determining up–down orientation and decrease their dependence on visual cues. There also appears to be significant reinterpretation of linear acceleration–induced otolithic input in the absence of the otoliths receiving head-tilt stimuli in space.[44] However, the character, magnitude, and time course of postflight perceptual responses are not fully consistent with the "central otolith reinterpretation" theory. Other mechanisms, such as central and peripheral nervous system changes, probably play a significant role as well.

SAS remains a problem in human spaceflight.[17]

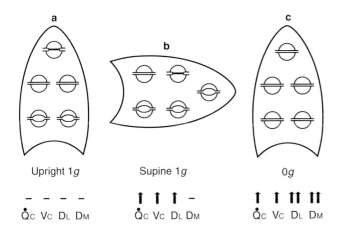

Fig. 34-6. A simple cartoon showing human alveolar–capillary relationships in (**a**) upright ($1g$) and (**b**) supine ($1g$) positions on Earth and (**c**) in microgravity ($0g$). On Earth, hydrostatic gradients alter pulmonary perfusion, and the superior regions of the lung in standing and supine subjects are relatively underperfused, as represented by the collapsed capillaries. In microgravity, all capillaries are well perfused and the effective capillary–alveolar surface area is greatly increased, leading to an augmented diffusing capacity of the lung. Pulmonary capillary blood flow ($\dot{Q}c$), pulmonary capillary blood volume (Vc), lung diffusing capacity (DL), and alveolar membrane diffusing capacity (DM) are reflected by the arrows showing relative changes (bars represent no change) in each experimental condition. Reproduced with permission from Prisk GK, Guy HJB, Elliott AR, Deutschman RA III, and West JB. Pulmonary diffusing capacity, capillary blood volume and cardiac output during sustained microgravity. *J Appl Physiol.* 1993;75:24.

A majority of astronauts experience symptoms that may include nausea, malaise, anorexia, and headaches in the first hours of spaceflight. About three

TABLE 34-1

CHANGES IN PULMONARY FUNCTION IN SPACE

Physiological Responses to Microgravity	No. of Subjects	Changes in Microgravity (In-Flight vs Preflight Standing Measurements)
Pulmonary Blood Flow		
Total pulmonary blood flow (cardiac output)	4	18% increase
Cardiac stroke volume	4	4% increase
Diffusing capacity (carbon monoxide)	4	28% increase
Pulmonary capillary blood volume	4	28% increase
Diffusing capacity of alveolar membrane	4	27% increase
Pulmonary blood flow distribution	7	More uniform but some inequality remained
Pulmonary Ventilation		
Respiration frequency	8	9% increase
Tidal volume	8	15% decrease
Alveolar ventilation	8	Unchanged
Total ventilation	8	Small decrease
Ventilatory distribution	7	More uniform but some inequality remained
Maximal peak expiratory flow rate	7	Decreased by 12.5% early in flight but then returned to normal
Pulmonary Gas Exchange		
O_2 uptake	8	Unchanged
CO_2 output	8	Unchanged
End-tidal P_{O_2}	8	Unchanged
End-tidal P_{O_2}	8	Small increase when $[CO_2]$ in spacecraft increased
Lung Volumes		
Functional residual capacity	4	15% decrease
Residual volume	4	18% decrease
Closing volume	7	Unchanged as measured by argon bolus

Adapted with permission from West JB, Elliott AR, Guy HJ, Prisk GK. Pulmonary function in space. *JAMA.* 1997;277(24):1959.

fourths will experience mild symptoms, whereas one fourth will experience more-severe symptoms, such as one or more episodes of vomiting, especially in the first day of flight. The symptoms generally subside within the first 24 to 72 hours on orbit, but they can be prolonged. Efforts to predict which astronauts will be affected by SAS have not succeeded. Age, gender, aerobic fitness level, prior aviation experience, and response to multiaxis, ground-based trainers (human centrifuges) are not accurate predictors.[45]

The etiology of SAS is not known, but the main theories are "sensory conflicts" and "fluid shifts." The former hypothesis states that discordant signals arising from visual, proprioceptive, and otolithic inputs produce the syndrome; the latter states that increased cerebral and otolithic perfusion and fluid content (ie, edema) cause the syndrome. Analogues such as "simulator" motion sickness show that neurovestibular sensory conflicts can produce symptoms similar to SAS. Direct evidence of cerebral edema in spaceflight is lacking, but intraocular pressures rise significantly in microgravity.[46] Also, many of the features of SAS, including headache, fatigue, nausea and vomiting, malaise, and slowed cognition, are consistent with the symptoms of cerebral edema. Our own unpublished transcranial doppler studies also lend support to changes in the intracerebral circulation. Neither hypothesis excludes the other and both mechanisms may play a role.

Treatment for SAS has been difficult, but since 1989, intramuscular promethazine has been the drug of choice in the Shuttle program.[47] Sedation on orbit has not been a problem despite intramuscular doses of 25 to 50 mg promethazine, and the drug has provided better relief than any previously tested drugs, including oral promethazine, scopolamine, dextroamphetamine, methylphenidate, and metochlopramide. Treatment with promethazine has minimized the operational impact of SAS. Testing on short parabolic flights suggests that astemizole will not be effective.[48] Potent, nonsedating, newer drugs such as ondansetron or granisetron have not yet been tested in spaceflight.

Musculoskeletal Unloading

Musculoskeletal changes are relatively minor during short-duration flights, but they represent a major challenge for missions of longer duration. Data from the National Aeronautics and Space Administration's (NASA's) Skylab flights suggest significant losses of bone and muscle mass despite aggressive exercise countermeasures.[49,50] Additional evidence of major decrements in both bone and muscle mass from the weight-bearing structures during long-duration MIR missions was published in 1996.[51] These data, gathered as part of a joint US–Russian study using computed tomography and and dual-energy X ray absorbancy (DEXA) scans, show continued tissue losses as the mission duration increases. No asymptote was reached for missions as long as 14.4 months (Table 34-2). These changes occurred despite extensive in-flight exercise programs of 1 to 2 hours daily, utilizing powered and unpowered treadmill and bicycle ergometers. Current exercise programs will probably not be sufficient to prevent significant, progressive bone loss during interplanetary travel. It remains to be determined whether high impact or pharmacological interventions or different exercise programs, including those focusing more on resistive than aerobic exercise, will suffice on future, long-duration missions.

Space Radiation

Radiation exposure for astronauts was reviewed by the National Academy of Sciences in 1993,[52] 1996,[53] and 1998.[54] These works provide in-depth discussion and extensive references, so only a brief overview will be provided here. Space radiation comes from three principal sources: galactic cosmic rays (approximately 87% protons, 12% helium ions, and 1% heavy ions)[55]; protons trapped in Earth's magnetosphere; and solar particle events (which are also composed of protons, but of much greater fluence than is found in galactic cosmic radiation).[56] Exposure in low-Earth orbit depends on orbital altitude, the magnitude and direction of Earth's magnetic field, solar flare activity, and shielding provided by the spacecraft. Substantial variation exists for each of these factors. Peaks in solar flare activity may occur at any time, but tend to follow approximately 11-year cycles. Increased solar flare activity can raise spacecraft radiation over 10-fold within a few hours. The most recent *solar maximum* occurred in the year 2000. Conversely, higher-energy particles increase during *solar minima*.

The physics of shielding is extremely complex and must take into account the types of incident radiation as well as the type and density of material of the shield. Gamma ray and proton shielding are relatively well understood and account for almost 2-fold changes in dosage at different locations in the International Space Station (ISS). High-energy particles, which are commonly found in interplanetary travel, remain highly problematic. Collisions of these high-energy particles with cells in the retina are responsible for the bright flashes (Cherenkov flashes) first reported by early astronauts and cosmonauts.[57] These particles also easily pass through traditional shield-

TABLE 34-2

MIR SPACE STATION: CHANGES* IN BONE MINERAL DENSITY AND LEAN BODY MASS

Body Region	Crew Members Studied	Mean	SD
Bone Mass Density			
Spine	18	−1.07[†]	0.63
Neck	18	−1.16[†]	0.85
Trochanter	18	−1.58[†]	0.98
Total	17	−0.35[†]	0.25
Pelvis	17	−1.35[†]	0.54
Arm	17	−0.04[†]	0.88
Leg	16	−0.34[†]	0.33
Lean Mass			
Leg	16	−1.00[†]	0.73
Arm	17	0.00	0.77
Total Lean	17	−0.57[†]	0.62
Total Fat	17	1.79	4.66

*Percentage per month, compared with baseline (preflight) measurements
[†]$P < .01$
SD: standard deviation
Adapted with permission from LeBlanc A, Schneider V, Shackelford L, et al. Bone mineral and lean tissue loss after long duration spaceflight [abstract]. *J Bone Miner Res.* 1996;11(suppl 1):S323.

ing materials such as aluminum and lead, producing a large range of secondary fragments including other nuclei, heavy fragments, and both protons and neutrons. In that setting, both primary and secondary radiation effects are important but poorly understood. The relative biological effects for such high-energy particles may be as much as 40-fold greater than for protons. The differential effects of acute versus chronic exposure and possible interactions of radiation with microgravity itself are likewise poorly understood.

Some evidence for spaceflight-induced chromosomal and cellular damage in humans has been reported.[58] The frequency of cellular changes is used to calculate bio-doses and seems to be in general agreement with other dosimetry methods. White blood cells from seven MIR cosmonauts were cultured after their flights. The X-ray equivalent dose was found to be below the cytogenetic detection level of 20 mGy in samples studied after flights of 2 to 3 weeks. After flights of 6 months' duration, the biological dose varied greatly among the cosmonauts, from 95 to 455 mGy equivalent dose (1 Gy ≈ 100 rad).

Spaceflight radiation dosage standards have been recommended, but the associated uncertainties are large.[59–61] The new recommendations for career dose limits, based on lifetime excess risk of cancer mortality, take into account age at first exposure and gender. The career limits range from 1.0 Sv (100 roentgen equivalents for man [rem]) for a 24-year-old woman to 4.0 Sv (400 rem) for a 55-year-old man, compared with the previous single limit of 4.0 Sv (400 rem). To decrease cataractogenesis, the career limit for the lens of the eye has been reduced from 6.0 Sv (600 rem) to 4.0 Sv (400 rem). Most astronauts can complete their careers without exceeding these recommended occupational exposure limits, but longer-duration flights and interplanetary travel will likely produce excessive exposures and could lead to fatalities if adequate shielding and effective radioprotectants are not developed. This remains an important area for aerospace medical research.

RETURN TO GRAVITY

Although it is generally agreed that physiological adaptation to microgravity is rapid and effective for full function in space, readaptation to Earth's gravity on return from space remains problematic and of major operational significance. The major problems associated with re-entry following orbital flights of up to 14 months are muscle weakness, vestibular disturbances, and orthostatic hypotension. A variety of

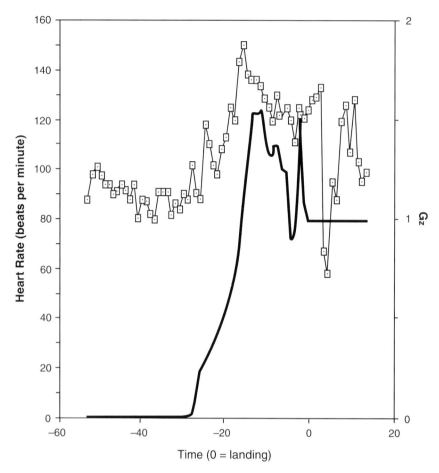

Fig. 34-7. An astronaut's heart rate (—☐—), measured via continuous electrocardiographic recording, and accelera-tion (Gz; ▬) are shown for a typical Shuttle re-entry period. A significant tachycardia is observed. Vasovagal episodes occurred just before, and more prominently, just after landing (time 0 = landing). Re-entry is characterized by hypovolemia, depressed baroreflexes, vestibular disturbances, and a significant heat load associated with both the launch-and-entry suits and a warm (35°C–36°C) cabin temperature. Reproduced with permission from Buckey JC Jr, Lane LD, Levine BD, et al. Orthostatic intolerance after space flight. *J Appl Physiol.* 1996;81:16.

visual and vestibular disturbances have been reported by returning astronauts and documented with de-tailed postflight testing.[62,63]

Bone and muscle wasting in-flight have already been described. Although there have been no post-flight fractures associated with loss of bone mass in humans, substantial muscle weakness and incoordi-nation have been noted. It is likely that this results from simple muscle atrophy as well as neuromuscu-lar changes postflight. Skylab leg volume data showed rapid reconstitution, from 10% below preflight vol-ume to approximately 5% below within 5 days of land-ing; but by 10 days after the flight, however, volumes were still below preflight levels.[50(p195)]

The absence of biopsy data precludes determina-tion of the time course and extent of recovery of bone mass. Also, it is completely unknown whether nor-malized bone and muscle mass also indicates normal

structure. Differences in trabecular structure and myo-neural junction numbers could persist despite normal-ized masses of bone and muscle.

Decreased orthostatic tolerance is a universal find-ing in astronauts exposed to microgravity for longer than a few days, although its magnitude has consid-erable interindividual variation. Skylab crews under-went serial orthostatic challenges with LBNP and showed decreased tolerance within 4 to 6 days on or-bit.[64] The greatest decrements were during the first 3 weeks of flight, with stability at a reduced level reached by 5 to 7 weeks in-flight. In-flight tolerance to LBNP seemed to be predictive of postflight toler-ance as well. More-recent data from the Spacelab Life Sciences missions show that after landing, almost two thirds of astronauts experience clinically significant orthostatic intolerance with 5 to 10 minutes of quiet standing.[65] Excessive lower extremity venous pooling does not appear to play a role, although excessive pooling in the abdomen and pelvis could be present. As noted previously, spaceflight produces hypovolemia, anemia, and baroreflex dysfunction, which contribute to significant orthostatic intolerance during re-entry and after landing (Figure 34-7). Extensive hemodynamic measurements during postflight orthostatic stress document a failure to increase total peripheral resistance appropriately. It is unknown whether this inadequate vasoconstriction is related to impaired baroreflex function, defective end-organ responsiveness, or both.

Aerobic exercise capacity appears to be well preserved in-flight, but there is a substantial decrease when it is measured immediately after the flight.[66–68] Elements of both muscle atrophy and poor neuromuscular coordination are undoubtedly present in this postflight deconditioning, but the main disability seems to stem from the cardiovascular dysfunction. Maximal heart rate is maintained, but stroke volume is reduced by almost 23%. Recovery is relatively rapid but varies with the length of the time on orbit.

Attempts to correct in-flight hypovolemia with saline ingestion immediately prior to re-entry have had limited success.[69] Despite careful hemodynamic measurements, no difference was found between those who did and those who did not undergo saline fluid loading prior to re-entry. The Russian space program uses in-flight LBNP and a high-salt diet prior to re-entry to retrain baroreflexes and volume load, but conclusive proof of efficacy in ameliorating orthostatic hypotension is lacking. A few attempts to use fludrocortisone to enhance volume replacement have likewise proven ineffective. The main countermeasure against orthostatic intolerance remains an abdominal or a lower-extremity pressure garment, or both. US astronauts use an anti-G suit (paradoxically, modified from the standard US Air Force G-suit) as part of the standard launch and entry suit (LES), and Russian cosmonauts utilize tight leg wrappings (called *Karkas)* to prevent lower-extremity venous pooling.

FUTURE MILITARY SPACE MISSIONS AND INTERPLANETARY EXPLORATION

At the present time, there is no official military role for humans in space, and most of the Department of Defense–supported Shuttle flights in the 1980s were for the launching of unmanned spacecraft. However, with improved launch capability, we can envision a number of types of future crewed missions that currently do not exist, the most obvious of which is reconnaissance. Both US and Russian flight experiments have examined observational abilities of humans in space, and claims have been made regarding abilities to detect subtle contrast changes over land and, perhaps even more so, over water.[70] Claims have also been made that the dynamic range of human vision and the ability to process unexpected information provide a significant advantage over the limited sensing spectra of many satellite systems, as was demonstrated during the Skylab missions. However, the broad geographical range of threat areas and the difficulties associated with keeping humans in the desired orbits appear to limit this application's military value. Most experts believe that for routine, anticipated, observation conditions, available technical means of data gathering offer adequate resolution at far less cost than human observation flights. In-flight repair of expensive sensing devices has already required human involvement, and the increasing costs and complexity of spacecraft make future repair missions likely. Current launch costs and the Shuttle's range, which is limited to low, equatorial Earth orbit, make repair by humans of most space systems—those in geostationary or polar orbits—impossible. However, newer launch systems and enormously expensive satellites could easily change the cost–benefit ratio in favor of more human repair missions, as has been done twice for the Hubble Space Telescope.

Development of an operational aerospace plane with appropriate lift vehicles would make short-notice "pop-up" (short-term, low-Earth-orbital) missions possible.[71] Crewed, transatmospheric vehicle flights could include emergency repairs of militarily important space assets, highly specialized reconnaissance missions, or even "insertion" flights that transport personnel to any spot on Earth within an hour or so. Rapid, relatively low-cost launch capability would almost certainly lead to a military role for humans in space but would simultaneously create significant physiological problems. The severe cardiovascular deconditioning associated with spaceflight would prevent the on-orbit stationing of specialists who could be returned to desired locations on Earth on short notice and be expected to function soon after landing. Likewise, brief orbital or suborbital pop-up missions might be complicated by vestibular symptoms associated with SAS. Our current knowledge of countermeasures for these basic problems remains suboptimal. Unless effective interventions are developed, future mission planners will continue to be limited in their ability to fully utilize the first few hours on orbit or on return to Earth immediately following spaceflight.

Spaceflights of long duration will be necessary if humans are to explore other planets. By the end of 1996, there had been 190 successful spaceflights (and 3 failed attempts) with 221 US astronauts, 83 Soviet or Russian cosmonauts, and 48 fliers from other countries.[72] Thirty-one of the 352 were women. The total days in space for humans was slightly over 17,000; Valery Polyakov, a Russian physician-cosmonaut holds the records for the longest flight, 437 days, as well as the most days in space, 678. These milestones will easily be surpassed when the ISS, now under construction, is used in part for systematic investigation of the biomedical challenges of exploration-class missions such as a proposed expedition to Mars, which might involve 6 to 12 months in transit each way and a stay of 1 to 2 years on the Red Planet. Such a voyage raises critical questions regarding human health and medical care in prolonged spaceflight and on return to planetary gravity. NASA's National Space Biomedical Research Institute (NSBRI) is charged with developing countermeasures against the deleterious effects of spaceflight, including problems observed in orbit and new difficulties associated with the remote, isolated conditions of an exploration-class mission. Validating the countermeasures is a formidable task, since even ISS will provide scientists with access to only limited numbers of subjects exposed to 0g for months rather than years.

Related issues include the willingness of astronauts to volunteer as subjects of medical studies and difficulties with protocol compliance in a remote operational setting. On the positive side, some of the research may find application to problems on Earth, including medical screening, training techniques, telemedicine, and rehabilitation. NSBRI has articulated 10 investigative themes, briefly summarized here[73]:

1. *Cardiovascular Alterations*
   Although spaceflight of any duration is known to produce orthostatic intolerance, neurovestibular readaptation-related problems, and an altered response to physical exertion, prolonged residence in 0g may lead to reduction of cardiac mass, increased susceptibility to arrhythmias, and possible unmasking of previously asymptomatic cardiovascular disease. Areas of investigation include identification and characterization of operationally significant medical problems as well as development of techniques for preflight screening, noninvasive onboard monitoring, and rehabilitation after landing.

2. *Muscle Changes*
   The muscle atrophy associated with spaceflight is viewed as a major threat to an exploration-class mission because the crew may be unable to deal with an emergency requiring muscular strength and may be prone to exertional muscle injury. Research will address mechanisms of muscle atrophy, response to muscle loading, and neuromuscular changes in 0g.

3. *Nutrition, Physical Fitness, and Rehabilitation*
   Astronauts in orbit lose muscle mass and strength, show significantly reduced aerobic capacity, and eat less than they do on Earth. Research in this area seeks an integrated approach to minimizing these changes during space missions and techniques for rehabilitation on return to Earth.

4. *Neurovestibular Adaptation*
   Research during the Shuttle era focused on problems associated with arrival in orbit due to changes in otolith function and the vestibulo-ocular reflex, as well as prediction of space sickness. Expedition-oriented research turns toward methods of preadaptation, improved drug countermeasures, the use of artificial gravity, and especially neurovestibular impairment and rehabilitation on return to a 1g field.

5. *Hematology, Immunology, and Infective Processes*
   In addition to the self-limited 10% reduction in plasma volume and RBC mass known to develop in orbit, interplanetary crews may be predisposed to secondary immunodeficiency due to a combination of stress, isolation, microbial contamination, nutritional deficit, and radiation exposure. Scientists seek to develop countermeasures for possible altered immune response, viral reactivation, and radiation-induced microbial mutation in flight.

6. *Bone Loss*
   Because bone loss in 0g progresses at a rate

of 1% to 2% per month indefinitely, astronauts could return from Mars with a 20% deficit. Major concerns include progressive osteoporosis and the associated problems of increased fracture risk and delayed bone healing, soft-tissue injury, and renal calculus formation. Research goals include screening out candidates at increased risk and optimizing environmental, nutritional, and hormonal conditions to minimize loss. Furthermore, astronauts must be given some assurance that recovery will occur following their retmastonurn to Earth.

7. *Radiation Effects*
Astronauts en route to Mars risk clinically significant exposure to radiation from galactic cosmic rays and high-energy solar particle showers. These types of radiation have not posed a major problem in low Earth orbit, and their bioeffects are not well understood. Studies with animals indicate that disruption of the function of the central nervous system is a possibility; other concerns are accumulating cellular pathology and carcinogenesis. Research in this area includes improved prediction of space radiation effects on human health, identification of appropriate biomarkers, and provision of effective shielding and pharmacological countermeasures.

8. *Human Performance, Sleep, and Chronobiology*
Crews in orbit have experienced chronic sleep disturbances due to stress and the artificial environment in which they live. Research focuses on methods of minimizing these effects as well as techniques for monitoring sleep and performance.

9. *Neurobehavioral and Psychosocial Factors*
Crew composition, leadership style, and communication with Earth posed significant difficulties aboard Russia's Mir space station but are only now receiving serious research attention. The prolonged isolation and close confinement of a mission to Mars will place extreme stress on individual function and group effectiveness; breakdown at either level could threaten crew performance and productivity and the safety of the mission. Research areas include crew selection, preflight training, and support mechanisms in flight.

10. *In-Flight Medical Care*
Medical emergencies and traumatic injury to crew members are real possibilities in the course of a long mission that offers no possibility of medical evacuation. Although the crew will likely include a physician, he or she cannot be expected to provide specialist knowledge in all areas. NSBRI is therefore investigating "smart medical systems," such as

- onboard computer systems for monitoring the crew, diagnosing problems, and assisting with surgical procedures, and
- communications systems designed to work within the effects of bandwidth limitations and the delay of up to 40 minutes between transmission of information from the spacecraft and the receipt of answers from Earth.

Many of the problems described by NSBRI relate to the absence of gravitational stress during spaceflight; experience aboard Russia's Mir space station shows that even vigorous exercise programs fail to prevent debility. Although artificial gravity on the scale seen in the motion picture *2001: A Space Odyssey*,[74] is unlikely to be provided by spacecraft in deep space, a more realistic possibility is development of a short-arm centrifuge combined with a cycle or other exercise device that would provide a Gz acceleration gradient sufficient to maintain at least partial adaptation to gravity. Such a device could be tested aboard the space station to optimize required workout schedules.

SUMMARY

Despite the relatively small number of flight opportunities, much has been learned about living and working in space. The knowledge gained has contributed to improved safety and performance on space missions and to a better understanding of human physiology on Earth. However, much work remains for the aeromedical military physicians of the future. We hope that readers will find aerospace physiology and medicine exciting and challenging as they provide support for flyers in this most unusual operational environment.

REFERENCES

1. Armstrong HG, Haber H, Strughold H. Aeromedical problems of space travel. *Journal of Aviation Medicine.* 1949;20:383–417.

2. Ley W. *Rockets and Space Travel.* New York, NY: Viking Press; 1949.

3. Waligora J, Sauer R, Bredt J. Spacecraft life support systems. In: Nicogossian A, Huntoon C, Pool S, eds. *Space Physiology and Medicine.* 2nd ed. Philadelphia, Pa: Lea & Febinger; 1989: 104–120.

4. Helmke C. *Advances in Soviet Extravehicular Activity (EVA) Suit Technology.* Washington, DC: Air Force Foreign Technology Division Bulletin. FTD-2660P-127/38-90; 16 Feb 1990.

5. Kelly GF, Coons DO, Carpentier WR. Medical aspects of Gemini extravehicular activities. *Aerospace Medicine.* 1968;39:611–615.

6. Waligora JM, Horrigan DJ Jr. Metabolic cost of extravehicular activities. In: Johnston RS, Dietlein F, eds. *Biomedical Results From Skylab.* Washington, DC: National Aeronautics and Space Administration; 1977: 395–399. NASA SP-377.

7. National Academy Press. *Guidelines for Developing Spacecraft Maximum Allowable Concentrations for Space Station Contaminants.* Washington, DC: National Academy Press; 1992.

8. Santy PA. *Choosing the Right Stuff: The Psychological Selection of Astronauts and Cosmonauts.* Westport, Conn: Praeger Press; 1994.

9. National Aeronautics and Space Administration. *Biomedical Results of Apollo.* Washington, DC: US Government Printing Office; 1975. NASA SP-368.

10. Berry CA. Medical legacy of Apollo. *Journal of Aviation Medicine.* 1974;45:1046–1057.

11. National Aeronautics and Space Administration. *The Apollo-Soyuz Test Project Medical Report.* Springfield, Va: National Technical Information Service; 1977. NASA SP-411.

12. Johnston RS, Dietlein F, eds. *Biomedical Results From Skylab.* Washington, DC: US Government Printing Office; 1977. NASA SP-377.

13. Berry CA. Medical legacy of Skylab as of May 9, 1974: The manned Skylab missions. *Aviat Space Environ Med.* 1976,47:418–424.

14. Hinghoffer-Szalkay HC. Physiology of cardiovascular, respiratory, interstitial, endocrine, immune, and muscular systems. In: Moore D, Bie P, Oser H, eds. *Biological and Medical Research in Space.* Berlin, Germany: Springer-Verlag; 1996: 107–153.

15. Blomqvist CG, Stone HL. Cardiovascular adjustments to gravitational stress. In: Shepard JT, Abboud FM, eds. *The Cardiovascular System.* Section 2, Vol 3. In: American Physiological Society. *Handbook of Physiology.* Bethesda Md: APS; 1983: 1025–1063.

16. Watenpaugh DE, Hargens AR. The cardiovascular system in microgravity. In: Fregly MJ, Blatteis CM, eds. *Environmental Physiology.* Section 4, Vol 1. In: American Physiological Society. *Handbook of Physiology.* New York, NY: Oxford University Press for APS; 1995: 631–674.

17. Davis JR, Vanderploeg JM, Santy PA, Jennings RT, Stewart DF. Space motion sickness during 24 flights of the Space Shuttle. *Aviat Space Environ Med.* 1988,59(12):1185–1189.

18. Vogel JM, Whittle MW, Smith MC Jr, Rambaut PC. Bone mineral measurement—Experiment M078. In: Johnson RS, Dietlein LF, Berry CA, eds. *Biomedical Results of Apollo.* Washington DC: National Aeronautics and Space Administration; 1975: 183–190. NASA SP368.

19. Thorton WE, Moore TP, Pool SL. Fluid shifts in weightlessness. *Aviat Space Environ Med.* 1987;58(suppl 9):A86–A90.

20. Moore TP, Thornton WE. Space Shuttle inflight and postflight fluid shifts measured by leg volume changes. *Aviat Space Environ Med.* 1987;58:A91–A96.

21. Watenpaugh DE, Buckey JC Jr, Lane LD, et al. Human leg blood flow and compliance during space flight [abstract]. *Bulletin of the American Society of Gravitational and Space Biology.* 1992;6:35.

22. Buckey JC Jr, Gaffney FA, Lane LD, Levine BD, Watenpaugh DE, Blomqvist CG. Central venous pressure in space. *N Engl J Med.* 1993;329:1853–1854.

23. Buckey JC Jr, Gaffney FA, Lane LD, et al. Central venous pressure in space. *J Appl Physiol.* 1996;81:19–25.

24. Foldager N, Andersen TAE, Jessen FB, et al. Central venous pressure during weightlessness in humans. In: Sahm PR, Keller MH, Schiewe B, eds. *Symposium on Scientific Results of the German Spacelab Mission D-2.* Norderney, Germany; 1994: 695–696.

25. Atkov OYu, Bednenko VS, Fomina GA. Ultrasound techniques in space medicine. *Aviat Space Environ Med.* 1987;58(9 pt 2):A69–A73.

26. Bungo MW, Goldwater DJ, Popp RL, Sandler H. Echocardiographic evaluation of Space Shuttle crew members. *J Appl Physiol.* 1987;62:278–283.

27. Eckberg DL, Fritsch JM. Influence of ten-day head-down bedrest on human carotid baroreceptor-cardiac reflex function. *Acta Physiol Scand.* 1992;144(suppl 604):69–76.

28. Fritsch-Yelle JM, Charles JB, Jones MM, Beightol LL, Eckberg DL. Space flight alters autonomic regulation of arterial pressure in humans. *J Appl Physiol.* 1994;77:1776–1783.

29. Leach CS, Alfrey CP, Suki WN, et al. Regulation of body fluid compartments during short-term space flight. *J Appl Physiol.* 1996;81:105–116.

30. Kimzey SL, Fischer CL, Johnson PC, Ritzmann SI, Mengel CE. Hematology and immunology studies. In: Johnson RS, Dietlein RS, Berry CA, eds. *Biomedical Results of Apollo.* Washington DC: National Aeronautics and Space Administration; 1975: 197–226. NASA SP368.

31. Alfrey CP, Udden MM, Leach-Huntoon CS, Driscoll T, Pickett MH. Control of red blood cell mass in space flight. *J Appl Physiol.* 1996;81:98–104.

32. Sawin CF, Nicogossian AE, Schachter AP, Rummel JA, Michel EL. Pulmonary function evaluation during and following Skylab Space Flights. In: Johnston, RS and Dietlein LF, eds. *Biomedical Results From Skylab.* Washington DC: National Aeronautics and Space Administration; 1977: 388–394. NASA SP-377.

33. West JB, Elliott AR, Guy HJ, Prisk GK. Pulmonary function in space. *JAMA.* 1997;277(24):1957–1961.

34. Prisk GK, Guy HJB, Elliott AR, Deutschman RA III, West JB. Pulmonary diffusing capacity, capillary blood volume and cardiac output during sustained microgravity. *J Appl Physiol.* 1993;75:15–26.

35. Guy HJB, Prisk GK, Elliott AR, Deutschman RA III, West JB. Inhomogeneity of pulmonary ventilation during sustained microgravity as determined by single-breath washouts. *J Appl Physiol.* 1994;76:1719–1729.

36. Prisk GK, Lauzon AM, Verbanck S, et al. Anomalous behavior of helium and sulfur hexafluoride during single-breath tests in sustained microgravity. *J Appl Physiol.* 1996;80:1126–1132.

37. Elliott AR, Prisk GK, Guy HJ, West JB. Lung volumes during sustained microgravity on Spacelab SLS-1. *J Appl Physiol.* 1994;77:2005–2014.

38. Grabiel A, Miller EF II, Homick JL. Experiment M131: Human vestibular function. In: Johnston, RS, Dietlein LF, eds. *Biomedical Results From Skylab.* Washington DC: National Aeronautics and Space Administration; 1977: 74–91. NASA SP-377.

39. Koslovskaya IB, Barmin VA, Keridich YV, Repin AA. The effects of real and simulated microgravity on vestibulo-oculomotor integration. *Physiologist.* 1985;28:S51–S56.

40. Young LR, Shelhamer M, Modestino S. MIT/Canadian vestibular experiments on the Spacelab-1 mission, II: Visual vestibular tilt interaction in weightlessness. *Exp Brain Res.* 1986;64:299–307.

41. Young LR, Shelhamer M. Microgravity enhances the relative contribution of visually-induced motion sensation. *Aviat Space Environ Med.* 1990;61:525–530.

42. Young LR, Mendoza JC, Groleau N, Wojcik PW. Tactile influences on astronaut visual spatial orientation: Human neurovestibular studies on SLS-2. *J Appl Physiol.* 1996;81:44–49.

43. Young LR, Oman CM, Watt GD, Money GD, Lichtenberg BK. Spatial orientation in weightlessness and readaptation to Earth's gravity. *Science.* 1984;225:205–208.

44. Parker DE, Reschke MF, Arrott AP, Homick JL, Lichtenberg BK. Otolith tilt-translation reinterpretation following prolonged weightlessness: Implications for pre-flight training. *Aviat Space Environ Med.* 1985;56:601–606.

45. Jennings RT, Davis JR, Santy PA. Comparison of aerobic fitness and space motion sickness during the Shuttle program. *Aviat Space Environ Med.* 1988;59:448–451.

46. Draeger J, Schwartz R, Stern C, Groenhoff S, Hechler B. Intraocular pressure in microgravity: Automatic self-tonometry during Spacelab mission D-2. In: Sahm PR, Keller MH, Schiewe B, eds. *Symposium on Scientific Results of the German Spacelab Mission D-2.* Norderney, Germany; 1994: 691–694.

47. Davis JR, Jennings RT, Beck BG, Bagian JP. Treatment efficacy of intramuscular promethazine for space motion sickness. *Aviat Space Environ Med.* 1993;64:230–233.

48. Kohl RL, Homick JL, Cintron N, Calkins DS. Lack of effects of astemizole on vestibular ocular reflex, motion sickness, and cognitive performance in man. *Aviat Space Environ Med.* 1987;58:1171–1174.

49. Smith MC Jr, Rambaut PC, Vogel JM, Whittle MW. Bone mineral measurement—Experiment M078. In: Johnston, RS, Dietlein LF, eds. *Biomedical Results From Skylab.* Washington DC: National Aeronautics and Space Administration; 1977: 183–190. NASA SP-377.

50. Thornton WE, Rummel JA. Muscular deconditioning and its prevention in space flight. In: Johnston, RS, Dietlein LF, eds. *Biomedical Results From Skylab.* Washington DC: National Aeronautics and Space Administration; 1977: 191–202. NASA SP-377.

51. LeBlanc A, Schneider V, Shackelford L, et al. Bone mineral and lean tissue loss after long duration spaceflight [abstract]. *J Bone Miner Res.* 1996;11(suppl 1):S323.

52. Space Studies Board, National Research Council. *Scientific Prerequisites for the Human Exploration of Space.* Washington, DC: National Academy Press; 1993.

53. Space Studies Board, National Research Council. *Radiation Hazards to Crews of Interplanetary Missions: Biological Issues and Research Strategies.* Washington, DC: National Academy Press; 1996.

54. Committee on Space Biology and Medicine, Space Studies Board, National Research Council. Radiation hazards. In: *A Strategy for Research in Space Biology and Medicine Into the Next Century.* Washington, DC: National Academy Press; 1998: Chap 11.

55. Simpson JA. In: Shapiro MM, ed. *Introduction to the Galactic Cosmic Radiation: Composition and Origin of Cosmic Rays.* Dordrecht, The Netherlands: Reidel Publishing; 1983.

56. Badhwar GD. The radiation environment in low-Earth orbit. *Radiat Res.* 1997;148(5 suppl):S3–S10. Review.

57. Fazio GG, Jelley JV, Charman WN. Generation of Cherenkov light flashes by cosmic radiation within the eyes of the Apollo astronauts. *Nature.* 1970;228:260–264.

58. Testard I, Ricoul M, Hoffschir F, et al. Radiation-induced chromosome damage in astronauts' lymphocytes. *Int J Radiat Biol.* 1996;70:403–411.

59. National Council on Radiation Protection and Measurements. *Guidance on Radiation Received in Space Activities: Recommendations of the National Council on Radiation Protection and Measurements.* Bethesda, Md: NCRP; 1989. NCRP Report 98.

60. Curtis SB, Nealy JE, Wilson JW. Risk cross sections and their application to risk estimation in the galactic cosmic-ray environment. *Radiat Res.* 1995;141:57–65.

61. Fry RJ, Nachtwey DS. Radiation protection guidelines for space missions. *Health Phys.* 1988;55:159–164.

62. Homick JL, Reschke MF, Miller EF II. The effects of prolonged exposure to weightlessness on postural equilibrium. In: Johnston, RS, Dietlein LF, eds. *Biomedical Results From Skylab.* Washington DC: National Aeronautics and Space Administration; 1977: 104–111. NASA SP-377.

63. Paloski WH, Reschke MF, Black FO, Doxey DD, Harm DL. Recovery of postural equilibrium control following space flight. *Ann N Y Acad Sci.* 1992;656:747–754.

64. Johnson RL, Hoffler GW, Nicogossian AE, Bergman SA Jr, Jackson MM. Lower body negative pressure: Third manned Skylab mission. In: Johnston, RS, Dietlein LF, eds. *Biomedical Results From Skylab.* Washington DC: National Aeronautics and Space Administration; 1977: 284–312. NASA SP-377.

65. Buckey JC Jr, Lane LD, Levine BD, et al. Orthostatic intolerance after spaceflight. *J Appl Physiol.* 1996;81:7–18.

66. Shykoff BE, Farhi LE, Olszwka AJ, et al. Cardiovascular response to submaximal exercise in sustained microgravity. *J Appl Physiol.* 1996;81:26–32.

67. Michel EL, Rummel JA, Sawin CF, Buderer MC, Lem JD. Results for Skylab medical experiment M171—Metabolic activity. In: Johnston, RS, Dietlein LF, eds. *Biomedical Results From Skylab.* Washington DC: National Aeronautics and Space Administration; 1977: 372–387. NASA SP-377.

68. Levine BD, Lane LD, Watenpaugh DE, Gaffney FA, Buckey JC, Blomqvist CG. Maximal exercise performance after adaptation to microgravity. *J Appl Physiol.* 1996;81:686–694.

69. Bungo MW, Charles JB, Johnson PC. Cardiovascular deconditioning during space flight and the use of saline as a countermeasure to orthostatic intolerance. *Aviat Space Environ Med.* 1985;56:985–990.

70. Helmke C. *Visual Capabilities in Space-USSR.* (U). Washington, DC: US Air Force. Air Force Technology Division Bulletin FTD-2660P-127/80-90; 22 May 1990.

71. Kuperman GG. *Information Requirements Analyses for Transatmospheric Vehicles.* San Antonio, Tex: Armstrong Laboratory. AL-TR-1992-0082.

72. Oberg J. Space engineer, Johnson Space Center, Houston, Tex, 1975–1997. Personal communication. See also www.jamesoberg.com.

73. The official website of the National Space Biomedical Research Institute is www.nsbri.org.

74. Kubrick S, director. *2001: A Space Odyssey* [motion picture]. Metro Goldwyn Mayer; 1968.

Chapter 35

MOTION SICKNESS

ALAN J. BENSON, MSc, MB, ChB, FRAeS[*]

[*]29 Coxheath Road, Church Crookham, Fleet, Hants GU13 0QQ, United Kingdom; formerly, Consultant in Aviation Medicine, Royal Air Force School of Aviation Medicine, Farnborough, Hampshire, United Kingdom; currently, Visiting Consultant in Aviation Medicine to the Royal Air Force Centre for Aviation Medicine, Henlow, Bedfordshire, United Kingdom

INTRODUCTION

Motion sickness, or kinetosis, is a condition characterized by pallor, nausea, and vomiting. It is brought about by exposure to real or apparent, unfamiliar motion to which the individual is not adapted. Many different motion environments lead to nausea and vomiting, and these are identified by terms such as seasickness, airsickness, carsickness, space sickness, simulator sickness, virtual reality sickness, ski sickness, and even camel and elephant sickness. Despite the apparent diversity of the causal stimuli, there are common features in the nature of the provocative motion stimuli and in the signs and symptoms evoked; all are manifestations of the motion sickness syndrome. Motion sickness is in certain respects a misnomer, for the word *sickness* carries the connotation of disease. The term obscures the fact that motion sickness is a normal response of a healthy individual to certain motion stimuli. Indeed, only the few who completely lack functional balance organs of the inner ear are truly immune.[1]

There are considerable differences among individuals in their susceptibility to motion sickness. For a particular motion environment, say that of a boat in rough seas, within a representative population some will be incapacitated by the motion, others will vomit from time to time but will carry out their allotted duties, and others will have no symptoms and no impediment other than that produced by the motion on their locomotor and postural activities (Figure 35-1). Because motion sickness can have an impact on operational effectiveness, the topic is of importance in the context of military medicine. Apart from the degradation of performance of trained personnel during land, sea, or air

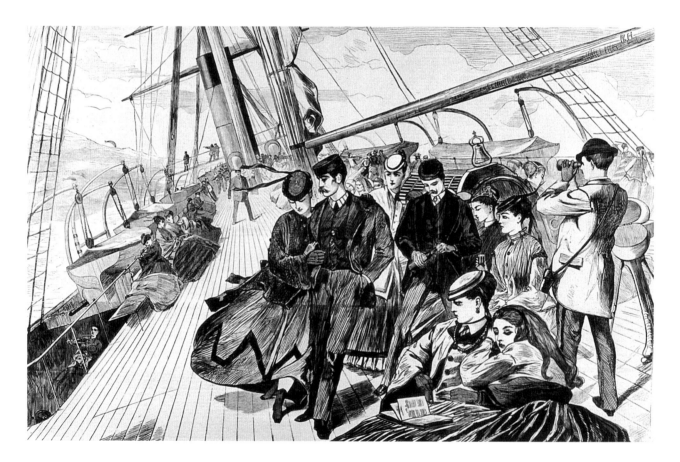

Fig. 35-1. Motion sickness is not unique to modern travelers. Winslow Homer's 1867 wood engraving entitled *Homeward Bound* portrays passengers (and crew, in the background) on the rolling deck of a ship on rough seas. The crew members that we can see seem relatively unaffected, in that they seem to be performing their duties. The passengers, on the other hand, seem to personify a spectrum of seasickness from miserable (the seated women and children along the left side of the ship) to few or no symptoms (the man at the right of the picture, perhaps looking at dolphins through binoculars). Wood engraving: Reproduced with permission from Sterling and Francine Clark Art Institute, Williamstown, Mass.

operations, motion sickness can cause attrition during training and interfere with the acquisition of skills.

Severe seasickness can also jeopardize the survival of those who have to escape to life rafts in rough seas.

SIGNS AND SYMPTOMS

On exposure to provocative motion of sufficient intensity and duration, the development of the motion sickness syndrome follows an orderly sequence, although there is considerable individual variability in the dominance of certain signs and symptoms.[2,3] This individual response pattern tends to be consistent and invariant of the causal motion environment.[4] The earliest symptom is typically an unfamiliar sensation of abdominal (mainly epigastric) discomfort, best described as *stomach awareness*. With continued exposure to the provocative motion, well-being deteriorates with the onset of nausea and may be preceded by a feeling of warmth and a desire to seek cool air. Some people experience skin flushing (vasodilation), but more commonly pallor and cold sweating are the harbingers of vomiting. Pallor is most apparent in the facial area and is a manifestation of heightened activity of the sympathetic nervous system. Sweating, another autonomic response, is usually confined to those areas of skin where thermal, as opposed to emotive, sweating occurs. Recordings of sweat production (Figure 35-2)

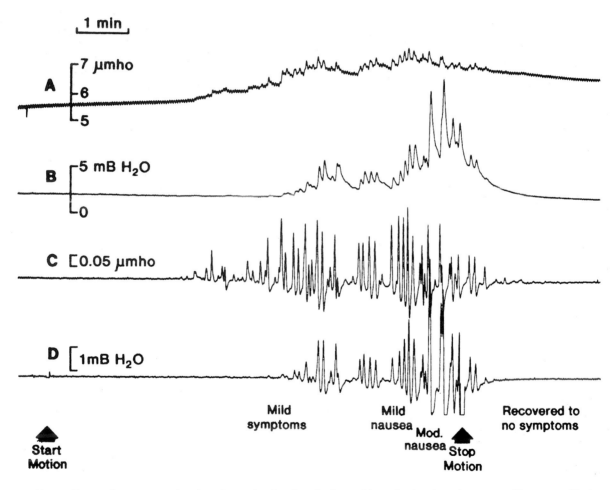

Fig. 35-2. Recordings of sweat production from the forehead of a subject during low-frequency linear oscillation. Tracings B and D show water vapor concentrations in an aspirated capsule on the forehead (DC-coupled in B and AC-coupled in D). Tracings A and C show skin conductance from forehead electrodes (DC-coupled in A and AC-coupled in C). Note both the progressive increase in sweating activity with increasing severity of symptoms and the rapid return to baseline after motion is stopped. Reproduced with permission from Golding JF. Phasic skin conductance activity and motion sickness. *Aviat Space Environ Med*. 1992;63:167.

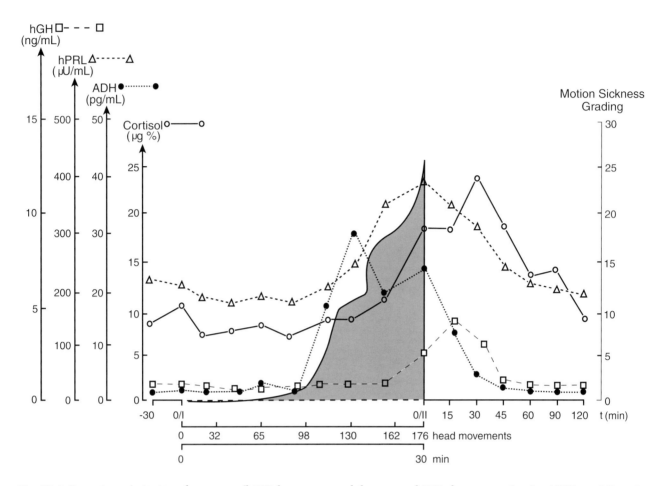

Fig. 35-3. Secretion of pituitary hormones (hGH: human growth hormone; hPRL: human prolactin; ADH: antidiuretic hormone) and cortisol in a subject in response to 30-minute cross-coupled (Coriolis) stimulation of increasing intensity (0/I to 0/II on the abscissa). The gray area, center, represents the development of motion sickness symptoms, which are scaled on the ordinate on the right. Reproduced with permission from Eversmann T, Gottsmann M, Uhlich E, Ulbrecht G, von Werder K, Scriba PC. Increased secretion of growth hormone, prolactin, antidiuretic hormone and cortisol induced by the stress of motion sickness. *Aviat Space Environ Med.* 1978;49:55.

show irregularly increasing sudomotor activity with pulses of sweat production that tend to accompany each wave of nausea.[5] Vomiting often brings some symptomatic relief, but with continued exposure, nausea again increases and culminates in vomiting or, if all gastric contents have been expelled, retching. This cyclical pattern of waxing and waning symptoms, recurrent vomiting and anorexia, may last for several days given continued exposure, as in storm conditions at sea or in the atypical force environment of space flight. However, most people in such circumstances adapt to the motion and are eventually symptom-free after 2 to 3 days.[6]

In addition to what may be identified as the cardinal signs and symptoms of motion sickness (ie, pallor, sweating, nausea, and vomiting), a number of other symptoms commonly, if not consistently, occur. Headache is a variable prodromal symptom, usually

frontal in distribution, and may be accompanied by an ill-defined dizziness. Other early symptoms are increased salivation, belching, and flatulence.

Changes in respiratory rhythm with sighing and yawning are not uncommon precursors to vomiting, and hyperventilation sometimes occurs, particularly in those who are anxious and apprehensive about the motion environment. In those exposed to motion of insufficient severity to evoke frank malaise, excessive drowsiness and extended duration of sleep may be the sole symptoms. The condition was first reported[7] in subjects living in a rotating room (in which head movements were provocative) and given the name *sopite syndrome* by the investigators. More-important changes in behavioral state are the apathy and depression that can accompany severe motion sickness and render the victims incapable or unwilling to carry out allotted duties or even to take basic steps to ensure the safety of themselves or their colleagues. An old adage holds that those aboard a boat in a storm first fear that the waves will wash them overboard; then after awhile, when motion sickness has taken hold, they wish that they *would* be washed overboard.

In addition to the symptoms experienced by those suffering from motion sickness, there are changes in physiological function that reflect alteration in the activity of the autonomic nervous system.[2,8] Motility and tonus of the stomach and gut decreases and bowel sounds (transduced by microphone or stethoscope) tend to disappear. Electrical activity of the gut (measured by the electrogastrogram, EGG) can be recorded by surface electrodes placed over the stomach. In those becoming motion sick, the EGG shows a reduction in amplitude and an increase in the basic electrical rhythm from the normal 3 cycles per minute to 5 to 7 cycles per minute.[9] The increase in frequency of the electrical activity seen on the EGG, termed tachygastria, correlates with the severity of symptoms and is associated with decreased gastric motility, as the EGG reflects pacemaker potentials of the stomach and not gastric contraction per se.

Cardiovascular changes are mainly confined to changes in vasomotor tone. The pallor caused by vasoconstriction of cutaneous vessels is accompanied by vasodilation of deeper vessels and increased muscle blood flow.[10] There may also be a modest elevation of heart rate and blood pressure, but these changes are variable and idiosyncratic and not highly correlated with the level of malaise.

Motion sickness is associated with increased excretion of anterior and posterior pituitary hormones. Most pronounced is the elevation of the antidiuretic hormone (ADH), which is responsible for the oliguria that accompanies motion sickness. Other pituitary hormones—notably adrenocorticotropic hormone, growth hormone, and prolactin—are also increased, although proportionately not to the same extent as ADH (Figure 35-3).[11] The change in secretion of pituitary hormones, in particular of ADH, correlates well with the severity of symptoms during both the motion challenge and recovery. Adrenal hormones, epinephrine and noradrenaline, are also elevated and, like the reduction in thyroid stimulating hormone, may be considered to be a nonspecific stress response.

ETIOLOGY

The pivotal role of the balance organ of the inner ear—the vestibular apparatus—in motion sickness has been recognized for more than a century, following the observation that some deaf-mutes are immune.[1] Subsequent efforts to evoke motion sickness in humans and animals deprived of vestibular function have consistently failed, and even partial destruction of vestibular receptors confers a degree of immunity, at least until central nervous system (CNS) compensation for the sensory loss has occurred.[12] The importance of the vestibular system in motion sickness led to the concept that the condition was due to overstimulation.[6] There was argument about the relative roles of stimulation of the receptors of the semicircular canals, which transduce angular movement of the head, and of stimulation of the otolith organs, which transduce linear motion and the orientation of the head to gravity (Figure 35-4). However, the overstimulation hypothesis is untenable, for some quite-strong motion stimuli (eg, those experienced by a rider of a galloping horse) are not provocative, whereas weaker stimuli (eg, those associated with head movement while turning slowly) can be highly nauseogenic. Furthermore, vestibular overstimulation does not account for the induction of motion sickness by purely visual stimuli in the absence of any motion of the observer and stimulation of vestibular receptors, as occurs in some static flight simulators or when

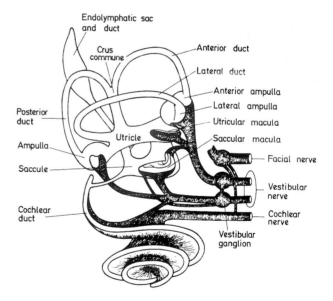

Fig. 35-4. The principal structures of the membranous labyrinth and its neural connections. Receptors in the ampulla of each semicircular duct are stimulated by angular accelerations acting in the plane of the duct. Receptors in the utricular and saccular maculae—the otolith organs—are stimulated by linear accelerations acting in the plane of the macula. Adapted with permission from Lindeman HH. Studies on the morphology of the sensory regions of the vestibular apparatus. *Ergebinsse der Anatomie und Entwicklungsgeschichte.* 1969;42:27.

watching dynamic scenes depicted on a large motion picture screen (Cinerama or Imax sickness). Nor does it account for the adaptation that occurs during continued or repeated exposure to provocative motion, nor the recurrence of symptoms on return to a familiar motion environment (eg, terrestrial) after having adapted to an atypical one (eg, weightlessness).

Neural Mismatch Theory

An alternative, and today widely accepted, explanation is that motion sickness is the response of the organism to discordant sensory information about bodily orientation and motion. The importance of *sensory conflict* as the principal etiologic factor was proposed more than a century ago,[13] but more cogently described by Guedry[14] and by Reason[15,16] in his neural mismatch, or sensory rearrangement, theory. Hypothesis would be a more appropriate term, as the neurophysiological substrate of the brain mechanisms proposed have not been elucidated, nor does Reason's theory provide a metric of neural mismatch that would allow a prediction

to be made of the nauseogenic potential of a given motion environment. Despite these deficiencies, neural mismatch is a unifying theory that permits the identification of different categories of mismatch that, in practice, are known to be provocative. However, it does not explain why humans, in common with many other animals (eg, monkeys, dogs, cats, even fish), respond to certain motion stimuli by vomiting. Emesis is clearly of benefit to an animal as a means of getting rid of ingested poison. Treisman[17] postulated that brainstem mechanisms subserving orientation and motion also detect neurophysiological dysfunction caused by a neurotoxin and initiate the teleologically beneficial response of vomiting. He further hypothesized that in motion sickness, vomiting occurs because this protective mechanism interprets conflicting sensory signals as neural dysfunction caused by poisoning. Support for this hypothesis comes from the demonstration that surgical removal of the vestibular apparatus abolished or reduced the emetic response to lobeline and L-dopa, whereas vomiting following the injection of apomorphine was unchanged.[18]

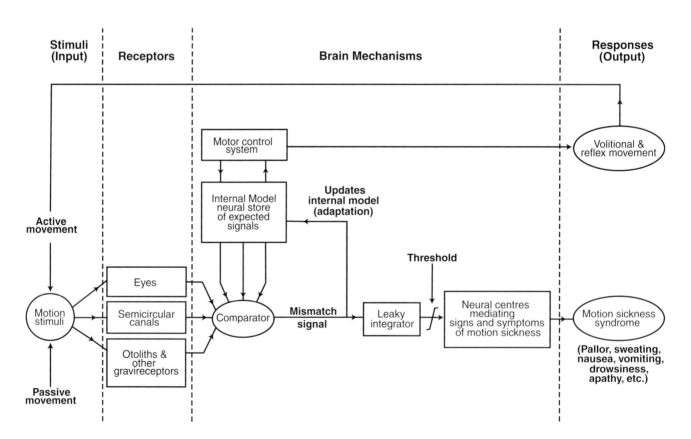

Fig. 35-5. A heuristic model of motor control, motion detection, and motion sickness based on the neural mismatch theory. Reproduced with permission from Benson AJ. Motion sickness. In: Dix MR, Hood JD, eds. *Vertigo*. Chichester, England: John Wiley & Sons, Ltd; 1984: 397.

The principal features of the neural mismatch theory are shown diagrammatically in Figure 35-5. Essential to the theory is the presence within the brain of a representation of afferent and efferent activity associated with bodily movement. This internal model is built up from information acquired during normal locomotor activity and the control of balance and posture. Afferent information about bodily orientation and movement comes from sensory organs stimulated by bodily motion, notably the eyes; the specialized receptors of the semicircular canals and otolith organs; and mechanoreceptors in the skin, capsules of joints, and muscles. These widely distributed receptors respond to forces acting on them and hence provide information about the orientation of the body to the gravitational vertical or, more precisely, to its orientation to the ambient gravito-inertial force. (In certain circumstances, as in aircraft in a coordinated turn, the resultant gravito-inertial force is not aligned with gravity and the otolith organs and the other mechanoreceptors no longer signal the orientation of head and body to the true vertical.)

An essential component of the neural mismatch theory is that any disparity between incoming signals from the sensory systems monitoring bodily motion and orientation, and the pattern of signals expected on the basis of past experience, leads to the generation of a mismatch signal. Transient mismatch is common during normal locomotor activity (eg, when one trips or is unexpectedly pushed); in such circumstances, the mismatch signal is used to initiate a corrective postural response. However, the presence of a sustained or repeated mismatch, as occurs on exposure to an unfamiliar motion environment, indicates that the internal model is inappropriate and requires modification.

It is postulated[15] that the mismatch signal brings about an updating of the internal model and, in a manner analogous to negative feedback, a reduction in the degree of mismatch. This mechanism—a primitive form of learning—underlies the process of adaptation to the atypical motion environment. The other postulated role of the mismatch signal is to excite neural centers that mediate the motion sickness syndrome. The nature of the coupling between the comparator and these neural centers is not known. Nevertheless, the relatively slow development of the syndrome and the persistence of malaise after withdrawal of the provocative stimulus suggest that there is some form of storage and progressive accumulation of the coupling agent; this is represented in Figure 35-5 by a leaky (or partial) integrator. A threshold is also required in this pathway to account for the acquisition of adaptation to

atypical motion without the development of malaise. The setting of this threshold and the time constants of the leaky integrator may play a part in determining an individual's susceptibility, although, as discussed below, other factors may be of greater importance.

Figure 35-6 represents the time course of the postulated mismatch signals on transfer from one motion environment to another. Inputs from sensory receptors accord with the internal model in the normal pedestrian environment, but a large mismatch signal occurs on initial exposure to a novel, unfamiliar environment. The mismatch signal slowly decays, probably with an exponential time course, as the internal model is updated. On reaching zero magnitude, the individual may be considered to have adapted to the atypical motion environment; new patterns of sensory–motor coordination will have been established, and signs and symptoms of motion sickness will have dissipated. On return to the familiar motion environment, mismatch again occurs because the internal model is no longer appropriate, and motion sickness may recur. This *mal de débarquement* (sickness of disembarkation) can also be accompanied by the persistence of patterns of postural control and sensory–motor coordination that were appropriate for life in the atypical environment but are inappropriate on return to the familiar. In addition, transient illusory sensations of motion may occur and be perceived either as self-motion or as motion of the visual scene. In general, readaptation proceeds more quickly than the initial adaptation to the atypical environment, because configurations of the internal model established by long experience are more readily retrieved (recalled from memory) than new ones acquired. By the same argument, adaptation to a motion environment to which a person had previously adapted is likely to be more rapid than on initial exposure, because copies are retained in memory.

In the diverse conditions in which motion sickness occurs, two main categories of neural mismatch can be identified according to the sensory systems involved. In the first, conflict is between motion cues provided by visual and inertial receptors. This will be referred to as visual–vestibular conflict, as the principal inertial receptors are those of the vestibular apparatus (although the contributions of nonvestibular mechanoreceptors, as discussed above, cannot be ignored). The second category of neural mismatch is between information provided by the semicircular canals and receptors stimulated by linear accelerations; for brevity, this is called canal–otolith conflict. In each of these cat-

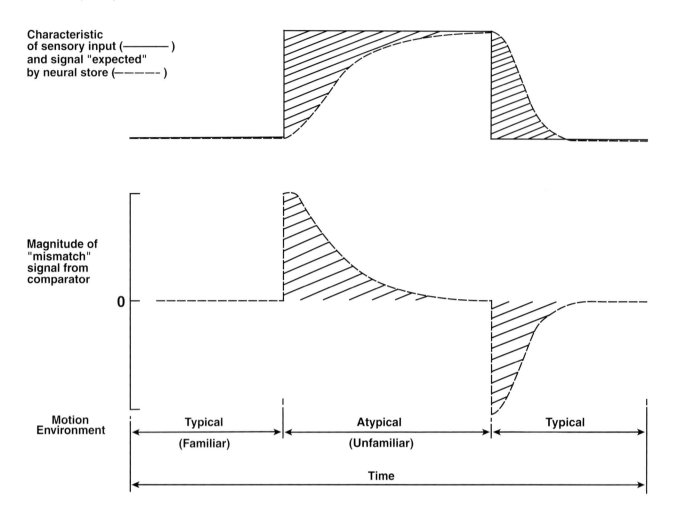

Fig. 35-6. The diagram illustrates both the time course and the magnitude of the mismatch signal, and changes in the internal model on exposure to a new and unfamiliar (atypical) motion environment and on return to the familiar (typical) environment. Adapted with permission from Reason JT, Brand JJ. *Motion Sickness.* London, England: Academic Press; 1975: 170.

egories, two types of neural mismatch can occur: Type 1 when both sensory systems concurrently signal contradictory or uncorrelated information, and Type 2 when one system signals information in the absence of the expected signal from the other system (Table 35-1). Readers should keep in mind, however, that most provocative motion environments involve more than one type of sensory conflict.

Visual–Vestibular Mismatch

Type 1. Uncorrelated visual and vestibular inputs are present when an observer on a moving vehicle cannot see an object or scene that provides stable orientational reference to the true vertical or horizontal. Vestibular and somatosensory receptors signal motion of the vehicle (whether a ship, aircraft, or land ve-

hicle), but if the occupant of the vehicle is using an unstabilized optical device, such as hand-held binoculars or an optical sight, some motion of the visual scene will not be correlated with vestibular information. Even minor changes in the perceived visual scene (eg, wearing eyeglasses with new lenses) can, in the presence of normal head movements, evoke mild symptoms of motion sickness. More dramatic distortion of vision produced by, for example, prisms that laterally reverse the visual scene (so that it moves to the right, rather than to the left, with a head movement to the right) can be highly provocative if the wearer of such a device executes head movements and attempts to walk about. Sickness induced by reading a hand-held map or book while being driven over rough roads or in turbulent flight is another example of Type 1 visual–vestibular conflict.

TABLE 35-1

CLASSIFICATION OF NEURAL MISMATCH IN PROVOCATIVE ENVIRONMENTS

Type	Category	
	Visual (A)/Vestibular (B)	Canal (A)/Otolith (B)
Type 1: A and B signals simultaneously give contradictory information	Watching waves from a ship Use of binoculars in a moving vehicle Making head movements when vision is distorted by an optical device Reading hand-held material in a moving vehicle Cross-coupled (Coriolis) stimulation Simulator sickness (moving base)	Making head movements while rotating about another axis (Coriolis, or cross-coupled, stimulation) Making head movements in an abnormal acceleration environment, which may be constant (eg, hyper- or hypogravity) or fluctuating (eg, linear oscillation) Space sickness (fast head movement) Vestibular disorders (eg, Ménière's disease, acute labyrinthitis, trauma)
Type 2a: A signals are received but expected B signals are absent	Simulator sickness (fixed base) Cinerama/Imax sickness Haunted swing[*] Circular linear vection	Space sickness (slow head movement) Pressure (alternobaric) vertigo Caloric stimulation of semicircular canals Vestibular disorders (eg, cupulolithiasis, round window fistula)
Type 2b: B signals are received but expected A signals are absent	Looking inside a moving vehicle without external visual reference Reading in a moving vehicle	Low-frequency (< 0.5 Hz) translational oscillation Rotating linear acceleration vector (eg, "barbecue-spit" rotation; rotation about an off-vertical axis)

[*]Haunted swing: a device in which the swing is stationary and the visual surround swings

Type 2a. Situations in which visual motion stimuli are not accompanied by commensurate and expected movement of the body can provoke Type 2a mismatch. However, severe symptoms are rarely engendered by the dynamic visual stimuli afforded by projected displays (Cinerama, Imax) or the computer-generated imagery of flight or road vehicle simulators. Visual stimuli that are meaningful to the observer and accord with previous real-world experience (eg, an aircraft entering a steep turn or an automobile decelerating hard) are most likely to provoke a response, but sickness can also be evoked by steady movement of nonrepresentational visual stimuli (eg, a pattern of bars or random spots). Such an *optokinetic* stimulus evokes an illusory sensation of turning, called circularvection, which, when not accompanied by concordant vestibular information, is a source of sensory mismatch.

Type 2b. The converse of Type 2a mismatch, Type 2b mismatch occurs when vestibular and other gravireceptors are stimulated by vehicular motion but the expected visual motion cues are absent. This type of conflict is present in all kinds of passive transportation wherein the occupant does not have a clear view of a stable, external, visual scene. Aboard ship in rough seas, an individual on deck with a good view of the horizon is less likely to suffer from seasickness than one who is below deck. The latter receives visual information only about his movement within the cabin and not the actual motion of the vessel as transduced by his nonvisual sensory systems. Sensory conflict is reduced by closing the eyes, which can increase tolerance to the provocative motion. Conversely, performance of a visual task decreases tolerance, especially if it involves visual search, such as the identification of targets on a map or radar display.[19] Tasks involving visual tracking of a moving target in the presence of whole-body motion have been shown in laboratory experiments[20] to be more provocative than when only a stationary target was observed.

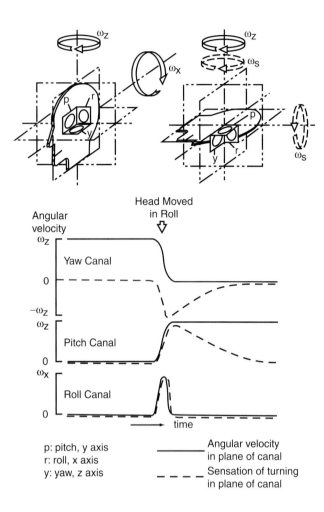

Head Moved in Roll

Angular velocity

Yaw Canal

Pitch Canal

Roll Canal

time

p: pitch, y axis
r: roll, x axis
y: yaw, z axis

——— Angular velocity in plane of canal

– – – Sensation of turning in plane of canal

Fig. 35-7. Cross–coupled (Coriolis) stimulation of the semicircular canals by a head movement of 90° in roll (x axis) having a maximum angular velocity of ω_x while also rotating at a constant velocity (ω_z) about a vertical axis. The six semicircular canals are represented by an idealized three-canal system (labeled y, p, and r in figure) orthogonally disposed to transduce angular movements of the head in the yaw (y), pitch (p), and roll (r) axes. The lower half of the figure shows the angular velocity, as a function of time, in the plane of each canal (———) and the sensation of turning (– – –) engendered by the angular stimulus. Note that in the steady state (ie, ω_z constant for 30 s or more), none of the canals signal rotation. However, when the head is moved in roll, the yaw canal is taken out of the plane of rotation and generates an illusory sensation of rotation about an Earth horizontal axis that is in conflict with information from the otoliths and other gravireceptors that signal a stable, left-ear-down, head position. Initially, the pitch canal signals veridically the vertical axis rotation of magnitude (ω_z), but as the speed of the vertical axis rotation is constant, the sensation decays, as does the erroneous sensation from the yaw canal. The plane of the roll canal does not change during the head movement, hence it is not influenced by the vertical axis rotation (ω_z) and it signals correctly the time course and angular velocity of the roll movement. Reproduced with permission from Benson AJ. Spatial disorientation: Common illusions. In: Ernsting J, Nicholson AN, Rainford DJ, eds. *Aviation Medicine*. 3rd ed. London, England: Butterworths; 1999: 445.

Intravestibular (Canal–Otolith) Mismatch

Vision is not essential for the induction of motion sickness, for the blind, like sighted individuals with eyes closed or in darkness, are susceptible.

Type 1. Type 1 neural mismatch, in which receptors of both the semicircular canal and the otolith organs each signal motion of the head, occurs when active or passive head movements are made in a vehicle that is turning, or is undergoing motion that exposes those aboard to an atypical force environment (ie, other than 1g vertical). When an angular head movement is made while exposed to sustained rotation about some other axis, the semicircular canals receive a cross-coupled, or Coriolis, stimulus. Figure 35-7 illustrates how three idealized orthogonal, semicircular canals are stimulated when a 90° head movement is made in *roll* (ie, movement about the front-to-back, or x, body axis) is made during a sustained turn in *yaw* (ie, the head-to-foot, or z, body axis). The head movement is correctly transduced by the roll canal, but the *pitch* (ie, the side-to-side, or y, body axis) and yaw canals expe-

rience changes in velocity, which give rise to erroneous sensations of turning in these planes and which take many seconds (typically 5–10 s) to decay. During the period the canals are generating *false* sensations, the otoliths provide *correct* information about the orientation, and the change in orientation, of the head with respect to gravity; there is, therefore, a mismatch that in practice can be highly provocative. In susceptible individuals, just one head tilt through 90° in roll, while rotating in yaw at 30 rpm, can evoke symptoms, even vomiting. In everyday life, however, such high rates of sustained rotation are rarely experienced outside the fairground or research laboratory. More commonly, sickness is induced by repeated head movements in a vehicle executing slow turns, with concomitant changes in the force environment.

Cross-coupled stimulation is not the only cause of neural mismatch associated with head movement. When the head is moved in an atypical force environment (ie, one in which the gravito-inertial force is greater or less than 1g [where g is a unit of acceleration equal to Earth's gravity, 9.81 m/s^2]), otolithic afferent information about the change in orientation of the head differs from that generated when the same head movement is made in the normal 1*g* environment. Neural mismatch occurs because the semicircular canals correctly transduce the angular movement of the head. Their sensitivity is but little, if at all, influenced by the force environment, whether this be the hypogravity of orbital flight or the hypergravity achieved by tight turns in combat aircraft.

The nausea, vomiting, and malaise suffered by those with acute vestibular disorders occur in the absence of motion and are, by definition, not motion sickness. Nevertheless, the signs and symptoms, often exacerbated by head movement, are in most respects identical to those of motion sickness, and they share a common etiology, namely a Type 1 mismatch of afferent signals from the canals and otoliths. For example, severe disturbance of afferent signals from vestibular receptors is associated with sudden unilateral loss of vestibular function by trauma or labyrinthectomy. Likewise, pathological processes such as Ménière's disease can cause a sudden change in the resting discharge of canal and otolithic receptors, an alteration of their stimulus response characteristic, or both.

Type 2a. Neural mismatch due to the absence of expected signals from the otoliths when the canals signal motion has been adduced as a primary cause of space sickness.[6,21] In weightlessness, movements of the head will be correctly transduced by the canals, but provided the head movement does not involve high angular accelerations, the linear acceleration of the otoliths will be insufficient to stimulate them, and a Type 2a intravestibular mismatch will occur. However, if an astronaut, for example, makes rapid head movements similar to those made on Earth, where angular accelerations of 400 degrees per second squared ($°/s^2$) to $500°/s^2$ are commonly achieved, the otoliths will be stimulated in an atypical manner and a Type 1 mismatch will occur.

Stimulation of semicircular canal receptors in the absence of concomitant otolithic stimulation can be caused by change in ambient pressure. During ascent, aircrew and divers sometimes experience sudden vertigo, hence the name *pressure* or *alternobaric vertigo*. The vertigo and associated nystagmus are commonly short-lived but in some individuals, symptoms may persist and be accompanied by nausea and malaise. Other conditions in which the canals are selectively stimulated are positional alcohol vertigo (PAV) and benign paroxysmal vertigo (BPV).[22] In both of these conditions, the semicircular canals may become sensitive to linear acceleration, and hence their orienta-

tion to gravity, owing to a change of density between the cupula and endolymph within the semicircular canals. The diffusion of alcohol from the blood into the cupula, rendering it less dense than the endolymph, may be responsible for the initial phase of PAV. The transient vertigo that occurs in BPV on moving the head to a right- or left-ear-down position has been attributed[23] to the lodgment of otoconial debris on the cupula (cupulolithiasis), which makes it more dense than the endolymph.

Type 2b. When signals from otolithic and somatosensory gravireceptors are not accompanied by the expected signals from the semicircular canals, Type 2b canal–otolith mismatch (the converse of Type 2a) occurs. Selective stimulation of the otoliths can readily be achieved by exposing an individual to rotation at a steady speed about a nonvertical axis. Once the effect of the initial angular acceleration has abated, the canals fail to signal rotation but the otoliths are stimulated by the continued reorientation of the head and body to gravity. Continuous rotation about an Earth-horizontal axis that is aligned with the z axis of the subject's body (as on a barbecue spit) is highly provocative, nausea being induced in most subjects within a few minutes when rotated at 10 rpm.[24] Otolithic stimulation produced by rotation of the specific force vector, as in barbecue spit rotation, is a feature of certain aerobatic maneuvers and fairground rides. Considerably more common are those situations in which motion sickness is induced by repetitive translational (linear) acceleration, such as is experienced aboard a heaving ship, an aircraft flying through turbulent air, or a motor vehicle that is repeatedly accelerated and braked.

A number of experiments carried out on vertical and horizontal oscillators, modified lifts, and parallel swings (reviewed by Guignard and McCauley[25] and Griffin[26]) demonstrated that the incidence of motion sickness bears an inverse relation to the frequency of oscillation (Figure 35-8). These laboratory studies accord with observations made in aircraft and ships. Aircraft with a high (0.8–0.9 Hz) natural frequency of response to turbulence produced less sickness than aircraft with a low (0.4 Hz) natural frequency. Similar observations have been made aboard ships,[27] and they accord with anecdotal reports that car sickness is more common in vehicles with a soft, low-frequency suspension than in those with firmer springing and a higher natural frequency.

The nature of the neural mismatch that causes motion sickness during linear oscillation at 0.2 Hz but not at 1 Hz is not immediately apparent. It may be explained[22] by consideration of the correlation of canal and otolithic activity established during normal

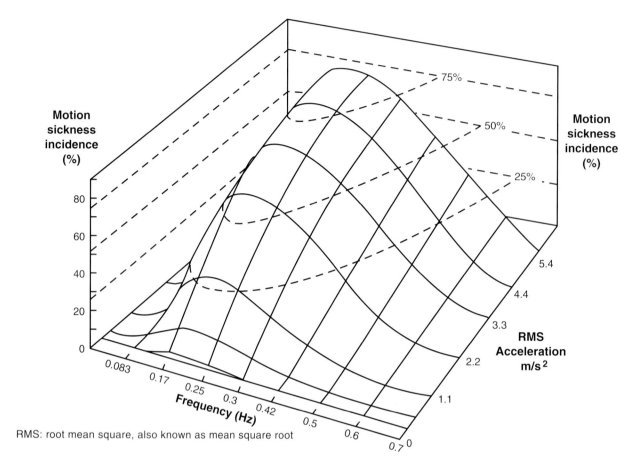

RMS: root mean square, also known as mean square root

Fig. 35-8. Oscillation about an earth-vertical axis at a frequency of about 0.2 Hz produces the highest incidence of motion sickness. At higher and lower frequencies the stimulus is progressively less provocative. The incidence of sickness increases as a function of the intensity of the oscillation, but even a stimulus having an RMS amplitude of less than 1 m/s^2 is provocative at 0.2 Hz. Adapted with permission from McCauley ME, Royal JW, Wylie CP, O'Hanlon JF, Mackie RR. *Motion Sickness Incidence: Exploratory Studies of Habituation, Pitch and Roll and the Refinement of a Mathematical Model.* Santa Barbara, Calif: Human Factors Research, Inc; 1976: 39. Technical Report 1733-2.

locomotor activities. The dominant frequencies of head motion during walking, running, jumping, and so forth lie in the range 0.5 to 10 Hz, so it is in this frequency domain that the canals and otoliths signal angular and linear motion in a dynamic but not necessarily correlated manner. At lower frequencies, however, a change in the head's orientation to gravity in the pitch and roll planes is signaled by the otoliths acting in their "static," position-sensing role, and the canals contemporaneously signal the angular movement. Thus, when otoliths and other gravireceptors are stimulated by a slowly changing force vector, the CNS expects concomitant and concordant information from the canals. During linear oscillation, the otoliths but not the canals are stimulated; Type 2b mismatch occurs and motion sickness may result.

An alternative explanation, although one still dependent on a mismatch between afferent information and that which the CNS expects to receive, was proposed by Stott.[28] He pointed out that during natural locomotor activity over periods of more than about 1 second, the average intensity of the linear acceleration of the head has a magnitude of 1*g* and therefore defines "downward." Conditions in which the otoliths and other gravireceptors signal slowly changing linear acceleration (eg, during linear oscillation at frequencies < 1 Hz) depart from the normal invariant pattern of sensory input and hence constitute a potentially provocative neural mismatch.

The well-defined inverse relation between the incidence of motion sickness and the frequency of linear oscillation implies the presence of a low-pass filter in either the comparator or the relay of the mismatch signal to the neural centers mediating the motion sickness syndrome. The characteristics of this postulated filter at frequencies below 0.2 Hz is a matter for conjecture. Sickness does not occur when stationary (ie, frequency = 0) in normal gravity but has a high incidence during "parabolic" flight, in which periods of 0g and 2g alternate at a frequency of about 0.05 Hz.[29] This, however, is a powerful stimulus and the gain of the low-pass filter is probably less than at 0.2 Hz. Flight experiments involving vertical oscillation at 0.1 Hz, with an acceleration of $\pm$ 0.3g, produced incapacitating motion sick-

ness when the investigator made head movements.[30] Provocation decreased as the period of oscillation increased and was insignificant at 0.02 Hz, $\pm$ 0.1g.

Etiologic Factors Affecting Incidence

The frequency and severity of symptoms in a group of people exposed to provocative motion is governed by a number of factors, of which the most important are the physical characteristics of the motion and the differences between individuals in their susceptibility to motion sickness.

Physical Characteristics of the Motion Stimulus

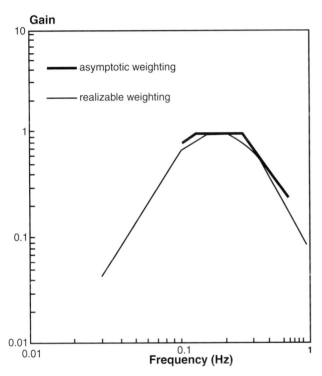

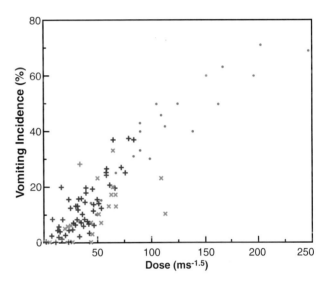

Fig. 35-9. Bode plot of the filter characteristic required to provide the frequency weighting (W_f) used to calculate the motion sickness dose value ($MSDV_z$) in the equation $MSDV_z = a \cdot W_f \cdot t^{1/2}$ (Equation 1 in the chapter). The graph shows a straight-line "asymptotic approximation" used to define the weighting function, as is required in the specification of measuring instruments, and the "realizable weighting" that can be achieved by conventional electronic filters. The weighting function has the characteristic of a band-pass filter with the greatest sensitivity in the octave 0.125–0.25 Hz with rapid attenuation in sensitivity at higher and lower frequencies. Reproduced with permission from Griffin MJ. Physical characteristics of stimuli provoking motion sickness. In: *Motion Sickness: Significance in Aerospace Operations and Prophylaxis.* Neuilly-sur-Seine, France: Advisory Group for Aerospace Research and Development, North Atlantic Treaty Organization. 1991; Paper 3:3-11. AGARD Lecture Series 175.

Fig. 35-10. Relation between motion dose, calculated in accordance with $MSDV_z = a \cdot W_f \cdot t^{1/2}$ (Equation 1 in the chapter), and the incidence of vomiting. The data points are from reports published by Alexander et al (1947, x) and McCauley et al (1976, •), who provoked sickness by vertical oscillation; and Lawther and Griffin (1986, +), who used data from ships' passengers on 6-hour voyages. Reproduced with permission from Lawther A, Griffin MJ. Prediction of the incidence of motion sickness from the magnitude, frequency and duration of vertical oscillation. *J Acoust Soc Am.* 1987;82:963.
x: Alexander SJ, Cotzin M, Klee JB, Wendt GR. Studies of motion sickness, XVI: The effects upon sickness rates of waves and varioius frequencies but identical acceleration. *J Exp Psychol.* 1947;37:440–447.
•: McCauley ME, Royal JW, Wylie CP, O'Hanlon JF, Mackie RR. *Motion Sickness Incidence: Exploratory Studies of Habituation, Pitch and Roll and the Refinement of a Mathematical Model.* Santa Barbara, Calif: Human Factors Research Inc; 1976. Technical Report 1733-2.
+: Lawther A, Griffin MJ. The motion of a ship at sea and the consequent motion sickness amongst passengers. *Ergonomics.* 1986;29:535–552.

The limited number of studies that have correlated the incidence of sickness with measures of the physical characteristics of the provocative motion confirm what is known from everyday experience, namely that the intensity, frequency, and duration of the motion are of prime importance. In most ships, aircraft, and land vehicles, there is motion with six degrees of freedom: three *angular* (pitch, roll, and yaw), and three *linear* (surge, heave, and sway). But in an extensive study in which ship motion was related to the incidence of sickness among passengers,[31] the best predictor of sickness was found to be the intensity of the linear acceleration of the vertical, z axis motion (heave) of the vessel, duly weighted for the frequency of the motion. Lawther and Griffin[31] proposed that the incidence of motion sickness for exposures of up to 6 hours could be predicted by the motion sickness dose value (MSDV$_z$), which is related to stimulus intensity and duration by the following formula (Equation 1):

1. $$\text{MSDV}_z = a \bullet W_f \bullet t^{1/2}$$

where *a* represents the root mean square (rms) heave acceleration in m/s^2, W_f represents a frequency weighting factor, and *t* represents the duration of exposure in seconds. The frequency weighting is based on laboratory experiments by O'Hanlon and McCauley[32] (see Figure 35-8) and takes the form shown in Figure 35-9. The greatest weight is given to frequency components in the octave 0.125 to 0.250 Hz, frequencies above and below this range being progressively attenuated. The time dependency of $t^{1/2}$ is also based on the McCauley experiments. These showed that for motion exposures of up to 2 hours, the incidence of sickness did not exhibit a linear relation to the duration of exposure but one that was better fitted by a power law function with an exponent of 0.5.

Lawther and Griffin[31] proposed a linear relation between the incidence of sickness and the MSDV$_z$ (Equation 2):

2. $$V = k \bullet \text{MSDV}_z$$

where *V* represents the predicted percentage incidence of vomiting and *k* represents a factor, estimated at one third, for the general population. Figure 35-10 shows the relation between MSDV and the incidence of vomiting in laboratory and field studies. Prediction of an "illness rating" (I) on a scale of 0 = "I feel all right," to 3 = "I feel dreadful" may also be made using the following formula (Equation 3):

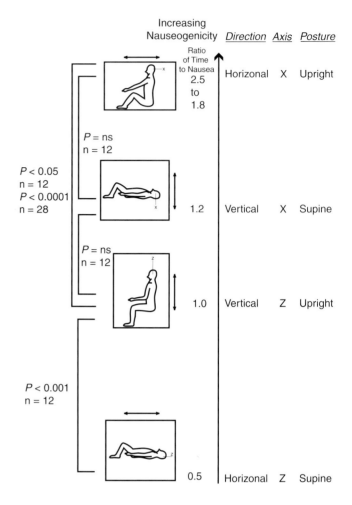

Fig. 35-11. Acceleration with the body in certain positions results in more-rapid onset of motion sickness. The nauseogenicity of a low-frequency linear oscillation varies with the posture of the subject (upright or supine) and the orientation to gravity of both the subject (horizontal or vertical) and the axis of motion (x or z). Statistical significance (*P*) of differences in nauseogenicity and numbers of subjects (n) used in each study are indicated along the brackets to the left of the figure. Reproduced with permission from Golding JF, Harvey HM, Stott JRR. Effects of motion direction, body axis, and posture on motion sickness induced by low frequency linear oscillation. *Aviat Space Environ Med.* 1995;66:1050.
ns: not significant

3. $$I = (0.045 \bullet V) + 0.1$$

The studies on which these three predictive formulas are based were confined to vertical, linear oscillation, principally acting in the head-to-foot (or z) body axis. The orientation of the body with respect to the direction of the linear motion can influence its nauseogenic potential, as can the direction of the

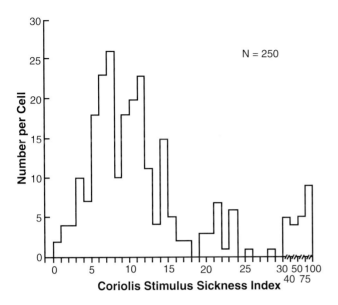

Fig. 35-12. Histogram showing the distribution, in 250 normal subjects, of susceptibility to motion sickness induced by cross-coupled (Coriolis) stimulation. The distribution of susceptibility is highly asymmetrical and perhaps bimodal. The measure of the magnitude of the stimulus (the Coriolis stimulus sickness index) is nonlinear, being a combination of the duration of exposure and the turntable speed, which increased with time. Note the presence of a small number of subjects who were highly resistant to the provocative stimulus. Reproduced from Miller EF, Graybiel A. The semicircular canals as a primary etiological factor in motion sickness. In: *Fourth Symposium on the Role of the Vestilinear Organs in Space Exploration.* Washington DC: National Aeronautics and Space Administration; 1970: 77. Report SP-187.

motion relative to the gravitational vertical. The findings of experiments[33] in which body orientation to gravity and to stimulus direction were systematically varied suggest that for a given intensity of low-frequency linear oscillation, the incidence of sickness is higher (*a*) when the stimulus acts in the x (antero–posterior) than in the z (head–foot) body axis and (*b*) when the individual is upright rather than supine. This is shown diagrammatically in Figure 35-11, in which the nauseogenicity of the stimuli is related to the z axis (ie, the vertical, upright condition).

Although there is some, albeit not consistent, evidence that restricting angular head movements in provocative motion environments reduces the incidence of sickness,[34,35] there is no support for the potentiation of a linear stimulus (typically vertical axis, heave motion) by concomitant angular rolling or pitching motions, such as occur aboard ship. These angular motions have frequency spectra with

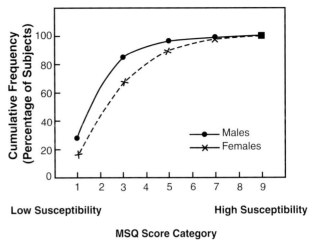

Fig. 35-13. Cumulative frequency distributions of the motion sickness questionnaire (MSQ) scores of 2,432 university students. The graph shows that the male students had a higher frequency of low MSQ scores than the female students, with median scores of 1.5 and 2.3 for men and women, respectively. Data source: Lentz JM, Collins WE. Motion sickness susceptibility and related behavioral characteristics in men and women. *Aviat Space Environ Med.* 1977;48:317.

peaks close to those of the dominant heave motion. Volitional or passive angular head movements made in the presence of such cyclical angular movements do not evoke erroneous cross-coupled (Coriolis) sensations, and they should not be provocative. Sustained angular motion, in which head movements are known to be provocative, does not commonly occur in transportation devices; notable exceptions, however, include aircraft in a steady turn, a spinning parachutist, or a tumbling space vehicle. The intensity of the sensations and the nauseogenic effect of an out-of-axis head movement depend on (*a*) the angle through which the head is moved and (*b*) a power law function of the steady rate of turn, having an exponent between 1.7 and 2.1.[36] Thus, a head movement made when turning at, say, 20°/s is roughly 4-fold more provocative than one made at 10°/s. As most individuals can make several large-amplitude head movements while rotating at 60°/s without becoming sick, we can infer that only the most sensitive are likely to suffer symptoms during sustained procedural turns in aircraft, as these rarely exceed 10°/s.

Individual Differences in Susceptibility

One notable feature of motion sickness is the

large difference between individuals in their susceptibility to provocative motion. On leaving harbor and heading into rough seas, some among those aboard develop symptoms and vomit within minutes, others tolerate the motion for half an hour or more, and a minority are unaffected. However, in extreme conditions the only people who will not succumb to motion sickness are those without functional vestibular systems.[1,17,37] The wide scatter in susceptibility is illustrated in Figure 35-12, which shows the number of subjects who developed significant signs and symptoms of motion sickness as a function of the intensity of a provocative crosscoupled (Coriolis) stimulus. Departure from a simple normal distribution is caused by a small, particularly resistant group of the population. It may be that the distribution in susceptibility is truly bimodal, but as the test employed a rotational stimulus that was increased incrementally, the high-tolerance tail of the distribution may be attributed to those subjects who had both low intrinsic susceptibility and the ability to adapt to the prolonged repetitive stimulus. Subjects with low tolerance had little opportunity to adapt before the test was terminated by the advent of their malaise. A bimodal distribution in susceptibility has, however, been adduced by Shepard and colleagues,[38] whose contention that susceptibility is a heritable trait is supported by the finding of differences in the α_2-adrenergic receptor gene in the subjects designated high- and low-susceptibles.

Susceptibility to motion sickness changes with age. Motion sickness is rare below the age of 2 years, but thereafter susceptibility increases to reach a peak between the ages of 4 and 12 years. Tolerance progressively increases over the next decade or so, so that beyond the age of 25 years, susceptibility is perhaps half of what it was at 17 to 19 years.[39] With increasing age, sensitivity declines further. The elderly are not, however, immune, as studies[27] of passengers in aircraft and ships have shown, but the reduction in sensitivity from that of the general population (ie, the value of k in Equation 2) has not been quantified.

A number of studies employing questionnaires show that women are more susceptible to motion sickness than men of the same age[6,40,41] (Figure 35-13). In passengers aboard a seagoing ferry, a higher incidence of seasickness was reported by female than by male passengers in the ratio of about 1.7:1 (ie, the value of k, in Equation 2 estimated at 0.33 for the general population, would be 0.25 for men and 0.42 for women).[27] The reason for this gender

difference is not known. It may be that women are more ready to report symptoms than men; on the other hand, hormonal factors may be significant, as women are reported to have higher susceptibility during their menses. In contrast, comparison of the incidence of space sickness and tolerance to ground-based provocative tests in male and female astronauts[42,43] has failed to show a gender difference; on average, the female astronauts had a slightly lower, albeit not significantly lower, incidence of space sickness than their male colleagues. Hormonal factors may also explain why men who had a high degree of aerobic fitness and, presumably, higher levels of endorphin, had a lower tolerance of provocative motion than those who had not participated in a physical training program.[44,45]

In a group of men or women of similar age and exposure to provocative motion, there are still large differences in susceptibility, differences that are largely enduring traits of the individual. With the known importance of the vestibular sensory system in motion sickness, we might have expected a correlation between measures of vestibular function and susceptibility. However, no clear relation having predictive power has been established despite numerous investigations (reviewed by Kennedy, Dunlap, and Fowlkes[46]). Interestingly, one of the few consistent findings was the presence of greater asymmetry in responses to caloric stimuli in those with a high susceptibility to seasickness and airsickness.[47,48]

As individual differences cannot be accounted for by differences in the transduction of bodily motion by receptor systems, they must be due to processes within the CNS. Reason and Graybiel[49] proposed that a large part of individual variation in susceptibility was due to the strength or weakness of three factors: (1) receptivity, (2) adaptability, and (3) the retention of adaptation. Receptivity refers to the internal scaling of sensory information. In terms of the motion sickness model, those who have high receptivity would be expected to have a more-intense mismatch signal and a higher susceptibility to motion sickness. Adaptability describes the rate at which an individual adapts, by updating the internal model, on exposure to an atypical motion environment. Those who adapt slowly will have a more-prolonged mismatch and are more likely to become sick than those who are fast adaptors. These concepts of receptivity and adaptability permit explanation of how a person may react on first exposure to provocative motion. His or her response on reexposure depends on how well the protective adaptation is retained (ie, on the degree of retentivity).

These three factors all influence susceptibility but are not of equal importance in an operational context. Evidence in an individual of high receptivity implies that sickness will occur on initial exposure to unfamiliar provocative motion, but if he or she is a fast adaptor and has high retentivity, then sickness is unlikely to be a persistent problem. Conversely, a person with low adaptability and poor retention is likely to suffer chronic motion sickness.

The idea that psychological factors are of prime importance in the etiology of motion sickness has had many advocates over the years, yet the weight of evidence (see reviews by Money,[2] Reason and Brand,[6] Mirabile,[39] and Tyler and Bard[50]) favors the conclusion that psychological factors and psychopathology play only a minor role in determining susceptibility. Nevertheless, there is experimental evidence[51] that mental stress and anxiety can heighten susceptibility. Attempts to correlate motion sickness susceptibility with psychological traits, as revealed by personality inventories, have yielded conflicting results, although significant correlations have been found in a number of tests (see reviews by Collins and Lentz[52]; Kennedy, Dunlap, and Fowlkes[46]; and Mirable[39]). In general, susceptible individuals are more prone to anxiety and have high neuroticism scores; in addition, they are more self-contained or introverted. The nonsusceptible tend to be tough and aggressive and are better able to cope with stress in a nonemotional manner.[52] Susceptible individuals, on the other hand, are more likely to manifest autonomic reactions (eg, increased heart rate, sweating) in stressful situations.

The extent to which these dimensions of personality are causally related to susceptibility is a matter for conjecture. The demonstration that introversion and neuroticism are associated with slow adaptation[49] suggest a possible mechanism for the lower tolerance found in individuals with high scores of these traits. Furthermore, a neurotic indi-

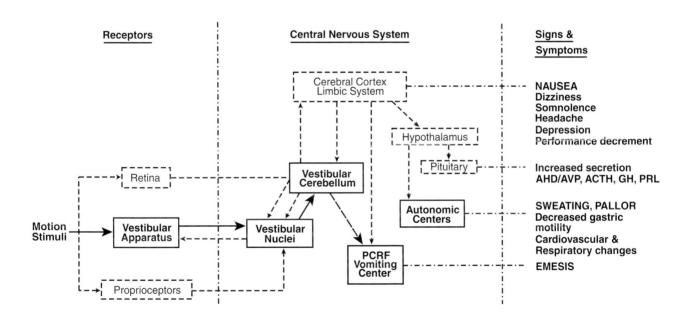

ACTH: adrenocorticotropic hormone
ADH/AVP: antidiuretic hormone/arginine vasopressin
GH: growth hormone
PCRF: parvicellular reticular formation
PRL: prolactin

Fig. 35-14. Neural structures involved in motion sickness. The bold-faced boxes and arrows indicate structures and pathways considered to be essential, whereas the broken boxes and arrows identify structures and pathways that can be involved in the development of the syndrome but are not essential. The dot-dash lines link the signs and symptoms with the neural structures thought to be involved. (They also guide the eye to indicate the separation of receptors from the central nervous system and the list of signs and symptoms.) Reproduced with permission from Benson AJ. Operational aviation medicine. In: Ernsting J, Nicholson AN, Rainford DJ, eds. *Aviation Medicine.* 3rd ed. London, England: Butterworths; 1999: 464.

vidual is more likely to be aroused and made anxious by what may be perceived as a life-threatening environment, such as aerobatic flight or storm conditions at sea. Heightened anxiety will degrade the acquisition of protective adaptation and may even prevent adaptation altogether.

NEURAL CENTERS AND PATHWAYS

Although the neural mismatch theory postulates certain neural processes within the CNS, it tells us little about which centers and pathways mediate the signs and symptoms of the motion sickness syndrome, nor about the process of adaptation. Knowledge about the neurophysiological mechanisms involved is far from complete, although some have been identified by experimental studies. Figure 35-14 summarizes the principal elements and pathways that are thought to be involved and relates them to the physiological and behavioral responses that characterize the motion sickness syndrome.

Essential for the development of motion sickness is the presence of a functional vestibular system, namely the semicircular canals and otolith organs in the membranous labyrinth and the vestibular nuclei. The importance of the vestibular projections to the cerebellar uvula and nodules is less certain. Early studies[53,54] indicated that ablation of these structures abolished swing sickness in dogs, but this was not confirmed by Miller and Wilson,[55] who demonstrated continued susceptibility of cats after large lesions of the cerebellar vermis were made.

The location of the mismatch comparator is a matter for conjecture, although it is most likely to lie in those structures where vestibular, visual, and proprioceptive signals converge, namely the vestibular nuclei and the cerebellum. The activity of cells in the second-order neurones of the vestibular nuclei can be influenced by optokinetic stimuli and by joint movement.[56] There is, however, no evidence to date for the presence of neurones that signal disparity of motion information. In contrast, Purkinje's cell activity of the flocculus of the cerebellum has been shown[57] to reflect the difference between retinal and vestibular signals of motion. The cerebellum is also of importance in adaptation to sensory rearrangements that typically evoke motion sickness. Removal of the vestibular cerebellar cortex prevents adaptive modification of vestibular–ocular control in animals whose vision was "reversed" by prisms[58] and inhibits habituation to vestibular stimuli.[59]

Supratentorial neural systems are not required for motion sickness to occur, as decerebrate animals retain their susceptibility. Nevertheless, the cerebral cortex is involved in the expression of symptoms (eg, nausea, dizziness, somnolence, and depression) and the establishment of aversive and conditioned responses to motion. Attention has also been directed toward the role of the telencephalic limbic system as another possible location for the identification of sensory mismatch and for the acquisition of protective adaptation.[60] The mesencephalic components are connected to visceral sensory centers in the reticular formation of the brainstem by both ascending and descending pathways. The latter probably play an important role in mediating the changes in autonomic activity, manifest as the vasoconstriction (pallor), sweating, and reduction in gastric motility that consistently occur in motion sickness. Involvement of the diencephalic component of the limbic system, the hypothalamus, must also be inferred from the increased secretion of pituitary and adrenal hormones found in subjects exposed to provocative motion stimuli.[11] It must be acknowledged, however, that ablation experiments[61] have shown that neither the hypothalamus nor the pituitary gland is essential for the induction of motion sickness.

The relatively slow development of the physiological correlates of motion sickness and the persistence of signs and symptoms after withdrawal of provocative motion suggest that the activation of autonomic centers and finally the act of vomiting are achieved by the accumulation of a neurohumoral agent released by the center or centers that identify sensory mismatch. Support for this concept came from experiments in which animals were rendered refractory to motion sickness when a plastic barrier was placed over the area postrema of the medulla or when the sylvian aqueduct was blocked. The findings are, however, not conclusive, and alternative explanations can be adduced (see Crampton[62] for a review of this topic). Furthermore, the role of the area postrema and its chemoreceptive trigger zone (CTZ), once thought to be essential for the emetic response in motion sickness, has been negated by careful ablation studies.[63] The CTZ is necessary for vomiting to be induced by various drugs, chemicals, and poisons, but it is not an essential component of the neural structures mediating motion sickness.

Emesis, a coordinated motor act involving contraction of the diaphragm and abdominal muscles, relaxation of the cardiac sphincter, and gastric stasis, appears to depend on the integrity of a zone of the parvicellular reticular formation (PCRF) in the medulla. Electrical stimulation in this area elicits vomiting as well as prodromal signs and led to its being identified as a central coordinating mechanism for emesis.[64] For convenience, the PCRF has been called a vomiting center, although this belies the fact that the area is not well localized.[55] The PCRF is located ventral to the vestibular nuclei and is traversed by an extensive vestibular commissural system. It also receives multiple descending afferents from cortical and subcortical structures, which would explain why an emetic response can be elicited by electrical stimulation of the frontal cortex, thalamus, amygdala, and limbic system structures.[65] The relevance of these centers for the development of motion sickness in humans is inchoate, like so much of our knowledge about the neurophysiological processes involved.

INCIDENCE OF MOTION SICKNESS

Airsickness

In military aviation, the incidence of airsickness is highest in student aviators during initial training flights. In US Navy flight officers, 74% of cadets reported experience of airsickness during basic training and 39% had vomited at least once; however, the incidence of sickness and vomiting fell during advanced training and was lower still in the Fleet Readiness squadron (Table 35-2).[66] Data from the Royal Air Force[67] indicate that 50% of navigators of high-performance aircraft suffered from airsickness during training, and some 39% of student pilots were also affected, symptoms being sufficiently severe in 15% to cause a training sortie to be modified or abandoned. In the Israeli Air Force, self-reports from flight cadets revealed that 46% experienced nausea at least once during their first five flights.[68]

Trained pilots rarely suffer from motion sickness when they control the aircraft's flight trajectory, although they may get sick, like other crew members and passengers, when they do not have hands-on control of the aircraft. A US Air Force study[69] revealed that 76% of aerial gunners and 57% of electronic warfare officers had experienced airsickness during operational duties. The highest incidence of airsickness appears to be among aviators engaged in hurricane-penetration flights. Severe turbulence caused symptoms in 90% of those with previous experience of such flights, whereas all of those who had not flown this type of sortie before were airsick, with one third reporting severe symptoms.[70] Airsickness is a relatively common problem among troops being transported by air when, for operational reasons, flight is at low level in turbulent conditions. A study of Mexican Air Force paratroopers[71] found that 64% of students were airsick on the first training flight (Figure 35-15), although the incidence fell steadily on consecutive daily flights; by the fifth day only 25% of the students were affected. Among trained paratroopers, 35% were airsick during a 1-day proficiency exercise. A recent study[72] of passengers on short hauls (average duration = 46 min) in small turboprop aircraft found that 0.5% vomited, 8.4% had nausea, and 16.2% felt ill.

Seasickness

TABLE 35-2

INCIDENCE OF AIRSICKNESS IN US NAVY STUDENT PILOTS

Training Phase	Students (N)	Sorties Flown (N)	Incidence of Airsickness (% of Sorties)		
			Symptomatic	Vomited	Performance Degraded
Basic	796	10,759	19.4	9.2	12.7
Advanced	543	9,299	11.9	4.9	4.2
Fleet Ready	372	8,325	7.6	3.0	3.6
Total—all phases	796	28,383	13.5	5.9	7.3

Adapted with permission from Hixson WC, Guedry FE, Lentz JM. Results of a longitudinal study of air sickness incidence during naval flight officer training. In: *Motion Sickness: Mechanism Prediction, Prevention and Treatment*. Neuilly-sur-Seine, France: Advisory Group for Aerospace Research and Development, North Atlantic Treaty Organization. 1984; Paper 30:4. AGARD Conference Proceedings 372.

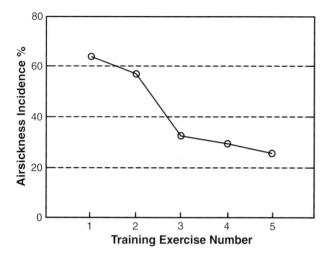

Fig. 35-15. Incidence of symptoms of airsickness in a group of 45 trainee paratroopers on consecutive daily exercises. The incidence of symptoms decreased more than 60% over the five daily training exercises, with the most dramatic change occuring between the second and third. Adapted with permission from Antuñano MJ, Hernandez JM. Incidence of airsickness among military parachutists. *Aviat Space Environ Med.* 1989;60:794.

The incidence of seasickness varies between a fraction of 1% to 100%. It depends primarily on the intensity of the motion stimulus and the extent to which those aboard the vessel are adapted to the motion. The motion stimulus is a function of the state of the sea and the size of the vessel and its sea-keeping properties.

In an extensive study[73] carried out aboard a 16,000-ton troop ship on trans-Atlantic crossings, the incidence of vomiting ranged from 20% to 41%. Similar sickness rates have been reported in other military transport ships (see review by Griffin[27]).

Questionnaires completed by sailors of the Royal Navy revealed that 70% had been seasick during their careers and that 42% had been sick in the past 12 months[73] (Table 35-3). These data also showed a relation between incidence of sickness and vessel size, which yielded a mathematical model that predicted sickness incidences of 67% to 29% as vessel size increased from 200 to 20,000 tons. These figures accord with an observed sickness rate of 62% of sailors in Israeli SAAR Missile Boats (300–500 tons).[74]

The motion of life rafts in rough seas is highly provocative and all but the most resistant succumb in storm conditions. In a life raft trial conducted in a wave tank, 55% of subjects had vomited and a further 21% were nauseated after 1 hour of exposure.[75] In totally enclosed, motor-propelled, survival craft (TEMPSC) used for escape from drilling rigs, seasickness occurred in more than 75% of the occupants. In one TEMPSC, all were sick except the coxswain, who was the only one who had a view out.[76]

Confirmation that the incidence of seasickness is positively correlated within the motion of the vessel—more specifically its linear, vertical acceleration—has come from a limited number of studies. The most extensive was carried out by Lawther and Griffin[31] and embraced data from 20,029 passengers aboard six ships, which varied in size from 67 m to 130 m (1,255–7,003 tons); two hovercraft; and one hydrofoil craft. The relation that they found between the motion dose ($MSDV_z$), calculated according to Equation 1, and the incidence of vomiting can be seen in Figure 35-10. Although there is still a good deal of scatter in the data, the positive correlation is highly significant, as is the relation between illness rating and $MSDV_z$.

The location of passengers and crew aboard ship can also materially influence the incidence of sick-

TABLE 35-3

INCIDENCE[*] OF SEASICKNESS AS A FUNCTION OF SEA STATE

Sea State	Frequency[†] of Sickness (%)			
	Always	Often	Occasionally	Not at all
Calm	0	0	4	94
Moderate	1	3	25	71
Rough	6	16	44	34

[*]Among 466 Royal Navy personnel aboard two ships: HMS *Gurkha* and HMS *Hermione*
[†]Percentage of sailors who had suffered seasickness during career: 70%; during past year: 42%
Adapted with permission from Pethybridge RJ, Davies JW, Walters JD. *A Pilot Study on the Incidence of Seasickness in RN Personnel on Two Ships.* Alverstoke, Hants, United Kingdom: Institute of Naval Medicine; 1978: 5. Report 55/78.

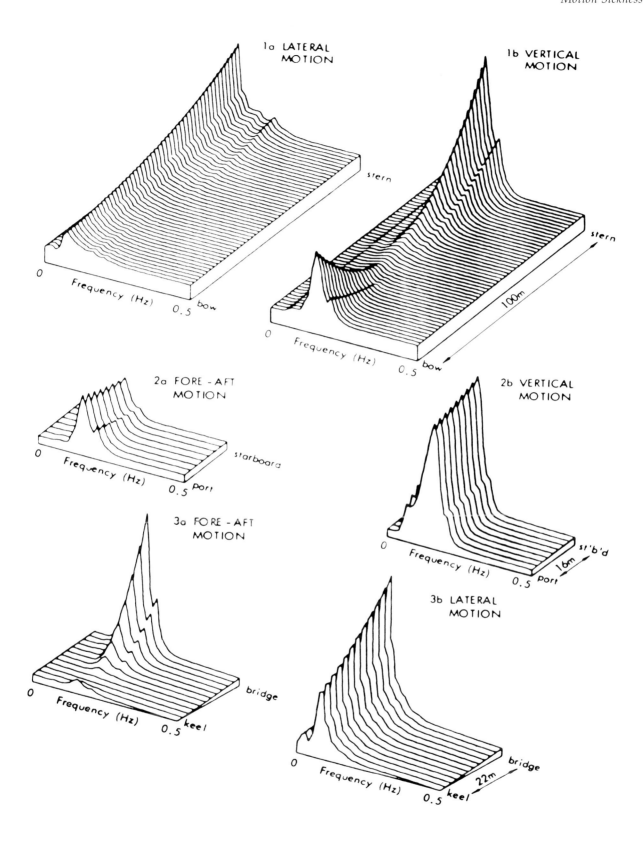

Fig. 35-16. Effect of location aboard ship on the magnitude of the motion stimulus. The graphs show the power spectra of the linear acceleration at incremental locations from bow to stern (1a and 1b), port to starboard (2a and 2b), and keel to bridge (3a and 3b). Reproduced with permission from Griffin MJ. Motion sickness. In: *Handbook of Human Vibration*. London, England: Academic Press; 1990: 314.

ness. Sickness was least among those quartered amidships, where the vertical motion is substantially less than at the bow or stern (Figure 35-16). Amidships, low in the ship, is clearly the most favorable position for minimizing the motion stimulus, but this benefit may be negated by loss of external, visual, orientational cues.

Simulator Sickness

The first reports of symptoms resembling motion sickness in pilots flying a helicopter simulator appeared in 1957. Nausea, vomiting, blurred vision, and other unpleasant symptoms tended to occur within the first 10 minutes of a simulator sortie and were experienced by 78% of those who flew the simulator. Over the ensuing 40 years, a number of studies have been conducted of what has come to be known as simulator sickness (see the review by Kennedy, Hettinger, and Lilenthal[77]). Some of the symptoms, commonly reported by those who fly aircraft simulators or drive tank and automobile simulators, are characteristic of the motion sickness that occurs in vehicular transportation (eg, airsickness, seasickness), notably, stomach awareness, nausea, vertigo, sweating, pallor, and drowsiness. However, severe nausea, vomiting and retching are rare. Other symptoms in

those who fly or drive simulators, but which are not common features of motion sickness, are eyestrain, blurred vision, and difficulty in focusing, which may be coupled with reports of headache, difficulty in concentrating, vertigo, and disorientation. The relative incidence of some of these symptoms in 10 US Navy flight simulators studied by Kennedy and colleagues[78] is shown in Table 35-4. The incidence of symptoms of simulator sickness varied from 10% to 60%. These figures embrace the incidence rates found in other flight simulators with synthetic displays of the external scene subtending large visual angles, most of which were equipped with a moving base to provide whole-body motion cues. The highest incidence of simulator sickness was found in a US Air Force air-to-air combat simulator, in which 88% of pilots had experienced one or more symptoms.

In addition to symptoms experienced during simulated flight, a number of postexposure effects have been described. These include disturbances of postural control, illusory sensations of motion, visual flash backs, disorientation, and dizziness. Typically, these sensory and motor disturbances are short lived and rarely last more than 12 hours, but some individuals have described delayed effects lasting up to several weeks.[77]

The incidence of simulator sickness is usually highest among student pilots with no prior experience of the simulator, and in most, the symptoms decrease with repeated exposure. In some studies,[79] pilots with extensive experience of the real aircraft but little of the simulator were most troubled during initial simulator flights. Reason and Brand[6] suggested in 1975 that the higher incidence in the experienced pilots is due to a greater disparity between motion cues that are provided by the visual display and motion base of the simulator, and those that their experience has led them to expect on executing particular flight maneuvers. The inexperienced pilots have a less structured internal model and expectancy of motion cues, so neural mismatch and the consequent motion sickness is accordingly less.

Virtual reality systems may be considered a particular type of visual simulation: one in which the observer sees only the external scene without any frame of reference, such as that provided by the aircraft cockpit in a flight simulator. In contemporary systems, the quality of the visual display—with regard to resolution, geometric distortion, and update lags—is inferior to that of flight simulators. As all of these factors have been implicated in the generation of the mismatch responsible for simulator sickness, it is to be expected that simulated movement through a virtual visual world will induce symptoms. One

TABLE 35-4

SYMPTOMS REPORTED BY PILOTS FOLLOWING SORTIES IN FLIGHT SIMULATORS*

Symptoms	Frequency (%)
"Motion Sickness"	
Drowsiness	26
Sweating	16
Nausea	10
Stomach awareness	8
Vertigo	5
"Eyestrain"	
Eyestrain	25
Headache	18
Difficulty in focusing	11
Difficulty in concentrating	10
Blurred vision	3

*Data based on 2,500 pilots' reports at 10 flight simulator facilities
Data source: Kennedy RS, Hettinger LJ, Lilienthal MG. Simulator sickness. In: Crampton GH, ed. *Motion and Space Sickness*. Boca Raton, Fla: CRC Press; 1990: 323.

study[80] found that of 150 subjects immersed for 20 minutes in a virtual reality system, 61% reported symptoms at some time during the test. Symptoms decreased after the exposure but were still present in 30% of the subjects 10 minutes after the visual display was removed. Nausea was the most significant symptom, followed by disorientation and oculomotor problems.

Space Motion Sickness

Since the first report by the cosmonaut G. S. Titov (who in 1961 was the first to experience sustained weightlessness in orbital flight) of seasickness-like symptoms on making head movements in the weightless environment of orbital flight, the occurrence of sickness in astronauts and cosmonauts during the first few days in orbit has been well documented. The incidence of what has come to be called *space sickness* (or *space adaptation syndrome*, a euphemism that does not subsume space sickness as just another form of motion sickness) has been well documented; the incidence for the first 20 years of space flight is summarized in Table 35-5. There was no report of sickness from astronauts in the small Mercury and Gemini capsules, but in the larger vehicles, where astronauts or cosmonauts could move about, many experienced symptoms. An analysis of space sickness in astronauts who flew in the Space Shuttle[42] (Table 35-6) revealed that 67% had symptoms, which were severe in 13%. On average, the incidence was slightly lower in astronauts on their second flight and was lower in female than in male astronauts, but neither of these differences is

TABLE 35-5

INCIDENCE OF SPACE MOTION SICKNESS IN ASTRONAUTS AND COSMONAUTS

Space Vehicles	Incidence (%)
USA	
Mercury	0
Gemini	0
Apollo	33
Skylab	56
Apollo–Soyuz Test Project	0
Shuttle	52
USSR	
Vostock	13
Voskhod	60
Soyuz/Salyut (1 & 4)	55
Apollo–Soyuz Test Project	0
Salyut 6	44
Salyut 7	40

Data source: Homick JL, Reschke, ME, Vanderploeg JM. Space adaptation syndrome: Incidence and operational implications for the space transportation system program. In: *Motion Sickness: Mechanism Prediction, Prevention and Treatment*. Neuilly-sur-Seine, France: Advisory Group for Aerospace Research and Development, North Atlantic Treaty Organization. 1984; Paper 36:36-2. AGARD Conference Proceedings 372.

TABLE 35-6

SPACE MOTION SICKNESS IN SPACE SHUTTLE ASTRONAUTS

Crew Member (Number)	Frequency (%) of Space Motion Sickness as a Function of Severity			
	None	Mild	Moderate	Severe
All (85)	33	30	24	13
Male (77)	30	33	23	14
Female (8)	63	12	25	0
Commander/Pilot (24)	3	29	25	13
Mission Specialist (41)	41	32	20	7
Payload Specialist (20)	15	30	30	25

Data source: Davis JR, Vanderploeg JM, Santy PA, Jennings RT, Stewart DF. Space motion sickness during 24 flights of the Space Shuttle. *Aviat Space Environ Med*. 1988;59:1186, 1187.

statistically significant.

Typically, astronauts report the onset of symptoms shortly after they begin moving about in the vehicle. With continued activity, stomach awareness and nausea usually precede vomiting, which, not infrequently, is projectile. Headache and anorexia are common, while the relative absences of cold sweating and pallor are the principal differences in the symptomatology of space sickness and that of terrestrial motion sickness. There are, however, more similarities than differences. Vomiting typically brings some transitory lessening of malaise; adaptation takes place over the first 2 to 4 days in weightlessness, after which time head movements can be made with impunity; drugs that are beneficial in motion sickness (eg, scopolamine, promethazine) also attenuate the symptoms of space motion sickness.[81,82]

Motion Sickness in Land Vehicles

Motion sickness in automobiles and buses is relatively common among the highly susceptible young and even some adults. A survey conducted on 3,256 passengers on coach journeys over a variety of routes in the United Kingdom with durations of 0.5 to 6.5 hours revealed that, overall, 22% felt "slightly unwell," 4% felt "quite ill," and 2% felt "absolutely dreadful." Nausea was reported by 13% of passengers, and 1.7% vomited.[83] There is a paucity of data on the incidence of sickness in automobiles and other land vehicles. Apart from one report[74] of motion sickness in tanks, in which 20% of subjects experienced nausea, only anecdotal and unquantified information supports the notion that motion sickness is a problem in fighting vehicles.

OPERATIONAL SIGNIFICANCE OF MOTION SICKNESS

Seasickness

The scientific literature does not convey a consistent picture of the effect of motion sickness on human performance.[74,84] Without doubt, the act of vomiting has a direct effect on performance, but this is transitory; some aviators and sailors maintain their ability to carry on their allotted tasks despite periodic vomiting. Others, however, in whom the classical signs and symptoms of motion sickness are less severe, are overcome by apathy and depression. Rolnick and Gordon[74] describe a *helplessness reaction,* which causes a decrement in performance through cognitive, emotional, and motivational deficits. Support for the dissociation of the nausea and depressive components of the motion sickness syndrome is afforded by the finding that decrement in performance at sea was not correlated with physiological signs of seasickness but was significantly correlated with feelings of helplessness.[74]

For those who suffer from severe seasickness in life rafts, the depression and erosion of motivation can impair the will to survive and to take positive steps to aid survival. In addition to these behavioral consequences, the dehydration and loss of electrolytes (metabolic alkalosis) brought about by repeated vomiting and retching can only reduce the ability of those in a life raft to withstand the privation, exposure, and other stresses of a hostile marine environment.

Airsickness

The principal operational impact of airsickness is in aviator training. As discussed above, there is a high incidence of airsickness in student pilots during initial flights. Fortunately, the majority adapt quite quickly, but there is a minority, estimated at 3% to 11%,[66,67] whose training is compromised because sorties have to be modified or curtailed. With continued airsickness, the student fails to make the required progress—sometimes interpreted as a lack of aptitude—and he or she is suspended from the training program. Yet airsickness is rarely given as a reason for rejection from training. Data from the air forces of the United States, France, and Belgium indicate that only 1% of students were removed because of airsickness when the overall attrition rate was on the order of 33%.[85] However, in a French Air Force study, of the 40 students who had consulted their flight medical officer because of airsickness, the attrition rate was 70%.[85]

Simulator Sickness

Simulator sickness, like sickness in actual flight, can interfere with training, although I am not aware of simulator sickness being so severe as to lead to removal of a student from flying training. However, the presence of malaise can direct the student's attention away from the task at hand and delay learning. Those who experience symptoms may individually or collectively develop a negative attitude toward simulation and may try to avoid further exposure in the simulator. Furthermore, behavior learned in the simulator to avoid symptoms, such as reducing head movements, may not be appropriate or safe behavior in actual flight.[86] Alteration of the simulator's motion-base dynamics to reduce provocative low-frequency components may also engender patterns of control behavior that do not transfer positively to the real aircraft. Flight safety may be compromised by simulator sickness aftereffects if the aviator pilots a real aircraft shortly after leaving the simulator. The presence of sensory disturbances (eg, disorientating sensations, flashbacks, and dizziness) may increase the likelihood of loss or inappropriate control and an orientation-error accident. On the ground, aftereffects are a potential hazard insofar as the disequilibrium could cause a fall and injury during normal locomotor activity, whereas sensory disturbances could interfere with the aviator's ability to drive an automobile safely.

Space Motion Sickness

Despite the extensive training of spaceflight crews and their high motivation to perform allotted tasks, those who become space sick suffer a degradation in performance. Vomiting interrupts ongoing activities, and the loss of well-being can have a deleterious effect on task performance. Awareness of the provocative nature of rapid head movements brings about a restriction of the amplitude and velocity of volitional head and body movements, which leads to tasks being performed more slowly. Those who experience severe symptoms tend to limit their activities to essential tasks and attempt to maintain a fixed orientation within the vehicle with good tactile support.[87]

Most astronauts' and cosmonauts' signs and symptoms of space motion sickness dissipate over the course of 2 to 4 days. Head movements can then be made with impunity, and the new patterns of sensory–motor integration, acquired as the space travelers adapt to weightlessness, allow tasks to be performed in an expedient manner, sometimes more efficiently than on Earth. Unfortunately, a small proportion of astronauts, perhaps cosmonauts too, fail to adapt fully. They continue to experience symptoms whenever provocative head and body movements are made, and their performance does not return to preflight levels.

Emesis within the space vehicle may be unpleasant for the individual who vomits and for nearby crew members, but it is not life-threatening. However, vomiting within the enclosed helmet and pressure suit worn during extravehicular activity (EVA) is potentially lethal. It is therefore essential that EVA is performed only by astronauts and cosmonauts who have adapted to weightlessness and are no longer space sick.

Mal de débarquement phenomena, notably disturbance of postural control, illusory sensations of bodily motion, dizziness, and nausea, have the potential to degrade performance during re-entry and landing. Most apparent is the disequilibrium that some astronauts experience on assuming an erect posture on leaving the spacecraft an hour or so after landing. Such individuals would be severely compromised if required to escape in an emergency on landing. Head movements can also be provocative on return to Earth, and in a few susceptible individuals can be sufficiently provocative to cause vomiting and significant incapacitation for a few days. The astronauts and cosmonauts who have serious mal de débarquement phenomena tend to be the same individuals who are badly affected by space sickness at the beginning of an orbital flight.

PREVENTION AND TREATMENT

The surest way to prevent motion sickness is to avoid exposure to provocative motion environments. Although this may be an option in civilian life—even if few are prepared to forego travel by car, airplane, or boat—it is not an option that is available to military personnel. Prevention, or at least reduction in the severity and incidence, of motion sickness may be achieved either by (*a*) lessening the intensity of the provocative stimulus or (*b*) increasing individual tolerance to provocative motion.

Reduction of Provocative Stimuli

Hull design can materially influence the response of a vessel to different sea states and the amplitude of motion in the critical 0.1- to 0.3-Hz frequency band.

Stabilization of the vessel in roll may make life more comfortable for those aboard, but it does little to reduce either heave acceleration or pitching movement, with their attendant high linear accelerations at bow and stern. In general, the larger the ship or aircraft, the lower the intensity of provocative motion; however, the ride quality of aircraft is governed by factors other than size.[27] Wing loading influences the response of the aircraft to turbulence, and control system characteristics determine the maximum vertical accelerations during automatic terrain following, although topographical features and ground speed govern the amplitude and frequency of the stimulus. The design of the suspension of fighting vehicles can influence ride quality and the frequency spectra of vertical motion, but the principal determinants of the motion stimuli to the occupants are the irregularity of the terrain and the manner in which the vehicle is driven (eg, rate of cornering, harshness of acceleration and braking).

Design factors relating to the occupants of the vehicle can also influence the incidence of motion sickness, such as the occupants' location and orientation to the dominant motion. Consideration should be given to the ability of those aboard to see out and obtain veridical, visual cues for orientation. Provision of adequate restraint can be important, as the restriction of head movement has been shown[34] to decrease the incidence of sickness in some situations.

Operator and Passengers

Those within a vehicle, whether in control or passengers, can adopt strategies that will reduce the intensity of provocative motion and sensory conflict and hence the likelihood of motion sickness. Those in control can, if operational constraints permit, steer a course that avoids the roughest seas, the most turbulent air, or the most irregular ground. They can also reduce the intensity of motion stimuli by making changes of speed and direction in a smooth and well-tempered manner. Passengers and others aboard who do not directly control the vehicle's motion trajectory may have the option to position themselves within the vehicle where the low-frequency heave acceleration is least (eg, aboard ship, near the center and low down; in aircraft, near the wing roots).

As noted above, restriction of head movements may or may not be advantageous in reducing the incidence of sickness produced by low-frequency, heave oscillation. There is no doubt, however, that head movements are provocative and should be avoided in the transient weightlessness of parabolic flight[29] and during the first few days of a space flight. The benefit of a recumbent posture at sea is also somewhat equivocal, but it is a common observation that those suffering from seasickness are more comfortable if made to lie down with the head supported. When recumbent, less postural activity is required, and conflicting visual cues are absent when the eyes are closed.[35]

Other behavioral measures can also reduce the incidence of motion sickness. Passengers and those who have to work in an enclosed cabin should, whenever feasible, avoid tasks involving prolonged visual search (eg, reading a map or book). Those able to see out should direct their visual attention to a stable orientational reference (eg, a distant point on the road ahead, or the horizon at sea); they

should not focus on nearby objects that may be in motion (eg, waves or other vehicles). It is also advantageous to be involved in tasks that minimize introspection and attention to bodily sensations. Best is the task of controlling the motion trajectory of the vehicle, for of those aboard, the skipper, driver, or pilot is the least likely to suffer motion sickness. For those not at the controls, involvement in some absorbing task, even singing, is better than preoccupation with endogenous sensations and self-pity.

Increasing Individual Tolerance

Adaptation

Some of the measures described above can be of immediate value to those exposed to provocative motion, but in the long term, adaptation is the most potent prophylactic. This is *nature's own cure* and, where practicable, acquiring protective adaptation is preferable to administering anti–motion sickness drugs to military personnel. The basic principle governing the acquisition and maintenance of protective adaptation is that there should be gradual and incremental exposure to progressively more-intense provocative motion. Adaptation, once achieved, should be maintained by regular and repeated exposure to the motion stimulus. Unfortunately, for most of the population at risk, the intensity and duration of exposure to provocative motion cannot be controlled, and so the acquisition and retention of adaptation cannot be optimized. Student aviators are a possible exception, for in this group steps can be taken to grade exposure to provocative flight maneuvers and to provide regular flight experience. Even so, not all aviators develop sufficient protective adaptation, and they have to be withdrawn from the flying program. Their withdrawal may be only temporary, for many aviators who continue to be troubled by airsickness can be helped by a treatment program of the type first employed by Dowd[88] and Dobie[67] in the 1960s.

This *desensitization therapy* typically involves a ground-based phase with twice-daily exposure to provocative, cross-coupled (Coriolis) stimulation of progressively increasing intensity. This is followed by a flying phase in which the process of incremental adaptation is continued by the progressive introduction of more-stressful and provocative flight maneuvers. Some flight medical officers have regarded vestibular adaptation as an essentially physiological process[89] and have not employed supportive psychotherapeutic procedures, such as cognitive–behavioral therapy, which Dobie and May[90] regard as an essential element of the program. There is experimental evidence[91] that autogenic feedback training (ie, a combination of biofeedback and autogenic therapy, which develops an individual's ability to control autonomic responses) can increase tolerance to provocative motion. However, the reduction in susceptibility achieved by autogenic therapy alone is inferior to that achieved when it is combined with incremental exposure to cross-coupled stimulation.[92,93]

Variants of desensitization therapy include the use of other adapting stimuli, such as vertical linear oscillation and moving visual patterns (optokinetic stimuli), in the belief that there will be better generalization of the adaptation to the flight environment than that achieved when only cross-coupled stimulation is employed in the ground-based phase of therapy.[89]

The literature on desensitization therapy (see reviews by Stott[35,92] and Dobie and May[90]) is confined to the treatment of flying personnel. It is in this group that the therapy is cost-effective: first, because of the financial investment in selection and training; and second, on return to flying, adaptation will likely be sustained by continued exposure to provocative flight maneuvers. There is anecdotal evidence of the successful desensitization of a chronically seasick sailor, but I am not aware of any systematic use of desensitization therapy on other military personnel. Apart from the cost of therapy, the irregularity of storm conditions at sea does not favor the maintenance of protective adaptation.

Acupressure and Acustimulation

Stimulation of the P6 (or Nei-Kuan) point on the anterior aspect of the wrist is believed by acupuncturists to be of prophylactic benefit in motion sickness. Commercially available elasticized bands, each with a plastic button that can apply steady pressure to the P6 point, have failed to show any benefit in controlled trials.[94–96] In contrast, acustimulation provided by cyclical manual pressure[96] or electrical stimulation[97] has had a statistically significant prophylactic effect. If these reports are substantiated by more-extensive field trials, acustimulation may become the method of choice for short-term prophylaxis, as there are no deleterious side effects such as those that arise with certain drugs.

Selection

In critical military tasks where motion sickness would impede mission effectiveness, personnel with low susceptibility can be selected. Reviewing the extensive literature on predictive tests, Kennedy, Dunlap, and Fowkles[46] conclude that assessment of susceptibility to motion sickness in an operational environment has the highest predictive validity. This is followed, in rank order, by laboratory provocative tests, motion sickness history, psychological factors (personality and perceptual style), and physiological measures (autonomic and sensory functions). Defense organizations in some countries (eg, France, Israel, the United Kingdom) employ an operational selection test for flying personnel. Candidates are exposed to provocative flight maneuvers, and only those who are not overcome by motion sickness are accepted for flight training. If there is no shortage of able candidates, this method of selection is acceptable, but wasteful: some, perhaps many, of those who become sick on initial exposure to unfamiliar motion may adapt quite adequately during subsequent flights. Although provocative tests, performed either in the operational environment or in laboratory simulations, give information about susceptibility at the time the test is performed, no well-validated test of the important attributes of adaptability and retentivity is available that would aid prediction.

When known to be used for selection, data from motion sickness questionnaires should also be treated with caution, as they are not always answered honestly. In the Royal Air Force, a questionnaire administered to candidates before selection for flying training yielded a history of motion sickness in 3.6%, but when the same confidential questionnaire was completed later by the same group, after they had been established in the flying training program, 59% gave an affirmative response.[67]

Drug Treatment

Over the years, many remedies have been recommended for the prophylaxis of motion sickness (reviewed by Reason and Brand[6]), but few have been proven in laboratory or field trials to be more effective than a placebo. The demonstration of therapeutic value is complicated by the need to control for a placebo effect. With motion sickness, the placebo effect can be large if the individual knows that he or she is taking a substance or following a procedure (eg, the application of pressure to the P6 point) with alleged therapeutic benefit. Trials also have to allow for differences between drugs in the mode of administration and in the rate of absorption and dosage, as well as to the timing, intensity, and duration of the provocative motion challenge.

Many drugs have been tested against motion sick-

TABLE 35-7

DOSAGE AND DURATION OF ACTION OF ANTI–MOTION SICKNESS DRUGS

Drug	Route	Adult Dose	Time of Onset	Duration of Action (h)
Scopolamine	oral	0.3–0.6 mg	30 min	4
Scopolamine	injection	0.1–0.2 mg	15 min	4
Scopolamine (Transderm Scop)	patch	one	6–8 h	72
Promethazine	oral	25–50 mg	2 h	15
Promethazine	injection	25 mg	15 min	15
Promethazine	suppository	25 mg	1 h	15
Dimenhydrinate	oral	50–100 mg	2 h	8
Dimenhydrinate	injection	50 mg	15 min	8
Cyclizine	oral	50 mg	2 h	6
Cyclizine	injection	50 mg	15 min	6
Meclizine	oral	25–50 mg	2 h	8
Buclizine	oral	50 mg	1 h	6
Cinnarizine	oral	15–30 mg	4 h	8

ness[98,99] but of those that are beneficial (Table 35-7), none provide complete protection and none is without side effect (see review by Stott[100]). Of the currently available drugs, the centrally active, muscarinic cholinergic antagonist, scopolamine (ie, *l*-hyoscine), is probably the most effective single drug. It is rapidly absorbed and reaches a peak concentration in the body at about 1 hour after ingestion but has a short half-life of 2.5 hours that limits its duration of action to about 4 hours. Side effects after ingestion of scopolamine in doses larger than 0.6 mg are frequent, particularly sedation, dry mouth, blurring of vision (due to impairment of accommodation), and lightheadedness. The drug is not well tolerated by children and should not be taken by the elderly, especially those with glaucoma or obstruction of the bladder neck. Side effects tend to be accentuated if the drug has to be taken repeatedly at 4- to 6-hour intervals for prolonged prophylaxis. With the scopolamine transdermal patch, protection can be provided for up to 72 hours after a patch has been applied to the skin behind the ear. The transdermal patch provides a loading dose of 200 μg of scopolamine and controlled release of the drug at 20 μg/h for up to 3 days. Therapeutic blood levels of scopolamine are not reached until 6 to 8 hours after application of the patch, so it is necessary either to anticipate the requirement for prophylaxis or, if more immediate protection is required, to take an oral dose of scopolamine when the patch is applied.

Scopolamine may be given by injection for the treatment of established motion sickness when vomiting and gastric stasis prevent or impede absorption of an orally administered drug. It should be noted that when injected, blood levels of the drug are 4- to 6-fold higher than when it is taken orally because there is no initial first pass through the liver, as occurs when the drug is absorbed from the gut.

Scopolamine, like atropine, has a broad affinity for the five muscarinic receptor subtypes that have so far been identified. With the availability of selective antimuscarinic drugs, there exists the possibility of targeting the neural processes of motion sickness without incurring the side effects produced by blockade of other muscarinic receptors. Studies[101] have shown that the unmarketed drug zamifenecin, which has high affinity for M_3 and M_5 receptors, is as effective as 0.6 mg scopolamine in increasing tolerance to cross-coupled stimulation in humans. On the other hand, the unmarketed drug idaverine, which has high affinity for M_2 and lower affinity for M_1 receptors, was without effect on motion sickness in cats.[102]

A number of drugs that were developed and marketed primarily for their antihistaminic properties have also been shown to be effective in motion sickness prophylaxis.[103,104] These are promethazine, dimenhydrinate, cyclizine, meclizine, and cinnarizine. All of these drugs can cross the blood–brain barrier and have some central anticholinergic activity as well as being histamine H_1-receptor antagonists. Both promethazine and meclizine have strong anticholinergic properties and a long duration of action (12–24 h). Dimenhydrinate, cyclizine, and cinnarizine are shorter acting and somewhat less effective than promethazine. All of these antihistaminic drugs cause drowsiness, promethazine and dimenhydrinate being the most sedative. Other side effects, dizziness, dry mouth, and blurred vision, which are attributable to the anticholinergic action of the drugs, occur but to a lesser extent than with scopolamine.

The central sympathomimetic (adrenergic) agent *d*-amphetamine phosphate was used empirically in combination with scopolamine for motion sickness prophylaxis in World War II. Yet not until the 1960s was amphetamine by itself shown to increase tolerance to provocative motion and also to have an additive effect in therapeutic effectiveness when combined at a dose of 5 to 10 mg with scopolamine or promethazine.[105] A further benefit was a reduction of some of the side effects of scopolamine, notably drowsiness and performance decrement, but dry mouth was increased. Unfortunately, *d*-amphetamine is a potentially addictive drug and is liable to abuse, so its general use in motion sickness prophylaxis cannot be justified. Ephedrine (15–30 mg) is almost as good as *d*-amphetamine in enhancing the efficacy of anti–motion sickness drugs and can be used in conjunction with scopolamine (0.6 mg) or promethazine (25 mg) when optimum protection of short or medium duration is required.

The observation that electroencephalographic changes in acute motion sickness have features in common with those that occur in minor epilepsy led to the experimental evaluation of the analeptic drug phenytoin for motion sickness prophylaxis. At plasma concentrations of 10 to 20 μg/mL (anticonvulsant therapeutic levels), the drug was highly effective in both laboratory and sea trials in increasing tolerance to provocative motion.[106,107] However, tests carried out 3 to 4 hours after a single 200-mg

dose of the drug showed only a slight increase in tolerance and no reduction in symptom score.[108] Phenytoin has a narrow therapeutic index, the relation between dose and plasma concentrations is nonlinear, and it has potentially serious side effects and drug interactions; accordingly, its general use for motion sickness prophylaxis is not recommended.

In concluding this review of prophylactic drugs, mention should be made of some drugs that are both widely used and effective in the treatment of nausea and vomiting but are without proven benefit in motion sickness. Examples are the phenothiazine, prochlorperazine; the dopamine antagonist, metoclopramide; and the $5HT_3$ receptor antagonist, ondansetron.

Treatment of Severe Motion Sickness and Vomiting

Individuals with severe symptoms and vomiting cannot benefit from orally administered anti–motion sickness drugs because of impaired absorption from the gastrointestinal tract due to gastric stasis and emesis. The preferred treatment is an intramuscular injection of promethazine (25–30 mg), although scopolamine, cyclizine, and dimenhydrinate may also be given by injection. Therapeutic blood levels of scopolamine are achieved through the buccal absorption of the drug,[109,110] and this offers an alternative, albeit slower, rate of drug delivery. Promethazine and cyclizine may also be administered by means of rectal suppositories.

Repeated vomiting and an attendant inability to retain ingested fluids carry a risk of dehydration and electrolyte imbalance, especially if potentiated by high insensible fluid loss, as in a hot environment. Usually, once vomiting is controlled, fluids can be replaced by mouth, but in those rare cases where vomiting has not been controlled, as can occur on board a life raft, an intravenous infusion of fluid and electrolytes may be necessary.

SUMMARY

Exposure to unfamiliar motion produces a syndrome consisting of pallor, nausea, and vomiting. Provocative stimuli may be produced in land vehicles, at sea, in the air, and during space flight. A related condition occurs in simulators ranging from large-screen movies to sophisticated virtual-reality laboratories. Susceptibility to motion sickness shows a large degree of variation within and between individuals and usually follows a reliable pattern, progressing from stomach awareness to

nausea, a feeling of warmth, flushing of the skin, and sweating before vomiting, which may offer transient relief from discomfort.

Motion sickness in all its manifestations depends on the vestibular apparatus of the inner ear. It is widely accepted today that symptoms result from mismatched sensory information regarding body orientation and motion. Normal locomotor activity produces an accustomed pattern of inputs from the eyes, the semicircular canals, and the otoliths, as well as gravireceptors in the musculoskeletal system. Trouble arises when there is a sustained disparity among these inputs. Two main categories of neural mismatch have been identified, representing (1) conflict between visual and vestibular receptors or (2) mismatch between the canals and the otoliths.

The incidence of motion sickness in a particular set of conditions can be traced to a combination of factors including the physical characteristics of the motion, innate susceptibility, and training or accustomization. Different problems typify airsickness, seasickness, simulator sickness, space motion sickness, and land transportation. Prevention may involve selection and training of resistant individuals, reduction in provocative stimuli, and progressive training programs. Pharmaceutical agents with varying mechanisms of action have been found to offer relief but may produce unacceptable side effects for military purposes.

REFERENCES

1. James W. The sense of dizziness in deaf-mutes. *Am J Otol*. 1882;4:239–254.

2. Money KE. Motion sickness. *Physiol Rev*. 1970;50:1–38.

3. Harm DL. Physiology of motion sickness symptoms. In: Crampton GH, ed. *Motion and Space Sickness*. Boca Raton, Fla: CRC Press; 1990: 153–178.

4. Cowings PS. Autogenic feedback training: A treatment for motion and space sickness. In: Crampton GH, ed. *Motion and Space Sickness*. Boca Raton, Fla: CRC Press; 1990: 313–390.

5. Golding JF. Phasic skin conductance activity and motion sickness. *Aviat Space Environ Med*. 1992;63:165–171.

6. Reason JT, Brand JJ. *Motion Sickness*. London, England: Academic Press; 1975.

7. Graybiel A, Knepton J. Sopite syndrome: A sometimes sole manifestation of motion sickness. *Aviat Space Environ Med*. 1976;47:873–882.

8. Hu S, McChesney KA, Bahl AM, Buchanan JB, Scozafava JE. Systematic investigation of physiological correlates of motion sickness induced by viewing an optokinetic rotating drum. *Aviat Space Environ Med*. 1999;70:759–765.

9. Stern RM, Koch KL, Leibowitz HW, Linblad IM, Shupert CL, Stewart WR. Tachygastria and motion sickness. *Aviat Space Environ Med*. 1985;56(11):1074–1077.

10. Johnson WH, Sunahara FA, Landolt JP. Motion sickness, vascular changes accompanying pseudo-Coriolis-induced nausea. *Aviat Space Environ Med*. 1993;64(5):367–369.

11. Eversmann T, Gottsmann M, Uhlich E, Ulbrecht G, von Werder K, Scriba PC. Increased secretion of growth hormone, prolactin, antidiuretic hormone and cortisol induced by the stress of motion sickness. *Aviat Space Environ Med*. 1978;49:53–57.

12. Igarashi M. Role of the vestilinear end organs in experimental motion sickness. In: Crampton GH, ed. *Motion and Space Sickness*. Boca Raton, Fla: CRC Press; 1990: 43–48.

13. Irwin JA. The pathology of sea sickness. *Lancet*. 1881;ii:907–909.

14. Guedry FE. Conflicting sensory orientation cues as a factor in motion sickness. In: *Fourth Symposium on the Role of the Vestibular Organs in Space Exploration*. Washington DC: National Aeronautics and Space Administration; 1970: 45–52. NASA Report SP-187.

15. Reason JT. Motion sickness: A special case of sensory rearrangement. *Adv Sci*. 1970;26:386–393.

16. Reason JT. Motion sickness adaptation: A neural mismatch model. *J Roy Soc Med*. 1978;71:819–829.

17. Treisman M. Motion sickness: An evolutionary hypothesis. *Science.* 1977;197:493–495.

18. Money KE, Cheung BS. Another function of the inner ear: Facilitation of the emetic response to poisons. *Aviat Space Environ Med.* 1983;54:208–211.

19. Guedry FE. Motion sickness and its relation to some forms of spatial orientation: Mechanisms and theory. In: *Motion Sickness: Significance in Aerospace Operations and Prophylaxis.* Neuilly-sur-Seine, France: Advisory Group for Aerospace Research and Development, North Atlantic Treaty Organization. 1991; Paper 2:1–30. AGARD Lecture Series LS 175.

20. Guedry FE, Benson AJ, Moore HJ. Influence of a visual display and frequency of whole-body angular oscillation on incidence of motion sickness. *Aviat Space Environ Med.* 1982;53:564–569.

21. Benson AJ. Possible mechanisms of motion and space sickness. In: *Life Sciences Research in Space.* Paris, France: European Space Agency; 1977: 101–108. Report SP-130.

22. Benson AJ. Motion sickness. In: Dix MR, Hood JD, eds. *Vertigo.* Chichester, England: John Wiley & Sons, Ltd; 1984: 391–425.

23. Schuknecht HL. Cupulolithiasis. *Arch Otolaryngol.* 1969;90:765–778.

24. Léger A, Money KE, Landolt, JP Cheung BS, Rodden BE. Motion sickness caused by rotations about Earth-horizontal and Earth-vertical axes. *J Appl Physiol.* 1981;50(3):469–477.

25. Guignard JC, McCauley ME. The accelerative stimulus for motion sickness. In: Crampton GH, ed. *Motion and Space Sickness.* Boca Raton, Fla: CRC Press; 1990: 123–152.

26. Griffin MJ. Physical characteristics of stimuli provoking motion sickness. In: *Motion Sickness: Significance in Aerospace Operations and Prophylaxis.* Neuilly-sur-Seine, France: Advisory Group for Aerospace Research and Development, North Atlantic Treaty Organization. 1991; Paper 3:1–32. AGARD Lecture Series 175.

27. Griffin MJ. Sea sickness. In: *Motion Sickness: Significance in Aerospace Operations and Prophylaxis.* Neuilly-sur-Seine, France: Advisory Group for Aerospace Research and Development, North Atlantic Treaty Organization. 1991; Paper 7;1–20. AGARD Lecture Series 175.

28. Stott JRR. Mechanisms and treatment of aviation sickness. In: Davis CJ, Lake-Rakaar GV, Grahame-Smith DG, eds. *Nausea and Vomiting: Mechanisms and Treatment.* Berlin, Germany: Springer-Verlag; 1986: 110–129.

29. Lackner JR, Graybiel A. Elicitation of motion sickness by head movements in the microgravity phase of parabolic flight maneuvers. *Aviat Space Environ Med.* 1984;55:513–520.

30. Melvill Jones G, Rolph R, Downing GH. Comparison of human subjective and oculomotor responses to sinusoidal vertical linear acceleration. *Acta Otolaryngol.* 1980;90:431–440.

31. Lawther A, Griffin MJ. Prediction of the incidence of motion sickness from the magnitude, frequency and duration of vertical oscillation. *J Acoust Soc Am.* 1987;82:957–966.

32. O'Hanlon JF, McCauley ME. Motion sickness incidence as a function of the frequency of vertical sinusoidal motion. *Aerosp Med.* 1974;45:366–369.

33. Golding JF, Harvey HM, Stott JRR. Effects of motion direction, body axis, and posture on motion sickness induced by low frequency linear oscillation. *Aviat Space Environ Med.* 1995;66:1046–1051.

34. Johnson WH, Mayne JW. Stimulus required to produce motion sickness: Restriction of head movements as a preventive of air sickness—Field studies of airborne troops. *J Aviat Med.* 1953;24:400–411.

35. Stott JRR. Prevention and treatment of motion sickness: Non-pharmacological therapy. In: *Motion Sickness:*

Significance in Aerospace Operations and Prophylaxis. Neuilly-sur-Seine, France: Advisory Group for Aerospace Research and Development, North Atlantic Treaty Organization. 1991; Paper 9:1–9. AGARD Lecture Series 175.

36. Miller EF, Graybiel A. The semicircular canals as a primary etiological factor in motion sickness. In: *Fourth Symposium on the Role of the Vestibular Organs in Space Exploration.* Washington DC: National Aeronautics and Space Administration; 1970: 69–82. Report SP-187.

37. Kellog RS, Kennedy RS, Graybiel A. Motion sickness symptomatology of labyrinthine defective and normal subjects during zero gravity maneuvers. *Aerosp Med.* 1965;36:315–318.

38. Shepard NT, Lockette W, Boismier T. Genetic predisposition to motion sickness. *Proc Bárány Soc Meeting.* Uppsala. 1994: 52.

39. Mirabile CS. Motion sickness susceptibility and behavior. In: Crampton GH, ed. *Motion and Space Sickness.* Boca Raton, Fla: CRC Press; 1990: 391–410.

40. Lentz JM, Collins WE. Motion sickness susceptibility and related behavioral characteristics in men and women. *Aviat Space Environ Med.* 1977;48:316–322.

41. Dobie T, McBride D, Dobie T Jr, May J. The effects of age and sex on susceptibility to motion sickness. *Aviat Space Environ Med.* 2001;72:13–20.

42. Davis JR, Vanderploeg JM, Santy PA, Jennings RT, Stewart DF. Space motion sickness during 24 flights of the Space Shuttle. *Aviat Space Environ Med.* 1988;59:1185–1189.

43. Reschke MF. Statistical prediction of space motion sickness. In: Crampton GH, ed. *Motion and Space Sickness.* Boca Raton, Fla: CRC Press; 1990: 263–316.

44. Banta GR, Ridley WC, McHugh J, Grisset JD, Guedry FE. Aerobic fitness and susceptibility to motion sickness. *Aviat Space Environ Med.* 1987;58:105–108.

45. Cheung BSK, Money KE, Jacobs I. Motion sickness susceptibility and aerobic fitness: A longitudinal study. *Aviat Space Environ Med.* 1990;61:201–204.

46. Kennedy RS, Dunlap WP, Fowlkes JE. Prediction of motion sickness susceptibility. In: Crampton GH, ed. *Motion and Space Sickness.* Boca Raton, Fla: CRC Press; 1990: 179-216.

47. Bles W, de Jong HAA, Oosterveld WS. Prediction of seasickness susceptibility. In: *Motion Sickness: Mechanisms, Prediction, Prevention and Treatment.* Neuilly-sur-Seine, France: Advisory Group for Aerospace Research and Development, North Atlantic Treaty Organization. 1984; Paper 27:1-6. AGARD Conference Proceedings 372.

48. Bles W, de Graff B, Bos JE. Vestibular examination in pilots susceptible to motion sickness. In: *The Clinical Basis for Aeromedical Decision Making.* Neuilly-sur-Seine, France: Advisory Group for Aerospace Research and Development, North Atlantic Treaty Organization. 1994; Paper 15:1–8. AGARD Conference Proceedings 553.

49. Reason J, Graybiel A. Factors contributing to motion sickness susceptibility: Adaptability and receptivity. In: *Predictability of Motion Sickness in the Selection of Pilots.* Neuilly-sur-Seine, France: Advisory Group for Aerospace Research and Development, North Atlantic Treaty Organization. 1973; Paper B4:1–15. AGARD Conference Proceedings 109.

50. Tyler DD, Bard P. Motion sickness. *Physiol Rev.* 1949;29:311–369.

51. Zwerling I. Psychological factors in susceptibility to motion sickness. *J Psychol.* 1947;23:219–239.

52. Collins WE, Lentz JM. Some psychological correlates of motion sickness susceptibility. *Aviat Space Environ Med.* 1977;48:587–594.

53. Bard P, Woolsey CN, Snider RS, Mountcastle VB, Bromiley RB. Delimitation of central nervous mechanisms involved in motion sickness. *Fed Proc.* 1947;6:72.

54. Wang SC, Chinn HI. Experimental motion sickness in dogs: Functional importance of chemoceptive emetic trigger zone. *Am J Physiol.* 1954;178:111–116.

55. Miller AD, Wilson VJ. "Vomiting center" reanalyzed: An electrical stimulation study. *Brain Res.* 1983;270:154–158.

56. Wilson VJ, Melvill Jones G. *Mammalian Vestibular Physiology.* New York, NY: Plenum Press; 1979.

57. Lisberger SG, Fuchs AF. Role of primate flocculus during rapid behavioral modification of vestibulo-ocular reflex. *J Neurophysiol.* 1978;41:733–763.

58. Robinson DA. Adaptative gain control of the vestibulo-ocular reflex by the cerebellum. *J Neurophysiol.* 1976;39:954–969.

59. Wolfe JW. Evidence for control of nystagmic habituation by folium-tuber vermis and fastigial nuclei. *Acta Otolaryngol.* 1968;suppl 231:1–48.

60. Kohl RL. Sensory conflict theory of space motion sickness: An anatomical location for the neuroconflict. *Aviat Space Environ Med.* 1983;54:464–465.

61. Money KE, Wood JD. Neural mechanisms underlying the symptomatology of motion sickness. In: *Fourth Symposium on the Role of the Vestibular Organs in Space Exploration.* Washington DC: National Aeronautics and Space Administration; 1970: 69–82. Report SP-187.

62. Crampton GH. Neurophysiology of motion sickness. In: Crampton GH, ed. *Motion and Space Sickness.* Boca Raton, Fla: CRC Press; 1990: 29–42.

63. Borison HL. A misconception of motion sickness leads to false therapeutic expectations. *Aviat Space Environ Med.* 1985;56:66–68.

64. Borison, HL, Wang SC. Functional localization of central coordinating mechanisms for emesis in cat. *J Neurophysiol.* 1949;12:305–313.

65. Brizzee KR. The central nervous connections involved in motion induced emesis. In: Crampton GH, ed. *Motion and Space Sickness.* Boca Raton, Fla: CRC Press; 1990: 9–27.

66. Hixson WC, Guedry FE, Lentz JM. Results of a longitudinal study of air sickness incidence during naval flight officer training. In: *Motion Sickness: Mechanism Prediction, Prevention and Treatment.* Neuilly-sur-Seine, France: Advisory Group for Aerospace Research and Development, North Atlantic Treaty Organization. 1984; Paper 30:1–13. AGARD Conference Proceedings 372.

67. Dobie TG. *Airsickness in Aircrew.* Neuilly-sur-Seine, France: Advisory Group for Aerospace Research and Development, North Atlantic Treaty Organization; 1974. AGARD Report 177.

68. Fox S, Arnon I. Motion sickness and anxiety. *Aviat Space Environ Med.* 1988;59(8):728–733.

69. Geeze DS, Pierson WP. Airsickness in B-52 crew members. *Mil Med.* 1986;151:628–629.

70. Kennedy RS, Moroney WF, Bale RM, Gregoire HG, Smith DG. Motion sickness symptomatology and performance decrements occasioned by hurricane penetrations in C-121, C130 and P-3 Navy aircraft. *Aerosp Med.* 1972;43:1235–1239.

71. Antuñano MJ, Hernandez JM. Incidence of airsickness among military parachutists. *Aviat Space Environ Med.* 1989;60:792–797.

72. Turner M, Griffin MJ, Holland I. Airsickness and aircraft motion during short-haul flights. *Aviat Space Environ Med.* 2000;71:1181–1189.

73. Pethybridge RJ, Davies JW, Walters JD. *A Pilot Study on the Incidence of Seasickness in RN Personnel on Two Ships.* Alverstoke, Hants, England: Institute of Naval Medicine; 1978. Report 55/78.

74. Rolnick A, Gordon CR. The effects of motion induced sickness on military performance. In: Gal R, Mangelsdorff AD, eds. *Handbook of Military Psychology.* Chichester, England: John Wiley & Sons; 1991: 279–293.

75. Brand JJ, Colquhoun WP, Perry WLM. Side effects of *l*-hyoscine and cyclizine studied by objective tests. *Aerosp Med.* 1968;39:999–1002.

76. Landolt JP, Light IM, Greenen MNI, Monaco C. Seasickness in totally enclosed motor propelled survival craft: Five offshore oil rig disasters. *Aviat Space Environ Med.* 1992;63:138–144.

77. Kennedy RS, Hettinger LJ, Lilienthal MG. Simulator sickness. In: Crampton GH, ed. *Motion and Space Sickness.* Boca Raton, Fla: CRC Press; 1990: 317–342.

78. Kennedy RS, Lilienthal MG, Berbaum KS, Baltzley DR, McCauley ME. *Symptomatology of Simulator Sickness in 10 US Navy Flight Simulators.* Orlando, Fla: Naval Systems Training Center. 1988. Report NTSC-TR-87-008.

79. Kennedy RS, Berbaum KS, Lilienthal MG, Dunlap WP, Mulligan BE, Funaro JF. *Guidelines for Alleviation of Simulator Sickness Symptomatology.* Orlando, Fla: Naval Systems Training Center. 1987. Report NTSC-TR-87-007.

80. Regan EC, Price KR. The frequency of occurrence and severity of side effects of immersion virtual reality. *Aviat Space Environ Med.* 1994;65:527–530.

81. Homick JL, Reschke ME, Vanderploeg JM. Space adaptation syndrome: Incidence and operational implications for the space transportation system program. In: *Motion Sickness: Mechanism Prediction, Prevention and Treatment.* Neuilly-sur-Seine, France: Advisory Group for Aerospace Research and Development, North Atlantic Treaty Organization. 1984; Paper 36:1–6. AGARD Conference Proceedings 372.

82. Oman CM, Lichtenberg BK, Money KE. Symptoms and signs of space motion sickness on Spacelab 1. In: Crampton GH, ed. *Motion and Space Sickness.* Boca Raton, Fla: CRC Press; 1990: 217–246.

83. Turner M. Driven to sickness? The effect of individual driving style on motion sickness occurrence. *Proceedings of the UK Informal Group Meeting on Human Response to Vibration.* 19–21 Sep 1994. Alverstoke, Hants, England: Institute of Naval Medicine; 1994: 1–13.

84. Hettinger, LJ, Kennedy RS, McCauley ME. Motion sickness and human performance. In: Crampton GH, ed. *Motion and Space Sickness.* Boca Raton, Fla: CRC Press; 1990: 411–441.

85. French, US, and Belgian air force data. Quoted by: Léger A. Signification opérationnelle des cinétoses pour l'air, l'espace et la survie en mer. In: *Motion Sickness: Significance in Aerospace Operations and Prophylaxis.* Neuilly-sur-Seine, France: Advisory Group for Aerospace Research and Development, North Atlantic Treaty Organization. 1991; Paper 4:1-8. AGARD Lecture Series LS 175.

86. Crowley JS. Simulator sickness: A problem for army aviation. *Aviat Space Environ Med.* 1987;58:355–357.

87. Oman CM, Lichtenberg BK, Money KE, McCoy RK. MIT/Canadian vestibular experiments on the Spacelab 1 Mission 4: Space motion sickness: Symptoms, stimuli and predictability. *Exp Brain Res.* 1986;64:316-334.

88. Dowd, PJ. Resistance to motion sickness through repeated exposure to Coriolis stimulation. *Aerosp Med.* 1965;36:452–455.

89. Bagshaw M, Stott JRR. The desensitization of chronically motion sick aircrew in the Royal Air Force. *Aviat Space Environ Med.* 1985;56:1144–1151.

90. Dobie TG, May JG. Cognitive-behavioral management of motion sickness. *Aviat Space Environ Med*. 1994;65(10 pt 2):C1–2. Review.

91. Cowings P, Toscano WB. The relationship of motion sickness susceptibility to learned autonomic control for symptom suppression. *Aviat Space Environ Med*. 1982;53:570–575.

92. Stott JRR. Adaptation to nauseogenic motion stimuli and its application in the treatment of airsickness. In: Crampton GH, ed. *Motion and Space Sickness*. Boca Raton, Fla: CRC Press; 1990: 373–390.

93. Jones DR, Levy RA, Gardner L, Marsh RW, Patterson JC. Self-control of psychophysiologic response to motion stress: Using biofeedback to treat airsickness. *Aviat Space Environ Med*. 1985;56:1152–1157.

94. Bruce DG, Golding JF, Hockenhull N, Pethybridge RJ. Acupressure and motion sickness. *Aviat Space Environ Med*. 1990;61:361–365.

95. Uijtdehaage SHJ, Salsgiver PJ, Stern RM, Koch KL. Acupressure fails to relieve symptoms of vection-induced motion sickness. Quoted by: Stott JRR. Prevention and treatment of motion sickness: Non-pharmacological therapy. In: *Motion Sickness: Significance in Aerospace Operations and Prophylaxis*. Neuilly-sur-Seine, France: Advisory Group for Aerospace Research and Development, North Atlantic Treaty Organization. 1991; Paper 9:1–9. AGARD Lecture Series 175.

96. Hu S, Stritzel R, Chandler A, Stern RM. P6 Acupressure reduces symptoms of vection-induced motion sickness. *Aviat Space Environ Med*. 1995;66:631–634.

97. Bertolucci LE, Didario B. Efficacy of a portable acustimulation device in controlling seasickness. *Aviat Space Environ Med*. 1995;66:1155–1158.

98. Graybiel A, Wood CD, Knepton J, Hoche JP, Perkins GF. Human assay of anti–motion sickness drugs. *Aviat Space Environ Med*. 1975;46:1107–1118.

99. Wood CD. Pharmacological countermeasures against motion sickness. In: Crampton GH, ed. *Motion and Space Sickness*. Boca Raton, Fla: CRC Press; 1990: 343–352.

100. Stott JRR. Management of acute and chronic motion sickness. In: *Motion Sickness: Significance in Aerospace Operations and Prophylaxis*. Neuilly-sur-Seine, France: Advisory Group for Aerospace Research and Development, North Atlantic Treaty Organization. 1991; Paper 11:1–7. AGARD Lecture Series LS 175.

101. Stott JRR, Golding JF. The effect of a selective muscarinic receptor antagonist and scopolamine on motion sickness, skin conductance and heart rate in humans. *J Physiol*. 1994;476:47P.

102. Lucot JB, van Charldorp KJ, Tulp MTM. Idaverine, an M_2- vs M_3-selective muscarinic antagonist, does not prevent motion sickness in cats. *Pharmacol Biochem Behav*. 1991;40:345–349.

103. Mitchelson E. Pharmacological agents affecting emesis, I: A review. *Drugs*. 1992;43:295–315.

104. Mitchelson E. Pharmacological agents affecting emesis, II: A review. *Drugs*. 1992;43:443–463.

105. Wood CD, Graybiel A. Evaluation of sixteen anti–motion sickness drugs under controlled laboratory conditions. *Aerosp Med*. 1968;39:1341–1344.

106. Chelen W, Kabrisky M, Hatsell C, Morales R, Fix E, Scott M. Use of phenytoin in the prevention of motion sickness. *Aviat Space Environ Med*. 1990;61:1022–1025.

107. Woodward D, Knox G, Myers J, Chelen W, Ferguson B. Phenytoin as a countermeasure for motion sickness in NASA maritime operations. *Aviat Space Environ Med*. 1993;64:363–366.

108. Stern RM, Uijtdehaage SHJ, Muth ER, Koch KL. Effects of phenytoin on vection-induced motion sickness and

gastric myoelectric activity. *Aviat Space Environ Med*. 1994;65:518–521.

109. Golding JF, Gosden E, Gerrel J. Scopolamine blood levels following buccal versus ingested tablets. *Aviat Space Environ Med*. 1991;62(6):521–526.

110. Norfleet WT, Degionni JJ, Calkins DS, et al. Treatment of motion sickness in parabolic flight with buccal scopolamine. *Aviat Space Environ Med*. 1992;63:46–51.

Chapter 36

PROTECTIVE UNIFORMS FOR NUCLEAR, BIOLOGICAL, AND CHEMICAL WARFARE: METABOLIC, THERMAL, RESPIRATORY, AND PSYCHOLOGICAL ISSUES

STEPHEN R. MUZA, PhD[*]; LOUIS E. BANDERET, PhD[†]; AND BRUCE CADARETTE, MS[‡]

[*]Research Physiologist, Thermal and Mountain Medicine Division
[†]Research Psychologist, Military Performance Division
[‡]Research Physiologist, Thermal and Mountain Medicine Division, US Army Research Institute of Environmental Medicine, Natick, Massachusetts 01760-5007

INTRODUCTION

Protective uniforms, in the broadest definition, describes every item of clothing or equipment worn by humans for protection from natural and man-made environments. Although clothing is an essential item for everyday human survival, the term protective uniform is usually reserved to describe individually worn garments and equipment designed to protect the wearer from extraordinary natural or man-made environmental extremes. In both military and civilian occupations, protective uniforms are routinely used to sustain the health and well-being of personnel performing activities in environments that pose hazards to human health. Protective uniforms fall into the following six general categories, each characterized by the nature of the hazard the uniform protects against:

1. cold weather (extreme cold weather clothing systems),
2. thermal, heat, and open flame (firefighting),
3. hazardous chemical agents, biological agents, or both (chemical–biological warfare, hazardous material cleanup),
4. ionizing radiation (nuclear power facilities, nuclear weapon fallout),
5. low-oxygen environments (aircrews, astronauts), and
6. ballistic projectiles (military operations, explosive ordinance disposal, law enforcement).

In each application, the protective uniform is designed to shield or isolate the user from specific hazards in the environment. Protective uniforms frequently encapsulate the wearer, creating a microenvironment within the uniform. Consequently, when wearing a protective uniform, the external environment, the nature of the barrier produced by the protective uniform, and the microenvironment within the uniform all contribute to the individual's physiological and psychological responses.

From the earliest days of warfare, combatants have used chemical and biological weapons against their opponents.[1] On the modern battlefield a soldier may be confronted with a wide array of chemical and biological weapons, as well as residual radioactivity from the detonation of nuclear weapons. Personal protection from these weapons requires that the soldier be isolated from the contaminated environment. This can be in the form of sealed shelters providing collective protection for small military units or via use of individual protective uniforms. Because the most widely used protective uniform in the military is for protection against nuclear, chemical, and biological weapons, this chapter focuses on that category of protective uniforms. Additional information about and illustrations of many of the protective items mentioned here are found in Chapter 16, Chemical Defense Equipment, and in particular its attachment, Psychological Problems Associated With Wearing Mission-Oriented Protective Posture Gear, in *Medical Aspects of Chemical and Biological Warfare,* another volume in the *Textbook of Military Medicine* series.[2]

The US Army refers to fighting on a battlefield on which nuclear–biological–chemical (NBC) hazards are present as *NBC operations.* To protect against these hazards, NBC protective garments (clothing, gloves, boots) and equipment (the mask) form a barrier between the user and the contaminated environment. However, the wearing of NBC protective clothing is accompanied by degradation in the performance of military operations.[3,4] The magnitude of the performance decrement depends on a complex interaction of human, mission (eg, uniform, equipment, and task), and environmental factors. In general, all protective uniforms increase the energy costs of performing work and impair the following human functions: biomechanics, thermal regulation, respiration, sensory perception, communications, eating and drinking, elimination of body wastes, and sleep. In concert, these stresses on physiological and psychological function degrade work performance and mission effectiveness. This chapter reviews these factors and discusses how they can impair the soldier's ability to perform military tasks and possible countermeasures to sustain performance.

PROTECTIVE UNIFORMS

Most modern NBC protective uniforms for combatants comprise five items:

1. a one- or two-piece overgarment that covers the torso and extremities,
2. overboots,
3. rubber gloves,
4. hood, and
5. a full-facial respiratory protective device, usually called a chemical–biological (CB) mask.

Depending on the environmental and operational situations, NBC overgarments may or may not be worn over the standard issue military utility uniform (ie, the combat fatigue, also called the battledress uniform, BDU) or other specialized uniforms (eg, flight suits). Protection against ballistic weapons or blunt impact is afforded by various styles of body armor and helmets. Although not considered part of the NBC protective uniform ensemble, body armor interacts with the protective uniform in a manner that may impair work performance. In the US military, the various levels of protection afforded by the NBC protective uniform are referred to as mission-oriented protective posture (MOPP), which has seven commonly encountered levels (Table 36-1). The concept behind MOPP levels is that the degree of NBC protection can be adjusted to the type and magnitude of the NBC threat. Furthermore, because the impairment of work performance increases with the degree of encapsulation, working in an intermediate MOPP level affords some NBC protection with less impairment of work performance.[5]

The current NBC protective uniform system provided to US military personnel is the battledress overgarment (BDO) with CB mask.[6] The BDO is a camouflaged, two-piece garment made with a nylon-and-cotton shell and an inner layer of charcoal-impregnated polyurethane foam. Drawstrings seal the BDO coat over the waist of the BDO trousers

(Figure 36-1). The wearer's feet are protected by vinyl overboots, the hands by butyl rubber gloves with cotton liners; the face is covered by the CB mask, and the scalp and neck by an attached butyl rubber hood. The BDO is engineered to protect the user from field concentrations of liquid, aerosol, and vapor chemical–biological warfare agents. The BDO protects through a combination of repelling an agent at the garment's surface, and absorbing and encapsulating the agent in an activated charcoal barrier. In environments where chemical or biological agents may exceed field concentrations, specialized protective uniforms, such as the Self-Contained Toxicological Protective Outfit (STEPO), which provides greater protection, may be used. The STEPO is a completely encapsulating, one-piece, protective garment, which can be worn for toxic chemical cleanup or by explosive ordnance disposal teams when chemical munitions are present. In situations where the NBC threat is low but still present, a chemical protective undergarment containing a charcoal layer worn under the BDU may provide a limited level of protection.[7–9]

Because the respiratory system's airways and lungs present the largest surface area of the body to the environment, inhalation is the most advantageous route for introducing NBC agents into the body. The CB mask is designed to protect the respiratory system, eyes, and face from NBC threats. In combination with a hood, it also protects the scalp, ears, and neck. Externally, a CB mask consists of a

TABLE 36-1

US ARMY CLASSIFICATION OF NUCLEAR–BIOLOGICAL–CHEMICAL PROTECTIVE UNIFORM ENSEMBLES[*]

NBC Protective Uniform Components	MOPP Ready	MOPP 0	MOPP 1	MOPP 2	MOPP 3	MOPP 4	Mask Only
CB Mask	Carried	Carried	Carried	Carried	Worn[†]	Worn	Worn
Overgarment	Ready	Available	Worn[†]	Worn[†]	Worn[†]	Worn	—
Vinyl Overboots	Ready	Available	Available	Worn	Worn	Worn	—
Gloves	Ready	Available	Available	Available	Available	Worn	—
Helmet Protective Cover	Ready	Available	Available	Worn	Worn	Worn	—
Chemical Protective Undergarment	Ready	Available	Worn[‡]	Worn[‡]	Worn[‡]	Worn[‡]	—

CB: chemical–biological; MOPP: mission-oriented protective posture
[*]Based on level of threat and degree of MOPP gear required
[†]In hot weather, coat or hood can be left open for ventilation
[‡]Chemical protective undergarment is worn under the battledress uniform, coveralls, and flight suit
Reproduced from US Department of the Army. *NBC Protection*. Washington, DC: DA; 1992: 2-4. Army Field Manual 3-4.

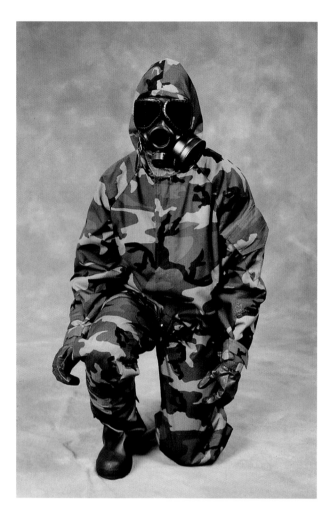

Fig. 36-1. A modern military nuclear, biological, and chemical (NBC) protective uniform (US Military Joint Service Lightweight Integrated Suit Technology Program, called the JSLIST). Note the total encapsulation of the individual at MOPP 4 (mission-oriented protective posture, level 4). From top to bottom, the NBC uniform components are the hood, US Army M40 Field Chemical–Biological (CB) protective mask, overgarment coat, overgarment trousers, rubber gloves, and vinyl overboots. Photograph: Courtesy of US Army Soldiers System Center, Natick, Mass.

facepiece and head harness, usually constructed of silicone rubber; transparent eyelenses; one or more voicemitters for transmitting the user's voice; one or more filter cartridges or a hose supplying filtered air; and a drinking tube, which allows the soldier to drink while wearing the mask (Figure 36-2). Internally, the CB mask is fitted with a nosecup, which isolates the oral and nasal openings from the eyes and eyelenses. Inlet and outlet valves on the nosecup direct filtered air into the respiratory system and prevent moist, exhaled air from flowing across the eyelenses and fogging them in cold weather.[10]

The standard NBC filter canister is designed to protect the user from field concentrations of CB agents and radioactive particles. The filter canister contains materials that capture and hold airborne particles, aerosols, and vapors. The filter does not alter the concentration of the atmospheric gases (oxygen, carbon dioxide, nitrogen) and does not absorb carbon monoxide gas. Thus, the standard military CB mask does not provide supplemental oxygen to sustain life in low-oxygen environments or protect against carbon monoxide poisoning. Typical construction materials include a high-efficiency particulate air (HEPA) filter made of either paper or glass wool, or both, to capture aerosols and particles, and activated (Whetlerized) charcoal to absorb organic compounds. With this filtering type of CB mask, soldiers must increase their breathing efforts to inhale air through the CB mask's filters and inspiratory ports.

In crew-served vehicles, a similar CB mask is frequently used, one that is supplied by a vehicle-powered blower with filtered air, thus alleviating the need for the wearer to generate airflow across the NBC filter. Vehicle-powered air blowers generally provide approximately 3 cu ft/min of filtered air to each crew member and are usually part of a vehicle-supplied microclimate cooling system, which also alleviates heat stress. Air-supplied CB masks may also be used aboard naval vessels, aircraft, and by ground-support vehicles that service civil engineering units that are performing repairs to airfield runways, roads, and bridges. The major limitation to the use of air-supplied CB masks is the availability of power for the blower motor; the uncertain power requirements limits the portability of air blowers and constrains the excursions of service personnel using such systems to the length of the umbilical line from the power source.

The NBC filters used in most current military CB masks present some potential problems to the user. Added resistance to airflow is the most significant problem, requiring increased breathing effort and producing various adverse respiratory sensations (ie, breathlessness). These filters occasionally produce ammonia, particularly in humid environments, which causes stinging, burning, and tightness of the chest that is only relieved when the wearer removes the CB mask. Also, inhalaion of the friable carbon is a possibility. Inhalation may produce deleterious health effects because Whetlerized carbon may contain copper, chromium, and silver, in addition to CB agent–contaminated carbon. Future NBC filters may avoid these potential problems by using zeolites and clathrate-like sorbents, which would capture organic agents by forming a cage around the toxic molecule.

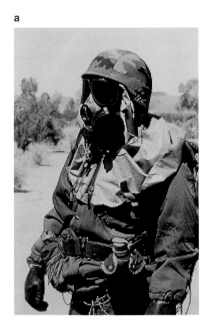
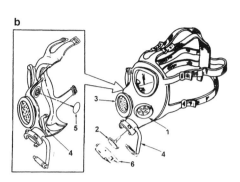
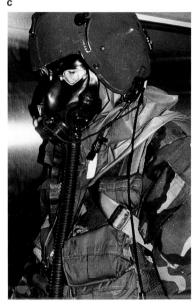

Fig. 36-2. (a) The soldier is wearing a US Army M40 Field Chemical–Biological (CB) protective mask with hood. **(b)** Mounted into the interior and exterior of the CB mask facepiece are (1) the inlet valve and filter canister connection, (2) the outlet valve, (3) the voicemitter, (4) the drinking tube, (5) the nosecup inlet valve, and (6) the outlet valve cover. **(c)** The pilot is wearing a US Army M43 Chemical–Biological (CB) mask and hood under the HGU-56p aviator helmet. The nuclear–biological–chemical (NBC) filter assembly is located near the pilot's waist. Note that the mask and eyepieces are contoured to interface with helmet-mounted heads-up displays. Photograph a: Courtesy of US Army Research Institute of Environmental Medicine, Natick, Mass. Drawing b: Department of the Army. *Operator's Manual for Chemical–Biological Mask: Field, M40.* Washington, DC: Headquarters, DA; June 1988: 2-2. Photograph c: Courtesy of US Army Aeromedical Research Laboratory, Fort Rucker, Ala.

BIOMEDICAL ASPECTS

Metabolic and Biomechanical Responses

Military occupational tasks can require a wide range of metabolic intensities, from slightly greater than rest to near maximal exercise. Many military tasks are physically demanding (see the Department of the Army's *Soldier's Manual of Common Tasks*[11] and *Military Occupational Specialties*,[12] both of which contain the Physical Task List). The wear and carriage of clothing, load carriage devices, and personal mission-related equipment all contribute to increasing the metabolic requirements of a work task. Several studies[13–16] have addressed the metabolic responses to multilayered garments. Routinely, NBC uniforms are worn over the service member's standard work uniform (ie, utility fatigue, BDU, aviator flight suit, or armored vehicle crew jumpsuit), creating a multilayered uniform.

Metabolic Rate Responses

Early studies of multilayered uniforms focused on cold weather garments. These studies found that the increase in metabolic rate for a given task was greater than would be predicted by the added weight of the garments alone, for which three possible explanations were proposed: increased weight on the extremities, hobbling, and friction between clothing layers.[13,14] It is well known that carrying a given weight on the hands or feet increases metabolic rate more than carrying that same weight on the torso.[17] However, only a small portion of the increased energy cost associated with wearing multilayer clothing is attributed to additional weight on the extremities.[13] This leaves hobbling and friction between clothing layers as the most likely explanations for increased metabolic rate when wearing multilayer clothing systems. Hobbling is the interference with joint movement caused by the bulkiness of the multilayer uniform. The friction produced between the clothing layers, which restricts body motion and increases the muscular force needed to accomplish a given body motion, contributes to the hobbling effect.[13,14] The change in center of gravity caused by the weight of the uniform may also contribute to the hobbling effect.[14]

Although early studies identified and measured the effect that multilayer arctic clothing ensembles have on energy costs, in general, extrapolation of these findings to all multilayer clothing ensembles is limited because only the bulkiest uniforms—arctic clothing—were studied, and energy costs were measured over a relatively narrow speed range of treadmill walking.

Two studies[15,16] evaluated the effect of NBC uniforms on energy costs of various tasks. One study[15] reported that wearing an NBC uniform (in the United Kingdom) increased the energy cost of a simple stepping task by approximately 9%. The authors estimated that each layer of clothing contributed 3% to 4% to the increased metabolic cost of the stepping task, even after they had accounted for the increased weight of the clothing.[15] A comprehensive study of the energy costs associated with performing a wide range of military occupational tasks in an NBC uniform was reported by Patton and associates.[16] Forty-two physical tasks were selected from the US Army's *Soldier's Manual of Common Tasks*[11] and the Physical Task List contained in AR 611-201, *Military Occupational Specialties*.[12] The physiological and perceptual responses of the test volunteers who performed each task were compared between the BDU and an NBC uniform (the BDO worn over the BDU; see Table 36-1). This study also evaluated the effects of gender on the physiological and perceptual responses on task performance in 36 of 42 tasks while wearing the NBC uniform.[16] The key findings of this study relating to energy expenditure are summarized in Table 36-2.

Patton and associates[16] found that wearing the NBC uniform over the BDU increased metabolic energy costs by more than 5% in 69% of the tasks performed by men and in 64% of the tasks performed by women. As the metabolic cost of a task increased (light to moderate to heavy), the effect of the NBC uniform on energy expenditure was greater. Furthermore, the effect of the NBC uniform on energy costs was larger in tasks requiring greater mobility (ie, load carriage). Although women worked at a greater percentage of their maximal oxygen uptakes ($\dot{V}O_2$max), the effect of the NBC uniform on energy cost was generally similar in men and women. The only gender difference noted was that women demonstrated a greater increase in metabolic costs in NBC uniforms in tasks requiring continuous mobility. The authors speculated that the hobbling effect of the NBC uniform may be greater in women than men due to women's smaller stature and weight. Consequently, the additional weight of the NBC uniform seems to impose a greater strain on women compared with men. A further possible explanation, not presented by the authors, is that the NBC uniforms may not have been sized and fitted appropriately to the female body.

TABLE 36-2

EFFECT OF WEARING THE NUCLEAR-BIOLOGICAL-CHEMICAL PROTECTIVE UNIFORM ON ENERGY COSTS OF VARIOUS MILITARY TASKS

Task Category	Men		Women	
	$\Delta\dot{V}O_2$	$\Delta\%$	$\Delta\dot{V}O_2$	$\Delta\%$
Light (< 325 W)	0.055 ± 0.011	8.1	0.041 ± 0.008	8.7
Moderate (325–500 W)	0.134 ± 0.022	12.6	0.145 ± 0.021	16.0
Heavy (> 500 W)	0.215 ± 0.019	11.3	0.183 ± 0.029	12.7
Stationary	0.051 ± 0.017	6.8	0.048 ± 0.011	7.8
Intermittent	0.108 ± 0.024	9.0	0.089 ± 0.015	10.1
Continuous	0.218 ± 0.017	14.3	0.202 ± 0.026	17.0

Mean ± SD increase in $\dot{V}O_2$ (L/min and percentage) between basic US Army battledress uniform, BDU (MOPP 0) and complete nuclear–biological–chemical (NBC) protective ensemble worn over the BDU (MOPP 4), by task category.
Task categories Stationary, Intermittent, and Continuous are based on the degree of whole-body mobility over a distance. Stationary: lift/lower tasks; Intermittent: lift/carry tasks; Continuous: load carriage tasks.
Adapted from Patton JF, Murphy M, Bidwell T, Mello R, Harp M. *Metabolic Cost of Military Physical Tasks in MOPP 0 and MOPP 4*. Natick, Mass: US Army Research Institute of Environmental Medicine; 1995: 21, 23. USARIEM Technical Report T95-9.

No study to date has attempted to address the contribution of each NBC uniform component (eg, gloves, overboots, overgarments) to the overall increase in energy cost. The finding that the NBC uniforms' greatest effect on metabolic cost was on tasks requiring mobility suggests that motion of the lower extremities was most hindered by the NBC uniform. Casual observations by various investigators suggest that loose-fitting overboots may be a significant source of increased energy cost with NBC uniforms. Without significantly altering the weight on the feet, an inappropriately large overboot may reduce traction, alter gait, or both, thus exacerbating the hobbling effect of the uniform.

Biomechanical Effects of NBC Uniforms

In addition to the increased energy costs of performing various tasks, the NBC protective uniform generally restricts the range of motion of the torso, head, and extremities.[18] Activities such as walking, running, dodging, and jumping are perceived to be more cumbersome in the NBC protective uniform. The US military NBC protective uniform can restrict head flexion as much as 20% in the ventral–dorsal plane and lateral rotation of the head by as much as 40% to 50%.[18,19] Such restrictions of head movements, caused principally by the CB mask, limit a soldier's normal visual scan; hence, more pronounced head movements are required to view the environment and to localize sound.[20]

Unfortunately, NBC protective uniforms also degrade manual dexterity, psychomotor coordination, and performance of many activities accomplished with the hands.[21] The rubber gloves distort the tactile sensations of various tools, equipment controls, keysets, and grip handles. Finger dexterity can be affected by as much as 30%, depending on the thickness of the gloves. Soldiers wearing thicker (0.44-mm) gloves required more time to accomplish simple keying tasks accurately.[22] Finger dexterity and visual–motor coordination degrade slightly by wearing the rubber handwear and mask.[18,23] Military pilots, keenly aware of the importance of tactile sensations from flight controls, are reluctant to wear the bulky gloves when flying an aircraft.[20]

In summary, several studies indicate that wearing NBC uniforms over a standard work uniform increases the metabolic cost of performing physical tasks, and that the increased energy costs are greatest in tasks requiring mobility. The potential for the hobbling effect and friction between cloth-ing layers of NBC uniforms to increase metabolic costs of military tasks underscores the importance of fitting service members with properly sized NBC garments and boots to minimize the increased energy costs associated with wearing these uniforms.

Thermoregulatory Responses

Heat stress is a major limitation to work performance and tolerance in NBC uniforms.[24–30] Aside from the fact that the protective uniform is significantly responsible for the thermal load on the wearer, the subsequent thermoregulatory responses and consequences of the heat strain are not unique to protective uniforms. Therefore, only aspects of managing heat stress directly attributable to work in NBC protective uniforms are addressed here.

As described earlier, to protect the wearer from a contaminated environment, the NBC protective uniform must provide a barrier between the wearer and that environment. This barrier creates a microclimate around the surface of the individual encapsulated in the NBC protective uniform. NBC protective uniforms have high insulating and low moisture permeability properties (Figure 36-3). The insulating property of a garment is measured by the *resistance* (Rc) to dry heat flow (conduction, convection, radiation), expressed in clo units (Equation 1):

$$(1) \qquad 1 \text{ clo} = 0.155°C \bullet m^2/W$$

The moisture permeability of a garment, also called the *evaporative resistance* (Re), is expressed as a ratio of the permeability index (Im) to the insulation (clo). The higher the evaporative resistance (Im/clo), the more potential a garment has for evaporative heat loss. When fully encapsulated in the US Army BDO, this NBC protective uniform has particularly low moisture permeability. Of particular note are the additive properties of an NBC uniform worn over the BDU, probably due to the air layers trapped between the garments. For example, compared with the complete NBC ensemble worn over a standard BDU, wearing the NBC uniform over only cotton underwear reduces the Rc by approximately 30% and increases the Re by approximately 3-fold. Several studies[7–9] have shown that wearing close-fitting NBC overgarments, thereby eliminating multiple air layers, would lower thermal insulation and increase moisture permeability, thus reducing heat strain.

The degree of thermal stress experienced when wearing an NBC protective uniform depends on the

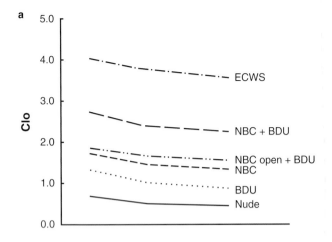

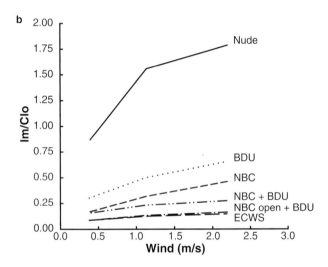

Fig. 36-3. Insulative (**a**) and moisture permeability (**b**) characteristics of a typical nuclear–biological–chemical (NBC) protective uniform and several representative military clothing ensembles. BDU: US Army battledress uniform; NBC open (ie, jacket unbuttoned) + BDU: open NBC overgarment worn over BDU; NBC + BDU: closed (ie, jacket buttoned) NBC uniform worn over BDU; ECWCS: extreme cold weather clothing system. Data sources: (1) Gonzales RR, Endrusick TL, Santee WR. Thermoregulatory responses to cold: Effects of handwear with multi-layer clothing. *J Appl Physiol.* 1998;69:1076–1082. (2) Gonzalez RR, Levell CA, Stroschein LA, Gonzalez JA, Pandolf KB. *Copper Manikin and Heat Strain Model Evaluations of Chemical Protective Ensembles for the Technical Cooperation Program.* Natick, Mass: US Army Research Institute of Environmental Medicine; 1993. USARIEM Technical Report T94-4.

environmental conditions (air temperature, humidity, radiant energy, and air velocity) and the rate of metabolic heat production. However, given the NBC uniform's resistance to heat dissipation, the most sig-

nificant factor determining the microclimate environment, and thus the thermal load on the service member, is the rate of metabolic heat production.[24,30] When the rate of metabolic heat production exceeds the rate of heat dissipation, metabolic heat is stored and body temperature rises (Figure 36-4). Generally, a cool, dry, ambient environment will facilitate metabolic heat dissipation at light physical work rates, and to a lesser degree as metabolic rate increases.[30] A simple way to assess the impact of ambient thermal conditions on physical activity in NBC uniforms is to use the wet bulb globe temperature (WBGT) index.[31] As a rule of thumb, wearing NBC protective uniforms adds approximately 10°F to the measured WBGT.[31] However, this recommended adjustment is based on field observations of physical work performance, not body heat storage.[32] Thus, adjusting the WBGT when wearing NBC uniforms should be done cautiously: although Technical Bulletin, Medical 507[31] states that the same approximately 10°F adjustment to the measured WBGT is applicable when wearing body armor, the actual adjustment is approximately 5°F.[32]

Because of the low moisture permeability of the NBC uniform, vapor loss from the skin (sweating) condenses on the skin and the internal surfaces of the protective uniform. Consequently, evaporative heat loss is greatly reduced, resulting in uncompensable heat stress.[28] Several options for reducing heat stress, and subsequently heat illness, in NBC protective uniforms have been suggested,[5,33] including (1) reduce the barrier by wearing the minimal level of protective clothing appropriate to the NBC threat, (2) reduce metabolic heat production, and (3) cool the microclimate by mechanical means. Owing to the power requirements of microclimate cooling systems, this manner of heat stress reduction is currently limited to crew-served vehicles and aircraft.

Military doctrine[5] provides commanders with methods for assessing the degree of NBC threat and determining the appropriate levels of protection. Minimizing the number of uniform layers or allowing service personnel to wear NBC uniforms open, or both, significantly enhance heat dissipation, thus increasing work capacity (see Figure 36-3). If the NBC threat requires total encapsulation within an NBC uniform, commanders can reduce heat casualties by employing mission-compatible preventive measures and medical support.

Because metabolic heat production is the main source of thermal stress in NBC uniforms, reducing metabolic intensity is the single most effective way of reducing heat illness in protective uniforms. The options are to work at a given metabolic inten-

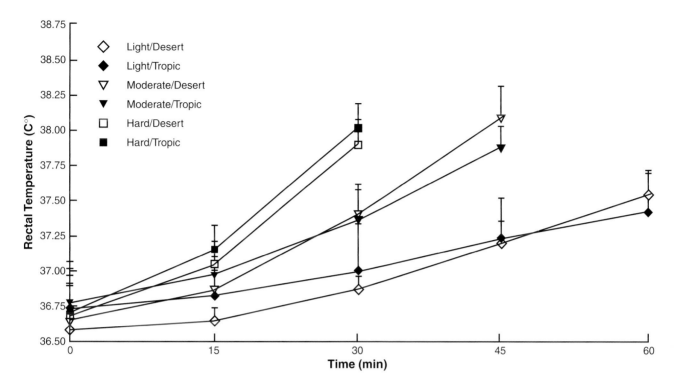

Fig. 36-4. Core body temperature response to physical work (light, ~ 300 W; moderate, ~ 430 W; and hard, ~ 600 W) in a nuclear–biological–chemical (NBC) protective uniform at MOPP 4 (mission-oriented protective posture, level 4) worn over cotton undergarments in desert (43°C, 20% rh) and tropic (35°C, 50% rh) environments. Note that when wearing the NBC protective uniform, core body temperature depends more on work rate than on ambient environmental conditions. Reproduced from Cadarette BS, Montain SJ, Kolka MA, Stroschein LA, Matthew WT, Sawka MN. *Evaluation of USARIEM Heat Strain Model: MOPP Level, Exercise Intensity in Desert and Tropic Climates.* Natick, Mass: US Army Research Institution of Environmental Medicine; 1996: 37. USARIEM Technical Report T96-4.

sity until exhaustion from heat strain occurs, or to decrease metabolic heat load by reducing work intensity and/or using rest periods to lower the time averaged metabolic rate. The use of work/rest cycles will increase tolerance times and decrease heat casualties, but the time required to perform a task will be increased. Using the prediction capability of the USARIEM Heat Strain Model,[34–36] the maximum single work period and work/rest cycle periods have been developed for a wide range of environmental conditions and work intensities. Tables 36-3 and 36-4[33] present maximum single work periods and work/rest cycles for a matrix of climatic conditions during daylight and nighttime operations.

The calculated work periods assume that the troops are fully hydrated, rested, and heat acclimatized, and that fewer than 5% heat casualties will result.[33] Adequate hydration is particularly difficult to achieve in NBC protective uniforms, given the barrier presented by the CB mask. Although most modern CB

masks have drinking tubes, they are cumbersome to use, and taking a drink requires expenditure of energy and time. Thus, if hypohydration is suspected, the work periods given in Tables 36-3 and 36-4 should be reduced.

For aircrews and other manned vehicles with clear canopies that expose the crew compartment to high radiant heat loads (the greenhouse effect), heat dissipation may not be possible even when metabolic heat production is low. The thermal strain is greatest when the aircraft is motionless on the ground and its onboard environmental control systems are shut down or at lower efficiency.[37–39] Typically, aircraft cockpits become cooler as the aircraft ascends into the lower temperatures of higher altitudes or cockpit ventilation is improved by the aircraft's forward motion. However, when wearing an aviator NBC protective uniform, body temperature may remain elevated for a long time after takeoff. This may cause crew performance decrements as well as diminished acceleration (G) tolerance.[38–40]

TABLE 36-3
WORK TIMES IN NUCLEAR-CHEMICAL-BIOLOGICAL PROTECTIVE UNIFORMS DURING DAYLIGHT OPERATIONS*

| WBGT (°F) | Ta | Maximum Single Work Period (minutes) | | | | | | | | Work/Rest Cycle (minutes of work per hour) | | | | | | | |
| | | NBC Uniform + Underwear | | | | NBC Uniform + BDU | | | | NBC Uniform + Underwear | | | | NBC Uniform + BDU | | | |
		VL	L	M	H	VL	L	M	H	VL	L	M	H	VL	L	M	H
78	82	NL	177	50	33	NL	155	49	32	NL	30	10	5	NL	25	10	5
80	84	NL	142	49	32	NL	131	48	32	NL	25	10	na	NL	20	10	na
82	87	NL	115	47	31	NL	110	46	30	NL	20	5	na	NL	15	na	na
84	89	NL	104	45	30	NL	100	45	30	NL	na	na	na	NL	na	na	na
86	91	NL	95	44	29	NL	93	44	29	NL	na	na	na	NL	na	na	na
88	94	NL	85	42	28	NL	83	42	27	NL	na	na	na	NL	na	na	na
90	96	NL	79	41	27	NL	78	41	27	NL	na	na	na	NL	na	na	na
92	98	NL	75	40	26	NL	74	40	26	NL	na	na	na	NL	na	na	na
94	100	NL	70	39	25	NL	70	39	25	NL	na	na	na	NL	na	na	na
96	103	203	65	37	23	194	65	37	23	na	na	na	na	na	na	na	na
98	105	141	62	36	22	140	62	36	22	na	na	na	na	na	na	na	na
100	107	118	59	35	21	118	59	35	21	na	na	na	na	na	na	na	na

*Assumptions used in generating this table: (1) service personnel are fully hydrated, rested, and acclimatized, (2) 50% relative humidity, (3) wind speed = 2 m/s, (4) clear skies, and (5) < 5% heat casualties.

BDU: battledress uniform
na: work/rest cycle not feasible
NL: no limit (continuous work possible)
Ta: ambient temperature (dry bulb, °F)
WBGT: wet bulb globe temperature (°F)

Work Intensities:
H: heavy (> 500 W)
M: moderate (325–500 W)
L: light (172–325 W)
VL: very light (105–175 W)

Adapted from Burr RE. *Heat Illness: A Handbook for Medical Officers.* Natick, Mass: US Army Research Institute of Environmental Medicine; 1991: 50, 54. USARIEM Technical Report T91-3.

TABLE 36-4

WORK TIMES IN NUCLEAR-CHEMICAL-BIOLOGICAL PROTECTIVE UNIFORMS DURING NIGHT OPERATIONS*

WBGT(°F)	Ta	Maximum Single Work Period (minutes)								Work/Rest Cycle (minutes of work per hour)							
		NBC Uniform + Underwear				NBC Uniform + BDU				NBC Uniform + Underwear				NBC Uniform + BDU			
		VL	L	M	H	VL	L	M	H	VL	L	M	H	VL	L	M	H
60	68	NL	NL	76	42	NL	NL	73	41	NL	NL	30	20	NL	NL	25	15
66	75	NL	NL	66	39	NL	NL	64	38	NL	NL	25	15	NL	NL	25	15
72	82	NL	NL	58	36	NL	NL	57	36	NL	NL	20	15	NL	NL	20	10
78	88	NL	NL	53	34	NL	NL	52	33	NL	NL	15	10	NL	NL	15	10
80	91	NL	NL	50	32	NL	NL	50	32	NL	NL	15	5	NL	NL	15	5
82	93	NL	206	49	32	NL	168	48	31	NL	30	10	5	NL	25	10	5
84	95	NL	144	47	31	NL	133	47	30	NL	25	10	na	NL	20	5	na
86	97	NL	121	46	30	NL	115	45	29	NL	15	5	na	NL	10	na	na
88	100	NL	100	44	28	NL	97	43	28	NL	na	na	na	NL	na	na	na
90	102	NL	91	43	27	NL	89	42	27	NL	na	na	na	NL	na	na	na
92	104	NL	83	41	26	NL	82	41	26	NL	na	na	na	NL	na	na	na
94	106	NL	77	40	25	NL	76	40	25	NL	na	na	na	NL	na	na	na

*Assumptions used in generating this table: (1) service personnel are fully hydrated, rested, and acclimatized, (2) 50% relative humidity, (3) wind speed = 2 m/s, (4) clear skies, and (5) < 5% heat casualties.

BDU: battledress uniform
na: work/rest cycle not feasible
NL: no limit (continuous work possible)
Ta: ambient temperature (dry bulb, °F)
WBGT: wet bulb globe temperature (°F)

Work Intensities:
H: heavy (> 500 W)
M: moderate (325–500 W)
L: light (172–325 W)
VL: very light (105–175 W)

Adapted from Burr RE. *Heat Illness: A Handbook for Medical Officers.* Natick, Mass: US Army Research Institute of Environmental Medicine; 1991: 58, 60. USARIEM Technical Report T91-3.

Paradoxically, G protection systems may contribute to the thermal strain by adding additional insulative layers to the aircrew uniform.[41]

Respiratory System Responses

Protective uniforms impede ventilation (ie, breathing) by adding three external loads to the respiratory system: (1) flow-dependent resistive loads, (2) volume-dependent elastic loads, and (3) dead space. Under normal conditions, breathing is opposed by two internal forces: *respiratory system resistance* and *elastance*. Respiratory system resistance is the sum of two internal resistive forces: airflow resistance and pulmonary tissue resistance, which is produced by the rubbing of the surfaces of the lung on the internal surface of the thorax. Airway resistance is the major contributor to total respiratory system resistance and is proportional to inspiratory and expiratory airflows. Airway resistance increases dramatically at the high airflow rates that are routinely obtained during moderate and higher intensity exercise. Resistance is expressed as a pressure drop (expressed in cm H_2O) per liter of airflow per second. The healthy adult has a total respiratory resistance of approximately 4 cm $H_2O/(L/s)$.[42]

Expansion of the thorax during inspiration is opposed by the elastic elements of the lung and the chest wall. Total respiratory system elastance is derived from the pressure–volume relaxation characteristics of the lung and the chest wall and is a measure of the "stiffness" of the respiratory system. Total respiratory system elastance increases as the volume of air inhaled increases. Total respiratory system elastance is expressed as the change in lung volume per change in pressure across the chest wall. A healthy adult has an average total respiratory system elastance, in the mid range of lung volume, of approximately 2% vital capacity (VC)/cm H_2O.[43]

Finally, although not a physical force opposing breathing, the respiratory system dead space (VDS) is the volume of air within the upper and lower airways that does not contribute to pulmonary gas exchange in the alveoli. This anatomical VDS is approximately 0.150 L in the adult. For effective gas exchange, the volume of air inhaled in each breath must be sufficiently large to fill the VDS, as well as an appropriate alveolar volume for pulmonary gas exchange.

Of the aforementioned loads imposed on the respiratory system by the NBC uniform, the CB mask contributes added resistance to airflow and increased dead space. The CB mask uses filter elements to remove chemical and particulate contaminants from inhaled air. By their very design, these filters increase airflow resistance. To separate the inspired and expired air pathways, CB masks utilize one-way valves and internal channels, which also impede airflow. The space within the CB mask nosecup adds dead space, which forces the wearer to increase his or her breathing. Finally, the NBC uniform garments, load carriage equipment, and body armor produce an external constraint on the chest wall separate from that imposed by the CB mask. These factors act independently and in concert to impair breathing; consequently, they impair performance of military operations.

CB Mask Airflow Resistance

The CB mask opposes breathing by applying a nonlinear, phasic, flow-resistive load. It is further defined as a passive load, as the respiratory muscles must develop forces to overcome the load. Although an early recognized limitation of the CB mask was its inspiratory and expiratory airflow resistance, the development of standards for acceptable levels of breathing resistance for CB masks did not occur until World War II. Even though common sense dictates that the added resistance to breathing should be kept as low as possible, increasing the filtering material at the inlet increases the protection a CB mask provides. Thus, every respiratory protective device, including CB masks, has a direct correlation between the degree of protection against CB agent penetration and the magnitude of added resistive load.

Studies by Silverman and colleagues[44] investigated the effects of breathing against added resistance while working at various rates on a cycle ergometer. These studies produced two major findings. First, added inspiratory resistance greater than 4.52 cm $H_2O/(L/s)$, in combination with expiratory resistance exceeding 2.90 cm $H_2O/(L/s)$, resulted in decreased submaximal oxygen uptake, minute ventilation ($\dot{V}E$) and physical endurance at work levels above 135 W. Second, they determined the mean airflow curves for external work rates up to 180 W, which they concluded probably represented the physiological limit for which respiratory protection should be provided. Their research also led to the standard practice of measuring CB mask airflow resistance at a steady state airflow rate of 85 L/min. These data provide the basis for most modern military CB mask design criteria and certification tests.

Subsequent studies sought to refine the maximum tolerable added resistance to breathing which a CB mask should impose on its wearer. Most notably, Bentley and colleagues[45] recognized that the peak negative intrathoracic pressure and respiratory work rate per liter of inhaled air were good predictors of subject discomfort (ie, dyspnea). Furthermore, they recognized that peak inspiratory airflows were approximately equal to 2.7 times the $\dot{V}_E$. (This latter finding is useful for estimating the appropriate steady state airflow rate of a blower-supplied CB mask system to match the ventilatory requirements of various physical activities). From these data, Bentley and colleagues[45] formulated a standard for acceptable CB mask resistance such that 90% of the population tested would not experience dyspnea. They determined that the pressure swing (peak exhalation pressure minus peak inhalation pressure) at the mouth should not exceed 17.0 cm H_2O.

A study by Lerman and colleagues[46] evaluated a range of inspiratory resistance from 0.3 to 4.6 cm $H_2O/(L/s)$ on physiological, psychological, and physical performance at a work rate equivalent to 80% of each subject's maximal oxygen uptake ($\dot{V}_{O_2}$max). At this work rate, all levels of added inspiratory resistance decreased exercise $\dot{V}_E$ (Figure 36-5) and exercise endurance. Thus, at this high but not uncommon level of physical work, any increase in the inspiratory resistance will impair $\dot{V}_E$ and physical work performance. Most sustained, self-paced work is performed at approximately 40% of $\dot{V}_{O_2}$max.[47] A study by Sulotto and colleagues[48] suggested that for prolonged work at this metabolic rate, the added resistance of the CB mask be such that maximal inspiratory pressures not exceed 2.0 cm H_2O. Assuming at approximately 40% $\dot{V}_{O_2}$ max that $\dot{V}_E$ will be approximately 40 L/min, then the inspiratory resistance would not exceed approximately 1.2 cm $H_2O/(L/s)$, using Sulotto's recommended guidelines.

During development of the current US Army field CB mask, the M40,[49] maximum permissible inspiratory and expiratory resistances were 3.88 and 1.84 cm $H_2O/(L/s)$, respectively, at a constant airflow of 1.42 L/s (85 L/min). However, as seen in the pressure–flow relationship for this mask (Figure 36-6), the relationship is not linear, and the apparent inspiratory resistance is nearly doubled at inspiratory flow rates higher than 4 L/s. Numerous studies have investigated the effects of added resistance applied to inspiration, expiration, or both during rest and exercise at various metabolic intensities. Many of these studies employed much larger

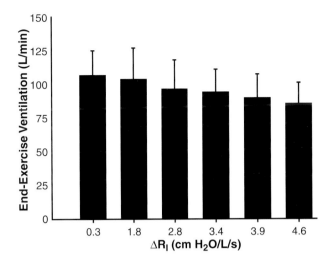

Fig. 36-5. The effect of increasing chemical–biological (CB) mask inspiratory resistance (ΔR_I) on exercise minute ventilation. In this experiment, the mask was commercially available respiratory protective device similar to a CB protective mask. Six filter canisters of varying airflow resistance were used. The exercise work rate (ie, level) was approximately 80% $\dot{V}_{O_2}$max. The three largest ΔR_I, right, are representative of filters common to CB masks. Data source: Lerman Y, Shefer A, Epstein Y, Keren G. External inspiratory resistance of protective respiratory devices: Effects on physical performance and respiratory function. *Am J Ind Med.* 1983;4:736, Table 3.

or smaller added resistance to breathing than is typical of CB masks [range: 2.5–6.0 cm $H_2O/(L/s)$]; thus, these studies are not directly relevant to ventilatory responses in NBC uniforms.

The following sections review breathing responses to added resistive loads comparable to those imposed by CB masks: their effects on respiratory system ventilatory capacities, energy costs and the work of breathing, and the pattern of breathing; and respiratory system limits to exercise, adaptation to wearing the CB mask, dead space in the CB mask, and the effects of the NBC uniform and individual equipment on breathing.

Effect of Resistive Loads on Respiratory System Ventilatory Capacities

The ventilatory, or breathing, capacity of the respiratory system is measured during various clearly defined breathing maneuvers, usually of maximal effort or short duration.[50] In clinical practice, pulmonary function tests are capable of evaluating restrictive and obstructive patterns of ventilatory dysfunction associated with pathophysiological conditions. These

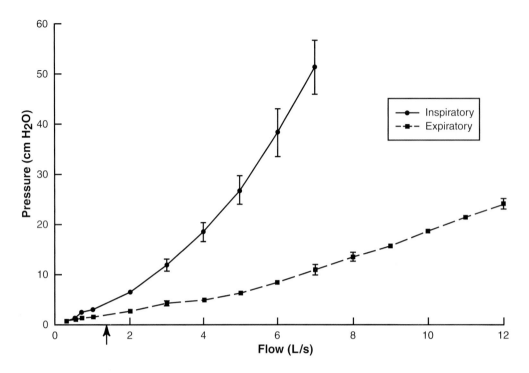

Fig. 36-6. Pressure-flow relationships of a US Army M40 Field Chemical–Biological (CB) protective mask with a C2 canister filter. All pressure drops were measured during steady state flows. The arrow indicates the standard flow rate (85 L/min) used to assess CB mask airflow resistance criteria. Note how the pressure drop across the inlet of the CB mask increases as a nonlinear function of flow.

same measures may be used to assess the impact of external loads imposed on the respiratory system. There are few published studies of the effects of a CB mask on maximal ventilatory capacities, as measured by standard pulmonary function tests.[51–53] The effects of a US Army M40 CB mask on pulmonary function of 15 healthy, male soldiers with normal pulmonary function is shown in Table 36-5.

In general, wearing a CB mask impairs an individual's normal pulmonary function. The pulmonary function tests that measure airflow characteristics, and are effort dependent, are more susceptible to reduction as a result of CB mask wear.[51] Furthermore, the inspiratory flows are impacted more than expiratory flows due to greater inspiratory verses expiratory resistance of the CB mask. Maximal lung volumes are not impacted by CB mask wear, because, in well-motivated subjects, maximum lung volumes are not flow-dependent. These effects on pulmonary function are visually apparent in the flow-volume loop of a healthy man with and without a CB mask (Figure 36-7). In this subject, the CB mask's impairment of inspiratory flows is clearly evident. On the other hand, the small added expiratory resistance may actually improve expiratory flow rates at the lower lung volumes (ie, $FEF_{25\%-75\%}$, or forced expired

flow, midexpiratory phase) by reducing the magnitude of the dynamic airway compression during the forced expiration. The overall impact of the CB mask on maximal ventilatory capacity is seen in the measured maximal voluntary ventilation (MVV). The MVV is a measure of the maximal volume of air an individual could breathe during a short (~15-s) period. The MVV represents the upper limit for exercise $\dot{V}_E$. When wearing the CB mask, the MVV is decreased by approximately 22%, due to the effort and flow-dependence of this breathing-capacity measurement. These results are similar to those reported in an earlier study of the M17A2 CB mask[52] and of a commercially available respiratory protective device[54] similar to the military CB mask.

The three studies mentioned above[51,52,54] also shed light on the value of conventional pulmonary function tests in assessing individual capability to use protective respiratory devices. In the three studies, the traditional benchmarks of pulmonary function—forced vital capacity (FVC) and forced expired volume in 1 second (FEV_1)—were not significantly affected by wear of a CB mask due to the relatively small added expiratory-flow resistance (compared with normal resistance associated with breathing without a mask). Only pulmonary function mea-

TABLE 36-5

EFFECT OF THE US ARMY M40 FIELD CHEMICAL–BIOLOGICAL PROTECTIVE MASK ON RESTING PULMONARY FUNCTION

PFT Variable	Clinical Mouthpiece and Nose Clip (Mean ± SD)	M40 CB Mask and C2 Filter Canister (Mean ± SD)	%Δ
FVC (L)	5.73 ± 0.90	5.66 ± 0.91	−1
FEV_1 (L)	4.65 ± 0.67	4.45 ± 0.69	−5
FEV_1 /FVC	0.82 ± 0.07	0.79 ± 0.08	−3
$FEF_{50\%}$ (L/s)	5.95 ± 1.51	5.20 ± 1.76	−12
$FIF_{50\%}$ (L/s)	7.38 ± 1.89	5.39 ± 0.78*	−23
$FEF_{50\%}/FIF_{50\%}$	0.84 ± 0.24	0.95 ± 0.24	+19
PEF (L/s)	8.96 ± 1.30	7.86 ± 1.92*	−12
PIF (L/s)	7.91 ± 1.64	5.71 ± 0.73*	−26
MVV (L/min)	188.9 ± 26.0	147.5 ± 24.1*	−22
TLC (L)	7.66 ± 1.34	7.61 ± 1.23	0
RV (L)	1.93 ± 0.89	1.96 ± 0.73	+10
FRC (L)	2.96 ± 0.77	3.09 ± 0.65	+7

*Significant difference from baseline ($P < .05$)
N = 15 male soldiers, aged 24 ± 5 y

$FEF_{50\%}$: forced expiratory flow, 50%
FEV_1: forced expiratory volume in 1 sec
$FIF_{50\%}$: forced inspiratory flow, 50%
FRC: functional residual capacity
FVC: forced vital capacity
MVV: maximum voluntary ventilation

PEF: peak expiratory flow
PFT: pulmonary function test
PIF: peak inspiratory flow
RV: residual volume
TLC: total lung capacity

Adapted from Muza SR, Banderet LE, Forte VA. *The Impact of the NBC Clothing Ensemble on Respiratory Function and Capacities During Rest and Exercise.* Natick, Mass: US Army Research Institute of Environmental Medicine; 1995: 17. USARIEM Technical Report T95-12.

sures of *inspiratory* flows were significantly impaired by CB mask wear. However, using pulmonary function measures of inspiratory performance may not be practical because many simple pulmonary function test instruments cannot measure inspiratory flows, and given the effort-dependent nature of inspiratory maneuvers, these measures are prone to greater variability, which can hinder their interpretation. Raven and colleagues[54] evaluated the effects of a respiratory protective mask in a large population that included individuals with above- and below-normal pulmonary function. Of particular note was their observation that the decrement in MVV was directly related to the individual's pulmonary function capability (Figure 36-8). Thus, individuals with the highest 15-second MVV without the mask experienced the greatest decrement with the mask on. Raven and colleagues[54] concluded that measurement of an individual's 15-second MVV while he or she is wearing a respiratory protective

mask can be used as a screening test for capability to perform work in a respiratory protective device.

Effect of Resistive Loads on Energy Costs and Work of Breathing

To breathe, the respiratory muscles must perform physical work. The total work of breathing is the sum of flow-resistive work, plus elastic work, plus chest wall deformation, plus gas compression, plus inertial work, plus negative work. At rest, during quiet breathing through the nose, the work of breathing is approximately 4 J/min (~ 0.5 J/$L_{\dot{V}_E}$).[55] As ventilation increases to meet the metabolic demands of exercise, the work of breathing progressively increases (Figure 36-9), approaching approximately 300 J/min at ventilations near 120 L/min (~ 2.5 J/$L_{\dot{V}_E}$). At rest, the oxygen cost of unobstructed breathing is approximately 1% to 2% of basal oxygen consumption (Table 36-6).[55] As ventilation increases to meet the metabolic demands of

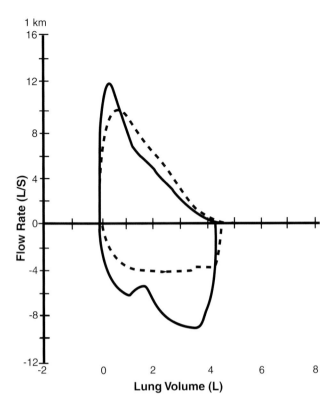

Fig. 36-7. Flow-volume loop of a healthy man with normal pulmonary function performed with standard clinical low resistance mouthpiece and nose clip (solid line) and the US Army M40 Field Chemical–Biological (CB) protective mask (dashed line). Data were obtained during single maximal effort forced expiratory and inspiratory efforts.

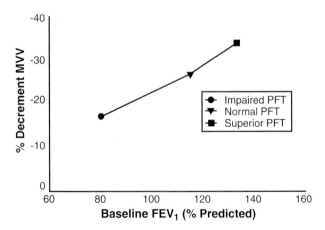

Fig. 36-8. Interaction between baseline pulmonary function (FEV$_1$) and decrement in maximal voluntary ventilation (MVV) induced by a commercially available respiratory protective device similar to a chemical–biological (CB) protective mask. PFT: pulmonary function test. Data source: Raven PB, Moss RF, Page K, Garmon R, Skaggs B. Clinical pulmonary function and industrial respirator wear. *Am Ind Hyg Assoc J.* 1981;42(12):899, Table 2.

physical work, respiratory muscle oxygen consumption increases hyperbolically.[56] However, if the oxygen cost of breathing is expressed as a function of respiratory work (O$_2$/J), less oxygen is consumed per unit work of breathing at the highest exercise ventilations, but the latter expression does not account for all the work of breathing, and thus the value of O$_2$/J is probably lower than reported.[57]

What is fundamentally important here is that the oxygen cost of breathing per unit of ventilation increases by 5- to 10-fold during heavy exercise, compared with rest. The greater cost of breathing at high levels of exercise ventilation (O$_2$/min/L$_{\dot{V}_E}$) may be the result of many factors, including

- increased flow-resistance associated with turbulence and dynamic airway compression,[58]
- increased respiratory muscle velocity of shortening,[59]

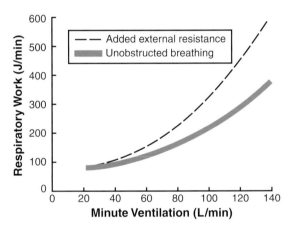

Fig. 36-9. Ventilatory work plotted as a function of minute ventilation. Unobstructed work of breathing[1,2,3] includes estimated work associated with chest wall distortion.[3] The estimated work of breathing with added resistance (~ 5.25 cm H$_2$O/L/s)[4] is calculated by adding the external work of the added resistance to the baseline unobstructed work of breathing. Thus, the estimated total work of breathing with the added resistance similar to that obtained from a typical chemical–biological (CB) protective mask does not include additional work caused by further chest wall distortion. Data sources: (1) Aaron EA, Johnson BD, Seow KC, Dempsey JA. Oxygen cost of exercise hyperpnea: Measurement. *J Appl Physiol.* 1992;72:1810–1817. (2) Johnson BD, Saupe KW, Dempsey JA. Mechanical constraints on exercise hyperpnea in endurance athletes. *J Appl Physiol.* 1992;73:874–886. (3) Goldman MD, Grimby G, Mead J. Mechanical work of breathing derived from rib cage and abdominal V-P partitioning. *J Appl Physiol.* 1976;41(5):752–763. (4) Demedts M, Anthonisen NR. Effects of increased external airway resistance during steady-state exercise. *J Appl Physiol.* 1973;35:361–366.

TABLE 36-6

THE OXYGEN COST OF UNOBSTRUCTED BREATHING FROM REST THROUGH MAXIMAL EXERCISE

Metabolic Rate	Rest	Mild to Moderate Exercise	Moderate to Heavy Exercise	Maximal Exercise
$\dot{V}_E$ (L/min)	< 20	63–79	79–117	117–147
mL O_2/min/L$\dot{V}_E$	~ 0.25–0.5	~ 1.80	~ 2.10	~ 2.85
mL O_2/J	~ 0.75	~ 1.4	—	~ 1.1

—: value not available

Data sources: (1) Roussos C, Campbell EJM. Respiratory muscle energetics. In: Macklem PT; Mead J, eds. *The Respiratory System*. In: Part 2, *Mechanics of Breathing*. Section 3, Vol 3. In: American Physiological Society. *Handbook of Physiology*. Baltimore, Md: Williams & Wilkins for APS; 1986: 481–509. (2) Aaron EA, Seow KC, Johnson BD, Dempsey JA. Oxygen cost of exercise hyperpnea: Implications for performance. *J Appl Physiol*. 1992;72:1818–1825.

- work done on the chest wall, producing distortion with no net external airflow,[60] and
- work done to decompress alveolar gas.[59]

Furthermore, as ventilation increases, expiratory muscles are recruited, which increases the oxygen cost of breathing. There is evidence that the efficiency of the expiratory muscles is approximately half that of the inspiratory muscles.[61] Thus, the oxygen cost of expiratory work is greater than that of inspiratory work. In healthy, fit individuals, the oxygen cost of breathing accounts for approximately 6% to 10% of the total body oxygen at exercise intensities between 75% and 100% of maximum.[57]

The external added airflow resistance imposed by a CB mask increases the work of breathing proportionally as ventilation increases (see Figure 36-9). Using a "respirator-type load" of unspecified magnitude, Harber and colleagues[62] reported that during progressive intensity exercise (O_2 range: 0.5–2.5 L/min), the increase in peak external inspiratory work was approximately 1.7-fold greater than the increase in average inspiratory work. Not illustrated in Figure 36-9 but nonetheless significant is the impact of the added external resistance on work done on chest wall distortion and alveolar gas decompression that may be expected as both the respiratory muscle force and the pattern of activation change to overcome the external resistive loads.[63–65] Many studies have measured the oxygen cost of breathing with externally applied airflow resistance. However, most of these studies employed added resistances much larger than those commonly found in CB masks. In general, these studies report that the oxygen cost of breathing is much greater during resistive loading than unobstructed

hyperpnea for the same amount of work done.[64,66,67] For example, Collett, Perry, and Engel[66] reported a linear relationship between respiratory muscle oxygen and external work of breathing (range: 10–137 J/min), with a slope of approximately 2.4 mL O_2/J across inspiratory resistance, ranging between 26 and 275 cm H_2O/(L/s) at inspiratory flow rates between 0.26 and 1.54 L/s. This study also found that the respiratory muscle oxygen consumption during inspiratory resistive loading is proportional to the inspiratory pressure generated against the load. Thus, given the typical pressure–flow characteristics of CB masks (see Figure 36-6), the oxygen cost of breathing will increase hyperbolically as minute ventilation increases.

Effect of Resistive Loads on Pattern of Breathing

When breathing is opposed by resistive loads, the ventilatory responses are regulated by the combined actions of mechanical load compensation intrinsic to the respiratory muscles (length–tension and force–velocity relationships) and neural reflexes.[68] In conscious humans, the ventilatory response to resistive loading is also modulated by neural responses mediated by conscious perception of the added load.[68,69] The literature is replete with reports of the effects of added flow-resistive loads on the pattern of breathing in normal healthy adults.[51,62,68,70–89] Four factors contribute to the subsequent ventilatory response:

1. the magnitude of the added resistive load;
2. whether the load is applied only to inspiration, expiration, or both;
3. the duration of the load; and

4. the background level of ventilation (ie, rest or exercise) when the load is presented.

Minute ventilation is commonly analyzed by its volume and timing components: tidal volume (V_T) and breathing frequency (f). However, this approach does not allow an analysis of the duration of the breath spent in inspiration (T_I) or expiration (T_E). A more informative approach is to partition $\dot{V}_E$ into its inspiratory flow rate and timing components. The mean inspiratory flow rate is the volume of inspiration divided by its time (V_I/T_I) and is a measure of inspiratory drive. The duty cycle is the ratio of time spent in inspiration to that of the total breathing cycle time (T_I/T_{TOT}) and represents the fraction of the respiratory cycle allocated to inspiration. During unobstructed breathing at rest, T_I/T_{TOT} is approximately 0.4, and V_I/T_I is proportional to the prevailing $\dot{V}_E$. With increasing $\dot{V}_E$ during exercise, the T_I/T_{TOT} increases to approximately 0.5, owing to the proportionally larger reduction in T_E than in T_I with increasing breathing frequency. The V_I/T_I increases in proportion to the exercise $\dot{V}_E$, consistent with the increased activity of the inspiratory muscles.[90] It is generally believed that both the pattern of breathing and the subsequent adjustments as $\dot{V}_E$ changes reflect an optimal adaptive regulation process by the *respiratory controller* (ie, the respiratory center in the brainstem) as it attempts to achieve some type of minimum work of breathing criterion.[91,92]

The typical ventilatory response to an added resistive load is to prolong the phase of the breath to which the load was applied.[82,87,93] Thus when a CB mask is worn, the pattern of breathing will reflect an increased T_I and T_I/T_{TOT}, a decreased V_I/T_I, and a possible decrease in T_E.[62,86,94,95] Depending on the prevailing $\dot{V}_E$ and the magnitude of the added resistive load, $\dot{V}_E$ may or may not be sustained at appropriate levels. This pattern of breathing reduces both the flow-resistive component of the work of breathing[86,91,92] and the adverse perception of the added load to breathing.[96,97] With the onset of exercise, the pattern of breathing during the ensuing hyperpnea—while wearing a CB mask or a comparable resistive load—does not demonstrate the usual adjustments observed during unobstructed breathing. Given the increased T_I/T_{TOT} due to the added inspiratory load, the usual increase in T_I/T_{TOT} as exercise $\dot{V}_E$ increases is diminished.[62,95] Likewise, the rise in the V_I/T_I is decreased when a CB mask is worn, particularly when the $\dot{V}_E$ exceeds approximately 40 L/min.[62,95] Thus, the added resistive load of a CB mask constrains the respiratory controller's adaptive regulation process.

Limits to Exercise When Using the CB Mask

Numerous studies have investigated the effects of added resistance applied to inspiration, expiration, or both, at various exercise intensities. A general finding of studies of added resistance to breathing, typical of many CB masks [range: 2.5–5.0 cm $H_2O/(L/s)$], is decreased exercise $\dot{V}_E$ and endurance time at metabolic rates greater than approximately 60% $\dot{V}O_2$max.[48,85,95,98–102] The reduction in $\dot{V}_E$ is usually directly proportional to the increase in resistance (see Figure 36-5). Usually the $\dot{V}O_2$max is reduced, but the relationship between oxygen uptake and submaximal workloads is not altered. The reduction in $\dot{V}O_2$max when breathing through the added resistance may be related to the increase of alveolar carbon dioxide subsequent to the relative hypoventilation.[46,98–100] At submaximal workloads, increased airflow resistance may decrease exercise endurance.[85,103,104] Even small increases in external airway resistance can negatively impact exercise endurance (Figure 36-10): simply *wearing* a CB mask—even with no filter elements—decreased exercise performance in healthy, fit soldiers during a high-intensity run.[85]

The physiological mechanisms by which added resistance to breathing impairs work performance are complex. Among the possible mechanisms are

- mechanical restrictions on ventilation,
- the increased metabolic cost of breathing,
- constraints on the pattern of breathing, and
- increased adverse respiratory load sensation.

Whatever the mechanism, ventilation may be sustained at adequate levels to meet metabolic demand right up to the premature cessation of the physical work task. Alternatively, hypoventilation may ensue, with consequent rise in partial pressure of arterial carbon dioxide ($PaCO_2$), which may contribute to subsequent task failure.[105]

In almost all healthy, fit individuals, unopposed breathing per se does not limit maximal aerobic exercise.[58,106] These individuals' maximal exercise $\dot{V}_E$ does not exceed their MVV, which represents the upper limit for exercise ventilation. The maximum sustained ventilatory capacity (MSVC) is the level of voluntary hyperpnea that could be maintained for prolonged (4–15 min) periods. The MSVC ranges from 55% to 80% of the MVV.[90,107] In normal adults, the maximal exercise $\dot{V}_E$ usually approaches only 70% to 80% of an individual's MVV,[108] a level corresponding to the MSVC. McCool and colleagues[109] observed that high rates of respiratory muscle oxy-

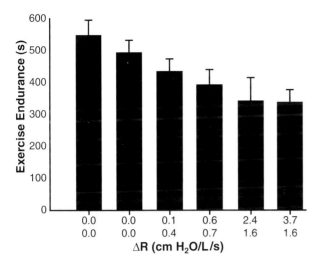

Fig. 36-10. Effect of US Army M9 and M17 Chemical–Biological (CB) protective masks with increasing inspiratory resistance on physical work endurance (running time); (~ 11 km/h at 0% to 6% grade. Each CB mask was modified to alter the magnitude of inspiratory resistance (upper ΔR values) and expiratory resistance (lower ΔR values). The bar on the left represents the "no mask" condition. Note that wearing the CB mask with no measureable airflow resistance (second bar from left) decreased exercise endurance. Data source: Stemler FW, Craig FN. Effects of respiratory equipment on endurance in hard work. *J Appl Physiol.* 1977;42(1):28–32.

gen consumption were associated with short respiratory muscle endurance times. Thus, maximal exercise $\dot{V}_E$ may be limited by (1) the development of respiratory muscle fatigue and (2) a protective mechanism within the respiratory controller that limits ventilation to retard development of respiratory muscle fatigue.[58,110,111] Consequently, any garments or equipment that decreases the maximal breathing capacity increases the risk of a ventilatory limitation to physical work.

There are no published measures of the effect of the CB mask on MSVC but, given the decreased MVV (see Table 36-5), it is reasonable to estimate that CB masks bring about a similar decrement in MSVC. Demedts and Anthonisen[99] observed that at each level of added resistance, maximum exercise $\dot{V}_E$ was approximately 70% of the MVV measured with that resistance. This suggests that the reduced maximal ventilatory capacity contributes to the decreased maximal exercise performance with CB mask use by lowering the threshold for development of respiratory muscle fatigue. Furthermore, just as the threshold ventilation for development of respiratory muscle fatigue is lowered, the added airflow resistance is *increasing* the respiratory

muscles' work and oxygen cost per unit of ventilation.[64,66,67] Thus, by simultaneously imposing both a constraint and a load on the respiratory muscles, the CB mask reduces respiratory muscle endurance and, subsequently, physical work capacity. Alternatively, in the absence of respiratory muscle fatigue, the greater oxygen cost of breathing through a CB mask may limit physical work by diverting a larger proportion of the cardiac output to the respiratory muscles,[67] thus limiting oxygen availability to the skeletal muscles that are performing the physical work.[58,111]

The CB mask also impairs ventilation through constraints imposed on the pattern of breathing. Usually, increases in respiratory frequency result from shortening of both the T_I and the T_E, although the latter is shortened proportionately more.[90] Given the CB mask's increased inspiratory flow resistance, studies[62,105,112] have shown that the limitation of ventilation during exerci se results from attempts to minimize the total work of breathing by reducing the T_E in order to prolong the T_I of each breath. Because CB masks produce their greatest resistance to breathing during inspiration, this strategy reduces inspiratory work while letting expiratory work increase slightly. Johnson and Berlin[112] demonstrated in 10 subjects that a minimum T_E of 0.66 seconds corresponded to the voluntary termination of exercise. However, Stemler and Craig[85] observed a variable T_E at the termination of exercise. They suggested that the minimal T_E attained is more a function of expiratory resistance than a general limitation on expiratory performance. Recognizing that the degree of constraint on T_I and T_E is proportional to the added airflow resistance to each phase, these data suggest that the CB mask restricts the range of pattern of breathing adjustments necessary for optimizing respiratory muscle efficiency.

Another, but not an exclusionary, hypothesis states that attempts to prolong T_I decrease the respiratory sensations associated with the development of the inspiratory muscle force.[113] Conscious humans demonstrate a wide range of psychophysical respiratory load sensitivity (ie, a given resistive load to breathing may be perceived to be of greater or lesser magnitude among individuals).[69] Harber and colleagues[114] found that healthy adults with high psychophysical respiratory load sensitivity did not tolerate physical work while breathing through a CB-masklike resistance as well as the subjects with low psychophysical load sensitivity. Likewise, in a study of healthy young soldiers, Muza, Levine, and Latzka[115] found a positive correlation between high perceptual sensitivity to added resistive loads and the score for the symptom "hard to breathe" during exercise while wearing a CB-style mask. Because the peak inspiratory pressure generated against the added inspiratory resistive load is the primary stimulus of the sensation of dyspnea[97,100,116] (shortness of breath), these studies suggest that subjects may alter their pattern of breathing to minimize adverse respiratory sensation associated with breathing against the added resistance of a CB mask. Cerretelli, Rajinder, and Farhi[100] suggested that when breathing against added resistance, exercise ventilation may consciously be restrained to confine the inspiratory and expiratory pressure swings to some internal limit. Thus, exercise ventilation through a CB mask may be limited by perceptual sensitivity to respiratory loads with consequent reduction in physical work capacity.

There is a wide range of psychophysical respiratory load sensitivity in the normal adult population. This mechanism may account for the large between-individual variability in soldiers of similar age and physical capability in the degree of their discomfort and tolerance to exercise attributed to use of the CB mask.[114,115] Another source of variability among normal healthy individuals is the wide range of ventilatory chemosensitivity.[117] Generally, the magnitude of an individual's ventilation per liter of carbon dioxide produced is directly related to his or her hypercapnic ventilatory responsiveness (HCVR).[98,118–120] The HCVR is a measure of the gain of an individual's respiratory control system to an increase in Pa_{CO_2}. Two studies[98,99] found that during exercise, when breathing was opposed by added resistance, subjects with low HCVR minimized their ventilatory effort and let their alveolar carbon dioxide rise; in contrast, those subjects who were most sensitive to carbon dioxide increased their respiratory work and maintained alveolar carbon dioxide near normal. Consequently, the latter subjects—by sustaining their $\dot{V}_E$ at levels appropriate to the metabolic demand of the exercise—demonstrated lower exercise endurance and tolerance to the added resistance. More recently, Muza and colleagues[95] reported that V_I/T_I was positively correlated to HCVR during moderate- to high-intensity exercise while breathing against added inspiratory resistance. These data suggest that individuals with high HCVR perform greater inspiratory muscle work compared with individuals with low HCVR. Thus, the exercise limitation imposed by added resistance to breathing depends both on the ventilatory limitations produced by the resistance per se and on the ventilatory chemosensitivity of the individual, which influences the level of respiratory muscle work performed to support the physical work task.[99]

Adaptation to Wearing the CB Mask

Because the respiratory muscles are skeletal muscles, they should respond like other skeletal muscles to appropriate strength- and endurance-training programs. Several studies[107,121–124] have evaluated respiratory muscle training protocols for their effectiveness in increasing ventilatory capacities and respiratory muscle endurance in healthy adults. A few[107,121,122] used sustained, normocarbic hyperpnea as the training stimulus because it most closely mimics the action of the respiratory muscles during exercise. One ventilatory muscle training program consisted of 30- to 45-minute training sessions conducted 5 days per week for 5 weeks. During each training session, subjects voluntarily ventilated to exhaustion at more than 81% of their pretraining MVV. Researchers found that this ventilatory muscle training program increased MVV and MSVC by approximately 14% (the 30-min training sessions) and approximately 18% (the 40-min sessions).[107] A similar training program, with the addition of added inspiratory resistance, resulted in greater increases in respiratory muscle endurance.[125]

Although respiratory muscle training can improve ventilatory capacities and endurance, this type of training requires monitoring and controlling alveolar ventilation and gases to maintain normocarbic conditions, and the appropriate ventilatory target. To achieve similar levels of ventilation during aerobic exercise would require sustaining near maximal aerobic exercise intensities for periods of time that exceed the endurance times for such exercise. One study[126] attempted to see if a program of daily, short (< 5 min), intense (80% $\dot{V}_{O_2}$max) exercise wearing a CB mask improved exercise tolerance in the mask. Although the findings demonstrated a slight improvement in exercise endurance, it was not statistically significant. The authors[126] reported that the pattern of breathing changed, resulting in reduced work of breathing. However, because the study lacked a control group, these results must be confirmed.

Two studies of the value of respiratory muscle training on aerobic exercise performance used a program of specific respiratory muscle training similar to that described above.[11] In a study[121] of sedentary adults, submaximal (~ 64 % $\dot{V}_{O_2}$max) cycle exercise endurance to exhaustion increased by approximately 50% following respiratory muscle training. However, another study[124] of moderately trained cyclists did not find an improvement in high-intensity cycle exercise performance following respiratory muscle training. Thus, from a physiological perspective, properly conducted respiratory muscle training will slightly increase ventilatory capacities and endurance, but a practical method of implementing this training is lacking. Moreover, whether respiratory muscle training will improve aerobic exercise performance in physically fit individuals during CB mask wear is inconclusive.

Additional Dead Space From the CB Mask

Each breath of air is composed of an anatomical dead space volume (non–gas-exchanging) and alveolar volume (gas-exchanging). A CB mask adds an external dead space to the wearers' anatomical dead space. At the end of an exhalation, the V_{DS} contains oxygen-depleted and carbon dioxide–enriched expired air. Consequently, this hypoxic, hypercapnic gas will be inhaled during the next inspiration before any fresh, filtered air can enter. Thus, added V_{DS} decreases the partial pressure of alveolar oxygen (P_{AO_2}) and increases the partial pressure of alveolar carbon dioxide (P_{ACO_2}), with corresponding changes in the arterial blood. Arterial hypercapnia is a potent ventilatory stimulus. Several studies measured the effect of added V_{DS} on ventilation during rest and exercise.[127–130] Bartlett, Hodgson, and Kollias[127] studied a range of V_{DS} (36–300 mL), encompassing the V_{DS} typical of many CB masks. They concluded that an added V_{DS} larger than 50 mL will increase $\dot{V}_E$, although they did not test a V_{DS} between 48 and 215 mL. Results of their study are illustrated in Figure 36-11. Added V_{DS} (215 or 300 mL) significantly increased $\dot{V}_E$ during rest and exercise. The added V_{DS} appeared to increase $\dot{V}_E$ more at rest than during exercise.

This latter observation may be of significance when personnel attempt to sleep while wearing a CB mask. During sleep, $\dot{V}_E$ decreases and P_{ACO_2} rises.[131] However, arousal from sleep may occur if P_{ACO_2} increases too much.[132] The V_{DS} of modern CB masks is generally between 150 and 300 mL.[94] Moreover, a poor seal of the mask's nose cup or internal partitions with the wearer's face can result in internal mask leaks, which may greatly increase the volume of the mask's V_{DS}. One study[133] observed that removing the nose cup of a CB-style mask increased $\dot{V}_E$ approximately 5% during mild exercise. Consequently, every CB mask imposes a V_{DS} load on respiration, to which the wearer must compensate by increasing ventilation.

Although by itself V_{DS} causes a compensatory

increase in $\dot{V}_E$, how V_{DS} interacts with the flow-resistive loads imposed by CB masks is less well known. Craig, Blevins, and Cummings[105] showed that an increase in inhaled carbon dioxide (mimicking added V_{DS}) was not well tolerated when combined with increased resistance. Harber and colleagues[130] reported the exercise ventilatory responses to imposition of V_{DS} and inspiratory and expiratory flow resistive loads, individually and in combination. During steady state exercise ($\dot{V}_{O_2}$ ~ 1.2 L/min), an added V_{DS} of 300 mL without added airflow resistance increased ventilation approximately 13%. However, added inspiratory flow resistance [5 cm $H_2O/(L/s)$] without added V_{DS} decreased exercise $\dot{V}_E$ approximately 20%. In combination with increased resistance, the added V_{DS} increased ventilatory effort and work of breathing, although $\dot{V}_E$ was not significantly different from the unloaded condition. Finally, the effects of V_{DS} on $\dot{V}_E$ tended to decrease as exercise intensity and $\dot{V}_E$ increased. This decreased effect of V_{DS} on exercise $\dot{V}_E$ is probably due to both a decreased V_{DS}/V_T ratio and the increased magnitude of the added flow-resistive load, which will rise proportionally with ventilation as exercise intensity increases. In summary, the results reported by Harber and colleagues[130] suggest that while added inspiratory flow resistance affects $\dot{V}_E$ more than added V_{DS}, the aversive effects of the added resistive load are accentuated by the added V_{DS}.

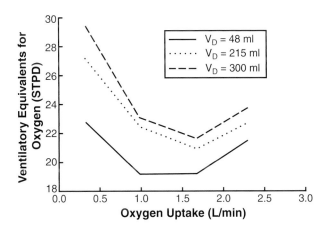

Fig. 36-11. The effect of adding volumes of external dead space (V_{DS}) on ventilation at metabolic rates ranging from rest to moderate-intensity exercise. As V_{DS} increases, ventilation increases to maintain appropriate level of alveolar ventilation. Note that the effect of added V_{DS} on ventilation is greatest at rest. Data source: Bartlett HL, Hodgson JL, Kollias J. Effect of respiratory valve dead space on pulmonary ventilation at rest and during exercise. *Med Sci Sports Exerc*. 1972;4:132–137.

The V_{DS} may be responsible for some of the be-tween-individual variability observed during CB mask use. Because the ventilatory sensitivity to carbon dioxide varies greatly among individuals, a given volume of external dead space can produce a wide range of ventilatory responses.

Effects of the NBC Uniform and Individual Equipment on Breathing

CB masks have usually been the focus of research relative to respiratory impairment associated with NBC ensemble to the exclusion of other components of the protective garment, load-carriage equipment systems, or both, that may interact and synergize impairment of respiratory function. Several studies[134–136] have demonstrated that load-carriage equipment systems worn over utility uniforms reduce MVV by approximately 10%. In a study[137] in which male soldiers walked on a treadmill at 35% to 65% peak oxygen uptake, the wearing of load-carriage equipment over the utility uniform caused increased sensations of breathlessness that accompanied a reduction in the inspired volume of each breath. However, $\dot{V}_E$ was maintained by increasing the rate of breathing. This pattern of breathing is a typical compensatory response to an elastic load.[138] In addition to changing the pattern of breathing, restricting the chest wall displacement requires increased respiratory muscle activity. Green, Mead, and Sears[139] reported that restricting rib cage expansion alone increased diaphragm electromyographic activity by nearly 50% at rest. Moreover, each additional layer of clothing worn increases the metabolic cost for walking,[13] further increasing ventilation and respiratory muscle activity.

In 1996, Muza, Banderet, and Forte[51] proposed that a portion of the ventilatory impairment when wearing NBC uniforms is the result of restricted motion of the chest wall (ie, increased elastance) caused by both the overlying protective clothing and load-carriage equipment. This combination would form an elastic load on the chest wall, which is usually compensated for by reducing the inspired volume of each breath and increasing the rate of breathing to maintain the desired minute ventilation.[87,138] However, as described above, the CB mask imposes a resistive load to breathing, which typically elicits (1) an increase of inspired volume and inspiratory duration and (2) decreased respiratory frequency[87] to reduce flow-resistive work. The CB mask also increases upper-airway dead space, which is typically compensated for by increasing inspired volume.[127,130] Thus, the ventilatory compen-

sations for increased dead space and inspiratory resistance are the opposite of those used when ventilation is opposed by a pure elastic load.

Muza, Banderet, and Forte[51] measured ventilatory performance in a variety of standard US Army uniforms, including the standard ground troop NBC uniform (US Army MOPP 4 with M40 CB mask and standard C2 filter canister). Over the NBC garment, the volunteers wore body armor (ground troop fragmentation protective vest) and load-bearing equipment (pistol belt with shoulder suspenders) that was configured with two full canteens and two ammunition carriers loaded with the equivalent of four 5.56-mm 30-round magazines. Compared with the loose-fitting physical training uniform, the NBC uniform configuration decreased MVV by approximately 25%, with nearly one fifth of this reduction attributed to the external load on the chest wall (Figure 36-12). As expected, the CB mask significantly decreased respiratory flows and had little impact on lung volumes (see Table 36-5). On the other hand, the overgarments and personal equipment significantly decreased maximal lung volumes by approximately 5% to 10% and potentiated the decrement in airflow.[51] Muza and colleagues speculated that the decreased lung volumes were caused by the "corsetlike" action of the combination of overgarments and personal equipment on the chest wall. Accordingly, they found that total respiratory system elastance was increased by approximately 16% in the NBC uniform–CB mask combination, compared with the standard US Army BDU. By comparison, assuming a normal adult value of 4 cm $H_2O/(L/s)$ for total respiratory resistance,[42] the M40 CB mask increases resistive opposition to breathing by approximately 85%. Nevertheless, wearing the NBC uniform overgarments and personal equipment increases the "stiffness" of the soldier's respiratory system, contributing to the decrease of MVV and most likely increasing the work of breathing.

Muza, Banderet, and Forte's study[51] also found that during submaximal treadmill exercise (~ 600 W), the exercise pattern of breathing was more influenced by the elastic forces opposing breathing than by the resistive forces. An approximately 8% smaller V_T during exercise while wearing the NBC overgarments and personal equipment was probably a compensation for the increased total respiratory system elastance. With a smaller V_T, $\dot{V}_E$ was maintained by a small increase in breathing rate. Although the NBC overgarments and personal equipment presented a smaller mechanical impairment on the respiratory system than the CB mask,

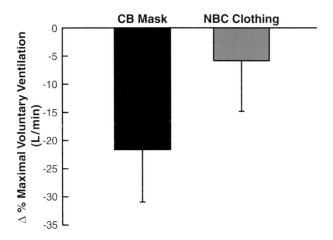

Fig. 36-12. The relative contributions of (left) the US Army M40 Chemical–Biological (CB) protective mask, presenting a flow-resistive load to breathing, and (right) nuclear–biological–chemical (NBC) overgarments with load-bearing equipment and body armor, presenting an elastic load to breathing, on decrement in maximal voluntary ventilation. Data source: Muza SR, Banderet LE, Forte VA. Effects of chemical defense clothing and individual equipment on ventilatory function and subjective reactions. *Aviat Space Environ Med.* 1996;67:1190–1197.

the subjects chose to adjust their pattern of breathing to compensate for this small elastic load rather than the larger resistive load opposing breathing. This suggests that elastic loads to breathing may not be subjectively tolerated as well as resistive loads (ie, the CB mask) and may be related to the fact that the psychological function for magnitude scaling of elastic loads is greater than for resistive loads.[140] Thus, although small, the constraint on the respiratory system imposed by external loading of the chest wall (NBC overgarments, body armor, load-carriage equipment) may, by its effect on the perception of respiratory sensations, present a significant mechanism for impairing exercise breathing and physical work performance.

CB Mask Effects on the Head and Face

The CB mask is likely to feel awkward and uncomfortable when it is put on for the first time or has been worn for only a few hours (cumulatively).[141–144] The initial reaction of many soldiers is that the mask, which weighs 1.0 to 1.5 kg, is heavy; when secured on the face and head, the weight of the mask is very noticeable. The mask and its interfacing surfaces and attaching straps also exert pressure on many areas of the head that are normally uncovered. If the straps are pulled too tight, sol-

diers may report that the straps seem to be cutting into their scalps. In field studies with troops, about 10% to 25% of soldiers reported headaches after wearing the mask a few hours.[141] This was especially true for younger soldiers who had little prior training or experience with NBC protective uniforms and equipment. They secured the straps on the mask too tightly in their attempt to create a good seal on the mask to protect themselves from simulated chemical agents. Fortunately, with practice and greater experience with the mask, such excessive tightening of the straps and many objectionable features of the mask can be minimized.[141,145]

Impaired Communications

Wearing the CB mask and hood hinders face-to-face transmission and reception of speech and radio and telephone communications. The CB mask and hood adversely affect speech intelligibility and amplitude.[19,146,147] Bensel, Teixeira, and Kaplan[19] demonstrated that listeners, unencumbered by CB mask or hood, only achieved a mean score of 65% on the Modified Rhyme Test when the person to whom they were listening wore either an M17 or an M40 CB mask. This score was less than the 75% level of acceptability for voice communications.[18] This finding is of concern because the newer M40 CB mask has two voice resonators (vs one in the M17) but still does not produce speech of adequate quality.

Thus, CB masks attenuate and distort speech; these degradations eliminate many of the tonal qualities of speech that indicate humor, joking, sarcasm, camaraderie, or a questioning attitude. Without relevant acoustical data in speech, less information and cues for behavior are available during informal or social communication. Likewise, the opportunity for misunderstanding mission communications or not hearing them is increased because of the sound-attenuating properties of the mask and hood.

Reduced Sensory Capabilities

CB masks often restrict visibility by blocking part of the visual field.[19,146,148,149] The newer M40 CB mask offers some advantages over the standard M17, but both respirators restrict vision significantly in the temporal and supernasal regions of the visual field, compared with viewing with no mask.[18] Especially at night, more head-turning movements are needed to see objects and receive information in the peripheral visual field.[20] Protective eye lens viewing ports affixed to the CB mask are usually made of flat, sturdy plastic, which contributes to visual parallax and distortion of important images during target detection and identification. Also, some regions in the pilot's visual field are obscured by the mask, a degradation of vision that can be critical during flight for helicopter pilots reading instrument panel indicators or looking for low-level flight hazards such as utility wires.[20]

There is also a practical problem of seeing through the CB mask when the lenses fog over, owing to exhaled moisture or an accumulation of perspiration inside the mask, creating a severe problem for a service member who must maintain good visual contact.[20] The moisture is not easily alleviated without breaking the mask-to-face seal to let the accumulation drain out the bottom of the mask. However, in certain crew-served weapon systems and aircraft, conditioned air can be circulated through the CB mask to minimize this problem.

The CB mask and filter system alters or eliminates olfactory cues, the "smells of the battlefield."[20(p267)] Personnel rely on detection of odors to indicate the status of diesel or electric motors and other equipment, to identify battlefield smokes and obscurants, and to detect the aroma of field food.

Degraded Optics From Prescription Insert Lenses

Soldiers who typically wear prescription eye wear (spectacles) should wear prescription insert lenses inside the CB mask. Getting corrective lens inserts for a CB mask has been a significant logistical problem, and even during field studies that involved the wearing of NBC protective uniforms, wearers of eyeglasses frequently do not have insert lenses for their CB masks.[141,143] Using a CB mask with insert lenses can be problematic, as the lenses are usually secured in a metal frame affixed on the lens well of the mask, and it is difficult to maintain the alignment of the lenses for comfortable visual acuity,[149] especially during visually demanding tasks such as rifle firing.[150] Furthermore, with prescription lens inserts in place, the lenses are more prone to fogging.

Various military occupational specialties (eg, aviation) involve tasks requiring exceptional visual functioning, even if it is achieved via use of prescriptive correction.[20] Because 20% to 30% of US Army aviators require optical correction,[151] the Army equipped its attack helicopter crews with extended-wear contact lenses so these pilots could have corrective lenses compatible with the aviator's CB mask and helmet-mounted display sighting systems. Unfortunately, some soldiers could not be fitted adequately with contact lenses because of presbyopia or astigmatism.[152]

Eating and Drinking

Although exploratory research has developed a means to supply soft food via tube feeding through the CB mask, a more popular alternative for personnel is to wait for the battle action to slow, doff the mask in a safe place, and eat solid food.[20] Few tube-feeding systems have been fielded. Drinking fluids, however, is critical to maintaining hydration during extended wearing of the NBC protective uniforms. Avoiding contaminants while drinking through the mask is difficult at best, but a new drinking-tube arrangement with snap-over connectors to affix to 2-qt water canteens protects both the mask and the water supply from contamination.[153]

Body Waste Management

The processes of urinating and defecating while wearing an NBC protective uniform are rarely written about.[20] It is difficult to eat and drink while wearing the CB mask; however, a regularized drinking regimen to protect against heat stress still requires periodic urination. NBC protective clothing, containing zippers and rear flaps, is poorly designed for waste elimination without the risk of compromising the protective capabilities of the uniform.[154] Most soldiers, when faced with the need to urinate or defecate during a training exercise in the presence of a simulated threat, simply unzip and void without fear of consequences. However, combatants exposed to an imminent chemical threat are likely to seek collective shelter (inside a vehicle or building) and only there doff portions of the clothing to meet this need.[20] Adequate provisions for special male and female hygiene are not accounted for in the present design of NBC protective clothing.

Sleep

It is difficult to sleep comfortably while wearing a CB mask.[20] Sleeping posture has to be carefully selected. When sleeping on one's side, for example, the somewhat rigid structure of the hard rubber mask may be displaced from its tight fit on the wearer's face. If the seal of the mask is compromised, the protective value of wearing the mask is sacrificed.

Although Lieberman and colleagues[155] noted that soldiers who slept in M40 masks tolerated them for most of the night, measurements with wrist-activity monitors indicated that soldiers required more time and found it more difficult to fall asleep when wearing the mask. Their sleep was significantly disturbed; length of time awake increased from 25 to 86 minutes per night, and the number of arousals increased from 8 to 20.

Depending on the integrity of the mask–face seal, protection provided by the mask against potential chemical agents varied among participants; some soldiers were protected throughout the night, others only intermittently.[155] On the other hand, when soldiers sleep on the ground or in armored vehicles, they frequently mention that the NBC protective uniform provides a certain amount of cushioning and warmth in cold weather.[20]

PSYCHOLOGICAL REACTIONS TO NBC PROTECTIVE UNIFORMS

Impact on the Young, Inexperienced Soldier

Younger (and therefore less experienced) soldiers are more impaired by NBC protective uniforms than are older soldiers.[141,143,144,156] Older, more experienced military personnel exhibit fewer symptoms and appear less anxious about training in NBC protective uniforms. It is thought that older service members have learned how to cope with many of the troublesome aspects of wearing NBC protective uniforms. The mask, hood, and other items of NBC protective uniforms present many aspects that are stressful; adaptation to and gradual experience with them is usually helpful.

Because many soldiers lack detailed familiarity with chemical and biological weapons, it is essential that they understand that the NBC protective uniforms issued to them *will* protect against chemicals on the battlefield.[145] This knowledge and understanding will do much to reduce fear, anxiety, and adverse reactions to the NBC protective uniform. Although familiarization training while wearing NBC protective uniforms varies widely in military units of all countries, most military forces effectively accomplish sufficient orientation through classroom didactic training, which usually includes photos of gruesome chemical wounds from past wars or industrial chemical accidents.[145] Students are assured that NBC protective uniforms, if used correctly, will protect them. Practical exercises usually include donning a CB mask and visiting a small enclosure filled with tear gas vapors. This demonstration helps recruits gain familiarity and confidence that the mask will protect them from airborne agents. Since the early 1980s, the US Army has conducted live nerve agent decontamination training for small numbers of chemical specialists in a controlled setting.[157]

Breathing and Its Psychological Effects

In response to the added breathing resistance imposed by CB masks (discussed above in the Effects of Resistive Loads subsections), altering physiological responses by conscious modification of the breathing pattern—such as attempting to breathe too little or too much—can lead to breathing distress, hyperventilation, shortness of breath, tremors, and claustrophobic reactions.[51,146] Many CB warfare agents provoke intense psychological concerns because they contaminate the air that we breathe to stay alive. Thus, NBC agents are linked to the most basic and urgent of all biological drives—the urge to breathe.[145] When troops who do not have NBC protective uniforms think about NBC agents, they may feel impotent and that nothing is within their control. Likewise, lack of confidence in their NBC protective clothing and equipment or their ability to use it may also evoke a profound sense of helplessness or hopelessness.[145]

Problems with breathing through a mask are also familiar to those in the civilian workforce (eg, firefighters) who wear respiratory protective devices.[158] Psychological anxiety encountered with such breathing resistance can be decreased through familiarity training with the CB mask. Troops should also practice sleeping in the mask after receiving advice on ways to avoid compromising the CB mask's protective seal and preventing respiratory distress or intermittent obstruction of breathing (sleep apnea) from occurring.[145] Performance of tasks requiring high aerobic power (eg, handling of ammunition) is hindered greatly by breathing resistance, as breathing is greater under high workload conditions.[112,159] Thus, more time is usually required to perform certain tasks when the CB mask is worn.

Maladaptive Psychological Reactions

Combat with CB weapons is likely to produce many more casualties with psychological stress than with actual CB injuries. That prediction reflects the adverse impact of fears and anxieties that troops experience in dealing with the threat of a CB-contaminated battlefield. In part, such anxieties are attributable to the insidious, ambiguous nature of many CB agents, which prompt fears of dying a hideous death on the battlefield. Maladaptive responses of soldiers to the battlefield include the psychological overreactions of hyperventilation, claustrophobia, gas-mask phobia, compulsive practices or obsessive concern with decontamination, congregating in safe or collective protection areas, finding excuses to never come out or let others into a safe space, and hoarding or stealing protective items. Underreactions to the chemical threat, such as psychological denial, fatalism, rationalization, or intellectualization, may also occur.[145] All of these prevent troops from taking adaptive actions or enacting useful countermeasures.

Muza, Banderet, and Forte[51] demonstrated that an NBC protective uniform evokes predictable psychological reactions such as anxiety, feelings of not getting enough air, and perceptions of abnormal breathing and of stress. For combatants, such concerns can be fueled by their lack of confidence in NBC protective uniforms and their inability to use them properly for protection.[141,143] Taylor[160] emphasized the benefits of coping strategies, relaxation techniques, good leadership, and training to decrease or prevent extreme fear and many adverse reactions. Education, training, and experience with NBC protective uniform can go a long way toward reducing these fears.[145,157,160]

Soldiers who spend lengthy training sessions garbed in NBC protective uniforms occasionally report loneliness, a distorted sense of time passage, and alterations in distance estimates.[20] For example, armor crews in MOPP 4, when approaching prominent terrain that narrows, "bunch up their vehicles" so they are five or six vehicles abreast waiting their turn to go through narrow terrain gaps.[20] This makes them an opportunistic high-value target, so that their risk of enemy attack from the air or from his artillery is greatly increased. At Fort Irwin, California, a National Training Center cadre sergeant stated:

> every group coming here for training does the same thing in MOPP IV, they bunch up their vehicles; ... it seems that they just want to feel closer together despite the obvious risks.[20(p274)]

Military history provides other illustrative examples and lessons regarding adverse psychological reactions. During World War I, when rumors suggested that new chemical agents could penetrate the gas masks, whole units fled after smelling an unfamiliar odor.[145] Units who were exhausted or demoralized were especially susceptible to panic. However, among the lessons from World War I was the suggestion that combat experience with the chemical threat often led to positive psychological

adaptation.[145] Training was developed to build confidence in the CB mask and motivate troops to use it. Gas-chamber training (using tear gas) during World War I had troops wearing their gas masks for more than 1 hour in the chamber before they took them off to experience the effects of a simulated chemical agent.[161] Newly assigned troops sometimes died in gas attacks if they lacked both adequate training and mentors, just as they were more likely to be victims of conventional weapons.[145] The survivors of chemical attacks were troops who had mastered the drill and tactics of chemical defense.

Accounts of maladaptive reactions during the 1990/91 Persian Gulf War include the following examples[145,162]:

- many soldiers who took no precautions with the CB mask and NBC protective uniforms when air (missile) alerts were sounded because prior alerts in the theater had been uneventful;
- a sergeant with gas-mask phobia who was evacuated to the United States;
- at least one case of inappropriate and premature atropine self-injection; and
- a physician who was barred from entering a collective protective shelter after an alert because fellow soldiers feared he would contaminate the shelter.

Another manifestation of maladaptive reactions is that troops may become obsessively concerned with decontamination procedures, which they then perform compulsively.[145] This consumes precious time needed for critical tasks and wastes scarce decontamination supplies. Excessive skin cleansing with decontamination solutions can cause rashes that might then be misinterpreted as confirmation of exposure to a chemical agent.

Civilian populations confronted with terrorist actions involving chemical agents also manifested maladaptive reactions. Newspapers and television in the United States reported (incorrectly) that 12 people were killed and 5,500 were "injured" during the March 1995 sarin nerve agent attack in the Tokyo, Japan, subway.[145,163] Findings from 5,110 victims of the sarin attack evaluated at hospitals in the first 24 hours document the overreactions and excessive concern that chemical warfare agents can create.[164] Overall, 73.9% of these so-called casualties showed no effects of exposure to nerve agent. These patients were instead the "worried well."

IMPACT ON MILITARY OPERATIONS

Sources of Information and Findings

Wearing NBC protective uniforms impairs the performance of several military tasks and limits soldiers' dexterity, mobility, communications, vision, and task endurance. It is important to try to specify and predict the impact that wearing NBC protective uniforms will have on military operations. Information comes from several sources[3,4] to help anticipate the impact of NBC protective uniforms on small-unit and large-scale military operations. Since the early 1980s, a variety of systematic programs were initiated to provide such information. Headley, Hudgens, and Cunningham[165] reviewed three military research programs involving field studies of soldiers wearing NBC protective uniforms in hot environments during extended operational military work scenarios, often 24 hours or longer, therefore including night operations. These studies[3,165,166] of military teams (military program titles: DO49, P²NBC² [Physiological and Psychological Effects of NBC and Extended Operations on Combat Vehicle Crew Performance], and CANE [Combined Arms in a Nuclear Environment]) were reviewed in great detail and included

- two-person teams performing cooperative tasks (eg, disassembling a tank engine for a DO49 project) while wearing an NBC protective uniform;
- about 20 different P²NBC² controlled scenarios with specific, crew-operated, military systems (eg, three to four crew members in tanks, self-propelled howitzers, and armored personnel carriers);
- five large-scale CANE tests, including a study of 40-person, platoon-sized military units performing infantry operations (ie, CANE I in 1986); and
- large, free-play operations of hundreds of soldiers (ie, CANE IIB in 1989) in tests of full, battalion-sized scenarios on simulated battlefields.

These field experiments demonstrated that although most standard military tasks can be performed satisfactorily, extra time is required to perform them in NBC protective uniforms.[20,167] High ambient temperatures and high work loads are especially detrimental to endurance in NBC protective uniforms.

Many measures of combat effectiveness degrade in MOPP 4, including[3,165,166]

- difficulty in locating and reporting enemy positions;
- poorly timed battle synchronization;
- engaging enemy forces at closer ranges than desirable;
- firing fewer primary weapons;
- lengthy time intervals to alternate battle positions; and
- general degradation in command, control, and communications.

These field studies, especially those engaging sizable numbers of soldiers carrying out military task scenarios on large stretches of terrain, tended to be exploratory and descriptive in nature.[165] They involved determining operational principles of practical importance to the military community, and some were noteworthy field demonstrations, but making trustworthy scientific extrapolation of findings from some of these studies is difficult. Some studies could be classified as indelicate experiments[168] because they incorporated many tenets of rigorous experimental design, but like many large man–machine system experiments,[169] they also involved numerous uncontrolled variables inherent in military field operations.[20] Frequently, good baseline performance data were not established before testing, and in some tests the presentation of experimental conditions was not counterbalanced.[3,170]

Despite such cautions, the overriding lessons of these studies[20] are

- that the present NBC protective uniforms used by the US military must be redesigned with more attention to human engineering factors, and
- that repetitious realistic training in NBC protective uniforms is essential to sustain performance on a CB contaminated battlefield.

Lessons learned, in particular, called for more-realistic training for military leaders at all levels to enhance understanding of how the behavior of individual soldiers changes within a unit when many soldiers are wearing NBC protective uniforms.[20]

Other information, especially on large-scale operations, results from efforts with operations research models. Military planners, combat developers, and tacticians use such models to help anticipate and prepare for threats envisioned on the next battlefield.[167]

Combat models involve aspects of offensive and defensive military operations and include safety analyses and projections of requirements concerning personnel, training, human factors, and survivability. Developing predictive models of soldier behavior on a dynamic battlefield is one of operations research's biggest challenges. Ramirez[167] emphasized what a daunting task it is to predict the outcome of many time- and task-linked sequential activities on a fluid, dynamic battlefield; it is particularly difficult when the combatants wear NBC protective uniforms intermittently. Useful, valid, predictive models must rely on reliable behavioral computer-accessible databases that can be used to foresee impacts of the battle theater on soldier performance.

Ramirez[167] described US Army and Air Force efforts to develop behavioral models of soldier performance while wearing NBC protective uniforms in simulated chemical warfare environments. Models to predict the times required to accomplish various military tasks and the debilitating psychological effects of wearing NBC protective uniforms are complex undertakings that are challenging to modify or verify. Early work in modeling concerned predictions of the time to complete or perform tasks by either individuals or small military units, then was extrapolated to larger units. Air Force and Army studies with an operations research approach yielded several useful insights[167]:

- The degradation in task performance varied with crew experience; larger degradations were usually associated with crews of less task experience.
- Performance of routine military tasks required 50% to 70% more time when crew members wore MOPP 4.
- Wearing NBC protective uniforms impeded performance of tasks requiring manual dexterity because of the encumbrance of the bulky NBC protective uniform.

The models also estimated the impact of dramatic heat effects on performance. Such models predicted heat-related casualties (heat exhaustion or heatstroke) resulting from sustained operations while wearing NBC protective uniforms in hot environments with little food and water.

Obtaining suitable quantitative data on large military units is a difficult and expensive proposition. Eventually, the US military, primarily the US Army, collected such data[3,165,171] to support computerized analyses and predictive modeling of unit performance in various chemical battlefield sce-

narios. From these and other data, Ramirez[167] devised a task taxonomy, which suggests some military tasks that do not require increased time to perform while wearing NBC protective uniforms, and ranges to tasks that take 3-fold longer to complete while wearing NBC protective uniforms. Tasks that are affected so dramatically by NBC protective uniforms are usually modified (redesigned) by the soldier or not completed at all.[167]

Use of actual data collected from soldiers can greatly increase the usefulness, robustness, and validity of operations research models. Such models can predict individual soldier and military unit performance, offer computer tools and cost-effective methods to designers of NBC protective clothing for evaluating new designs, enable testers of equipment to better perform their evaluations, and provide battlefield planners with tactical insights for deployment of forces.[167]

Soldier Readiness and Training

In combat involving chemical warfare agents during World War I, psychological stressors caused more casualties than did chemical injuries.[172] In a remarkable instance involving 281 casualties of gas attacks who were evaluated at a field hospital, 68%[172(p65)] showed no signs of chemical injuries. In this situation, two[172(p65)] psychological (stress) casualties were noted for each actual chemical injury. Such statistics of medical casualties may even underestimate the total number of dysfunctional stress cases because they do not include troops who bolted in panic at the threat of gas attack, unless those troops were subsequently evacuated for medical care. Panic reactions were triggered by many events.[172,173] Units who were exhausted or demoralized were especially susceptible to panic. Stokes and Banderet[145] emphasized that if soldiers are not prepared for chemical warfare and experienced with the CB mask and NBC protective uniforms, the number of ineffective soldiers will be much greater. The wearing of NBC protective uniforms and the thoughts or sights of chemical warfare provoke many stressors, some largely psychological, which should be mastered through training, drill, and familiarization with NBC protective clothing and the CB mask.[145]

Military units experience a high turnover of personnel. Therefore, to ensure that they are adequately trained to use their NBC protective uniforms, troops should train frequently in their NBC protective uniforms on common military tasks and, as well, in larger-scale team scenarios in which they practice working together.[20] Because NBC protective uniforms usually encumber movement, breathing, heat exchange, and mission performance (especially during heavy physical work in high ambient temperatures), it is important that training be conducted under realistic conditions for maximal transfer of training. Lack of experience with the CB mask and NBC protective clothing are good predictors of soldiers who most likely will experience difficulties or terminate during a field training exercise. As discussed above in this chapter, soldiers with corrected vision who do not have prescription inserts for their CB masks are vulnerable when wearing NBC protective uniforms,[141,143] and therefore the logistical system should address their specific needs for individual prescription eyewear.

Intensive training to do critical tasks in NBC protective uniforms can promote confidence, reduce adverse emotions, and better prepare all forces to fight successfully on a contaminated battlefield.[20] Today's multimedia training technologies provide many low-cost, sophisticated, high-technology alternatives for training that can be used to present information and scenarios in militarily relevant ways that troops will enjoy and learn from. Many such multimedia training systems are interactive and the level of complexity can be adjusted, providing troops with training for combat situations with more alternatives and fewer static options. Training must be realistic for maximum benefits to result, and realistic training could reduce some adverse emotional effects and even help alleviate some performance impairments associated with NBC protective uniforms. Today, the tactical play of many Army field exercises (eg, National Training Center, Joint Readiness Training Center) provides much greater feedback and realism as warfighters practice skills and acquire "lessons learned"—lessons that are better gained in training than in combat.[174]

As concerns about the likelihood of terrorist actions involving chemical and biological agents in large cities persist,[175–178] the orientation and training of federal, state, and local officials and first-responders are essential so that the mass casualty effects of terrorist attacks can be managed optimally.[179] Holloway, Norwood, and Fullerton[175] emphasize the importance of realistic training for medical personnel so they can experience the numbers and types of casualties and to see how such disruption will create unprecedented demands within medical facilities. Lessons learned from simulations or realistic training in the impact of chemical and biological attacks should benefit agencies that will provide services and assistance to casualties[179]; service providers and public officials will then be better able to anticipate how terrorist attacks would perturb and disrupt public facilities, essential services, and life styles of those in the affected city.[175,179]

Difficulty Identifying Friend or Foe

A psychological complaint is that the CB mask and NBC protective uniform make everyone look identical and hide the usual cues by which we recognize team members, leaders, and followers.[145] When all combatants are garbed in MOPP 4–level NBC protective uniforms, identification is difficult largely because characteristics such as hair, skin color, stature, and body shape are disguised or not visible.[20] Furthermore, voices are distorted and their distinctive tonal qualities are masked. Many military units therefore resort to supplemental identifying markings on the ensemble and to hand signals to ensure visual feedback in intraunit communication.[145] Distinctive symbols are sometimes added to the face part of the hood to represent the team, unit, rank, and individual soldier.[180] However, symbols placed on the mask must not compromise durability, camouflage, operational security, and public sensibilities.

In warfare and in training, when the enemy is difficult to distinguish from others, fratricide and other tragic mistakes can result.[3,165,166] Such situations, like trying to recognize and identify soldiers in NBC protective uniforms, are very stressful because cues normally used to identify fellow soldiers and leaders are no longer available or reliable.

OPTIMIZING TRADE-OFFS IN FUTURE NBC PROTECTIVE UNIFORMS

In the future, warfare will be highly mobile and often fought in urban and suburban areas. Combat will be dynamic and require initiative and actions by teams or individuals to cope with fast-moving, changing situations and sites of resistance. Currently, NBC protective uniforms of the US military protect troops from many NBC threats; however, as this chapter emphasizes, NBC protective uniforms also impose performance, physical, and psychological liabilities for the combatants who wear NBC protective clothing.

Evolving doctrine, training, and advances in materiel should optimize practices associated with wearing NBC protective uniforms and find new ways to reduce the limitations of such protective clothing so that troops can function effectively on future NBC-contaminated battlefields. The current (published in 1992, revised in 1996) manual for NBC protection for the US Army and Marines[5] devotes one page to describing a mask-only posture and variations to the standard protective postures. This brief section in the manual emphasizes the need for greater flexibility in the use of protective uniforms and protective postures and that much more is required. A more-extensive effort would involve computer modeling with salient variables to investigate, such as

- the NBC weapons capabilities of different countries,
- other countries' ways of deploying NBC weapons,
- likely theaters of combat and their climates,
- types of NBC agents (respiratory vs skin-penetrating),
- protection from varied components of NBC protective uniforms, and
- expected missions.

Such iterations could synthesize expert information on risks and the likelihood of respiratory and skin-contact threats, the protection that components of NBC protective uniforms such as the CB mask or a lighter-weight overgarment would offer for special situations, and the increased comfort and performance that would be realized from the use of light-weight NBC protective clothing or CB masks with less inspiratory resistance. Such an effort could also facilitate reexamination of current procedures and assumptions of application of MOPP gear and ensure that NBC protective uniforms of the future sustain military performance and offer optimal protection against the NBC threat.

NBC Protective Uniforms of the Future

Much is known about the effects of NBC protective uniforms (eg, their effects on the soldier's respiration, thermoregulation, ambulatory mobility, manual dexterity, and sensorimotor and psychomotor performance).[20] Considerable data describe degrading effects of NBC protective uniforms on visibility, communications, and respiration. Most proposals call for significant improvements in human engineering of the encapsulated microenvironment of NBC protective uniforms. Many such enhancements will come as developments in future technologies become mature enough for implemen-

tation. Parallel efforts are also being made to minimize the effects of chemical or biological agents in other ways.[180] The Defense Advanced Research Projects Agency (DARPA), an agency that has funded defense-related engineering and novel electronics applications for over 30 years, is encouraging and funding projects that seem highly unusual, such as placing an "electronic canary" on a silicon chip to detect a wide variety of CB agents, immunizations that would offer general protection against classes of noxious CB agents rather than protection against a specific threat (eg, smallpox), and skin creams or ingested substances that would provide protection against many noxious agents. Significant advances in detection or prevention against NBC threats would reduce requirements for protective uniforms of the future.

Several biomechanical restrictions imposed by NBC protective uniforms might be lessened if protective-level design criteria could be made slightly less stringent when applied to select military scenarios (eg, quick offense vs slow defense) or to functional specialties (eg, aviators, armor crewmen, infantrymen). This might lead to adopting several alternative inventories of NBC protective uniform systems.[20] Operational doctrine, regarding the use of NBC protective uniforms at the unit level, might be improved if local commanders had more flexibility in determining what MOPP level their troops would assume during operations.[20,145] Each of these notions is described below.

Systems View: Human Engineering

It is essential that an improved NBC protective uniform be designed and evaluated as a "soldier protective system."[18,20] This approach includes accounting for the interactions of NBC protective uniforms with different environments, crucial equipment interfaces such as optical sighting systems, and critical military operational tasks. Bensel[181] provided an important perspective for systems design with her outline of the characteristics of NBC protective uniforms and associated equipment; the physiological and mechanical effects they impose; and her commentary on soldier differences and the influences of leadership, cohesion, and training. Her perspective was similar to and reinforced that proposed by Taylor.[160] Johnson and colleagues[182] offered an equipment-performance rating scheme for CB masks to permit decisions involving trade-offs, an approach that could be adapted to evaluate components of NBC protective uniforms such as gloves, boots, and overgarments. Multinational cooperative programs are now prevalent to address these important issues.

CB Mask

The CB mask is implicated as the primary NBC protective uniform item responsible for negative psychological reactions among soldiers and for much of the operational performance degradation.[18,20,145,181] Design changes should include reduced resistance to breathing, improved visibility through the mask, an easy system for use with prescription lenses, an antifogging system, enhanced speech intelligibility through innovative use of electronic technologies, a better interface of the mask with other equipment, especially optic sights, and easier access to food and drink.[20]

Protective Overgarments

Extensive redesign of NBC protective uniforms is required to improve gross body movement and fine psychomotor control while wearing the suit. Lightweight protective materials that impose less heat burden also should be integrated with personal, wearable cooling devices or a source of cool, conditioned air from a vehicle.[20] Other desiderata include thinner handwear to provide adequate tactile feel and features to permit easier donning and doffing, compatibility with sleeping, and a convenient means of voiding excess perspiration and exhaled moisture resulting during work in excessive heat.[20] Special attention will need to be given to waste elimination and personal hygiene so that soldiers can utilize these uniforms and capabilities rapidly, conveniently, and in a manner acceptable to all users.[154]

Lightweight Protective Uniforms

Developmental programs of North Atlantic Treaty Organization (NATO) forces and other western nations strive to devise suitable, lightweight NBC protective uniforms with less risk of heat stress. McLellan and colleagues[8,183] described Canadian efforts to evaluate protective clothing ensembles, designed by the Canadians and the French, that are worn directly over the skin or, at most, over underpants and shirt, eliminating the usual utility uniform worn under an NBC protective uniform. In a similar program, Levine and colleagues[7] described one of a series of tests to evaluate chemical protective undergarments designed in the United States.

Such developments undoubtedly will find their way into the design of an integrated protective ensemble, which might offer modular clothing and equipment systems for combat ground troops.

Cadarette and colleagues[184] evaluated the first components of such a system and published the associated physiological data. The four branches of the US military presently collaborate on a Joint Service Lightweight Integrated Suit (JSLIST) technology program to produce lighter and less-bulky protective uniforms.[185] Using recent improvements in carbon absorber technology, the Australians claimed that their CB suit, developed to provide protection against liquid and vapor chemical agents, significantly reduced heat strain in tropical environments.[9]

Individual Cooling Systems

Military laboratories in the United States have experimented with varied personal microclimate cooling systems worn under the NBC protective uniform.[186] Banta and Braun[187] used ice vests in high-heat environments to reduce heat strain of helicopter pilots based on US Navy carriers. Ice cooling is generally less effective than air or liquid cooling. Although the wearer can move about without being tethered, ice cooling necessitates repeated access to ice, so it may be suitable only for short-term work.[188]

More frequently, liquid-cooled or air-cooled vests are worn under NBC protective uniforms.[186,189–193] Both systems have benefits and limitations. Air cooling can increase tolerance time 4-fold, whereas circulation of hot ambient air provides little cooling and may be dangerous. Air cooling is less efficient, however, than liquid cooling, because the specific heat of air is lower. Liquid cooling is more effective in reducing heat strain at light-to-moderate work loads when applied on large body surfaces (eg, on the thighs during lower-body exercise). However, if overcooling results, discomfort may occur due to cutaneous vasoconstriction. Also, liquid-cooled systems are heavy and require excessive maintenance, and the flow of coolant can be interrupted if the tubes are pinched or bent.

Temperature-conditioning technologies that use liquid- or air-cooled systems are especially promising for use by crews in armored vehicles, helicopters, or airplanes with access to suitable power sources. Cadarette and colleagues[194] demonstrated the utility of air-cooled microclimate vests and ventilated facepieces for armor personnel in desert and tropic environments; Thornton and colleagues[195,196] explored the use of liquid- and air-cooled microclimate cooling systems for helicopter pilots; and, for the ground soldier, Masadi, Kinney, and Blackwell[191] evaluated liquid-cooled vests in which the coolant was chilled by ice packs carried on the back. These investigators found that batteries for electric-powered, portable air-conditioning systems added too much weight to an infantryman's backpack. Also, although such self-contained systems provide substantial body cooling, the reduction in heat is not adequate under highly stressful conditions.[184,197]

It may be necessary to select the best cooling system for crew-served vehicles and other situations on a case-by-case basis. For ground-based and other personnel who do not have access to a power source, much more design work needs to be done on portable cooling systems, including lightweight batteries or alternate sources of power for microclimate cooling systems that are carried by the soldier on his back.[20] Improving cooling systems will increase comfort, allowing soldiers to perform more efficiently for longer durations in toxic chemical environments.

Adopting More Than One Type of NBC Protective Uniform

US military forces and others train for deployment to combat theaters anywhere in the world. These theaters vary dramatically in terms of their climatic conditions, the enemy to be engaged, the type of military operation, and the tasks performed by the soldier. Reardon and colleagues[198,199] evaluated 14 US Army aviators in a UH-60 simulator and compared their flight performances, physiological parameters, and moods, for two different flight uniforms (standard aviator uniform or NBC protective uniform, MOPP 4, with aviation life-support equipment vest and the laminated ballistic plate) and two environmental conditions (21°C, 50% relative humidity [rh]; or 38°C, 50% rh). Personnel who wore NBC protective clothing and associated flight equipment in a hot cockpit showed decreased flight performance, increased physiological parameters (heart rate, core body temperature, and dehydration), and heightened symptoms of heat stress (nausea, dizziness, headache, and thirst). These two studies suggest that helicopter pilots do not tolerate high ambient temperatures in the cockpit well when they must also wear NBC protective uniforms during flight.

Caldwell[200] surveyed 148 Army personnel after the Desert Storm phase of the Persian Gulf War (1991) to describe wear compatibility and logistical problems associated with NBC protective uniforms during desert combat. Helicopter pilots frequently commented that NBC protective uniforms were incompatible with night-vision goggles or with head-up displays (8%), were bulky or heavy (6%), were

unavailable in the quantities required or that the expected usefulness was exceeded (5%), presented mask-related problems (4%); and that the NBC protective overboots were incompatible with flying (4%). From this survey, it is evident that NBC protective uniforms were somewhat incompatible with both the mission and the special equipment associated with flying a helicopter. No doubt similar stories could be told by armor, mechanized infantry forces, and others.

The many constraints that NBC protective uniforms impose seem in part attributable to a logistical scheme of providing a single, standardized design: NBC protective uniforms with thick layers of protective materials.[20,145] This strategy provides maximum personal protection to all combatants. US military field tests of NBC protective uniforms (eg, P^2NBC^2 in the mid to late 1980s) often set goals for participants to wear NBC protective uniforms for 3 days or more at the MOPP 4 level.[20,165] Such testing told much about what soldiers can and cannot do in studies of endurance. In future conflicts, it is unlikely that our forces will be wearing the maximal protection NBC protective uniform (MOPP 4) for several days at a time. Given the enormous distances covered in an open desert by today's fast-moving armor and air forces (eg, the 100-hour war of Desert Storm), it is also unlikely that any military force could keep an open battlefield continuously bathed in CB agents long enough to prohibit vehicle-mounted forces from navigating their way out of danger.[20]

Perhaps, therefore, the military supply system should provide multiple NBC protective uniforms, including lighter-weight clothing, which might provide less absolute protection but allow greater personal mobility for fast movement on a fluid battlefield. If multiple NBC protective uniforms were adopted, that decision might permit better optimization of the characteristics of an NBC protective uniform to the military mission (environment and threat), and better matching of NBC protective uniforms with the soldier and the tasks that he or she performs (eg, US Army Rangers or Light Infantry on a ground reconnaissance mission vs a driver in a vehicle or a pilot in a high-performance aircraft). Although the strategy of having several sets of NBC protective uniforms will increase developmental costs, inventory requirements, and distribution efforts for the military, the US military already issues numerous other uniforms and clothing systems and issues several different versions of the CB mask for infantry, aviators, and tankers.[20,145] It seems to make sense in the case of NBC protective uniforms as well.

Adaptive Doctrine for Lowest Feasible Protective Posture

Military doctrine should support training and fighting whenever possible at the lowest safe MOPP level so that adverse effects of NBC protective uniforms can be minimized. Because not all enemies have the same chemical capabilities, tactical situations determine the likelihood that specific chemicals will be used; environmental conditions influence chemical agent effectiveness; and differing mission requirements dictate how much NBC protective uniforms will compromise soldier performance.[20,145] In any event, the employment of NBC protective uniforms in combat is a calculated risk, matching the level of personal protection from NBC warfare agents against adverse effects of the uniform on soldier health, performance, and psychological well-being.

The greatest performance-limiting factor of NBC protective uniforms is excessive buildup of metabolic heat during work in hot environments. If more training with lower protective postures (eg, MOPP 1, 2, and 3) is to occur, military doctrine must guide and specify conditions under which training is appropriate. It should also establish how decisions are to be made with regard to changes toward more- or less-restrictive protective postures in training and in combat. The decision logic must be communicated so forces involved understand the ground rules at both the centralized command level and the unit level, where local protective conditions might differ from those of other units. These concepts should be practiced so troops learn to operate confidently and comfortably in training, and in combat situations, at lower levels of protective posture.[20,145]

SUMMARY

NBC warfare protective uniforms encapsulate the wearer, producing a barrier to the ambient environment and simultaneously creating a microenvironment within the uniform. Protective uniforms may impair essential human functions. The energy cost of performing tasks, particularly tasks requiring mobility, is increased when wearing an NBC protective uniform. The higher metabolic rate is associated with both the added weight of the protective uniform and the friction produced by the multiple layers of garments. Furthermore, the bulky NBC protective uniform limits the range of motion around body joints and reduces manual dexterity, thus increasing the difficulty and accuracy of relatively simple tasks. These impediments can be reduced by wearing the fewest layers of clothing possible and fitting service members with properly sized NBC overgarments, boots, and gloves.

Heat stress is a major limitation to work performance and tolerance in NBC uniforms. NBC protective uniforms have high insulating and low moisture-permeability properties. Heat stress, and subsequently heat illness, in NBC protective uniforms can be decreased by (1) reducing the barrier by wearing the lowest MOPP level appropriate to the NBC threat, (2) decreasing metabolic heat production, or (3) cooling the service member by mechanical means. Because metabolic heat production is the main source of thermal stress in NBC uniforms, reducing it is the most effective way to reduce heat illness in protective uniforms. The use of work/rest cycles will increase tolerance times and decrease heat casualties but will also increase the time required to perform tasks.

Protective uniforms impede breathing by adding three external loads to the respiratory system: (1) flow-dependent resistive loads, (2) dead space, and (3) volume-dependent elastic loads. The CB mask opposes breathing by applying a nonlinear, phasic, flow-resistive load, which decreases maximal breathing capacity while simultaneously increasing the work of breathing. The increased intrathoracic forces generated to breathe against the CB mask heighten the perception of adverse respiratory sensations (eg, breathlessness). The added external dead space of the CB mask increases ventilatory effort and the work of breathing. The NBC uniform overgarments, load-carriage equipment, and body armor produce an external constraint on the chest wall separate from that imposed by the CB mask. These factors interact to impair breathing and consequently the performance of military operations. Respiratory problems can be managed by using moderate work rates and by frequent training in the CB mask to become familiar with the respiratory sensations associated with it.

The NBC protective uniform also reduces sensory capabilities and impairs bodily functions. Gloves impair tactile sensations. The CB mask and hood restrict the visual field, impair hearing, distort speech, and eliminate olfactory clues. NBC protective uniforms make eating, drinking, eliminating body wastes, and sleeping difficult. Through-the-mask tube drinking systems are commonplace but time-consuming to use, and the possible risk of contamination may deter service members from drinking as frequently as they should. Elimination of body wastes while wearing the NBC protective uniform is cumbersome at best. These functions are easier if performed in in a collective shelter. It is difficult to sleep comfortably while wearing a CB mask; in protective clothing, personnel require more time to fall asleep and once asleep are more likely to awaken spontaneously.

In combat with CB weapons, many more casualties with psychological stress than actual CB injuries are likely. This prediction reflects the adverse impact of fears and anxieties that troops experience in dealing with the threat of a CB contaminated battlefield. Maladaptive responses include hyperventilation, claustrophobia, gas-mask phobia, and compulsive practices or obsessive concern with decontamination, congregating in safe or collective protection areas, finding excuses to never come out or let others into a safe space, and hoarding or stealing protective items. Psychological denial, fatalism, rationalization, and intellectualization may also occur; all prevent troops from taking adaptive actions or enacting useful countermeasures. These responses are more common in younger and less-experienced soldiers than in older ones. Because many soldiers lack detailed familiarity with CB weapons, it is essential that they understand that the NBC protective uniforms issued to them will protect against chemicals on the battlefield. This will do much to reduce

fear, anxiety, and adverse reactions to NBC protective uniform. Many field experiments have demonstrated that most standard military tasks can be performed satisfactorily in NBC protective uniforms, but extra time is required to perform them. Adaptation and gradual experience with NBC protective uniforms and equipment is usually helpful. Younger, less-experienced soldiers are more impaired by NBC protective uniforms than are older soldiers. Older military personnel exhibit fewer symptoms and appear less anxious about training in NBC protective uniforms.

Because personnel in military units turn over frequently, all troops should train frequently in their NBC protective uniforms on common military tasks and, as well, in larger-scale team scenarios in which they practice working together. Intensive training to do critical tasks in NBC protective uniforms can promote confidence, reduce adverse emotions, and better prepare all forces to fight successfully on a contaminated battlefield.

Future doctrine, advances in protective uniforms, and training should strive to develop new ways to reduce the limitations of NBC protective uniforms so that troops can function effectively on future NBC-contaminated battlefields.

ACKNOWLEDGMENT

The authors acknowledge and recognize the intellectual, scientific, and collegial contributions of Colonel Gerald P. Krueger, MSC, US Army (Ret), and Colonel James W. Stokes, MC, US Army, to the psychological aspects of this manuscript. We thank Allyson Nolan, Patricia Bremner, and Pam Dotter, US Army Natick Technical Library, for their continued commitment to provide expert information for this and other manuscripts. We appreciate the encouragement and support of our Division Chiefs, Dr J. Patton and Dr M. Sawka. We also recognize the varied contributions of Sergeant S. Carson, Jennifer Collins, and Specialists M. Horne and E. DeJesus to this effort.

REFERENCES

1. Christopher GW, Cieslak TJ, Pavlin JA, Eitzen EM. Biological warfare: A historical perspective. *JAMA.* 1997;278:412–417.

2. Sidell FR, Takafujk ET, Franz DR. *Medical Aspects of Chemical and Biological Warfare.* In: Zajtchuk R, Bellamy RF. *Textbook of Military Medicine.* Washington, DC: Washington, DC: US Department of the Army, Office of The Surgeon General, Borden Institute; 1997: 361–396.

3. Taylor HL, Orlansky J. The effects of wearing protective chemical warfare combat clothing on human performance. *Aviat Space Environ Med.* 1993;64:A1–A41.

4. Banderet LE, Blewett W, Gonzalez RR, et al. *Proceedings of a Symposium—Consequences of Wearing the Chemical Protective Ensemble: Illustrative Assessment Approaches.* Natick, Mass: US Army Research Institute of Environmental Medicine; 1992. USARIEM Technical Report T9-92.

5. US Department of the Army. *NBC Protection.* Washington, DC: DA; 1992. Army Field Manual 3-4.

6. Bensel CK, Santee WR. Climate and clothing. In: Salvendy G, ed. *Handbook of Human Factors and Ergonomics.* 2nd ed. New York, NY: John Wiley & Sons; 1997: 909–934.

7. Levine L, Quigley MD, Latzka WA, Cadarette BS, Kolka MA. *Thermal Strain in Soldiers Wearing a Chemical Protective Undergarment: Results From a Laboratory Study and a Field Study.* Natick, Mass: US Army Research Institute of Environmental Medicine; 1993. USARIEM Technical Report T2-93.

8. McLellan TM, Bell DG, Dix JK. Heat strain with combat clothing worn over a chemical defense (CD) vapor protective layer. *Aviat Space Environ Med.* 1994;65:757–763.

9. Amos D, Hansen R. The physiological strain induced by a new low burden chemical protective ensemble. *Aviat Space Environ Med.* 1997;68:126–131.

10. US Department of the Army. *Operator's Manual for Chemical-Biological Mask: Field, M40.* Washington, DC; 1988. Technical Manual 3-4240-300-10-1.

11. US Department of the Army. *Soldier's Manual of Common Tasks, Skill Level 1.* Washington, DC: DA; 1990. STP 21-1-SMCT.

12. US Department of the Army. *Military Occupational Specialties.* Washington, DC: DA; 1978. Army Regulation 611-201.

13. Teitlebaum A, Goldman RF. Increased energy cost with multiple clothing layers. *J Appl Physiol.* 1972;32:743–744.

14. Amor AF, Vogel JA, Worsley DE. *The Energy Cost of Wearing Multilayer Clothing.* Farnborough, England: Royal Aircraft Establishment; 1973. Technical Report 18/73.

15. Duggan A. Energy cost of stepping in protective clothing ensembles. *Ergonomics.* 1988;31:3–11.

16. Patton JF, Murphy M, Bidwell T, Mello R, Harp M. *Metabolic Cost of Military Physical Tasks in MOPP 0 and MOPP 4.* Natick, Mass: US Army Research Institute of Environmental Medicine; 1995. USARIEM Technical Report T95-9.

17. Soule RG, Goldman RF. Energy cost of loads carried on the head, hands or feet. *J Appl Physiol.* 1969;27:687–690.

18. Bensel CK. Soldier performance and functionality: Impact of chemical protective clothing. *Military Psychology.* 1997;9:287–300.

19. Bensel CK, Teixeira RA, Kaplan DB. *The Effects of Two Chemical Protective Clothing Systems on the Visual Field, Speech Intelligibility, Body Mobility, and Psychomotor Coordination of Men.* Natick, Mass: US Army Natick Research, Development and Engineering Center; 1992. Technical Report TR-92-025.

20. Krueger GP, Banderet LE. Effects of chemical protective clothing on military performance: A review of the issues. *Military Psychology.* 1997;9:255–286.

21. Kobrick JL, Johnson RF, McMenemy DJ. *Nerve Agent Antidotes and Heat Exposure: Summary of Effects on Task Performance of Soldiers Wearing BDU and MOPP-IV Clothing Systems.* Natick, Mass: US Army Research Institute of Environmental Medicine; 1988. USARIEM Technical Report T1-89.

22. Bensel CK. The effects of various thicknesses of chemical protective gloves on manual dexterity. *Ergonomics.* 1993;36:687–696.

23. Bensel CK, Teixeira RA, Kaplan DB. *The Effects of US Army Chemical Protective Clothing on Speech Intelligibility, Visual Field, Body Mobility and Psychomotor Coordination of Men.* Natick, Mass: US Army Natick Research, Development and Engineering Center; 1987. Technical Report TR-87-037.

24. Goldman RF. Tolerance time for work in the heat when wearing CBR protective clothing. *Mil Med.* 1963;128:776–786.

25. Montain SJ, Sawka MN, Cadarette BS, Quigley MD, McKay JM. Physiological tolerance to uncompensable heat stress: Effects of exercise intensity, protective clothing, and climate. *J Appl Physiol.* 1994;77:216–222.

26. Joy RJT, Goldman RF. A method of relating physiology and military performance: A study of some effects of vapor barrier clothing in a hot climate. *Mil Med.* 1968;133:458–470.

27. McLellan TM, Jacobs I, Bain JB. Influence of temperature and metabolic rate on work performance with Canadian forces NBC clothing. *Aviat Space Environ Med.* 1993;64:587–594.

28. Kraning KK, Gonzalez RR. Physiological consequences of intermittent exercise during compensable and uncompensable heat stress. *J Appl Physiol.* 1991;71:2138–2145.

29. McLellan TM, Jacobs I, Bain JB. Continuous vs intermittent work with Canadian forces NBC clothing. *Aviat Space Environ Med.* 1993;64:595–598.

30. McLellan TM, Jacobs I, Bain JB. Influence of temperature and metabolic rate on work performance with Canadian forces NBC clothing. *Aviat Space Environ Med.* 1993;64:587–594.

31. US Department of the Army. *Occupational and Environmental Health: Prevention, Treatment and Control of Heat Injury.* Washington, DC: DA; 1980. Technical Bulletin, Medical 507.

32. Goldman RF. Chief Scientist, Comfort Technology, Inc, 45 Fox Hill Road, Framingham, Mass; former Director, Military Ergonomics Division, US Army Research Institute of Environmental Medicine, Natick, Mass. Personal communication, 1997.

33. Burr RE. *Heat Illness: A Handbook for Medical Officers.* Natick, Mass: US Army Research Institute of Environmental Medicine; 1991. USARIEM Technical Report T91-3.

34. Cadarette BS, Montain SJ, Kolka MA, Stroschein LA, Matthew WT, Sawka MN. *Evaluation of USARIEM Heat Strain Model: MOPP Level, Exercise Intensity in Desert and Tropic Climates.* Natick, Mass: US Army Research Institution of Environmental Medicine; 1996. USARIEM Technical Report T96-4.

35. Givoni B, Goldman RF. Predicting effects of heat acclimatization on heart rate and rectal temperature. *J Appl Physiol.* 1973;35:875–879.

36. Givoni B, Goldman RF. Predicting rectal temperature response to work, environment, and clothing. *J Appl Physiol.* 1972;32(6):812–822.

37. Nunneley SA, Flick CF. Heat stress in the A-10 cockpit: Flights over desert. *Aviat Space Environ Med.* 1981;52:513–516.

38. Nunneley SA, Myhre LG. Physiological effects of solar heat load in a fighter cockpit. *Aviat Space Environ Med.* 1976;47:969–973.

39. Nunneley SA, Stribley RF, Allan JR. Heat stress in front and rear cockpits of F-4 aircraft. *Aviat Space Environ Med.* 1981;52:287–290.

40. Thornton R, Caldwell JL. The physiological consequences of simulated helicopter flight in NBC protective equipment. *Aviat Space Environ Med.* 1993;64:69–73.

41. Sowood PJ, O'Connor EM. Thermal strain and G protection associated with wearing an enhanced anti-G protection system in a warm climate. *Aviat Space Environ Med.* 1994;65:992–998.

42. DuBois AB. Resistance to breathing. In: Fenn WO, Rahn H, eds. *Respiration.* In: Section 3, Vol 1. American Physiological Society. *Handbook of Physiology.* Baltimore, Md: Williams & Wilkins for APS; 1964: 451–462.

43. Agostoni E, Mead J. Statics of the respiratory system. In: Fenn WO, Rahn H, eds. *Respiration.* In: Section 3, Vol 1. American Physiological Society. *Handbook of Physiology.* Baltimore, Md: Williams & Wilkins for APS; 1964: 387–409.

44. Silverman L, Lee G, Plotkin T, Sawyers LA, Yancey AR. Airflow measurements on human subjects with and without respiratory resistance at several work rates. *Am Ind Hyg Assoc J.* 1951;3:461–478.

45. Bentley RA, Griffin OG, Love RG, Muir DCF, Sweetland KF. Acceptable levels for breathing resistance of respiratory apparatus. *Arch Environ Health.* 1973;27:273–280.

46. Lerman Y, Shefer A, Epstein Y, Keren G. External inspiratory resistance of protective respiratory devices: Effects on physical performance and respiratory function. *Am J Ind Med*. 1983;4:733–740.

47. Levine L, Evans WJ, Winsmann FR, Pandolf KB. Prolonged self-paced hard physical exercise comparing trained and untrained men. *Ergonomics*. 1982;25(5):393–400.

48. Sulotto F, Romano C, Dori S, Piolatto G, Chiesa A, Ciacco C. The prediction of recommended energy expenditure for an 8 h work-day using an air-purifying respiratory. *Ergonomics*. 1993;36:1479–1487.

49. Wold NP, Steelman J. *Development Test II (PQT-G) of XM30 Series Protective Masks and Accessories*. Dugway, Utah: US Army Dugway Proving Ground; 1984. Technical Report DPG-FR-203.

50. American Thoracic Society: Medical Section of the American Lung Association. Standardization of spirometry: 1994 update. *Am J Respir Crit Care Med*. 1995;152:1107–1136.

51. Muza SR, Banderet LE, Forte VA. Effects of chemical defense clothing and individual equipment on ventilatory function and subjective reactions. *Aviat Space Environ Med*. 1996;67:1190–1197.

52. Kelly TL, Yeager JA, Sucec AA, Englund CE, Smith DA. *The Effect of the M17A2 Mask on Spirometry Values in Healthy Subjects*. San Diego, Calif: US Naval Health Research Center; 1987. Technical Report 87-39.

53. Muza SR, Banderet LE, Forte VA. *The Impact of the NBC Clothing Ensemble on Respiratory Function and Capacities During Rest and Exercise*. Natick, Mass: US Army Research Institute of Environmental Medicine; 1995. USARIEM Technical Report T95-12.

54. Raven PB, Moss RF, Page K, Garmon R, Skaggs B. Clinical pulmonary function and industrial respirator wear. *Am Ind Hyg Assoc J*. 1981;42(12):897–903.

55. Roussos C, Campbell EJM. Respiratory muscle energetics. In: Macklem PT; Mead J, eds. *The Respiratory System*. In: Part 2, *Mechanics of Breathing*. Section 3, Vol 3. In: American Physiological Society. *Handbook of Physiology*. Baltimore, Md: Williams & Wilkins for APS; 1986: 481–509.

56. Aaron EA, Seow KC, Johnson BD, Dempsey JA. Oxygen cost of exercise hyperpnea: Implications for performance. *J Appl Physiol*. 1992;72:1818–1825.

57. Aaron EA, Johnson BD, Seow KC, Dempsey JA. Oxygen cost of exercise hyperpnea: Measurement. *J Appl Physiol*. 1992;72:1810–1817.

58. Johnson BD, Saupe KW, Dempsey JA. Mechanical constraints on exercise hyperpnea in endurance athletes. *J Appl Physiol*. 1992;73:874–886.

59. McCool FD, McCann DR, Leith DE, Hoppin FG Jr. Pressure-flow effects on endurance of inspiratory muscles. *J Appl Physiol*. 1986;60(1):299–303.

60. Goldman MD, Grimby G, Mead J. Mechanical work of breathing derived from rib cage and abdominal V-P partitioning. *J Appl Physiol*. 1976;41(5):752–763.

61. Dodd DS, Yarom J, Loring SH, Engel LA. O_2 cost of inspiratory and expiratory resistive loading in humans. *J Appl Physiol*. 1988;65:2518–2523.

62. Harber P, Shimozaki S, Barrett T, Fine G. Effect of exercise level on ventilatory adaptation to respirator use. *J Occup Med*. 1990;32:1042–1046.

63. Sampson MG, De Troyer A. Role of intercostal muscles in the rib cage distortions produced by inspiratory loads. *J Appl Physiol*. 1982;52:517–523.

64. McGregor M, Becklake MK. The relationship of oxygen cost of breathing to respiratory mechanical work and respiratory force. *J Clin Invest*. 1961;40:971–980.

65. Agostoni E, Mognoni P. Deformation of the chest wall during breathing efforts. *J Appl Physiol.* 1966;21:1827–1832.

66. Collett PW, Perry C, Engel LA. Pressure-time product, flow and oxygen cost of resistive breathing in humans. *J Appl Physiol.* 1985;58:1263–1272.

67. Robertson CHJ, Pagel MA, Johnson RLJ. The distribution of blood flow, oxygen consumption, and work output among the respiratory muscles during unobstructed hyperventilation. *J Clin Invest.* 1977;59:43–50.

68. Axen K, Haas SS, Haas F, Gaudino D, Haas A. Ventilatory adjustments during sustained mechanical loading in conscious humans. *J Appl Physiol.* 1983;55(4):1211–1218.

69. Zechman FW, Wiley RL. Afferent inputs to breathing: Respiratory sensations. In: Fishman AP, Cherniack NS, Widdicombe JG, Geiger SR, eds. *The Respiratory System.* In: Section 3. American Physiological Society. *Handbook of Physiology.* Baltimore, Md: Williams & Wilkins for APS; 1986: 449–474.

70. Cherniack NS, Milic-Emili J. Mechanical aspects of loaded breathing. In: Roussos C, Macklem PT, eds. *The Thorax.* New York, NY: Marcel Dekker, Inc; 1985: 751–786.

71. Daubenspeck JA, Bennett FM. Immediate human breathing pattern responses to loads near the perceptual threshold. *J Appl Physiol.* 1983;55(4):1160–1166.

72. Deno NS, Kamon E, Kiser DM. Physiological responses to resistance breathing during short and prolonged exercise. *Am Ind Hyg Assoc J.* 1981;42:616–623.

73. El-Manshawi A, Killian KJ, Summers E, Jones NL. Breathlessness during exercise with and without resistive loading. *J Appl Physiol.* 1986;61:896–905.

74. Flook V, Kelman GR. Submaximal exercise with increased inspiratory resistance to breathing. *J Appl Physiol.* 1973;35:379–384.

75. Gothe B, Cherniack NS. Effects of expiratory loading on respiration in humans. *J Appl Physiol.* 1980;49(4):601–608.

76. Haxhiu MA, Cherniack NS, Altose MD, Kelsen SG. Effect of respiratory loading on the relationship between occlusion pressure and diaphragm EMG during hypoxia and hypercapnia. *Am Rev Respir Dis.* 1983;127:185–188.

77. Iber C, Berssenbrugge A, Skatrud JB, Dempsey JA. Ventilatory adaptations to resistive loading during wakefulness and non-REM sleep. *J Appl Physiol.* 1982;52(3):607–614.

78. Lopata M, Onal E, Evanich MJ, Lourenco RV. Respiratory neuromuscular response to CO_2 rebreathing with inspiratory flow resistance in humans. *Respir Physiol.* 1980;39:95–110.

79. Martin RR, Wilson JE, Ross WRD, Anthonisen NR. The effect of added external resistance on regional pulmonary filling and emptying sequences. *Can J Physiol Pharmacol.* 1971;49(5):406–411.

80. Mengeot PM, Bates JHT, Martin JG. Effect of mechanical loading on displacements of chest wall during breathing in humans. *J Appl Physiol.* 1985;58:477–484.

81. Pardy RL, Bye PTP. Diaphragmatic fatigue in normoxia and hyperoxia. *J Appl Physiol.* 1985;58(3):738–742.

82. Pope H, Holloway R, Campbell EJM. The effects of elastic and resistive loading of inspiration on the breathing of conscious man. *Respir Physiol.* 1968;4:363–372.

83. Scharf SM, Bark H, Heimer D, Cohen A, Macklem PT. "Second wind" during inspiratory loading. *Med Sci Sports Exerc.* 1984;16(1):87–91.

84. Shannon R, Zechman FW. The reflex and mechanical response of the inspiratory muscles to an increased airflow resistance. *Respir Physiol.* 1972;16:51–69.

85. Stemler FW, Craig FN. Effects of respiratory equipment on endurance in hard work. *J Appl Physiol.* 1977;42(1):28–32.

86. Zin WA, Rossi A, Milic-Emili J. Model analysis of respiratory responses to inspiratory resistive loads. *J Appl Physiol.* 1983;55(5):1565–1573.

87. Milic-Emili J, Zin WA. Breathing responses to imposed mechanical loads. In: Fishman AP, Cherniack NS, Widdicombe JG, Geiger SR, eds. In: *The Respiratory System.* In: Section 3. American Physiological Society. *Handbook of Physiology.* Baltimore, Md: Williams & Wilkins for APS; 1986: 751–769.

88. Findlay IN, Gillen G, Cunningham AD, Elliott AT, Aitchison T, Dargie HJ. A comparison of isometric exercise, cold pressor stimulation and dynamic exercise in patients with coronary heart disease. *Eur Heart J.* 1988;9:657–664.

89. Georgopoulos D, Berezanski D, Anthonisen NR. Effect of dichloroacetate on ventilatory response to sustained hypoxia in normal adults. *Respir Physiol.* 1990;82:115–122.

90. Whipp BJ, Pardy RL. Breathing during exercise. In: Macklem PT; Mead J, eds. *The Respiratory System.* In: Part 2, *Mechanics of Breathing.* Section 3, Vol 3. In: American Physiological Society. *Handbook of Physiology.* Baltimore, Md: Williams & Wilkins for APS; 1986: 605–629.

91. Grodins FS, Yamashiro SM. Control of ventilation. In: West J, ed. *Control of Ventilation in Bioengineering Aspects of the Lung.* New York, NY: Marcel Dekker, Inc. 1977: 543–552.

92. Yamashiro SM, Grodins FS. Respiratory cycle optimization in exercise. *J Appl Physiol.* 1973;35:522–525.

93. Zechman F, Hall FG, Hull WE. Effects of graded resistance to tracheal airflow in man. *J Appl Physiol.* 1957;10(3):356–362.

94. Louhevaara V. Physiological effects associated with the use of respiratory protective devices. *Scand J Work Environ Health.* 1984;10:275–281.

95. Muza SR, Levine L, Latzka WA, Sawka MN. Inspiratory resistance effects on exercise breathing pattern relationships to chemoresponsiveness. *Int J Sports Med.* 1996;17:344–350.

96. Killian KJ, Bucens DD, Campbell EJM. Effect of breathing patterns on the perceived magnitude of added loads to breathing. *J Appl Physiol.* 1982;52(3):578–584.

97. Burki NK. Effects of bronchodilation on magnitude estimation of added resistive loads in asthmatic subjects. *Am Rev Respir Dis.* 1984;129:225–229.

98. D'Urzo AD, Chapman KR, Rebuck AS. Effect of inspiratory resistive loading on control of ventilation during progressive exercise. *J Appl Physiol.* 1987;62:134–140.

99. Demedts M, Anthonisen NR. Effects of increased external airway resistance during steady-state exercise. *J Appl Physiol.* 1973;35:361–366.

100. Cerretelli P, Rajinder S, Farhi LE. Effect of increased airway resistance on ventilation and gas exchange during exercise. *J Appl Physiol.* 1969;27:597–600.

101. Hermansen L, Vokac Z, Lereim P. Respiratory and circulatory response to added airflow resistance during exercise. *Ergonomics.* 1972;15:15–24.

102. Jetté M, Thoden J, Livingstone S. Physiological effects of inspiratory resistance on progressive aerobic work. *Eur J Appl Physiol.* 1990;60:65–70.

103. Craig FN, Blevins WV, Froehlich HL. *Training to Improve Endurance in Exhausting Work of Men Wearing Protective Masks: A Review and Some Preliminary Experiments.* Edgewood Arsenal, Md: US Army Medical Research Laboratory; 1971. Technical Report AD 729787.

104. Craig FN, Stemler FW. *Respiratory Resistance and the Endurance of Men Working Under Thermal Stress.* Aberdeen Proving Ground, Md: US Army Armament Command; 1975. Technical Report EB-TR-75025.

105. Craig FN, Blevins WV, Cummings EG. Exhausting work limited by external resistance and inhalation of carbon dioxide. *J Appl Physiol.* 1970;29(6):847–851.

106. Dempsey JA. Is the lung built for exercise? *Med Sci Sports Exerc.* 1986;18:143–155.

107. Leith DE, Bradley MD. Ventilatory muscle strength and endurance training. *J Appl Physiol.* 1976;41:508–516.

108. Wasserman K, Hansen JE, Sue DY, Whipp BJ. Normal values. In: *Principles of Exercise Testing and Interpretation.* Philadelphia, Pa: Lea & Febiger; 1987: 72–86.

109. McCool FD, Tzelepis G, Leith DE, Hoppin FG Jr. Oxygen cost of breathing during fatiguing inspiratory resistive loads. *J Appl Physiol.* 1989;66(5):2045–2055.

110. Bai TR, Rabinovitich BJ, Prady RL. Near maximal voluntary hyperpnea and ventilatory muscle function. *J Appl Physiol.* 1984;57:1742–1748.

111. Bye PTP, Esau SA, Walley KR, Macklem PT, Pardy RL. Ventilatory muscles during exercise in air and oxygen in normal men. *J Appl Physiol.* 1984;56:464–471.

112. Johnson AT, Berlin HM. Exhalation time characterizing exhaustion while wearing respiratory protective masks. *Am Ind Hyg Assoc J.* 1974;35:463–467.

113. Altose MD, Zechman FWJ. Loaded breathing: Load compensation and respiratory sensation. *Fed Proc.* 1986;45(2):114–122.

114. Harber P, Shimozaki S, Barrett T, Loisides P. Relationship of subjective tolerance of respirator loads to physiologic effects and psychophysical load sensitivity. *J Occup Med.* 1989;31:681–686.

115. Muza SR, Levine L, Latzka WA. *Respiratory Chemosensitivity and Resistive Load Sensation on Ventilatory Control During Exercise.* Natick, Mass: US Army Research Institute of Environmental Medicine; 1990. USARIEM Technical Report T14-90.

116. Altose MD, Dimarco AF, Gottfried SB, Strohl KP. The sensation of respiratory muscle force. *Am Rev Respir Dis.* 1982;126:807–811.

117. Hirshman CA, McCullough RE, Weil JV. Normal values for hypoxic and hypercapnic ventilatory drives in man. *J Appl Physiol.* 1975;38:1095–1098.

118. Mahler DA, Moritz ED, Loke J. Ventilatory responses at rest and during exercise in marathon runners. *J Appl Physiol.* 1982;52:388–392.

119. Martin BJ, Weil JV, Sparks KE, McCullough RE, Grover RF. Exercise ventilation correlates positively with ventilatory chemoresponsiveness. *J Appl Physiol.* 1978;45:557–564.

120. Rebuck AS, Read J. Patterns of ventilatory response to carbon dioxide during recovery from severe asthma. *Clin Sci.* 1971;41:13–21.

121. Boutellier U, Piwko P. The respiratory system as an exercise limiting factor in normal sedentary subjects. *Eur J Appl Physiol.* 1992;64:145–152.

122. Bradley ME, Leith DE. Ventilatory muscle training and the oxygen cost of sustained hyperpnea. *J Appl Physiol.* 1978;45(6):885–892.

123. Fanta CH, Leith DE, Brown R. Maximal shortening of inspiratory muscles: Effect of training. *J Appl Physiol.* 1983;54(6):1618–1623.

124. Morgan DW, Kohrt WM, Bates BJ, Skinner JS. Effects of respiratory muscle endurance training on ventilatory and endurance performance of moderately trained cyclists. *Int J Sports Med.* 1987;8:88–93.

125. Leith DE, Philip B, Gabel RA, Feldman H, Fencl V. Ventilatory muscle training and ventilatory control. *Am Rev Respir Dis.* 1979;119:99–100.

126. Epstein Y, Keren G, Lerman Y, Shefer A. Physiological and psychological adaptation to respiratory protective devices. *Aviat Space Environ Med.* 1982;53(7):663–665.

127. Bartlett HL, Hodgson JL, Kollias J. Effect of respiratory valve dead space on pulmonary ventilation at rest and during exercise. *Med Sci Sports Exerc.* 1972;4:132–137.

128. Jones NL, Levine GB, Robertson DG, Epstein SW. The effect of added dead space on the pulmonary response to exercise. *Respiration.* 1971;28:389–398.

129. Kelman GR, Watson WS. Effect of added dead space on pulmonary ventilation during sub-maximal steady-state exercise. *Q J Exp Physiol.* 1973;58:305–313.

130. Harber P, Shimozaki S, Barrett T, Losides P, Fine G. Effects of respirator dead space, inspiratory resistance, and expiratory resistance ventilatory loads. *Am J Ind Med.* 1989;16:189–198.

131. Gothe B, Altose MD, Goldman MD, Cherniack NS. Effect of quiet sleep on resting and CO_2 stimulated breathing in humans. *J Appl Physiol.* 1981;50(4):724–730.

132. Berthon-Jones M, Sullivan CE. Ventilation and arousal responses to hypercapnia in normal sleeping humans. *J Appl Physiol.* 1984;37(1):59–67.

133. Harber P, Beck J, Brown C, Luo J. Physiologic and subjective effects of respirator mask type. *Am Ind Hyg Assoc J.* 1991;52:357–362.

134. Muza SR, Latzka WA, Epstein Y, Pandolf KB. Load carriage induced alterations of pulmonary function. *Int J Ind Ergonomics.* 1989;3:221–227.

135. Legg SJ. Influence of body armour on pulmonary function. *Ergonomics.* 1988;31:349–353.

136. Legg SJ, Mahanty A. Comparisons of five modes of carrying a load close to the trunk. *Ergonomics.* 1985;28:1653–1660.

137. Muza SR, Quigley MD, Prusaczyk WK, Sawka MN. Influence of backpack wear on ventilation and acid–base equilibrium during exercise. US Army Research Institute of Environmental Medicine, Natick, Mass; 1993. Unpublished results.

138. Agostoni E, D'Angelo E, Piolini M. Breathing pattern in men during inspiratory elastic loads. *Respir Physiol.* 1978;34:279–293.

139. Green M, Mead J, Sears TA. Muscle activity during chest wall restriction and positive pressure breathing in man. *Respir Physiol.* 1978;35:283–300.

140. Killian KJ, Mahutte CK, Campbell EJM. Magnitude scaling of externally added loads to breathing. *Am Rev Respir Dis.* 1981;123:12–15.

141. Blewett W, Redmond D, Popp K, Harrah D, Kirven L, Banderet LE. *A P^{2}NBC^2 Report: Detailed Equipment Decontamination Operations.* Aberdeen Proving Ground, Md: Chemical Research, Development and Engineering Center; 1992. Technical Report CRDEC-TR-330.

142. Brooks FR, Ebner DG, Xenakis SN, Balson PM. Psychological reactions during chemical warfare training. *Mil Med.* 1983;148:232–235.

143. Carter BJ, Cammermeyer M. Human responses to simulated chemical warfare training in US Army reserve personnel. *Mil Med.* 1989;154:281–288.

144. Munro I, Rauch TM, Banderet LE, Lussier AR, Tharion WJ, Shukitt-Hale B. *Psychological Effects of Sustained Operations in a Simulated NBC Environment on M1 Tank Crews.* Natick, Mass: US Army Research Institute of Environmental Medicine; 1987. USARIEM Technical Report T26-87.

145. Stokes JW, Banderet LE. Psychological aspects of chemical defense and warfare. *Military Psychology.* 1997;9:395–415.

146. Muza SR. *A Review of Biomedical Aspects of CB Masks and Their Relationship to Military Performance.* Natick, Mass: US Army Research Institute of Environmental Medicine; 1986. USARIEM Technical Report T1-87.

147. Garinther GR, Hodge DC. *Effect of the M25 Protective Mask and Hood on Speech Intelligibility and Voice Level.* Aberdeen Proving Ground, Md: US Army Human Engineering Laboratory; 1987. Technical Report Tech Memo 19-87.

148. Harrah D. *Binocular Scanning Performance for Soldiers Wearing Protective Masks—2.* Aberdeen Proving Ground, Md: US Army Human Engineering Laboratory; 1985. Technical Report Tech Memo 14-85.

149. McAlister WH, Buckingham RS. A comparison of the visual field restrictions with the M17 series protective mask and the MCU-2/P chemical biological mask. *Mil Med.* 1993;158:266–269.

150. Harrah D, McMahon R, Stemann KM, Kirven L. *HEL Evaluation of Vision-Corrective Inserts for the M40 Protective Mask.* Aberdeen Proving Ground, Md: US Army Human Engineering Laboratory; 1991. Technical Report 4-91.

151. Wildzunas RM. Visual performance effects and user acceptance of the M43A1 aviation protective mask frontserts. *Aviat Space Environ Med.* 1995;66:1136–1143.

152. Lattimore MR, Cornum RLS. *The Use of Extended Wear Contact Lenses in the Aviation Environment: An Army Wide Study.* Fort Rucker, Ala: US Army Aeromedical Research Laboratory; 1992. Technical Report 92-35.

153. Szlyk PC, Tharion WJ, Francesconi RP, et al. *Effects of a Modified Through-Mask Drinking System (MDS) on Fluid Intake During Exercise in Chemical Protective Gear.* Natick, Mass: US Army Research Institute of Environmental Medicine; 1989. USARIEM Technical Report T1-90.

154. Cardello AV, Darsch G, Fitzgerald C, Gleason S, Teixeira RA. Nutrient, waste management, and hygiene systems for chemical protective suits. *Mil Med.* 1991;156:211–215.

155. Lieberman HR, Mays MZ, Shukitt-Hale B, Chinn KSK, Tharion WJ. Effects of sleeping in a chemical protective mask on sleep quality and cognitive performance. *Aviat Space Environ Med.* 1996;67:841–848.

156. Blewett W, Redmond D, Seitzinger AT, Fatkin L, Banderet LE. *A P^2NBC^2 Report: Light Division Night Decontamination Operations.* Aberdeen Proving Ground, Md: Chemical Research, Development and Engineering Center; 1993. Technical Report ERDEC-TR-087.

157. Fatkin L, Hudgens GA. *Stress Perceptions of Soldiers Participating in Training at the Chemical Defense Training Facility: The Mediating Effects of Motivation, Experience, and Confidence Level.* Aberdeen Proving Ground, Md: US Army Human Engineering Laboratory; 1994. Technical Report ARL-TR-365.

158. Morgan WP. Psychological problems associated with the wearing of industrial respirators: A review. *Am Ind Hyg Assoc J.* 1983;44(9):671–676.

159. Van De Linde FJG. Loss of performance by wearing a respirator does not increase during a 22.5-hour wearing period. *Aviat Space Environ Med.* 1988;59:273–277.

160. Taylor BJ. *Psychological Reactions to Encapsulation in Protective Ensemble: Identifying the Problems, Offering Some Solutions.* Canberra, Australia: 1st Psychological Research Unit; 1993. Technical Report 2-93.

161. Haber LF. *The Poisonous Cloud: Chemical Warfare in the First World War.* Oxford, England: Clarendon Press; 1986.

162. O'Brien LS, Payne RG. Prevention and management of panic in personnel facing a chemical threat: Lessons from the Gulf War. *J R Army Medical Corps.* 1993;139:41–45.

163. Altman L. Nerve gas that felled Tokyo subway riders said to be one of the most lethal known. *New York Times.* 1995;21 Mar:A13.

164. Lillibridge SR, Liddle JA, Leffingwell SS, Sidell FS. *Report of the American Delegation to Japan.* Atlanta, Ga: Centers for Disease Control and Prevention; 1995.

165. Headley DB, Hudgens GA, Cunningham D. The operational impact of chemical protective clothing on field task performance during military operations. *Military Psychology.* 1997;9:359–374.

166. Draper ES, Lombardi JJ. *Combined Arms in a Nuclear/Chemical Environment Force Development Testing and Experimentation: CANE FDTE Summary Evaluation Report, Phase 1.* Fort McClellan, Ala: US Army Chemical School; 1986.

167. Ramirez T. Modeling military task performance for Army and Air Force personnel wearing chemical protective clothing. *Military Psychology.* 1997;9:375–393.

168. Sinaiko HW, Belden TG. The indelicate experiment. In: Spiegel J, Walker DE, eds. *Second Congress on the Information System Sciences.* Washington, DC: Spartan Books; 1965: 343–348.

169. Parsons HM. *Man–Machine System Experiments.* Baltimore, Md: The Johns Hopkins University Press; 1972.

170. Montgomery JR. *Maintenance Operations in Mission-Oriented Protective Posture IV (MOPP IV).* Dugway, Utah: US Army Dugway Proving Ground; 1987.

171. Driskell JE, Guy W, Saunders T, Wheeler W. *Performance Degradation Assessment for Operations in Chemical/Biological Environments.* Dugway, Utah: US Army Dugway Proving Ground; 1992. Technical Report DPG/JOD-92/030.

172. Gilchrist HL. Field arrangements for gas defense and the care of gas casualties. In: Weed FW, McAfee AM, eds. *Medical Aspects of Gas Warfare.* Vol 14. In: Bancroft WD, Bradley HC, Eyster JAE, et al, eds. *The Medical Department of the United States Army in the World War.* Washington, DC: Office of the Surgeon General, Medical Department, US Department of the Army; 1926: 59–80.

173. Newhouse P. Neuropsychiatric aspects of chemical warfare. In: Belenky G, ed. *Contemporary Studies in Combat Psychiatry.* Westport, Conn: Greenwood Press. 1987: 185–202.

174. Gourley SR. Ready or not: Preparing for the chemical onslaught. *Jane's International Defense Review.* 1997;30:65–69.

175. Holloway HC, Norwood AE, Fullerton CS. The threat of biological weapons: Prophylaxis and mitigation of psychological and social consequences. *JAMA.* 1997;278:425–427.

176. Simon JD. Biological terrorism: Preparing to meet the threat. *JAMA.* 1997;278:428–430.

177. Tucker JB. National health and medical services response to incidents of chemical and biological terrorism. *JAMA.* 1997;278:362–368.

178. Franz DR, Jahrling PB, Friedlander AM. Clinical recognition and management of patients exposed to biological warfare agents. *JAMA.* 1997;278:399–411.

179. Bayles F. Boston finds out how ready it is for terror attack. *USA Today.* 1997;15 Sep:5A.

180. Stephenson J. Pentagon-funded research takes aim at agents of biological warfare. *JAMA.* 1997;278:373–375.

181. Bensel CK. *Psychological Aspects of Nuclear, Biological and Chemical Protection of Military Personnel.* Washington, DC: The Technical Cooperation Program, Subgroup U: Human Resources and Performance; 1994. Technical Report SGU-94-007.

182. Johnson AT, Grove CM, Weiss RA. Mask performance rating table for specific military tasks. *Mil Med.* 1993;158:665–670.

183. McLellan TM. Heat strain while wearing the current Canadian or a new hot-weather French NBC protective clothing ensemble. *Aviat Space Environ Med.* 1996;67:1057–1062.

184. Cadarette BS, Quigley MD, McKay JM, Kolka MA, Sawka MN. *Physiological Evaluation of the Soldier Integrated Protective Ensemble (SIPE) Clothing System.* Natick, Mass: US Army Research Institute of Environmental Medicine; 1993. USARIEM Technical Report T3-93.

185. Bomalaski SH, Hengst R, Constable SH. *Thermal Stress in Seven Types of Chemical Defense Ensembles During Moderate Exercise in Hot Environments.* Brooks Air Force Base, Tex: US Air Force Armstrong Laboratories; 1993. Technical Report 1992-141.

186. Pandolf KB, Allan AE, Gonzalez RR, Sawka MN, Stroschein LA, Young AJ. Chemical warfare protective clothing: Identification of performance limitations and their possible solution. In: Asfour SS, ed. *Trends in Ergonomics/Human Factors IV.* North Holland: Elsevier Science Publishers, BV; 1987: 397–404.

187. Banta GR, Braun DE. Heat strain during at-sea helicopter operations and the effect of passive microclimate cooling. *Aviat Space Environ Med.* 1992;63:881–885.

188. Derion T, Pozos RS. *A Review of Microclimate Cooling Systems in the Chemical, Biological, Radiological Environment.* San Diego, Calif: US Naval Health Research Center; 1993. Technical Report NHRC 93-23.

189. Bomalaski SH, Chen YT, Constable SH. Continuous and intermittent personal microclimate cooling strategies. *Aviat Space Environ Med.* 1995;66:745–750.

190. Fonseca GF. *Effectiveness of Five Water-Cooled Undergarments in Reducing Heat Stress of Vehicle Crewmen Operating in a Hot Wet or Hot Dry Environment.* Natick, Mass: US Army Research Institute of Environmental Medicine; 1981. USARIEM Technical Report T2-81.

191. Masadi R, Kinney RF, Blackwell C. *Evaluation of Five Commercial Microclimate Cooling Systems for Military Use.* Natick, Mass: US Army Natick Research, Development and Engineering Center; 1991.

192. Pimental NA, Cosimini HM, Sawka MN, Wenger CB. Effectiveness of an air-cooled vest using selected air temperature and humidity combinations. *Aviat Space Environ Med.* 1987;58:119–124.

193. Vallerand AL, Michas RD, Frim J, Ackles KN. Heat balance in subjects wearing protective clothing with a liquid- or air-cooled vest. *Aviat Space Environ Med.* 1991;62:383–391.

194. Cadarette BS, Pimental NA, Levell CA, Bogart JE, Sawka MN. *Thermal Responses of Tank Crewman Operating With Microclimate Cooling Under Simulated NBC Conditions in the Desert and Tropics.* Natick, Mass: US Army Research Institute of Environmental Medicine; 1986. USARIEM Technical Report T7-86.

195. Thornton R, Caldwell JA, Guardiani F, Pearson J. *Effects of Microclimate Cooling on Physiology and Performance While Flying the UH-60 Helicoptor Flight Simulator in NBC Conditions in a Controlled Heat Environment.* Fort Rucker, Ala: US Army Aeromedical Research Laboratory; 1992. Technical Report 92-32.

196. Caldwell JL, Caldwell JA, Salter CA. Effects of chemical protective clothing and heat stress on Army helicopter pilot performance. *Military Psychology.* 1997;9:315–328.

197. Constable SH. *USAF Physiological Studies of Personal Microclimate Cooling: A Review.* Brooks Air Force Base, Tex: US Air Force Armstrong Laboratory; 1993. Technical Report 1993-30.

198. Reardon MJ, Smythe NI, Omer J, et al. *Effects of Heat Stress and an Encumbered Aviator Uniform on Flight Performance in a UH-60 Helicopter Simulator.* Fort Rucker, Ala: US Army Aeromedical Research Laboratory; 1997. Technical Report 97-12.

199. Reardon MJ, Smythe NI, Omer J, et al. *Physiological and Psychological Effects of Thermally Stressful UH-60 Helicopter Simulator Cockpit Conditions on Aviators Wearing Standard and Encumbered Flight Uniforms.* Fort Rucker, Ala: US Army Aeromedical Research Laboratory; 1997. Technical Report 97-06.

200. Caldwell JA. A brief survey of chemical defense, crew rest, and heat stress/physical training issues related to Operation Desert Storm. *Mil Med.* 1992;157:275–281.

Chapter 37

MEDICAL SUPPORT OF SPECIAL OPERATIONS

FRANK K. BUTLER, JR, MD[*]

*Captain, Medical Corps, US Navy, Naval Special Warfare Command, Detachment Pensacola, Department of Ophthalmology (Code 65), Naval
Hospital, Pensacola, Florida 32512

INTRODUCTION

The term *special operations* as applied to the military of the United States is used to describe a variety of missions carried out by highly select units from the Army, Navy, and Air Force. Historically, individuals in these units are subjected to rigorous selection and training in preparation for missions that are often extremely physically demanding and carried out with limited support from larger conventional forces. Special Operations Forces (SOF) units employ many highly specialized infiltration techniques in the conduct of their arduous missions, which may result in uncommon physiological problems and present unique challenges in the management of casualties. Providing optimal medical support to these units requires a detailed understanding of their organizational structure, the nature of the missions, the medical administrative tasks that must be addressed, and the management of combat trauma in this special environment. These issues have not previously been addressed in a single, comprehensive document. This chapter is designed to meet that need.

Command Structures of the US Military Special Operations Units

Although the US military has a rich history of small, highly trained units operating either behind enemy lines or in advance of the main forces, the configuration of SOF as it exists today is a relatively new one. The failure of the attempted rescue of the Americans held hostage in our embassy in Iran in 1980 is etched into the national memory. The ensuing investigations into the reasons for the failure at Desert One revealed a lack of interoperability of the special operations units involved that led to the decision that a single, unified command that controlled all SOF units would help prevent such occurrences in the future. In October 1986, the US Congress passed legislation calling for the creation of a unified command.

Before the needs for medical support of the special operations units of the various military services can be discussed, however, it is well to review the organization of the US government's unified command and the interconnectedness of its constituent parts. The president, and below him the secretary of defense, both of whom are advised by the chairman of the joint chiefs of staff, control nine unified commands, which are organized by (1) geographical areas and (2) function (Figure 37-1). The US Special Operations Command (USSOCOM) is one of the four unified commands that are based on a specific function. When the United States becomes a combatant in an armed conflict, the SOF units that will participate in that conflict are assigned (or "chopped") to the commander-in-chief (CINC) of the involved geographical command. There are five geographical unified commands:

1. US Atlantic Command (the Atlantic Ocean and the Caribbean),
2. US Central Command (Asia, the Middle East, and India),
3. US European Command (Europe and Africa),
4. US Pacific Command (the Pacific Ocean and its islands), and
5. US Southern Command (Central and South America).

USSOCOM was established on 16 April 1987.[1] This command is located at MacDill Air Force Base, Tampa, Florida. The CINC is a four-star flag officer, and the deputy commander is a three-star position. The senior medical officer in the special operations community is the USSOCOM command surgeon, who is an O-6. USSOCOM has approximately 47,000 active duty and reserve personnel from the Army, Navy, and Air Force. The organization of the USSOCOM is shown in Figure 37-2.[2]

The service components of USSOCOM—the Army, Navy, and Air Force commands—are discussed below. In addition, a triservice element—the Joint Special Operations Command (JSOC) has as its charter the development of joint operating doctrine.

US Army Special Operations Command

The Army component of USSOCOM is the US Army Special Operations Command (USASOC) and is by far the largest of the three service components. USASOC's command structure (Figure 37-3) consists of the Army Special Forces Command, the John F. Kennedy (JFK) Special Warfare Center and School, the Civil Affairs and Psychological Operations Command, the 75th Ranger Regiment, the 160th Special Operations Aviation Regiment, and the Special Operations Support Command. USASOC is located in Fort Bragg, North Carolina, the traditional home of the Army Special Forces.

The Army Special Forces Command is further divided into seven Special Forces (SF) groups. Each group of approximately 1,400 soldiers is divided into three battalions, with each battalion having

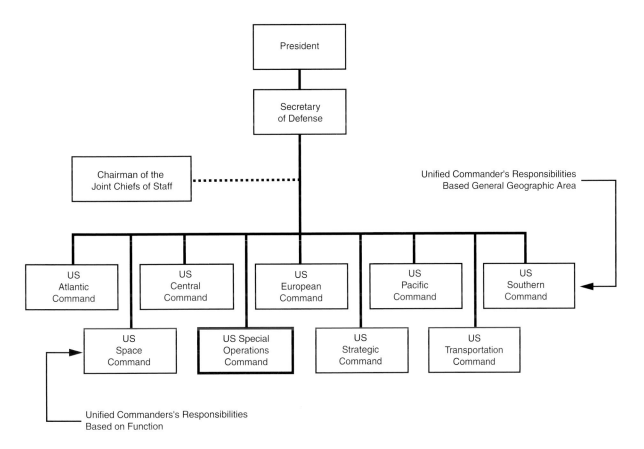

Fig. 37-1. United States Unified Command structure

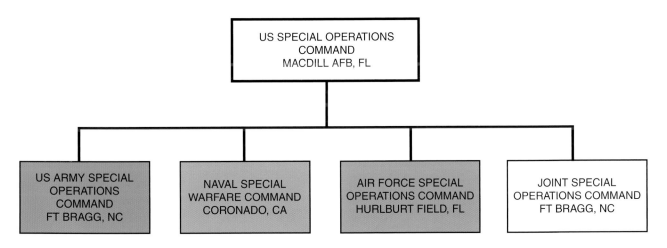

Fig. 37-2. United States Special Operations Command (USSOCOM) organizational chart

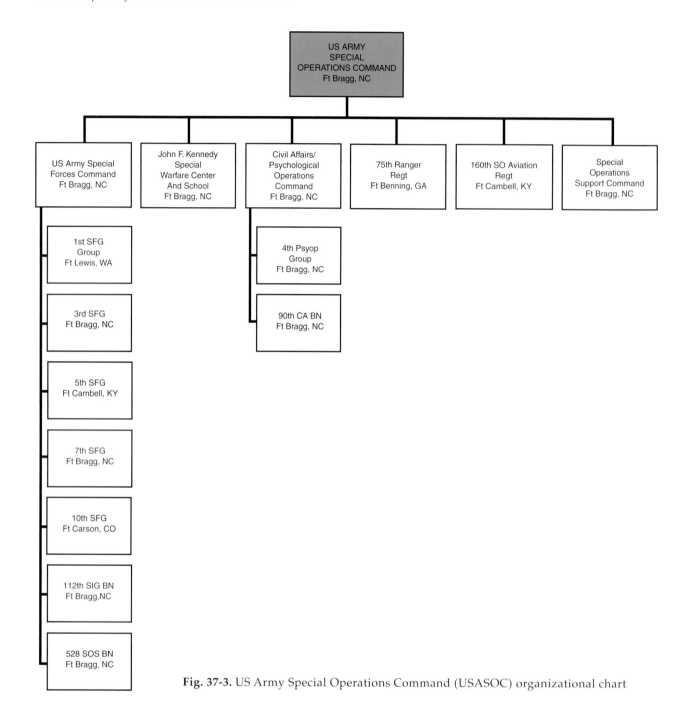

Fig. 37-3. US Army Special Operations Command (USASOC) organizational chart

three companies and each company having six A-teams (Operating Detachments Alpha, ODAs). The A-team is the basic operating unit in SF and comprises two officers and 10 senior enlisted men. Each company usually has one of its six teams qualified in high-altitude, low-opening (HALO) parachute operations and another qualified in self-contained underwater breathing apparatus (scuba) operations.[3] All officers and noncommissioned officers assigned to A-teams have passed the highly selective Special Forces As-sessment and Selection course and the Qualification, or "Q," course taught at the JFK Center. In addition, they are all language qualified. SF A-teams are espe-cially well qualified for Foreign Internal Defense mis-sions (discussed below) but may be used for a wide variety of other special operations missions as well.

The 160th Special Operations Aviation Regiment (SOAR) supports SOF worldwide with their specially modified OH-60 (Little Birds), MH-60, and MH-47 helicopters.[1,4] Nicknamed the Night Stalkers, the

160th SOAR has its headquarters and two battalions in Fort Campbell, Kentucky, and another battalion at Hunter Army Airfield in Savannah, Georgia.[4]

The 75th Ranger Regiment is headquartered in Fort Benning, Georgia, and comprises the First Battalion (Hunter Army Airfield, Savannah, Georgia), the Second Battalion (Fort Lewis, Washington), and the Third Battalion (Fort Benning, Georgia).[5] Rangers have earned their designation at the challenging 9-week Ranger Qualification course. Enjoying a well-deserved reputation as the finest light infantry in the world, Ranger battalions have approximately 580 soldiers each, with each battalion having three rifle companies of 152 Rangers each and a headquarters company.[5] The Rangers are usually the SOF unit of choice when large assaults must be made against well-defended fixed targets.

The Civil Affairs and Psychological Operations Command, located at Fort Bragg, provides expertise in linking the SOF field commanders to the civil authorities in the operating area and in disseminating truthful information to foreign audiences in support of US policy and national objectives.[6] The seventh USASOC command, the Special Operations Support Command, is also located at Fort Bragg. It provides administrative and logistical support for the other major USASOC commands.

Naval Special Warfare Command

The Navy component of USSOCOM is the Naval Special Warfare Command (NAVSPECWARCOM), which is headquartered in Coronado, California, and is divided into six subordinate commands (Figure 37-4). Naval Special Warfare (NSW) Groups One and Two are based, respectively, in Coronado and in Norfolk, Virginia. Each of these groups contains three SEAL (*sea, air, land*) teams and a SEAL delivery vehicle (SDV) team.[7] They also contain a number of subsidiary NSW Units, which are headquarters elements positioned in various locations outside the continental United States. The individual SEAL teams are divided into 10 operating platoons, each composed of two officers and 14 enlisted men.[2] SEAL platoons

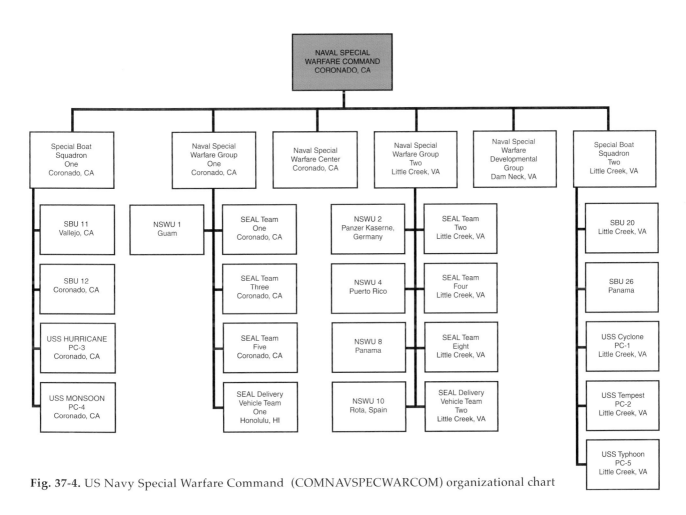

Fig. 37-4. US Navy Special Warfare Command (COMNAVSPECWARCOM) organizational chart

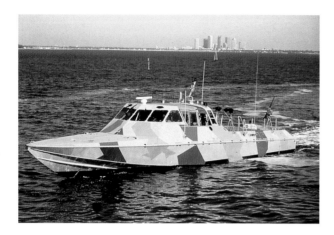

Fig. 37-5. The Mk V Special Operations Craft. Photograph: Courtesy of US Special Operations Command, MacDill Air Force Base, Tampa, Fla.

usually operate independently and are employed to carry out any of the wide variety of special operations missions discussed later in this chapter, especially those that entail a maritime element.

The SDV teams conduct combat swimmer operations using small, open-submersible SDVs. SDVs allow personnel and ordnance to be transported to target areas farther and faster than is possible with free-swimming divers. SDVs are typically transported to operating areas in dry deck shelter (DDS) complexes, which are fitted onto modified fast-attack and ballistic missile submarines.

Two other subordinate NAVSPECWARCOM commands, Special Boat Squadrons One and Two, are also based in Coronado and Norfolk and are the parent commands for the various craft that support SEAL operations. These craft include several sizes of rigid-hull inflatable boats (RHIBs), several types of high-speed boats (HSBs), the Mark V Special Operations Craft (Figure 37-5), and the 170-ft Cyclone-class patrol coastal craft (PCs).[2]

Another command, The Naval Special Warfare Development Group, is located in Dam Neck, Virginia, and provides centralized management for testing, evaluating, and developing current and emerging technology applicable to NSW forces.[7]

All NSW unit commanding officers, platoon personnel, and SDV pilots and navigators are SEAL operators. SEAL operators have successfully completed the demanding 26-week Basic Underwater Demolition/SEAL (BUD/S) training course conducted at the sixth NAVSPECWARCOM major command, the Naval Special Warfare Center in Coronado, California (Figure 37-6). Although the Underwater Demolition teams have now all been redesignated SEAL teams, the Underwater Demolition component in the course name has been retained as a reminder of the SEALs' origins. The Special Warfare designator, or Trident, is not awarded until operators have also successfully passed a probationary period with an operational SEAL or SDV team. The Naval Special Warfare Center also conducts advanced as well as basic training for NSW personnel.

a
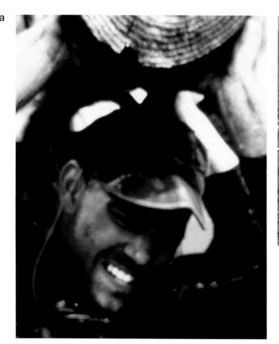

b
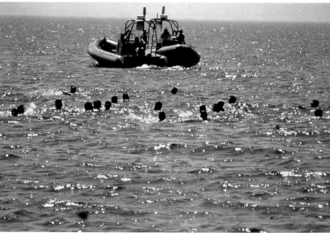

Fig. 37-6. Basic Underwater Demolition/SEALS (BUD/S) training: (**a**) physical training with a log (Log PT) develops teamwork; (**b**) surface training swim. Photographs: Courtesy of US Special Operations Command, MacDill Air Force Base, Tampa, Fla.

Air Force Special Operations Command

The Air Force Special Operations Command (AFSOC) is headquartered at Hurlburt Air Force Base, Florida. As shown in Figure 37-7, it has four constituent parts: the 16th Special Operations Wing, the 18th Flight Test Squadron, the 720th Special Tactics Group, and the Air Force Special Operations School.

The primary AFSOC operational command is the 16th Special Operations Wing (SOW). The 16th SOW is further divided into a number of special operations squadrons (SOSs), which are organized by the type of aircraft flown. The basic C-130 airframe is modified into several different variations.[8] The AC-130U/H Spectre (16th SOS) is designed to serve primarily as a gunfire-support aircraft. The MC-130E and MC-130H Combat Talon aircraft (8th and 15th SOS) accomplish a variety of missions, including long-range insertion of SOF, resupply of ground forces in the field, gunfire support, and communications support. The HC-130 N/P Combat Shadow (9th SOS) provides an airborne refueling capability for SOF rotary-wing aircraft. The MH-53J Pave Low (20th SOS) and MH-60G Pave Hawk (55th SOS) are helicopters that can insert and extract SOF, provide limited gunfire support, and conduct combat search and rescue operations. The Pave Low aircraft has a longer operating range than the smaller Pave Hawk. AFSOC has one operational squadron, the 6th SOS, whose primary mission is to provide aviation-related foreign internal defense (Figure 37-8).

AFSOC also has administrative control of two operational groups, the 352nd in Mildenhall, United Kingdom, and the 353rd in Kadena, Japan. Each of

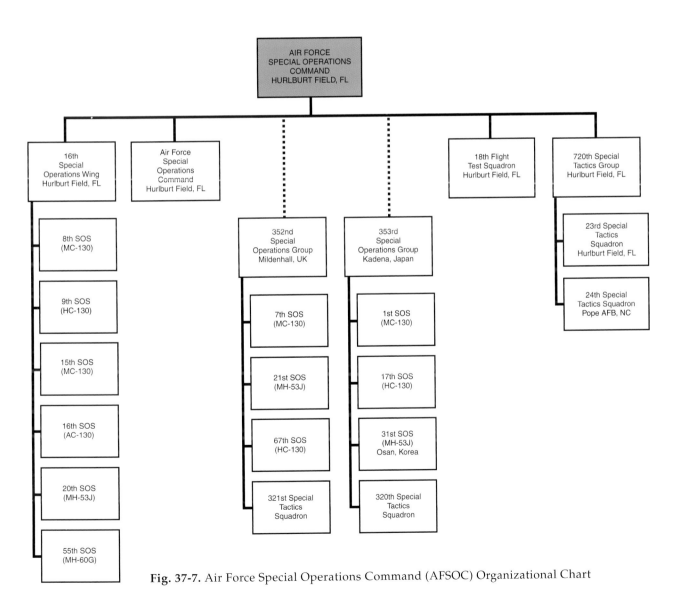

Fig. 37-7. Air Force Special Operations Command (AFSOC) Organizational Chart

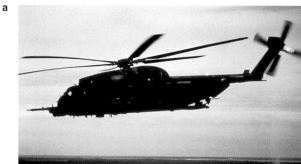

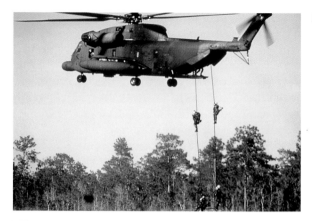

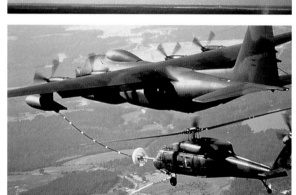

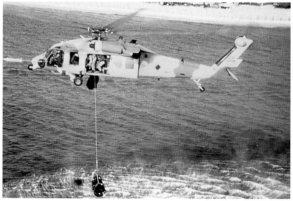

Fig. 37-8. (**a**) Air Force Special Operations Command (AFSOC) MH-53J Pave Low in flight. (**b**) US Army Special Operations Forces (SOF) troops fast-roping from an AFSOC MH-53J Pave Low aircraft. (**c**) AFSOC HC-130 Combat Shadow refuels a Pave Hawk. (**d**) AFSOC MH-60 Pave Hawk conducts a search-and-rescue mission. Photographs: Courtesy of US Special Operations Command, MacDill Air Force Base, Tampa, Fla.

these groups is subdivided into four SOSs.

The second AFSOC command, the Air Force Special Operations School, is located at Hurlburt Field and conducts a variety of courses to educate US and Allied military personnel in the geopolitical, psychological, sociological, and military considerations of US Air Force and Joint Special Operations.[9]

The third AFSOC command is the 18th Flight Test Squadron (FTS), also located at Hurlburt Field. This command is responsible for testing and evaluating proposed Air Force special operations and combat rescue aircraft and associated equipment.[10] The 18th Flight Test Squadron also develops and evaluates new tactics for AFSOC use.

The fourth AFSOC command is the 720th Special Tactics Group. The group has two squadrons, the 23rd STS at Hurlburt and the 24th STS at Fort Bragg, North Carolina. Squadrons are also attached to the 352nd and 353rd wings[11] and comprise small units called special tactics teams. These teams contain two specially trained types of individuals:

- combat controllers, who are air traffic controllers trained to survey, mark, and control airfields in austere and nonpermissive environments and to designate targets for air interdiction and close air support; and
- pararescuemen, also known as PJs, who are, like the SF medics and SEAL corpsmen, emergency trauma specialists and combatants combined.

Special tactics personnel are trained in military free-fall parachuting, open- and closed-circuit scuba, and airmobile employment methods.[11]

Types of Special Operations Missions

USSOCOM forces conduct a wide variety of missions during armed conflicts and peacetime.[2] Although SOF combat operations are often carried out in support of conventional forces, special operations missions typically involve relatively small force elements operating clandestinely in areas that are geographically remote from main bodies of conventional forces. SOF missions include all of the following[2]:

- Amphibious Warfare: direct action operations launched from the sea by naval and landing forces against a hostile or potentially hostile shore. These operations include preassault cover and diversionary operations, surf observation, hydrographic reconnaissance, and obstacle clearance.
- Civil Affairs: advise and assist commanders in establishing and maintaining relations among military forces, civilian authorities (both governmental and nongovernmental), and the civilian population in an area of operation.
- Coastal Patrol and Interdiction: a special reconnaissance activity in coastal regions involving area denial, interdiction, support, and intelligence. These operations are designed to halt or limit the enemy's warfighting capability by denying movement of vital resources over coastal and riverine lines of communication.
- Combat Search and Rescue: search and rescue missions conducted to recover distressed personnel during wartime and contingency operations.
- Counterdrug: active measures taken to detect, monitor, and counter the production, sale, trafficking, and use of illegal drugs.
- Counterproliferation: measures undertaken to combat the proliferation of weapons of mass destruction.
- Counterterrorism: both defensive and offensive measures undertaken to oppose and prevent terrorist activities.
- Direct Action: short-duration strikes and other small-scale offensives by SOF to seize, destroy, capture, recover, or inflict damage on designated personnel or material.

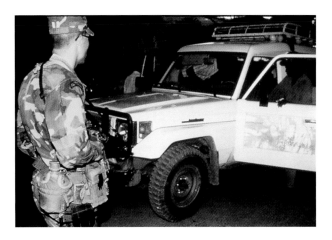

Fig. 37-9. Operations Other Than War: US Army Special Operations Forces (SOF) personnel conduct vehicle inspections in Haiti during Operation Restore Democracy. Photograph: Courtesy of US Special Operations Command, MacDill Air Force Base, Tampa, Fla.

- Foreign Internal Defense and Civic Action: missions that provide assistance to another country to help free and protect its citizens from subversion, lawlessness, and insurgency.
- Humanitarian Assistance: missions conducted to prevent or reduce pain, hunger, or loss of life resulting from natural or man-made disasters or endemic conditions.
- Operations Other Than War (OOTW): if we consider direct action missions to be at one end of a spectrum and humanitarian assistance operations at the other, then OOTW comprise the midpoint of the continuum. Examples of OOTW include providing security for the humanitarian famine relief effort in Somalia and augmenting local police and militia forces during Operation Restore Democracy in Haiti (Figure 37-9). Ideally, these missions are carried out without the use of arms, but volatile tactical environments (eg, Somalia) may quickly turn OOTW into direct actions.

INITIAL TRAINING IN MEDICINE OF SPECIAL OPERATIONS MEDICAL PERSONNEL

This chapter is being written at a major turning point in the history of SOF medical training, as the Joint Special Operations Medical Training Center (JSOMTC) at Fort Bragg, North Carolina, began operations in July 1996. The JSOMTC will conduct most SOF Combat Medical Training courses in the future. For completeness, the current training at the JSOMTC and the medical training prior to 1996 will

both be described.

The JSOMTC is a subordinate command of the JFK Special Warfare Center and School in Fort Bragg, North Carolina. The primary course taught at this institution is the Special Forces Medical Sergeant (SFMS) course. This course is divided into two segments. The first, the Special Operations Combat Medic (SOCM) course, is 24 weeks long and provides basic combat trauma training for SOF combat medical personnel. The course includes anatomy and physiology, the American College of Surgeons' Advanced Trauma Life Support (ATLS) course, pharmacology, and Emergency Medical Technician–Paramedic (EMT-P) training. All SEAL corpsmen, SF medics, and Air Force PJs attend this course before being assigned to an operational unit.

The second segment of the SFMS course is the Advanced Special Operations Combat Medic (ADSOCM) course, which in 20 weeks covers advanced anatomy and physiology, pharmacology, infectious disease, and trauma care. SF medics attend this course and earn their 18 Delta qualification before being assigned to an operational SF unit. SEAL corpsmen are designated Navy Enlisted Code (NEC) 8492s after completing the SOCM course and are assigned to an operational unit. They return later in their careers to attend the ADSOCM course, where they earn the Navy NEC 8491. Air Force combat medical personnel are not currently anticipated to attend ADSOCM, although this issue is under re-

view at the time this chapter is being written.

The medical dean of the JSOMTC is an Army O-6 medical officer and is responsible for recommending policy on medical training issues to the commander. In addition, a senior Army O-5 or O-6 line officer is responsible for administration and personnel. Both officers report to a flag officer (and/or his staff) at the next-higher echelon.[12]

Enlisted Medical Personnel

Army Medics

Special Forces 18 Delta Medics. Special Forces combat medics are known as 18 Deltas and earn this distinction by successfully completing the SFMS course (Figure 37-10). The first phase of this year-long course was previously conducted at Fort Sam Houston, San Antonio, Texas, and the second phase conducted at Fort Bragg. The 18 Delta candidates must be E-5 or higher and have passed the Special Forces Assessment and Selection course as well as

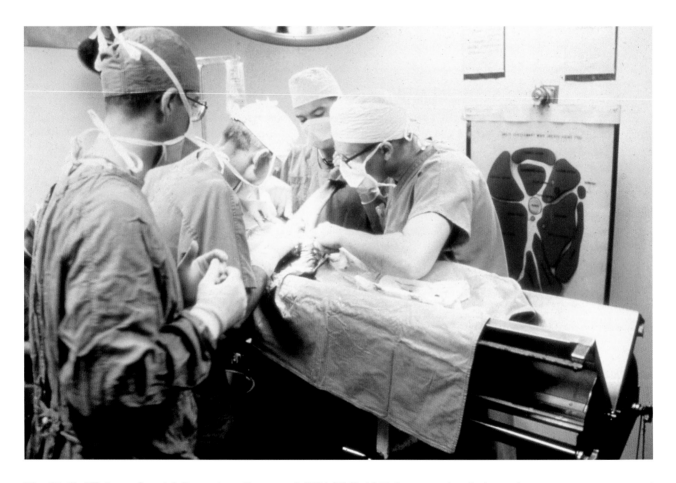

Fig. 37-10. US Army Special Operations Command (USASOC) 18-Deltas practice their combat trauma management skills. Photograph: Courtesy of US Special Operations Command, MacDill Air Force Base, Tampa, Fla.

the SF Qualification course. After completing the SFMS course, Special Forces medics are able to function independently, as defined by USASOC Regulation 350-9. They next report to a Special Forces Group where they are assigned to an operational A-team. Two medics are usually assigned to each team.

Ranger Medics. Ranger medics, who hold the Army Medical Occupational Specialty designator 91B, provide tactical medical support for the units of the 75th Ranger Battalion. They also attend the SOCM course taught at the JSOMTC in Fort Bragg. As SOCM graduates, they are all EMT-P qualified. One Ranger medic is assigned to each 40-man platoon. The training a Ranger medic receives does not include providing sick call care in garrison, so they receive on-the-job training in these skills at their units. Although completion of Ranger training is not a prerequisite for the Ranger medic, many of these individuals attend Ranger School while assigned to their units.

Navy SEAL Corpsmen

In the past, medical training for SEAL corpsmen began at the Navy Corpsman A School at Great Lakes, Chicago, Illinois, or San Diego, California, where students received 12 weeks of basic instruction in anatomy, physiology, nursing care, intravenous therapy techniques, pharmacology, and other general medical topics. This school was often followed by a tour in a hospital prior to receiving orders to BUD/S training. Corpsman A School may now be omitted if a BUD/S graduate subsequently attends the SOCM course, as would normally be the case. The corpsman receives no extra medical training during his 26 weeks at BUD/S, but is subjected to the same combination of selection and training as others in the course. After completing their SEAL training, corpsmen remain at the Naval Special Warfare Center for an extra 3 weeks of Special Operations Technician (SOT) training, where they receive additional training in the recognition and treatment of diving medical disorders and in the operation and maintenance of recompression chambers. Still prior to reporting to an operational SEAL team, the new SEAL corpsman attends Jump School at Fort Benning, Georgia.

In the past, SEAL corpsmen then went to Fort Sam Houston, Texas, to receive instruction in trauma care adapted from the 18 Delta course, but this training has now been replaced by the SOCM course. The corpsman then reports to his first operational SEAL team, where he is usually assigned as one of the two corpsmen in a SEAL platoon.

As noted previously, SEAL corpsmen who have taken only the 18 Delta Trauma Module or the SOCM are designated as NEC 8492s and have a more-limited scope of practice than SF 18 Deltas. Some SEAL corpsmen return to finish the remainder of the 18 Delta course and receive the NEC 8491 designation. These individuals may function as Independent Duty corpsmen. SEAL units may also have Diving Medical Technicians (DMTs) and other non-SEAL operator corpsmen attached to provide noncombat medical care.

Air Force Medics

AFSOC enlisted medical personnel are currently of three types. The first is the Medical Service Specialist, Air Force Specialty Code (AFSC) 4N0X1. Medical service specialists attend a 13-week Phase 1 School at Sheppard Air Force Base in Wichita Falls, Texas, followed by an additional 8 weeks at a Phase 2 training site. The medical service specialist course provides instruction in basic anatomy, physiology, cardiopulmonary resuscitation, nursing care, and clinical medicine. Graduates are qualified as EMT-Basic on completion of this course. The second type of medic is the Aeromedical Service Specialist, AFSC 4F0X1. Aeromedical service specialists attend a 12-week course at Brooks Air Force Base, San Antonio, Texas, where they receive instruction in many of the topics noted for medical service specialists as well as altitude physiology, flight medicine, and aviation physical standards. After finishing these schools, they receive an initial assignment to a hospital, clinic, or operational wing. Once they have achieved the rank of E-5 and have reached a minimum skill level of 5 by completing the Air Force Career Development course, they are eligible for assignment to AFSOC.

Prior to arriving at AFSOC, both types of specialists must also have taken the 10-week Independent Duty Medical Technician course at Sheppard Air Force Base and the 7-week Aeromedical Evacuation Technician course at Brooks Air Force Base. Both types of specialists are therefore EMT-Intravenous qualified and able to function as independent care providers on arrival at AFSOC. EMT-Paramedic training is conducted on an individual basis after arrival at AFSOC. Flight physicals and routine flight crew healthcare are provided by aeromedical service specialists under the supervision of the flight surgeon, with each squadron usually having one flight surgeon and two aeromedical service specialists. Medical service specialists are assigned to clinics or other fixed medical treatment facilities (MTFs). Both aeromedical service specialists and medical specialists may provide in-flight medical care in AFSOC aircraft but neither has the training in small arms and tactics to act as a combatant outside the aircraft when necessary to rescue downed aircrews.

That duty is the province of the third type of Air Force medical care provider, the pararescueman (PJ). The PJs first go to the 10-week Pararescue Indoctrination course at Lackland Air Force Base, San Antonio, Texas. Also known as "OL-H", for operating location H, this course is physically demanding and has a high attrition rate. After the successful completion of the Pararescue Indoctrination course, the candidate then goes to Jump School at Fort Benning (3 wk), Survival School at Fairchild Air Force Base, Spokane, Washington (3 wk), Military Free-Fall Parachute School at Fort Benning (4 wk), Special Forces Combat Diver School, Key West, Florida (4 wk), and the 26-week Pararescue School at Kirtland Air Force Base in Albuquerque, New Mexico. This course provides training in trauma care (EMT-Paramedic) as well as weapons, rescue techniques, and small-unit tactics. Although they do receive in-hospital experience in trauma care and endotracheal intubation, PJs do not attend Independent Duty Medical Technician School and their scope of practice is limited to trauma care. On completion of their training, they are assigned to the Special Tactics Teams and are considered primarily combat medics, much like a SEAL 8492.

Medical Officers

Army SOF Physicians

Not surprisingly, the three component services also vary considerably in their methods of training physicians to provide medical support for special operations. A first-tour Army SOF physician is usually assigned to an SOF unit following his internship. There is no formally required additional training before being assigned to an Army SOF unit, but medical officers often obtain tropical medicine training at Walter Reed Army Medical Center, Washington, DC (4 wk), the classroom phase of the diving medical officer (DMO) course at the Naval Diving and Salvage Training Center in Panama City, Florida (3 wk), airborne training at Fort Benning, Georgia (3 wk), and Army Flight Surgeon training at Fort Rucker, Alabama (6 wk). Training is usually done en route to the SOF command but may be done after reporting.

Most first-tour medical officers are captains and are assigned to an SF or Ranger battalion. These initial tours typically last 2 to 3 years, after which the physician returns for a residency in a clinical specialty. Medical billets at the group level or higher are usually filled by a senior major who has returned to a SOF billet after completing a residency and spending a tour practicing that specialty. Some SOF medical officers may get a chance to attend Ranger training, but they do not generally go to the SF qualification course. The senior physician in USASOC is the USASOC Command Surgeon, who is a senior O-5 or O-6.

Naval Special Warfare Diving Medical Officers

All NSW billets except for the single medical officer at each of the two special boat squadrons are filled by physicians who have successfully completed the Navy Undersea Medical Officer (UMO) course, which encompasses diving, submarine, and Special Warfare medicine. The submarine and Special Warfare medicine portions of the course (12 wk) are taught at the Naval Undersea Medical Institute in Groton, Connecticut, and the diving medicine portion (9 wk) is taught at the Naval Diving and Salvage Training Center in Panama City, Florida. On completion of the course, the DMO qualification is granted automatically, but designation as a submarine medical officer and UMO requires passing a submarine qualification exam, the completion of a thesis, and at least 30 days of service aboard a submarine. The physicians attending this course have usually just finished their internship, although some senior medical officers at the O-5 and O-6 level who are already board certified elect to attend.

Currently, three medical officers are at each of the two NSW Groups, two at the NSW Center, two at COMNAVSPECWARCOM (the commander's headquarters unit of NAVSPECWARCOM) and two at the NSW Development Group. After an initial tour in NSW, most medical officers return to residency training, although some of the individuals who have previously completed residencies may elect to stay for multiple tours in NSW. NSW DMOs do not go through BUD/S training. The senior physician in NSW is the COMNAVSPECWARCOM Force Medical Officer, who is a senior O-5 or O-6.

Air Force Special Operations Command Flight Surgeons

AFSOC Flight Surgeons have all been through the Aerospace Medicine Primary course, which is 8 weeks long and is taught at Brooks Air Force Base, in San Antonio, Texas. AFSOC has three operational flight medicine units; they are located in the 16th

SOW at Hurlburt Field, Florida; the 352nd Special Operations Group (SOG) at Mildenhall, England; and the 353rd SOG at Kadena Air Force Base, Okinawa. Each unit consists of a Senior (O-4/O-5) Flight Surgeon who has completed the 3-year Resident in Aerospace Medicine course at Brooks Air Force Base, several basic-trained flight surgeons

(O-3/O-4), a medical service corps officer (O-3), and medical technicians (medical service specialists and aeromedical service specialists.) Squadrons have a medical element that consists of an O-3 flight surgeon and two aeromedical technicians. The senior physician in AFSOC is the AFSOC Command Surgeon, who is usually a senior O-5 or O-6.

ROUTINE MEDICAL SUPPORT OF SPECIAL OPERATIONS FORCES

When SOF units are not engaged in a conflict, they are engaged in a continuing cycle of training and operational exercises. SOF medical personnel play a critical part in helping their units maintain their operational readiness. In this setting, the need to care for combat casualties is not routinely encountered but the functions noted below are.

Primary Healthcare

SOF medical personnel must be able to deal with the routine problems encountered in providing healthcare and periodic physicals to a group of generally healthy, young and (lest we forget the colonels and the master chiefs) not-so-young individuals. The establishment of efficient and well-run sick call procedures for SOF units is essential. It is generally expected that most primary medical care for active duty SOF personnel will be provided by the medical personnel organic to the unit if at all possible. Care for dependents is less common, and pediatric and obstetrical–gynecological care may be best accomplished at a clinic that deals routinely with patients in these special categories. SOF medical personnel should work to establish a rapport with the local referral MTF so that consults to that facility will be handled promptly. It may be worthwhile to visit the facility periodically with a senior line commander and to invite the hospital or clinic leadership to visit the SOF compound for a demonstration of SOF missions and capabilities.

Sports Medicine

Navy SEALs, Army Special Forces and Rangers, and Air Force Special Tactics Teams are required to maintain extremely high levels of physical fitness to perform the many physically demanding activities encountered in their operations. This requirement necessitates a heavy emphasis on both strength and aerobic physical training in SOF units. Associated with these rigorous training schedules is a high incidence of traumatic and overuse musculoskeletal injuries. If these exercise-related injuries are not accurately diagnosed and treated with the most effective therapeu-

tic measures available, unnecessarily long recovery periods may result. These delays may have detrimental effects on both the unit's operational readiness and the long-term health of the service member.

To ensure that the best possible care is obtained for these injuries, a proactive sports medicine program should (*a*) be a high priority of every SOF major command and (*b*) consist of a self-contained rehabilitation facility and regular supervision by physical therapists, physical therapy technicians, or athletic trainers. Most internships provide relatively little instruction and training in sports medicine. Unless they are already trained in sports medicine, SOF physicians should receive supplemental training in this area shortly after they report for duty. In addition, a periodic visit by a sports medicine specialist to examine difficult diagnostic or therapeutic patients is helpful. On-site specialty care can be obtained through personal liaison with the appropriate MTF or by contracting for civilian consultants.

Flight Medicine

Many SOF medical officers are assigned to units with aircraft and aircrews. These medical officers must perform the careful periodic flight physicals required for aircrews, make recommendations about crew suitability to fly after acute minor illnesses or injuries, and provide input to line commanders about the physiological aspects of flight operations as required.

Occupational Medicine

SOF medical personnel deal with many occupational medicine issues. For example,

- the requirement for extensive small-arms training entails a substantial risk of noise-induced hearing loss if an aggressive hearing conservation program is not implemented;
- the need to conduct prolonged training evolutions in harsh environments may result in heat or cold injury if reasonable guide-

lines for preventing such injuries are not established and followed; and

- live-fire exercises in confined spaces present the potential for exposure to elevated ambient lead levels.

SOF medical personnel must be alert for the presence of such hazards and implement whatever measures are needed to reduce the risk and monitor the well-being of their units.

Medical Readiness

Shifts in national defense policy, a changing worldwide geopolitical picture, and advances in medical care create a constantly evolving environment for SOF; physicians and senior enlisted medical personnel must monitor changes in these areas and evaluate the ability of their personnel and equipment resources to meet their units' medical needs in light of these changes. Long-range planning for medical requirements is conducted through each component's Program Objective Memorandum (POM) process. The POM process, however, requires several years of lead time. More immediate medical needs may be addressed at the command level with Operations and Maintenance (O&M) funds. Needed purchases should be documented with memoranda to the unit commander. If the command needs to acquire medical equipment before the POM can provide it, the unit commander may elect to use O&M funds for these purchases. At all times, it is important to maintain a prioritized list of proposed equipment purchases; this list is often very useful as the end of the fiscal year approaches.

Diving Medicine

Physicians assigned to units with combat swimmers, such as SEAL teams, scuba-capable SF teams, and Air Force Combat Control Teams, must be able to deal with problems relating to diving medicine. Special needs of divers in SOF include fitness-to-dive evaluations and the recognition and treatment of diving disorders. Navy guidelines for physical standards for divers are found in the *Manual of the Medical Department*.[13] Medical supervision of SDV/DDS operations is a specialized area of diving medicine and will be addressed separately in the following section.

Most SOF diving operations are conducted with closed-circuit scuba. These underwater breathing apparatuses (UBAs) recycle the diver's exhaled gas through a carbon dioxide absorbent canister rather than allowing the exhaled gas to escape to sea. Compared with conventional open-circuit scuba, closed-circuit scuba has the following advantages:

- increased operating times; since all of the oxygen carried is available for metabolism, operations of up to 3 hours or longer can be carried out with a single small gas cylinder;
- the lack of escaping bubbles allows for clandestine diving operations to be conducted without the threat of compromise that results from a trail of bubbles rising to the surface; and
- closed-circuit UBAs can be designed with very low acoustical and magnetic signatures, which are critical in Explosive Ordnance Disposal operations.

Disadvantages include

- greatly increased cost of equipment, both in acquisition and maintenance;
- added diving complexity, with resultant increased training requirements; and
- increased risk of diving accidents.

The two main types of closed-circuit scuba are (1) closed-circuit oxygen, in which only a single bottle of compressed oxygen is used, and (2) closed-circuit mixed-gas, which employs a bottle of pure oxygen and a second bottle filled with either air or oxygen mixed with helium (heliox). Both types of closed-circuit UBAs use a canister filled with carbon dioxide absorbent to remove the carbon dioxide from expired air.

The closed-circuit oxygen UBA currently used by the US military is the Draeger LAR V Mk 28 Mod 2 (Figure 37-11). This rig is worn over the chest and abdomen of the diver, with the breathing bag and the canister contained in a fiberglass shell and the oxygen bottle attached to the bottom of the UBA. The LAR V offers the advantages of being very light (25 lb) and mechanically simple. The primary disadvantage of closed-circuit oxygen as compared with closed-circuit mixed-gas scuba is the depth limitations imposed by the risk of central nervous system oxygen toxicity. This is often not a significant problem in SEAL diving operations because many combat swimmer missions require only a dive depth sufficient to provide concealment at night.

The Mk 16 UBA is a closed-circuit mixed gas UBA, which uses a microprocessor to control the partial pressure of oxygen at 0.75 atmospheres absolute (atm). It contains two high-pressure gas bottles: one for oxygen and one for a diluent

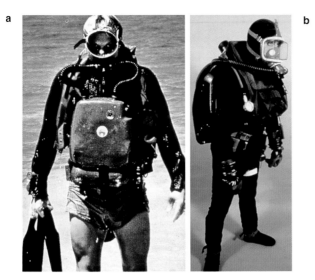

Fig. 37-11. (**a**) A US Navy SEAL (*sea*, *air*, *land*) diver is wearing the Draeger LAR V underwater breathing apparatus (UBA). (**b**) A SEAL diver is dressed in an Mk 16 UBA. Photograph: Courtesy of US Special Operations Command, MacDill Air Force Base, Tampa, Fla.

gas (either air or a heliox mix). As oxygen is consumed, three sensors in the breathing loop detect the falling partial pressure of oxygen (Po_2) and activate the oxygen-addition valve. The diver is able to monitor the status of his Po_2 on both a face mask–mounted primary display as well as a secondary display. Both gas bottles; the microprocessor; the breathing bag; and a large, circular carbon dioxide absorbent canister are all enclosed in a fiberglass casing worn on the diver's back. A manual bypass valve is available to add additional oxygen or diluent gas to the UBA if necessary. The large, well-insulated carbon dioxide absorbent canister on the Mk 16 achieves excellent operating durations, ranging from 100 to 400 minutes depending on the water temperature, dive depth, and gas used. Testing with Sofnolime in a resting diver scenario has produced even longer canister durations (currently classified) for SDV operations.

SEAL Delivery Vehicle and Dry Deck Shelter Operations

Operations involving SEAL Delivery Vehicles (SDVs) and Dry Deck Shelters (DDSs) provide a number of unique challenges for NSW physicians and diving medical technicians. Special decompression techniques are required for these operations.[14] Many SDV operations require use of both air and nitrox mixtures on the same dive. Calculation of decompression for these profiles may be done in several ways:

- The Combat Swimmer Multi-Level Dive (CSMD) procedures were developed by Thalmann and Butler[15] at the Navy Experimental Diving Unit (NEDU) in Panama City, Florida, in 1983 and have been used by the SDV teams since then. These procedures allow more precise calculation of the decompression obligation for long, multilevel dives by dividing the dive into transit periods (≤ 30 ft) and downward excursions (> 30 ft). These procedures are based on the 1957 Navy air tables and assume that the diver is breathing air at shallow depths; for depths greater than 70 feet of seawater (fsw) on the Mk 16, the equivalent air depth is calculated and used. This procedure does not allow the diver to receive decompression credit for the higher Po_2 of the Mk 16 during decompression stops but still results in substantial decompression savings, because the diver is not required to decompress as though the entire bottom time were spent at the deepest depth attained on the dive.
- The Naval Special Warfare Dive Planner was developed at the Naval Medical Research Institute (NMRI), Bethesda, Maryland, in 1993. This program uses a laptop computer version of the NMRI maximum likelihood nitrox decompression algorithm that has been approved by the Naval Sea Systems Command (NAVSEA) for use in SDV operations. The divers follow the CSMD procedures until they return to the launching submarine. At that point, they provide the DMO and Diving Supervisor with their dive profile. The profile is entered into the Dive Planner program and a customized decompression schedule calculated. The two primary benefits of the Dive Planner are that (1) it is able to give the diver credit for the long periods spent breathing from the Mk 16 at shallow depths and (2) it is able to provide decompression schedules for either air, Mk 16, or oxygen decompression. Version 6.0 of the Dive Planner software, which was approved by NAVSEA in June 1996, allows the DMO to track the decompression obligation for several dives simultaneously. The Dive Planner is the preferred method for calculating the decompression obligation for repetitive or long bottom-time dives because of its increased conservatism on this type of dive profile.

The DDS is a unique diving system with the potential for presenting medical personnel who support DDS operations with novel and complicated casualty situations (Figure 37-12). Some general guidelines concerning medical support of DDS operations and management have been issued for use by NSW DMOs.[16] The DMO should remain at the submarine control throughout DDS launch and recovery operations. In general, management of a medical emergency in the DDS consists of four phases:

1. Immediate movement of the casualty to the bubble.
2. Equalization of the transfer trunk to the hangar depth and transfer of the casualty to the transfer trunk.
3. The transfer trunk is drained to the appropriate level and the casualty is then moved to either the chamber or the submarine as indicated by his condition.
4. Definitive medical treatment is implemented.

Specific examples of the types of emergencies that may be encountered in the DDS environment and suggested management plans for each are found in the *Dry Deck Shelter Medical Emergency Procedures*.[16]

Medical Sustainment Training

SOF corpsmen, medics, and physicians require ongoing training in a wide variety of subjects. This training may be accomplished through lectures, practical skills refresher training, hospital or ambulance rotations, correspondence courses, or the Special Operations Interactive Medical Training Program discussed below in this chapter. As part of the EMT-P recertification process, all EMT-P–qualified individuals in SOF must attend the SOF Medical Sustainment course that is taught at Fort Bragg every 2 years.

Ensuring the Quality and Scope of Healthcare

Changes in the American healthcare delivery system are also impacting on the practice of medicine in SOF. One of the most significant changes in the last decade for healthcare professionals has been the imposition of more-stringent credentialing procedures. The goal of the credentialing process is to ensure that each individual healthcare provider has been properly trained to deliver the types of healthcare services that he or she wishes to provide. Not unlike military hospitals, SOF units must ensure that credentialing of physicians is accomplished in accordance with each component's medical department instructions. USASOC and AFSOC currently have their physicians credentialed at the

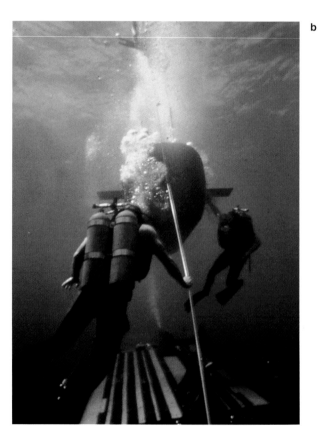

Fig. 37-12. (a) A Dry Deck Shelter (DDS) is being installed onto a host submarine. **(b)** US Navy SEAL (*sea, air, land*) divers launch a SEAL delivery vehicle (SDV) from the DDS. Photographs: Courtesy of US Special Operations Command, MacDill Air Force Base, Tampa, Fla.

nearest hospital. NAVSPECWARCOM credentials its physicians through its own process, with the commander being the credentialing authority and the force medical officer administering the program.

Establishing the scope of care for nonphysician providers is more complex because of the various types of nonphysician medical training and interservice differences. Guidance for these issues is found in the Navy OPNAV and BUMED 6400.1 series of instructions and in USASOC Regulation 350-9.

Quality assurance is another process designed to ensure that the quality of healthcare delivered by SOF medical providers meets high standards. This process typically consists of reviewing a number of charts for each provider every month to check for appropriateness and proper documentation of care. Quality assurance procedures are also enumerated by the respective components in service-specific directives. Patterns of deficiencies identified in these reviews call for focused refresher training in the areas indicated.

IN-THEATER MEDICAL SUPPORT

Predeployment Preparation

Preparation for a combat deployment requires that SOF medical officers and senior enlisted personnel ensure that their deploying forces have adequately addressed area-specific medical intelligence, immunizations, medical equipment, the threat assessment for weapons of mass destruction, and predeployment training for medical personnel.

Area-Specific Medical Intelligence

The US Army Research Institute for Environmental Medicine (USARIEM), Natick, Massachusetts, publishes medical information summaries for areas of the world that are identified as potential locations for armed conflicts that may involve US forces. The medical officer should contact USARIEM (DSN: 256-4811; commercial telephone: 508-233-4509) to see if such a publication is available for the area to which the unit will be deploying.

Another source of medical intelligence about a specific region is the Armed Forces Medical Intelligence Center (AFMIC), Fort Detrick, Maryland, whose information about worldwide medical conditions and facilities is especially detailed and current. Much of this information is classified and not available in USARIEM publications. AFMIC can be contacted at DSN: 343-7603.

Immunizations

SOF units typically have an ongoing program of vaccinations and immunizations for their personnel. Once a specific area is identified as a deployment location, the immunization status of the personnel scheduled for deployment should be reviewed immediately. Potential sources of information about required immunizations are the service-specific preventive medicine units; the Centers

for Disease Control and Prevention, Atlanta, Georgia; the office of the theater CINC surgeon; AFMIC; and service-specific directives.

Medical Equipment

Another important aspect of predeployment planning is to review the service-specific list of medical equipment that the physicians, corpsmen, and medics should have available to them. Because logistics are often initially problematic in-theater, it is important to ensure that the deploying forces have sufficient medical supplies to last for at least the number of days specified in the theater or the CINC operation plan. Medical equipment and supplies should include both combat casualty care equipment and supplies needed to care for the significant numbers of disease and nonbattle injuries (DNBI) that are encountered by deployed troops. These conditions include musculoskeletal injuries, as troops strive to maintain their physical readiness in-theater; acute gastroenteritis, as the troops make the acquaintance of the local enteric pathogens; the ubiquitous upper respiratory infections; and other infectious diseases specific to the area.

An adequate supply of medications to treat these and the other expected sick call maladies should be deployed with the SOF units to ensure that their medical readiness does not suffer as the transition to theater operations is effected. Every medication to be sent in-theater should be reviewed to ensure that the expiration date on medications or sterility has not passed. Medical reference sources that will be needed by the deployed medical personnel should be obtained and packed. Weight-efficient CD-ROM–based reference materials should be used if possible. The microprocessors used to support the CD-ROM–based medical references can also be used to support the medical tracking systems described below in this chapter.

Nuclear–Biological–Chemical Warfare Threat Assessment

The threat assessment data from AFMIC with respect to the theater nuclear–biological–chemical (NBC) warfare threat should be reviewed. Many SOF units do not routinely train in the use of NBC protective clothing, monitoring techniques, and decontamination procedures. If a significant threat is anticipated from these agents in the impending conflict, then procurement of the appropriate protective clothing and monitoring devices should be coordinated by the medical department prior to deployment and training conducted in their use.

Predeployment Medical Training

The final aspect of predeployment preparation is to conduct focused training for the medical personnel who will be going in-theater. Training should consist primarily of a review of the factual information and technical skills necessary to care for SOF operators injured in combat as well as training in the disease entities particular to the mission area.

In-Theater Procedures and Facilities

Ideally, each SOF component service should have at least one medical officer assigned to the task element commander. In addition, a senior SOF medical officer should be assigned to the Joint Special Operations Task Force (JSOTF) staff. Combat Casualty Transport Teams should be identified, and, if not organic to the SOF units deployed, then assigned as augmentation medical forces.[17]

Once the SOF contingent has left the United States and arrives in-theater, mobility, communications, and other aspects of unit operations will initially be somewhat disorganized. The approach outlined below provides a sequence of measures that the medical officer or senior enlisted medical person can undertake to set up a smoothly functioning medical department. The likelihood of being able to accomplish all the steps outlined below just as they are described is probably small, but the paragraphs below will at least offer some thoughts as to the items that need to be addressed.

Senior Theater Medical Officer

The Senior Theater Medical Officer may be the CINC Surgeon or the Joint Task Force Surgeon. The senior SOF medical officer assigned to the staff of the JSOTF commander should contact and preferably meet with this individual to ensure that SOF medical planning is consistent with the theater CINC operation plan. Issues that need to be addressed include casualty evacuation procedures for both combat injuries and DNBI, medical resupply, and appropriate theater preventive medicine measures. A coordination visit to the SOF compound by the Senior Theater Medical Officer may be helpful in demonstrating some of the unique aspects of planning battlefield casualty evacuation for SOF units.

Combat Casualty Evacuation Procedures

An appropriate plan to evacuate SOF casualties that occur in combat must be developed. Evacuation of SOF casualties from the battlefield (CASEVAC; the term "CASEVAC" should be used to describe the evacuation of casualties instead of the commonly used "MEDEVAC," because the Air Force uses MEDEVAC to describe noncombat medical transport) will most often be accomplished by AFSOC tactical rotary-wing air assets, but—depending on the operations to be conducted—may be accomplished with maritime craft, desert assault vehicles, or mobility assets provided by conventional forces. Determination of the assets that are to be used must be coordinated with the staff of the JSOTF commander. The potential CASEVAC assets should be visited and consideration of a number of issues considered: What is the best Combat Casualty Transport Team for that asset? What medical treatment and equipment are appropriate to each potential asset? How will casualties be loaded into the asset and best arranged for treatment? These issues should addressed promptly after the SOF contingent arrives in-theater.

Other details must be reviewed in particular for each mission: How will the SOF unit contact the CASEVAC asset, with primary and with back-up communications? In what general area will the force be operating? Geographical location is an important factor in deciding which MTF casualties should be evacuated to. How many personnel will be going on the mission? The JSOTF medical officer and the Combat Casualty Transport Teams need to know at least some of the details of any mission that takes place in-theater for which the possibility of casualty evacuation exists. Rehearsal of representative CASEVACs is invaluable in refining both operating techniques with the CASEVAC assets and coordination with the receiving MTF.

Medical Treatment Facility Coordination

As part of the development of casualty evacuation procedures, the senior SOF medical officer should visit the theater MTFs that may receive SOF casualties. Items to be reviewed at the MTF include casualty evacuation procedures, communications, and medical and surgical services offered. Probably the most important aspect of the visit is to identify several individuals to serve as points of contact if the SOF unit has casualties to send there, and to ensure that a reliable means of contacting these individuals is available. Cellular phones, very high-frequency radio, or satellite pagers may all be possibilities.

Sick Call Facilities

Another high-priority item in-theater is the establishment of a medical treatment capability in the SOF compound. Medical equipment and supplies should be secured in an environment that will prevent damage from rain, heat, or cold and will prevent unauthorized use. Treatment tables should be obtained or improvised and the best possible lighting, climate control, and cleanliness arrangements should be made. Unit sick call hours and procedures should be announced and maintained.

Hyperbaric Treatment Facility

If the SOF unit has a diving mission, coordination must be established with the nearest hyperbaric chamber in much the same manner as that described for the MTF. This may be difficult in many remote areas. Navy diving commands such as the Navy Experimental Diving Unit (DSN: 436-4351; commercial telephone: 850-234-4351) may be helpful in locating the nearest chamber. Civilian diving organizations such as the Diver's Alert Network, Durham, North Carolina (commercial telephone: 919-684-8111), or The Undersea and Hyperbaric Medical Society, Kensington, Maryland (commercial telephone: 301-942-2980), may also be able to provide assistance. If there is no in-theater chamber that can be reached reliably by casualty evacuation assets, and if diving operations are anticipated during the conflict, then coordination with the JSOTF staff should be made to have a transportable recompression chamber (TRC) deployed to the theater.

Wartime Diving Medicine

Diving procedures for the Navy and other US armed services are established by the Supervisor of Diving and Salvage at the Naval Sea Systems Command, usually based on the testing and recommendations of the NEDU. These procedures are described in the *US Navy Diving Manual*,[18] with interim changes transmitted by letter or message. Areas that impact directly on NSW diving operations are the oxygen-exposure limits, closed-circuit scuba canister operating limits, and decompression procedures.

During peacetime diving operations these guidelines are followed meticulously. In the setting of armed conflicts, however, operational exigencies may require that SOF combat swimmers go beyond the standards of accepted peacetime military diving practice. Special Warfare DMOs may be called on to advise operational commanders about the magnitude of hazard entailed in their swimmers' exceeding peacetime guidelines.

Take, for example, a proposed mission that requires a closed-circuit oxygen dive deeper or longer than allowed by the current US Navy limits.[18] What is the risk of a diver's having a convulsion if a more-severe oxygen exposure is attempted? How can the risk of oxygen toxicity be reduced for these divers? The DMO can use the information found in previous oxygen toxicity and Draeger LAR V purging studies[19–29] to provide risk estimations to his line commanders. Another potential source of questions in wartime NSW combat swimmer operations relates to operating times of the carbon dioxide canister. Both the Mk 16 and the Draeger LAR V UBAs have carbon dioxide absorbent canister operating limits that have been established through careful testing at EDU. These limits are not exceeded during peacetime NSW diving missions. On a combat operation, however, if an unexpected problem causes a delay during the mission, would the diver be more at risk from continuing to breathe from the UBA after reaching the end of the canister operating limit, or from surfacing in a hostile harbor? Information on closed-circuit UBA canister durations is found in a number of EDU reports[30–40] and may be of great use to the DMO in answering questions of this nature.

All of the references mentioned in this section are available to the in-theater DMO on the Special Operations Computer-Assisted Medical Reference System, which is described below. This CD-ROM–based information source is an important item for medical officers in-theater and a microprocessor with a CD-ROM capability should be standard equipment for medical officers supporting SOF operations in a conflict.

Additional Medical Support Measures

Medical Logistics. A medical resupply system must be established quickly after arriving in-theater. Resupply procedures should be spelled out in the theater operation plan, but reliable resupply of all necessary items of medical equipment may require coordination with the SOF parent units or other sources of support.

Preventive Medicine. Preventive medicine measures are an important aspect of in-theater medical support. Sanitation and hygiene inspections should be conducted to ensure that the deployed forces have the safest living and messing spaces possible. The medical department will need to help administer programs such as the successful planned rehydration efforts designed to help prevent heat injuries

in the Persian Gulf War (1990/91). Medical officers should be aggressive in making recommendations to line commanders regarding such issues as thermal stress and sleep hygiene, since both of these areas may have a direct impact on operational success.

Medical Surveillance. A microprocessor-based system for tracking SOF DNBI as well as combat casualties should be established and maintained. DNBI often account for the loss of more combat troops than do combat casualties, and collection of epidemiological data might help to reduce these losses.

Continued Medical Training. Continued training in combat casualty care should be conducted in-theater. Additional training topics should include preventive medicine and the disease entities specific to the operating area.

TACTICAL COMBAT CASUALTY CARE IN SPECIAL OPERATIONS

The issue of tactical combat casualty care in the SOF environment has been addressed in a recent paper.[17] Trauma care training for SOF physicians, corpsmen and medics has historically been based primarily on the principles taught in the ATLS course.[41] ATLS provides a standardized approach to the management of trauma and has proven very successful when used in the setting of a hospital emergency department. The value of at least some aspects of ATLS in the prehospital setting, however, has been questioned.[42–64]

The importance of the prehospital phase in caring for combat casualties is evident from the fact that approximately 90% of combat deaths occur on the battlefield before the casualty reaches an MTF.[65] The standard ATLS course makes no mention of the exigencies of combat care, and the perceived shortcomings of ATLS in the combat environment have been addressed by military medical authors.[61,66–70] The need to make significant modifications to the principles of care taught in ATLS is obvious when considering the complicating effect of factors that occur in special operations, such as darkness, enemy fire, medical equipment limitations, longer evacuation times, and the unique problems entailed in transporting SOF combat casualties.[17]

These observations do not imply any shortcomings in the ATLS course. The ATLS course is well accepted as the standard of care once the patient reaches the emergency department of an MTF. Problems arise only as the military attempts to extrapolate the ATLS principles of care from the emergency department into the battlefield setting. This is an environment for which ATLS was clearly not designed and that needs to have

its own standards of care. This section is designed to help address that need.

Stages of Care

It is useful to consider the management of casualties that occur during Direct Action SOF missions as being divided into three distinct phases[17]:

1. Care under fire: the care rendered by the medic or corpsman at the scene of the injury, while he and the casualty are still under effective hostile fire. Available medical equipment is limited to that carried by each operator on the mission or by the corpsman or medic in his medical pack.

2. Tactical field care: the care rendered by the medic or corpsman once he and the casualty are no longer under effective hostile fire. The term also applies to situations in which an injury has occurred on a mission but no hostile fire has occurred. Available medical equipment is limited to that carried into the field by mission personnel. The time prior to evacuation to an MTF may range from a few minutes to many hours.

3. Combat casualty evacuation (CASEVAC) care: care rendered once the casualty (and usually the rest of the mission personnel) have been picked up by an aircraft, vehicle, or boat. Additional personnel and medical equipment that have been prestaged in these rescue assets should be available at this stage of casualty management.

Basic Tactical Combat Casualty Care Plan

Having identified the three phases of casualty management in the SOF tactical setting, the next step is to outline in a general way the care appropriate to each phase. A basic tactical casualty management plan, consisting of a generic sequence of steps that will often require modification for specific SOF casualty scenarios, is important as a starting point from which development of individualized scenario-based management plans can begin. A detailed rationale for the steps outlined in the basic management plan for each of these stages of care has been presented.[17] A few of the major differences between this management plan and ATLS will be reviewed here.

Care Under Fire

A minimal amount of medical care should be attempted while the casualty and corpsman or medic are actually under effective hostile fire (Exhibit 37-1). The use of a tourniquet to manage life-threatening extremity hemorrhage is encouraged, however, because hemorrhage from extremity wounds is the leading cause of preventable death on the battlefield and was the cause of death in more than 2,500 casualties in the Vietnam War who had no other injuries.[71]

There is no requirement to immobilize the cervical spine prior to moving a casualty out of a firefight if he has a penetrating neck or head wound. Arishita, Vayer, and Bellamy[42] examined the value of cervical spine immobilization in penetrating neck injuries in Vietnam and found that in only 1.4% of patients with penetrating neck injuries would immobilization of the cervical spine have been of possible benefit. The risk of additional hostile fire injuries to both casualty and rescuer while immobilization is being attempted poses a much more significant threat than damage to the spinal cord from failure to immobilize the neck.[42]

Tactical Field Care and Combat Casualty Evacuation Care

If a casualty with traumatic wounds is found to be in cardiopulmonary arrest on the battlefield as a result of blast or penetrating trauma, attempts at resuscitation are not appropriate.[17] Prehospital resuscitation of trauma victims in cardiac arrest has been found to be futile even in the urban setting where the victim is in close proximity to trauma centers. One study[72] reported no survivors among 138 trauma victims who suffered a prehospital cardiac arrest in whom resuscitation was attempted. Only in nontraumatic disorders (eg, hypothermia, near-drowning, electrocution) should cardiopulmonary resuscitation be performed.

The airways of unconscious casualties should be opened with the chin-lift or jaw thrust maneuvers (Exhibits 37-2 and 37-3). In these patients, if spontaneous respirations are present and respiratory distress is absent, a nasopharyngeal airway is the airway of choice. The two main advantages of this device are that it is better tolerated than an oropharyngeal airway should the patient regain consciousness and that it is less likely to be dislodged during transport.[17]

Should an airway obstruction develop or persist despite the use of a nasopharyngeal airway, a more-definitive airway is required. The ability of experienced paramedical personnel to master the technique of endotracheal intubation has been well documented.[44,45,73–82] This technique may be more difficult to accomplish in the SOF tactical care setting, however,[17] and cricothyroidotomy is probably a better next step for most SOF combat medics and corpsmen. This procedure has been reported to be safe and effective in trauma victims.[83] It may well be the only feasible alternative for any potential intubationist when the casualty has sustained maxillofacial wounds in which blood or disrupted anatomy precludes visualization of the vocal cords.[61,83] This procedure is not without complica-

---

EXHIBIT 37-1

BASIC SPECIAL OPERATIONS FORCES TACTICAL CASUALTY MANAGEMENT PLAN

Phase 1: Care Under Fire

1. The casualty remains engaged as a combatant if possible

2. Return fire as directed or required

3. Try to keep from getting shot

4. Try to keep the casualty from sustaining additional wounds

5. Stop any life-threatening external hemorrhage with a tourniquet

6. Take the casualty with you when you leave

EXHIBIT 37-2

BASIC SPECIAL OPERATIONS FORCES TACTICAL COMBAT CASUALTY CARE PLAN

Phase 2: Tactical Field Care

1. Airway management

   - Chin-lift or jaw-thrust

   - For an unconscious casualty without airway obstruction: nasopharyngeal airway

   - For an unconscious casualty with airway obstruction: cricothyroidotomy

   - Cervical spine immobilization is not necessary for casualties with penetrating head or neck trauma

2. Breathing: consider tension pneumothorax and decompress with needle thoracostomy if a casualty has unilateral penetrating chest trauma and progressive respiratory distress

3. Circulation (Bleeding): consider removing tourniquet and controlling bleeding with direct pressure, if feasible

4. Establish intravenous (IV) access: start an 18-gauge IV line or saline lock

5. Initiate fluid resuscitation:

   - For controlled hemorrhage without shock: no fluids necessary

   - For controlled hemorrhage with shock: administer 1 L Hespan (6% hydroxyethylstarch, manufactured by Du Pont Pharmaceuticals, Wilmington, Del)

   - For uncontrolled (intraabdominal or thoracic) hemorrhage: no IV fluid resuscitation unless the casualty exhibits a decreased state of consciousness. In this instance, administer 500 mL Hespan initially. A second 500 mL may be given if needed, but 1 L should generally be the maximum volume infused.

6. Inspect and dress wound

7. Check for additional wounds

8. Administer analgesia as necessary: morphine: 5 mg (administered IV); wait 10 min; repeat as necessary

9. Splint fractures and recheck pulse

10. Initiate antibiotic therapy: cefoxitin: 2 g (slow IV push, over 3–5 min) for penetrating abdominal trauma, massive soft-tissue damage, open fractures, grossly contaminated wounds, or long delays before casualty evacuation.

11. Cardiopulmonary resuscitation should not be attempted in the Tactical Field Care phase on casualties who are in cardiac arrest as a result of penetrating or blunt trauma sustained in combat.

---

tions,[84,85] but SOF corpsmen and medics are all trained in this technique, and a prepackaged SOF cricothyroidotomy kit that contains the equipment for an over-the-wire technique has been developed at Walter Reed Army Institute of Research, Washington, DC, and approved by the FDA.

A presumptive diagnosis of tension pneumothorax should be made when progressive, severe respiratory distress develops in the setting of unilateral penetrating chest trauma. The diagnosis of tension pneumothorax on the battlefield should not rely on such clinical signs as breath sounds, tracheal shift, and hyperresonance to percussion because these signs may not always be present[86]; even if they are, they may be exceedingly difficult to appreciate on the battlefield. A casualty with penetrating chest trauma will generally have some degree of hemothorax or pneumothorax as a result of his primary wound, and the additional trauma caused by a needle thoracostomy would not be expected to significantly worsen his condition should he not actually have a tension pneumothorax.[82] All SOF corpsmen and medics are trained in this technique and should perform it without hesitation in this setting.

Paramedics are authorized to perform needle thoracostomy in some civilian emergency medical

EXHIBIT 37-3

BASIC SPECIAL OPERATIONS FORCES TACTICAL COMBAT CASUALTY CARE PLAN

Phase 3: Combat Casualty Evacuation (CASEVAC) Care

1. Airway management
   - Chin-lift or jaw-thrust
   - For an unconscious casualty without airway obstruction: nasopharyngeal airway, endotracheal intubation, Combitube (mfg by Sheridan Catheter Corp, Argyle, NY) or laryngeal mask airway
   - For an unconscious casualty with airway obstruction: cricothyroidotomy if endotracheal intubation or other airway devices are unsuccessful

2. Breathing
   - Consider tension pneumothorax and decompress with needle thoracostomy if the casualty has unilateral penetrating chest trauma and progressive respiratory distress
   - Consider chest tube insertion if a suspected tension pneumothorax is not relieved by needle thoracostomy
   - Administer oxygen, if available

3. Circulation (Bleeding): consider removing tourniquets and using direct pressure to control bleeding if possible

4. Establish intravenous (IV) access; start an 18-gauge IV line or saline lock if not already done

5. Initiate fluid resuscitation:
   - For casualty with no hemorrhage or controlled hemorrhage without shock, administer lactated Ringer's solution IV at 250 mL/h
   - For casualty with controlled hemorrhage with shock, initially administer 1 L (IV) Hespan (6% hydroxyethylstarch, mfg by Du Pont Pharmaceuticals, Wilmington, Del)
   - For casualty with uncontrolled (intraabdominal or thoracic) hemorrhage: no IV fluid resuscitation unless the casualty exhibits a decreased state of consciousness. In this instance, administer 500 mL Hespan initially. A second 500 mL may be given if needed, but 1 L should generally be the maximum volume infused.
   - For casualty with head wound: administer Hespan IV at minimal flow to maintain infusion unless hemorrhagic shock is concurrent

6. Monitoring: institute electronic monitoring of heart rate, blood pressure, and hemoglobin oxygen saturation

7. Inspect and dress wounds if not already done

8. Check for additional wounds

9. Administer analgesia as necessary: morphine: 5 mg IV; wait 10 minutes; repeat as necessary

10. Splint fractures and recheck pulse

11. Initiate antibiotic therapy, if not already given: cefoxitin: 2 g (slow IV push, over 3–5 min) for penetrating abdominal trauma, massive soft-tissue damage, open fractures, grossly contaminated wounds, or long delays before casualty evacuation

services,[77,82] but chest tubes are not recommended in this phase of care.[17] Tube thoracostomy is generally not part of the paramedic's scope of care in civilian EMS settings,[77,82] nor were any studies found that address the use of this procedure by corpsmen and medics on the battlefield.

Although standard trauma care involves starting two large-bore (14- or 16-gauge) intravenous catheters,[41] the use of an 18-gauge catheter is preferred in the field because of the increased ease of starting.[17] The larger catheters are needed to rapidly administer large volumes of blood products, but this is not a factor in the tactical setting because blood products will not be available. Crystalloid solutions can be administered rapidly through the 18-gauge catheters.[87,88] Although larger-bore catheters may need to be started on arrival at an MTF, prehospital intravenous infusions are often discontinued on arrival because of concern about battlefield contamination of the intravenous site.[89]

Despite its frequent use, the benefit of prehospital fluid resuscitation in trauma victims has not been established.[45–47,49–51,53,55,58,60,61,64,90] The beneficial effect from crystalloid and colloid fluid resuscitation in hemorrhagic shock has been demonstrated largely on animal models where the volume of hemorrhage is controlled experimentally and resuscitation is initiated after the hemorrhage has been stopped.[60,62] In uncontrolled hemorrhagic shock models, the animal data are clear that when there is an unrepaired vascular injury, aggressive fluid resuscitation is associated with either no improvement in survival or increased mortality.[48,49,55,56–60,62–64,91–96] This lack of benefit is presumably due to interference with vasoconstriction and hemostasis while the body attempts to adjust to the loss of blood volume and develop a thrombus at the bleeding site. Several studies noted that only after previously uncontrolled hemorrhage was stopped did fluid resuscitation prove to be of benefit.[95–97]

Three studies have addressed this issue in humans. First, a large study of 6,855 trauma patients found that although hypotension was associated with a significantly higher mortality rate, the administration of prehospital intravenous fluids did not influence this rate.[53] Second, a retrospective analysis of patients with ruptured abdominal aortic aneurysms showed a survival rate of 30% for patients who were treated with aggressive preoperative colloid fluid replacement; in contrast, there was a 77% survival rate for patients in whom fluid resuscitation was withheld until the time of operative repair.[98] Crawford, the author of that study, strongly recommended that fluid resuscitation be withheld until the time of surgery in these patients. And third, a large prospective trial examining this issue in 598 victims of penetrating torso trauma was recently published by Bickell and colleagues.[43,52] They found that aggressive prehospital fluid resuscitation of patients with penetrating wounds of the chest and abdomen was associated with a poorer outcome than that seen in patients for whom aggressive volume replacement was withheld until the time of surgical repair. Although confirmation of these findings in other randomized, prospective studies has not yet been obtained, no human studies were found that demonstrated any benefit from fluid replacement in patients with ongoing hemorrhage, and battlefield casualties with penetrating abdominal or thoracic trauma must be presumed to have ongoing hemorrhage prior to surgical repair of their injuries.

If fluid resuscitation is required for controlled hemorrhagic shock in the tactical field care phase, Hespan (6% hydroxyethylstarch, mfg by Du Pont Pharmaceuticals, Wilmington, Del) is recommended as an alternative to lactated Ringer's (LR) solution.[17] LR solution is a crystalloid, which means that its primary osmotically active particle is sodium. Since the distribution of sodium is the entire extracellular fluid compartment, LR solution moves rapidly from the intravascular space to the extravascular space. This fluid shift has significant implications for fluid resuscitation. One hour after 1 L of LR solution has been infused into a trauma patient, only 200 mL of that volume remains in the intravascular space to replace lost blood volume.[17] This is not a problem in the civilian setting, as the typical time for transport of the patient to the hospital in an ambulance is less than 15 minutes,[52,53] and once the patient has arrived at the hospital, infusion of blood products and surgical repair can be initiated rapidly. In the military setting, however, where several hours or more typically elapse before a casualty arrives at an MTF, effective volume resuscitation may be difficult to achieve with LR solution.

In contrast, the large hetastarch molecule in Hespan is retained in the intravascular space and no fluid is lost to the interstitium. Hespan actually draws fluid into the vascular space from the interstitium, such that an infusion of 500 mL of Hespan results in an intravascular volume expansion of almost 800 mL,[99] and this effect is sustained for 8 hours or longer.[100] In addition to providing more effective expansion of the intravascular volume, a significant reduction in the weight of medical equipment is achieved by carrying Hespan instead of LR solution into the field: 4 L of LR weighs almost 9 lb, while the 500 mL of Hespan needed to achieve a similar sustained intravascular volume expansion weighs just over 1 lb.[17] Although concerns have been voiced about coagulopathies and changes in immune function associated with the use of Hespan,[63,101–104] these effects are not seen with infusion of 1,500 mL or less.[103–105] Several studies have found Hespan to be a safe and effective alternative to LR solution for resuscitating patients with controlled hemorrhagic shock.[106,107] Hespan is also believed to be an acceptable alternative to LR solution for intraoperative fluid replacement.[108]

If the casualty is conscious and requires analgesia, it should be achieved with morphine, preferably administered intravenously.[17] This mode of administration allows for much more rapid onset of analgesia and for more effective titration of dosage than intramuscular administration. An initial dose of 5 mg is given and repeated at 10-minute intervals until adequate analgesia is achieved.

Infection is an important late cause of morbidity and mortality in wounds sustained on the battlefield. Cefoxitin (2 g, administered intravenously) is an accepted monotherapeutic agent for empirical treatment of abdominal sepsis[109] and should be given without delay to all casualties with penetrating abdominal trauma.[61,110,111] Cefoxitin is effective against Gram-positive aerobes (except some *Enterococcus* spp) and Gram-negative aerobes (except some *Pseudomonas* spp). It also has good activity against anaerobes (including *Bacteroides* and *Clostridium* spp). Because it is effective against the clostridial species that cause myonecrosis, cefoxitin is also recommended for casualties who sustain wounds with massive soft-tissue damage,[111] grossly contaminated wounds, open fractures, or those for whom a long delay until CASEVAC is anticipated.[112]

Scenario-Specific Tactical Combat Casualty Care Plans

The basic management plan described above provides a starting point from which to discuss the management of specific casualties, but, as mentioned above, a great many additional considerations may come into play. This section describes one approach to planning for casualties on such missions.

Combat Operations

A number of approaches or infiltration techniques may be part of SOF combat missions (Exhibit 37-4). A casualty with a specific hostile fire injury is then imposed into one of the elements in the mission scenario (Exhibit 37-5). Hostile fire is not the only possible source of injuries to SOF personnel on missions, however, so combat injuries that occur in a hostile environment but are not caused by enemy action must also be considered (Exhibit 37-6). If the mission is sustained for several days, the onset of acute medical conditions (eg, diarrhea, cough, allergic rhinitis, sneezing, vomiting) as well as sprains, fractures, and environmental injuries such as heatstroke are also possible. A mild cold with frequent sneezing or coughing or a severely sprained ankle may be minor annoyances in the usual course of events, but can lead to mission compromise and the loss of an entire patrol if the problem occurs, for example, on the second day of a 5-day sustained mission and is not effectively treated.

EXHIBIT 37-4

ELEMENTS OF SPECIAL OPERATIONS FORCES COMBAT OPERATIONS

1. Closed-circuit self-contained underwater breathing apparatus (scuba) diving

2. Dry Deck Shelter (DDS) launch and recovery

3. Helicopter cast (ie, jumping from a moving, airborne helicopter into the water) and recovery

4. High-speed boat transits

5. Surface swimming

6. Parachute insertions

7. Fast rope or helicopter rappel insertions

8. SEAL Delivery Vehicle (SDV) transits

9. Small-unit land warfare

10. Small boat transits

11. Submarine lock-outs and lock-ins

12. Winter warfare patrols

13. Helicopter transits

14. Fixed-wing aircraft transits

Another variable that must be considered is the number of casualties. A management plan may work very well for a casualty scenario that entails only one casualty but not at all for a scenario in which 6 members of a 12-man patrol are casualties. Yet another major variable is the outcome of the engagement in which the casualty is sustained (Exhibit 37-7). If hostile fire is incompletely suppressed or if the SOF unit is overpowered, managing the unit's casualties may be difficult or impossible. Other casualty variables must also be anticipated (Exhibit 37-8). A variety of casualty scenarios can be developed for SOF combat missions by using different combinations of the variables found in Exhibits 37-4 through 37-8. Several representative SOF casualty scenarios are presented in Exhibit 37-9.

Foreign Internal Defense and Civic Action

Medical support of foreign internal defense and civic action missions poses a different set of challenges than combat missions.[113] SOF medical personnel may have to function in areas devoid of sophisticated diagnostic equipment, specialty con-

EXHIBIT 37-5

REPRESENTATIVE WOUNDS THAT CAN OCCUR UNDER HOSTILE FIRE

1. Penetrating head trauma

2. Maxillofacial trauma with potential airway compromise

3. Penetrating chest trauma

4. Penetrating chest trauma with hemothorax and shock

5. Penetrating chest trauma with tension pneumothorax

6. Penetrating abdominal trauma without shock

7. Penetrating abdominal trauma with shock

8. Penetrating upper extremity trauma with hemorrhage

9. Penetrating lower extremity trauma with hemorrhage

10. Traumatic amputation

11. Penetrating neck trauma with massive external hemorrhage

12. Penetrating neck trauma without external hemorrhage

13. Burns

14. Blast trauma

15. Multiple shrapnel trauma

EXHIBIT 37-6

REPRESENTATIVE NON–HOSTILE FIRE COMBAT INJURIES*

1. Minor but debilitating extremity orthopedic trauma (severe ankle sprain or shoulder dislocation)

2. Major extremity orthopedic trauma (open fracture or fracture-dislocation)

3. Snakebite

4. Fall from a significant distance with unconsciousness

5. Fall from a significant distance with neck or back pain

6. Hypothermia

7. Hypoxia

8. Oxygen toxicity

9. Near-drowning

10. Severe jellyfish envenomation

11. Severe insect envenomation

12. Shark attack

13. Decompression sickness

*Injuries occurring in a hostile environment but not due to enemy action

EXHIBIT 37-8

OTHER CASUALTY VARIABLES

1. When in the mission was the casualty wounded?

2. What will be lost if the mission is aborted?

3. What is the extraction plan?

4. Can casualty evacuation (CASEVAC) occur at the casualty's location?

5. Is the casualty a corpsman or medic?

6. What is the weight of the casualty?

7. What is the risk to other operators or support personnel?

8. How critical is time-to-CASEVAC to the casualty's survival?

9. Is the mission a day or night operation?

EXHIBIT 37-7

REPRESENTATIVE OUTCOMES OF SPECIAL OPERATIONS ENGAGEMENTS

1. Hostiles (ie, enemy combatants) are all dead or withdrawn from the engagement

2. Standoff, with both sides firing from cover

3. Hostile force has fire superiority but organized withdrawal is possible; non-casualties outnumber casualties

4. Hostile force has fire superiority; no chance for organized withdrawal because of volume of fire or number of casualties

5. Friendly forces are defeated and overrun

EXHIBIT 37-9

REPRESENTATIVE SPECIAL OPERATIONS CASUALTY SCENARIOS

Underwater Explosion Scenario

- Ship attack
- Launch from coastal patrol craft 12 miles out
- One-hour transit in two Zodiacs (ie, inflatable boats)
- Seven swim pairs using Draeger LAR V closed-circuit oxygen underwater breathing apparatus (UBA)
- Zodiacs get to 1 mile from the harbor
- Water temperature 78°F; divers in wet suits
- Surface swim for half mile, then purge UBA and submerge
- Underwater explosion occurs while divers are under target ship
- One diver unconscious; other member of swim pair conscious

Oxygen Toxicity Scenario

- Ship attack
- Launch from coastal patrol craft 12 miles out
- One-hour transit in two Zodiacs
- Seven swim pairs using Draeger LAR V
- Zodiacs get to 1 mile from the harbor
- Water temperature 78°F; divers in wet suits
- Surface swim for half mile, then purge UBA and submerge
- Very clear, still night; transit depth 25 ft
- Diver notes that buddy is disoriented and confused with arm twitching

SEAL Delivery Vehicle Scenario

- Two SEAL Delivery Vehicles (SDVs) launched from Dry Deck Shelter (DDS)
- Two-hour transit to beach
- Target is a heavily defended harbor in a bay
- Water temperature 43°F; divers in dry suits
- Air temperature 35°F
- Boats bottomed (ie, grounded) for across-the-beach radio beacon placement
- Swim to shore using Draeger LAR V
- One man shot in the chest at the objective
- Hostile forces in pursuit as team begins to extract

Parachute Insertion Injury Scenario

- Twelve-man Special Forces team
- Interdiction operation for weapons convoy
- Night static line jump made from C-130 aircraft
- Four-mile patrol over rocky terrain to objective
- Planned helicopter extraction near target
- One jumper's canopy collapses 40 ft above the drop zone
- Open facial fractures with blood and teeth in the oropharynx
- Bilateral ankle fractures
- Open angulated fracture of the left femur

Snakebite Scenario

- Twelve-man Special Forces team
- Planned interdiction operation in arid, mountainous Middle Eastern terrain
- Two hostile trucks carrying surface-to-air missiles (SAMs) expected in several hours
- Estimated hostile strength is 10 men with automatic weapons in two armored personnel carriers (APCs)
- Helicopter insertion and extraction
- Six-mile patrol to target; can extract close to anticipated contact site
- While patrol is in position, one team member is bitten on the leg by an unidentified snake
- Over the next 5 minutes, the injured man becomes dizzy and confused
- Target convoy expected in 1 to 2 hours

Acute Gastroenteritis Scenario

- Twelve-man Special Forces team
- Dropped into unfriendly Middle Eastern country
- Four-day SCUD missile hunt
- Planned helicopter extraction at end of operation
- Lost communications: no casualty evacuation (CASEVAC) or extraction plan changes possible
- Patrolling in moderately populated area
- Two patrol members develop severe diarrhea and stomach cramps

sultations, modern surgical facilities, and adequate supplies of medications. In addition, the population being treated is often ravaged by the debilitating effects of malnutrition and chronic disease.[114] Cultural differences can make seemingly simple steps complex in their implementation. One report[115] documents the difficulty encountered by Air Force personnel trying to control an outbreak of rabies by using poisoned meat to rid the area of stray dogs. The local Buddhist spiritual leader required that two equal-sized pieces of meat (one poisoned and one not) be put out, thus giving the rabid dogs a choice. The same report discusses the difficulty in prescribing medications to a populace that not only speaks a different language from the healthcare provider but also often reads not at all. In such a setting, how do we ensure that the patients will remember the appropriate dosages and intervals for their medications?

Adequate quantities of medicines, vitamins, and medical supplies to treat the expected diseases must be determined and taken into the area with the SOF unit deployed. The providers' scope of care should be carefully outlined and procedures established for handling emergency cases that fall outside that prescribed scope of care. Both action and failure to act may have unfavorable consequences, so a careful examination of the medical ethics and the political realities of such dilemmas must be accomplished by the planners before the medical provider leaves for the mission.

The Department of Defense has a growing telemedicine capability that may be of some use in this environment. Foreign internal defense missions require a maximal effort to teach and train the populace in medical and preventive measures that they can implement themselves, because the presence of the US advisors must be assumed to be only temporary. First World medical care provided for a brief time is of little benefit if the population subsequently returns to its baseline state of healthcare. Before deployment, medical personnel must be familiar with the elements of the local culture and religion that are likely to impact on healthcare.

A final consideration is to provide the medical personnel on the mission with clear instructions on how to document and follow-up on human rights violations that may be encountered in rendering care to the local population.[115] Violations committed by the current power structure may be encountered. Immediate confrontation with the local authorities may result in a rapid breakdown in relations, so this eventuality in particular should be planned for in advance.

Humanitarian Assistance

Humanitarian assistance missions are often undertaken after another country has been ravaged by an armed conflict or a natural disaster. Such natural disasters often have more devastating effects in underdeveloped countries than in First World nations. An example is the cyclone that struck southeastern Bangladesh in 1991 with 160-knot winds and a 6-m storm surge, resulting in the loss of more than 140,000 lives.[116]

SOF personnel assisting on relief efforts such as this will typically have to contend with most of the considerations described above for foreign internal defense and civic action missions, but in addition will have the superimposed effects of the conflict or natural disaster. Some of the additional considerations in this circumstance are the need to provide security for personnel, equipment, and medications, as medical teams try to render care to what may be an impossibly large number of patients. Deployable clinics and medical facilities should be used as extensively as possible. Preventive medicine measures (eg, obtaining potable water, establishing adequate sanitation facilities) are a very high priority in caring for the victims of natural disasters and armed conflicts.[116] SOF efforts in such undertakings will have to be coordinated with theater medical personnel and other agencies involved with international relief efforts.

Operations Other Than War

Planning for medical support of OOTW may present the greatest challenge of all to SOF medical personnel, as OOTW may include elements of several other missions—from tactical combat casualty care to foreign internal defense to humanitarian medical assistance. SOF medical personnel may have to shift rapidly from rendering care to friendly foreign personnel to flying into a gunfight to evacuate multiple combat casualties. The potential for this rapid change in conditions was dramatically illustrated in the SOF actions during Operation Restore Hope in Somalia, in which a planned humanitarian relief effort quickly turned into a direct action combat situation.

Aspects of Postdeployment Medicine

Medical Afteraction Reports

After the conflict or mission has ended and SOF units return to business as usual, a thorough medical afteraction report should be written to provide documentation of the successes and failures of the medical aspects of the operation so that the military medical community may learn from both. There is no better method available in the military with which to bring about needed changes in medical equipment, manning, and training than a well-written afteraction report that identifies specific deficiencies in our current system and suggests appropriate changes with which to remedy these problems.

A case in point is the casualty evacuation experience in Mogadishu, Somalia, during Operation Restore Hope (1992). Narrow streets and rocket-propelled grenade fire made helicopter evacuation impractical. This observation has great importance for future urban warfare mission planners.

Disease Surveillance

Disease surveillance is critically important for individuals returning from a theater conflict, as they may be subject to large assortment of infectious diseases that are not frequently seen in the United States. These disorders may not be diagnosed promptly if a high index of suspicion is not maintained by the SOF medical officers.

BIOMEDICAL RESEARCH

In 1991, the Naval Special Warfare Command established a Biomedical Research Program to conduct biomedical studies designed to better safeguard the health of its operators and to identify possible biomedical enhancements to the probability of mission success. This program addressed a wide range of biomedical issues that were believed to be important to members of the SEAL community, who operate in a variety of hazardous environments (Figure 37-13). The results obtained from these studies were useful enough that funding for the program has significantly increased since 1991, and USSOCOM has expanded the scope of the program to address the biomedical research requirements of the Army and Air Force Special Operations Commands and the Joint Special Operations Command, as well. All of the reports generated from USSOCOM biomedical research projects are incorporated into the Special Operations Computer-Assisted Medical Reference System (SOCAMRS) each year as they become available so that they will available to medical officers and combat medical personnel in-theater and to future gen-

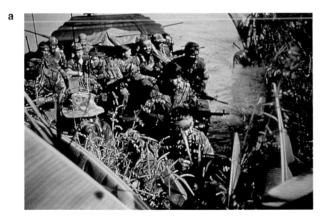

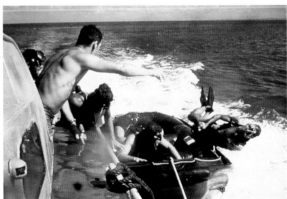

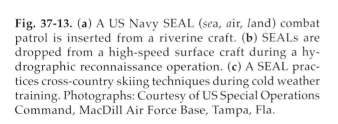

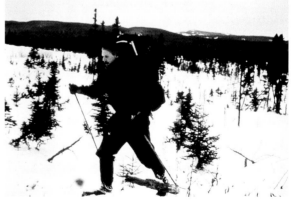

Fig. 37-13. (a) A US Navy SEAL (*sea, air, land*) combat patrol is inserted from a riverine craft. (b) SEALs are dropped from a high-speed surface craft during a hydrographic reconnaissance operation. (c) A SEAL practices cross-country skiing techniques during cold weather training. Photographs: Courtesy of US Special Operations Command, MacDill Air Force Base, Tampa, Fla.

erations of SOF medical personnel. Some of the areas in which biomedical research has benefited the conduct of special operations are discussed below.

Medical Aspects of Mission Planning

The SOCAMRS is a customized CD-ROM designed to provide SOF physicians, corpsmen, and medics with a single comprehensive reference source that contains the entire spectrum of specialized information required to provide medical support to special operations. The SOCAMRS is updated each year and delivered to all SOF commands in sufficient quantities for every physician, corpsman, and medic to have his own copy. Customized and updated versions of this CD are prepared each year. The information contained on the 1996 5th edition of the SOCAMRS,[117] for example, includes

- approximately 1,000 clinical articles and research reports on various topics related to the conduct of special operations;
- the current edition of the *US Navy Diving Manual*;
- review materials for the American Heart Association's Advanced Cardiac Life Support (ACLS) and Basic Life Support (BLS) courses, and the ATLS course;
- the *Special Forces Medical Handbook*;
- the *Navy General Medical Officer's Guide*;
- area-specific medical information manuals on Southwest Asia, Somalia, and Croatia, prepared by the US Army Institute for Environmental Medicine;
- a guide to Tactical Combat Care in Special Operations[17];
- the Combat Swimmer Multi-Level Dive procedures[15];
- the *Dry Deck Shelter Medical Emergency Procedures*[16]; and
- triservice manuals on the management of NBC warfare casualties.

Medical Sustainment Training

Special operations corpsmen and medics are required to maintain a wide variety of both medical and operational skills. Intense unit training schedules often require medical personnel to be away from their command a great deal of the time and make the scheduling of group medical training classes very difficult. This problem was addressed by the Naval Health Research Center in San Diego, California, in a 3-year research effort, which has resulted in the development of the Special Operations

Interactive Medical Training Program (SOIMTP). This program contains instruction modules on 18 different medical topics such as diving medicine, tropical medicine, NBC warfare, combat casualty management, and ATLS. The modules have been written by physicians and senior enlisted medical personnel attached to special operations units and the program is contained on a CD-ROM. The SOIMTP provides both a training and a testing capability. The program has been approved by the Navy for the granting of continuing education unit credits, allowing formally recognized sustainment training to be accomplished by SOF medical personnel anywhere that a personal computer is available.

Casualty Management

Medical training for special operations corpsmen and medics has historically been based primarily on nationally recognized courses (ATLS and Emergency Medical Technician) that have been developed to train physicians and paramedics in the principles of trauma care as it would be delivered in a hospital emergency department or by ambulance attendants. These courses were supplemented by training in a field environment but did not address many of the factors that will be encountered on the special operations battlefield, such as hostile fire, medical equipment limitations, CASEVAC availability, and integration of casualty management into the tactical considerations regarding mission completion. As noted above in this chapter, this research has resulted in a management plan for combat trauma that is more appropriate for the battlefield. More specific scenario-based research into combat trauma management plans is currently ongoing.

The Special Operations CD-ROM Medical Translator, developed at the Naval Operational Medical Institute, Pensacola, Florida, allows a medical provider to conduct an interview with a non-English-speaking patient through the use of medical phrase menus contained on a laptop microprocessor with a sound board. The questions are presented to the patient in his own language and phrased so that the requested information is conveyed through nonverbal responses to the physician or corpsman. The 1995 version of this program contains 43 languages and more than 2,000 medical phrases. This program has already proven itself to be of great benefit in rendering care to victims of the conflict in the former Yugoslavia and to Special Forces medical personnel preparing for Foreign Internal Defense missions. Additional information on this device is available from SOF component medical departments or the Naval Operational Medical Institute.

Nutrition and Hydration

Preventing degradation of physical and mental performance during the conduct of long, stressful training and combat missions is of considerable importance to the special operations community. Ensuring that SEAL operators achieve the optimal nutrition and hydration status possible before and during physically arduous missions is a critical element in minimizing performance decrements. In 1992, a research project was undertaken to develop a nutrition guide for SEALs that would incorporate current scientific information regarding both the performance-enhancing and the long-term health aspects of nutrition into an understandable training manual. After an extensive review of the scientific literature on nutrition, hydration, and food supplements was conducted, the research was summarized and published in 1994 as *The Navy SEAL Nutrition Guide*.[118] This manual, which presents the material in a format which is easily understood by SEALs and other SOF operators, has been the most widely disseminated medical publication in the history of special operations.

Exercise and Mission-Related Physiology

When, if ever, can a SEAL dive after having had cataract surgery or a corneal transplant? Can a Special Forces combat swimmer dive with glaucoma or after having had a retinal detachment? A number of such questions have been asked but surprisingly little information was available to help ophthalmologists and DMOs make these decisions. This issue was addressed in 1994 and the resultant major review published in 1995 in the journal *Survey of Ophthalmology*.[119] Only approximately 10 such major reviews are published in the ophthalmology literature each year, so this paper was a significant contribution that has been of considerable use to the civilian diving community as well.

A study examining methods by which to quantify SOF mission-related performance was undertaken at NMRI in 1992 to determine which performance factors are most critical to mission success in special operations and to identify the best measures with which to quantitate these elements of performance. The investigators used extensive interviews with SOF operators to identify the performance factors they believed to be the most important to the successful completion of a variety of SOF missions. Then the investigators designed a battery of cognitive and physical tests to measure these factors. These tests are now being used in USSOCOM physiological studies that seek to identify decre-

ments in performance associated with physiological stressors such as sleep deprivation or thermal stress. The tests will also be used to evaluate the efficacy of proposed interventions to improve SOF performance, such as food supplements, thermal protective garments, or pharmacological agents.

Decompression

An in-house NSW update to the CSMD procedures was completed in 1992 and subsequently approved by NAVSEA; the following improvements to the original CSMD procedures were incorporated:

- increased the maximum operational depth using the Mk 16 UBA from 70 fsw to 110 fsw;
- greatly improved the unplanned excursion procedures;
- allowed use of the Surface Interval Credit Table[18] to decrease the repetitive group designator during the overland or surface phases of operations;
- added provisions for altitude diving and flying after diving; and
- improved and simplified the CSMD worksheet.

A new nitrox decompression model based on the statistical principle of maximum likelihood as applied to the probability of suffering an episode of decompression sickness was developed at NMRI. This computer model allows for the precise calculation of decompression obligation for the very long, multilevel, multigas dives that are often necessary in SDV operations. A laptop version of this model was approved by NAVSEA for use in SDV/DDS operations on 16 May 1994. Called the NSW Dive Planner (mentioned above), this computer model was the first Navy use of such a device to calculate decompression for operational dives. Use of the Dive Planner has substantially reduced or eliminated the decompression required after many SDV/DDS dives.

As a follow-on project to the NSW Dive Planner, NMRI examined the use of 100% oxygen breathing in the DDS complex to reduce decompression time in the event of a SEAL operator suffering a traumatic injury or hypothermia during an operation and needing to be evacuated from the DDS complex as soon as possible. This NMRI study demonstrated that breathing 100% oxygen at a depth of 40 feet in a dry recompression chamber allows the total air decompression time as calculated by the NSW Dive Planner to be reduced by 80%. The Emergency Oxygen Decompression Procedures[120] have now been approved by NAVSEA for use in DDS/SDV operations.

Life-Support Technology

In 1990, the NSW community began to plan to acquire the Mk 16 for use in SDV operations. At that time, the operating limits of the Mk 16 canister were based on testing that studied free-swimming divers; they were thought to be too restrictive for SDV operations in which the divers had a lower oxygen consumption. In December 1990, COMNAVSPECWARCOM requested that NAVSEA task NEDU to retest the Mk 16 under conditions more appropriate for SDV operations. This study resulted in new Mk 16 canister limits for SDV operations. The increases vary for different water temperatures, but for most conditions, the canister limits were almost doubled, allowing for much longer SDV operations using the Mk 16.

SUMMARY

Medical support of special operations requires both a variety of specialized medical skills and that those skills be correctly applied to the unique training and mission scenarios encountered in special operations. Failure to recognize this fact may result in avoidable loss of lives and mission failures. Medical personnel must understand fully the demanding and difficult nature of SOF missions, and SOF line commanders must understand the unique contributions that adequately prepared medical personnel can make to the health of their force and the success of their operations.

SOF physicians, corpsmen, medics, and PJs have recently redefined combat casualty care in the tactical environment. AFSOC flight surgeons are currently supervising the critical altitude decompression sickness research needed to allow the new CV-22 Osprey aircraft to achieve its desired operating profile. SOF medical personnel have made invaluable contributions to special operations in the US military since their inception and will continue to provide the SOF warrior with the medical support he needs to help him meet the challenges of his unique profession.

ACKNOWLEDGMENT

The author expresses his appreciation to the following individuals in the SOF medical community for their assistance in the preparation of this chapter: Colonel Dick Smerz, USSOCOM; Captain Steve Giebner and Master Chief Andy Knoch, COMNAVSPECWARCOM; Lieutenant Colonel Dick Tenglin and Mr. Bob Clayton, USASOC; Lieutenant Colonel Doug Wilcox, AFSOC; and Commander Mike Wilkinson, JSOMTC.

REFERENCES

1. US Special Operations Command. *United States Special Operations Command Fact Sheet.* Tampa, Fla: USSOCOM Public Affairs Office; 1994.

2. US Special Operations Command. *United States Special Operations Forces—Posture Statement.* Tampa, Fla: USSOCOM Public Affairs Publication; 1996.

3. US Army Special Operations Command. *The Special Forces A-Team.* Fort Bragg, NC: USASOC Public Affairs Office Publication; 1994.

4. US Army Special Operations Command. *Army SOF Aviation.* Fort Bragg, NC: USASOC Public Affairs Office Publication; 1994.

5. US Army Special Operations Command. *The 75th Ranger Regiment.* Fort Bragg, NC: USASOC Public Affairs Office Publication; 1994.

6. US Army Special Operations Command. *An Army Special Operations Forces Primer.* Fort Bragg, NC: USASOC Public Affairs Office Publication; 1994.

7. Naval Special Warfare Command. *Naval Special Warfare Command Fact File.* Coronado, Calif: COMNAVSPECWARCOM Public Affairs Office Publication; 1993.

8. US Air Force Special Operations Command. *Fact Sheet: Air Force Special Operations Command.* Hurlburt Field, Fla: AFSOC Public Affairs Office Publication; 1994.

9. US Air Force Special Operations Command. *Fact Sheet: US Air Force Special Operations School.* Hurlburt Field, Fla: AFSOC Public Affairs Office Publication; 1994.

10. US Air Force Special Operations Command. *Fact Sheet: 18th Flight Test Squadron.* Hurlburt Field, Fla: AFSOC Public Affairs Office Publication; 1995.

11. US Air Force Special Operations Command. *Fact Sheet: Air Force Special Tactics Teams.* Hurlburt Field, Fla: AFSOC Public Affairs Office Publication; 1994.

12. Cloonan C. Colonel, Medical Corps, US Army; Professor and Chairman, Department of Military and Emergency Medicine, F. Edward Hébert School of Medicine, Uniformed Services University of the Health Sciences, 4301 Jones Bridge Road, Bethesda, Maryland 20814-3799; formerly, Medical Dean, Joint Special Operations Medical Training Center, Fort Bragg, North Carolina. Personal communication, 17 September 2001.

13. US Department of the Navy. *Manual of the Medical Department.* Washington, DC: Chief, Bureau of Medicine and Surgery Publication; 1995. Change 111, Chap 15.

14. Butler FK, Smith DJ. US Navy diving equipment and techniques. In: Bove AA, ed. *Bove and Davis' Diving Medicine.* 3rd ed. Philadelphia, Pa: Saunders; 1997: 372–387.

15. Thalmann ED, Butler FK. *A Procedure for Doing Multi-Level Dives Using Repetitive Groups.* Panama City Beach, Fla: US Navy Experimental Diving Unit; 1983. EDU Report 13-83.

16. Commander, Naval Special Warfare Command. *Dry Deck Shelter Medical Emergency Procedures.* Coronado, Calif: NAVSPECWARCOM. Letter, 21 January 1993.

17. Butler FK, Hagmann J, Butler EG. Tactical combat casualty care in special operations. *Mil Med.* 1996;161(suppl):1–16.

18. Commander, Naval Sea Systems Command, US Department of the Navy. *US Navy Diving Manual.* SS521-Ag-PRO-010. Washington, DC: Naval Sea Systems Command. Rev 4 (20 Jan 1999); Change A (1 Mar 2001). NAVSEA 0994-LP-100-3199.

19. Butler FK, Thalmann ED. Central nervous system oxygen toxicity in closed circuit SCUBA divers. In: Bachrach AJ, Matzen MM, eds. *Underwater Physiology 8: Proceedings of the 8th Symposium on Underwater Physiology.* Bethesda, Md: Undersea Medical Society; 1984: 15–30.

20. Butler FK. *Closed-Circuit Oxygen Diving.* Panama City Beach, Fla: US Navy Experimental Diving Unit; 1985. EDU Report 7–85.

21. Butler FK, Thalmann ED. Central nervous system oxygen toxicity in closed circuit SCUBA divers, II. *Undersea Biomed Res.* 1986;13:193–223.

22. Butler FK. *Central Nervous System Oxygen Toxicity in Closed Circuit SCUBA Divers, III.* Panama City Beach, Fla: US Navy Experimental Diving Unit; 1986. EDU Report 5-86.

23. Butler FK. *Purging Procedures for the Draeger LAR V Underwater Breathing Apparatus.* Panama City Beach, Fla: US Navy Experimental Diving Unit; 1984. EDU Report 5-84.

24. Butler FK. *Underwater Purging Procedures for the Draeger LAR V UBA.* Panama City Beach, Fla: US Navy Experimental Diving Unit; 1986. EDU Report 6-86.

25. Harabin AL, Survanshi SS, Homer LD. *A Model for Predicting Central Nervous System Toxicity From Hyperbaric Oxygen Exposure in Man: Effects of Immersion, Exercise, and Old and New Data.* Bethesda, Md: Naval Medical Research Institute; 1994. NMRI Report 94-03.

26. Lanphier EH, Dwyer JV. *Diving With Self-Contained Underwater Operating Apparatus.* Washington, DC: US Navy Experimental Diving Unit; 1954. US Navy Experimental Diving Unit Report 11-54.

27. Donald KW. Oxygen poisoning in man, I. *Br Med J.* 1947;1:667–672.

28. Donald KW. Oxygen poisoning in man, II. *Br Med J.* 1947;1:712–717.

29. Yarborough OD, Welham W, Brinton ES, Behnke AR. *Symptoms of Oxygen Poisoning and Limits of Tolerance at Rest and at Work.* Washington, DC: US Navy Experimental Diving Unit; 1947. EDU Report 1-47.

30. Middleton JR, Thalmann ED. *Standardized NEDU Unmanned UBA Test Procedures and Performance Goals.* Panama City Beach, Fla: US Navy Experimental Diving Unit; 1981. EDU Report 3-81.

31. Clarke J, Russell K, Crepeau L. *MK 16 Canister Limits for SDV Operations.* Panama City Beach, Fla: US Navy Experimental Diving Unit; 1993. EDU Report 2-93.

32. Knafelc ME. *Mk 15 Mod 0 Alternate Carbon Dioxide Absorbent Materials.* Panama City Beach, Fla: US Navy Experimental Diving Unit; 1987. EDU Report 11-87.

33. Keith JS. *Unmanned Evaluation of the US Navy MK 15 and Modified MK 15 Closed-Circuit UBA.* Panama City Beach, Fla: US Navy Experimental Diving Unit; 1984. EDU Report 10-84.

34. Zumrick JL. *Manned Evaluation of the MK 15 UBA Canister Duration in 13 Degrees C Water Using a Resting Diver Scenario.* Panama City Beach, Fla: US Navy Experimental Diving Unit; 1984. EDU Report 2-84.

35. Crepeau LJ. LAR V Canister Duration Limits for HP Sodasorband L-Grade Sofnolime. Panama City Beach, Fla: US Navy Experimental Diving Unit; 1994. EDU Report 1-94.

36. Presswood CG. *Unmanned Evaluation of Five Carbon Dioxide Absorbents Which Were Frozen Prior to Use With the Draeger LAR V UBA.* Panama City Beach, Fla: US Navy Experimental Diving Unit; 1986. EDU Report 3-86.

37. Middleton JR, Keith JS. *Unmanned Evaluation of Six Carbon Dioxide Absorbents With the Draeger LAR V UBA.* Panama City Beach, Fla: US Navy Experimental Diving Unit; 1985. EDU Report 4-85.

38. Giedraitis RB. *Recommended Storage Time Following Prepacking UBA MK 16 Mod 0 With HP Sodasorb.* Panama City Beach, Fla: US Navy Experimental Diving Unit; 1992. EDU Technical Memorandum 92-06.

39. Knafelc ME. *Mk 16 Mod 0 Underwater Breathing Apparatus: Manned and Unmanned Canister Duration.* Panama City Beach, Fla: US Navy Experimental Diving Unit; 1986. EDU Report 9-86.

40. Zumrick JL. *Manned Evaluation of the EX 15 Mod 1 UBA Carbon Dioxide Absorbent Canister.* Panama City Beach, Fla: US Navy Experimental Diving Unit; 1986. EDU Report 4-86.

41. Committee on Trauma, American College of Surgeons. *Advanced Trauma Life Support Program for Physicians: Instructor Manual.* 5th ed. Chicago, Ill: American College of Surgeons; 1993.

42. Arishita GI, Vayer JS, Bellamy RF. Cervical spine immobilization of penetrating neck wounds in a hostile environment. *J Trauma.* 1989;29:332–337.

43. Bickell WH, Wall MJ, Pepe PE, et al. Immediate versus delayed fluid resuscitation for hypotensive patients with penetrating torso injuries. *N Engl J Med.* 1994;331:1105–1109.

44. Honigman B, Rohwder K, Moore EE, et al. Prehospital advanced trauma life support for penetrating cardiac wounds. *Ann Emerg Med.* 1990;19:145–150.

45. Smith JP, Bodai BI. The urban paramedic's scope of practice. *JAMA.* 1985;253:544–548.

46. Smith JP, Bodai BI, Hill AS, et al. Prehospital stabilization of critically injured patients: A failed concept. *J Trauma.* 1985;25:65–70.

47. Dronen SC, Stern S, Baldursson J, et al. Improved outcome with early blood administration in a near-fatal model of porcine hemorrhagic shock. *Am J Emerg Med.* 1992;10:533–537.

48. Stern SA, Dronen SC, Birrer P, et al. Effect of blood pressure on hemorrhage volume and survival in a near-fatal hemorrhage model incorporating a vascular injury. *Ann Emerg Med.* 1993;22:155–163.

49. Chudnofsky CR, Dronen SC, Syverud SA, et al. Early versus late fluid resuscitation: Lack of effect in porcine hemorrhagic shock. *Ann Emerg Med.* 1989;18:122–126.

50. Bickell WH. Are victims of injury sometimes victimized by attempts at fluid resuscitation? *Ann Emerg Med.* 1993;22:225–226.

51. Chudnofsky CR, Dronen SC, Syverud SA, et al. Intravenous fluid therapy in the prehospital management of hemorrhagic shock: Improved outcome with hypertonic saline/6% Dextran 70 in a swine model. *Am J Emerg Med.* 1989;7:357–363.

52. Martin RR, Bickell WH, Pepe PE, et al. Prospective evaluation of preoperative fluid resuscitation in hypotensive patients with penetrating truncal injury: A preliminary report. *J Trauma.* 1992;33:354–361.

53. Kaweski SM, Sise MJ, Virgilio RW. The effect of prehospital fluids on survival in trauma patients. *J Trauma.* 1990;30:1215–1218.

54. Gross D, Landau EH, Klin B, et al. Treatment of uncontrolled hemorrhagic shock with hypertonic saline solution. *Surg Gynecol Obstet.* 1990;170:106–112.

55. Deakin CD, Hicks IR. AB or ABC: Pre-hospital fluid management in major trauma. *J Accid Emerg Med.* 1994;11:154–157.

56. Bickell WH, Bruttig SP, Millnamow GA, et al. Use of hypertonic saline/Dextran versus lactated ringer's solution as a resuscitation fluid after uncontrolled aortic hemorrhage in anesthetized swine. *Ann Emerg Med.* 1992;21:1077–1085.

57. Dontigny L. Small-volume resuscitation. *Can J Surg.* 1992;35(1):31–33.

58. Krausz MM, Bar-Ziv M, Rabinovici R, et al. "Scoop and run" or stabilize hemorrhagic shock with normal saline or small-volume hypertonic saline? *J Trauma.* 1992;33:6–10.

59. Gross D, Landau EH, Assalia A, et al. Is hypertonic saline resuscitation safe in uncontrolled hemorrhagic shock? *J Trauma.* 1988;28:751–756.

60. Kowalenko J, Stern S, Dronen S, et al. Improved outcome with hypotensive resuscitation of uncontrolled hemorrhagic shock in a swine model. *J Trauma.* 1992;33:349–353.

61. Zajtchuk R, Jenkins DP, Bellamy RF, eds. *Combat Casualty Care Guidelines: Operation Desert Storm.* Washington, DC: Department of the Army, Office of The Surgeon General, and Borden Institute; 1991.

62. Krausz MM, Klemm O, Amstislavsky T, et al. The effect of heat load and dehydration on hypertonic saline solution treatment on uncontrolled hemorrhagic shock. *J Trauma.* 1995;38:747–752.

63. Napolitano LM. Resuscitation following trauma and hemorrhagic shock: Is hydroxyethyl starch safe? *Crit Care Med*. 1995;23:795–796.

64. Krausz MM. Controversies in shock research: Hypertonic Resuscitation—Pros and cons. *Shock*. 1995;3:69–72.

65. Bellamy RF. The causes of death in conventional land warfare: Implications for combat casualty care research. *Mil Med*. 1984;149:55–62.

66. Bellamy RF. How shall we train for combat casualty care? *Mil Med*. 1987;152:617–622.

67. Baker MS. Advanced Trauma Life Support: Is it adequate stand-alone training for military medicine? *Mil Med*. 1994;159:587–590.

68. Wiedeman JE, Jennings SA. Applying ATLS to the Gulf War. *Mil Med*. 1993;158:121–126.

69. Heiskell LE, Carmona RH. Tactical emergency medical services: An emerging subspecialty of emergency medicine. *Ann Emerg Med*. 1994;23:778–785.

70. Ekblad GS. Training medics for the combat environment of tomorrow. *Mil Med*. 1990;155:232–234.

71. Maughon JS. An inquiry into the nature of wounds resulting in killed in action in Vietnam. *Mil Med*. 1970;135:8–13.

72. Rosemurgy AS, Norris PA, Olson SM, et al. Prehospital cardiac arrest: The cost of futility. *J Trauma*. 1993;35:468–473.

73. Sladen A. Emergency endotracheal intubation: Who can—Who should? *Chest*. 1979;75:535–536.

74. Stewart RD, Paris PM, Winter PM, et al. Field endotracheal intubation by paramedical personnel: success rates and complications. *Chest*. 1984;85:341–345.

75. Jacobs LM, Berrizbeitia LD, Bennet B, et al. Endotracheal intubation in the prehospital phase of emergency medical care. *JAMA*. 1983;250:2175–2177.

76. Pointer JE. Clinical Characteristics of paramedics' performance of endotracheal intubation. *J Emerg Med*. 1988;6:505–509.

77. Lavery RF, Doran J, Tortella BJ, et al. A survey of advanced life support practices in the United States. *Prehospital Disaster Med*. 1992;7:144–150.

78. DeLeo BC. Endotracheal intubation by rescue squad personnel. *Heart Lung*. 1977;6:851–854.

79. Stratton SJ, Kane G, Gunter CS, et al. Prospective study of manikin-only versus manikin and human subject endotracheal intubation training of paramedics. *Ann Emerg Med*. 1991;20:1314–1318.

80. Trooskin SZ, Rabinowitz S, Eldridge C, et al. Teaching endotracheal intubation using animals and cadavers. *Prehospital Disaster Med*. 1992;7:179–182.

81. Stewart RD, Paris PM, Pelton GH, et al. Effect of varied training techniques on field endotracheal intubation success rates. *Ann Emerg Med*. 1984;13:1032–1036.

82. Cameron PA, Flett K, Kaan E, et al. Helicopter retrieval of primary trauma patients by a paramedic helicopter service. *Aust N Z J Surg*. 1993;63:790–797.

83. Salvino CK, Dries D, Gamelli R, et al. Emergency cricothyroidotomy in trauma victims. *J Trauma*. 1993;34:503–505.

84. McGill J, Clinton JE, Ruiz E. Cricothyrotomy in the emergency department. *Ann Emerg Med*. 1982;11:361–364.

85. Erlandson MJ, Clinton JE, Ruiz E, et al. Cricothyrotomy in the emergency department revisited. *J Emerg Med*. 1989;7:115–118.

86. Mines D. Needle thoracostomy fails to detect a fatal tension pneumothorax. *Ann Emerg Med*. 1993;22:863–866.

87. Aeder MI, Crowe JP, Rhodes RS, et al. Technical limitations in the rapid infusion of intravenous fluids. *Ann Emerg Med*. 1985;14:307–310.

88. Hoelzer MF. Recent advances in intravenous therapy. *Emerg Med Clin North Am*. 1986;4:487–500.

89. Lawrence DW, Lauro AJ. Complications from IV therapy: Results from field-started and emergency department-started IV's compared. *Ann Emerg Med*. 1988;17:314–317.

90. Kramer GC, Perron PR, Lindsey DC, et al. Small volume resuscitation with hypertonic saline dextran solution. *Surgery*. 1986;100:239–245.

91. Shaftan GW, Chiu C, Dennis C, et al. Fundamentals of physiological control of arterial hemorrhage. *Surgery*. 1965;58:851–856.

92. Milles G, Koucky CJ, Zacheis HG. Experimental uncontrolled arterial hemorrhage. *Surgery*. 1966;60:434–442.

93. Krausz MM, Horne Y, Gross D. The combined effect of small-volume hypertonic saline and normal saline in uncontrolled hemorrhagic shock. *Surg Gynecol Obstet*. 1992;174:363–368.

94. Bickell WH, Bruttig SP, Wade CE. Hemodynamic response to abdominal aortotomy in anesthetized swine. *Circ Shock*. 1989;28:321–332.

95. Landau EH, Gross D, Assalia A, et al. Treatment of uncontrolled hemorrhagic shock by hypertonic saline and external counterpressure. *Ann Emerg Med*. 1989;18:1039–1043.

96. Rabinovici R, Krausz MM, Feurstein G. Control of bleeding is essential for a successful treatment of hemorrhagic shock with 7.5 percent NaCl solution. *Surg Gynecol Obstet*. 1991;173:98–106.

97. Landau EH, Gross D, Assalia A, et al. Hypertonic saline infusion in hemorrhagic shock treated by military antishock trousers (MAST) in awake sheep. *Crit Care Med*. 1993;21:1554–1561.

98. Crawford, ES. Ruptured abdominal aortic aneurysm [editorial]. *J Vasc Surg*. 1991;13:348–350.

99. Marino PL. Colloid and crystalloid resuscitation. In: *The ICU Book*. Malvern, Pa: Lea & Febiger; 1991: 205–216.

100. Mortelmans Y, Merckx E, van Nerom C, et al: Effect of an equal volume replacement with 500 cc 6% hydroxyethyl starch on the blood and plasma volume of healthy volunteers. *Eur J Anaesthesiol*. 1995;12:259–264.

101. Lucas CE, Denis R, Ledgerwood AM, et al. The effects of Hespan on serum and lymphatic albumin, globulin, and coagulant protein. *Ann Surg*. 1988;207:416–420.

102. Sanfelippo MJ, Suberviola PD, Geimer NF. Development of a von Willebrand–like syndrome after prolonged use of hydroxyethyl starch. *Am J Clin Path*. 1987;88:653–655.

103. Strauss RG. Review of the effects of hydroxyethyl starch on the blood coagulation system. *Transfusion*. 1981;21:299–302.

104. Dalrymple-Hay MB, Aitchison R, Collins P, et al. Hydroxyethyl starch-induced acquired Von Willebrand's disease. *Clin Lab Haematol*. 1992;14:209–211.

105. Macintyre E, Mackie IJ, Ho D, et al. The haemostatic effects of hydroxyethyl starch (HES) used as a volume expander. *Intensive Care Med*. 1985;11:300–303.

106. Falk. Choice of fluid in hemorrhagic shock. *Crit Care Clin*. 1992;330–338.

107. Shatney CH, Krishnapradad D, Militello PR, et al. Efficacy of hetastarch in the resuscitation of patients with multisystem trauma and shock. *Arch Surg.* 1983;118:804–809.

108. Ratner LE, Smith GW. Intraoperative fluid management. *Surg Clin North Am.* 1993;73:229–241.

109. Shands JW. Empiric antibiotic therapy of abdominal sepsis and serious perioperative infections. *Surg Clin North Am.* 1993;73:291–306.

110. The Medical Letter, Inc. *The Medical Letter Handbook of Antimicrobial Therapy.* New Rochelle, NY: The Medical Letter, Inc; 1994: 53.

111. Bowen TE, Bellamy RF, eds. *Emergency War Surgery NATO Handbook.* 2nd rev US ed. Washington, DC: Department of Defense, Government Printing Office; 1988: 175.

112. Ordog GJ, Sheppard GF, Wasserberger JS, et al. Infection in minor gunshot wounds. *J Trauma.* 1993;34:358–365.

113. Luz JA, DePauw JW, Gaydos JC, Hooper RR, Legters LJ. The role of military medicine in military civic action. *Mil Med.* 1993;158:362–366.

114. Blount BW, Krober MS, Gloyd SS, Kozakowski M, Casey L. Nutritional status of rural Bolivian children. *Mil Med.* 1993;158:367–370.

115. Geiger HJ, Cook-Deegan RM. The role of physicians in conflicts and humanitarian crises. *JAMA.* 1993;270:616–620.

116. Sharp TW, Yip R, Malone JD. US military forces and emergency international humanitarian assistance. *JAMA.* 1994;272;5:386–390.

117. US Naval Special Warfare Command. Special Operations Computer-Assisted Medical Reference System, Coronado, Calif: NAVSPECWARCOM; 1996.

118. Deuster P, Singh A, Pelletier P. *The Navy SEAL Nutrition Guide.* Bethesda, Md: Uniformed Services University of the Health Sciences; 1994.

119. Butler FK. Diving and hyperbaric ophthalmology. *Surv Ophthalmol.* 1995;39(5):347-366.

120. Naval Medical Research Institute. *Emergency Oxygen Decompression Procedures Using the NSW Dive Planner.* NAVSEA LTR, 8 June 1995.

RECOMMENDED READING

Commander of the Special Operations Command, Office of the Command Surgeon, et al. *Special Operations Forces Medical Handbook.* Jackson, Wyo: Teton NewMedia; 2001.

Committee on Trauma, American College of Surgeons. *Advanced Trauma Life Support Program for Physicians: Instructor Manual.* 5th ed. Chicago, Ill: American College of Surgeons; 1993.

Cummins RO. *Advanced Cardiac Life Support: ACLS Provider Manual.* Dallas, Tex: American Heart Association; 2001.

Department of the Navy. *General Medical Officer Manual.* Washington, DC: Bureau of Medicine and Surgery, DN; 2000. NAVMED P-5134. Available at http://www.vnh.org.

Stapleton ER, Aufderheide TP, Hazinski MF, Cummins RO, eds. *Basic Life Support for Healthcare Providers.* Dallas, Tex: American Heart Association; 2001.

US Department of the Navy. *US Navy Diving Manual.* SS521-Ag-PRO-010. Washington, DC: Naval Sea Systems Command. Rev 4 (20 Jan 1999); Change A (1 Mar 2001). NAVSEA 0994-LP-100-3199.

Chapter 38

ORGANIZATIONAL, PSYCHOLOGICAL, AND TRAINING ASPECTS OF SPECIAL OPERATIONS FORCES

WILLIAM KEITH PRUSACZYK, PhD[*]; AND GLENN M. GOLDBERG, PhD[†]

[*]Science and Technology Program Manager, Warfighter Protection, Future Naval Capability, Office of Naval Research, Arlington, Virginia 22217
[†]Commander, US Navy; Naval Special Warfare Development Group, Virginia Beach, Virginia 23461

INTRODUCTION

This overview of special operations provides an operational framework within which the reader may come to appreciate some of the differences between the conduct of special operations and of conventional warfare. The chapter also provides information about how the special operations combatant is selected and trained for service in the highly specialized units. Further, the chapter provides some insight into the operational stressors that these select individuals encounter during their training and real-world operations, including some of the physical risks, operational techniques, and modes of employment. More importantly for the medical community, it illustrates how the warfighters in special operations units, with the requisite independence from friendly support, make the demands on the Special Operations Forces (SOF) medical care providers unique in military medicine.

Members of SOF are often misunderstood—not only by the civilian community but also by others in the military. In the past, they often encountered the mistrust of conventional force commanders, who thought of SOF as difficult-to-control, trouble-causing renegades and rogues. In fact, during the planning phase (Operation Desert Shield) of the 1990/91 Persian Gulf War, leaders of the unified command were at first reluctant to fully employ the capabilities of the SOF units at their disposal. These misgivings were quickly dispelled by the decisive actions of the SOF units that performed the preliminary and initial operations of that 100-hour conflict.

The skilled combatants of SOF frequently carry out training and missions in great secrecy, adding to the mystery that surrounds them. Perhaps it is the image of highly unconventional warriors carrying out seemingly impossible operations, cloaked in secrecy, that propagates the aura. Still, the armed forces of nearly every country have units that are highly specialized, from Argentina's 601 and 602 Commando companies to Zimbabwe's Parachute brigade. These highly trained units carry out some of the most difficult missions required of military forces in service to their country.

There are, in fact, so many specialized military units that there is some disagreement on which should be properly called SOF. In the United States, for example, the Federal Bureau of Investigation's hostage rescue team and the Army's 82nd and 101st Airborne divisions could arguably be called SOF units. It is not the purpose of this chapter, however, to discuss the full range of SOF units operating in this country or in others around the world. This chapter focuses on organizations in the US military service that are undeniably SOF units. These include the Army Special Forces (SF, also known as the Green Berets) and Rangers, the Naval Special Warfare (NSW) Units (Sea-Air-Land [SEAL] teams and Special Boat Units), the Air Force Special Operations Forces (Pararescue [PJ] and Combat Controller teams), and the Marine Corps Marine Expeditionary Units (Special Operations Capable) [MEU(SOC)] and Surveillance, Reconnaissance, and Intelligence Group (SRIG) (including elements from Force Reconnaissance, Air Naval Gunfire Liaison Companies [ANGLICO], Communications, and support units).

The fundamental differences between SOF and conventional military operations are rooted not only in the way these operations are conducted but also in the reasons for which they are conducted. The Joint Chiefs of Staff's *Doctrine for Joint Special Operations* defines special operations "direct action" missions as those that are

> conducted by specially organized, trained, and equipped military and paramilitary forces to achieve military, political, economic, or psychological objectives by unconventional military means in hostile, denied, or politically sensitive areas.[1(Chap I, p1)]

These operations may be conducted during peacetime or wartime, but they

> differ from conventional operations in degree of physical and political risk, operational techniques, mode of employment, independence from friendly support, and dependence on detailed operational intelligence and indigenous assets.[1(Chap I, p1)]

Today, the US SOF are trained and deployed in support of theater combatant commands to ensure that the objectives of our national security policy are met in peacetime as well as wartime. As national security policies have evolved, and with a reduced potential for major multinational military conflicts, a greater emphasis has been placed on SOF peacekeeping actions. As a result, the various theater commands' requirements for SOF have expanded in the areas of peacekeeping and managing actions for low-intensity conflict. Today, about half of the US SOF are trained or deployed to meet potential warfighting requirements. The other half are conducting training to provide a forward presence in regions of the world where peace is considered key to US national interests.[2] One of the distinct advantages of conducting special operations lies in the flexibility with which the small units may be employed. This chapter describes some of the organizational and operational characteristics of SOF that allows them the required flexibility.

Interested readers may find useful the extensive list of publications related to the training and operations of US SOF at the end of this chapter (see Attachment).

THEORY AND ORGANIZATION OF SPECIAL OPERATIONS

Although in his classic treatise, *On War,* von Clausewitz[3] asserted that an army's most effective weapon is a superior number of combatants, modern unconventional forces conducting special operations depend on what Navy SEAL Commander William McRaven calls *"relative* superiority."[4(p4)] To achieve relative superiority, a numerically inferior force works rapidly to gain a decisive military advantage over what is often a well-defended, numerically superior force. The processes by which that small force gains relative superiority illustrate the differences between SOF and conventional forces in their tactics and modes of operation.

Six key principles are involved in achieving and, when required, maintaining relative superiority (Exhibit 38-1). These principles, which form the foundation for SOF unit military actions, are (1) simplicity, (2) speed, (3) repetition (or rehearsal) (Exhibit 38-2), (4) surprise, (5) security, and (6) specificity of purpose.[4(pp11–23)] The integration of these six principles, when properly executed, results in relative superiority favoring the small SOF unit. If, however, any of the six principles are compromised, the military advantage may shift rapidly to the opposing forces.

SOF have five primary missions: (1) direct action, (2) special reconnaissance, (3) unconventional warfare, (4) foreign internal defense, and (5) counterterrorism (Exhibit 38-3). Although these missions do not cover the full range of actions that SOF are prepared to conduct, they are common to SOF unit mission capabilities. (Also see Chapter 37, Medical Support of Special Operations, for a fuller discussion of the various missions.)

EXHIBIT 38-1

SIX PRINCIPLES BY WHICH SPECIAL OPERATIONS FORCES ACHIEVE AND MAINTAIN RELATIVE SUPERIORITY

---

1. *Simplicity* of action allows the small special operations forces (SOF) units to direct the limited manpower available in a small unit to a point where each unit member can focus on the action to be performed. This is in contrast to the operations of conventional forces that often depend on a complex series of actions with large numbers of combatants performing coordinated maneuvers. Simplicity reduces the number of contingencies on which an operation depends.

2. *Speed* permits the SOF unit to infiltrate an area that may be heavily defended by a larger force, perform the operation, and then exfiltrate before the enemy realizes the size of the attacking force and regroup for a counterattack. Speed and maneuverability are primary advantages small SOF units have over larger conventional forces.

3. *Rehearsal,* or practice, enables the SOF unit to capitalize on and effectively employ the principles of simplicity and speed. The more frequently an action is rehearsed, the more "reflexive" each operator's actions become. Sufficient rehearsal can turn even the most complex actions into a finely honed tactical skill.

4. *Surprise* is one of the SOF unit's most potent weapons. The small unit may achieve relative superiority rapidly only if there is an element of surprise for the enemy force. Without this surprise, the smaller SOF unit's actions can be severely, if not fatally, compromised.

5. *Security* is paramount to achieving the required element of surprise. SOF mission planning and rehearsal must be conducted in such a way that the enemy is completely unaware of the action to be undertaken. Any hope of attaining relative superiority disappears if security is breached.

6. *Specificity of purpose* allows the small unit to focus on a limited number of objectives. Attempting to achieve too many objectives in a single action compromises the element of surprise for later objectives in that mission, thereby placing the SOF unit, and the overall mission, at increased risk of failure.

United States Special Operations Command

By the mid 1980s, each service branch had established and was maintaining an independent SOF structure under that service's direct control. The lack of centralized command and control resulted in problems with several SOF missions conducted in the late 1970s and early 1980s. One such mission— in fact, *the* mission that prompted congressional and presidential action—was the ill-fated joint service attempt to rescue the American hostages held in Iran. As a result of these failures, the US Congress directed the president of the United States and the Department of Defense (DoD)[5] to establish a joint special operations command for the purpose of ensuring the combat readiness of the assigned SOF units. (Please see Chapter 37, Medical Support of Special Operations, for additional discussion.)

In response to the congressional mandate, DoD established the United States Special Operations Command (USSOCOM) in April 1987. The organization was established to provide a unified com-

---

EXHIBIT 38-2

ARCTIC OPERATIONS: A SEAL OUT OF WATER

I was a member of a SEAL squad that inserted into the wooded hills north of Fairbanks, Alaska. Our target, a simulated fuel depot, lay 4,000 m ahead, a distance that would normally have required only 6 hours of patrolling through the 3-foot base of wet snow to cover. The monotonous rolling hills offered no distinct landmarks for navigation. Disembarking the helicopter at the exact insertion point was critical, as all land navigation (pacing on compass bearings) would have to rely on this starting point. Unfortunately, the pilots set down several thousand meters north of the intended insertion point. Our squad set off in search of a target that wasn't there.

After 4 or 5 hours of humping and careful pacing, we calculated our position to be within 1,000 m of the target and decided to rest for the next hour until darkness fell. Most of the squad had anticipated that this direct action mission would require a maximum of 8 or 10 hours in the field and thus had packed light. Over the next hour, an inch and a half of heavy, wet snow fell and soaked our outer garments. A hasty decision was made to move on despite the fact that no one had eaten in the last 10 hours. The squad, although very fit, was now cold and hungry. With the flawed idea that the target was nearly in sight and the mission only an hour or two from completion, we pressed on. Little did we know that we were moving further and further away from the target and our extraction point. After another 2 hours, the paceman picked up the pace and we were 500 m beyond the expected target site. We believed that surely the target must be just over the next hill.

We now had been in the field for 10 hours and had not eaten for 12 hours. We were wet through and through, and fatigue and frustration were starting to take their toll. Our communications man, who was bearing a disproportionate amount of weight, looked the worst. After another hour of searching for the target, we determined we had been inserted in the wrong spot. Any hope of finding the target was soon lost.

Critical mistakes had been made all along, but now it seemed that all reason was lost. Despite protests from the corpsman to bivouac, hydrate, and take on sustenance, the squad leader immediately decided to return to the insertion point, where the Chinook helicopter would pick us up. After an hour of retracing our steps, the radioman became ataxic and collapsed with hypothermia. Fortunately, our corpsman had a clear enough mind to recognize the potential for disaster and directed the squad to erect a tent. He placed the injured squad member in a dry sleeping bag with another alert squad member. By the time a casualty evacuation (CASEVAC) helicopter arrived (within 1 h), there were three more casualties with cold injuries. All three were extracted and then CASEVACed via jungle penetrator (ie, a forest canopy penetrator). They were treated and returned to full duty within 24 hours.

The mistakes made by the squad are obvious but, unfortunately, far too common. Severe climates are never forgiving, and disregard for basic hydration and caloric needs almost always results in senseless injury or death.

Prepared especially for this textbook by Lieutenant Commander Kevin Walters, MC, USN, a SEAL who is currently assigned to the medical department of the Naval Special Warfare Center, Coronado, California. After many years as a Naval Special Warfare operator, Lieutenant Commander Walters obtained his medical degree from the Uniformed Services University of the Health Sciences, Bethesda, Maryland.

mand structure responsible for triservice SOF operations. At that time, USSOCOM inherited most of its force structure from existing SOF units in the three services. Between 1988 and 1994 USSOCOM's organic assets increased while DoD's overall personnel and funding levels were decreasing. This uneven distribution reflected the changing needs of national security in response to our dynamic global defense requirements.

At the time that USSOCOM was established, the Marine Corps elected not to participate in the organizational structure. Instead, the Corps chose to maintain an autonomous special operations capability. Marine Expeditionary Units (Special Operations Capable) (MEU-SOC) and Surveillance, Reconnaissance, and Intelligence Group (SRIG) both use personnel from the Marine Corps's own highly skilled Force Reconnaissance, Air Naval Gunfire Liaison Company (ANGLICO) and support units. To ensure coordination for joint operations, however, the Marine Corps maintains a detachment at USSOCOM.

USSOCOM is headquartered at MacDill Air Force Base, Florida. Its mission is to provide command and control and to establish training requirements for all SOF units under its command. It provides SOF manpower ready for rapid deployment in support of the other eight unified commands. To accomplish this task, USSOCOM is directly responsible for developing doctrine, tactics, techniques and procedures; conducting specialized instruction; ensuring interoperability of equipment and forces; and developing or acquiring equipment or conducting research to address unique SOF needs. The latter is accomplished through the Special Operations Center, which is also located at MacDill Air Force Base, Florida.

The major subordinate commands of USSOCOM include the Joint Special Operations Command and the special operations commands of the Army, Air Force, and Navy. The special operations of the Marine Corps is separate from the USSOCOM.

Joint Special Operations Command

The Joint Special Operations Command (JSOC), Fort Bragg, North Carolina, is responsible for analyzing joint special operations requirements and techniques, developing plans for training and exercises, and for establishing tactics.

EXHIBIT 38-3

FIVE PRIMARY MISSIONS OF SPECIAL OPERATIONS FORCES

1. *Direct action* (DA) missions are typically of short duration and limited scope, involving overt or covert operations. The purpose of DA is to capture, disable, or destroy enemy assets or personnel considered of strategic importance. The goals are achieved through the use of raids, ambushes, or direct assaults on targets in hostile or denied territory. DA may be used in support of conventional forces by providing targeting for precision munitions, deception operations, or mine emplacement.

2. *Special reconnaissance* (SR) missions are conducted to provide local or theater commanders with information critical to operational objectives. The actions provide direct information on enemy strength and location, terrain features, weather, hydrography, or other information needed by commanders. These missions can also provide direct verification of information provided by other intelligence sources, or provide postaction information on the effectiveness of conventional assaults.

3. *Unconventional warfare* (UW) is probably the mission most commonly associated with the actions of special operations forces (SOF). These missions include a wide variety of military and paramilitary activities and are typically conducted covertly or clandestinely. The actions taken to accomplish the missions may include guerilla warfare, including long-duration activities. They are frequently conducted by indigenous forces that are trained, equipped, and supported by SOF.

4. *Foreign internal defense* (FID) missions are conducted by SOF to provide training and assistance to friendly indigenous forces or developing host nations. This assistance can take the form of technical assistance to military or civil forces; humanitarian aid; and the fostering of internal economic, political, or social stability.

5. *Counterterrorism* (CT) missions have become increasingly visible to the public with the increase in international terrorism. The actions are offensive in nature and are designed to prevent or react to incidents of terrorism. These activities are most frequently directed and performed by the specialized units in the SOF community.

US Army Special Operations Command

The US Army Special Operations Command (USASOC), also located at Fort Bragg, has primary responsibility for the United States–based Army SOF commands, both active and reserve. The Army SOF units include Special Forces (SF, also known as the Green Berets), Rangers, Special Operations Aviation Regiment (Airborne) (SOAR), Psychological Operations (PSYOP), and Civil Affairs (CA). In addition, the command is responsible for select special mission and support units assigned to it by the secretary of defense. USASOC currently has about 30,000 active and reserve personnel in the command.

Special Forces. Army SF units are organized into seven groups. Of these, five are active duty and two are National Guard groups (Table 38-1). Each group is responsible for operations conducted in a different region of the world.

The groups are organized, trained, and equipped to conduct the five primary special operations missions (see Exhibit 38-3). In addition, SF soldiers train, advise, and assist host nation military or paramilitary forces. In addition to the five primary missions, SF soldiers engage in Coalition Warfare/Support (CWS) and Humanitarian and Civic Action (HCA). These additional tasks take full advantage of the language skills and cultural training that are a hallmark of SF training. There are currently about 6,000 active duty SF soldiers, with another 2,000 in the National Guard units.

Special Operations Aviation Regiment (Airborne). The 160th SOAR is organized into one active duty regiment comprised of three battalions, with a detachment in Panama and one National Guard battalion. The 1st and 2nd battalions are headquartered at Fort Campbell, Kentucky, and the 3rd battalion at Hunter Army Airfield, Georgia. SOAR units act as a dedicated specialty force for aviation support of other SOF units. The units' missions include offensive attack, insertion, extraction, and resupply of SOF personnel. They also provide aerial security, medical evacuation, electronic warfare, mine dispersal, and command and control support.

Psychological Operations. Army PSYOP forces are organized into one active duty and three reserve groups. Their mission is to examine, evaluate, and prepare strategies designed to influence the attitudes and behaviors of the civilian and military personnel of foreign populations. They operate with conventional forces and other SOF, both foreign and domestic, to advise and assist host nations in support of special operations missions. The size of the PSYOP groups varies in personnel number and in the type of subordinate units, based on the mission requirements.

Civil Affairs. CA consists of 1 active duty battalion; 5 reserve headquarters, comprised of 3 commands and 9 brigades; and 24 reserve battalions. The units function principally to foster favorable relationships between foreign governments and populations and the US military in those countries. CA also assists ongoing military operations in those countries by conducting population and refugee assistance and providing support to other US agencies in the area. The CA reserve units provide professional civilian skills unavailable in the active duty unit, engineering, law enforcement, magisterial, and other civil functions.

Battalion Support Company. The battalion provides intelligence, combat service, and signal support to the forward-deployed SF teams. The intelligence detachment may deploy teams with the operational A-Teams of the SF (discussed below in the Special Operations Tactical Units section) to provide intelligence and electronic warfare support. The service detachment provides unit-level supply and maintenance services for the battalion. A signal detachment provides communications between the forward operating base and the operating detachment. There is also a medical section to provide support to the forward operating base.

TABLE 38-1

US ARMY SPECIAL FORCES GROUPS (AIRBORNE)

Group	Home Base	Area of Operations
1st SFG(A)[*]	Ft Lewis, Wash	Pacific and eastern Asia
3rd SFG(A)[*]	Ft Bragg, NC	Western Africa and Caribbean
5th SFG(A)[*]	Ft Campbell, Ky	Southwest Asia and northeast Africa
7th SFG(A)[*]	Ft Bragg, NC	Central and South America
10th SFG(A)[*]	Ft Carson, Colo	Europe and western Asia
19th SFG(A)[†]	Camp Williams, Utah	Asia
20th SFG(A)[†]	Birmingham, Ala	Europe and western Asia

[*]active duty
[†]National Guard

Rangers. The Rangers are organized into a single regiment, the 75th Ranger Regiment, comprising a headquarters company and three operational battalions, with a total of approximately 1,600 qualified soldiers. At present, there are no reserve Ranger units. The Rangers are organized and trained to perform as rapidly deployable, airborne, light infantry units. The units are organized, trained, and equipped to conduct joint strike operations; however, when needed, they can operate as light infantry, supporting conventional forces during operations.

US Air Force Special Operations Command

The US Air Force Special Operations Command (AFSOC), Hurlburt Field, Florida, has one Special Operations Wing, two Special Operations Groups, and one Special Tactics Group in its active duty force. There are also one Special Operations Wing and one Special Operations Group as AFSOC reserve components. The command has approximately 9,500 reserve and active duty personnel (Table 38-2).

The command's primary missions are to organize, train, and equip its units, but it may also train, assist, and advise the air forces of other nations in support of foreign internal defense missions. The command operates uniquely equipped fixed- and rotary-wing aircraft for missions that include inserting, extracting, and resupplying SOF personnel;

TABLE 38-2

AIR FORCE SPECIAL OPERATIONS COMMANDS AND ACTIVITIES

Major Command and Headquarters	Region of Responsibility	Component Squadrons	Craft/Activity
16th Special Operations Wing, Hurlburt Field, Fla	North America, South America, the Middle East, and Northeast Africa	4th Special Operations Squadron (SOS)	AC-130U Spectre gunship
		6th SOS	FID
		8th SOS	
		9th SOS	HC-130P/N Combat Shadow
		15th SOS	MC-130 Combat Talon II
		16th SOS	AC-130H Spectre gunship
		20th SOS	MH-53J Pave Low III
		55th SOS	MH-60G Pave Hawk
352nd Special Operations Group, Royal Air Force Mildenhall, United Kingdom	Africa and Europe (including much of the territory of the former USSR)	7th SOS	MC-130H Combat Talon II
		21st SOS	MH-53J Pave Low III
		67th SOS	HC-130P/N Combat Shadow
		321st Special Tactics Squadron (STS)	Combat Controller Team (CCT) and Pararescue (PJ)
353rd Special Operations Group, Kadena AFB, Japan	Southeast Asia, Australia, and the Pacific Islands	1st SOS	MC-130H Combat Talon II
		17th SOS	HC-130P/N Combat Shadow
		31st SOS	MH-53J Pave Low
		320th STS	CCT and PJ
720th Special Tactics Group, Hurlburt Field, Fla	N/A	21st STS	CCT and PJ
		22nd STS	
		23rd STS	
		24th STS	
58th Special Operations Wing, Kirtland AFB, NM	N/A	N/A	CCT and PJ

aerial fire support; refueling; and psychological operations. Its aircraft are capable of operating in hostile airspace, at low altitudes, under cover of darkness, and in adverse weather conditions in collaboration with Army and Navy SOF. Specially trained personnel in AFSOC operating primarily on the ground include the Combat Controller Teams and the Pararescue (PJ). The command also includes a Tactical Air Control Party SOF and the Special Operations Weather Team.

AFSOC specialized aircraft and capabilities include the fixed-wing AC-130U and AC-130H Spectre gunships, the HC-130P/N Combat Shadow, and the MC-130E Combat Talon II. The AC-130U and AC-130H Spectre gunships are specially modified C-130 airframes used to provide all-weather close air support of SOF missions, reconnaissance, and aerial interdiction. The HC-130P/N is a tanker that can provide worldwide capability for the other airships in the inventory. In addition to aerial refueling of the MH-53J and the MH-60G, the HC-130P/N can resupply SOF through airdrops. The MC-130E Combat Talon II is used to provide support for unconventional warfare and other SOF missions.

The rotary-winged aircraft at AFSOC disposal include the MH-53J Pave Low II and the MH-60G Pave Hawk. These aircraft are capable of all-weather, day or night, low-level penetration, and are used for infiltration and exfiltration, resupply, and fire support for SOF on the ground. In addition, the Pave Hawk adds long-range capability, making it useful for combat rescue.

Naval Special Warfare Command

The Naval Special Warfare Command (NAVSPECWARCOM), Coronado, California, consists of two Naval Special Warfare (NSW) Groups, one located in Coronado (NSWG-One) and one in Little Creek, Virginia (NSWG-Two). There are two Special Boat Squadrons collocated with the NSW Groups. Each group is composed of three SEAL teams, one SEAL Delivery Vehicle (SDV) team, and supporting special warfare units. Each Special Boat Squadron includes subordinate Special Boat Units (SBU). SBU-12 (Coronado, Calif) is under the command of Special Boat Squadron One in Coronado, while SBU-20 (Little Creek, Va), SBU-22 (New Orleans, La), and SBU-26 (Panama) fall under Special Boat Squadron Two, Little Creek. NSW forces deployed outside the continental United States receive forward support from permanent NSW units located in Guam; Stuttgart, Germany; Rota, Spain; Puerto Rico; and Panama. NAVSPECWARCOM has

a manning status of about 5,500 active duty and reserve personnel.

The six active duty SEAL teams are organized into headquarters elements and ten 12- to 16-man operational platoons. Navy SEALs are organized, trained, and equipped to conduct the five primary SOF missions. Although maritime and riverine operations are undisputedly the SEALs' specialty, they are fully capable of operating in terrestrial and aerial operations. SEALs may also be used to provide direct support during conventional Navy and Marine Corps maritime operations. Each team has a world region of responsibility for SOF actions (Table 38-3).

Marine Corps

Marine Expeditionary Unit (Special Operations Capable)

While not falling within the command structure of USSOCOM, a Marine Expeditionary Unit (Special Operations Capable) [MEU(SOC)] has many of the same missions as the SOF units; hence, we will describe them here. A MEU is composed of a Marine Battalion Ground Combat Element (GCE), an Aviation Combat Element (ACE), and a MEU Service Support Group (MSSG). The ground force is an artillery-reinforced infantry battalion including light armor and amphibious assault vehicles forming a battalion landing team (BLT). Among the BLTs is a Force Reconnaissance (Force Recon) platoon.

TABLE 38-3

US NAVY SEAL TEAMS: HOME BASE AND REGION OF RESPONSIBILITY

Unit	Home Base	Region of Responsibility
Naval Special Warfare Group One		
SEAL Team 1	Coronado, Calif	Southeast Asia
SEAL Team 3	Coronado, Calif	Middle East
SEAL Team 5	Coronado, Calif	Pacific Rim, Asia
Naval Special Warfare Group Two		
SEAL Team 2	Little Creek, Va	Northern Europe
SEAL Team 4	Little Creek, Va	South America
SEAL Team 8	Little Creek, Va	Africa

The aviation element is an augmented Marine Medium Helicopter Squadron. Additional rotary-winged aircraft include the CH-53E Super Stallion, CH-46E Sea Knight, UH-1N Huey, and AH-1W Super Cobra. The aviation element also may include fixed-wing aircraft for mission support. Notable among the fixed-wing craft is the AV-8B Harrier, or jump jet, and the KC-130 transport plane. The MSSG maintains, among other capabilities, logistics, maintenance, engineering, and medical services. A command element provides command and control for the three other elements of the MEU(SOC).

The MEU is unique to Marine Corps operations, in that the ACE and GCE are combined with the MSSG under a single commander. The flexibility of a combined air/ground task force provides the ability to organize rapidly for operations under a wide variety of combat situations. Having the MSSG providing the sustenance and support capability with the combat battalion means that the MEU(SOC) can accomplish its mission rapidly, setting the stage for any follow-on elements. To achieve the SOC status, a unit must successfully complete and demonstrate excellence in a rigorous evaluation process with field capability demonstrations. Prior to deployment, a MEU conducts training in 29 areas ranging from humanitarian assistance to the traditional techniques of amphibious warfare. The MEU(SOC) receives further training in special operations missions.

There are currently seven MEU(SOC)s; the 11th, 13th, and 15th are based at Camp Pendelton, California; the 22nd, 24th, and 26th at Camp Lejeune, North Carolina; and the 31st at Okinawa, Japan. A typical MEU(SOC) has a complement of approximately 2,100 Marines and sailors. Of the overall force, the Command Element is manned by 250 Marines and Sailors, the GCE by 1,150, the ACE by 450, and the CSSE by 250.

Surveillance, Reconnaissance, and Intelligence Group

Within the Marine Expeditionary Force (MEF), the major service components are Ground Combat Element (GCE), Air Combat Element (ACE), Combat Service Support Element (CSSE), and a Surveillance, Reconnaissance, and Intelligence Group (SRIG). As does the MEU(SOC), a SRIG contains elements from specialized Marine Corps units. SRIG Headquarters directs the action of personnel from a Force Reconnaissance Company, an Air Naval Gunfire Liaison Company (ANGLICO), an Intelligence Company, a Communications Company, and a Headquarters and Service Company. These elements are brought together and trained prior to deployment. The Fleet Marine Forces formed the SRIGs to bring together under one commander the resources necessary to meet the operational and tactical commander's needs. This action facilitated the integration of command and control, communications, computing, and intelligence (C4I) resources at the tactical level.

PSYCHOLOGICAL ASSESSMENT OF SPECIAL OPERATIONS GROUPS

There are numerous reasons to utilize psychological methods to assess personnel applying to work in special operations units. By definition, such personnel will be tasked to do things that require not only great physical ability and highly specialized skill but also the personality qualities that allow them to effectively utilize these skills in stressful situations. While physical stressors are generally accepted, intense psychological stressors, which are not necessarily either widely understood or accepted, nonetheless also exist. Special operations personnel may be expected to spend extended periods performing important missions in harsh and hostile environments that may quickly change, and that may present unprecedented challenges. Furthermore, while in such an environment the operators (ie, individual members of SOF) must generally apply their skills at a superior level of performance in order to succeed or even survive. Under such circumstances, psychological and interpersonal factors may become as important as one's physical abilities or technical expertise.

Methods of assessing the psychological status of special operations personnel were developed initially in the United States during World War II when it became apparent such a need existed. Although the methods have been improved on over the years, the challenge of predicting an individual's "real-world" performance remains.

Psychological assessment methods attempt to provide unique data not readily obtainable through other methods. However, psychological assessment is but one component of an overall screening and selection process and must always be viewed within the context of other available information. Although the challenges of using psychological assessment techniques for selection are many, so are the benefits. For if such methods are used to help select personnel best suited for special operations roles, an organization may have a better chance of succeeding in carrying out high stake/high risk missions with a reduction in potential liabilities. In the words of Sun Tzu, a Chinese general and military theorist who lived about 500 BC,

> He who knows the enemy and himself will never in a hundred battles be at risk; ... He who knows neither the enemy nor himself will be at risk in every battle.[6]

Historical Beginnings of US Special Operations Selection

Although psychological assessment methods were being implemented as early as World War I in an effort to reduce battlefield psychiatric casualties, the first US organization to utilize psychological assessment methods for the selection of special operations personnel was the Office of Strategic Services, or OSS.[7] The OSS was a World War II wartime agency that was unlike any other in United States history.[8] It was created in 1941 to conduct various forms of unconventional warfare such as intelligence collection, espionage, subversion, and psychological warfare.[7] Because its purposes were so varied, agents selected into the OSS could be expected to perform a wide range of roles, often under dangerous circumstances. For example, whereas one function was to establish intelligence-gathering networks in the US and abroad, another function involved carrying out destructive missions in enemy-occupied territory and working with the underground. Most of these activities were quite novel for the OSS agents being recruited. For some assignments it was difficult even to know the job description in advance, or what the situation was like prior to arrival at an assignment, which might be at a remote overseas location. Not surprisingly, many agents experienced significant difficulty in adapting to such high levels of stress.

Along with reports from the field expressing concern over the quality of individuals selected for difficult missions, Medical Branch records of the OSS indicate that 52 acute psychiatric casualties among the personnel who should be removed from duty. This figure represents approximately 0.29% of the total (all of whom were nonassessed) OSS personnel.[8] This finding led to the decision in 1943 to develop assessment procedures that included a significant psychological component, so as to improve the chances of selecting agents who would be better suited to endure the extreme stress of their assignments.

About the same time, an OSS official who had visited the War Office Selection Board in Great Brit-

ain reported that a British psychological–psychiatric assessment unit was successfully screening British officer candidates, and a recommendation was made to develop a similar OSS unit.[7] The screening program implemented by the OSS did in fact seem to be useful. At one assessment location (Station S), of a total of 2,373 people evaluated, only two (0.04%) developed emotional problems severe enough to warrant removal from duty.[8] The results are even more impressive when we consider that, of the two individuals, one was not recommended for OSS service by the screening staff but was selected anyway; and the other was recommended under the condition that he be closely watched and used only if concerns expressed by the assessment staff seemed unjustified. Although at a second screening site (Area W) the percentage of candidates assessed who developed significant emotional problems (0.20%) was higher than that obtained at Station S, the percentage obtained at Area W is still lower than the overall 0.26% for the OSS.

Although psychological screening methods were being utilized by the US in World War I and fairly extensively in Germany prior to World War II, the methods used by the OSS represent the first US attempt to systematically screen special operations personnel. While not perfect, the assessment techniques used by the OSS were an ambitious and fairly successful effort to utilize scientific psychological research methods for the purposes of systematic evaluation; they are the precursors to many psychological assessment procedures currently used in special operations assessment and selection.

Goals of Psychological Assessment for Personnel Selection

As noted above, psychological assessment is but one component of a special operations selection process that draws from numerous data sources. In this regard, the psychologist is in the role of a consultant rather than a decision maker. The final decisions regarding selection of SOF personnel are almost always made by senior special operations personnel.

While it is true that methods of psychological assessment often can provide valuable information to assist in making a decision about selection, psychological assessment alone cannot begin to provide all of the information necessary. For example, although psychological assessment may indicate that certain Special Forces applicants are intelligent and highly tolerant of stress, it cannot indicate if they have the physical capabilities or technical aptitude to meet the required standards. Conversely, even though psychological assessment may raise concerns about an individual, there may be a "real life" record of superior performance that outweighs such concerns.

On the other hand, psychological assessment can often provide the type of information that can help to predict the performance of special operations candidates (eg, their level of flexibility in adapting to changing or unexpected challenges, their ability to manage sensitive interpersonal situations). Similarly, such an assessment can help determine how responsibly and maturely the candidates live their personal lives, a consideration that may have direct relevance to professional reliability.

In that the information obtained through psychological assessment methods must be viewed in conjunction with other available sources of data (eg, performance history, supervisor and peer recommendations, technical expertise), the assessment should provide unique data (eg, personality and interpersonal strengths and/or weaknesses) that are not readily available through other sources and that can assist in the selection process. For example, whereas review of an applicant's service record or observation of a candidate performing a task may reveal certain abilities, or lack of abilities, psychological testing and interviewing can reveal personality traits, work values, and interpersonal qualities that may influence an applicant's performance in general, and yet be difficult to discern through other methods without long-term contact with that individual. Once obtained, the information can be compared with other sources of information to help round out a selection team's knowledge of an applicant. Furthermore, because psychological assessment methods can often be conducted in group settings and are neither expensive nor time consuming, they can provide such information in a cost- and time-efficient manner.

In terms of the goals of psychological assessment for personnel selection, a basic distinction is made between "screening-out" versus "screening-in." Screening-out has been described as the process of weeding out applicants who cannot meet the minimum standards for the job,[9] especially when the applicant pool may be large and the processing costs are high.[10] In contrast, the objective of screening-in is to identify the most desirable applicants based on the qualities, abilities, or both, believed to be related to successful performance.[9]

From a special operations perspective, the goal of screening-out is to identify individuals who have an extremely low likelihood of successfully com-

pleting a selection program. This is done by assessing the variables that are associated with performance or adjustment problems. If identified early in the selection process, a decision may be made not to have such individuals participate in the more costly and risky aspects of a special operations selection program. From a psychological assessment perspective, some common criteria for screening-out include evidence of significant character pathology, emotional problems, poor interpersonal skills, low stress tolerance, and limited intelligence.

Screening-in, on the other hand, attempts to identify the characteristics that are associated with successful performance and adjustment. This approach can be used to identify applicants who not only have a higher probability of passing a selection program but who also possess qualities that are valued in special operations personnel. In addition, a screening-in approach can be used to identify individuals who have the characteristics or abilities that are associated with better performance at specific types of tasks. This is not, however, an attempt to identify a specific profile for the "perfect" candidate. There is no ideal special operations profile, and variety among personnel allows for individual strengths to emerge. Furthermore, heterogeneity among personnel often leads to creative improvements in how things are done.

From a practical standpoint, it is usually much easier to identify characteristics that will predict problems than it is to determine the "perfect model soldier,"[7] especially when no measure of attributes can account for all of the variance in job performance.[9] Furthermore, it is impossible to determine in advance exactly what type of performance will be required in a situation, or what other variables may influence the outcome. In reality, both screening-in and screening-out methods may be used together, along with other components of the assessment and selection process.

Challenges of Psychological Assessment for Selection

The challenges of accurate psychological assessment for SOF personnel selection are many. Basically, an attempt is being made to identify qualities that can predict future performance. This presents an immense challenge, considering that we are dealing with a multitude of fluid and unpredictable variables. Although psychological assessment methods can provide accurate information about a person, they cannot predict with complete accuracy how an individual will respond or perform in every type of situation. An individual may perform differently depending on his or her physical or emotional state, or on the type of information or perception held about their situation at the moment in which he or she must perform. Clearly, these are variables that are difficult to control for during an assessment.

In addition, we can never underestimate the situational component that personnel face. Personnel assessed in one context may be required to perform in a completely different—and alien—situation. This may involve not only environmental changes (eg, climate, geography, threat of harm) but also social, cultural and language, and consequential differences between the setting in which they were assessed and that in which they must act.

Finally, even comprehensive psychological assessment methods can provide but a sampling (albeit an important one) of the whole individual. Although psychological testing can reveal much information, it certainly cannot tell us everything about an individual, or how that individual will act in every type of situation. Even when psychological assessment methods are linked to performance criteria in a selection or training program, there is never a perfect correlation between psychological information and performance. Even if such an amazing feat were possible, it would still be impossible to assess an individual's response to every type of challenge. Despite these challenges—or perhaps because of them—special operations assessment methods have continued to evolve and improve in their efforts to identify the factors that are most likely to influence performance in a variety of situations.

One of the basic challenges in an assessment program is knowing what to assess, or, to state it differently, what are we attempting to screen-out or screen-in? Certainly one source of guidance for this is experienced special operations personnel, who have a fairly clear idea of what they are looking for in an applicant. Consider the following portion of a memorandum written by a Navy SEAL in a leadership position following a discussion on personnel screening with the author:

> The personal traits we want are HONESTY, seeks CHALLENGES, will take calculated RISKS (RISK/ OPPORTUNITY are different sides of the same coin). I'll pay lip service to COURAGE because I think that quality exists in all the guys. We don't want guys who have large mood swings (combative) when they drink. Extreme introverts don't fit in well, nor do men that place blame on other factors and won't accept responsibility for their shortcomings. We don't want guys that have endless excuses for problems. Guys that are extremely "anal retentive" and value order above all else do not seem to do well either, because they have a hard time dealing with disorder and chaos.

(Later, the writer of the memorandum also emphasized the need for a sense of humor.)

While not the results of a scientific study, these comments are based on the memorandum writer's years of personal experience in special operations, and although additional qualities may be added to these, it is doubtful that anyone in the field of special operations would disagree with any of those given. In fact, these comments are consistent with the findings of an empirical study[11] that examined the personality traits of SEALs. This study compared the personality traits of SEALs with non-SEAL adult males, and found that SEALs score higher on measures of excitement-seeking behavior, assertiveness, activity interests, openness, and conscientiousness, and lower on measures of emotional vulnerability and depression. Consider the comments in the memorandum excerpt with those of the study's authors, who describe typical Navy SEALs as

> calm, hardy, secure, and not prone to excessive psychological stress ... rarely impulsive ... prefer being in large groups ... seek excitement and stimulation and prefer complex and dangerous environments ... very reliable.[11(p13)]

Extensive research conducted with Army SOF focused on the qualities of their personnel and determined which qualities are more likely to lead to success (Exhibit 38-4).[12] This research, like the Navy's, certainly dispels any stereotypes of special operations personnel as "crazy commandos" and instead conveys the impression of highly trained professionals. Several methods are used that allow for the assessment of qualities associated with success in special operations. To begin with, a "mission analysis" may be carried out to determine what the requirements of a mission are likely to be.[12] As pointed out by the OSS assessment staff, a lack of knowledge concerning job requirements was one of the chief causes of prediction error concerning those personnel screened.[8]

Following that, personnel attributes associated with mission success must be identified,[12] quite often through the use of psychological tests or self-report questionnaires. Conversely, attributes and abilities that predict failure at training tasks and challenges similar to those likely to be encountered in a real-world special operations environment must also be identified. Some of this information is

---

EXHIBIT 38-4

DESIRABLE PSYCHOLOGICAL QUALITIES FOR SUCCESS IN US ARMY SPECIAL OPERATIONS FORCES

- Organizational skills

- Trainability

- Situational awareness

- Ability to make complex discriminations and decisions

- Personal adaptability

- Resistance to stress

- Dependability, determination, and stability

- Physical endurance and specialized military skills

---

available through an applicant's service record (eg, the Armed Forces Vocational Aptitude Battery and physical readiness scores).

Psychological information is generally obtained by administering tests and questionnaires to applicants prior to entering a selection or training program, and then later analyzing these data statistically to identify the qualities that are associated with success or failure. For example, one study[13] examining psychological factors associated with passing Basic Underwater Demolition/SEALS (BUD/S) training discovered several differences between those trainees who complete training and those who drop out. Those who completed BUD/S scored higher on measures of self-perception of athletic and physical abilities, as well as measures of self-esteem/confidence and lack of anxiety, cordiality/even-temperedness, a disposition toward being helpful and courteous, and leadership ability, including planning and decision making skills. Similarly, preliminary findings from a study[14] in progress on BUD/S trainees suggest that trainees with even suggestive evidence of psychopathology or stress vulnerability on psychological testing are much more likely to fail training, as are those who report a significant history of family dysfunction.

The use of instruments such as psychological tests has been termed the "elementalistic" approach, whereas an "organismic" approach assesses performance on training challenges designed to simulate those likely to be encountered in special operations missions. In reality, these two approaches are often combined today, just as they were by the OSS assessment staff.[8,15] Possible strengths or weaknesses identified through testing can be watched for while applicants confront performance challenges.

The final component of the selection process generally entails some type of selection board that considers all of the available information. As noted above, the final decision regarding selection is made by experienced SOF personnel. Research with Army SOF has shown that such a process results in the selection of personnel who have a high probability of success, including a 95% rate of success in training following selection and a 99% success rate during operational assignments.[12]

SPECIAL OPERATIONS RECRUIT TRAINING

SOF missions require the operators to be in peak physical condition as well as to be tactically and technically skilled. Studies of Army and Navy SOF show that the operators are highly aerobically fit, with peak oxygen uptakes of 53 ± 4 mL/kg/min for Army SF[16] and approximately 59 ± 5 mL/min for Navy SEALs.[17,18] Those in training to become SEALs are even more aerobically fit than are the operators; Beckett, Goforth, and Hodgdon[17] reported a peak aerobic capacity of 62 ± 4 mL/kg/ for recent graduates from the Navy's BUD/S training.

US Army Special Operations Forces

The US Army SOF comprise five main organizational units. (1) Army *Special Forces* plan, prepare for, and when directed, deploy to conduct unconventional warfare, foreign internal defense, special reconnaissance, and direct actions in support of US national policy objectives within designated areas of responsibility. (2) *Rangers* are the special light infantry units for conducting special operations. The missions include attacks to temporarily seize and secure key objectives. Like their Special Forces counterparts, Rangers infiltrate an area by land, sea, or air. (3) The *160th Special Operations Aviation Regiment* is a unique unit providing support to SOF worldwide. The capabilities of the aviation units include inserting, resupplying, and extracting US and Allied SOF personnel. They also assist in SOF search and rescue, and they provide airborne command and control and fire support. (4) *Psychological Operations* disseminates information in support of US goals and objectives. (5) *Civil Affairs* units prevent civilian interference with tactical operations, assist commanders in discharging their responsibilities toward the civilian population, providing liaison with civilian governments and nongovernmental organizations.

Special Forces

Training for Special Forces consists of two courses: the first deals with assessment and selection, the second with qualification. Each course is subdivided into several phases.

Special Forces Assessment and Selection (SFAS) Course. The purpose of the 3-week SFAS course is to identify soldiers (E-4 and above) who have the potential for completing SF training. The SFAS course consists of two distinct phases. During the first phase, instructors assess the soldiers' overall physical fitness and motivation. Perhaps more importantly, this phase gives the instructors an opportunity to evaluate the individual soldier's ability to cope with stresses imposed on them during the assessment activities.

In this first phase, soldiers will undergo psychological tests as well as tests of physical fitness, swimming ability, run and march times, and orienteering. Following completion of this phase, an evaluation board, with input from the instructors, determines which candidates are qualified to continue into the second phase.

The second phase of SFAS emphasizes individual leadership ability and the ability to work as part of an operational team. At the end of the 3 weeks, on completion of this phase, a board meets to evaluate the soldier's performance. Here soldiers are selected or deselected for continuation in training.

Special Forces Qualification Course (SFQC). SFQC is composed of Individual Skills, Military Occupational Specialty (MOS) Training, and a Collective Training phase. The course ranges in duration from 24 to 55 weeks, depending on the candidates' MOS. Individual Skills are taught over the 40-day course conducted at Fort Bragg. Training includes small-unit patrolling tactics and land navigation.

For the MOS Training portion of the SFQC, each soldier engages in specialty training based on the individual's aptitude and (occasionally) aspirations. MOS Training is 24 weeks for Detachment Commander (18A), Weapons Sergeant (18B), and Engineer Sergeant (18C). The Communications Sergeant (18E) course is 32 weeks; and the Medical Sergeant (18D) course is 57 weeks, during which the medics receive instruction in many advanced medical procedures.

Training culminates with a 38-day deployment to the Nicholas Rowe Special Forces Training Center near Fort Bragg. During this period, students are trained in air operations and unconventional warfare techniques. There, the SF candidates engage in the Robin Sage Field Training Exercise, wherein each candidate demonstrates his military skills as a member of an A-Team. The first 5 days are spent with the A-Team in isolation, at which time the teams plan their operation. On day 6, the students make an airborne insertion into a fictitious country, link up with other detachments, and begin execution of the operation. The instructors place the students in realistic situations where each will be allowed to demonstrate his skills and abilities. Those who successfully complete the exercise will receive the coveted Green Beret of the Army SF soldier.

Special Operations Aviation Regiment

Only the best-qualified Army aviators are selected for the 160th SOAR. All soldiers selected for the SOAR, commissioned officers and enlisted, attend the Basic Mission Qualifications course. The Officers Qualification course is 14 weeks long, whereas the Enlisted Qualification Course is just 3 weeks. After the qualification courses, SOAR personnel can achieve two other levels of qualification. The Fully Mission Qualified level is 12 to 18 months, and the Flight Lead qualification requires 36 to 48 months of additional training. The high level of training of SOAR aviators is required, given the mission requirements of the SOF operations in which they engage.

Ranger

The Ranger course is 65 days in length and is designed to provide the Ranger candidate with tough, realistic training. During the course, training averages 19.5 hours per day, 7 days per week, with a minimum of classroom instruction. Training is divided into three phases, each conducted at a different location. During the three phases, students are under the constant stress of nearly continuous operations, physical demands, mental challenges, and restricted dietary intake. The course is designed to force each candidate to physical, mental, and emotional limits. The course can take a substantial physical toll on the candidates.[19] In all phases, leadership is stressed and any candidate may be called on to become a small-unit leader at any time during training.

"Benning Phase" is 17 days long and is conducted by the Ranger Training Brigade at Fort Benning,

Georgia. This phase is designed to develop the basic military skills of a small-unit leader and to enhance the physical and mental endurance required for completing the course. This phase includes instruction in land navigation skills, airborne operations, and survival training (including environmental and medical aspects). (For additional information, see Exhibit 17-1, Ranger Training Incident Report, in Chapter 17, Cold Water Immersion, in *Medical Aspects of Harsh Environments, Volume 1.*[20] (One of the authors of this chapter [WKP] served as the first Subject Matter Expert for the Office of the Under Secretary of the Army, providing a review of the conditions that lead to the deaths of the Ranger candidates.) Also during Benning Phase, candidates receive instruction in combat operations to prepare them for reconnaissance and direct action missions.

The second phase of training, the "Mountain Phase," occurs in the mountains of northern Georgia near the town of Dahloniga. Here candidates continue developing the skills required to conduct small-unit operations in mountainous terrain. Training during this phase includes ambush, air assault, rappelling, and rock climbing. The phase culminates in a field training exercise in which the candidate must apply all of his acquired knowledge and skills.

The third phase of Ranger training occurs at Eglin Air Force Base, Florida. This experience allows the Ranger candidate to develop the skills required for small-unit operations in a jungle and swamp environment. Techniques learned during this phase include small boat operations, stream and swamp crossing, air assault operations, and survival skills. During an 8-day field training exercise under live-fire conditions, the candidates can apply all of the combat survival and leadership skills accrued during the previous training.

On graduation, the Ranger has developed the skills required of a SOF unit leader. He can plan, organize, execute small-unit operations; perform demolition actions, ambush, and long-range operations; and execute the required infiltration and exfiltration operations by sea, air, and land as required.

US Air Force Special Operations Command

AFSOC is an Air Force major command and constitutes the Air Force component of the unified USSOCOM. AFSOC operational forces consist of uniquely equipped fixed- and rotary-wing aircraft operated by highly trained aircrew. This command's primary missions include insertion and extraction, resupply, aerial fire support, refueling, combat search and rescue, and PSYOPS. AFSOC forces are available for worldwide deployment (as a unit motto says, "anytime, anywhere"). Unit assignment to regional unified commands promotes the conduct of the full spectrum of principal special operations missions.

Only the most qualified airmen serve in AFSOC units. Each of the different airframes in AFSOC service requires highly specialized technical training to operate and maintain. Perhaps the most physically demanding specialties are the PJ and Combat Controller teams, and this chapter focuses on the intense training that personnel in these specialties undergo. Much of the basic training indoctrination course occurs during 12 weeks at Lackland Air Force Base, Texas, in what is known as Operating Location–Hotel (OL-H). Advanced PJ training is conducted at Kirtland Air Force Base, New Mexico. Before beginning training, each candidate has demonstrated his physical capabilities in a Physical Ability and Stamina Test (PAST). The PAST is conducted over a 3-hour period during which the candidate must demonstrate proficiencies in surface and underwater swimming, running, and calisthenics. The PAST is a physically rigorous screening tool, allowing only the most physically fit to continue in training.

Operating Location–Hotel (OL-H). This training element is divided into two phases. The first phase is a 4-week section called Initial Familiarization Training (IFT). This phase consists of progressively demanding physical conditioning combined with water skills and confidence building. Academic skills taught during IFT include diving physiology and physics. Progress checks are done weekly to ensure skill advancement during this phase. The remainder of OL-H consists of team training. Physical training continues to grow more intense, with weekly evaluations of physical advancement and of underwater confidence skills. The physical training is so intense that a large proportion of students drop from training due to physical injury.[21]

Scuba School. Following OL-H, successfully advancing candidates attend the Special Forces Underwater Operations Combat Diver Course at Key West, Florida. The course consists of 4 weeks of didactic and practical instruction in diving. Here the students continue physical conditioning, but they also get advanced instruction in open- and closed-circuit diving. They learn, among other things, about underwater navigation, diving physics and physiology, dive tables, hazardous marine life, antiswimmer systems, and altitude diving.

Airborne School. Following successful completion of the Scuba School, candidates attend the Army's 3-week Airborne School at Fort Benning.

Here they are taught the basics of military parachuting while continuing to undergo rigorous physical training.

USAF Survival School. The 17-day Survival School, conducted at Fairchild Air Force Base, Washington, is designed to promote survival-skills training to aircrew. The USAF Survival School provides PJ candidates—along with USAF personnel in other high-risk positions—academic and practical information on survival, evasion, rescue, and escape.

USAF Water Survival School. Held at Naval Air Station Pensacola, Florida, the 4-day USAF Water Survival School provides instruction in the basics of flotation devices, water parachute landing and survival, airframe safety, parasailing, helicopter hoist recovery, and raft survival and safety. The purpose of the course is to promote skill development and proficiency in the basics of military water survival requirements.

Pararescue School. The PJ School is located at Kirtland Air Force Base, New Mexico. The 24 weeks of training are divided into four sections: medical, field operations and tactics, tactics, and air operations. During the medical section, the candidate receives advanced medical training, reaching the level of Emergency Medical Technician–Paramedic (EMT-P). The field operations section includes training in foraging, signaling and communications, land navigation, mountain operations, and search and rescue. The tactics section trains each PJ candidate with the information and experience to conduct small-unit operations in hostile territory. The final phase of PJ School, the air operations section, consists of training in crew coordination, aerial search techniques, and aircraft operations. As part of the air operations section, the candidates learn advanced parachuting techniques, fast roping, rappelling, hoisting, and water deployment and recovery. Each phase of training is capped by a field training exercise in which the candidates practice the skills they have learned in real-world situations. Graduation from the School allows the successful candidate to wear the coveted maroon beret of an Air Force PJ.

Naval Special Warfare

Naval Special Warfare Command is one of the most responsive, versatile, and effective forces available to the commanders in chief of the unified commands. The command's authorized manning is about 2,300 SEALs and 600 Special Warfare Combatant Crewmen (SWCC). The primary mission areas of NSW are unconventional warfare, direct action, special reconnaissance, and foreign internal defense, but the command also conducts security assistance, counterdrug operations, personnel recovery, and hydrographic reconnaissance. With the ability to conduct operations at sea, on land, and in the air, NSW comprises ready forces for any environment.

Sea, Air, Land (SEAL) and Basic Underwater Demolition/SEAL (BUD/S) Training

SEAL is an acronym for the modes of *sea-air-land* infiltration, exfiltration, and operations. All sailors aspiring to be SEALs must go through a 26-week program of Basic Underwater Demolition/SEAL (BUD/S) instruction. They may receive additional training before reporting to a SEAL team. BUD/S training is conducted at the Naval Special Warfare Center, Coronado, California. The highly demanding physical training required at BUD/S leads to a large number of overuse injuries.[22] The training requires that the individual be physically and mentally fit prior to entering training, characteristics that are developed throughout training.[23] The training is intentionally demanding and difficult, developing confidence in the individual's abilities and those of his classmates.

BUD/S is divided into three phases. All BUD/S students have passed an entrance physical fitness test that includes swimming. First Phase (Physical Conditioning) is designed for progressive physical conditioning that builds on the entry fitness level. The phase is 9 weeks long and consists of calisthenics, running, swimming, and team-building—all physically demanding drills. The emphasis throughout BUD/S is on teamwork. Early in training, students are divided into 6-man boat crews. Everything that students at BUD/S do is centered around the boat crew. The first 4 weeks of First Phase are designed to prepare the students for the physical and mental demands of the fifth week, known as Motivational Week (and unofficially as "Hell Week").

Hell Week consists of 5.5 days, during which students conduct continuous activities that require both military skills and team-building drills. Students receive about 2 hours of sleep a night, and the threat of hypothermia is a constant companion. Hours are spent going into and out of chilling ocean water while the students engage in nearly constant physical activity. Most of the attrition at BUD/S occurs by the end of Hell Week. The remaining 3 weeks of First Phase are primarily devoted to continued physical conditioning and learning the techniques of hydroreconnaissance, or beach and littoral survey, a major function performed in preparation for amphibious landings.

Second Phase (Diving) is 7 weeks long with a primary focus on learning open- and closed-circuit scuba techniques. Students learn the techniques of operating the LAR V Draeger rebreathing system. They also begin to develop the techniques that will be required for combat swimmer operations, including underwater navigation, survival, and rescue skills. During Second Phase there is a continued emphasis on physical conditioning. Second Phase culminates with a 5.5-mile open-ocean swim that challenges the student to demonstrate his physical capabilities and endurance.[24] The swim is conducted to confirm the confidence and physical skills that must be exhibited to successfully complete this phase. At the end of this phase, the student is a qualified combat swimmer.

Third Phase (Land Warfare) consists of 9 weeks of instruction in SOF military operations and tactics. The first 6 weeks are spent learning small-unit tactics, rappelling, land navigation, the use of explosive ordnance, and weapons. The final 3 weeks of Third Phase are spent on San Clemente Island, California. In this relatively isolated environment, the students practice the skills learned during the mainland portion of the phase.

Following graduation from BUD/S, SEAL candidates attend the 3-week Army Airborne School at Fort Benning to become jump qualified. Prior to 1997, the corpsmen received advanced medical training at the Army's 30-week 18D Combat Medic Course at Fort Sam Houston, Texas. Beginning in 1997, corpsmen attend the 6-month Special Operations Medical Training Course at the JFK Special Warfare Center at Fort Bragg before being attached to a SEAL team. Those who are going on the SDV teams complete an additional 10 weeks of training at the Naval Special Warfare Center's SDV School. These students engage in didactic training, training in the high-fidelity SDV simulator (Navy Training Device 21D3), and open-water training in the SDV.

Once assigned to a SEAL team, all BUD/S graduates will undergo further SEAL Tactical Training (STT). This consists of approximately 4 to 6 months of tactical training taught by team members so they can not only assess the level of skill of the individual but also to teach the advanced skills necessary to be a member of the SEAL team. On successful completion of STT, the candidate will be able to pin on the badge of a SEAL-qualified combatant, the "Budweiser" (so-called because it resembles the logo of the Anheuser-Busch company).

SEAL Delivery Vehicle

The SEAL Delivery Vehicle (SDV) is a small, wet submersible operated by a two-man crew: a pilot and navigator pair. The SDV provides a stand-off platform for covert delivery of combat swimmers or for actions conducted by the pilot and navigator pair. The course for basic training of SDV personnel occurs at the Naval Special Warfare Center, Coronado, California. Over the duration of the course, students spend approximately 7 weeks in didactic instruction, operation of the high-fidelity SDV simulator (Navy Training Device 21D3), and training in the SDV during open-water operations. The technical skill required to be an SDV operator is enormous, because the operators must perform the complex required tasks under difficult operational conditions.[25] These operators receive additional instruction in the use of the MK-16 closed-circuit breathing device. On graduation, the students are assigned to one of the two SDV teams.

Small-Craft Combatants

Although Small-Craft Combatants have not gone through BUD/S training and will not wear the SEAL trident, they are integral to NSW operations and will ultimately be assigned to one of the Special Boat Units (SBU). Basic training is conducted at the Special Warfare Combatant Crewmember (SWCC) School, Coronado, California. This course of instruction is a separate curriculum taught by personnel at the NSW Center. The course was initiated in 1992 with 6 weeks of instruction, expanded to 9 weeks in 1995 (10 including Week 0, which provides basic indoctrination). Students are instructed in the three core areas of physical fitness/water safety skills, basic crewmember skills, and basic SWCC warfare skills. Personnel receive instruction in tactics and operations required for seamless integration into NSW missions. Crewmembers are trained in the basics of boat handling and operations using the 10-m Rigid-Hull Inflatable Boat (RIB) and the Combat Rubber Raiding Craft (CRRC).

On graduation from SWCC, the crewmembers are assigned to a unit to continue their instruction. At the unit, they enter SWCC-Individual (SWCC-I). Over the course of several months, personnel are assigned to a boat detachment. It is at the SBU that they learn all aspects of maintenance and operations of a single type of watercraft.

Marine Corps Force Reconnaissance

There are many different reconnaissance qualifications within the Marine Corps, including the Light Armored Reconnaissance (LAR), Amphibious Reconnaissance, and, perhaps the best known, Force Reconnaissance (Force Recon). Those considered for Force Recon usually have an Infantry or Communications MOS in the Marine Corps, or are Navy Corpsmen. They are required to have a first-class rating on the Marine Corps physical fitness test and must be certified by their commanding officers as qualified to attend. Typically, those recommended for the course from the infantry are sergeants (E-5) or very senior corporals (E-4), or are lance corporals (E-3) from communications.

Each Recon company sets it own standards for recruiting and testing. A typical qualification process for the 1st Force Recon includes a 48-hour indoctrination program. The program includes back-to-back obstacle-course runs; a 500-m swim, and 30 minutes of treading water in full battle dress uniform; and two physical fitness tests: a 20-mile forced march followed by a 3- to 4-mile timed run with a rucksack. Being physically able to complete the program is only the first step. On the afternoon of the second day, prospective candidates are interviewed by the company executive officer and commanding officer. Often, the attitude displayed during the physically demanding tests and the interview will determine selection.

Reconnaissance Indoctrination Platoon. Individuals selected as prospective Force Recon personnel are first assigned to a Reconnaissance Indoctrination Platoon (RIP). Here they are introduced to the mission of the Force Recon and continue to engage in demanding physical training. The Marines or sailors assigned to the RIP stay there until they are deselected, quit, or are selected to attend the Amphibious Reconnaissance School.

Amphibious Reconnaissance School. From the RIP, prospective Force Recon personnel can attend the 9-week Amphibious Reconnaissance School (ARS) at either Little Creek, Virginia, or Coronado, California. During the course, candidates are taught skills in communications, fire support, patrolling, sketching and photography, demolitions, helicopter insertion and extraction, small-boat handling, and hydrographic and beach reconnaissance. On completion of ARS, the graduate is assigned a 0321 MOS, that of Reconnaissance Marine.

Following ARS, these Marines can attend other military specialty schools. Among the schools available are the Army Airborne and Freefall schools; the Special Operations Dive School; Survival, Escape, Evasion, and Reconnaissance School; Scout Sniper School; Jungle Environment Survival Training; and Army Pathfinder School.

SPECIAL OPERATIONS TACTICAL UNITS

US Army Special Operations

The basic tactical operating unit in Army Special Operations is the Special Forces Operational Detachment-Alpha, or the A-Team. Each SF company is composed of six A-Teams, units of 12 men led by a captain (O-3) as detachment commander, with a warrant officer second in command as the executive officer. The remaining members of the A-Team are noncommissioned officers (E-6 and higher). Team members are cross-trained in each of five basic areas: weapons, engineering and demolition, medicine, communications, and operations and intelligence. All members are trained in at least one additional language. Each of the basic areas is staffed by two noncommissioned officers, one with primary responsibility for that area of expertise and the other acting as an assistant. This provides redundancy for each of the capabilities. The A-Teams' capabilities include the ability to infiltrate and exfiltrate by means of air, sea, or land (further described below in the section entitled Infiltration and Exfiltration Techniques); operate behind enemy lines for extended periods with minimal external support; and organize, equip, and train indigenous forces. They also train, advise, and assist US and other allied forces and agencies. Within an SF company, one of the A-Teams is trained in combat diving and one in free-fall parachuting.

The A-Teams members are well equipped to perform their assigned duties. The communications equipment they operate provides the capability for satellite transmissions, global positioning systems, and secure communications. The medical equipment includes, among other items, kits for emergency field surgery, sterilizers, and resuscitators. In addition to the standard kits for each specialty, A-Team members carry mission-specific auxiliary equipment. The A-Teams that are combat diving qualified use both open- and closed-circuit (LAR V Draeger) systems for aquatic operations (see Chapter 31, Military Diving Operations and Medical Support, for additional information on the open- and closed-circuit scuba systems, including the LAR V Draeger rebreathing system).

Naval Special Warfare

SEALs

Although the uniquely capable SEALs undeniably excel in underwater operations, they are also fully capable of operating in all areas of operation. Prusaczyk and colleagues[26] reported the high degree of complexity that goes into SEAL missions. The physical demands of a mission or mission segment can be great, and even simple mission segments can be made more difficult by the demands of all the segments that preceded it.

A SEAL team is composed of approximately 30 officers and 200 enlisted men. From these are formed approximately eight platoons, each in various stages of training and deployment. Two corpsmen are assigned to each platoon. At an operational level, SEALs have multiple operational units to be used during training and missions. Beginning at BUD/S, SEALs train to work with a swim buddy to form a "dive pair." Given the hostility of the underwater environment, it is critical that each diver has a companion who knows his "buddy's" location and functional capabilities. Training for SEAL teams is conducted at the platoon level with 12 to 16 members. A SEAL platoon comprises two officers (the senior is an O-3), one chief petty officer (E-6), and thirteen enlisted. Primary responsibilities in a platoon are determined by the positions held in a patrol (eg, point man, patrol leader, radioman, gunner, corpsman, and rear security).

Overall planning and execution depends on department leadership (eg, diving, air operations, and ordnance/demolition). The senior enlisted man in the platoon is the chief petty officer, with the second-most senior enlisted the leading petty officer, who is in charge of the day-to-day management of the enlisted platoon members. As operational requirements dictate, the platoon is divided into eight-member squads. The squad is then broken into four-man fire teams. SEAL platoons have a training cycle that includes a 12- or 18-month training "work-up," followed by a 6-month deployment in an operational "combat ready" status at one of the NSW units or detachments.

Combat swimmers operate in dive pairs, much as they were trained at BUD/S. The two SEALs forming the dive pair are the "driver" and the "navigator." Using an illuminated compass and watch, the navigator assures that the dive pair will arrive at the predetermined location at the designated time. The driver, attached to the navigator by a lanyard, observes the surroundings for underwater obstacles, surface craft, or other unanticipated obstacles to mission success.

SDVs are operated by a pilot–navigator pair. Although many of the SDVs functions are jointly managed during an operation, each position has primary responsibilities. It is the pilot's responsibility to "fly" the craft. He must operate the craft so that on-course indicators are followed. He is responsible for maintaining the craft's depth, altitude (from the bottom), and heading. The navigator is responsible for ensuring that the craft avoids obstacles, both expected and unexpected, using Obstacle Avoidance Sonar. Crew coordination is necessary for successful mission completion. The SDV may carry additional operators, equipment, or ordnance as needed for the mission.

Special Boat Units

Although most SBU operators are not SEALs, the theory of having redundancy in operational units carries over from the SEAL platoon. Operations are usually conducted with boat pairs. The operational requirements determine which of the numerous types of craft are selected. The crew of these crafts typically includes a coxswain in charge of boat operations, a navigator, and an engineer, although the exact crew composition depends on the vessel class and the operational requirements. The Combatant Crewmember teams most often are trained on and stay with one class of vessel, developing the required knowledge of performance characteristics and capabilities, maintenance, and operations. They coordinate closely with the SEAL teams to provide tactical support as required to complete the missions.

Marine Corps Force Reconnaissance

The mission of Force Recon is to conduct amphibious, deep ground reconnaissance and surveillance, and limited scale raids for the Marine Expeditionary Force, or the Joint Task Force. The basic operating unit is the Recon team, which is organized within a Force Recon company. A Force Recon company typically has 12 officers and 145 enlisted. Within the company are a Company Headquarters, a Supply Service platoon, and six Recon platoons. Headquarters conducts overall command and control through operations and communications sections. The Supply Service platoon provides supply, mess, medical, motor transport, and equipment repair. Each Recon platoon has a Headquarters platoon and three four-man Recon teams. A Force Recon company normally operates under the cognizance of a Marine Air Ground Task Force G-2/S-2 (Intelligence) for its reconnaissance and surveillance requirements and the G-3/S-3 (Operations) for offensive missions.

INFILTRATION AND EXFILTRATION TECHNIQUES

As mentioned above, the theory of relative superiority[4] suggests that beginning an operation unobserved is one of the elements critical to achieving mission success (see Exhibit 38-1), and conducting an operation completely unobserved often is the most desirable goal. In the words of Sun Tzu (who emphasized surprise, mobility, flexibility, and deception[27]):

> Attack where [the enemy] is not prepared; go by way of places where it would never occur to him you would go.[6]

While not always necessary, it is highly desirable that the technique work at night. Because of the requirements of special operations and the similarity of missions and training, many of these techniques are common to the SOF units, while others are uniquely based on mission capabilities and requirements. The methods of insertion and extraction are highly diverse, owing to the diversity of mission requirements and operational conditions. They are integral parts of the mission and critical to mission success. Only those that are more frequently employed by SOF are mentioned below.

The infiltration and exfiltration techniques of SOF personnel may be broadly categorized on the primary mode of transportation and requirement for action; the seven most common methods are (1) fully terrestrial, (2) fully aquatic, (3) fully aerial, (4) aerial to terrestrial, (5) aerial to aquatic, (6) terrestrial to aerial, and (7) aquatic to aerial. As mission requirements dictate, the full infiltration and exfiltration procedure may require combinations of techniques that may be used independently for insertion and extraction. There are many potential combinations of techniques; those presented here are, of necessity, not inclusive, but they represent some of the common methods by which SOF personnel reach and are removed from the area of operations. A hallmark of SOF is the ability to reach the target and perform the operation despite seemingly impossible odds against success.

It is contrary to USSOCOM policy to release details of insertion and extraction techniques. Readers should understand, however, that the physical demands of the techniques can be great; they may involve transporting loads of up to, and occasionally exceeding, 55 kg of operational materiel. The medical consequences and injuries associated with some of these techniques have been documented.[28,29]

SPECIAL OPERATIONS FORCES MEDICINE

Few medical procedures are unique to the special operations medical community. The treatments used for combat injuries incurred during special operations missions, in general, do not differ from those used in the treatment of casualties of conventional warfare. However, the extraction of casualties is notable in one respect. In fact, a key phrase from *Publication on Special Operations* points out that the unique requirement of special operations casualty handling is the "independence from friendly support."[1(Chap I, p1)]

Until 1997, Army and Navy SOF medics and corpsmen were trained at the Army's 18D Special Forces Medical Sergeant course held at Fort Sam Houston (31 wk) and the JFK Special Warfare Center and School at Fort Bragg (15 wk). During the 46-week-long course, they were educated in such medical skills as providing anesthesia; basic recognition and treatment of cardiovascular; dental; eye, ear, nose, and throat; and orthopedic problems; and basic trauma medicine and surgery. They also received instruction in handling environmental and nuclear–biological–chemical problems, psychiatric and neurological problems, and veterinary medicine.[30,31] The training they received made them among the most skilled medical care providers outside the Medical Corps.

In 1997, Special Operations Combat Medic (SOCM) and Advanced Special Operations Combat Medic (ASOCM) courses were established to provide a common training course for all SOF enlisted medical care providers. The 24-week SOCM course provides training to EMT Paramedic certification. The ASOCM course provides an additional 20 weeks of training. Enlisted medical care providers from the Army SF and Ranger, AFSOC PJs, NSW SEALs, and Marine Corps Force Reconnaissance attend the SOCM course, with Army SF, SEALs, and Reconnaissance personnel continuing their training with the ASOCM course. The courses are currently held four times each year.

SUMMARY

This chapter provides a broad overview of the organizational, psychological, and training aspects of the United States's special operations. Each of the service-specific SOF organizations can boast of special skills that make them unique among the warfighter communities, but they must also be prepared for joint operations; hence the USSOCOM.

A general goal of psychological assessment is to provide unique information about a special operations candidate in a cost- and time-efficient manner. This information, when viewed in conjunction with other sources of data, attempts to predict how an applicant will perform in a special operations role. Special operations selection programs within the United States have continued to evolve since their inception within the selection programs developed by the OSS. Psychological methods are but one component of the screening and selection process, and attempt to provide unique data in a cost- and time-efficient manner, which can help to screen-out undesirable applicants, or screen-in those who are best qualified. This is generally done by identify-ing those factors that have been found to be associated with performance success or failure at tasks relevant to special operations missions. A great challenge for any assessment and selection program involves the attempt to use limited data to predict "real world" performance that will take place in an unpredictable environment. Despite this challenge, assessment methods can greatly assist in the challenge of selecting the most qualified personnel for special operations programs.

Special operations stands apart from conventional warfare in the unique physical and technical requirements placed on the SOF operator. With the changing global political climate, the role that SOF personnel play in maintaining national security will be ever increasing, with a concomitant increase in the technical, technological, physical, and emotional demands placed on the operators. It is critical that both the military and the civilian communities understand and appreciate the importance of SOF in maintaining national and international peace and security.

REFERENCES

1. Joint Chiefs of Staff. *Publication on Special Operations*. Washington, DC: Department of Defense; 17 Apr 1998: Chap I: 2–4. Joint Publication 3-05. Available at www.dtic.mil/doctrine.

2. Report to the Chairman, Committee on Armed Services, House of Representatives. *Special Operations Forces—Force Structure and Readiness Issues*. Washington, DC: Special Operations Forces; 1994. GAO/NSIAD-94-105.

3. von Clausewitz C. *On War*. Howard M, Paret P, trans. Princeton NJ: Princeton University Press; 1976.

4. McRaven WH. *Spec Ops, Case Studies in Special Operations Warfare: Theory and Practice*. Novato, Calif: Presidio Press; 1995.

5. Public Law 99-661.

6. Giles L, trans-ed. *Sun Tzu on The Art of War*. The Project Gutenberg Etext of *The Art of War* by Sun Tzu. May 1994 [Etext 132].

7. Banks LM. *The Office of Strategic Services Psychological Selection Program* [master's thesis]. Fort Leavenworth, Kan: US Army Command and General Staff College; 1995.

8. The OSS Assessment Staff. *Assessment Of Men*. New York, NY: Rinehart & Co; 1948.

9. Leake SA. Basic issues in the psychological screening of sensitive classes: Screening-in versus screening-out. Paper presented at the 1st annual Med-Tox Conference for Psychological Screening and Physical Ability Testing of Police, Firefighters, and Corrections; November, 1988; Santa Ana, Calif.

10. Hogan R, Hogan J, Roberts BW. Personality measurement and employment decisions. *Am Psychol*. 1996;51(5):469–477.

11. Braun DE, Prusaczyk WK, Goforth HW Jr, Pratt NC. *Personality Profiles of US Navy Sea-Air-Land (SEAL) Personnel*. San Diego, Calif: Naval Health Research Center; 1993. NHRC Technical Report 94-8.

12. Carlin TM, Sanders M. Soldier of the future: Assessment and selection of Force XXI. *Spec Warfare*. 1996;9(2):16–21.

13. McDonald MA, Norton BA, Hodgdon MS. Training success in US Navy Special Forces. *Aviat Space Environ Med*. 1990;61:548–554.

14. Vickers RR, PhD, Research Psychologist, Human Performance Department, Naval Health Research Center, San Diego, Calif. Personal communication, 1996.

15. Young S. A short history of SF assessment and selection. *Spec Warfare*. 1996;9(2):22–27.

16. Sawka M, Young AJ, Rock PB, et al. Altitude acclimatization and blood volume: Effects of exogenous erythrocyte volume expansion. *J Appl Physiol*. 1996;81(2):636–642.

17. Beckett MB, Goforth HW Jr, Hodgdon JA. *Physical Fitness of US Navy Special Forces Team Members and Trainees*. San Diego, Calif: Naval Health Research Center; 1989. NHRC Technical Report 89-29.

18. Jacobs I, Prusaczyk WK. Unpublished data, 1993–1994.

19. Moore RJ, Friedl KE, Kramer TR, et al. *Changes in Soldier Nutritional Status and Immune Function During the Ranger Training Course*. Natick, Mass: US Army Research Institute of Environmental Medicine; 1992. USARIEM Technical Report T13-92.

20. Pandolf K, Burr RE, Wenger CB, Pozos RS, eds. *Medical Aspects of Harsh Environments, Volume 1*. In: Zajtchuk R, Bellamy RF, eds. *Textbook of Military Medicine*. Washington, DC: Department of the Army, Office of The Surgeon General, and Borden Institute; 2001 (in press). Available at www.armymedicine.army.mil/history.

21. Hammer D. AFSOC Force Surgeon, San Antonio, Tex. Personal communication, 1996.

22. Shwayhat AF, Linenger JM. *Profiles of Exercise History and Overuse Injuries Among US Navy SEAL Recruits*. San Diego, Calif: Naval Health Research Center; 1993. NHRC Technical Report 93-3.

23. McDonald DG, Norton JP, Hodgdon JA. Determinants and Effects of Training Success in US Navy Special Forces. San Diego, Calif: Naval Health Research Center; 1988. NHRC Technical Report 88-34.

24. Prusaczyk WK, Goforth HW Jr, Sopchick T, Griffith P, Schneider K. *Thermal and Physiological Responses of Basic Underwater Demolition/SEAL (BUD/S) Students to a 5.5-Mile Open-Ocean Swim*. San Diego, Calif: Naval Health Research Center; 1993. NHRC Technical Report 93-27.

25. Prusaczyk WK, Stuster JW, Goforth HW Jr. *An Analysis of Critical Tasks and Abilities of SEAL Delivery Vehicle (SDV) Crew Positions (C)*. San Diego, Calif: Naval Health Research Center; 1995. NHRC Technical Report 95-20.

26. Prusaczyk WK, Stuster JW, Goforth HW Jr, Sopchick Smith T, Meyer LT. *Physical Demands of US Navy Sea-Air-Land (SEAL) Operations*. San Diego, Calif: Naval Health Research Center; 1995. NHRC Technical Report 95-24.

27. Dupuy TN, Johnson C, Bongard DL. *Harper Encyclopedia of Military Biography*. New York, NY: HarperCollinsPublishers; 1992: 720.

28. Kragh JF, Taylor DC. Fast-roping injuries among Army Rangers: A retrospective survey of an elite airborne battalion. *Mil Med*. 1995;160(6):277–279.

29. Miser WF, Doukas WC, Lillegard WA. Injuries and illnesses incurred by an Army Ranger unit during Operation Just Cause. *Mil Med*. 1995;160(8):373–380.

30. Moloff AL, Bettencourt B. The special forces medic: Unique training for a unique mission. *Mil Med*. 1992;157(2):74–76.

31. Hasbarger JA, Culclasure TF. Special Forces medical sergeants (18 Delta) recertification. *Mil Med*. 1994;159(1):7–9.

Chapter 38: ATTACHMENT

SELECTED PUBLICATIONS RELATED TO SPECIAL OPERATIONS FORCES TRAINING AND OPERATIONS

Prepared for this textbook by William Keith Prusaczyk, PhD, and Glenn M. Goldberg, PhD.

Army Special Forces–Related Publications:

FM 21-76	*Survival.* 05 June 1992.
FM 31-19	*Military Free-Fall Parachuting Tactics, Techniques, and Procedures.* 18 February 1993.
FM 31-20	*Doctrine for Special Forces Operations.* 20 April 1990.
FM 31-20-3	*Foreign Internal Defense Tactics, Techniques, and Procedures for Special Forces.* 20 September 1994.
FM 31-20-5	*Special Reconnaissance Tactics, Techniques, and Procedures for Special Forces.* 23 March 1993.
FM 31-71	*Northern Operations.* 21 June 1971.
FM 33-1	*Psychological Operations.* 18 February 1993.
FM 33-1-1	*Psychological Operations Techniques and Procedures.* 05 May 1994.
FM 34-36	*Special Operations Forces Intelligence and Electronic Warfare.* 30 Sep 1991.
FM 41-5	*Joint Manual for Civil Affairs.* 18 November 1966.
FM 41-10	*Civil Affairs Operations.* 11 January 1993.
GTA 31-1-2	*Detachment Mission Planning Guide.* 01 August 1993.
GTA 41-1-1	*Civil Affairs Information Planning Guide.* 01 September 1994.
ARTEP 33-705-MTP	*Mission Training Plan for a Psychological Operations Battalion Headquarters.* 23 October 1989.
ARTEP 33-707-30-MTP	*Mission Training Plan for a Psychological Operations Regional Support Company.* 01 October 1994.
ARTEP 33-708-30-MTP	*Mission Training Plan for a Psychological Operations Tactical Support Company.*
ARTEP 41-701-30-MTP	*Mission Training Plan for a Headquarters and Headquarters Company, Civil Affairs Command.* 31 December 1993.
ARTEP 41-702-30-MTP	*Mission Training Plan for a Headquarters and Headquarters Company, Civil Affairs Brigade.* 02 September 1993.
ARTEP 41-705-MTP	*Mission Training Plan for a Civil Affairs Battalion (GP).* 22 March 1992.
ARTEP 41-707-30-MTP	*Mission Training Plan for a Detachment (General Support), Civil Affairs Battalion (GP).* 19 March 1993.
ARTEP 41-715-MTP	*Mission Training Plan for a Civil Affairs Battalion (FID/UW).* 20 April 1992.
ARTEP 41-717-30-MTP	*Mission Training Plan for a Detachment (General Support), Civil Affairs Battalion (Foreign Internal Defense/Unconventional Warfare).* 30 September 1993.
ARTEP 41-718-30-MTP	*Mission Training Plan for a Detachment (Direct Support), Civil Affairs Battalion (Foreign Internal Defense/Unconventional Warfare).* 30 September 1993.

STP 31-18-SM-TG	*Soldier's Manual and Trainer's Guide Cmf18 Special Forces Basic Tasks Skill Levels 3 and 4.*
STP 31-18B34-SM-TG	*Soldier's Manual/Trainer's Guide MOS 18b Special Forces Weapons Sergeant Skill Levels 3/4. 05 October 1990.*
STP 31-18C34-SM-TG	*Soldier's Manual and Trainer's Guide MOS 18c Special Forces Engineer Sergeant Skill Level 3 and 4. 05 October 1990.*
STP 31-18E34-SM-TG (FD)	*Soldier's Manual and Trainer's Guide MOS 18e Special Forces Communications Sergeant Skill Levels 3 and 4. 20 September 1994.*
STP 31-18F4-SM-TG	*Field Manual Focus: An Infantryman's Guide to Combat in Built-Up Areas.*

Training Publications Recommended by the Ranger Training Brigade, Fort Benning, Georgia:

FM 5-20	*Camouflage, Basic Principles.*
FM 5-25	*Explosives and Demolitions.*
FM 7-8	*Infantry Platoon and Squad.*
FM 7-9	MTP *Mission Training Plan for the Infantry Rifle Platoon and Squad.*
FM 7-10	*The Infantry Rifle Company.*
FM 7-20	*The Infantry Battalion.*
FM 7-85	*Ranger Unit Operations and Training.*
FM 21-11	*First Aid for Soldiers.*
FM 21-20	*Physical Readiness Training.*
FM 21-26	*Map Reading.*
FM 21-75	*Combat Skills of the Soldier.*
FM 21-76	*Survival, Evasion and Escape.*
SH 21-76	*Ranger Handbook.*
FM 21-150	*Combatives.*
FM 22-100	*Military Leadership.*
FM 22-101	*Counseling.*
FM 25-100	*Training the Force.*
FM 30-5	*Combat Intelligence.*
FM 90-3	*Desert Operations.*
TC 21-24	*Rappelling.*
TC 90-6-1	*Military Mountaineering.*
TC 621-1	*Evasion and Escape Training.*
TM 9-1005-224-10	*Operating Manual M60 Mg.*

TM 9-1005-249-10	*Operating Manual M16 Rifle.*
TM 9-1010-221-10	*Operating Manual 40mm Grenade Launcher M203.*
TM 11-5855-203-13	*Individual Weapons.*
STP 7-11BCHM14-SM-TG	*Soldiers Manual and Trainers Guide.*
STP 21-1 SMCT	*Soldiers Manual of Common Tasks, Skill Level 1.*
STP 21-24 SMCT	*Soldiers Manual of Common Tasks, Skill Level 2 through 4.*
ARTEP 7-8 DRILL	*Battle Drills for the Infantry Rifle Platoon and Squad.*

Ranger-, Special Forces-, and Light Infantry-Related Publications:

FM 7-92	*Infantry Reconnaissance Platoon and Squad (Airborne, Air Assault, Light Infantry). 23 Dec 1992.*
FM 7-93	*Long-Range Surveillance Unit Operations. 3 Oct 1995.*
FM 7-98	*Operations in a Low Intensity Conflict. 19 Oct 1992.*
FM 17-98	*Scout Platoon. Supersedes FM 17-98, 7 Oct 87, 9 Sep 1994.*
FM 20-3	*Camouflage.*
FM 23-10	*Sniper Training. 17 Aug 1994.*
FM 57-38	*Pathfinder Operations. 9 Apr 1993.*
FM 90-13	*River Crossing Operations.*

Air Operations-Related Publications:

FM 1-108	*Doctrine for Army Special Operations Aviation Forces. 3 Nov 1993.*
FM 1-112	*Tactics, Techniques, and Procedures for the Attack Helicopter Battalion. 21 Feb 1991.*
FM 1-113	*Assault Helicopter Battalion. 28 Oct 1986.*
FM 1-114	*Tactics, Techniques, and Procedures for the Regimental Aviation Squadron. 20 Feb 1991.*
FM 1-116	*Tactics, Techniques, and Procedures for the Air Cavalry/Reconnaissance Troop. 20 Feb 1991.*
FM 57-220	*Static Line Parachuting Techniques and Training.*
FM 5-125	*Rigging Techniques, Procedures, and Applications. 3 Oct 1995*
FM 10-500-1	*Airdrop Support Operations in a Theater of Operations. 19 Jun 1991*
FM 10-500-7	*Airdrop Derigging and Recovery Procedures. 20 Sep 1994*

Intelligence Operations-Related Publications:

FM 34-60	*Counterintelligence.*
FM 34-1	*Intelligence and Electronic Warfare Operations. Supersedes FM 34-1, 2 Jul 87, 27 Sep 1994.*
FM 34-2-1	*Tactics, Techniques, and Procedures for Reconnaissance and Surveillance and Intelligence Support to Counterreconnaissance. 19 Jun 1991.*

FM 34-8   *Combat Commander's Handbook on Intelligence.* 28 Sep 1992.

Selected Naval Health Research Center (NHRC) Technical Reports Related to Special Operations Forces:

Beckett MB, Goforth HW, Hodgdon JA. *Physical Fitness of US Navy Special Forces Team Members and Trainees.* San Diego, Calif: Naval Health Research Center; 1989. NHRC Technical Report 89-29.

Beckett MB, Hodgdon JA. *Heat Production and Optimal Cooling for Navy Special Warfare Divers.* San Diego, Calif: Naval Health Research Center; 1992. NHRC Technical Report 91-23.

Braun DE, Prusaczyk WK, Goforth HW Jr, Pratt NC. *Personality Profiles of US Navy Sea-Air-Land (SEAL) Personnel.* San Diego, Calif: Naval Health Research Center; 1994. NHRC Technical Report 94-8.

Burton HD, Banks WW, Schultz EE, Berghage TE. *An Inventory of Wargaming Models for Special Warfare: Candidate Applications for the Infusion of Human Performance Data.* San Diego, Calif: Naval Health Research Center; 1989. NHRC Technical Report 89-60.

Hermansen LA, Butler FK, Flinn S, Noyes LD. *(1995) Naval Special Warfare Computer-Aided Corpsman Training Program (Version 1.0)–Multiple Choice Items.* San Diego, Calif: Naval Health Research Center; 1994. NHRC Technical Document 94-3C.

Hodgdon JA, Goforth HW Jr, Hilderbrand RL. *Biochemical Responses of Navy Special Warfare Personnel to Carbohydrate Loading and Physical Performance.* San Diego, Calif: Naval Health Research Center; 1983. NHRC Technical Report 82-3.

Jacobs I, Prusaczyk WK, Goforth HW Jr. *Muscle Glycogen, Fiber Type, Aerobic Fitness, and Anaerobic Capacity of West Coast US Navy Sea-Air-Land Personnel (SEALS).* San Diego, Calif: Naval Health Research Center; 1993. NHRC Technical Report 92-10.

Jacobs I, Prusaczyk WK, Goforth HW Jr. *Adaptations to Three Weeks of Aerobic/Anaerobic Training in West Coast US Navy Sea-Air Land Personnel (SEALs).* San Diego, Calif: Naval Health Research Center; 1995. NHRC Technical Report 94-28.

Kelly T, Assmus J, Shillcutt C, Goforth HW Jr. *The Use of Tobacco Products Among Naval Special Warfare Personnel.* San Diego, Calif: Naval Health Research Center; 1993. NHRC Technical Report 92-16.

McDonald DG, Norton JP, Hodgdon JA. *Determinants and Effects of Training Success in US Navy Special Forces.* San Diego, Calif: Naval Health Research Center; 1988. NHRC Technical Report 88-34.

Meyer, LT; J Moore, T Sopchick-Smith, & A Friedlander Naval Special Warfare Sports Medicine Conference Proceedings. San Diego, Calif: Naval Health Research Center; 1995. NHRC Technical Document 95-4D.

Meyer LT, Smith TS Friedlander AL. *Expert Panel Review of Naval Special Warfare Calisthenics: Sports Medicine Conference Summary.* San Diego, Calif: Naval Health Research Center; 1995. NHRC Technical Document 95-5E.

Naitoh P, Kelly TL, Goforth HW Jr. *Sleep During SEAL Delivery Vehicle (SDV)/Dry Dock Shelter Exercises Analyzed by a Graphic Approach.* San Diego, Calif: Naval Health Research Center; 1995. NHRC Technical Report 94-30.

Naitoh P, Kelly T. *Sleep Management User's Guide for Special Operations Personnel.* San Diego, Calif: Naval Health Research Center; 1993. NHRC Technical Report 92-28.

Prusaczyk WK, Goforth HW Jr, Nelson ML. *Physical Training Activities of East Coast US Navy SEALs.* San Diego, Calif: Naval Health Research Center; 1995. NHRC Technical Report 94-24.

Prusaczyk WK, Goforth HW Jr, Nelson ML. *Characteristics of Physical Training Activities of West Coast US Navy Sea-Air-Land Personnel (SEALs).* San Diego, Calif: Naval Health Research Center; 1993. NHRC Technical Report 90-35.

Prusaczyk WK, Goforth HW Jr, Sopchick T, Griffith P, Schneider K. *Thermal and Physiological Responses of Basic Underwater Demolition/SEAL (BUD/S) Students to a 5.5-Mile Open-Ocean Swim.* San Diego, Calif: Naval Health Research Center; 1994. NHRC Technical Report 93-27.

Prusaczyk WK, Stuster JW, Goforth HW Jr, Sopchick Smith T, Meyer LT. *Physical Demands of US Navy Sea-Air-Land (SEAL) Operations.* San Diego, Calif: Naval Health Research Center; 1995. NHRC Technical Report 95-24.

Prusaczyk WK, Stuster JW, Goforth HW Jr. *An Analysis of Critical Tasks and Abilities of SEAL Delivery Vehicle (SDV) Crew Positions (C).* San Diego, Calif: Naval Health Research Center; 1995. NHRC Technical Report 95-20.

Shwayhat AF, Linenger JM. *Profiles of Exercise History and Overuse Injuries Among US Navy SEAL Recruits.* San Diego, Calif: Naval Health Research Center; 1994. NHRC Technical Report 93-3.

Selected US Army Research Institute of Environmental Medicine (USARIEM) Publications Related to Special Operations Forces:

Fairbrother B, Shippee RL, Askew EW, et al. *Nutritional Assessment of Soldiers During the Special Forces Assessment and Selection Course.* Natick, Mass: US Army Research Institute of Environmental Medicine; 1995. USARIEM Technical Report T95-22.

Jezior D, Arsenault J. *Nutritional and Immunological Assessment of Ranger Students With Increased Caloric Intake.* Natick, Mass: US Army Research Institute of Environmental Medicine; 1995. USARIEM Technical Report T95-5.

Moore RJ, Friedl KE, Kramer TR, et al. *Changes in Soldier Nutritional Status and Immune Function During the Ranger Training Course.* Natick, Mass: US Army Research Institute of Environmental Medicine; 1992. USARIEM Technical Report T13-92.

Selected Nonfiction Reading Related to Special Operations Forces:

Adams J. *Secret Armies: The Full Story of the SAS, Delta Force and Spetsnaz.* Hutchinson & Co. ISBN 0-330-30661-8.

Bank A. *From OSS to Green Berets.* Novato, Calif: Presidio Press; 1987.

Barker GT. *A Concise History of US Army Special Operations Forces.* Tampa, Fla: Anglo-American Publishing Co; 1993.

Beaumont R. *Special Operations and Elite Units, 1939–1988.* New York, NY: Greenwood Press.

Beckwith CA, Knox D. *Delta Force.* San Diego, Calif: Harcourt Brace Jovanovich; 1983.

Bosiljevac, TL. *SEALs: UDT/SEAL Operations in Vietnam.* Ballantine Books. ISBN 0-8041-0722-X.

Chinnery PD. *Air Commando: Inside the Air Force Special Operations Command.* St Martin's Paperbacks. ISBN 0-312-95881-1.

Collins JM. *Green Berets, SEALs and Spetsnaz.* Washington, DC: Pergamon-Brassey; 1987. ISBN 0-099-035747-4.

Cummings DJ. *The Men Behind the Trident: SEAL Team One in Vietnam.* Naval Institute Press. ISBN 1-55750-139-4.

Fane FD, Moore D. *The Naked Warriors: The Story of the US Navy's Frogmen.* Naval Institute Press. ISBN 1-55750-266-8.

Halberstadt H. *Green Berets.* Novato, Calif: Presidio Press; 1988.

Kelly FJ. *US Army Special Forces, 1961-1971: Vietnam Studies.* Washington, DC: US Government Printing Office; 1973.

Kelly O. *Brave Men, Dark Waters: The Untold Story of the Navy SEALs.* Novato, Calif: Presidio Press; 1982.

Kelly O. *From a Dark Sky: The Story of US Air Force Special Operations.* Novato, Calif: Presidio Press; 1996. ISBN 0-89141-520-3.

Kelly O. *Never Fight Fair! Navy SEALs' Stories of Combat and Adventure.* Novato, Calif: Presidio Press; 1995. ISBN 0-89141-519-X.

Landau A, Landau F. *Airborne Rangers*. Motorbooks International. ISBN 0-87938-606-1.

McRaven WH. *SPEC OPS: Case Studies in Special Operations Warfare: Theory and Practice*. Novato, Calif: Presidio Press; 1995. ISBN 0-98141-544-0 (hardcover) and 0-89141-600-5 (paperback).

Padden I. *US Army Special Forces*. New York, NY: Bantam Books; 1995.

Rottman GL. *US Army Special Forces, 1952-1984*. London, England: Osprey; 1985.

Simpson CM. *Inside the Green Berets: The First Thirty Years*. Novato, Calif: Presidio Press; 1983.

Simpson CM. *Inside the Green Berets: The Story of US Army Special Forces*. Berkley, Calif. ISBN 0-425-09146-5.

Stanton SL. *Green Beret at War*. Novato, Calif: Presidio Press; 1985.

Sutherland IDW. Special Forces of the United States Army, 1952–1982. San Jose, Calif: R. James Bender Publishing; 1990.

Thompson L. *US Special Forces 1941-1987*. New York, NY: Blandford Press; 1987.

Time–Life Books. *Special Forces and Missions*. Alexandria, Va: Time–Life Books; 1990. ISBN 0-8094-8600-8.

Waller D. *The Commandos*. New York, NY: Simon & Schuster. ISBN 0-671-78717-9.

Walmer, M. *An Illustrated Guide to Modern Elite Forces*. Prentice Hall Press. ISBN 0-668-06064-6.

Watson J, Dockery K. *Point Man*. William Morrow. ISBN 0-688-12212-4.

ABBREVIATIONS AND ACRONYMS

2,3 DPG: 2,3 diphosphoglycerate
5-LO: 5-lipoxygenase

A

ABG: arterial blood gas
abs: absolute
ACE: angiotensin-converting enzyme
ACE: Aviation Combat Element
ACh: acetylcholine
ACLS: Advanced Cardiac Life Support
ADH: antidiuretic hormone
ADSOCM: Advanced Special Operations Combat Medic
AFMIC: Armed Forces Medical Intelligence Center
AFSC: Air Force Specialty Code
AFSOC: Air Force Special Operations Command
AGE: arterial gas embolism
AMP: adenosine monophosphate
AMREE: American Medical Research Expedition to Everest
AMS: acute mountain sickness
AMS-C: AMS-Cerebral
ANGLICO: Air Naval Gunfire Liaison Companies
ANP: atrial natriuretic peptide
ANVIS: Aviator Night Vision Imaging System
ARDS: acute respiratory distress syndrome
ARS: Amphibious Reconnaissance School
ASOCM: Advanced Special Operations Combat Medic
ata: atmosphere absolute
ATLS: Advanced Trauma Life Support
ATP: adenosine 5'-triphosphate
ATPase: adenosine triphosphatase
ATPD: ambient temperature and pressure, dry
AVP: arginine vasopressin

B

BAL: bronchoalveolar lavage
BC: buoyancy compensator
BDO: battledress overgarment
BDS: battle dressing station
BDU: battledress uniform; also called the combat fatigue
BLS: Basic Life Support
BLT: battalion landing team
BMR: basal metabolic rate
BPV: benign paroxysmal vertigo
BTPS: *body temperature, ambient pressure, and saturated with water vapor*
BUD/S: Basic Underwater Demolition/SEALS

C

C.O.: cardiac output
C: Celsius
CA: Civil Affairs
CAGE: cerebral arterial gas embolism
CANE: Combined Arms in a Nuclear Environment
CaO_2: arterial oxygen content
CASEVAC: casualty evacuation
CB: chemical–biological
CBF: cerebral blood flow
CCTV: closed-circuit television
CINC: commander-in-chief
CNS: central nervous system
CO: carbon monoxide
COMNAVSPECWARCOM: commander's headquarters unit of NAVSPECWARCOM
COPD: chronic obstructive pulmonary disease

CPO: Chief Petty Officer
CPP: cerebral perfusion pressure
CRRC: Combat Rubber Raiding Craft
CSF: cerebrospinal fluid
CSMD: Combat Swimmer Multi-Level Dive
CSSE: Combat Service Support Element
CT: computed tomography
CTZ: chemoreceptive trigger zone
CVP: central venous pressure
CVR: cerebrovascular resistance
CWS: Coalition Warfare/Support

D

D: diopter
DAN: Divers Alert Network
DARPA: Defense Advanced Research Projects Agency
DC: Damage Control
DCI: decompression illness
DCS: decompression sickness
DDC: Deck Decompression Chamber
DDS: dry deck shelter
DEXA: dual-energy X-ray absorbancy
D_{LCO}: diffusing capacity of lung for carbon monoxide
D_{LO_2}: lung diffusion capacity for oxygen
$D_{LO_2}max$: maximal lung diffusion capacity for oxygen
DMO: Diving Medical Officer
DMT: Diving Medical Technician
DNBI: disease and nonbattle injuries
DoD: Department of Defense
DOW: died of wounds
DSRV: Deep Submergence Rescue Vehicle
DVT: deep venous thrombosis

E

EAN: enriched air nitrox
ECG: electrocardiogram
EEG: electroencephalography
EGG: electrogastrogram
ELAM-1: endothelial leukocyte adhesion
EM: electron microscopy
EMT-P: Emergency Medical Technician–Paramedic
EMU: Extravehicular Maneuvering Unit
EOD: Explosive Ordnance Disposal
EPAP: expiratory positive airway pressure
ESQ: Environmental Symptoms Questionnaire
EVA: extravehicular activity

F

F: Fahrenheit
FEV_1: forced expired volume in 1 second
FIO_2: fraction of inspired oxygen
fsw: feet of seawater
FTS: Flight Test Squadron
FVC: forced vital capacity

G

G: acceleration, for convenience
g: gauge
g: SI unit of gravity
GABA: γ-aminobutyric acid
GCE: Ground Combat Element
G-LOC: acceleration-induced loss of consciousness
G-measles: petechiae

Gx: front-to-back acceleration vector
Gy: side-to-side acceleration vector
Gz: head-to-foot acceleration vector

H

HACE: high-altitude cerebral edema
HALO: high-altitude, low-opening
HAPE: high-altitude pulmonary edema
HAPE-S: HAPE-susceptible
HAR: high-altitude retinopathy
HARH: high-altitude retinal hemorrhage
HCA: Humanitarian and Civic Action
HCVR: hypercapnic ventilatory response
HEPA: high-efficiency particulate air
HIV: human immunodeficiency virus
HPNS: high-pressure nervous syndrome
HPV: hypoxic pulmonary vasoconstriction
HPVR: hypoxic pulmonary vasopressor response
HSB: high-speed boat
HTE: high terrestrial elevation
HVR: hypoxic ventilatory response

I

ICAO: International Civil Aviation Organization
IFT: Initial Familiarization Training
IOP: intraocular pressure
ISS: International Space Station

J

JFK: John F. Kennedy
JSLIST: Joint Service Lightweight Integrated Suit
JSOC: Joint Special Operations Command
JSOMTC: Joint Special Operations Medical Training Center
JSOTF: Joint Special Operations Task Force

K

K: Kelvin
KIA: killed in action

L

LAR: Light Armored Reconnaissance
LBNP: lower-body negative pressure
LES: launch and entry suit
LOC: loss of consciousness
LOX: liquid oxygen
LR: lactated Ringer's
LTB_4: leukotriene B_4

M

MDSU: Mobile Diving and Salvage Units
MECO: main-engine cutoff
MEDEVAC: medical evacuation
MEF: Marine Expeditionary Force
MEU(SOC): Marine Corps Marine Expeditionary Units
  (Special Operations Capable)
MIA: missing in action
Mk: Mark
MO: Medical Officer
MOPP: mission-oriented protective posture
MOS: military occupational specialty
MRI: magnetic resonance imaging
$MSDV_z$: motion sickness dose value
MSOC: molecular sieve oxygen concentrating (system)
MSSG: MEU Service Support Group

MSVC: maximum sustained ventilatory capacity
msw: meters of seawater
MTF: medical treatment facility
MVV: maximal voluntary ventilation

N

NADH: nicotanamide adenine dinucleotide (reduced form)
NASA: National Aeronautics and Space Administration
NATO: North Atlantic Treaty Organization
NAVSEA: Naval Sea Systems Command
NAVSPECWARCOM: Naval Special Warfare Command
NBC: nuclear–biological–chemical
NDSTC: Navy Diving and Salvage Training Center
NEC: Navy Enlisted Code
NEDU: Navy Experimental Diving Unit
NEPMU: Naval Environmental and Preventive Medicine Unit
NMRI: Naval Medical Research Institute
NOAA: National Oceanic and Atmospheric Administration
NSBRI: National Space Biomedical Research Institute
NSW: Naval Special Warfare
NSWC: Naval Special Warfare Center
NSWG: Naval Special Warfare Group
NUMI: Naval Undersea Medicine Institute

O

O+M: Operations and Maintenance
ODC: oxyhemoglobin dissociation curve
OOTW: operations other than war
OSS: Office of Strategic Services

P

P^2NBC^2: Physiological and Psychological Effects of NBC and
  Extended Operations on Combat Vehicle Crew Performance
P_{ACO_2}: partial pressure of alveolar carbon dioxide
P_{aCO_2}: partial pressure of arterial carbon dioxide
P_{AH_2O}: partial pressure of alveolar water vapor
P_{AN_2}: partial pressure of alveolar nitrogen
$P_{AO_2} - P_{aO_2}$: alveolar–arterial oxygen tension difference
P_{AO_2}: partial pressure of alveolar oxygen
P_{aO_2}: partial pressure of arterial oxygen
PAP: pulmonary arterial pressure
PAST: Physical Ability and Stamina Test
PAV: positional alcohol vertigo
P_B: barometric pressure
PBA: PPB for altitude
PBG: positive-pressure breathing during acceleration
PCRF: parvicellular reticular formation
PE: pulmonary embolus
PEEP: positive end-expiratory pressure
P_{ETCO_2}: end-tidal partial pressure of carbon dioxide
P_{ETO_2}: end-tidal partial pressure of oxygen
P_{H_2O}: partial pressure of water vapor
PHC: portable hyperbaric chamber
P_{IO_2}: partial pressure of oxygen in the inspired gas
PJ: pararescueman
PML: portable medical locker
P_{O_2}: partial pressure of oxygen
POM: Program Objective Memorandum
PPB: positive-pressure breathing
ppmv: parts per million by volume
PRK: photorefractive keratectomy
psia: pounds per square inch absolute
PSYOP: Psychological Operations
PTC: Personnel Transfer Capsule
P_{vO_2}: partial pressure of venous oxygen

Q

Q (course): Qualification (course)

R

RBC: red blood cell
RD: rapid decompression
REM: rapid eye movement
RHIB: rigid-hull inflatable boat
RIP: Reconnaissance Indoctrination Platoon
RK: radial keratotomy
rms: root mean square

S

Sa_{O_2}: arterial oxygen saturation
SAS: space adaptation syndrome
SBU: Special Boat Units
scuba: self-contained underwater breathing apparatus
SDV: SEAL Delivery Vehicle
SEAL: *sea, air, land*
SEV: surface equivalent
SF: Special Forces, also known as the Green Berets
SFAS: Special Forces Assessment and Selection
SFMS: Special Forces Medical Sergeant
SFQC: Special Forces Qualification Course
SI: Système International d'Unités, the International System of Units
SLS: Spacelab Life Sciences
SOAR: Special Operations Aviation Regiment
SOCAMRS: Special Operations Computer-Assisted Medical Reference System
SOCM: Special Operations Combat Medic
SOF: Special Operations Forces
SOG: Special Operations Group
SOIMTP: Special Operations Interactive Medical Training Program
sonar: *so*und *na*vigation *a*nd *r*anging
SOS: Special Operations Squadron
SOT: Special Operations Technician
SOW: Special Operations Wing
SRC: Submarine Rescue Chamber
SRIG: Surveillance, Reconnaissance, and Intelligence Group
SRS: slow-reacting substance
SRS-A: slow-reacting substance of anaphylaxis
STD: sexually transmitted disease
STEPO: Self-Contained Toxicological Protective Outfit
STPD: *s*tandard conditions of *t*emperature (0°C), *p*ressure (760 mm Hg), and *d*ry
STT: SEAL Tactical Training
sur-DO_2: surface decompression with oxygen
SWCC: Special Warfare Combatant Crewmember

T

T_3: triiodothyronine
T_4: thyroxine
T_E: tidal expiration
TEMPSC: totally enclosed, motor-propelled, survival craft
T_I: tidal inspiration
TIA: transient ischemic attack
TOW: tube-launched, optically tracked, wire-guided
TRC: transportable recompression chamber
TSH: thyroid stimulating hormone
TUC: Time of Useful Consciousness
TxB_2: thromboxane B_2

U

UBA: underwater breathing apparatus
UCT: Underwater Construction Team
UDM: Underwater Decompression Monitor
UMO: Undersea Medical Officer
UPTD: unit pulmonary toxicity dose
USARIEM: US Army Research Institute of Environmental Medicine
USASOC: US Army Special Operations Command
USSOCOM: US Special Operations Command
UV: ultraviolet

V

V_A: alveolar ventilation
VC: vital capacity
$\dot{V}_{CO_2}/\dot{V}_{O_2}$: respiratory quotient
$\dot{V}_{CO_2}$: volume of carbon dioxide
V_{DS}: volume of respiratory system dead space
V_E: ventilation expired
$\dot{V}_E$: ventilation expired, volume per unit time
$\dot{V}_E/\dot{Q}$: ratio of the rates of ventilation and perfusion
VI: volume of inspiration
VNH: Virtual Naval Hospital
$\dot{V}_{O_2}max$: maximal oxygen consumption, or uptake
VOT: Voice Onset Time
V_T: tidal volume
$\dot{V}/\dot{Q}$: ventilation–perfusion ratio

W

WBGT: wet bulb globe temperature
WIA: wounded in action

X

XO: Executive Officer

H